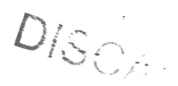

Principles of
Gender-Specific
Medicine

Principles of Gender-Specific Medicine

Volume 2

Edited by

Marianne J. Legato, MD

Section Editors:

John P. Bilezikian, MD
William Byne, MD, PhD
Ann M. Coulston, MS, RD
Kevin C. Fleming, MD
Scott M. Hammer, MD
Robyn G. Karlstadt, MD
Robert G. Lahita, MD, PhD
George M. Lazarus, MD, FAAP
Lauri Romanzi, MD
Janice B. Schwartz, MD
Amy Tiersten, MD
David R. Trawick, MD, PhD

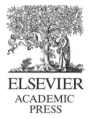

ELSEVIER
ACADEMIC
PRESS

AMSTERDAM • BOSTON • HEIDELBERG • LONDON
NEW YORK • OXFORD • PARIS • SAN DIEGO
SAN FRANCISCO • SINGAPORE • SYDNEY • TOKYO

Elsevier Academic Press
525 B Street, Suite 1900, San Diego, California 92101-4495, USA
84 Theobald's Road, London WC1X 8RR, UK

This book is printed on acid-free paper. ∞

Library of Congress Cataloging-in-Publication Data
Application submitted.

British Library Cataloguing in Publication Data
A catalogue record for this book is available from the British Library

ISBN: 0-12-440905-9 (set)
ISBN: 0-12-440906-7 (volume 1)
ISBN: 0-12-440907-5 (volume 2)

For all information on all Academic Press publications
visit our Web site at books.Elsevier.com

Printed in the United States of America
04 05 06 07 08 09   9 8 7 6 5 4 3 2 1

We dedicate this textbook to Doctor Thomas Q. Morris, with profound admiration for the astonishing variety and uniform excellence of his contributions to medicine over the course of a fifty-year career. His insights, wisdom, and, above all, his personal integrity and virtue made him uniquely valuable to us all.

Contents

SECTION 6
Reproductive Biology
Lauri Romanzi

Volume 2

SECTION 7
Oncology
Amy Tiersten

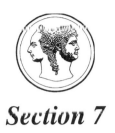

Section 7

ONCOLOGY

Amy Tiersten, MD

Associate Professor of Medicine, New York University School of Medicine, New York, NY

Cancer is the second leading cause of mortality in the United States after heart disease. Years of epidemiologic observation has taught us that certain cancers are more common according to gender; however, there are a paucity of studies addressing why this may be the case. Reasons for these differences are clearly complex, and results of studies are often inconsistent.

Of course, there are truly gender specific cancers such as prostate cancer, testicular cancer, and ovarian cancer. It is not clear why cancer of the testis is predominantly germ cell in origin, whereas most ovarian tumors are epithelial in origin. Breast cancer is nearly a gender-specific cancer; although it is rare in men, when it does occur it is fundamentally identical to female breast cancer in behavior with few exceptions. Gastrointestinal malignancies, primary brain tumors, and hematologic malignancies are all more common among men. It is well understood that both breast and prostate cancer are linked to levels of sex hormones and are treated in part by changing the levels of these hormones. Although in the case of breast cancer, we understand the importance of estrogen and progesterone receptors, in other cancers we are only just learning that these receptors and hormonal milieu may play a role as well.

Other factors that may explain why certain cancers are more common according to gender, such as differences in exposures (e.g., occupational exposures) versus true biologic differences in susceptibility, are only just beginning to be explored. In addition, the association of certain malignancies with other disease states, such as chronic inflammatory conditions, may add to our knowledge base.

Does the fact that women are more likely to see physicians, thereby making screening programs easier to implement among females, help explain some of the differences we see? Clearly issues such as access to health care, income, and education level contribute to issues related to cancer screening.

What about the different effects of treatment according to gender? We are learning more about the long-term effects of hormonal alteration and gender-related differences in response to treatment such as sexual dysfunction, osteoporosis, and cognitive function.

This section is a first attempt to explore what is currently known regarding these issues. It is our hope that more information could translate into greater therapeutic options and ultimately into strategies for early detection and prevention.

57

Gender Differences in Hematologic Malignancies

GWEN L. NICHOLS, MD
Columbia University, College of Physicians and Surgeons, New York, NY

I. Hematologic Malignancies: Gender Differences and Environmental Factors

There are consistent gender differences in the incidence of all hematologic malignancies in adults including acute and chronic leukemias, Hodgkin's disease (HD) and non-Hodgkin's lymphoma (NHL), and multiple myeloma (MM). Such gender differences, although small, are consistent. Males have a greater risk of hematologic malignancies. Acute myelogenous leukemia (AML) ratios M/F are 1.6:1, acute lymphocytic leukemia (ALL) 1.4:1, chronic myelogenous leukemia (CML) 1.7:1, and chronic lymphocytic leukemia (CLL) 1.7:1. Hairy cell leukemia has the most dramatic male predominance 3.3:1 and MM the least at 1.4:1 [1]. NHL incidence is also increased in males ranging from 1.5:1 to 1.7:1 overall, with less skewing among follicular (low-grade) lymphomas and greater male predominance in diffuse (intermediate) and high-grade lymphomas 1.8:1 to 2.3:1 [2]. The most recent American Cancer Society (ACS) update of cancer statistics from the Surveillance, Epidemiology and End Results (SEER) data shows a continued male predominance in the hematologic malignancies [3] for which there is no straightforward explanation. Because the etiology for most hematologic neoplasms remains obscure, studying these gender differences in cancer incidence may lead to insights into cancer causation. Only a limited number of studies have looked at gender and occupational exposures as a primary analysis, as opposed to gender as part of a subset analysis. For instance, studies that have looked at women and occupation have found new connections to particular occupations and cancer incidence in women [4,5]. Such studies deserve separate analysis. Because these studies are of limited number, and because environment may play a role in the development of hematologic malignancies, occupations that are traditionally skewed toward one gender provide clues for the male predominance in hematologic malignancies. Only through this type of study can we determine if there are true differential predispositions or sensitivities to the development of hematologic malignancies between the sexes.

A. Non-Hodgkin's Lymphomas

There has been a dramatic increase in the incidence of NHLs during the second half of the 20th century. This has occurred during a period when the incidence of HD has remained stable or decreased, suggesting that detection does not account for the change. NHL is now 5th in cancer incidence in the United States. The recent cancer statistics update from the ACS shows that the rapid increase in lymphoma incidence during the late 20th century may be tailing off but confirms the continued male predominance. The SEER data 1979 to 1998, on which these statistics are based [6], further defines that the incidence of NHL in males appears to be leveling off, whereas female incidence continues to increase [3]. The SEER data give credence to the hypothesis that environmental exposures, particularly in the workplace, may account for a proportion of NHL cases. With larger numbers of women entering the workplace during the second half of the 20th century, and presumably being exposed to similar carcinogens, gender differences in environmental exposures are likely to decrease. The literature contains a large number of articles suggesting potential environmental factors in lymphomagenesis including pesticides, chemicals, radiation, and viruses (reviewed in [7,8]).

1. Pesticides

NHLs have been linked to chemical exposures [9–13], in particular pesticides, particularly in the farming and agricultural professions [14]. Exposure to livestock in farming and meat processing has also been associated with increased risk of NHL [14]. Over a time similar to that of the increase in NHL there has been a dramatic increase in the use of pesticides, which has only decreased slightly within the last decade (reviewed in [2]). A dose-response effect on NHL incidence has been suggested among farmers who apply herbicides themselves [9,11–13,15,16]. In light of this data for a dose-response effect, the usual farm exposure for women and men may differ, with males more likely to perform as direct appliers of pesticides. The increase may not be due to gender-specific sensitivity, because studies of women in agricultural professions also show an increased risk of NHL and other tumors [5].

2. Agent Orange

The association of particular classes of herbicide exposure and NHL has prompted considerable attention to herbicide exposure during military service in Vietnam. Agent Orange, which contains the carcinogen 2,3,7,8-tetrachlorodibenzo-para-dioxin, has been an environmental exposure subject to heated debates both in the medical and lay press. Although there appears to be an increased incidence of NHL among Vietnam veterans as compared with an age-matched population [17,18], a specific association with exposure to Agent Orange has not been definitively shown. Quantitation of exposure is difficult because of latency, unknown degree of exposure, and multiple potential chemical exposures in military personnel. More significant testing both of exposure levels in Vietnamese nationals and in U.S. service personnel may yield more conclusive results [19]. Studies that include Vietnamese nationals may also yield information regarding female exposure and risk, because the bulk of potentially exposed military personnel among Vietnam veterans are male. The increase in NHL in Vietnam era veterans has not been sufficiently explained by available data.

3. Radiation

The type, dose, and length of exposure to radiation appears to determine the likelihood of development of radiation-related NHL. Evidence for this risk comes from accidental, occupational, and therapeutic exposures. An increased number of lymphomas have been seen after exposure to the radioactive imaging agent Thorotrast [20]. Thorotrast, used clinically from 1930 to 1950, is a thorium dioxide colloid. The major site of deposition of this radionuclide is the reticuloendothelial system and skeleton. Therapeutic use led to continued radioactive exposure from thorium dioxide of life-long alpha-particle irradiation [20]. This low-level, long-term radiation exposure has been associated with an increase in all hematologic malignancies except CLL and an increase in sarcomas and hepatic neoplasms. These studies included both males and females, but data were not analyzed specifically for differences in incidence based on gender or dose/gender relationships. Higher level, shorter term therapeutic x-ray exposure for treatment of ankylosing spondylitis (a disease that preferentially affects males) has also been associated with a significant increase in NHL [21].

In studies of atomic bomb survivors, NHL rates increased over background incidence about 3% per year over 20 years of study. This is similar to the rate of increase in NHL seen in the U.S. population over the same time period, making the association of NHL with higher dose radiation less clear cut [22]. The risk from lower levels of radiation exposure in the workplace, predominantly gamma-particle irradiation, also remains controversial. Until the end of the 20th century, occupations that involved radiation exposures in the workplace (nuclear industry, laboratory, therapeutic radiation) were predominantly male. Therefore, most studies showed male-only changes in NHL risk. Studies of exposure at nuclear facilities, suggested primarily an increase in leukemia and MM rather than NHL [23,24]. None of these studies addressed the question of nuclear workplace exposures in women.

4. Viruses (Human Immunodeficiency Virus)

Infection with the human immunodeficiency virus (HIV) has been associated with more than a 60-fold increase in the incidence of NHL as compared with the general population [25]. With the advent of highly active antiretroviral therapy (HAART), the incidence of acquired immunodeficiency syndrome (AIDS)-related primary central nervous system NHL has decreased [26,27]. Although controversy exists [28], several authors have seen a decrease in all NHL secondary to HIV after HAART [26,29]. There is also improvement in survival in HIV-related lymphoma patients, with the improvement in immunologic status and ability to tolerate effective chemotherapy seen after the development of HAART. It has been estimated that HIV-associated NHL may account for an excess of up to 2700 cases of NHL per year [25] before the advent of effective antiretroviral therapy, but this accounts for only a small percentage of the estimated 54,000 new cases of NHL in the United States anticipated in 2002. HIV-related disease was initially skewed toward males. Currently the fastest growing population for new HIV exposure

is heterosexual females. With the changing demographics of HIV infection, the male predominance in HIV-related NHL is also likely to change, and this will be evident over the next several decades. Only then will differences in gender sensitivity become apparent if they exist.

B. Myeloma

A number of environmental and occupational exposures have been associated with the development of MM (reviewed in [30–33]). These include a wide range of occupations that are not always consistent from study to study including painters, teachers (both male and female), metalworkers, farmers, and chemical workers.

1. Radiation

Myeloma has been associated with whole body ionizing radiation exposure particularly during older age in case-control studies performed with workers at nuclear facilities [23]. Similar associations have been seen in uranium-processing regions (not just workers but people living in proximity to a power plant) [24]. These studies, although suggestive, are far from definitive or controlled, and, again, the exposure of workers was almost exclusively in males. How this data translates to women or the population in general is much less clear, in particular after ambient radiation exposure or diagnostic x-rays [34].

2. Hair Dyes

Hair dyes, which may be carcinogenic in animal models, have been studied for their potential to increase the risk of hematologic malignancies in humans. Women are more likely than men to regularly use permanent hair dyes, and a gender difference on this basis would be expected if the exposure truly increased risk. Although many studies have shown a small increase in NHL and MM in women with long-time use of dark-colored permanent hair dyes, this association appears to be small and does not hold up for male hairdressers [15,35–37]. A recent case-control study suggests an increased NHL risk in women using hair dyes prior to 1980 [37a].

3. Breast Implants

Although many studies have questioned the role that breast implants may play in impeding mammography and, therefore, the observation of breast cancer (reviewed in [38]), another major concern is the body's immunologic reaction to silicone in breast implants. This includes the deterioration of the capsule over time, which allows leakage of silicone into tissues. Long-term effects of different types of implants are also a concern, including an increased incidence of rheumatologic/inflammatory diseases and immunologic disturbances, potentially leading to an increased incidence of other cancer types. This association has yet to be conclusively shown [39]. Because there is a linkage between chronic inflammation and lymphoma, this raises a concern that would differentially affect females. No conclusive studies have defined any risk of either cancer or rheumatologic disease after breast implants. Concerns regarding the risk of monoclonal gammopathy and MM after implants have also been raised [40], although the data currently remain purely speculative.

C. Leukemia

A number of environmental factors have been linked to the development of leukemia. Because acute leukemias are rare, many reports are studies of leukemia clusters or large surveys of cancer in general, which, although suggestive, are not conclusive [30,41]. Although the risk of leukemia from exposure to a number of environmental factors remains hypothetical because of the small numbers, it is quite clear that both radiation exposure and exposures to organic solvents may be associated with the development of leukemia.

1. Radiation

Radiation's clearest environmental affect is leukemia. The incidence of hematopoietic malignancies among atomic bomb survivors has been analyzed through the late 1980s with dosimetry estimates. There is strong evidence for radiation-induced ALL, AML, and CML but not acute T-cell leukemia or CLL in survivors, and an estimated 20% of excess deaths after the atomic bombs were due to leukemia. There appears to be a dose-response relationship between radiation and leukemia risk. Risk for leukemia rises rapidly after exposure and decreases over time. Interestingly, this varies both by sex and age at exposure (older survivors have an excess risk that decreases less rapidly). Risk for women appeared to be less, but the risk for women decreased less rapidly with time than did the risk for men. For CML the risks over time decreased rapidly but this also differed by sex, with men having a high initial peak and rapid decrease whereas women's risk, although lower, remained constant over a longer period [14]. These findings suggest a number of theoretical explanations. There may be gender-based differences in genomic stability or sensitivity to DNA damage. These differences might account for the lower risk for leukemic DNA damage after radiation in women. The longer time of risk in response to radiation damage for women versus men suggests potential gender-specific differences in DNA repair after damage. These mechanisms remain to be elucidated.

Thorotrast studies also confirmed an excess of leukemia after radiation exposure, which was first seen after a median latency of 5 years. This risk continued throughout the exposed person's lifetime [20]. As in the atomic bomb survivor studies, the incidence of CLL after thorotrast exposure was unchanged compared with the other leukemias. The Swedish thorotrast study broke down incidence of leukemia by gender and found that males had a higher incidence of leukemia after exposure to thorotrast than females (SIR 7.1 vs 4.5, respectively). The numbers were too small to confirm any differences in the time or period of risk between males and females. Although females received a slightly lower dose of thorotrast overall, this did not completely explain the lower incidence of leukemia after thorotrast exposure in females. These studies also suggest a different sensitivity to radiation-induced hematopoietic cell damage between the sexes and the phenomenon is worthy of further study.

2. Chemicals

Exposure to organic solvents has been associated with the development of leukemia, in particular AML [42–44]. This has primarily been seen in relation to commercial and industrial/occupational exposure, although household exposures (e.g., paints) have been associated with childhood ALL [45]. These studies, which review exposure in the chemical industry, have predominantly shown exposure of males.

3. Other Exposures

The debate both in the popular press and the literature about magnetic field exposure and leukemia has yet to be confirmed although suggestive studies for occupational-level exposure and leukemia exist [46]. This has prompted evaluation of the levels of exposure seen in a number of occupations, including those of traditionally female occupations [47]. A study designed to evaluate the work environment of job categories typically held by women was prompted by an earlier study of mothers of children with ALL and the mothers' occupations. These included textile machine operators, cashiers, and bakery workers. No definitive conclusions can be made, but these thorough analyses of exposures by sex are needed to provide any validity to epidemiologic data. These studies are hampered by small numbers of patients who develop leukemia and the likely contribution of multiple factors in its development.

II. Hematologic Malignancies: Gender Differences in Predisposing Medical Conditions

Gender differences in both the underlying illness and the types of treatment needed may play a role in the development of hematologic malignancies. Pregnancy, as a sex-specific condition, also may affect both incidence and treatment of hematologic malignancies.

A. Rheumatologic Illnesses and Hematologic Malignancies

The risk of lymphoma is increased in patients with chronic inflammatory conditions, in particular in autoimmune disorders. Many of the most common rheumatologic diseases affect women disproportionately. Rheumatoid arthritis (RA), systemic lupus erythematosus (SLE), and Sjögren's syndrome are predominantly diseases of women. In North America it is estimated that SLE affects women six to eight times more than men, RA affects women three times more than men, and primary Sjögren's syndrome is 90% female. Immunosuppression, whether iatrogenic (i.e., after organ transplantation), congenital, or postinfectious (HIV), has been associated with an increased incidence of hematologic malignancies, and there is an increased incidence of hematologic malignancies in patients with autoimmune diseases. The question is whether autoimmune diseases themselves or the immunosuppressive therapies used to treat these disorders are most critical for the increased incidence of hematologic malignancies.

Many case reports and retrospective analyses provide evidence for an increased incidence of NHL in association with rheumatologic disorders including RA, Sjögren's syndrome, and SLE [48,49] (Table 57-1). Although the majority of these studies are retrospective and small in size, they are consistent in their findings of increased incidence of hematologic malignancies, particularly NHL, most notably in the female-predominant primary Sjögren's syndrome. This is almost exclusively a female risk for NHL, because studies that included secondary Sjögren's syndrome (and some male patients) showed a lesser risk. There are no firm statistics because Sjögren's is so rare in males. Secondary Sjögren's has a greater than 50% lower risk of NHL. Most of the available studies are outlined in Table 57-1, and none of the Sjögren's studies break out whether males developed NHL. Many do not even mention gender and other studies are all female. Chronic inflammation and its associated immune dysregulation clearly predispose to the development of NHL. Although no comparative trials are available, none of the studies showed a clear increase in hematologic malignancies associated with any of the common treatments of rheumatologic disease including chemotherapeutics and gold (see Table 57-1).

Celiac disease, gluten-sensitive enteropathy, is also associated with an increased incidence of NHL, in particular T-cell lymphomas of the gastrointestinal tract [50]. This disease also has a female predominance, which lends credence to the association of inflammatory disorders, immune dysregulation, and NHL. However, the association of inflammatory disorders and NHL is not unique to women, because Behçet's disease, a rare male-predominant inflammatory disease, is also associated with lymphoid malignancies [51]. The small numbers of patients with this disorder make the association difficult to characterize further. The degree to which sex truly plays a role in the development of malignancy in patients with rheumatologic illnesses versus being a reflection only of the gender differences in incidence of rheumatologic disease is an area for further study.

B. Therapy-related Leukemias

Chemotherapy, when used to treat a primary malignancy, may predispose to the development of secondary or therapy-related damage to the normal bone marrow stem cells. Using standard dose chemotherapy, exposure to alkylating agents has been associated with the development of therapy-related leukemia (t-AML) and abnormalities of chromosomes 5 and 7 [52]. The use of topoisomerase II inhibitors, including doxorubicin, has been associated with t-AML; translocations of chromosome 11q23, the mixed lineage leukemia (MLL) gene [53], have

Table 57-1
Risk of NHL in Rheumatologic Diseases

Disease	# pts.	Sex	# Dev. NHL	Subtype	RX	Reference
Sjögren's	62	F	4/62 (6.4%)	2 diffuse mixed, small and large cleaved, 2 LCL	n.a.	Pariente et al
RA	11,683	3750 M, 7933 F	SIR 1.5–2.6 both males and females	NHL	n.a.	Gridley et al
Sjögren's	250	n.a.	60 LPD, 12 NHL	60 LPD (41, MG, 4 pseudo, 12 NHL 3 other)	n.a.	Sugai et al
RA	610	n.a.	increased risk NHL, leukemia	n.a.	signif. with gold treatment	Bendix et al
SLE	276	n.a.	180/276 NHL	n.a.	not assoc. with CSP, various RX	Sultan et al
Sjögren's	110	107 F	3 NHL	n.a.	higher than ref pop. none in men	Pertovaara et al
Sjögren's	331	318 F, 13 M	9 NHL all female	extranodal	no immunosupp., no XRT	Valesini et al
Sjögren's/RA	1385/9469	119F, 192 M/7757 F, 1712 M	SIR 8.7 primary, 4.5 secondary, 2.2 RA	25 (16 NHL, 2 HD, 4 AL, 3 MM)/58 (34 NHL, 4 HD, 12 AL, 8 MM)	n.a.	Kauppi et al
Sjögren's	80	n.a.	6 NHL	extranodal	n.a.	Gannot et al
Sjögren's	250	n.a.	4/250	2 NHL, 1 AILD, 1 MM	n.a.	Dong et al
SLE	1,585	1300 F, 277 M	8 NHL 1.5 expected	extranodal	n.a.	Mellemkjaer et al
Sjögren's	55	n.a.	5 NHL 9%	n.a.	n.a.	Zufferey et al
SLE	724	627 F, 97 M	24 NHL (4.1 fold increase)	n.a.	no assoc. with cytotoxic RX	Abu-Shakra et al

HD, Hodgkin's disease (HD); MM, multiple myeloma; NHL, non-Hodgkin's lymphoma; RA, Rheumatoid arthritis; SLE, systemic lupus erythematosus. (From Abu-Shakra M, Gladman DD, Urowitz MB. [1996]. Malignancy in systemic lupus erythematosus. *Arthritis Rheum.* 39:1050–1054; Bendix G, Bjelle A, Holmberg E. [1995]. Cancer morbidity in rheumatoid arthritis patients treated with Proresid or parenteral gold. *Scand J Rheumatol.* 24:79–84; Dong Y, Zhao Y, Zeng X, Sun D. [1998]. Primary Sjögren's syndrome and its lymphoid malignancy: A report of four cases. *Chin Med J [Engl].* 111:218–219; Gannot G, Lancaster HE, Fox PC. [2000]. Clinical course of primary Sjögren's syndrome: Salivary, oral, and serologic aspects. *J Rheumatol.* 27:1905–1909; Gridley G, McLaughlin JK, Ekbom A *et al.* [1993]. Incidence of cancer among patients with rheumatoid arthritis. *J Natl Cancer Inst.* 85:307–311; Kauppi M, Pukkala E, Isomaki H. [1997]. Elevated incidence of hematologic malignancies in patients with Sjögren's syndrome compared with patients with rheumatoid arthritis [Finland]. *Cancer Causes Control.* 8:201–204; Mellemkjaer L, Andersen V, Linet MS *et al.* [1997]. Non-Hodgkin's lymphoma and other cancers among a cohort of patients with systemic lupus erythematosus. *Arthritis Rheum.* 40:761–768; Pariente D, Anaya JM, Combe B *et al.* [1992]. Non-Hodgkin's lymphoma associated with primary Sjögren's syndrome. *Eur J Med.* 1:337–342; Pertovaara M, Pukkala E, Laippala P *et al.* [2001]. A longitudinal cohort study of Finnish patients with primary Sjögren's syndrome: Clinical, immunological, and epidemiological aspects. *Ann Rheum Dis.* 60:467–472; Sugai S, Saito I, Masaki Y *et al.* [1994]. Rearrangement of the rheumatoid factor-related patients with Sjögren's syndrome. *Clin Immunol Immunopathol.* 72:181–186; Sultan SM, Ioannou Y, Isenberg DA. [2000]. Is there an association of malignancy with systemic lupus erythematosus? An analysis of 276 patients under long-term review. *Rheumatology [Oxford].* 39:1147–1152; Valesini G, Priori R, Bavoillot D *et al.* [1997]. Differential risk of non-Hodgkin's lymphoma in Italian patients with primary Sjögren's syndrome. *J Rheumatol.* 24:2376–2380; and Zufferey P, Meyer OC, Grossin M, Kahn MF. [1995]. Primary Sjögren's syndrome [SS] and malignant lymphoma. A retrospective cohort study of 55 patients with SS. *Scand J Rheumatol.* 24: 342–345.)
LPD, lymphoproliferative disease; LCL, large cell lymphoma; MG, monoclonal gammopathy; AL, acute leukemia; CSP, cyclosporine; XRT, X-ray therapy (radiation therapy); AILD, angioimmunoblastic lymphadenopathy with dysplasia.

been attributed to the use of this agent. The median time from exposure to onset of AML is 5 to 7 years after alkylating agents; however, onset may be measured in months after topoisomerase II inhibitors. Therapy-related leukemias are in general refractory to conventional treatment and are associated with poor survival [54]. There are significant gender-based differences in a number of malignancies, and the risk of therapy-related leukemias is directly related to the likelihood of receiving more leukemogenic treatments. Alkylating agents, nitrosoureas and procarbazine appear to have the highest leukemogenic potential, and this may be potentiated by the concomitant exposure to radiation therapy.

Among patients at risk for t-AML, those with HD are the most extensively studied, because of a major impact of alkylating agents included in common chemotherapy schedules. Patients treated for HD, have a 20- to 40-fold increased risk of developing t-AML, correlated with the number of mechlorethamine-containing cycles given and possibly with splenectomy and greater age. In the Gruppo Italiano Malattie Ematologiche dell'Adulto (GIMEMA) archive more than 50% of patients with secondary AML have breast cancer, NHL, or HD [55,56]. In particular, HD patients who received mechlorethamine, oncovin, procarbazine, prednisone (MOPP) chemotherapy with or without radiation had a significant risk of t-AML likely secondary to the mechlorethamine (nitrogen mustard) and procarbazine, both of which are alkylating agents. Current chemotherapy regimens use less of these agents, in the hope of avoiding this complication. However, because the latency for development of t-AML may be considerable, it is unclear what the risk of t-AML will be after treatment with adriamycin, bleomycin, vinblastine, dacarbazine (ABVD), which is a regimen with less DNA alkylation. This risk appears to affect males and females equally, although more males are at risk.

Treatment for NHL also produces a risk for t-AML because of extensive use of alkylating agents and topoisomerase II inhibitors in common chemotherapy regimens. In MM and ALL the determinants of risk of t-AML are the dose of melphalan and of epipodophyllotoxin, respectively. Patients with breast, ovarian, and testicular neoplasms are also at risk, in particular if treated with alkylating agents and topoisomerase II inhibitors. Generally, patients with NHL or breast or testicular cancer experience a lower, albeit significant, risk of developing t-AML (2- to 15-fold increased risk) than those with HD treated with MOPP. Epipodophyllotoxins appear to be the most important factor for t-AML in patients treated for testicular cancer. Following cumulative doses of etoposide greater than $2 \, g/m^2$ for germ cell tumors, the risk of t-AML has been reported at 1.3% and may increase with longer follow-up [57]. Adjuvant cyclophosphamide, methotrexate, and 5-FU therapy in breast cancer patients does not appear to increase risk significantly as compared with the general population. A higher incidence of t-MDS in breast cancer has been linked to combined radiation and alkylating agents [58] and the use of more leukemogenic alkylating agents such as melphalan [59]. The extent of the leukemogenic potential of anthracyclines in adjuvant breast cancer regimens remains to be defined. Several studies indicate that higher dose adjuvant regimens, which include epirubicin, and those using mitoxantrone may have a higher risk of t-AML [60–64]. Breast cancer is both common and almost uniquely female and poses a risk to a greater number of patients than the much rarer male testicular cancer. The risk of t-AML after treatment for NHL appears to affect males and females equally, although more males are at risk.

High dose chemotherapy and autologous stem cell transplantation may also pose an increased risk of t-AML. After stem cell transplantation for lymphomas, there appears to be a substantial risk of t-AML, with studies showing 2 to 20% at 5 to 6 years [65–68]. However, because the risk of t-AML after conventional therapy for NHL may be quite high, the added risk posed by the use of high-dose chemo-radiotherapy is not clear, because prior therapy appears to play a large role [69]. The incidence of t-AML after autologous stem cell transplantation for breast cancer appears to be lower than for lymphoma, although the number of patients currently at risk is smaller, long-term survival is less likely, and length of follow-up for these patients is shorter. Again, prior therapy appears to play a substantial role in the development of t-AML [70–72]. Those diseases for which transplantation may be offered as a therapeutic option differ in incidence by gender and, therefore, pose a differential risk of this complication.

C. Pregnancy and Hematologic Malignancies

Cancer is the second leading cause of death in women during their reproductive years, affecting an estimated 0.1% of all pregnancies [73]. The presentation of hematologic malignancies during pregnancy is rare but presents a challenge to both patients and oncologists. Because pregnancy is associated with altered levels of female sex hormones not found in males or nulliparous females, hormonal effects of pregnancy might be important in understanding the male predominance of hematologic malignancies. Recent studies have begun to examine whether pregnancy protects against the development of some hematologic malignancies [74]. No firm conclusions can yet be drawn. Hodgkin's disease and acute leukemias are among the most common malignant neoplasms in women of reproductive age. There is no evidence that pregnancy alters the prognosis of these malignancies, but pregnancy may significantly affect the course of treatment that may be given and may delay diagnosis [75]. Cancer treatment may also significantly affect fetal outcome. Although hematologic neoplasms rarely affect the pregnancy directly, indirect effects may be multiple including anemia, thrombocytopenia, coagulopathy, and placental infiltration. (The teratogenic effects of chemotherapeutic agents, particularly in the first trimester of pregnancy, are well documented in animals and humans [76,77]. Later in pregnancy many chemotherapeutic agents may be used without apparent change in fetal outcome [78–80]. Because the incidence of these diseases in pregnant women is small, controlled trials cannot be performed, and case histories provide the most reliable source of data to determine the best treatment options. Likewise, the long-term effects on development of children exposed *in utero* to chemotherapeutic agents comes from case reports [81–85].

1. Leukemia

Surprisingly, there is little evidence to support that leukemia during pregnancy is associated with an adverse fetal outcome [78]. Although intrauterine growth retardation, low birth weight, prematurity, and congenital deformities have been reported resulting from leukemia alone [86–88], the greater contribution to adverse fetal outcome appears to be due to the leukemia treatment rather than the leukemia itself. Leukemic cells may invade the placenta, although this complication appears to be rare [89]. Disseminated intravascular coagulation associated with leukemia and infectious complications may cause placental thrombosis and hemorrhage leading to placental insufficiency. A case of vertical transmission of a monocytic leukemia has been reported, although this appears to be exceedingly rare [90]. Acute leukemia is rapidly fatal if untreated, and chemotherapy often must be given in an attempt to save the life of the mother. Many of the common acute leukemia therapies pose substantial risk during early pregnancy, particularly folate antagonists [81]. Anthracyclines and cytarabine, mainstays of the treatment of AML, have not been associated with significant teratogenicity, particularly when used after the first trimester of pregnancy [82]. All-trans retinoic acid, used in the treatment of acute promyelocytic leukemia may pose a risk of vitamin A toxicity to the fetus although it has been successfully used in pregnancy [88,91–95].

Chronic leukemias are generally diseases that affect non–reproductive age females, and CLL is rarely seen in pregnancy [96,97]. CML occurs occasionally but can be treated palliatively with hydroxyurea, a synthesis inhibitor, or with leukapheresis if needed until delivery. Alpha-interferon has also been safely used later in pregnancy [98–101]. CML and other myeloproliferative disorders also hold some risk for coagulation-related adverse outcomes during pregnancy [102]. Gleevec, imatinib mesylate (Novartis), a new small molecule tyrosine kinase inhibitor, has no information available to date concerning its safety in pregnancy.

2. Lymphoma

Lymphoma is the fourth most frequent cancer diagnosed in pregnant females [103] with the largest proportion being HD. NHL is generally a disease of older adults, with a mean age of presentation of older than 50 years. There are less than 100 cases of NHL peripregnancy reported in the literature [104] because this disease more frequently occurs in women after their reproductive years. Reviews suggest that pregnancy may be associated with more aggressive forms of lymphoma including the Burkitt's subtype and may also be associated with extra-lymphatic involvement, a worse prognostic factor. Although hormonal effects may be the cause for these more aggressive lymphoma subtypes, younger patients, regardless of pregnancy, are more likely to present with aggressive histology. The role of female gender remains unclear because there are too few cases to be conclusive about whether pregnancy influences the histology or presentation of NHL. Staging and treatment are certainly affected by pregnancy. Aggressive NHL cannot be palliated with survival of the mother, if presentation is early in pregnancy. Therefore, chemotherapy often must be undertaken despite risk to the fetus [105]. The risks of particular chemotherapies during pregnancy has been studied, and some guidelines can be made as to the likelihood of damage during specific times in pregnancy with specific chemotherapeutic agents [76]. Radiation may also be part of definitive therapy for NHL. Risks to the fetus can be reduced by appropriate shielding; however,

congenital anomalies and microcephaly remain a concern, particularly with pelvic irradiation early in pregnancy [106].

Hodgkin's disease is more common than NHL during pregnancy. Some patients with HD have localized disease, which can be treated with local radiation until completion of the pregnancy. Later in pregnancy, chemotherapy can be successfully given without apparent risk to the fetus [107]. Retrospective studies have looked at female sex hormones and reproductive history in patients with HD to see if female hormones might be protective, which might explain the male predominance in this disease [108]. Associations between parity, age at first birth, and the risk of developing HD were evaluated in 917 cases of HD in women and five randomly selected age-matched controls. A nonsignificant risk reduction of HD was found in parous compared with nulliparous women, with some evidence of an increased risk with late age at first birth in women younger than age 45 at HD diagnosis. However, no statistically significant role was found for hormonal changes of pregnancy being protective against the development of HD.

III. Gender-related Differences in Response to Treatment

Gender-related differences in response to therapy have long been a part of prognostic categorization in the hematologic malignancies. Only recently have underlying explanations for these differences begun to be explored.

A. Stem Cell Transplantation

Gender differences appear to play a role in the incidence of graft-versus-host disease (GVHD), and therefore the morbidity of allogeneic stem cell transplantation. In human leukocyte antigen (HLA)-matched sibling allogeneic transplantation there is a consistent increase in acute and chronic GVHD with female or multiparous donors, particularly if the recipient is male. After recipient age, sex-mismatch of transplants and donor alloimmunization (either through prior pregnancy or transfusion) are the two most frequent factors predicting GVHD [109–111]. Multiparous female donors have shown a higher rate of chronic GVHD in transplants including those from unrelated donors [112], although this finding has not been consistent in all studies [113]. The presumed mechanism of this GVHD is a change in the T-cell repertoire by exposure to additional foreign HLA antigens or a change from naïve to memory T cells. The exposure of the mother during childbirth to paternal HLA antigens is hypothesized to be the source of this change in T-cell reactivity.

B. Leukemia

In ALL there is a tendency toward higher remission rates for female patients in most adult series (reviewed in [114]), and survival in males is generally inferior. This is not explained by male testicular relapse, which occurs rarely in adults. Some authors have found more complex chromosomal abnormalities in men, which are a poor prognostic factor [115], although this finding has not been consistent. In AML, gender differences in treatment response are less striking. Age and chromosomal abnormalities are more significant prognostic factors, and they do not clearly differ between the genders. A tempting hypothesis is increased sensitivity or more likelihood in males of toxic exposures causing chromosomal damage that leads to leukemia; however, it has no clear scientific verification.

C. Hodgkin's Disease

In HD, female sex has been shown to be a positive prognostic factor generally attributed to a more favorable subtype (nodular sclerosing), which is more frequent in women, and diagnosis at an earlier stage of disease among females (reviewed in reference 114). Gender itself is not an independent prognostic factor, but it is associated with favorable differences in presentation. Gender-related differences in presenting nodal location and subtype in HD have lead investigators to suggest gender-related differences in risk factors for the development of HD [116] In young adults with HD, social class appears to modify risk leading to hypotheses about infectious etiologies, which do not clearly differ according to gender. Parity appears to be protective against the nodular sclerosing subtype of HD [117], and the greater increase for females in the incidence of young-adult nodular sclerosis in recent years may reflect the impact of trends toward later childbearing and lower parity. As mentioned previously, the potentially protective role of female sex hormones has yet to be fully explored in this disease, and there is no ready explanation for subtype differences between males and females. Side effects after treatment of HD may also differ in a gender-related fashion. Cardiopulmonary sequelae after treatment of HD have been found to a greater extent in female patients independent of treatment or other risk factors [118], leading to questions about gender-based differences in inflammation, organ sensitivity, and/or response to tissue damage.

IV. Conclusions

Gender-based differences in the hematologic malignancies in risk, incidence, treatment response, and side effects have only recently begun to be explored. Although gender-differences in experimental carcinogenesis after chemical exposures are often attributed to hormonal factors, there is little evidence to inform scientists of how they operate to produce human hematologic cancers. Certainly there is little evidence for hormonal differences alone as factors in leukemogenesis or lymphomagenesis, but there is little or no research on which to base conclusions. Considerable epidemiologic data are available to suggest the importance of environmental exposures in the gender differences seen in the incidence of hematologic malignancies. There is as yet little experimental evidence available to determine whether differences are due to time/degree of exposure or true differential susceptibilities between the sexes. Recent decreases in gender differences, particularly in the NHLs at a time when there are more women in traditionally male occupations, suggests that occupation is more relevant than gender. Likewise, there are data suggesting a possible beneficial effect of childbearing on the risk of developing some of the hematologic malignancies. Increases in the incidence for females over the last decade, particularly in the lymphomas, may also reflect the later childbearing and lower parity of women in the United States over this time period. Clearly there are differences in presentation and incidence of hematologic malignancies between males and females that have no ready explanation. Recently the *Journal of the National Cancer Institute* has called for more analysis of sex and ethnicity both in clinical and epidemiologic studies [119]. From this review it is clear how much we still need to explore.

V. Suggestions for Further Investigations

- Are occupational exposures to potentially carcinogenic agents pointing out true differences in gender sensitivities to the development of hematologic malignancies or only differential exposures by gender differences in the workplace?
- How can the gender-specific differences in development of leukemias after radiation exposure be explained? Does differential degree and time course of risk suggest gender-specific differences in sensitivity to DNA damage and repair?
- What is the true connection between rheumatologic illness and the development of lymphomas? Can collaborative gender-specific studies between hematologists/oncologists and rheumatologists/immunologists help us determine some fundamental understanding of immune alterations and the development of hematologic malignancies?

References

1. Hernandez JA, Land KJ, McKenna RW. (1995). *Cancer*. 75:381–394.
2. Groves FD, Linet MS, Travis LB, Devesa SS. (2000). *J Natl Cancer Inst*. 92:1240–1251.
3. Jemal A, Thomas A, Murray T, Thun M. (2002). *CA Cancer J Clin*. 52:23–47.
4. Robinson CF, Walker JT. (1999). *Am J Ind Med*. 36:186–192.
5. McDuffie HH. (1994). *J Occup Med*. 36:1240–1246.
6. Ries LAG, Eisner MP, Kosary CL *et al*. (2001). Bethesda, MD: National Cancer Institute.
7. Pearce N, Bethwaite P. (1992). *Cancer Res*. 52:5496s–5500s.
8. Baris D, Zahm SH. (2000). *Curr Opin Oncol*. 12:383–394.
9. Zheng T, Zahm SH, Cantor KP *et al*. (2001). *J Occup Environ Med*. 43:641–649.
10. Zahm SH, Blair A. (1992). *Cancer Res*. 52:5485s–5488s.
11. Waddell BL, Zahm SH, Baris D *et al*. (2001). *Cancer Causes Control*. 12:509–517.
12. Mao Y, Hu J, Ugnat AM, White K. (2000). *Ann Oncol*. 11(Suppl 1):69–73.
13. Hardell L, Eriksson M. (1999). *Cancer*. 85:1353–1360.
14. Amadori D, Nanni O, Falcini F *et al*. (1995). *Occup Environ Med*. 52:374–379.
15. Hartge P, Devesa SS. (1992). *Cancer Res*. 52:5566s–5569s.
16. McDuffie HH, Pahwa P, McLaughlin JR *et al*. (2001). *Cancer Epidemiol Biomarkers Prev*. 10:1155–1163.
17. (1990). *Arch Intern Med*. 150:2473–2483.
18. Dalager NA, Kang HK, Burt VL, Weatherbee L. (1991). *J Occup Med*. 33:774–779.
19. Kramarova E, Kogevinas M, Anh CT *et al*. (1998). *Environ Health Perspect*. 106(Suppl 2):671–678.
20. van Kaick G, Dalheimer A, Hornik S *et al*. (1999). *Radiat Res*. 152:S64–S71.
21. Weiss HA, Darby SC, Doll R. (1994). *Int J Cancer*. 59:327–338.
22. Preston DL, Kusumi S, Tomonaga M *et al*. (1994). *Radiat Res*. 137:S68–S97.
23. Wing S, Richardson D, Wolf S *et al*. (2000). *Ann Epidemiol*. 10:144–153.
24. Lopez-Abente G, Aragones N, Pollan M *et al*. (1999). *Cancer Epidemiol Biomarkers Prev*. 8:925–934.
25. Rabkin CS, Biggar RJ, Horm JW. (1991). *Int J Cancer*. 47:692–696.
26. Kirk O, Pedersen C, Cozzi-Lepri A *et al*. (2001). *Blood*. 98:3406–3412.
27. Tirelli U, Bernardi D, Spina M, Vaccher E. (2002). *Crit Rev Oncol Hematol*. 41:299–315.
28. Levine AM, Seneviratne L, Tulpule A. (2001). *Oncology (Huntingt)*. 15:629–639; discussion 639–640, 645–646.
29. Besson C, Goubar A, Gabarre J *et al*. (2001). *Blood*. 98:2339–2344.

30. Costantini AS, Miligi L, Kriebel D et al. (2001). Epidemiology. 12:78–87.
31. Demers PA, Vaughan TL, Koepsell TD et al. (1993). Am J Ind Med. 23:629–639.
32. Figgs LW, Dosemeci M, Blair A. (1994). J Occup Med. 36:1210–1221.
33. Heineman EF, Olsen JH, Pottern LM et al. (1992). Cancer Causes Control. 3:555–568.
34. Hatcher JL, Baris D, Olshan AF et al. (2001). Cancer Causes Control. 12:755–761.
35. Shibata A, Sasaki R, Hamajima N, Aoki K. (1990). Nippon Ketsueki Gakkai Zasshi. 53:116–118.
36. Altekruse SF, Henley SJ, Thun MJ. (1999). Cancer Causes Control. 10:617–625.
37. Grodstein F, Hennekens CH, Colditz GA et al. (1994). J Natl Cancer Inst. 86:1466–1470.
37a. Zhang Y, Holford TR, Leaderer B et al. (2004). Hair-coloring product use and risk of non-Hodgkin's lymphoma: a population-based case-control study in Connecticut. Am J Epidemiol. 159:148–154.
38. Brinton LA, Brown SL. (1997). J Natl Cancer Inst. 89:1341–1349.
39. Tugwell P, Wells G, Peterson J et al. (2001). Arthritis Rheum. 44: 2477–2484.
40. Karlson EW, Tanasijevic M, Hankinson SE et al. (2001). Arch Intern Med. 161:864–867.
41. Loomis DP, Savitz DA. (1991). Am J Ind Med. 19:509–521.
42. Lynge E, Anttila A, Hemminki K. (1997). Cancer Causes Control. 8:406–419.
43. Duarte-Davidson R, Courage C, Rushton L, Levy L. (2001). Occup Environ Med. 58:2–13.
44. Albin M, Bjork J, Welinder H et al. (2000). Scand J Work Environ Health. 26:482–491.
45. Freedman DM, Stewart P, Kleinerman RA et al. (2001). Am J Public Health. 91:564–567.
46. Kilian PH, Skrzypek S, Becker N, Havemann K. (2001). Leuk Res. 25:839–845.
47. Deadman JE, Infante-Rivard C. (2002). Am J Epidemiol. 155:368–378.
48. Pettersson T, Pukkala E, Teppo L, Friman C. (1992). Ann Rheum Dis. 51:437–439.
49. Kojima M, Nakamura S, Futamura N et al. (1997). Jpn J Clin Oncol. 27:84–90.
50. Catassi C, Fabiani E, Corrao G et al. (2002). JAMA. 287:1413–1419.
51. Cengiz M, Altundag MK, Zorlu AF et al. (2001). Clin Rheumatol. 20:239–244.
52. Le Beau MM, Albain KS, Larson RA et al. (1986). J Clin Oncol. 4:325–345.
53. Pedersen-Bjergaard J, Sigsgaard TC, Nielsen D et al. (1992). J Clin Oncol. 10:1444–1451.
54. Pedersen-Bjergaard J, Andersen MK, Christiansen DH. (2000). Blood. 95:3273–3279.
55. Leone G, Mele L, Pulsoni A et al. (1999). Haematologica. 84:937–945.
56. Leone G, Voso MT, Sica S et al. (2001). Leuk Lymphoma. 41:255–276.
57. Kollmannsberger C, Beyer J, Droz JP et al. (1998). J Clin Oncol. 16:3386–3391.
58. Diamandidou E, Buzdar AU, Smith TL et al. (1996). J Clin Oncol. 14:2722–2730.
59. Curtis RE, Boice JD, Stovall M et al. (1992). N Engl J Med. 326:1745–1751.
60. Fisher B, Anderson S, DeCillis A et al. (1999). J Clin Oncol. 17:3374–3388.
61. Bergh J, Wiklund T, Erikstein B et al. (2000). Lancet. 356:1384–1391.
62. Carli PM, Sgro C, Parchin-Geneste N et al. (2000). Leukemia. 14:1014–1017.
63. Chaplain G, Milan C, Sgro C et al. (2000). J Clin Oncol. 18:2836–2842.
64. Linassier C, Barin C, Calais G et al. (2000). Ann Oncol. 11:1289–1294.
65. Stone RM, Neuberg D, Soiffer R et al. (1994). J Clin Oncol. 12:2535–2542.
66. Miller JS, Arthur DC, Litz CE et al. (1994). Blood. 83:3780–3786.
67. Milligan DW, Ruiz De Elvira MC, Kolb HJ et al. (1999). Br J Haematol. 106:1020–1026.
68. Micallef IN, Lillington DM, Apostolidis J et al. (2000). J Clin Oncol. 18:947–955.
69. Krishnan A, Bhatia S, Slovak ML et al. (2000). Blood. 95:1588–1593.
70. Laughlin MJ, McGaughey DS, Crews JR et al. (1998). J Clin Oncol. 16:1008–1012.

71. Roman-Unfer S, Bitran JD, Hanauer S et al. (1995). Bone Marrow Transplant. 16:163–168.
72. Nichols G, deCastro K, Wei L-X et al. (2002). Leukemia. 16:1673–1679.
73. Weisz B, Schiff E, Lishner M. (2001). Hum Reprod Update. 7:384–393.
74. Ekstrom K, Wuu J, Hsieh CC et al. (2002). Cancer Causes Control. 13:47–53.
75. Lambe M, Ekbom A. (1995). BMJ. 311:1607–1608.
76. Ebert U, Loffler H, Kirch W. (1997). Pharmacol Ther. 74:207–220.
77. Zemlickis D, Lishner M, Erlich R, Koren G. (1993). Teratog Carcinog Mutagen. 13:139–143.
78. Peleg D, Ben-Ami M. (1998). Obstet Gynecol Clin North Am. 25:365–383.
79. Doll DC, Ringenberg QS, Yarbro JW. (1989). Semin Oncol. 16:337–346.
80. Sadural E, Smith LG. (1995). Clin Obst Gynecol. 38:535–546.
81. Brell J, Kalaycio M. (2000). Semin Oncol. 27:667–677.
82. Caligiuri MA, Mayer RJ. (1989). Semin Oncol. 16:388–396.
83. Greenlund LJ, Letendre L, Tefferi A. (2001). Leuk Lymphoma. 41:571–577.
84. Zuazu J, Julia A, Sierra J et al. (1991). Cancer. 67:703–709.
85. Partridge AH, Garber JE. (2000). Semin Oncol. 27:712–726.
86. Achtari C, Hohlfeld P. (2000). Am J Obstet Gynecol. 183:511–512.
87. Garcia L, Valcarcel M, Santiago-Borrero PJ. (1999). J Perinatol. 19:230–233.
88. Terada Y, Shindo T, Endoh A et al. (1997). Leukemia. 11:454–455.
89. Sheikh SS, Khalifa MA, Marley EF et al. (1996). Int J Gynecol Pathol. 15:363–366.
90. Osada S, Horibe K, Oiwa K et al. (1990). Cancer. 65:1146–1149.
91. Delgado-Lamas JL, Garces-Ruiz OM. (2000). Hematology. 4:415–418.
92. Harrison P, Chipping P, Fothergill GA. (1994). Br J Haematol. 86:681–682.
93. Hoffman MA, Wiernik PH, Kleiner GJ. (1995). Cancer. 76: 2237–2241.
94. Nakamura K, Dan K, Iwakiri R et al. (1995). Ann Hematol. 71:263–264.
95. Stentoft J, Lanng-Nielsen J, Hvidman LE. (1994). Leukemia. 8:1585–1588.
96. Welsh TM, Thompson J, Lim S. (2000). Leukemia. 14:1155.
97. Chrisomalis L, Baxi LV, Heller D. (1996). Am J Obstet Gynecol. 175: 1381–1382.
98. Haggstrom J, Adriansson M, Hybbinette T et al. (1996). Eur J Haematol. 57:101–102.
99. Lipton JH, Derzko CM, Curtis J. (1996). Hematol Oncol. 14:119–122.
100. Kuroiwa M, Gondo H, Ashida K et al. (1998). Am J Hematol. 59:101–102.
101. Mubarak AA, Kakil IR, Awidi A et al. (2002). Am J Hematol. 69:115–118.
102. Griesshammer M, Bergmann L, Pearson T. (1998). Baillieres Clin Haematol. 11:859–874.
103. Haas JF. (1984). Int J Cancer. 34:229–235.
104. Ward FT, Weiss RB. (1989). Semin Oncol. 16:397–409.
105. Pohlman B, Macklis RM. (2000). Semin Oncol. 27:657–666.
106. Greskovich JF Jr, Macklis RM. (2000). Semin Oncol. 27:633–645.
107. Anselmo AP, Cavalieri E, Enrici RM et al. (1999). Fetal Diagn Ther. 14:102–105.
108. Lambe M, Hsieh CC, Tsaih SW et al. (1998). Cancer Epidemiol Biomarkers Prev. 7:831–834.
109. Weisdorf D, Hakke R, Blazar B et al. (1991). Transplantation. 51: 1197–1203.
110. Nash RA, Pepe MS, Storb R et al. (1992). Blood. 80:1838–1845.
111. Carlens S, Ringden O, Remberger M et al. (1998). Bone Marrow Transplant. 22:755–761.
112. Kollman C, Howe CW, Anasetti C et al. (2001). Blood. 98:2043–2051.
113. Przepiorka D, Smith TL, Folloder J et al. (1999). Blood. 94:1465–1470.
114. Wiernik P. (1995). In Neoplastic Diseases of the Blood, 3rd Edition (Wiernik PH, Canellos GP, Dutcher J, Kyle RA, eds.). New York: Elsevier Science.
115. Li YS, Khalid G, Hayhoe FG. (1983). Scand J Haematol. 30:265–277.
116. Brandt L, Brandt J, Olsson H et al. (2001). Acta Oncol. 40:479–484.
117. Glaser SL, Jarrett RF. (1996). Baillieres Clin Haematol. 9:401–416.
118. Lund MB, Kongerud J, Boe J et al. (1996). Ann Oncol. 7:257–264.
119. Arnold K. (2000). J Natl Cancer Inst. 92:15–16.

58

Effects of Hormone Deprivation in Survivors of Breast and Prostate Cancer

DAWN HERSHMAN, MD, MS, ELLEN RITCHIE, MD, AND ZACHARY ROSNER

Department of Medicine and the Herbert Irving Comprehensive Cancer Center, College of Physicians and Surgeons, Columbia University, New York, NY

I. Introduction

Cancers specific to gender—prostate cancer and breast cancer—are among the most successfully treated malignancies with the largest numbers of survivors. As the number of cancer survivors grow, the long-term side effects of treatment play an increasingly prominent role in the routine care of these patients. The issues facing cancer survivors are unique, and many of the side effects of treatment have not been adequately studied by the medical community. This chapter offers a review of the issues faced by cancer survivors, and information about the evaluation and treatment of conditions affecting the quality of life (QOL) of these patients.

Breast cancer is the most commonly diagnosed cancer in women, with 182,000 new cases per year [1]. More than 2 million women in the United States today are breast cancer survivors [2]. Because the number of women diagnosed with invasive and noninvasive breast cancer is increasing and the number of women who die each year from breast cancer has decreased modestly [3], the number of breast cancer survivors is likely to increase even more. This is particularly true for women diagnosed with early-stage breast cancer, who have a life expectancy similar to that of age-matched controls [3].

Prostate cancer is the most common malignancy in men, with 180,000 new cases diagnosed each year. Similar to breast cancer patients in many ways, most men are diagnosed with early-stage disease and have a life expectancy similar to that of age-matched controls. Approximately 80% of patients are diagnosed with locoregional disease and the overall 5-year survival is more than 90%. Many of the patients diagnosed with prostate cancer are elderly and have other co-morbid illness that contribute to overall mortality and play a prominent role in treatment decisions [4].

There are many issues facing survivors of breast and prostate cancer treatment with implications for the ongoing primary care of these patients. Many of these issues center on hormonal changes associated with the cancer treatment and require special attention to the conditions caused by sex hormone deprivation. Breast cancer treatment frequently causes premature ovarian failure, which results in prolonged estrogen deprivation and thereby increases the risks of osteoporosis, cardiovascular disease, menopausal symptoms, cognitive dysfunction, and weight gain.

For men with prostate cancer, bilateral orchiectomy or hormonal therapy with gonadotropin-releasing hormone (GnRH) agonists are the standard of care for patients with metastatic disease. Evidence suggests that earlier hormone therapy may prolong survival in these patients. Although androgen deprivation therapy is successful at controlling prostate cancer, there are both short- and long-term consequences to this therapy. Short-term side effects include hot flashes and decreased libido; long-term consequences include decline in muscle mass, gynecomastia, osteoporosis, and QOL [5].

II. Vasomotor Instability

Vasomotor instability is a constellation of symptoms including hot flashes, sweats, nausea, palpitations, and insomnia that can be caused by treatment of breast and prostate cancer. For many patients, these symptoms are a significant clinical problem. They can affect the QOL of women and men who have been treated for breast or prostate cancer and can affect compliance with therapy and satisfaction with treatment decisions. The causes of vasomotor symptoms in these patients is thought to be related to abrupt androgen and estrogen losses caused by surgery, radiation therapy, chemotherapy, and hormonal therapy.

The effort to quantify the degree of distress caused by these symptoms in relation to other side effects of treatment is not simple because it involves finding an objective way to measure the subjective responses of patients to their treatment. In other words, it is difficult to scientifically verify the presence or absence of these symptoms. This subject was addressed in a paper by Sloan *et al* from the Mayo Clinic [6]. This group has developed a validated instrument to measure these symptoms. Participants record their perceptions and the frequency and severity of their symptoms in a diary. Reviewers then quantitate the patient's diary entries and responses. Using feedback from patient diaries, the group records the effect of various treatments on hot flashes and other vasomotor symptoms. The investigators feel that their instrument to measure response to treatment is valid but caution that the large placebo effect observed in their experience must be considered when evaluating the results of clinical trials and when considering anecdotal reports of response to new potential therapies. In addition, when evaluating treatment arms of clinical trials of various agents used to treat vasomotor symptoms, the baseline frequency and intensity of these symptoms often differs between the different treatment arms, making interpretation of response rates sometimes difficult to interpret.

A. Breast

Breast cancer therapy influences the timing of the onset of menopause. On average, menopause occurs in the United States at age 51. Adjuvant chemotherapy is frequently associated with either temporary or permanent amenorrhea, which results from direct toxicity to the ovary. The incidence of chemotherapy-induced ovarian failure depends on the chemotherapy regimen, the cumulative dose (especially of alkylating agents such as cyclophosphamide), and the age of the patients. Chemotherapy-induced ovarian failure causes changes similar to those seen in natural menopause: diminished circulating levels of estrogen and progesterone and elevated levels of follicle-stimulating hormone and luteinizing hormone. Because there is a rapid change in hormonal levels, symptoms can be more severe than those associated with the more gradual decline in estrogen levels seen in normal aging. Women treated for breast cancer who are closest to the age of natural menopause (50 to 60 years of age) often experience the highest rate of symptoms, which suggest that the natural age-related symptoms of menopause are exacerbated by adjuvant therapy but are not entirely caused by it. As in men, most likely the abruptness of the loss of estrogen during the treatment of breast cancer is what contributes to the vasomotor symptoms and other symptoms of menopause.

The vasomotor symptoms, which are so prominent in breast cancer survivors, are not only caused by the abrupt onset of menopause but are exacerbated by hormonal treatments for breast cancer, in particular tamoxifen, which is a mixed estrogen agonist and antagonist. Patients treated with hormonal therapy alone are less likely to experience premature ovarian failure or early menopause but are likely to experience many of the symptoms associated with menopause such as hot flashes, night sweats, nausea, and vaginal symptoms. Women who have received previous hormonal replacement therapy or who have had severe hot flashes during natural menopause are at a greater risk for hot flashes with tamoxifen. Vasomotor symptoms often become less severe after several months of tamoxifen therapy.

The treatments for the vasomotor symptoms in women do not differ substantially from those given to men treated for prostate cancer. Hormonal agents are an effective treatment for hot flashes in women; however, hormone replacement therapy (HRT) is controversial even in patients who do not have a history or risk factors for the development of breast cancer. A recent study of HRT in normal women was stopped early because the adverse effects of hormonal treatment (including increased risk of development of breast cancer) outweighed the potential benefits of therapy. HRT historically has been contraindicated because of the relationship between estrogen exposure and breast cancer and because antiestrogen therapy prevents the recurrence and the development of cancer in the contralateral breast. Actual data on the risk of breast cancer recurrence on HRT is limited, given that studies done on this subject have been retrospective and small and involved selected patients with a lower risk of breast cancer recurrence. Given that this is the case, HRT is not recommended for survivors of breast cancer because of the possible risks of disease recurrence and of death from breast cancer in women using this therapy for symptomatic relief.

Megesterol acetate (Megace) is a progestin that is also an agent used to treat breast cancer in certain circumstances. Although it is an effective treatment for hot flashes, because it is a hormone with receptors on breast tissue, there is a risk of disease exacerbation in women taking this drug. For this reason, this is not generally recommended for treatment of hot flashes.

Antidepressant drugs such as fluoxetine, venlafaxine, and paroxetine are used to treat hot flashes in women with some success [7–9]. All of these drugs have been tested in clinical trials and shown to have a statistically significant effect decreasing the frequency and intensity of hot flashes as compared with placebo. Clonidine, an antihypertensive, has been used to treat hot flashes in breast cancer survivors but with limited efficacy and substantial side effects.

Vitamin E has been shown to have a minimal benefit in clinical outcome over placebo in treating hot flashes [10]. Soy phytoestrogens in daily tablet doses have been tested and shown to give no improvement in symptoms as compared with placebo [11]. Given the strong placebo effect in the clinical trials of drugs used to treat vasomotor symptoms, anecdotal reports of effective agents sold over-the-counter need to be treated with caution.

B. Prostate

Androgen deprivation is the most effective treatment for metastatic cancer of the prostate. This can be achieved surgically with bilateral orchiectomy or with hormonal therapy. In some series of patients up to 70% of men who had either surgery or hormonal therapy reported hot flashes [12]. Unlike women who go through menopause, in men the physiologic decreases in testosterone associated with aging rarely cause hot flashes. The level to which testosterone must be suppressed for hot flashes to occur in not known. It is not clear whether it is the abruptness of the drop in testosterone levels or the degree to which these levels are dropped in the treatment of prostate cancer that leads to symptoms. Also unclear is whether it is testosterone alone or the drop in estrogen levels in men that contribute to the problem.

In a study of men who had regrets in their choice of treatment for metastatic prostate cancer, two thirds reported having hot flashes and one third reported having nausea. Most were satisfied with their treatment decisions, but 23% expressed regret at their treatment choice and wished they had chosen another treatment modality [12]. In comparing the men who were satisfied with their treatment and those who were not, the two groups reported hot flashes, nausea, and breast tenderness at nearly the same rate. Those who expressed regret were not significantly more distressed by the vasomotor symptoms than those who were satisfied with their treatment decisions.

In a study of 421 men who had received diagnoses of prostate cancer, those that expressed dissatisfaction with the effects of their treatments felt that urinary problems were associated with the most discomfort followed by sexual symptoms [13]. In another survey of 1583 patients, urinary problems were found to cause the most dissatisfaction [14]. Vasomotor symptoms were not prominent causes of dissatisfaction in either of these groups, although they were mentioned as a side effect of treatment that caused regret of treatment choice.

There are a number of different drugs that have been used to treat hot flashes in men. Historically, estrogens and estrogen-related drugs have been used to treat this symptom [15–17]. Their use is limited by the tendency of estrogens to increase the risk of cardiovascular morbidity and for the difficulties of administration including parenteral administration of diethylstilbestrol

(DES) (oral DES is not commercially available). There have been investigations of transdermal estrogens in men, which appear to improve symptoms of hot flashes, but larger studies are necessary to assess the safety and cardiac effects of this therapy and the effectiveness of this preparation [16].

Megestrol acetate (Megace) in low doses (40 mg/day) was found in a placebo-controlled clinical trial to reduce hot flashes by 87% [18]. However, there are case reports of progression of prostate cancer in patients who have used this drug to suppress hot flashes during androgen ablation therapy [19]. This possibility may limit the use of this drug to treat vasomotor symptoms and warrants further investigation to assess this effect.

Venlafaxine (Effexor) is an antidepressant that inhibits neuronal serotonin and norepinephrine uptake [20]. In a small clinical trail of 16 patients, 63% had greater than a 50% decrease in the frequency and severity of hot flashes by the 4th week of treatment. This therapy was well tolerated by the participants, and a larger clinical trial is currently ongoing.

Clonidine (Catapres), an antihypertensive drug, can be given orally or as a patch. Trials have shown some effectiveness of this drug with 10 to 20% reduction in symptoms as compared with placebo [21]. However, there were substantial side effects given that the ability of this drug to relieve symptoms was limited. Other proposed drugs include vitamin E and soy phytoestrogens, but there are no clinical trial data in men to support the effectiveness of these drugs.

III. Osteoporosis

Another effect of abrupt hormone deprivation in breast and prostate cancer survivors is the development of osteoporosis during therapy and afterward. This affects both women and men and can have a significant impact on QOL as breast and prostate cancer survivors age. At present, monitoring of bone mineral density (BMD) and treatment for bone loss during therapy are not the standard of care for patients undergoing treatment for breast and prostate cancer. An increasing body of evidence documents the dangers of substantial bone loss during therapy for these cancers and suggests that the primary care of these patients should include the measurement of BMD and adequate treatment for bone loss.

A. Breast

Women with a history of premenopausal breast cancer have higher than average rates of bone loss and fracture [22,23]. Women with a history of nonmetastatic breast cancer have been found to have a risk of vertebral fractures nearly five times that of the general population [23]. Bone loss is greatest in women who become amenorrheic as a result of chemotherapy, suggesting that estrogen deficiency is an important etiologic factor. A cross-sectional study of 27 breast cancer survivors reported that the BMD of women who became amenorrheic was 14% lower than that of cycling women [22]. Two studies have evaluated lumbar spine (LS) BMD in women before and after chemotherapy for localized breast cancer. At 2 years, bone loss ranged from 4.4% in one study to 5.9% in the other. Bone loss was as high as 9.5% in women who had become amenorrheic during chemotherapy [24,25]. Another study compared 44 women with

breast cancer who were treated with adjuvant chemotherapy and 44 who were not. Treated women had a decrease in total body BMD of 1.29 g/cm^2 compared with 1.12 g/cm^2 in the untreated group p 0.03, (using a Lunar DPY scanner). Again, the loss was particularly great in women who became amenorrheic as a result of chemotherapy [26]. Preliminary results presented in May 2001 report total body bone loss of >5% in premenopausal women treated with the bisphosphonate Zoladex (p < 0.01) in an effort to prevent bone loss [27].

Considerable data support the concept that estrogen administration reduces bone turnover and the rate of bone loss [28] and substantially increases BMD in postmenopausal women [29]. Estrogen use is associated with a reduced risk of vertebral and possibly hip fracture [30]. As soon as estrogen is discontinued, however, BMD begins to decline at a rate similar to that observed before initiation of therapy [31]. For women with a history of breast cancer, the use of estrogen to prevent bone loss is contraindicated because the risk of breast cancer may be increased or hastened by the administration of estrogen agonists.

Adjuvant tamoxifen therapy has been shown to preserve bone density in postmenopausal women with breast cancer [32,33]. Resorption of bone was lower in women treated with tamoxifen compared with those who received placebo [33]. However, in premenopausal women tamoxifen therapy has been associated with varying levels of bone loss. The mean annual loss in lumbar BMD per year over the 3-year study period in tamoxifen-treated compliant women who remained premenopausal throughout the study period was 1.44% (1.88% calculated on an intent-to-treat basis), compared with a small gain of 0.24% per annum for women on placebo (p<0.001) [34]. Other selective estrogen receptor inhibitors, such as raloxifene, also reduce the risk of fractures from osteoporosis in postmenopausal women. The effects of these agents in premenopausal women are currently unknown [35].

Bisphosphonates are pyrophosphate analogues that avidly adsorb to bone surfaces. They reduce bone turnover by specifically inhibiting osteoclastic bone resorption and have demonstrated therapeutic efficacy in the treatments of hypercalcemia of malignancy, lytic bone disease associated with multiple myeloma, and mixed lytic and blastic bone metastases associated with breast cancer [36–44]. The precise mechanism by which bisphosphonates inhibit osteoclast function is not fully understood but may include a direct toxic effect on mature osteoclasts, an inhibition of osteoclast production from precursor cells, and an impairment of osteoclast chemotaxis to sites of active bone [45].

The ability of intravenous bisphosphonates to restore bone has been documented in patients with either breast cancer or multiple myeloma with osteolytic lesions. An 11% increase in LS BMD was noted in the group of patients receiving zoledronic acid 2 or 4 mg. Zoledronic acid at 4 mg was most effective in reducing the skeletal morbidity rate [46].

In early-stage breast cancer, the oral bisphosphonate clodronate has been evaluated in two British studies [25,47]. Among these patients, most of whom received chemotherapy and/or hormonal therapy, a randomized, placebo-controlled trial found that oral clodronate, taken for 2 years, was efficacious in preventing bone loss. By 1 year BMD had fallen by 2.20% in the placebo group and risen by 0.18% in the clodronate group (mean difference of 2.38%). The mean difference between the clodronate and placebo subjects was greater among perimenopausal than among premenopausal women (4.08% vs 2.48%) [25]. In a second trial restricted to premenopausal women receiving chemotherapy with cyclophosphamide, methotrexate, 5FU (CMF), the clodronate and placebo groups differed in LS BMD by 3% at 1 year and by 3.7% at 2 years (p<0.01). Among patients who developed ovarian failure, the LS bone loss in the clodronate group was 5.9% compared with 9.5% in the placebo group (p<0.001) [24]. In both groups, the treatment was well tolerated, and there were no differences in adverse events.

B. Prostate

Men rendered testosterone-deficient during therapy for prostate cancer have biochemical evidence of increased bone resorption, sustain gradual but significant bone loss, and are at increased risk for fragility fractures over the long-term compared with normal men. The trend toward early initiation of androgen deprivation therapy may result in increased bone mineral loss over time.

In a recent cross-sectional study, BMD, biochemical markers of bone turnover, and body composition were measured in 60 men with prostate cancer (19 receiving GnRH therapy and 41 eugonadal). Bone mineral density was also measured in 197 community-living healthy controls of similar age. Bone mineral density was significantly lower at the lateral spine (0.69 ± 0.17 vs $0.83 \pm 0.20\,\text{g/cm}^2$; p<0.01), total hip [TH] (0.94 ± 0.14 vs $1.05 \pm 0.16\,\text{g/cm}^2$; p<0.05), and forearm ($0.67 \pm 0.11$ vs $0.78 \pm 0.07\,\text{g/cm}^2$; p<0.01) in men receiving GnRH therapy compared with the eugonadal men with prostate cancer. Bone mineral density was similar in eugonadal men with prostate cancer and healthy controls. Bone resorption (as measured by urinary N-telopeptide [NTX]) and formation (as measured by bone-specific alkaline phosphatase [BSAP]) markers were elevated in men receiving GnRH therapy compared with eugonadal men with prostate cancer [48]. Therefore, men with prostate cancer receiving androgen deprivation therapy have significantly decreased BMD and increased bone turnover, placing them at increased risk of fracture.

Bone loss in men with both prostate cancer and benign prostatic hypertrophy receiving hormone ablation therapy has also been evaluated in several longitudinal studies [49–53]. At 1 year, the loss in BMD at the LS ranges from 3.1 to 10% and the loss in femoral neck (FN) BMD varies from 3.8 to 8.4%. The studies are small and the degree of bone loss is variable, but all report significant bone loss.

The pathogenesis of increased bone turnover, bone loss, and fracture in men on GnRH agonists is incompletely understood. Traditionally, estrogen was considered to be the major gonadal steroid regulating bone metabolism in women, and testosterone was thought to play the same role in men. However, recent evidence suggests that estrogen is the dominant sex steroid regulating bone resorption in men [54], as it does in women [55]. Because most estrogen in men is derived from peripheral conversion of testosterone to estradiol, androgen ablation therapy also results in estrogen deficiency. New data suggest that the increased bone turnover and bone loss associated with GnRH therapy may be related, at least in part, to estrogen deficiency [56–58].

These observations have aroused great interest in the therapeutic potential of antiresorptive therapy with bisphosphonates in the prevention and therapy of osteoporosis in this clinical setting. Pamidronate has recently been reported to prevent bone loss at the TH and LS in men with prostate cancer receiving androgen ablation therapy [59]. Bone mineral density of men receiving leuprolide alone fell by 3.3% at the LS, 2.1% at the trochanter, and 1.8% at the TH. BMD did not change at any site in men who received leuprolide plus pamidronate (60 mg intravenous every 3 months).

IV. Sexual Dysfunction

Sexual dysfunction is a prominent side effect of treatment for breast and prostate cancer. Mastectomy and lumpectomy can change the self-image of a woman and can effect enjoyment of sexual life. There also is compelling evidence that women who have been treated with chemotherapy have ongoing dissatisfaction with their sexual life. The reasons for this are not well understood, and more research must be done to determine the causes.

Men undergoing therapy for prostate cancer often are left with urinary incontinence and impotence after surgery and/or radiation treatment. Ongoing therapy for more advanced disease with hormone deprivation therapy causes erectile dysfunction and a lack of sexual drive. These side effects of treatment can have a strong impact on the QOL experienced by cancer survivors.

Patients suffering from these complaints may be embarrassed or hesitant to discuss these problems with their physicians. In taking care of these patients, physicians must be aware of these problems and must ask cancer survivors about symptoms. There are treatments for some causes of sexual dysfunction. As the numbers of breast and prostate cancer survivors grow, more attention must be paid to the problem by the research community with the hope that more devices and medications can be added to the arsenal of treatments.

A. Breast

The effects of breast cancer treatment with surgery, chemotherapy, radiation, and hormonal therapies in conjunction with the psychologic anguish of having a diagnosis of cancer and of having survived a potentially life-threatening illness can have significant impact on a woman's sexual functioning.

Although breast-conserving surgical procedures have shown benefits over mastectomy when it comes to body image [60,61], most studies have found no difference between lumpectomy and mastectomy in terms of their effects on sexual functioning [62,63]. One study that examined sexual function retrospectively by giving questionnaires 4 years after surgery found that women who received a partial mastectomy were better able to experience pleasure during intercourse than those who received immediate reconstructive surgery. In this study, no difference was reported in body image, satisfaction with relationships, or sexual life [64]. A review by Schover [65] in 1994 found that despite the expectation that changes in breast appearance would have more devastating effects on a woman's sexuality, no difference was found between psychologic distress, marital satisfaction, and sexual frequency. Some studies suggest that age may be a significant factor in a patient's self-image and that partial mastectomies may have a more beneficial effect on QOL for younger women. In these studies, however, the relationship of self-image to sexual dysfunction is not entirely clear [66].

More than surgery type or radiation therapy, chemotherapy and endocrine therapy appear to have the most significant effects on sexual functioning. Among breast cancer survivors in a health-related QOL study, women who received chemotherapy were found to have the highest level of sexual dysfunction [67]. One study comparing women who received nonpharmacologic treatment with those who received chemotherapy or hormonal therapy found that 7 years after treatment chemotherapy patients were 5.7 times more likely to report vaginal dryness, 3.0 times more likely to report decreased libido, 5.5 times more likely to report increased pain during intercourse, and 7.1 times more likely to report difficulty achieving orgasm [68]. Another study confirmed these findings by noting that chemotherapy treatment was found to be a predictor of a woman's sexual health status [69].

The effects of chemotherapy on sexual functioning may decrease with time. One study comparing the effects of adjuvant CMF chemotherapy to no adjuvant chemotherapy 10 years after treatment found no difference in sexual functioning between those who received treatment and those who did not [62,70]. More research into the long-term effects of chemotherapy on sexual functioning is needed.

Treatment of breast cancer using the GnRH agonist Zoladex in combination with tamoxifen was found to increase sexual dysfunction in comparison to patients treated with Zoladex alone. The reason for this is not clear. In this same study, tamoxifen as a single agent did not appear to produce sexual dysfunction, but patients treated with combination chemotherapy had continued sexual dysfunction over time [71]. Other studies have found no connection between tamoxifen and sexual functioning [72]. Clinical investigations have not yet clarified whether hormonal agents contribute to sexual dysfunction. Symptoms associated with tamoxifen use such as vaginal dryness would appear to contribute to sexual dysfunction, but studies so far have not clarified that this is the case. Investigations suggest that chemotherapy is most strongly linked to sexual dysfunction after treatment and that women treated with chemotherapy are at highest risk for ongoing dissatisfaction with their sexual lives.

B. Prostate

One of the major side effects of prostate cancer treatment is sexual dysfunction. Radical prostatectomy, radiation treatment, and brachytherapy have all been associated with impotence either immediately after the treatment or developing over time after therapy. There are some studies that suggest a better outcome with brachytherapy: ultrasound guided transperineal brachytherapy was less damaging to vascular bundles than other therapies [73]; and another study found that initial potency after brachytherapy was high but that it declined over 3 to 6 years [74]. From the studies of brachytherapy in comparison with other modes of treatment with surgery and radiation, it is not clear that brachytherapy is clearly better at preserving erectile function [75]. All forms of therapy for local-regional disease are associated with erectile dysfunction and hence sexual malfunction.

For more advanced disease, androgen deprivation therapy caused by orchiectomy or the use of GnRH agonists is associated with sexual dysfunction. A study comparing men receiving medical castration using GnRH agonists, men who were post-prostatectomy but were not receiving androgen deprivation therapy, and healthy men was done to examine the effects of hormone treatments on a number of QOL measures. Patients who received androgen therapy for at least 12 months were found to have significant sexual dysfunction [76]. The relationship between androgen levels and sexual function is not entirely clear because the causes for this problem are multifactorial and can be related to a number of different causes including nerve damage, psychologic state, and vascular damage. Testosterone appears, however, to have significant effects on a number of indicators of sexual function [77].

Erectile dysfunction after radical prostatectomy is common despite the prevalence of nerve-sparing techniques. When compared to non–nerve sparing techniques, nerve-sparing techniques were found to have a significantly positive effect on sexual function with 50% of patients who received nerve-sparing radical prostatectomy having spontaneous erectile activity after treatment [78]. Even after nerve-sparing techniques, however, sexual dysfunction is still a problem for about 40% of patients [79]. In some series of patients who have undergone radical prostatectomy, erectile dysfunction has been found in up to 90% of patients [80].

Treatment of prostate cancer using three-dimensional conformal radiation therapy has shown that such radiation can reduce sexual potency significantly from baseline [81]. The incidence of sexual dysfunction and impotence can increase over time after treatment with radiation therapy. Although alternative treatments to radical prostatectomy aim to preserve erectile function, it is not clear that other modalities are superior to surgery in this regard over time.

Urinary incontinence often is associated with prostate cancer treatments and can have a significant effect on a patient's sexual life. Other urinary symptoms after prostate cancer treatment include nocturia, hesitancy, frequency, and dysuria. An observational study conducted in Japan found that daily urinary leakage was common in 30% of patients treated with radical prostatectomy [82]. Similarly, urinary incontinence was found to be a common problem along with sexual dysfunction in patients treated with brachytherapy and external beam radiation [83]. A study by Marsh and Lepor [84] found that a continence score could be used at the time of catheter removal to help predict the likelihood that the patient will suffer from urinary incontinence. The same study found that most men regained significant urinary continence. In one study, surgical patients have two times the rate of urinary incontinence than do patients treated with radiation [85]. To control urinary incontinence many men wear pads to protect from leakage. Some patients have an artificial urinary sphincter surgically implanted to help prevent leakage. Other possibilities for treatment include collagen injection therapy and the male bulbourethral sling [86].

There are a number of treatments for the erectile dysfunction caused by therapies for prostate cancer that can improve sexual dysfunction. These modalities include oral drugs, intraurethral alprostadil, vacuum devices, intracavernous injections, and penile prostheses [87].

Sildenafil citrate (Viagra) has been found to greatly aid men suffering from erectile dysfunction after treatment for prostate cancer. A study of sildenafil on men who had erectile dysfunction resulting from external beam radiotherapy found that the average score on the International Index of Erectile Function questionnaire increased from baseline in men receiving sildenafil and minimal side effects were seen [88]. This has been supported by another study noting that 71% of patients with erectile dysfunction treated with sildenafil were able to maintain an erection after treatment [89]. For this medication to be effective, nerve endings must be intact because nitric oxide from nerve endings are involved in stimulating smooth muscle to cause an erection [90]. When nerve endings have been damaged by surgery or radiation therapy, this treatment will not be effective.

Vacuum erection devices are also an option for men suffering from erectile dysfunction after treatment for prostate cancer. Some problems associated with the use of a vacuum device are the need for practice in using the device and lack of appeal to some patients. Side effects include pain during ejaculation, bruising, and numbness [90]. The devices, however, are safe enough to be sold over-the-counter and do not require a prescription.

Penile prostheses are also an option for treatment of sexual dysfunction and come in two forms, inflatable and noninflatable. Three-piece inflatable prostheses come closest to normal erectile function having the ability to alternate between flaccid and erect levels and providing girth expansion. One of the most common problems associated with penile prostheses is postsurgical infection, which may require additional surgery and a significant delay in implantation. Inflatable prostheses seem to give more satisfaction overall than noninflatable ones [91].

A number of newer medications are currently in phase 3 trials that may also help men for whom sildenafil does not work. These drugs include oral phentolamine, apomorphine, newer phosphodiesterase type-5 inhibitors, and topical agents [92]. Intraurethral injections, such as the MUSE system, are available but very difficult to use and often painful [90]. The main factor in choosing a system should be ease of use and minimum number of side effects. This is an active area of research with promise for new drugs in the future to treat erectile dysfunction.

V. Depression

Among the most serious ongoing side effects of cancer treatment is depression. The causes for this can be complex: the diagnosis of a serious, life-threatening illness; the side effects of treatment with surgery, radiation, and chemotherapy; the effect on family and friends of treatment; and the survival of the illness when others have not been so fortunate. The depression can be an effect of circumstance—such as chemotherapy treatment or recovery from surgery—and will pass as the condition improves or the chemotherapy ends. It also can be ongoing with serious consequences for a patient's QOL. Physicians

taking care of these patients need to be aware that many patients experience depression at some point during their treatment and recovery and that questions relating to this problem needs to be addressed frequently. Many treatments exist for this problems and can have an impact as great as therapies for the cancer in patients' overall experience of life.

A. Breast

Depression in survivors of breast cancer has been found to be significantly higher than in the general population [93]. Similarly, studies have shown that chemotherapy treatment can have a profound effect on a cancer survivor's degree of depression. One study comparing the long-term psychologic effects on survivors of childhood leukemia, Hodgkin's disease, and non-Hodgkin's lymphoma found that exposure to chemotherapy was a predictor of depressive symptomology [94]. Chemotherapy has been reported to cause more psychologic distress when compared with other forms of breast cancer treatment [64]. One study comparing 3 weeks of radiotherapy, 1 year of chemotherapy, and radiotherapy followed by chemotherapy found depressive symptoms become significantly worse in patients treated with chemotherapy for more than 13 months. Until 13 months, however, little difference was found in levels of depression, and the authors suggest restricting chemotherapy to 6 months to minimize this discrepancy [95]. In a study of psychosocial morbidity among breast cancer patients, chemotherapy was among the factors associated with increased depression [96].

The effect of tamoxifen on depression is still being debated. One review found that depression had been correlated to greater degrees of depression and recommended further investigation into the association of the hormone with mood [97]. One study found that women treated with tamoxifen for 8 months had higher levels of depression ($p<0.05$) [98]. One argument for the association of tamoxifen with depression is based on the theory that it acts as an antagonist in the central nervous system (CNS). According to this theory, estrogen can have effects on serotonin receptor density and stimulation of serotonin receptors within the brain. Competitive inhibition of estrogen by tamoxifen may change serotonin receptor density and decrease stimulation causing depression [97]. Despite some studies associating tamoxifen with mood changes, recent reports from the National Surgical Adjuvant Breast and Bowel Project's Breast Cancer Prevention (P-1) Randomized Study have found tamoxifen to have no effect on overall depression based on measurements using the CES-D depression questionnaire [99–101].

When comparing modes of cancer treatment and the association with depression, there is little benefit in choosing a lumpectomy over a mastectomy [64]. Although some past reports have found trends suggesting mastectomy to have more significant psychologic effects [102,103], recent reports have found little difference in QOL between patients who choose mastectomy and lumpectomy [60,61,66]. Some reports suggest that allowing women to participate in choosing the type of surgery to be done will help then psychologically accept the consequences of their surgical treatment with less distress and depression [63,104]. Younger women with breast cancer appear to be more at risk for the development of depression during therapy or after treatment. Studies have shown a higher prevalence of depressive symptoms in younger women, which may be due to a number of factors [96,105].

Treatments for depression among cancer survivors include individual counseling with a trained professional and group therapy sessions and support groups. Breast cancer support programs have been found to positively influence breast cancer survivors' QOL [106]. Supportive behavior by health care providers and strong social support can greatly help patients who have survived chemotherapy [107]. For patients who prefer alternative modes of therapy, one report found similar results from a complementary and alternative medicine group as with a standard group support program [108]. Antidepressant medications may also be appropriate in helping patients who are suffering from depression.

B. Prostate

Prostate cancer patients, like many other cancer patients, suffer from depressive symptoms as a result of their diagnosis and their treatment choice. Whether the cause of depression is in the diagnosis of the disease or in the treatment choice is not clear and not easy to delineate in clinical trials. The significant side effects of treatment—incontinence, erectile dysfunction, vasomotor effects, gynecomastia—can all have a profound effect on QOL and certainly contribute to the depressive symptoms in these patients.

Depression also may be associated with suppressed levels of testosterone. Some studies suggest that there is a positive correlation between testosterone levels and the severity of a patient's depression; however, the literature is not definitive. Studies examining low testosterone levels in men have been primarily based on men who are hypogonadal or elderly men who are experiencing a decline in their testosterone levels as they age, not on men who have prostate cancer. Depressed elderly men have been observed to have the lowest testosterone levels, and testosterone has been considered for treatment of depressed hypogonadal elderly men who do not respond to regular antidepressants, although the efficacy of this therapy has yet to be established [109]. A number of studies have found that testosterone treatments are beneficial for depressed hypogonadal men but not necessarily in eugonadal men [109–111]. A study assessing sexual function in eugonadal men with erectile dysfunction who were treated with testosterone concluded that, although testosterone had an effect on sexual function in these men, no difference in mood could be observed [112].

Treatment of depression for prostate cancer survivors is similar to treatment for breast cancer survivors. Social networks of support and positive relationships with health care providers can have a significant impact on a survivor's depression level. Self-help groups help prostate cancer survivors to meet with others and gather helpful information about their disease in a supportive environment [113]. Pharmacologic treatment with antidepressants also are indicated in select patients.

VI. Cognitive Decline

As more patients survive cancer, there is greater interest in the medical community as to whether treatment with chemotherapy, hormonal agents, and radiation effect long-term cognitive skills. Other problems associated with cancer therapy, including depression, fatigue, and other psychologic problems, can affect cognitive skill and can complicate the assessment of cognitive decline. Also complicating the assessment of this problem are the effects of normal aging. Many breast and prostate cancer patients are diagnosed at older ages and declines noticed over time may have occurred if they had not had therapy. There are many ongoing questions about the role of cancer therapy in cognitive decline and this is an area of active research.

A. Breast

There are several studies of the long-term cognitive effects of cancer treatment on patients. Cognitive impairments have been reported for many of the chemotherapy agents commonly used in treatment protocols [114]. In a study of 50 medical oncology patients who were treated for a variety of non-CNS malignancies, a significant association between cognitive impairment and a wide range of chemotherapeutic agents was reported. The neurotoxicity of various chemotherapeutic agents is not fully understood. Several chemotherapeutic agents that are thought to be unable to pass through the blood-brain-barrier, may lead to CNS neurotoxicity when administered in frequent doses [115,116]. The mechanism by which this toxicity occurs is unclear but may be related to metabolic by-products, vascular injury, direct parenchymal injury, and/or immunologically induced vasculitis [117].

To date, only a small number of studies have focused specifically on cognitive functioning in women treated with adjuvant chemotherapy for breast cancer, and none have been reported evaluating declining cognitive functioning in men with prostate cancer. Most of the studies of cognitive effects of chemotherapy are limited by cross-sectional methodologies or simple correlational analyses. Using a battery of neuropsychologic tests to examine cognitive functioning in women with stages I and II breast cancer treated with adjuvant chemotherapy, 21 of 28 women were moderately impaired on one or more tests, independent of depression and type of chemotherapy. One study links cognitive impairment to the duration of chemotherapy treatment [118].

Studies of patients have found that cognitive impairments were most substantial in the patients following conventional treatment with high-dose chemotherapy and stem cell transplant [119]. Cognitive impairment was independent of anxiety, depression, fatigue, and time since treatment [120]. In addition, they found a low correlation between subjective complaints of cognitive problems and objective cognitive deficits.

From the time of cancer diagnosis through the post-treatment readjustment period, cancer patients face a variety of physical and psychosocial challenges. Throughout this period, factors such as anxiety, depression, fatigue, and poor sleep quality are prevalent [121,122]. Cognitive symptoms experienced by patients may or may not be correlated with objectively measured cognitive deficits. In breast cancer patients, correlations with true cognitive deficits and other factors such as anxiety, depression, fatigue, and poor sleep quality have been observed before treatment [123]; after surgery [124,125]; and after chemotherapy [126]. Although the findings have been mixed, they suggest that psychologic distress, fatigue, or poor sleep quality may also affect cognitive function.

There are data suggesting that estrogen may enhance certain areas of cognitive functioning [127]. Therefore, it is possible that suppression of estrogen levels may account declines in cognitive functioning. No studies, however, have adequately differentiated these effects from the specific effects of chemotherapy. Research is currently ongoing to assess the role of estrogen in cognitive function and the connection of low levels of estrogen to Alzheimer's disease and other causes of cognitive decline.

B. Prostate

Definitive studies have yet to be conducted on the effects of chemotherapy on cognitive functioning in men receiving treatment for prostate cancer. However, research into the effects of hormones, such as testosterone, on the cognitive functioning of men is an active area of interest. Research on the role of testosterone and estrogen in cognitive skills may further the understanding of the effects of hormone deprivation therapies on men with prostate cancer.

A number of studies have been done in recent years examining the effects of testosterone on the cognitive functioning of older men. It has been observed that blood levels of testosterone decrease in men as they age [111], coinciding with a decrease in cognitive functioning as men age. Although some studies have found that men with lower testosterone performed better on spatial ability tests [128], a positive correlation between testosterone and spatial ability has been shown when serum testosterone levels, salivary testosterone levels, and 5-dihydrotestosterone (DHT) are within normal physiologic range in college-aged men [129]. Janowsky, Oviatt, and Orwoll [130] found that when testosterone levels are increased to 150% of normal levels, a significant increase in spatial cognition abilities is observed. These findings support a curvilinear relationship between testosterone and spatial cognition in which both extremes inhibit spatial cognitive abilities. Further research into the effects of "andropause," the decrease in testosterone levels with age, may help to elucidate some of the problems faced by men receiving GnRH agonists or other forms of antiandrogen therapy.

The effects of testosterone on cognitive functioning are far from definite. It has been proposed in a number of studies that the suspected curvilinear relationship of testosterone and spatial cognition is related to the aromatization of testosterone into estrogen in the brain [128,130]. The effect would be that higher than normal testosterone levels would cause a decrease in the production of estradiol, which has been found to decrease spatial abilities [111]. In menopausal women, estrogen replacement therapy has been seen to improve verbal memory [131–133], and testosterone's effects on estradiol levels may be the reason for changes in cognitive function with testosterone treatments.

Other studies have suggested that the ratio of testosterone to estrogen may be responsible for differences in working memory [134]. This may have significant implications for men receiving hormonal therapy for prostate cancer because this therapy may change sex hormone proportions. The role of sex hormones was also examined in terms of hormone cycles showing variations in cognitive functions based on hormone fluctuation [135]. Whether such an effect is seen in men who are hypogonadal because of

prostate treatment is unknown, and the extent of such effects in such men is questionable.

Most of the evidence suggests that there is some connection between testosterone levels and cognition, but determining the extent to which cognition is impaired has been particularly difficult. If the effects of hormones on cognition do turn out to be significant, further research is required to determine what methods are applicable to aid men who experience such cognitive declines after being treated with hormone therapies. Hopefully, with increasing interest in over-the-counter androgens such as dehydroepiandrosterone (DHEA) and androstenedione and increasing numbers of prostate cancer survivors, the long-term effects of androgen deprivation on cognitive functioning will continue to be investigated.

VII. Conclusion

Breast cancer and prostate cancer are two of the most common gender-specific malignancies. Their survival rates are comparable, and both cancers are treatable when diagnosed in the early stages. In addition, both cancers are linked to levels of sex hormones and are treated in part by changing the levels of those hormones. Understanding the long-term effects of hormonal alterations is essential. With regard to QOL issues, breast and prostate cancer treatments have very similar effects. Parallel effects of cancer treatment can be seen in issues of vasomotor instability, osteoporosis, sexual functioning, cognitive functioning, and depression. The adverse effects on QOL are connected to hormonal effects caused by treatment.

As the population of breast and prostate cancer survivors grows, it is increasingly important to evaluate survivors' QOL after treatment and look into how we can treat and minimize adverse effects. More research into the role of sex hormones has the potential to revolutionize how the medical community responds to post-treatment problems in cognition, depression, sexual dysfunction, and other side effects of treatment. Hopefully, more research will be available in the coming years to more easily predict the effects of hormonal treatments on cancer patients and to treat the more debilitating side effects. Similarly, more research into the effects of treatment on different patient populations would also be valuable. For a number of QOL issues, such as depression or sexual functioning, it appears that age can be a significant factor in determining how likely it is that the patient will be negatively affected. Further research will help physicians to prepare patients for potential changes in their QOL and to be more prepared to help patients when they observe such effects.

Understanding the effects of chemotherapy on QOL issues may also provide a significant benefit for cancer survivors. By understanding the long-term effects of chemotherapy, we may better be able to prevent or treat problems and minimize suffering. As more patients survive cancer, a better understanding of the long-term chemotherapy consequences will allow physicians to select drugs that have minimal adverse effects.

Most importantly, however, the medical community must be prepared to help patients cope with QOL problems that result from their treatments. Understanding the physiologic and psychologic effects of cancer treatment will allow doctors to better relate to their patients and provide them with more complete treatments.

VIII. Suggestions for Further Investigations

- More research on how to combat the effects of hormone depletion caused by aging and cancer treatment—better medications for vasomotor symptoms and sexual symptoms.
- More research investigating therapies for bone loss and osteoporosis caused by disease, drugs and aging.
- More research on the neurologic effects of chemotherapy on cancer patients affecting mood and cognitive function with new treatments to reduce these effects.
- A greater understanding in the medical community about how to provide primary care to survivors of cancer treatment.

References

1. Greenlee RT, Murray T, Bolden S *et al.* (2000). Cancer statistics, 2000. *CA Cancer J Clin.* 50:7–33.
2. Hewitt M, Breen N, Devesa S. (1999). Cancer prevalence and survivorship issues: Analyses of the 1992 National Health Interview Survey. *J Natl Cancer Inst.* 91:1480–1486.
3. Wingo PA, Ries LA, Parker SL *et al.* (1998). Long-term cancer patient survival in the United States. *Cancer Epidemiol Biomarkers Prev.* 7:271–282.
4. McPherson CP, Swenson KK, Kjellberg J. (2001). Quality of life in patients with prostate cancer. *Semin Oncol Nurs.* 17:138–146.
5. Herr HW, Kornblith AB, Ofman U. (1993). A comparison of the quality of life of patients with metastatic prostate cancer who received or did not receive hormonal therapy. *Cancer.* 71:1143–1150.
6. Sloan JA, Loprinzi CL, Novotny PJ *et al.* (2001). Methodologic lessons learned from hot flash studies. *J Clin Oncol.* 19:4280–4290.
7. Loprinzi CL, Sloan JA, Perez EA *et al.* (2002). Phase III evaluation of fluoxetine for treatment of hot flashes. *J Clin Oncol.* 20:1578–1583.
8. Stearns V, Yamauchi H, Hayes DF. (1998). Circulating tumor markers in breast cancer: Accepted utilities and novel prospects. *Breast Cancer Res Treat.* 52: 239–259.
9. Loprinzi CL, Sloan JA, Perez EA *et al.* (1999). Preliminary data from a randomized evaluation of fluoxetine for treating hot flashes in breast cancer survivors. *Breast Cancer Res Treat.* 57:34–36.
10. Barton DL, Loprinzi CL, Quella SK *et al.* (1998). Prospective evaluation of vitamin E for hot flashes in breast cancer survivors. *J Clin Oncol.* 16:495–500.
11. Quella SK, Loprinzi CL, Barton DL *et al.* (2000). Evaluation of soy phytoestrogens for the treatment of hot flashes in breast cancer survivors: A North Central Cancer Treatment Group Trial. *J Clin Oncol.* 18:1068–1074.
12. Clark JA, Wray NP, Ashton CM. (2001). Living with treatment decisions: Regrets and quality of life among men treated for metastatic prostate cancer. *J Clin Oncol.* 19:72–80.
13. Miles BJ, Giesler B, Kattan MW. (1999). Recall and attitudes in patients with prostate cancer. *Urology.* 53:169–174.
14. Carvalhal GF, Smith DS, Ramos C *et al.* (1999). Correlates of dissatisfaction with treatment in patients with prostate cancer diagnosed through screening. *J Urol.* 162:113 118.
15. Cox RL, Crawford ED. (1995). Estrogens in the treatment of prostate cancer. *J Urol.* 154:1991–1998.
16. Gerber GS, Zagaja GP, Ray PS *et al.* (2000). Transdermal estrogen in the treatment of hot flushes in men with prostate cancer. *Urology.* 55:97–101.
17. Spetz AC, Hammar M, Lindberg B *et al.* (2001). Prospective evaluation of hot flashes during treatment with parenteral estrogen or complete androgen ablation for metastatic carcinoma of the prostate. *J Urol.* 166:517–520.
18. Loprinzi CL, Michalak JC, Quella SK *et al.* (1994). Megestrol acetate for the prevention of hot flashes. *N Engl J Med.* 331:347–352.
19. Sartor O, Eastham JA. (1999). Progressive prostate cancer associated with use of megestrol acetate administered for control of hot flashes. *South Med J.* 92:415–416.
20. Quella SK, Loprinzi CL, Sloan J *et al.* (1999). Pilot evaluation of venlafaxine for the treatment of hot flashes in men undergoing androgen ablation therapy for prostate cancer. *J Urol.* 162:98–102.
21. Loprinzi CL, Goldberg RM, O'Fallon JR *et al.* (1994). Transdermal clonidine for ameliorating post-orchiectomy hot flashes. *J Urol.* 151:634–636.
22. Bruning PF, Pit MJ, de Jong-Bakker M *et al.* (1990). Bone mineral density after adjuvant chemotherapy for premenopausal breast cancer. *Br J Cancer.* 61:308–310.
23. Kanis JA, McCloskey EV, Powles T *et al.* (1999). A high incidence of vertebral fracture in women with breast cancer. *Br J Cancer.* 79:1179–1181.
24. Saarto T, Blomqvist C, Valimaki M *et al.* (1997). Clodronate improves bone mineral density in post-menopausal breast cancer patients treated with adjuvant antioestrogens. *Br J Cancer.* 75:602–605.
25. Powles TJ, McCloskey E, Paterson AH *et al.* (1998). Oral clodronate and reduction in loss of bone mineral density in women with operable primary breast cancer. *J Natl Cancer Inst.* 90:704–708.
26. Headley JA, Theriault RL, LeBlanc AD *et al.* (1998). Pilot study of bone mineral density in breast cancer patients treated with adjuvant chemotherapy. *Cancer Invest.* 16:6–11.
27. Sverrisdottir A, Fornander T, Rutqvist L. (May, 2001). Bone mineral density is premenopausal patients in a randomized trial of adjuvant endocrine therapy (ZIPP TRIAL), American Society of Clinical Oncology. San Francisco.
28. Riis BJ, Overgaard K, Christiansen C. (1995). Biochemical markers of bone turnover to monitor the bone response to postmenopausal hormone replacement therapy. *Osteoporos Int.* 5:276–280.
29. Lindsay R, Cosman F. (1990). Estrogen in prevention and treatment of osteoporosis. *Ann N Y Acad Sci.* 592:326–333.
30. Cauley JA, Seeley DG, Ensrud K *et al.* (1995). Estrogen replacement therapy and fractures in older women. Study of Osteoporotic Fractures Research Group. *Ann Intern Med.* 122:9–16.
31. Lindsay R, Hart DM, MacLean A *et al.* (1978). Bone response to termination of oestrogen treatment. *Lancet.* 1(8078):1325–1327.
32. Love RR, Mazess RB, Barden HS *et al.* (1992). Effects of tamoxifen on bone mineral density in postmenopausal women with breast cancer. *N Engl J Med.* 326:852–856.
33. Love RR, Barden HS, Mazess RB *et al.* (1994). Effect of tamoxifen on lumbar spine bone mineral density in postmenopausal women after 5 years. *Arch Intern Med.* 154:2585–2588.
34. Powles TJ, Hickish T, Kanis JA *et al.* (1996). Effect of tamoxifen on bone mineral density measured by dual energy x ray absorptiometry in healthy premenopausal and postmenopausal women. *J Clin Oncol.* 14:78–84.
35. Ettinger B, Black DM, Mitlak BH *et al.* (1999). Reduction of vertebral fracture risk in postmenopausal women with osteoporosis treated with raloxifene: Results from a 3-year randomized clinical trial. Multiple Outcomes of Raloxifene Evaluation (MORE) Investigators. *JAMA.* 282:637–645.
36. Delmas PD. (1996). Zoledronate. *Br J Clin Pract Suppl.* 87:15, discussion 22.
37. Green J. (1996). Zoledronate: The preclinical pharmacology. *Br J Clin Pract Suppl.* 87:16–18, discussion 22.
38. Lipton A. (1996). Zoledronate in the treatment of osteolytic bone metastases. *Br J Clin Pract Suppl.* 87:21, discussion 22.
39. Siris E. (1996). Zoledronate in the treatment of Paget's disease. *Br J Clin Pract Suppl.* 87:19–20, discussion 22.
40. Body JJ. (1997). Clinical research update: Zoledronate. *Cancer.* 80: 1699–1701.
41. Binkley N, Kimmel D, Bruner J *et al.* Zoledronate prevents the development of absolute osteopenia following ovariectomy in adult rhesus monkeys. *J Bone Miner Res.* 13:1775–1782.
42. Pataki A, Muller K, Green JR *et al.* (1997). Effects of short-term treatment with the bisphosphonates zoledronate and pamidronate on rat bone: A comparative histomorphometric study on the cancellous bone formed before, during, and after treatment. *Anat Rec.* 249:458–468.
43. Muller K, Wiesenberg I, Jaeggi K *et al.* (1998). Effects of the bisphosphonate zoledronate on bone loss in the ovariectomized and in the adjuvant arthritic rat. *Arzneimittelforschung.* 48:81–86.
44. Body JJ, Lortholary A, Romieu G *et al.* (1999). A dose-finding study of zoledronate in hypercalcemic cancer patients. *J Bone Miner Res.* 14: 1557–1561.
45. Flanagan AM, Chambers TJ. (1991). Inhibition of bone resorption by bisphosphonates: Interactions between bisphosphonates, osteoclasts, and bone. *Calcif Tissue Int.* 49:407–415.
46. Berenson J. (August, 1999). Phase II trial of zoledronate vs pamidronate in multiple myeloma and breast cancer patients with osteolytic lesions. Second North American Symposium on Skeletal Complications of Malignancy. Montreal, Canada.
47. Kanis JA, Powles T, Paterson AH *et al.* (1996). Clodronate decreases the frequency of skeletal metastases in women with breast cancer. *Bone.* 19: 663–667.

48. Stoch SA, Parker RA, Chen L *et al*. (2001). Bone loss in men with prostate cancer treated with gonadotropin-releasing hormone agonists. *J Clin Endocrinol Metab*. 86:2787–2791.

49. Maillefert JF, Sibilia J, Michel F *et al*. (1999). Bone mineral density in men treated with synthetic gonadotropin-releasing hormone agonists for prostatic carcinoma. *J Urol*. 161:1219–1222.

50. Daniell HW, Dunn SR, Ferguson DW *et al*. (2000). Progressive osteoporosis during androgen deprivation therapy for prostate cancer. *J Urol*. 163: 181–186.

51. Diamond T, Campbell J, Bryant C *et al*. (1998). The effect of combined androgen blockade on bone turnover and bone mineral densities in men treated for prostate carcinoma: Longitudinal evaluation and response to intermittent cyclic etidronate therapy. *Cancer*. 83:1561–1566.

52. Eriksson S, Eriksson A, Stege R *et al*. (1995). Bone mineral density in patients with prostatic cancer treated with orchidectomy and with estrogens. *Calcif Tissue Int*. 57:97–99.

53. Goldray D, Weisman Y, Jaccard N *et al*. (1993). Decreased bone density in elderly men treated with the gonadotropin-releasing hormone agonist decapeptyl (D-Trp6-GnRH). *J Clin Endocrinol Metab*. 76:288–290.

54. Falahati-Nini A, Riggs BL, Atkinson EJ *et al*. (2000). Relative contributions of testosterone and estrogen in regulating bone resorption and formation in normal elderly men. *J Clin Invest*. 106:1553–1560.

55. The Writing Group for the PEPI (1996). Effects of hormone therapy on bone mineral density: Results from the postmenopausal estrogen/progestin interventions (PEPI) trial. *JAMA*. 276:1389–1396.

56. Khosla S, Melton LJ 3rd, Atkinson EJ *et al*. (1998). Relationship of serum sex steroid levels and bone turnover markers with bone mineral density in men and women: A key role for bioavailable estrogen. *J Clin Endocrinol Metab*. 83:2266–2274.

57. Khosla S, Melton LJ 3rd, Atkinson EJ *et al*. (2001). Relationship of serum sex steroid levels to longitudinal changes in bone density in young versus elderly men. *J Clin Endocrinol Metab*. 86:3555–3561.

58. Finkelstein JS, Klibanski A, Arnold AL *et al*. (1998). Prevention of estrogen deficiency-related bone loss with human parathyroid hormone-(1–34): A randomized controlled trial. *JAMA*. 280:1067–1073.

59. Smith MR, McGovern FJ, Zietman AL *et al*. (2001). Pamidronate to prevent bone loss during androgen-deprivation therapy for prostate cancer. *N Engl J Med*. 345:948–955.

60. Wapnir IL, Cody RP, Greco RS. (1999). Subtle differences in quality of life after breast cancer surgery. *Ann Surg Oncol*. 6:359–366.

61. Ganz PA, Schag AC, Lee JJ *et al*. (1992). Breast conservation versus mastectomy. Is there a difference in psychological adjustment or quality of life in the year after surgery? *Cancer*. 69:1729–1738.

62. Thors CL, Broeckel JA, Jacobsen PB. (2001). Sexual functioning in breast cancer survivors. *Cancer Control*. 8:442–448.

63. Fallowfield LJ, Hall A, Maguire GP *et al*. (1990). Psychological outcomes of different treatment policies in women with early breast cancer outside a clinical trial. *BMJ*. 301:575–580.

64. Schover LR, Yetman RJ, Tuason LJ *et al*. (1995). Partial mastectomy and breast reconstruction. A comparison of their effects on psychosocial adjustment, body image, and sexuality. *Cancer*. 75:54–64.

65. Schover LR. (1994). Sexuality and body image in younger women with breast cancer. *J Natl Cancer Inst Monogr*. 16:177–182.

66. Dorval M, Maunsell E, Deschenes L *et al*. (1998). Type of mastectomy and quality of life for long term breast carcinoma survivors. *Cancer*. 83: 2130–2138.

67. Ganz PA, Rowland JH, Desmond K *et al*. (1998). Life after breast cancer: Understanding women's health-related quality of life and sexual functioning. *J Clin Oncol*. 16:501–514.

68. Young-McCaughan S. (1996). Sexual functioning in women with breast cancer after treatment with adjuvant therapy. *Cancer Nurs*. 19:308–319.

69. Ganz PA, Desmond KA, Belin TR *et al*. (1999). Predictors of sexual health in women after a breast cancer diagnosis. *J Clin Oncol*. 17:2371–2380.

70. Joly F, Espie M, Marty M *et al*. (2000). Long-term quality of life in premenopausal women with node-negative localized breast cancer treated with or without adjuvant chemotherapy. *Br J Cancer*. 83:577–582.

71. Berglund G, Nystedt M, Bolund C *et al*. (2001). Effect of endocrine treatment on sexuality in premenopausal breast cancer patients: A prospective randomized study. *J Clin Oncol*. 19:2788–2796.

72. Fallowfield L, Fleissig A, Edwards R *et al*. (2001). Tamoxifen for the prevention of breast cancer: Psychosocial impact on women participating in two randomized controlled trials. *J Clin Oncol*. 19:1885–1892.

73. Stock RG, Stone NN, Iannuzzi C. (1996). Sexual potency following interactive ultrasound-guided brachytherapy for prostate cancer. *Int J Radiat Oncol Biol Phys*. 35:267–272.

74. Stock RG, Kao J, Stone NN. (2001). Penile erectile function after permanent radioactive seed implantation for treatment of prostate cancer. *J Urol*. 165:436–439.

75. Wei JT, Dunn RL, Sandler HM *et al*. (2002). Comprehensive comparison of health-related quality of life after contemporary therapies for localized prostate cancer. *J Clin Oncol*. 20:557–566.

76. Basaria S, Lieb J, Tang AM *et al*. (2002). Long-term effects of androgen deprivation therapy in prostate cancer patients. *Clin Endocrinol (Oxf)*. 56: 779–786.

77. Basaria S, Dobs AS. (1999). Risks versus benefits of testosterone therapy in elderly men. *Drugs Aging*. 15:131–142.

78. Gralnek D, Wessells H, Cui H *et al*. (2000). Differences in sexual function and quality of life after nerve sparing and nonnerve sparing radical retropubic prostatectomy. *J Urol*. 163:1166–1169, discussion 1169–1170.

79. Kawanishi Y, Lee KS, Kimura K *et al*. (2001). Effect of radical retropubic prostatectomy on erectile function, evaluated before and after surgery using colour Doppler ultrasonography and nocturnal penile tumescence monitoring. *BJU Int*. 88:244–247.

80. Zippe CD, Raina R, Thukral M *et al*. (2001). Management of erectile dysfunction following radical prostatectomy. *Curr Urol Rep*. 2:495–503.

81. Chen CT, Valicenti RK, Lu J *et al*. (2001). Does hormonal therapy influence sexual function in men receiving 3D conformal radiation therapy for prostate cancer? *Int J Radiat Oncol Biol Phys*. 50:591–595.

82. Homma Y, Kawabe K, Hayashi K. (1998). Urologic morbidity and its influence on global satisfaction with treatment outcome after radical prostatectomy for prostate cancer. *Int J Urol*. 5:556–561.

83. Joly F, Brune D, Couette JE *et al*. (1998). Health-related quality of life and sequelae in patients treated with brachytherapy and external beam irradiation for localized prostate cancer. *Ann Oncol*. 9:751–757.

84. Marsh DW, Lepor H. (2001). Predicting continence following radical prostatectomy. *Curr Urol Rep*. 2:248–252.

85. Grise P, Thurman S. (2001). Urinary incontinence following treatment of localized prostate cancer. *Cancer Control*. 8:532–539.

86. MacDiarmid SA. (2001). Incontinence after radical prostatectomy: Pathophysiology and management. *Curr Urol Rep*. 2:209–213.

87. Teloken C. (2001). Management of erectile dysfunction secondary to treatment for localized prostate cancer. *Cancer Control*. 8:540–545.

88. Incrocci L, Slob AK, Levendag PC. (2002). Sexual (dys)function after radiotherapy for prostate cancer: A review. *Int J Radiat Oncol Biol Phys*. 52: 681–693.

89. Kedia S, Zippe CD, Agarwal A *et al*. (1999). Treatment of erectile dysfunction with sildenafil citrate (Viagra) after radiation therapy for prostate cancer. *Urology*. 54:308–312.

90. Mulcahy JJ. (2000). Erectile function after radical prostatectomy. *Semin Urol Oncol*. 18:71–75.

91. Montague D. (2002). Nonpharmacologic treatment of erectile dysfunction. *Rev Urol*. 4(Suppl 3):S9–S16.

92. Carson CC. (2000). Oral and injectable medications for the treatment of erectile dysfunction. *Curr Urol Rep*. 1:307–312.

93. Broeckel JA, Jacobsen PB, Balducci L *et al*. (2000). Quality of life after adjuvant chemotherapy for breast cancer. *Breast Cancer Res Treat*. 62: 141–150.

94. Zebrack BJ, Zeltzer LK, Whitton J *et al*. (2002). Psychological outcomes in long-term survivors of childhood leukemia, Hodgkin's disease, and non-Hodgkin's lymphoma: A report from the Childhood Cancer Survivor Study. *Pediatrics*. 110:42–52.

95. Hughson AV, Cooper AF, McArdle CS *et al*. (1986). Psychological impact of adjuvant chemotherapy in the first two years after mastectomy. *BMJ (Clin Res Ed)*. 293:1268–1271.

96. Hughson AV, Cooper AF, McArdle CS *et al*. (1998). Psychosocial consequences of mastectomy: Levels of morbidity and associated factors. *J Psychosom Res*. 32:383–391.

97. Thompson DS, Spanier CA, Vogel VG. (1999). The relationship between tamoxifen, estrogen, and depressive symptoms. *Breast J*. 5:375–382.

98. Shariff S, Cumming CE, Lees A *et al*. (1995). Mood disorder in women with early breast cancer taking tamoxifen, an estradiol receptor antagonist. An expected or unexpected effect? *Ann N Y Acad Sci*. 761:365–368.

99. Day R. (2001). Quality of life and tamoxifen in a breast cancer prevention trial: A summary of findings from the NSABP P-1 study. National Surgical Adjuvant Breast and Bowel Project. *Ann N Y Acad Sci*. 949:143–150.

100. Day R, Ganz PA, Costantino JP. (2001). Tamoxifen and depression: More evidence from the National Surgical Adjuvant Breast and Bowel Project's Breast Cancer Prevention (P-1) Randomized Study. *J Natl Cancer Inst.* 93:1615–1623.

101. Ganz PA. (2001). Impact of tamoxifen adjuvant therapy on symptoms, functioning, and quality of life. *J Natl Cancer Inst Monogr.* 30:130–134.

102. Holmberg L, Omne-Ponten M, Burns T *et al.* (1989). Psychosocial adjustment after mastectomy and breast-conserving treatment. Cancer. 64:969–974.

103. McArdle JM, Hughson AV, McArdle CS. (1990). Reduced psychological morbidity after breast conservation. *Br J Surg.* 77:1221–1223.

104. Maguire P. (1989). Breast conservation versus mastectomy: Psychological considerations. *Semin Surg Oncol.* 5:137–144.

105. Wenzel LB, Fairclough DL, Brady MJ *et al.* (1999). Age-related differences in the quality of life of breast carcinoma patients after treatment. Cancer. 86:1768–1774.

106. Ashbury FD, Cameron C, Mercer SL *et al.* (1998). One-on-one peer support and quality of life for breast cancer patients. *Patient Educ Couns.* 35:89–100.

107. Lee CO. (1997). Quality of life and breast cancer survivors. Psychosocial and treatment issues. *Cancer Pract.* 5;309–316.

108. Targ EF, Levine EG. (2002). The efficacy of a mind-body-spirit group for women with breast cancer: A randomized controlled trial. *Gen Hosp Psychiatry.* 24:238–248.

109. Margolese HC. (2000). The male menopause and mood: Testosterone decline and depression in the aging male—Is there a link? *J Geriatr Psychiatry Neurol.* 13:93–101.

110. Wang C, Swedloff RS, Iranmanesh A *et al.* (2000). Transdermal testosterone gel improves sexual function, mood, muscle strength, and body composition parameters in hypogonadal men. Testosterone Gel Study Group. *J Clin Endocrinol Metab.* 85:2839–2853.

111. Bhasin S, Buckwalter JG. (2001). Testosterone supplementation in older men: A rational idea whose time has not yet come. *J Androl.* 22:718–731.

112. Schiavi RC, White D, Mandeli J *et al.* (1997). Effect of testosterone administration on sexual behavior and mood in men with erectile dysfunction. *Arch Sex Behav.* 26:231–241.

113. Kaps EC. (1994). The role of the support group, "Us Too". Cancer. 74:2188–2189.

114. Silberfarb PM. (1983). Chemotherapy and cognitive defects in cancer patients. *Annu Rev Med.* 34:35–46.

115. Kaasa S, Olsnes BT, Mastekaasa A. (1988). Neuropsychological evaluation of patients with inoperable non-small cell lung cancer treated with combination chemotherapy or radiotherapy. *Acta Oncol.* 27:241–246.

116. Neuwelt EA, Glasberg M, Frenkel E *et al.* (1983). Neurotoxicity of chemotherapeutic agents after blood-brain barrier modification: Neuropathological studies. *Ann Neurol.* 14:316–324.

117. Ahles TA, Saykin A. (2001). Cognitive effects of standard-dose chemotherapy in patients with cancer. *Cancer Invest.* 19:812–820.

118. Wieneke M, Dienst E. (1995). Neuropsychological assessment of cognitive functioning following chemotherapy for breast cancer. *Psycho-Oncology.* 4:61–66.

119. van Dam FS, Schagen SB, Muller MJ *et al.* (1998). Impairment of cognitive function in women receiving adjuvant treatment for high-risk breast cancer: High-dose versus standard-dose chemotherapy. *J Natl Cancer Inst.* 90:210–218.

120. Brezden CB, Phillips KA, Abdolell M *et al.* (2000). Cognitive function in breast cancer patients receiving adjuvant chemotherapy. *J Clin Oncol.* 18:2695–2701.

121. Cull A, Hay C, Love SB *et al.* (1996). What do cancer patients mean when they complain of concentration and memory problems? *Br J Cancer.* 74;1674–1679

122. Bower JE, Ganz PA, Desmond KA *et al.* (2000). Fatigue in breast cancer survivors. Occurrence, correlates, and impact on quality of life. *J Clin Oncol.* 18:743–753.

123. Cimprich B. (1999). Pretreatment symptom distress in women newly diagnosed with breast cancer. *Cancer Nurs.* 22:185–194, quiz 195.

124. Cimprich B. (1992). Attentional fatigue following breast cancer surgery. *Res Nurs Health.* 15:199–207.

125. Shimozuma K, Ganz PA, Petersen L *et al.* (1999). Quality of life in the first year after breast cancer surgery: Rehabilitation needs and patterns of recovery. *Breast Cancer Res Treat.* 56:45–57.

126. Schagen SB, van Dam FS, Muller MJ *et al.* (1999). Cognitive deficits after postoperative adjuvant chemotherapy for breast carcinoma. Cancer. 85:640–650.

127. Sherwin BB. (1988). Estrogen and/or androgen replacement therapy and cognitive functioning in surgically menopausal women. *Psychoneuroendocrinology.* 13:345–357.

128. Gouchie C, Kimura D. (1991). The relationship between testosterone levels and cognitive ability patterns. *Psychoneuroendocrinology.* 16:323–334.

129. Christiansen K, Knussmann R. (1987). Sex hormones and cognitive functioning in men. *Neuropsychobiology.* 18:27–36.

130. Janowsky JS, Oviatt SK, Orwoll ES. (1994). Testosterone influences spatial cognition in older men. *Behav Neurosci.* 108:325–332.

131. Phillips SM, Sherwin BB. (1992). Effects of estrogen on memory function in surgically menopausal women. *Psychoneuroendocrinology.* 17:485–495.

132. Kampen DL, Sherwin BB. (1994). Estrogen use and verbal memory in healthy postmenopausal women. *Obstet Gynecol.* 83:979–983.

133. Fedor-Freybergh P. (1977). The influence of oestrogens on the wellbeing and mental performance in climacteric and postmenopausal women. *Acta Obstet Gynecol Scand Suppl.* 64:1–91.

134. Janowsky JS, Chavez B, Orwoll E. (2000). Sex steroids modify working memory. *J Cogn Neurosci.* 12:407–414.

135. Sanders G, Sjodin M, de Chastelaine M. (2002). On the elusive nature of sex differences in cognition: Hormonal influences contributing to within-sex variation. *Arch Sex Behav.* 31:145–152.

59

The Difference Between Male and Female Breast Cancer

MEREDITH SELLECK, MD* AND AMY TIERSTEN, MD**

*New York Presbyterian Hospital, College of Physicians and Surgeons, Columbia University, New York, NY
**Associate Professor of Medicine, New York University School of Medicine, New York, NY

I. Introduction

Breast cancer develops in both men and women. It is the most commonly diagnosed malignancy in women resulting in immense socioeconomic ramifications. In men, breast cancer is rare. Is this disease biologically different in men and women? Or is it similar between the sexes with the same etiologic, prognostic, and clinical features? Emerging data suggest that breast cancer in men is fundamentally identical to breast cancer in women with few exceptions. This chapter explores the classic features of breast cancer in both sexes highlighting the differences and more often the similarities between them.

II. Anatomy and Development

Both men and women have breasts; however, the rate of breast carcinoma is much higher in women. This is due, in part, to the anatomic differences between them. Breast tissue is well developed only in women. The female breast consists of some 15 to 20 lobules of glandular tissue that form the functional units of the breast. Each lobule is drained by a lactiferous duct, which opens on the nipple. Deep to the areola, each duct enlarges to form a lactiferous sinus in which milk can accumulate. The lobules are connected and supported by various amounts of fibrous connective tissue and adipose tissue. It is these stromal elements that comprise the majority of the breast volume in the nonlactational state.

Male and female breasts are similar at birth consisting of a small number of rudimentary branching ducts beneath the nipple-areola complex. They diverge at the time of puberty. In males, development ceases. In females there is continued growth and branching of the lactiferous ducts and increased adipose and stromal tissue. As a result, progressive enlargement of the breasts occurs. Eventually, the terminal ducts give rise to saccular buds from which secretory glands develop during pregnancy. After lactation ceases, there is glandular atrophy and once again the stromal elements are the predominant component of the breast.

III. Epidemiology

The health of women is significantly affected by breast cancer. It represents 31% of all cancers diagnosed and 15% of all cancer deaths in women [1]. There were an estimated 193,700 cases diagnosed in the United States in 2001 with 40,600 deaths [1]. It is the second leading cause of death in women after lung cancer. Through age 85 the lifetime risk of being diagnosed with breast cancer for an American women is 12.5%, or 1 in 8. This is in contrast to men in whom breast cancer is a rare disease. Male breast cancer accounts for less than 1% of malignancies

diagnosed in men with an estimated 1600 cases and 400 deaths diagnosed in 2001 in the United States [1].

Although the incidence of female breast cancer remained approximately level during the 1990s, the number of new cases per year increased 1.4 times from 1987 to 1997 [1–3]. There is evidence to support an increase in male breast cancer as well. According to the SEER database of the National Cancer Institute, the estimated numbers of male breast cancer cases expected in the United States are rising. Since 1987 the annual number of breast cancer cases in males has increased 1.6 times [4,5]. In a retrospective review of 217 cases of male breast cancer obtained from tumor registries at 18 institutions between 1953 to 1995, the number of cases registered annually increased progressively [4]. Fifty of the cases were diagnosed after 1986 (Fig. 59-1). This increase is likely multifactorial, influenced by the proliferation of tumor registries, increased use of urban health care facilities, and perhaps by a true rise in the incidence of the disease. In addition, the increased awareness and public education regarding breast carcinoma and screening directed toward women may play a role in the recognition of this disease by men and their doctors.

Female breast cancer incidence and mortality rates vary between countries and to a lesser extent within different areas of the United States [6]. The incidence is highest in the United States and Northern Europe and is lowest in Asia. There are many studies reported in the literature showing that the incidence rises as people emigrate from a country of low risk to one of high risk and correlates with the recency of migration [6]. This suggests that lifestyle and environment of the geographical destination influences breast cancer risk. The overall ratio of female to male breast cancer in most white Western countries

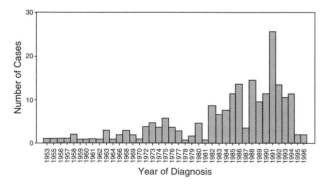

Fig. 59-1 Male breast carcinoma by year of diagnosis. The majority were diagnosed after 1981. (From Donegan NL, Redlich P, Lang P, Gall M. [1998]. Carcinoma of the breast in males. A multiinstitutional study. *Cancer.* 83:498–509.)

is 100:1. The incidence rate of male breast cancer in most populations for which data is available is one or less case per 100,000 [7]. Muir *et al* [8] report that the highest incidence for male breast cancer occurs in Brazil at a rate of 3.4 cases per 100,000 versus Columbia, Singapore, Hungary, and Japan where the incidence is much lower at 0.1 cases per 100,000. The effect of migration on the incidence of male breast cancer has not been explored likely because of the rarity of this disease.

IV. Risk Factors

Breast cancer in females has been extensively studied. The medical community and the community at large has been informed of the known factors that may increase a woman's risk for this disease. Because breast cancer is a rarity in males, much less data have accumulated. Therefore, risk factors in general remain uncertain. There are some epidemiologic studies that have afforded some insight into this disease. Various hormonal, lifestyle, and genetic factors reported to play a role in the development of breast carcinoma are described in the following sections. However, most individuals of either gender who develop breast cancer have no apparent risk factor for the disease, and most male patients have no detectable hormonal imbalances [9].

A. Reproductive and Hormonal

In epidemiologic studies, a woman's reproductive history has been consistently shown to contribute to the risk of developing breast cancer underscoring the role of the hormonal milieu in normal and abnormal breast development. Early menarche, shorter cycle length, nulliparity or low parity, and late menopause are several reproductive variables that increase a woman's risk for developing breast cancer. After menopause, adipose tissue becomes the major source of estrogen and obese, postmenopausal women have higher levels of endogenous estrogen and a higher risk of developing cancer [6].

Exogenous estrogen use in the form of oral contraceptives use and the risk of subsequent breast cancer is an important concern of women. The Nurses' Health Study examined more than 3000 cases of breast cancer diagnosed prospectively between 1976 to 1992. At the start of the study, 46% of women reported past or current use of oral contraceptive pills. In sum, they found no increased risk of breast cancer associated with the use or duration of use of oral contraceptives. No conclusions could be drawn, however, for women younger than 40 because there were too few cases of breast cancer in that age group [10]. Other studies have suggested a risk for developing breast cancer in women who use oral contraceptives when they are younger than 35 years. In a case-control study of women between the ages of 20 through 44 years, which examined 1648 cases of breast cancer and 1505 controls, the relative risk (RR) for breast cancer development was 1.3 in oral contraceptive users younger than age 45. The RR increased to 1.7 in users younger than 35 years and up to 2.2 in women using the pill for more than 10 years [11]. This slight increase in RR is unlikely to translate into large differences in attributable risk because the incidence of breast cancer is so low in this population. The data regarding postmenopausal hormone replacement therapy have

also been examined in many epidemiologic studies, several meta-analyses, and a large pooled analysis [6]. There appears to be a consensus in the literature that there is no increase in risk of breast cancer in users compared with those who never used hormone replacement therapy. In general, this observation reflects women who used hormones in the past and for a short period of time. The studies do suggest that postmenopausal hormone use increases the risk of breast cancer in two subgroups of users: users of long duration and current users [6]. In the pooled analysis that combined the results of 51 epidemiologic studies, a statistically significant association was observed between breast cancer risk and current or recent users of hormone replacement that escalated with increasing duration of use. For example, the RR of current users as compared with women who never used hormone replacement was 1.08 for 1 to 4 years of use, 1.31 for 5 to 9 years, 1.24 for 10 to 14 years, and 1.56 for 15 or more years of use [12].

The hormonal influence on breast cancer risk in men has also been described. Conditions that result in relative estrogen excess or lack of androgens have been linked to cases of male breast cancer in epidemiologic studies. The strongest risk factor for developing male breast cancer is Klinefelter's syndrome, a condition that results from the inheritance of an additional X chromosome. Affected males have atrophic testes resulting in low plasma levels of testosterone. Their circulating levels of gonadotropins (follicle- stimulating hormone and luteinizing hormone) remain high, thus exposing them to a high estrogen-testosterone ratio. These men have a 50 times higher rate of developing breast cancer than those with no genetic abnormality and may account for up to 3% of male breast cancers [13–15]. Other conditions affecting the testes have also been reported to increase risk, including mumps orchitis, undescended testes, or testicular injury [7]. This too may suggest a hormonal association; however, it remains unclear if testosterone levels are actually abnormal at the time of breast cancer diagnosis in these men [7].

Chronic liver disease leading to cirrhosis may predispose males to the development of breast cancer [16,17]. The diseased liver and its altered metabolism lead to a hyperestrogenic state promoting the growth of breast tissue and subsequent risk of malignant transformation. Gynecomastia is frequently present in male breast cancer tumor specimens. The role of gynecomastia in breast cancer is controversial. It may impart an increased risk for the development of breast cancer or simply serves as a marker for an underlying hyperestrogenic state [18]. Exogenous estrogens have also been implicated in this disease. There have been reports of transsexuals developing breast cancer and reports of breast cancer in men receiving treatment for prostate cancer [9].

B. Dietary and Environmental

The causal relationship between dietary fat consumption and breast cancer remains controversial. This hypothesis is based on the observation that breast cancer mortality rates are highest in countries where the national per capita fat consumption is high [6]. This correlation is confounded by many other variables also present in these generally affluent Western countries such as low parity, late age at first birth, greater body fat, and lower levels of physical activity. There have been several prospective cohort studies examining this issue and in those with over 200 incident cases of breast cancer there was no association seen with dietary fat intake [19–24]. Hunter et al [25] published a pooled analysis of 4980 cases of breast cancer in 337,819 women and again no association was observed between intake of total, saturated, monounsaturated, or polyunsaturated fat and risk of breast cancer. What does appear to play an important but complex role in the causation of breast cancer is energy balance. High-energy intake in relation to expenditure accelerates growth and the onset of menstruation. If this positive balance continues it can lead to weight gain later in life and overall increases a woman's risk of subsequent breast cancer [6].

Other dietary factors including, vitamins, fiber, alcohol consumption, and caffeine, and the role they play in the development of breast cancer have also been thoroughly explored in women. It appears that alcohol intake is the best-established specific dietary risk factor for breast cancer in women [26]. The studies performed to examine this relationship, all of which were controlled for other major breast cancer risk factors, consistently support the existence of a positive association between alcohol consumption and risk of breast cancer in women. In addition, it has been shown that moderate alcohol consumption of approximately two drinks per day has been shown to increase estrogen levels providing a mechanism by which breast cancer risk might be increased [27].

Clearly, there are numerous studies examining female breast cancer and potential risk factors for this disease. Through these efforts, an abundance of knowledge has been gained. It remains less clear which of these established or potential risk factors plays a role in the development of male breast cancer. There have been some reported case-control studies in the literature that attempt to further define this issue. For example, Rosenblatt et al investigated the relationship between food and beverage consumption and the development of breast cancer in men in a report of 220 cases of male breast cancer and 291 controls [28]. No trends in risk were observed with increasing intakes of specific food, with the exception of citrus fruits. The authors conclude that dietary factors are unlikely to be strong determinants of breast cancer in men [28]. Another case-control study obtained demographic and dietary information from next-of-kin interviews of 178 men who had died of breast cancer and 512 male controls. This study suggested that obesity increases the risk of male breast cancer [29].

C. Genetics

Several genes that are associated with a high lifetime risk of breast cancer in females have been identified in the past decade. These genes appear responsible for 5 to 10% of all breast cancer cases [30]. Two such susceptibility genes are BRCA1 located on chromosome 17 and BRCA2 on chromosome 13. Mutations in both genes predispose to earlier onset and increase risk of female breast cancer, but the risk profile and risk of cancers at other sites differs between the two genes [30]. Studies by the Breast Cancer Linkage Consortium (BCLC) have shown that both genes increase the risk of female breast cancer to 80 to 85% by the age of 80 [31,32]. For ovarian cancer, BRCA1 confers a 60% lifetime risk and BRCA2 a 27% risk [32]. Both genes are also now thought to increase the risk of prostate cancer, and

BRCA2 has been associated with a variety of other malignant disorders as well, including male breast cancer [33].

BRCA2 mutations are thought to be associated with a 6% lifetime risk of male breast cancer representing a 100-fold increased RR over the general population [33]. One report by Couch et al [34] analyzed 50 cases of male breast cancer for BRCA2 mutations. The mutation was found in 14% of the cases, but these were men who had a significant family history of breast cancer. The prevalence of BRCA2 mutations in male breast cancer cases unselected for family history has been reported by Friedman et al [35]. This study demonstrated a 4% prevalence of BRCA2 mutations. The data remain inconclusive mainly because male breast cancer is an infrequent occurrence and even more difficult to study in the context of an inheritable familial disease. Only 16 families of two or more cases of male breast cancer have been reported in the literature in the last 100 years [36]. Over half of these families had other types of cancers, and nine reported cases of female breast cancer. In a recent report examining 94 cases of male breast cancer, there were 9.37 excess cases of breast cancer in female first-degree relatives of which only one was accounted for by BRCA2 [37]. The authors concluded that BRCA2 accounts for approximately 15% of the excess risk. The possibility of additional male breast cancer susceptibility genes is suggested and remains an area of active investigation. To date, two families have been identified with a germ-line mutation of the androgen receptor gene, and this may be a very rare cause of inherited male breast cancer [38,39].

V. Clinical Factors and Diagnosis

Breast cancer in males generally occurs a decade later than breast cancer in females with a mean age of presentation ranging from 60 to 65 [9]. The presenting symptom in most patients is a nontender, palpable mass that is centrally located 70 to 90% of the time [9]. Because of the proximity of breast ducts to the skin, other manifestations, such as, nipple retraction, fixation, ulceration, edema, and discharge can also occur frequently in men [40]. Serosanguineous or bloody discharge from the male breast is associated with malignancy in 75% of the cases and should always be investigated by biopsy [9,41]. When bloody discharge occurs from the female breast it is most commonly due to a benign papillary adenoma. Axillary adenopathy suspicious for metastatic disease is clinically detected in 40 to 55% of male patients at diagnosis. Bilateral breast cancer occurs much less frequently in males than in females and is reported to be in the range of 1.4 to 1.9% [41]. This is likely due to the lack of lobular differentiation in men because it is frequently the lobular forms of cancer that present with multicentric and bilateral disease.

Both male and female breast cancers are staged according to the American Joint Committee Clinical Staging System (AJCC), which is based on tumor size, axillary lymph node involvement, and evidence of distant metastases. In general, breast cancer in men presents at a later stage than the disease in women [18,42,43]. This has been attributed to a delay in diagnosis. The older series reported a mean duration of symptoms anywhere between 14 to 21 months suggesting a lack of recognition of this uncommon entity by men and their physicians [9]. One of the largest retrospective series included 215 cases of male breast cancer from 1953 to 1995 [4]. In this study the average duration of symptoms was 10.2 months. Over time, this appeared to improve as reflected by a decrease in the mean tumor size from 2.87 cm to 2.42 cm during two time periods analyzed (1953 to 1985 and 1986 to 1995) [4]. AJCC TMN staging was available for 155 of these cases (72%). Stage I represented 19%, stage II was 46%, and stages III and IV accounted for 13% and 14% of the cases, respectively [4]. Another series of 104 men with breast cancer reported by Borgen et al compared the stage at presentation of the male patients to a female cohort treated at the same time [18]. They found a preponderance of stage III tumors in the male group. Between 1975 to 1990, there were 95 male breast cancer cases: 17% of these were stage 0, 27% stage I, 33% stage II, and 22% stage III. In a female cohort of 932 patients who presented to a single institution in 1989 there were 18% with stage 0 disease, 32% with stage I disease, 39% with stage II disease, and only 6% with stage III disease [18].

In the evaluation of suspected female breast disease, mammography plays a pivotal and well-accepted role. In addition, when used as a screening tool in asymptomatic, older women it has been shown to reduce mortality from breast cancer by 30% [44]. The role of mammography in male breast disease is much less defined. Ideally it would serve to distinguish benign from malignant processes; however, there is no consensus to date on its utility in this capacity. Evans et al [45] attempted to define the diagnostic accuracy of mammography in evaluation of male breast disease. Using 104 mammograms categorized into malignant, benign, gynecomastia, or normal and comparing them to definitive tissue diagnoses they determined a sensitivity of 92%, specificity of 90%, positive predictive value of 55%, and a negative predictive value of 99% for mammography in diagnosis of malignant disease. In this series, 11 of 12 breast cancers in men were detected by mammography; 6 of the cases had concurrent gynecomastia. The one case that was not detected was obscured by the presence of coexisting gynecomastia [45]. Although this study addresses the accuracy of mammography, other factors such as history and physical examination (PE) clearly play a role in making the diagnosis and cannot be replaced by a single test. Many investigators argue that the algorithm in diagnosing male breast disease should involve PE followed by biopsy when needed with mammography reserved for excluding contralateral malignant disease [18,46]. In addition, because of the rare nature of male breast cancer, screening mammography is not advocated for the general male population.

Vetto et al [46] studied the combination of PE and fine needle aspiration (FNA) with or without mammography as an alternative approach to surgical biopsy in the diagnosis of breast masses in men. They looked at 51 consecutive men with unilateral breast masses and using these tools scored them as benign or malignant. All tests were benign in 38 cases and no cancers subsequently developed. In six cases, the tests were suspicious and open biopsy confirmed malignancy. There were seven cases in which PE and FNA were not in agreement, so open biopsy was performed leading to a diagnosis of benign disease. Mammography, which was performed in 13 of the cases, added no further information. They concluded that the combination of FNA and PE is diagnostically accurate and

when used appropriately can avoid unnecessary biopsies for benign disease [46].

VI. Pathologic Features

Similarly to its female counterpart, the most common histology of male breast cancer is infiltrating ductal carcinoma. Because of the lack of lobules in the male breast, lobular carcinoma is very uncommon but has been reported in the literature [47]. In women, this histology accounts for 5 to 10% of the cases [48]. In situ ductal carcinoma is seen in 20 to 25% of female breast cancer cases. In men, the percentage is much less ranging from 0 to 17% [49]. There are many pathologic subtypes used to describe female breast cancer—medullary, mucinous, squamous, papillary, and adenocystic—and in general all of these have also been reported in men [7].

Estrogen receptor (ER) and progesterone receptor (PR) status is routine in the pathologic evaluation of female breast cancer. One, or both, is positive in 60 to 70% of the cases [48]. From the literature there seems to be a consensus that hormone receptors are even more frequently encountered in male breast tumors. There have now been several published series that reported an ER and/or PR positivity rate in male breast tumors of greater than 90% [40,50]. In other published reports the rate is slightly lower ranging between 70 to 90% [41].

The study of molecular markers including protooncogenes, cell cycle regulatory proteins, and markers of apoptosis have led to new insights into the biology of female breast cancer. The HER-2/neu protein is a transmembrane receptor protein with tyrosine kinase activity involved in normal cell growth and division. HER-2 overexpression, usually secondary to gene amplification, is seen in 20 to 30% of invasive females breast cancers and is associated with a poorer outcome and shortened survival [51]. The two methods used to assess HER-2/neu status include immunohistochemistry and fluorescence in situ hybridization (FISH); these are routinely used in the evaluation of female breast tumors. Another molecular marker shown to have clinical implications in female breast cancer is p53. Somatic p53 mutations and p53 protein overexpression have been correlated to prognostic factors such as high tumor grade, negative ER status, and poorer prognosis [52,53]. Much less is known about the presence and prognostic significance of these molecular markers in males with breast cancer although data are emerging [54,55]. Table 59-1 highlights rates of Her-2 neu overexpression in various series of male breast cancer reported

Table 59-1
Rates of Her-2 neu Positivity in Male Breast Cancer Reported in the Literature

Author	No. of Cases	Her-2 neu
Wick et al [54]	10	30%
Clark et al [55]	15	13.3%
Rayson et al [50]	76	29%
Joshe et al [43]	17	41%
Andre et al [91]	82	12%
Shpitz et al [52]	26	39%
Pich et al [56]	50	56%

Table 59-2
Survival Rates Based on Axillary Lymph Node Status in Males with Breast Cancer

Author	No. Patients	Nodal Status	5-Year Survival	5-Year DSS	10-Year Survival	10-Year DSS
Cutuli *et al* [86]	308	Positive	63%	67%	28%	39%
		Negative	82%	93%	58%	77%
Guinee *et al* [60]	224	Positive	NR	65–73%	NR	14–44%*
		Negative		90%		84%
Borgen *et al* [18}	104	Positive	60%	NR	NR	NR
		Negative	100%			
Herman *et al* [58]	45	Positive	59.6%	NR	58.3%	NR
		Negative	87.4%		28.6%	
McLachlan *et al* [59]	66	Positive	55%	NR	NR	NR
		Negative	81%			

*Ranges depending on number of involved nodes (1–3 or ≥4)
NR, not reported.

in the literature. In a series of 111 male breast cancer patients from the Mayo Clinic, tumor samples were analyzed for the presence of various markers. Androgen receptor was almost uniformly present, positive in 95% of the cases. HER-2 was positive in 29% and p53 in 21% of the cases. The cell cycle regulatory protein cyclin D1, which is expressed in approximately 50% of female breast tumors, was also present in 58% of male cases. Shpitz *et al* [52] in a report of 26 male breast cancer patients found that p53 and HER-2/neu were expressed in 46% and 39%, respectively. They found no correlation between the presence of these biomarkers and adverse clinical features or survival. This is in contrary to a report by Pich *et al* [56]. They retrospectively reviewed 50 male patients with breast carcinoma and found that c-erbB-2 and p53 protein overexpression significantly correlated with a worse prognosis. The rate of c-erb2-b positivity was 56% in their series.

VII. Prognostic Factors

Prognostic factors are those measurements available at the time of diagnosis that are associated with disease free or overall survival and can often be used to predict the natural history of the tumor. Optimizing treatment based on prognostic factors plays an important role in the management of female breast cancer. The standard prognostic factors currently applied in new cases of breast cancer include axillary lymph node status, histologic subtype, tumor size, nuclear grade, hormone receptor status, measures of proliferation, and newer molecular markers such as HER-2 overexpression. Of these, the presence or absence of metastatic carcinoma in the axillary lymph nodes is the most powerful prognostic factor for patients with primary breast cancer. A direct relationship between the number of nodes involved and clinical outcome has been demonstrated [57]. There are a number of reports in male breast cancer that also correlate outcome with nodal involvement (Table 59-2) [58,59]. Guinee et al. [60] after reviewing 335 cases of male breast cancer over a 20-year period found 10-year survival to be 84% for patients with histologically negative nodes, 44% if one to three nodes were positive, and 14% in those patients with more than four positive nodes. Five-year survival in male

Table 59-3
Five-Year Survival in Men Based on Stage Reported in the Literature

Author	N	Stage I	Stage II	Stage III	Stage IV
Borgen *et al* [18]	104	83%	70%	74%	NR
Donegan *et al* [4]	155	85%	60%	30%	<10%
Joshe *et al* [43]	46	100%	83%	60%	25%

NR, not reported.

Table 59-4
Ten-Year Relative Survival Rates in Women Undergoing Local and Adjuvant Treatment

Stage of Disease	10-Year Survival
0	95%
I	88%
II	66%
III	36%
IV	7%

(CA. [1999]. *Cancer J Clin.* 49:145–158.)

breast cancer declines with increasing stage of disease (Table 59-3). This is similar to what is seen in females (Table 59-4).

Of the other prognostic factors frequently considered in female breast cancer, controversy exists over their usefulness in male breast cancer cases. There are numerous series in the literature addressing these issues, but, because of the rarity of male breast cancer, none of them are large enough or designed appropriately to evaluate potential molecular or pathologic markers as prognostic indicators.

VIII. Treatment

A. Surgical Management

The mainstay of managing earlier stage breast cancer is surgical removal of the tumor. In women, both modified radical mastectomy and lumpectomy with radiation are equivalent approaches [61]. This differs in men. Because of the lack of breast tissue and central location of most tumors, breast conservation is not a viable option and modified radical mastectomy is the standard surgical approach [7]. The transition to the modified radical mastectomy in men was based on the equivalent outcomes to radical mastectomy seen with this approach in women [7].

Lymph node sampling is an integral part in the initial surgical management of breast cancer. Whether or not the lymph nodes are involved is one of the major prognostic factors in this disease, and knowing the status of the axillary lymph nodes is critical in guiding further management of the patient. The appropriate extent of axillary dissection has been defined on either the basis of the number of nodes removed or the anatomic location of the nodes [57]. Using the pectoralis minor muscle, the axillary lymph nodes can be divided into three anatomic locations (Fig. 59-2). Several investigators have studied the involvement of nodes in the upper axilla when lower lymph nodes are tumor free to determine the accuracy of the dissection. In general, when both level I and II nodes are negative, isolated disease in level III nodes is present in only a small percentage of cases. The rates of positive level II lymph nodes when level I has no disease are more variable ranging anywhere from 1.5 to 29% [62–67]. The National Institutes of Health in a consensus conference in 1991 stated that a level I and II anatomic dissection is the preferred operation [68]. Unfortunately, there are a number of morbidities associated with this operation including seroma formation, shoulder dysfunction, loss of sensation or paresthesias, and upper extremity edema. In particular, lymphedema can affect 10 to 25% of patients who undergo axillary dissection,

and it can be a chronic and disabling problem for which there are limited therapies [69].

To avoid these complications a less invasive procedure, sentinel lymph node biopsy (SLNB), is under investigation in women with small primary tumors who statistically have the lowest risk for lymph node involvement. Although not yet standard practice this procedure is quickly becoming a widely implemented technique for evaluating the axilla in women. Men with breast cancer face the same potential complications as women after a classic lymph node dissection. In a study reported from Memorial Sloan-Kettering Cancer Center, Port *et al* [69] retrospectively reviewed 16 cases of male breast cancer that were treated with a SLNB. Fifteen of the 16 men had T1 tumors with a mean size of 1.3 cm. They found that in 15 of the men the sentinel lymph node was successfully identified. Five (33.3%) of the men had a positive result. Two of these were on frozen section, and the men underwent immediate complete dissection yielding further positive lymph nodes. The other three were on pathologic review and sectioning; two of these men agreed to further surgery and the subsequent lymph nodes had no metastatic carcinoma [69]. Although the number of men in this study was limited, it suggests that in men with small primary tumors SLNB can be as successful as it is in women with the appropriate surgical expertise.

B. Adjuvant Systemic Therapy

Unfortunately, despite adequate removal of the tumor and regional lymphatics, recent surgical series still produce a 10-year disease free survival rate of 50%. Thirty percent of node-negative and 75% of node-positive patients eventually have recurrences and die of their disease when surgery is the only therapeutic modality [70]. Adjuvant systemic therapy, which is given after the primary surgery to kill or inhibit clinically occult micrometastases, has been extensively studied in women. Physicians can draw on data consisting of many randomized clinical trials with extensive follow-up to assist in counseling and treating their female patients with breast cancer. It has been well established that the use of cytotoxic chemotherapy and/or endocrine therapy in the adjuvant setting improves long-term survival of women with breast cancer [70].

In men, the low incidence of breast carcinoma precludes the development and completion of clinical trials to assess the efficacy of adjuvant therapy. Therefore, the standard treatment of male breast cancer has generally been extrapolated from the treatment used in women. Most men have ER and/or PR positive tumors; therefore, adjuvant tamoxifen is recommended. In a report by Ribeiro *et al* [71] 39 male patients who received tamoxifen were compared with a historical control group. Overall survival and disease-free survival at 5 years were higher in the group that received tamoxifen (61% vs 44% and 56% vs 28%). The most common side effects of tamoxifen include decreased libido, weight gain, hot flashes, and mood alterations. More men have been shown to discontinue the drug as compared with females because of side effects [72].

Experience with chemotherapy in male breast cancer is very limited. There are two studies reported in the literature using adjuvant cyclophosphamide, methotrexate, and 5-fluorouracil (CMF) chemotherapy in men with stage II or III disease comparing them

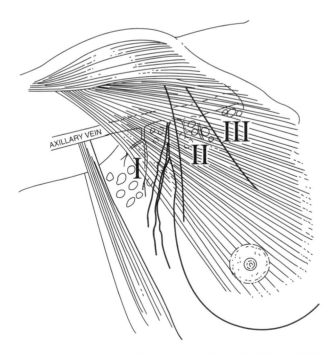

Fig. 59-2 Axillary lymph nodes by level. Levels I (low axilla), II (midaxilla), and III (apex of the axilla) defined in relation to the pectoralis minor muscle. (From Clark G. [2000]. Prognosis and Predictive Factors. In *Diseases of the Breast* [Harris JR, ed.], p. 489. Philadelphia: Lippincott Williams & Wilkins.)

to untreated historical controls. Both studies suggested a survival benefit with the use of CMF chemotherapy [73,74].

C. Radiation Therapy

Radiation therapy has been used in the treatment of breast cancer since the early 1990s [75]. Initially it was used in the treatment of chest wall recurrences or advanced disease, but, currently, it plays an integral role in managing women after lumpectomy and in postmastectomy patients who are at high risk for local recurrence. There are no clinical trials available in male breast cancer patients to evaluate the role of postoperative radiotherapy. In several series, radiation appeared to reduce postmastectomy recurrence in men but had no obvious impact on survival [76]. Given that the data in women do show a survival advantage, it would seem prudent to extrapolate this to the male patient with breast cancer [77,78].

D. Treatment of Metastatic Disease

Despite continued advances in the surgical and adjuvant management of breast cancer, 20 to 30% of patients will relapse. In addition, 1 to 5% will present initially with metastatic disease [79]. Stage IV breast cancer treatment varies little between the sexes. Both women and men can be treated with hormonal manipulation, cytotoxic chemotherapy, or both with similar responses.

Because the goal of treatment in metastatic disease is palliation of symptoms while maintaining quality of life, most clinicians tailor therapy to obtain responses with the least toxicity. For hormone receptor positive patients, endocrine therapy plays an important role. Traditionally, tamoxifen is usually the agent of first choice. Second-line and even third-line endocrine therapies include estrogen deprivation therapy in premenopausal women, either by oophorectomy or a luteinizing hormone-releasing hormone agonist, selective aromatase inhibitors (SAIs), and progestational agents such as megestrol acetate. Recently published studies have now shown that SAIs are superior to tamoxifen in hormone receptor positive postmenopausal women as first-line therapy [80,81]. In men, the newer SAIs have not been studied, and tamoxifen remains the endocrine treatment of choice for metastatic disease. Most breast cancers in men express ER and response rates as high as 81% have been reported to tamoxifen [7].

Breast cancer in considered one of the most chemosensitive solid tumors. Previously untreated patients receiving chemotherapy for metastatic disease have a significant chance of responding and therefore benefiting. This benefit comes at the expense of greater toxicity that must be considered with each patient before embarking on a new therapy. There are many active agents for this disease with documented single-agent response rates of greater than 20% and frequently much higher [79]. The most commonly used agents include the anthracyclines, particularly doxorubicin; cyclophosphamide; methotrexate; 5-fluorouracil and its oral derivatives; taxanes; and the vinca alkaloids among others. The use of these chemotherapeutic agents in metastatic disease has been well studied in women. The same cannot be said of men with breast cancer. The literature contains only anecdotal reports describing the

activity of chemotherapy in male breast cancer [82]. In general, treatment guidelines for men are similar to those used for women.

The newest approach to managing metastatic breast cancer is targeted therapy. Trastuzumab is a recombinant monoclonal antibody against HER2, which, as previously discussed, is overexpressed in 20 to 30% of breast cancer and portends a worse prognosis. Trastuzumab when used alone in HER2-overexpressing metastatic breast cancer is well tolerated and produces durable objective responses [83]. A randomized controlled study was conducted in women with metastatic HER2-overexpressing breast cancer comparing trastuzumab plus chemotherapy with chemotherapy alone. The addition of trastuzumab to chemotherapy was associated with an improved disease-free and overall survival [51]. It has become an important addition to the management of female metastatic breast carcinoma. HER-2 status has also been evaluated in male breast cancer [84]. The rates of overexpression are variable in the published series, and trastuzumab as a treatment modality has not been investigated.

The rarity of male breast cancer poses a significant impediment to the prospective study of treatment options in this disease. In general, recommendations have primarily been based on successes seen in clinical trials of females with breast cancer.

IX. Prognosis and Survival

Male breast cancer is classically described as having a poorer prognosis than female breast cancer suggesting that, in males, it is a more aggressive disease. However, evidence is accumulating that suggests that the disease is biologically similar in the two genders. Despite this, a poorer survival in men is a consistent finding [4]. This has been attributed to a delay in diagnosis, later stage at presentation, anatomic factors, and an older age at diagnosis with an increase in non-breast cancer related deaths that is seen in most series of male breast cancer [4,43,85].

Because of the older age at diagnosis, many of these patients have comorbidities and deaths unrelated to breast cancer. Guinee et al [56] reported on 335 male patients, 83 (47%) of the 178 deaths were due to causes other than breast cancer. In another paper comprising 397 cases of male breast cancer, 39.5% of the deaths were unrelated to breast cancer [86].

The prognosis for male breast cancer has been described as worse or similar to that of age- and stage-matched women [42,43,60,86–89]. In a comparative study using data from the National Cancer Data Base of 4755 men and 624,174 women, 3627 pairs of men and women with breast cancer were matched for age, stage, and demographics. Age-corrected relative survival was equivalent for men and women with stage 0, I, and II disease. The survival curves diverge for stage III and IV disease; men showed worse 5-year survival rates than women, although this did not reach statistical significance [87]. This is in contrast to a study by Borgen et al [89]. They compared the survival of 58 men with breast cancer to that of 174 women who were matched for stage and age at diagnosis [89]. All patients had stage I or II disease and were treated with mastectomy and axillary dissection. He found breast cancer survival at 10 years to be similar between the genders (Fig. 59-3). After stratification by nodal status, survival differences between men and women were more pronounced in the positive-node patients (Fig. 59-4)

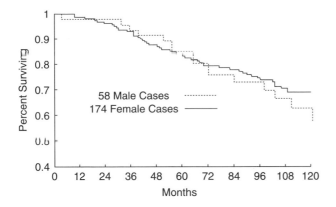

Fig. 59-3 Breast cancer survival of 58 male and 174 female breast cancer patients. (From Borgen P, Senie R, McKinnon W, Rosen P. [1997]. Carcinoma of the male breast: Analysis of prognosis compared with matched female patients. *Ann Surg Oncol.* 4:385–388.)

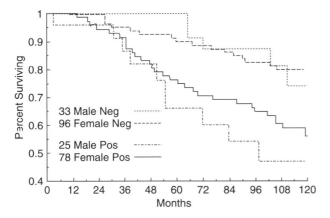

Fig. 59-4 Breast cancer survival of 58 male and 174 female breast cancer patients according to nodal status at diagnosis. (From Borgen P, Senie R, McKinnon W, Rosen P. [1997]. Carcinoma of the male breast: Analysis of prognosis compared with matched female patients. *Ann Surg Oncol.* 4:385–388.)

but did not reach statistical significance [89]. Another matched study was performed in the United Kingdom by Willsher *et al* [90]. Forty-one male patients and 123 female patients with invasive cancer were matched for age, pathologic size and grade of the primary tumor, and pathologic lymph node status. The authors also found no statistical difference in disease-free or overall survival between the groups. When these patients were compared with more than 3000 unmatched women with breast cancer treated at the same time, both the male and female matched groups had a worse outcome (Fig. 59-5). The authors suggested that this difference and the worse outcome in general with male breast cancer patients is due to a difference in the distribution of prognostic factors. In this case, there was a preponderance of grade 3 tumors, which were seen in 73% of the cases [90].

In summary, it appears that breast cancer is a similar disease in men and women. Despite the clear disparity in the incidence of breast cancer between the sexes, once it occurs in either a man

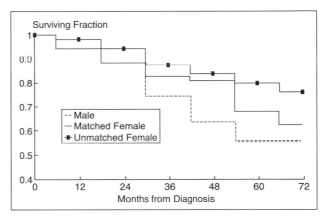

Fig. 59-5 Survival curves for male and matched female patients with breast cancer showing no significant difference (p=0.27). Compared with an unmatched female series, both the male patients (p=0.0003) and matched female patients (p=0.0006) have a worse outcome. (From Willsher P, Leach I, Ellis I *et al.* [1997]. A comparison outcome of male breast cancer with female breast cancer. *Am J Surg.* 173:185–188.)

or woman, its clinical presentation, pathologic appearance, response to treatment, and overall prognosis are not that different. Given that breast cancer in women is a prevalent disease and the second leading cause of cancer-related death, there is a great socioeconomic burden. This has led to extensive research into this disease. The risk factors, prognostic factors, and treatment algorithm have all been thoroughly explored, and clinicians have resources to draw on when treating their female patients. This is the major difference between the sexes. Breast cancer is a rarity in males; therefore, it is much less studied. Most knowledge and treatment approaches for this disease in males comes from the extrapolation of information about female patients with breast cancer.

X. Suggestions for Further Investigations

- Many advances in the appropriate treatment of female breast cancer have come from the use of prognostic stratification based on the biologic parameters of the individual tumors; prospective studies would help further define these variables in male breast cancer.
- Newer hormonal and targeted biologic agents such as aromatase inhibitors and trastuzumab have advanced the treatment of female breast cancer; however, their role in male breast cancer has yet to be defined.

References

1. Greenlee RH, Hill-Harmon M, Murray T, Thun M. (2001). Cancer Statistics, 2001. *CA Cancer J Clin.* 51:15–36.
2. Parker SL, Tong T, Bolden S, Wingo PA. (1997). Cancer Statistics, 1997. *CA Cancer J Clin.* 47:5–27.
3. Silverberg E, Lubera J. (1987). Cancer Statistics, 1987. *CA Cancer J Clin.* 37:2–19.
4. Donegan WL. Redlich P, Lang P, Gall M. (1998). Carcinoma of the breast in males, a multiinstitutional study. *Cancer.* 83:408–509.
5. Statistics. (1998). *SEER cancer statistics review, 1973–1995.* Bethesda, MD: US National Cancer Institute.

6. Willett W, Rockhill B, Hankinson S *et al.* (2000). Epidemiology and Assessing and Managing Risk. In *Diseases of the Breast* (Harris JR, ed.), pp. 175–220. Philadelphia: Lippincott Williams & Wilkins.

7. Gradisher W. (2000). Male Breast Cancer. In *Diseases of the Breast* (Harris JR, ed.), pp. 661–667. Philadelphia: Lippincott Williams & Wilkins.

8. Muir C, Waterhouse J, Mack T *et al.* (1987). Cancer Incidence in Five Continents. In *Cancer*, vol. 5. Lyon, France: International Agency for Research on Cancer Scientific Publications.

9. Ravandi-Kashani F, Hayes TG. (1998). Male breast cancer: A review of the literature. *Eur J Cancer.* 34:1341–1347.

10. Hankinson SE, Colditz GA, Manson JE *et al.* (1997). A prospective study of oral contraceptive use and risk of breast cancer (Nurses' Health Study, United States). *Cancer Causes Control.* 8(1):65–72.

11. Brinton LA, Daling JR, Liff JM *et al.* (1995). Oral contraceptives and breast cancer risk among younger women. *J Natl Cancer Inst.* 87:827–835.

12. Collaborative Group on Hormonal Factors in Breast Cancer. (1997). Breast cancer and hormone replacement therapy: Collaborative reanalysis of data from 51 epidemiological studies of 52,705 women with breast cancer and 108,411 women without breast cancer. *Lancet.* 350:1047–1059.

13. Harnden R, McLean N, Langlands AO. (1971). Carcinoma of the breast and Klinefelter's syndrome. *J Med Genet.* 8:460.

14. Scheike O, Visfeldt J, Peterson B. (1973). Breast carcinoma in association with Klinefelter's syndrome. *Acta Pathol Microbiol Scand.* 81:352.

15. Hultborn R, Hanson C, Kopf I, Verbiene I *et al.* (1997). Prevalence of Klinefelter's syndrome in male breast cancer patients. *Anticancer Res.* 17:4293.

16. Lenfant-Pejovic MH, Milka-Cabanne N, Bouchardy C, Auquier A. (1990). Risk factors for male breast cancer: A Franco-Swiss case-control study. *Int J Cancer.* 45:660.

17. Sorensen HT, Friis S, Olsen JH *et al.* (1998). Risk of breast cancer in men with liver cirrhosis. *Am J Gastroenterol.* 93:231.

18. Borgen PI, Wong GY, Vlamis V *et al.* (1992). Current management of male breast cancer. A review of 104 cases. *Ann Surg.* 215:451–457, discussion 457–459.

19. Kushi LH, Sellers TA, Potter JD *et al.* (1992). Dietary fat and postmenopausal breast cancer. *J Natl Cancer Inst.* 84:1092–1099.

20. Graham S, Hellman R, Marshall J *et al.* (1991). Nutritional epidemiology of postmenopausal breast cancer in western New York. *Am J Epidemiol.* 134:552–566.

21. Howe GR, Friedenreich CM, Jain M *et al.* (1991). A cohort study of fat intake and risk of breast cancer. *J Natl Cancer Inst.* 83:336–340.

22. Mills PK, Deeson WL, Phillips RL *et al.* (1989). Dietary habits and breast cancer incidence among Seventh-day Adventists. *Cancer.* 64:582–590.

23. van den Brandt PA, Vantveer P, Goldbohm RA *et al.* (1993). A prospective cohort study on dietary fat and the risk of postmenopausal breast cancer. *Cancer Res.* 53:75–82.

24. Wolk A, Bergstrom R, Hunter D *et al.* (1998). A prospective study of association of monounsaturated fat and other types of fat with risk of breast cancer. *Arch Intern Med.* 158:41–45.

25. Hunter DJ, Spiegalman D, Adami HO *et al.* (1996). Cohort studies of fat intake and the risk of breast cancer. *N Engl J Med.* 334:356–361.

26. Smith-Warner SA, Spiegelman D, Yaun SS *et al.* (1998). Alcohol and breast cancer in women: A pooled analysis of cohort studies. *JAMA.* 279:535–540.

27. Reichman ME, Judd JT, Longscope C *et al.* (1993). Effects of alcohol consumption on plasma and urinary hormone concentrations in premenopausal women. *J Natl Cancer Inst.* 85:722–727.

28. Rosenblatt KA, Thomas DB, Jimenez LM *et al.* (1999). The relationship between diet and breast cancer in men (United States). *Cancer Causes Control.* 10:107–113.

29. Hsing AW, McLaughlan JK, Cocco P *et al.* (1998). Risk factors for male breast cancer (United States). *Cancer Causes Control.* 9:269–275.

30. Eeles R, Powles T. (2000). Chemoprevention options for BRCA1 and BRCA2 mutation carriers. *J Clin Oncol.* 18(21s):93s–99s.

31. Ford D, Easton D, Peto J. (1995). Estimates of the gene frequency and its contribution to breast and ovarian cancer incidence. *Am J Hum Genet.* 57:1457–1462.

32. Ford D, Easton D, Stratton MR. (1998). Genetic heterogeneity and penetrance analysis of the BRCA1 and BRCA2 genes in breast cancer families. *Am J Hum Genet.* 62:676–689.

33. Breast Cancer Linkage Consortium. (1999). Carrier risks in BRCA2 mutation carriers. *J Natl Cancer Inst.* 91.1310–1316.

34. Couch FJ, Fario LM, Deshano ML *et al.* (1996). BRCA2 germline mutations in male breast cancer cases and breast cancer families. *Nat Genet.* 13:123–125.

35. Friedman LS, Gayther SA, Kurosaki T *et al.* (1997). Mutation analysis of BRCA 1 and BRCA2 in a male breast cancer population. *Nat Genet.* 60(2):313–319.

36. DeMichele A, Weber B. (2000). Inherited Genetic Factors. In *Diseases of the Breast* (Harris JR, ed.), pp. 221–236. Philadelphia: Lippincott Williams & Wilkins.

37. Basham VM, Lipscombe JM, Ward JM *et al.* (2002). BRCA1 and BRCA2 mutations in a population-based study of male breast cancer. *Breast Cancer Res.* 4:R2.

38. Wooster R, Mangion J, Eeles R *et al.* (1992). A germline mutation in the androgen receptor gene in two brothers with breast cancer and Reifenstein syndrome. *Nat Genet.* 2:132.

39. Labaccaro J, Lombroso S, Belon C. (1993). Male breast cancer and the androgen receptor gene [letter]. *Nat Genet.* 5:109.

40. Donegan WL, Redlich PN. (1996). Breast cancer in men. *Surg Clin North Am.* 76:343.

41. Carmalt H, Mann L, Kennedy C *et al.* (1998). Carcinoma of the male breast: A review and recommendations for management. *Aust N Z J Surg.* 68:712–715.

42. Salvadori B, Saccozzi R, Manzari A *et al.* (1994). Prognosis of breast cancer in males: An analysis of 170 cases. *Eur J Cancer.* 30A:930–935.

43. Joshe M, Lee A, Loda M *et al.* (1996). Male breast carcinoma: An evaluation of prognostic factors contributing to a poorer outcome. *Cancer.* 77:490–498.

44. Shapiro S. (1977). Evidence on screening for breast cancer from a randomized trial. *Cancer.* 39(6 Suppl):2772–2782.

45. Evans G, Anthony T, Appelbaum A *et al.* (2001). The diagnostic accuracy of mammography in the evaluation of male breast disease. *Am J Surg.* 181:96–100.

46. Vetto J, Schmidt W, Pommier R *et al.* (1998). Accurate and cost-effective evaluation of breast masses in males. *Am J Surg.* 175:383–387.

47. Michaels BM, Nunn CR, Roses DF. (1994). Lobular carcinoma of the male breast. *Surgery.* 115:402.

48. Schnitt S, Guidi A. (2000). Pathology of Invasive Breast Cancer. In *Diseases of the Breast* (Harris JR, ed.), pp. 425–470. Philadelphia: Lippincott Williams & Wilkins.

49. Camus MG, Joshi MG, Mackarem G *et al.* (1994). Ductal carcinoma in situ of the male breast. *Cancer.* 83:154.

50. Rayson D, Erlichman C, Suman VJ *et al.* (1998). Molecular markers in male breast carcinoma. *Cancer.* 83:1947.

51. Slamon DJ, Leylano-Jones B, Shak S *et al.* (2001). Use of chemotherapy plus a monoclonal antibody against HER2 for metastatic breast cancer that overexpresses HER2. *N Engl J Med.* 344:783–792.

52. Shpitz B, Bornstein Y, Sternberg A *et al.* (2000). Angiogenesis, p53, and c-erbB-2 immunoreactivity and clinicopathological features in male breast cancer. *J Surg Oncol.* 75:252–257.

53. Caleffi M, Teague MW, Jensen RA *et al.* (1994). p53 gene mutations and steroid receptor status in breast cancer. clinicopathological correlation and prognostic assessment. *Cancer.* 73:2147–2156.

54. Wick M, Sayadi H, Ritter J *et al.* (1999). Low stage carcinoma of the male breast. *Am J Clin Pathol.* 111:59–69.

55. Clark J, Nguyen P, Jaszcz W *et al.* (2000). Prognostic variables in male breast cancer. *Am Surg.* 66:502–510.

56. Pich A, Margaria E, Chiusa L. (2000). Oncogenes and male breast carcinoma: c-erbB-2 and p53 coexpression predicts a poor survival. *J Clin Oncol.* 18:2948–2956.

57. Clark G. (2000). Prognosis and Predictive Factors. In *Diseases of the Breast* (Harris JR, ed.), pp. 489–514. Philadelphia: Lippincott Williams & Wilkins.

58. Herman K, Lobaziewicz W, Skotnicki P *et al.* (2000). Male breast cancer. Does the prognosis differ compared to female? *Neoplasma.* 47(3):191–195.

59. McLachlan SA, Etuchman C, Liu FF *et al.* (1996). Male breast cancer: An 11 year review of 66 patients. *Breast Cancer Res Treat.* 40(3):225–230.

60. Guinee VF, Olsson H, Moller T *et al.* (1993). The prognosis of breast cancer in males. A report of 335 cases. *Cancer.* 71:154–160.

61. Fisher B, Redmond C, Poissen R *et al.* (1989). Eight-year results of a randomized clinical trial comparing total mastectomy and lumpectomy with or without irradiation in the treatment of breast cancer. *N Engl J Med.* 320:822–828.

62. Rosen PP, Lesser ML, Kinne DW *et al.* (1983). Discontinuous or "skip" metastases in breast carcinoma. Analysis of 1228 axillary dissections. *Ann Surg.* 197:276–283.

63. Veronesi U, Rilke F, Lvini A *et al.* (1987). Distribution of axillary node metastases by level of invasion. An analysis of 539 cases. *Cancer.* 59:682–687.

64. Smith JA 3rd, Gamez-Araujo JJ, Gallager HS *et al.* (1977). Carcinoma of the breast: Analysis of total lymph node involvement versus level of metastasis. *Cancer.* 39:527–532.

65. Danforth DN Jr, Findlay PA, McDonald HD *et al.* (1986). Complete axillary lymph node dissection for stage I-II carcinoma of the breast. *J Clin Oncol.* 4:655–662.

66. Chevinsky AH, Ferrara J, James AG *et al.* (1990). Prospective evaluation of clinical and pathologic detection of axillary metastases in patients with carcinoma of the breast. *Surgery.* 108:612–617, discussion 617–618.

67. Pigott J, Nichols R, Maddox WA *et al.* (1984). Metastases to the upper levels of the axillary nodes in carcinoma of the breast and its implications for nodal sampling procedures. *Surg Gynecol Obstet,* 158:255–259

68. National Institutes of Health Consensus Conference. (1991). Treatment of early stage breast cancer. *JAMA.* 265:391.

69. Port E, Fey J, Cody HS, Borgen P. (2000). Sentinel lymph node biopsy in patients with male breast carcinoma. *Cancer.* 91:319–323.

70. Osborne CK, Ravdin PM. Adjuvant Systemic Therapy of Primary Breast Cancer. In *Diseases of the Breast* (Harris JR, ed.), pp. 599–632. Philadelphia: Lippincott Williams & Wilkins.

71. Ribeiro G, Swindell R. (1992). Adjuvant tamoxifen for male breast cancer (MBC). *Br J Cancer.* 65:252–254.

72. Anelli TF, Anelli A, Tran KN *et al.* (1994). Tamoxifen is associated with a high rate of treatment-limiting symptoms in male breast cancer patients. *Cancer.* 74:74.

73. Patel HZ 2nd, Buzdar AU, Hortobagyi GN. (1989). Role of adjuvant chemotherapy in male breast cancer. *Cancer.* 64:1583–1585.

74. Bagley CS, Wesley MN, Young RC, Lippman ME. (1987). Adjuvant chemotherapy in males with cancer of the breast. *Am J Clin Oncol.* 10:55.

75. Lichter A, Pierce L. (2000). Techniques of Radiation Therapy. In *Diseases of the Breast* (Harris JR, ed.), pp. 589–598. Philadelphia: Lippincott Williams & Wilkins.

76. Schuchardt U, Sergenschmiedt MH, Kirschner MJ *et al.* (1996). Adjuvant radiotherapy for breast carcinoma in men: A 20 year clinical experience. *Am J Clin Oncol.* 19:330.

77. Overgaard M, Hansen PS, Overgaard J *et al.* (1997). Postoperative radiotherapy in high risk premenopausal women with breast cancer who receive adjuvant chemotherapy. Danish Breast Cancer cooperative Group 82 b trial. *N Engl J Med.* 337:949.

78. Ragaz J, Jackson SM, Le N *et al.* (1997). Adjuvant radiotherapy and chemotherapy in node-positive women with breast cancer. *N Engl J Med.* 337:956.

79. Ellis M, Hayes D, Lippman M. Treatment of Metastatic Breast Cancer. In *Diseases of the Breast* (Harris JR, ed.). Philadelphia: Lippincott Williams & Wilkins.

80. Nabholtz JM, Buzdar A, Pollak M *et al.* (2000). Anastrozole is superior to tamoxifen as first-line therapy for advanced breast cancer in postmenopausal women: Results of a North American multicenter randomized trial. Arimidex Study Group. *J Clin Oncol.* 18:3758–3767.

81. Mouridsen H, Bershanovich M, Sun Y *et al.* (2001). Superior efficacy of letrozole versus tamoxifen as first-line therapy for postmenopausal women with advanced breast cancer: Results of a phase III study of the International Letrozole Breast Cancer Group. *J Clin Oncol.* 19:2596–2606.

82. Jaiyesimi IA, Buzdar AU, Sahin AA, Ross MA. (1992). Carcinoma of the male breast. *Ann Intern Med.* 117:771–777.

83. Cobleigh M, Vogel C, Tripathy D *et al.* (1999). Multinational study of the efficacy and safety of humanized anti-HER2 monoclonal antibody in women who have HER2-overexpressing metastatic breast cancer that has progressed after chemotherapy for metastatic disease. *J Clin Oncol.* 17:2639–2648.

84. Bloom K, Govil H, Gattuso P, Reddy V, Francescatti D. (2001). Status of HER2 in male and female breast carcinoma. *Am J Surg.* 182:389–392.

85. Meijer-van Gelder ME, Look MP, Bolt-De-Vries J *et al.* (2001). Clinical relevance of biologic factors in male breast cancer. *Breast Cancer Res Treat.* 68:249–260.

86. Cutuli B, Lacroze M, Dilhuydy JM *et al.* (1995). Male breast cancer: Results of the treatments and prognostic factors in 397 cases. *Eur J Cancer.* 31A:1960–1964.

87. Scott-Conner CE, Jochimsen PR, Menck AR *et al.* (1999). An analysis of male and female breast cancer treatment and survival among demographically identical pairs of patients. *Surgery.* 126:775–780, discussion 780–781.

88. Winchester DJ. (1996). Male breast cancer. *Semin Surg Oncol.* 12:364–369.

89. Borgen P, Senie R, McKinnon W, Rosen P. (1997). Carcinoma of the male breast: Analysis of prognosis compared with matched female patients. *Ann Surg Oncol.* 4:385–388.

90. Willsher P, Leach I, Ellis I *et al.* (1997). A comparison outcome of male breast cancer with female breast cancer. *Am J Surg.* 173:185–188.

91. Andre S, Fonseca I. (2001). Male breast cancer: A reappraisal of clinical and biologic indicators of prognosis. *Acta Oncol.* 40:472–478.

60

Difference in the Germ Cell Tumors of the Reproductive Tract in Men and Women

TATJANA KOLEVSKA, MD, MS* AND AMY TIERSTEN, MD**

*Department of Medicine, Division of Medical Oncology and Hematology, Kaiser Permanente Medical Center, Vallejo, CA
**Associate Professor of Medicine, New York University School of Medicine, New York, NY

Germ cells (primordial cells) are cells stored in the male and female reproductive tracts (testis and ovary) that carry the reproductive machinery of both sexes. A unique characteristic of these cells is that they divide by meiosis retaining only half of the cell chromosomes (haploid); thus, when the male sperm cell and female ovum join, the resulting human embryo has normal diploid somatic cell number of chromosomes. Although they have the same function and originate from the same cells, their development, number, maturation, and pathology are very different in men and women.

Germ cell tumors (GCTs) constitute a remarkably heterogeneous group of neoplasms that can arise from the germ cells in the gonads (testis and ovary) or in extragonadal sites (mainly in the sacrococcygeal region, retroperitoneum, mediastinum, and central nervous system). An estimated 7000 new cases (6900 testis, 100 ovarian) and 300 deaths caused by GCTs of all primary sites were reported in the United States in 2000 and their incidence appears to be increasing [1].

Despite their common origin, germ cells can cause very different tumors in men and women. They are uncommon in women, representing less than 5% of all ovarian neoplasms [2]. Most ovarian carcinomas are epithelial in origin, accounting for more than 90% of the estimated 25,000 new cases of ovarian cancer diagnosed per year in the United States. The pathogenesis, clinical presentation, treatment, and outcome of ovarian germ cell and epithelial cancer are very different. In this chapter we concentrate on the GCTs. On the other hand, cancer of the testis is predominantly germ cell and is the most common solid tumor in men between the ages of 20 and 35. To understand this significant difference in GCTs between sexes it is necessary to describe the difference in germ cell development. The main differences between male and female germ cells are presented on Table 60-1.

I. Origin of Germ Cells

Primordial germ cells arise in the endoderm of the embryonic yolk sac, allantois, and hindgut of the male and female embryo. The germ cells migrate and multiply through the wall of the midgut to the genital ridge at 4 to 5 weeks of gestation. The migration proceeds along the paravertebral gonadal ridge in caudal to cranial direction. Germ cells arrested in this migration are thought to be the source of the extragonadal GCTs in both sexes, including the sacrococcygeal region, retroperitoneum, mediastinum, and pineal and suprasellar area [3]. The midline location of the paravertebral gonadal ridge explains the near midline location of most extragonadal GCTs. The reasons for

Table 60-1
Characteristics of Germ Cells in Men and Women During the Human Lifetime

Time	Characteristic	Men	Women
Prenatal			
Origin	Endoderm	+	+
5 weeks	Migration to genital ridge	+	+
8 weeks	Duct formation		
	Müllerian	–	+
	Wolffian	+	–
24 weeks	Number of germ cells	Millions	1 Million
Birth	Cell division		
	Mitosis	+	+
	Meiosis	+	+
	Number of germ cells	Millions	400,000
Postnatal			
Until puberty	Cell division		
	Mitosis	Present	–
	Meiosis	Present	–
Lifetime	Cell division		
	Mitosis	+	–
	Meiosis	+	–
	Number of germ cells	Millions	400

migration arrest of germ cells are unknown. Before the eighth week of gestation, the sex of the embryo cannot be recognized [4]. Appropriately, this period is termed the indifferent phase of sexual development. After 8 weeks of gestation the embryo acquires two duct systems within the primitive kidney. The Müllerian duct forms female internal reproductive organs, and the wolffian duct gives rise to the male reproductive organs.

A. Embryologic Development and Maturation of Germ Cells in Men

The germ cells are incorporated in the developing gonad around the eighth week of gestation, when they are termed the gonocytes [4]. They differentiate into spermatogonia during the second and third trimester of pregnancy. In the postnatal testis, the spermatogonial cells undergo a series of mitotic divisions leading to the development of type A, intermediate type, and type B spermatogonia. The type B spermatogonium undergoes meiosis followed by mitosis, resulting in four haploid cells that develop into spermatids and spermatozoa. Apoptotic or programmed cell death plays an important role during the development of the sperm cells by regulating the number of surviving cells in relation to the availability of growth factors. It is apparent that male germ cells divide and undergo apoptosis at a high rate during the entire male life. The high rate of turnaround (mitosis and apoptosis) is thought to be the main reason for mistakes in the DNA control and the high rate of development of testicular tumors. Ovarian GCTs develop rarely because the germ cells stop dividing early in the female embryonic development.

B. Embryologic Development and Maturation of Germ Cells in Women

The germ cells incorporated in the developing ovary multiply at high rate, and, by 24 weeks of gestation, there are 7 million oogonia in the primitive ovaries. They continue to multiply, but most die by apoptosis, so that only about 1 million primary oocytes are left at birth [4]. These decrease to about 400,000 by puberty. The surviving oogonia are arrested at the prophase of meiosis. Completion of the first division of meiosis does not occur until the time of ovulation. Only about 400 of these oocytes actually mature and are released by ovulation in a woman's lifetime; the others undergo apoptosis and die at various stages of development. In contrast to the situation in the male, female germ cells stop dividing by mitosis during prenatal life. As mentioned previously that may be the reason for the low rate of development of ovarian GCTs.

II. Gender Differences in the Epidemiology of Germ Cell Tumors

A. Childhood Germ Cell Tumors

In contrast to the rarity of GCTs in adult females, ovarian tumors account for approximately 25% of all (male and female) pediatric GCTs. Also both benign and malignant extragonadal GCTs are more frequent in girls. The reason for this difference in unclear. One possibility is that female germ cells undergo most of their divisions and apoptosis early in human life, so the chances of malignant transformation of their genome is highest during this period. In contrast to female cells, male germ cells divide and mature during the male's entire life.

The peak incidence of ovarian GCTs is 10 years of age [5]. Most of these tumors are benign mature cystic teratomas, although nearly one third contain malignant elements. In contrast to adult ovarian tumors, malignancies of epithelial or stromal cell origin are uncommon in girls. The most common pediatric ovarian neoplasias are dysgerminomas and yolk sac tumors. Immature teratomas account for approximately 10% of ovarian masses [6].

Testicular tumors make up approximately 10% of all pediatric GCTs. In contrast to ovarian tumors, most male GCTs are

Table 60-2

Characteristics of Adult Gonadal Male and Female Germ Cell Tumors

Characteristic of Germ Cell Tumors	Male	Female
Cell origin	Germ cells	Germ cells
Incidence in young adults	High	Low
12p chromosome copies	Increased	Unknown
Cyclin D2 overexpression	Present	Unknown
Main clinical symptom	Testicular mass	Nonspecific
Response to chemotherapy	High	High

malignant (80%), characteristically containing yolk sac elements [5]. Pediatric testicular GCTs follow a bimodal age distribution, occurring in very young children and in adolescent boys. Boys with yolk sac tumors of the testis have been diagnosed with additional anomalies including inguinal hernia, double ureter, ectopic kidney, and renal agenesis [7].

Extragonadal GCTs are more frequent in girls and are usually located in the presacral and sacrococcygeal region. Most of them are teratomas, and they are usually diagnosed at birth or during the first month of life [8].

B. Adult Germ Cell Tumors

As mentioned previously GCTs are rare in adult females. Of an estimated 7000 new cases of GCTs per year in the United States, 98% are testicular [1]. In contrast to pediatric ovarian tumors, GCTs of the ovary are much less common then epithelial ovarian neoplasms in the adult female. They represent 3% of all ovarian cancers in Western countries. They almost always occur in younger women, and their peak incidence is in the early 20s. An increased incidence of GCTs is found in Asians and Africans, and these tumors represent as many as 15% of all ovarian cancers in these populations [2]. The reasons for this racial difference in GCT development in females are unclear.

Germ cell tumors are the most common solid tumors in men between ages of 20 and 35 years. In contrast to GCTs in adult females, male GCTs have two modal peaks: ages 25 to 40 and approximately age 60 [1]. The incidence of testicular GCTs in the United States is 6900. In contrast to ovarian tumors, GCTs of the testis are more common in young whites with ratios between whites and African Americans in the U.S. military of 40:1 (annual incidence) [9]. In African Americans, GCTs behave similarly to those of the general population.

The main differences between gonadal male and female GCTs are presented in Table 60-2.

Extragonadal GCTs are very rare in adults representing only 1 to 5% of all GCTs [10]. The mediastinum is the most common site for their development. In adults, benign GCTs have no gender predilection. Malignant extragonadal GCTs in contrast occur almost exclusively in men [11]. They are commonly diagnosed in the third decade of life, but tumors in patients as old as 60 years have been reported. The incidence of these neoplasms is equal in all races.

III. Biology and Risk Factors for Germ Cell Tumors—Are They Gender Specific?

A. Biology and Risk Factors of Male Germ Cell Tumors

Cytogenetic and molecular genetic analysis of male GCTs has yielded important data relevant to the understanding of the mechanism of germ cell malignant transformation.

Virtually 100% of male GCTs show the same abnormal increased number of copies of the 12 p chromosome [12]. This chromosome marker is present in the first recognizable stage of GCTs—carcinoma in situ—suggesting that this abnormality may be the earliest genetic change in the development of GCTs [13]. The most likely driver gene candidate for GCTs development in this 12 p region is the cyclin D2 gene that regulates phosphorylation of pRB protein and control the G1-S cell cycle checkpoint. Disruption of this checkpoint through overexpression of cyclin D2 is known to be one of the important pathways in human tumor development [14]. Immunohistochemical analysis of normal testis germ cells and GCTs also suggest that cyclin D2 plays a major role in the development of GCTs because it is only occasionally expressed in the normal testis, whereas most aberrant germ cells in carcinoma in situ and GCTs overexpress cyclin D2 [15].

Two models of origin of GCTs have been proposed. Skakkebaek et al [16,17] suggested that germ cell kit receptor/stem cell factor paracrine loop dysregulation leads to uncontrolled proliferation of gonocytes on gonadotrophin stimulation during postnatal life and puberty. A second model proposed by Chaganti et al [18] suggested that aberrant chromatid exchange events during meiotic crossing over may lead to increase 12 p copy number and overexpression of cyclin D2 [18]. Germ cells containing unrepaired DNA breaks that would normally undergo apoptosis, in the presence of increased concentration of cyclin D2, may block a p 53-dependent apoptotic response and lead to reinitiation of cell-cycle, genomic instability and neoplastic transformation of the germ cells [19]. Because testicular germ cells undergo many more meiotic divisions than ovarian germ cells the chances of the previously described mistakes are much higher in men. That may be one of the reasons for higher incidence of GCTs in men.

The strongest risk factor for male GCTs is previous history of testicular cancer. It represents a 500-fold increase in incidence compared with the normal male population [20]. Cryptorchidism increases the risk 20- to 40-fold compared with normal counterparts. Genetic abnormalities such as Klinefelter's and Down syndromes have been reported to increase the risk for GCTs. Weak association with GCTs was suggested for diethylstilbestrol in utero exposure and Agent Orange exposure. Prior trauma, elevated scrotal temperature (secondary to use of thermal underwear), and recurrent exercises that impact the scrotum such as horseback and motorcycle riding do not appear to be related to the development of testicular cancer.

B. Biology of Female Germ Cell Tumors

Perhaps because of their rare occurrence, female GCTs were much less studied in the past. Very little is known about their biology and risk factors. It is not currently known if female GCTs overexpress cyclin D2, if they have an abnormal increase in copy number of the 12 p chromosome as GCTs in the male

do, and if they originate in carcinoma in situ lesions. It is not known with certainty why adult female GCTs are much less common than male GCTs. Several theories mentioned previously, based on knowledge about male GCTs, are currently being investigated [12].

Because female germ cells have a very different speed of maturation than do male germ cells and because they do not multiply in female's postnatal life, study of the female adult GCTs may give answers about the behavior and the mechanisms of malignant transformation of all germ cells.

Very little is known about the risk factors for female GCTs. There are few reports in the literature about familial ovarian germ cell cancers, but the genes and the pathogenesis of these tumors are largely unknown [21]. Several families have been reported in which both males and females have been diagnosed with malignant GCTs [21]. Given the similar histology of testicular and ovarian GCTs, and the presence of both tumor types in several reported families, it is possible that these tumors may arise from a common genetic etiology.

C. Origin of Extragonadal Germ Cell Tumors

Most of extragonadal GCTs in men and women occur in the mediastinum, retroperitoneum, and the pineal gland. Most adult patients with malignant extragonadal GCTs are male [10]. Retroperitoneal tumors are generally considered to be metastasis of primary gonadal lesions, whereas the origin of primary mediastinal and pineal lesions has been a matter of speculation. The view that suggests that tumors in these locations are the result of local transformation of germ cells misplaced during embryogenesis is questioned by the failure of multiple researchers to identify evidence of the presence of any misplaced germ cells in human and murine embryos [22]. Cytogenetic studies showed that extragonadal GCTs are not different from gonadal GCTs in the pattern of differentiation and have no specific chromosomal aberrations or incidence of recurring breakpoints [23,24]. On the bases of these observations, an alternative suggestion was made that extragonadal GCTs represent reverse migration of occult germ cell carcinoma in situ of the gonads and may be gonadal in origin. These tumors are very rare, and there are no studies so far about possible gender differences in their biology.

IV. Histology of Germ Cell Tumors

Although very different in their incidence, male and female GCTs have very similar histologic features. Female GCTs are divided into dysgerminomas and nondysgerminomas (endodermal sinus tumor, embryonal carcinoma, teratoma, and choriocarcinoma). Male GCTs are divided into seminomas and nonseminomas (endodermal sinus tumor, embryonal carcinoma, teratoma, and choriocarcinoma).

Seminoma and dysgerminoma cells are large with abundant cytoplasm and areas arranged in sheets with trophoblastic giant cells producing human chorionic gonadotropin. The prognosis of both is favorable compared with nonseminomas and nondysgerminomas.

Nonseminomas (testicular) and nondysgerminomas (ovary) have worse prognosis than seminomas and dysgerminomas in both sexes. They have very different histology and produce different tumor markers than seminomas and dysgerminomas. Choriocarcinoma produces high levels of beta-human chorionic gonadotropin (hCG), and endodermal sinus tumors produce alpha fetoprotein (AFP).

It is important to emphasize that, in the presence of even a minimal amount of the more malignant tumor type in either a man or a woman, the whole neoplasm should be classified as the more malignant tumor type and treated as such (nonseminoma in a man and nondysgerminoma in a woman).

V. Gender Differences in Clinical Presentation of Germ Cell Tumors

Because gonadal germ cells have different locations in men and women their clinical presentation is very different. The location of extragonadal GCTs is the same in both sexes, and their clinical characteristics are similar.

A. Clinical Features of Male Germ Cell Tumors

Clinical presentation of male GCTs is usually that of a painless, swollen testicle, sometimes with distinct palpable masses. Often, there is a sensation of heaviness, although pain is less frequent. Men with metastatic disease can have back pain from retroperitoneal lymphadenopathy. Symptoms from other metastatic sites such as hemoptysis from lung metastasis are rare. Gynecomastia can sometimes be seen in patients with a very high beta-hCG. Low sperm counts are associated with GCTs, and a diagnosis can result from investigation of infertility.

B. Clinical Features of Female Germ Cell Tumors

Abdominal pain, pelvic fullness, and urinary symptoms are common in women with GCTs of the ovary. In a minority of patients (approximately 10%), abdominal pain can be severe, usually the result of hemorrhage, rupture, or torsion of the tumor. Abdominal distension can also be a symptom and often is associated with ascites.

C. Clinical Features of Extragonadal Germ Cell Tumors

In both men and women, primary mediastinal GCTs can present with symptoms of local compression such as superior vena cava syndrome, dysphagia, cough, or dyspnea.

Pineal GCTs are very rare, representing 0.5% of all intracranial tumors [25]. Neurologic signs and symptoms are caused by obstructive hydrocephalus and involvement of ocular pathways in both men and women. Major symptoms are headache, nausea and vomiting, lethargy, and diplopia. The major ocular manifestation is paralysis of conjugate gaze (Parinaud's syndrome).

VI. Diagnosis of Male and Female Germ Cell Tumors

Male and female gonadal GCTs are anatomically situated very differently and have different clinical presentation as mentioned previously, and their diagnosis requires different approaches. The metastatic workup is similar, because the biology of these tumors in men and women is alike.

All men with testicular mass or pain should have an immediate testicular ultrasound. Occasionally when indicated, a short course of antibiotics for possible epididymitis or orchitis is given before the ultrasound. Testicular biopsy and scrotal orchiectomy are rarely indicated, because of the risk of tumor seeding of the scrotum and possible inguinal and pelvis metastasis from retroperitoneal lymphatic and vascular drainage [26]. Radical inguinal orchiectomy in which the spermatic cord is ligated at the internal ring is the procedure of choice.

Women with a palpable adnexal mass should have evaluation with ultrasound. All adnexal masses of 8 cm or larger require surgical exploration [2].

Mediastinal extragonadal GCT in both sexes is most often detected on chest x-ray examination as an anterior (95%) or posterior (5%) mediastinal mass [10].

Staging workup in men and women for gonadal and extragonadal GCTs should include complete blood count, serum lactate dehydrogenase (LDH), alfa fetoprotein (AFP), beta subunit human chorionic gonadotropin (beta-hCG), computed tomography (CT) scans of the abdomen and pelvis, and chest x-ray examination. If the chest x-ray film is abnormal or there is evidence of abdominal or pelvic lymphadenopathy, CT of the chest should be performed. If neurologic findings are present, a CT or magnetic resonance imaging (MRI) scan of the brain is done [26].

VII. Treatment of Male and Female Germ Cell Tumors

Because of the different locations of the GCTs in men and women the initial surgical therapy is very different. Because of the similar biology, male and female GCTs tumors have very similar sensitivity to chemotherapy and radiation. Thus, multiple chemotherapy regimens tested on the more prevalent testicular GCTs were adopted for treatment of ovarian GCTs.

The staging systems for male and female GCTs are very different. The female GCTs are staged in the same way as the more prevalent epithelial ovarian neoplasms, according to the Federation of Gynecology and Obstetrics (FIGO) (Table 60-3). Male germ cell cancer is staged by the tumor, nodal, metastasis (TNM) system (Table 60-4).

Table 60-3
FIGO Staging System for Ovarian Cancer

Stage	Characteristics
I	Growth limited to the ovaries
II	Growth involving one or both ovaries with pelvic extension
III	Tumor involving one or both ovaries with peritoneal implants outside the pelvis and/or positive retroperitoneal or inguinal lymph nodes; superficial liver metastasis; tumor is limited to the pelvis but with histologically verified malignant extension to the small bowel or omentum
IV	Growth involving one or both ovaries with distant metastasis

FIGO, International Federation of Gynecology and Obstetrics.

Table 60-4
TNM Staging System for Testicular Cancer

TNM Stage	Description
I	N0 Disease confined to the testis and peritesticular tissue
II	N1, N2a Fewer than six positive lymph nodes without extension into retroperitoneal fat, no node >2 cm
	N2b Six or more positive lymph nodes, well encapsulated and/or retroperitoneal fat extension; any node >2 cm
	N3 Any node >5 cm
III	Disseminated disease (lung, liver, bone, or supradiaphragmatic spread)

TNM, tumor, lymph nodes, metastasis.

A. Male Seminomas and Female Dysgerminomas

Seminomas and dysgerminomas share many biologic similarities that make them very responsive to both radiation and chemotherapy.

1. Treatment of Stage I Seminomas and Dysgerminomas

Very early (stage I) disease is defined as no lymph node involvement and growth limited to one gonad (ovary or testis) [2,26]. For these patients, surgery is the initial therapeutic approach for both sexes. In females, classic surgical staging standard for all ovarian cancers is performed that includes transverse incision, inspection of the peritoneal cavity, histologic examination of the peritoneal washings, random biopsies, and oophorectomy. Although dysgerminomas frequently spread to the contralateral ovary, bilateral oophorectomy is not routinely necessary because postoperative chemotherapy is curative and fertility can be preserved [2]. Initial intervention for testicular cancer is radical inguinal nerve-sparing orchiectomy [26].

Surveillance would appear to be a reasonable approach for patients with stage I seminomas and stage IA dysgerminomas because 80% of both men and women will be cured with surgery alone [26–28]. However, because surveillance requires frequent abdominal CT scans and the progression is usually not associated with symptoms until the tumor burden is large, most groups have discontinued surveillance protocols in lieu of prophylactic radiotherapy to the draining lymphatics or chemotherapy [26].

2. Treatment of Stage II Seminomas and Dysgerminoma

Stage II disease is defined as growth involving one or both ovaries with pelvic extension (uterus, fallopian tubes, positive peritoneal washings, tumor on the surface of the ovaries, ruptured capsule, malignant cells in the ascites) but no lymph node involvement for dysgerminoma and disease involving the testis and abdominal lymph nodes without distant metastasis for seminoma. Dysgerminoma is currently staged the same as all other epithelial tumors of the ovary, so spread of the tumor to the lymph nodes represents stage III disease. This difference in the staging of tumors with identical biology creates confusion in the possible transfer of knowledge established for the management of the more frequent seminomas to the management of dysgerminomas.

Male patients with seminoma and infradiaphragmatic adenopathy of less than 5 cm are treated with postsurgical radiotherapy alone, whereas those with larger lymph nodes are treated with platinum-based chemotherapy [29].

For females with dysgerminoma strict guidelines were not established, so the current approach is to give postsurgical cisplatin-based chemotherapy for both stage II and III disease [2].

3. Treatment of Advanced Seminoma and Dysgerminoma

Patients with stage III seminomas have disseminated disease (lung, liver, bone, or supradiaphragmatic spread). Advanced dysgerminoma is called stage IV and includes growth in the distant metastatic sites (lungs, liver, brain).

Chemotherapy is the treatment of choice for patients with advanced seminoma and dysgerminoma. The regimen used for both sexes is bleomycin, 30 IU/week on days 2, 9, and 16; VP16 100 mg/m^2 on days 1 to 5; and cisplatin 20 mg/m^2 on days 1 to 5 given every 21 days (BEP). This regimen is very effective in both seminoma and dysgerminoma with a complete response rate of greater than 90% in most studies in both sexes [30]. The management of patients with bulky disease after chemotherapy (residual mass >3 cm) is somewhat controversial. Some investigators suggest radiotherapy or surgical removal, but in one study relapse rate of 10 to 15% in patients with residual masses was found with or without postchemotherapy surgery or radiotherapy [26].

B. Male Nonseminomas and Female Nondysgerminomas

1. Male Nonseminomas

Because female nondysgerminomas are very rare and their staging is very different from the nonseminomas they are described separately. However, the biology of these tumors is very similar and to find answers to our therapeutic questions in the future, we may need to define a common staging system and conduct clinical trials involving both men and women.

Stage I nonseminomas are treated with surgery alone and close follow-up [26]. For stage II patients with tumors measuring 3 cm or less, primary radical lymph node dissection is considered standard. For stage II patients with masses larger than 3 cm primary platinum-based chemotherapy is used. For low-risk patients with stage III disease (low AFP, nonmediastinal primary, or no nonpulmonary visceral metastasis) BEP chemotherapy is used with a greater than 90% cure rate. If the mass persists 4 to 6 weeks postchemotherapy with normal serum markers, surgical resection is used [31]. If the tumor still contains cancer cells, two additional cycles of cisplatin are given. For high-risk patients (high AFP, mediastinal primary site, or presence of nonpulmonary visceral metastasis) platinum-based chemotherapy, radiation, and resection are used with a cure rate of less than 50%. New experimental therapies for these patients include ifosfamide, high-dose chemotherapy and bone marrow transplant, paclitaxel, and gemcitabine.

2. *Female Nondysgerminoma*

Most female nondysgerminomas irrespective of the stage are treated with surgery and chemotherapy.

Immature teratomas of grade I and stage I are treated with surgery alone. All other women with this type of tumor are treated with surgery and BEP combination chemotherapy. This chemotherapy regimen was studied and established in patients with testicular cancer [28,30].

Endodermal sinus tumors are treated with surgical resection and chemotherapy regardless of the extent of the tumor on initial surgery [32]. Survival rates increased dramatically with the introduction of platinum-based chemotherapy in which a response rate of approximately 60% is seen.

Embryonal carcinoma and nongestational choriocarcinoma are extremely rare, and the recommended treatment is surgical resection and platinum-based chemotherapy [32].

VIII. Suggestions for Further Investigations

Germ cells are one of the rare cell types in the human body that have the same embryonal origin and function in both sexes but go through very different development, environment, and hormone stimulation during the lifetime of an individual. Despite the very different proliferation rate of these cells in men and women (very high in men, none after birth in women) the tumors arising from them have very similar biologic characteristics.

Is the reason for the high frequency of germ cell testicular cancers compared with ovarian GCTs because of the very high proliferative rate and the much higher chance of a "genetic mistake" in males? Because adult testicular cancer is much more frequent than ovarian GCTs, it was studied in the past in much more detail. However, exploring the reasons for rare ovarian GCTs in females might help answer many questions about the etiology, behavior, and management of these tumors in general. Some of the questions that need further studies in the future are as follows:

- Is the specific genetic finding for male GCTs I(12 p), present in female GCTs?
- Is cyclin D2 overexpressed in the normal and neoplastic female germ cells?
- Should investigators develop a similar staging system for male and female GCTs so that clinical studies may be conducted and knowledge about GCTs may be used more effectively?

References

1. Greenlee RT, Murray T, Bolden S *et al.* (2000). Cancer statistics 2000. *CA Cancer J Clin.* 50:7.
2. Ozols FO, Scwartz PE, Eifel PJ. (2000). Ovarian Cancer, Fallopian Tube Carcinoma, and Peritoneal Carcinoma. In *Cancer Principles & Practice of Oncology* (DeVita VT Jr, ed.), pp. 1597–1628. Philadelphia, Lippincott Williams & Wilkins.
3. Pinkerton CR. (1997). Malignant germ cell tumors in childhood. *Eur J Cancer.* 33:895.
4. Lingappa VR. (2003). Disorders of the Female Reproductive Tract. In *Pathophysiology of Disease* (McPhee S, ed.), pp. 612–642. Columbus, OH, McGraw-Hill.
5. Ebb DH, Green MD, Shamberger CR, Tarbell NJ. (2001). Solid Tumors of Childhood. In *Cancer Principles & Practice of Oncology* (DeVita VT Jr, ed.), pp. 2169–2202. Philadelphia, Lippincott Williams & Wilkins.
6. Gobel V, Calaminus G, Engert J *et al.* (1998). Teratomas of infancy and childhood. *Med Ped Oncol.* 31:8.
7. Birch JM, Marsden HB, Swindell R. (1982). Pre-natal factors in the origin of germ cell tumors of childhood. *Carcinogenesis.* 3:75.
8. Altman RP, Randolph JG, Lilly JR. (1974). Sacrococcygeal teratoma: American Academy of Pediatrics Surgical Section survey–1973. *J Pediatr Surg.* 9:389.
9. Daniels JL, Stutzman R, McLeod D. (1981). A comparison of testicular tumors in black and white patients. *J Urol.* 125.341.
10. Kuhn M, Weissbach L. (1985). Localization, incidence, diagnosis and treatment of extratesticular germ cell tumors. *Urol Int.* 40:166.
11. Luna M, Valenzuela-Tamariz J. (1976). Germ cell tumors of the mediastinum: Postmortem findings. *Am J Clin Pathol.* 65:450.
12. Chaganti RSK, Houldsworth J. (2000). Genetics and biology of adult human germ cell tumors. *Cancer Res.* 60:1475.
13. Vos A, Oosterhuis JW, de Jong B *et al.* (1990). Cytogenetics of carcinoma in situ of the testis. *Cancer Genet Cytogenet.* 46:75.
14. Weinberg RA. (1995). The retinoblastoma protein and cell cycle control. *Cell.* 81:323.
15. Houldsworth J, Reuter V, Bosl GJ *et al.* (1997). Aberrant expression of cyclin D2 is an early event in human male germ cell tumorigenesis. *Cell Growth Differ.* 8:293.
16. Skakkebaek NE, Rajpert-de Meyts E, Jorgensen N *et al.* (1998). Germ cell cancer and disorders of spermatogenesis: an environmental connection? *Acta Pathol Microbiol Immunol Scand.* 106:3.
17. Skakkebaek NE, Berthelsen JG, Giwercman A *et al.* (1987). Carcinoma in situ of the testis: Possible origin from gonocytes and precursors of all types of germ cell tumors except spermatocytoma. *Int J Androl.* 10:19.
18. Chaganti RSK, Houldsworth J. (1998). The cytogenetic theory of the pathogenesis of human adult male germ cell tumors. *Acta Pathol Microbiol Immunol Scand.* 106:80.
19. Schwartz D, Goldfinger N, Kam Z *et al.* (1999). p53 control low DNA damage-dependent premeiotic checkpoint and facilitates DNA repair during spermatogenesis. *Cell Growth Differ.* 10:665.
20. van der Maase H, Specht L, Jacobsen GK *et al.* (1993). Surveillance following orchiectomy for stage I seminoma of the testis. *Eur J Cancer.* 29A:1931.
21. Stettner A, Hartenbach EM, Schink JC *et al.* (1999). Familial ovarian germ cell cancer: Report and review. *Am J Med Genet.* 84:43.
22. Witschi E. (1948). Migration of the germ cells of human embryos from the yolk sac to the primitive gonadal folds. *Contr Embryol Carnegie Inst.* 32:67.
23. Wylie C. (1999). Germ cells. *Cell.* 96:165.
24. Chaganti RSK, Rodriguez E, Mathew S. (1994). Origin of adult male mediastinal germ cell tumors. *Lancet.* 343:1130.
25. Hoffman HJ. (1987). Pineal region tumors. *Prog Exp Tumor Res.* 30:281.
26. Loehrer PJ, Ahlering TE, Pollack A. (2001). Testicular Cancer. In *Cancer Management: A Multidisciplinary Approach*, 3rd Edition (Pazdur R, Coia LR, Hoskins W, Wagman L, eds.), pp. 383–403. New York, The Oncology Group.
27. Williams SD. (1994). Current management of ovarian germ cell tumors. *Semin Oncol.* 8:53.
28. Williams SD. (1998). Ovarian germ cell tumors: An update. *Semin Oncol.* 25:407.
29. Dosmann MA, Zagars GK. (1993). Postorchiectomy radiotherapy for stages I and II testicular seminoma. *Int J Radiat Oncol Biol Phys.* 26:381.
30. Williams SD, Blessing JA, Hatch KD *et al.* (1991). Chemotherapy for advanced dysgerminoma: Trials of the GOG. *J Clin Oncol.* 9:1950.
31. Einhorn LH. (1994). Salvage therapy for germ cell tumors. *Semin Oncol.* 21:47.
32. Williams S, Blessing JA, Liao SY *et al.* (1994). Adjuvant therapy of ovarian germ cell tumors with cisplatin, etoposide, and bleomycin: A trial of GOG. *J Clin Oncol.* 12:701.

61

Gender and Gastrointestinal Malignancies: Incidence and Response to Treatment

KYRIAKOS PAPADOPOULOS, MD
Columbia University College of Physicians and Surgeons, New York, NY

Gender is a predictor of incidence and mortality in patients with gastrointestinal (GI) malignancies, with lower incidence and mortality in women than men for most GI cancers worldwide [1]. Surveillance, Epidemiology, and End Results (SEER) derived age-adjusted incidence and mortality rates of GI malignancies in the United States are shown in Table 61-1 [2]. Biologic factors and differences in exposure to risk factors may contribute to these differences. This chapter reviews the epidemiology and treatment of upper and lower GI malignancies, with particular emphasis on gender-related factors contributing to both pathogenesis and response to and side effects of therapy.

I. Upper Gastrointestinal Malignancies

A. Esophageal Cancer

Esophageal cancer caused approximately 12,600 deaths in 2002 in the United States [3]. There is both gender and racial disparity in incidence and mortality. Esophageal cancer is four times more frequent in males than females and twice as common in blacks than whites. Both squamous and adenocarcinoma of the esophagus have been associated with cigarettes and alcohol consumption [4,5]. The incidence of adenocarcinoma has surpassed squamous carcinoma in white males [6]. Men with gastroesophageal reflux are twice as likely as women to have Barrett's esophagus [7], and there is a strong link between gastroesophageal reflux, Barrett's esophagus, and adenocarcinoma of the esophagus [8].

1. Treatment of Esophageal Cancer

A multidisciplinary team approach is essential for optimal treatment of patients with esophageal cancer. Early-stage esophageal cancer can be treated by surgical resection alone or combined chemotherapy and radiation [9]. The overall 5-year survival rates are similar, and a randomized trial comparing these modalities is unlikely to be undertaken. Factors such as facilities, local expertise, and patient preference will determine which approach is selected. Patients with locally advanced esophageal cancer benefit from combination chemoradiation therapy as compared with radiation alone, with a 5-year survival rate of 26% [10]. Advanced disease can be palliated with local dilatation and stenting. Although there is no standard chemotherapy regimen for metastatic disease, encouraging results are reported with newer drugs such as the taxanes and irinotecan combined with cisplatin [11].

B. Gastric Cancer

Despite a decline in incidence and mortality in most countries, gastric cancer remains one of the most common malignancies worldwide. Overall, gastric cancer occurs twice as frequently in men than in women, and there is evidence for familial predisposition. Incidence varies with age, and the stomach cancer related mortality for young Japanese women between 20 to 40 years is higher relative to young men [12]. This suggests some possible contributing effect of sex hormones, but studies of reproductive history and the effects of sex hormones on the incidence of gastric cancer have been inconsistent in their conclusions, particularly with respect to the influence of age at menarche and menopause [13,14]. Assessment of reproductive factors separately in premenopausal and postmenopausal women and by histology and anatomic site of occurrence in the stomach may help clarify the influence of female hormones on gastric carcinogenesis [15]. *Helicobacter pylori* has been implicated in the pathogenesis of gastric cancer [16]; dietary and environmental factors playing a significant role, as evidenced by the marked difference in incidence in different regions of the world.

1. Treatment of Gastric Cancer

Patients with localized gastric cancer are candidates for surgical resection. There is ongoing debate regarding the most appropriate surgical procedure for curative resection. Multicenter European trials have not shown benefit in survival at 5 years from extended lymphadenectomy [17,18]. With respect to postsurgical adjuvant therapy, results of a recent randomized trial show survival benefit and a reduction in local disease recurrence with adjuvant radiation and 5-fluorouracil (5-FU) chemotherapy compared with surgery alone [19]. Toxicity is nonetheless significant, and the 4-year survival for patients remains dismal at less than

Table 61-1

Incidence and Mortality Age-adjusted Rates for Gastrointestinal Malignancies in the United States (1992–1999) [2]

Tumor Type	Incidence/100,000		Mortality/100,000	
	Male	Female	Male	Female
Esophageal	7.5	2.1	7.5	1.8
Stomach	13.0	6.1	7.1	3.5
Pancreas	12.3	9.7	12.2	9.3
Gallbladder	0.9	1.5	0.5	0.9
Liver and biliary	8.3	3.3	6.5	2.9
Colon/rectum	63.4	46.2	26.3	18.5

50%. There was no difference in the effect of therapy according to gender [19]. No particular multidrug regimen has proven superior in the treatment of advanced gastric cancer, and there does not appear to be any difference in treatment efficacy according to gender for metastatic gastric cancer [20]. The result of randomized trials incorporating newer agents such as docetaxel and irinotecan are awaited.

C. Pancreatic Cancer

Pancreatic cancer caused almost 30,000 deaths in 2002 in the United States [3]. It remains one of the most lethal malignancies with most patients dead within 6 months of diagnosis and fewer than 4% of patients surviving 5 years. The incidence of pancreatic cancer is slightly higher in men than in women, and the cancer is related to environmental exposures. About 30% of pancreatic cancers are attributed to smoking [21,22]. Aspirin use appears to decrease by half the risk of pancreatic cancer in postmenopausal white women [23]. Obesity [24] and *H. pylori* infestation [25] may increase the risk of pancreatic cancer for unclear reasons, but alcohol and caffeine do not increase the risk [26]. Heredity accounts for about 5% of pancreatic cancers. Some familial cases of pancreatic cancer are associated with hereditary nonpolyposis colorectal cancer (HNPCC) with abnormal DNA repair genes [27], and BRCA2 associated familial breast cancer [28].

1. Treatment of Pancreatic Cancer

Pancreatic cancer rarely presents early. Fewer than 10% of patients with pancreatic cancer are considered for surgical resection of the tumor. After surgery or if surgery is not possible, combination chemotherapy and radiation therapy has been used, a common regimen being 5-FU with 4500 cGy of radiation therapy to the tumor bed. This improves the survival from 10.9 to 21 months in patients where the tumor is resected [29]. The recent European Study Group for Pancreatic Cancer (ESPAC) study shows no survival benefit for adjuvant chemoradiation therapy, but a potential benefit for adjuvant chemotherapy in resectable pancreatic cancer. There is no gender difference in survival in this study [30]. 5-Fluorouracil plus 4000 cGy of radiation therapy increases the median survival in patients with locally advanced pancreatic cancer from 5.5 months to 10 months [31].

For patients with advanced pancreatic cancer, standard chemotherapy agents have only been marginally effective. Gemcitabine chemotherapy is the standard of care. The phase III trials showing a benefit to therapy in patients with unresectable disease or stage IV disease randomized treatment between gemcitabine and 5-FU and showed an 18% 1-year survival for gemcitabine, compared with a 2% 1-year survival for 5-FU [32]. Combination therapies with gemcitabine and platinum-based drugs, 5-FU based drugs, or taxanes are being evaluated to determine if these combinations improve survival [33,34].

D. Hepatobiliary Cancer

Hepatocellular carcinoma (HCC) is the fourth leading cause of cancer deaths worldwide, accounting for almost half a million deaths per year [1]. The overall incidence of HCC is three times higher in men than in women and twice as common in blacks than whites in the United States. Chronic hepatitis B and hepatitis C infections, which occur more frequently in men, are significant risk factors for HCC. Differences in the rates of cigarette smoking and alcohol consumption may also account for some of the gender difference in incidence, but these data are not consistent [35,36]. Sex hormones may play a role, because increased parity is a significant risk factor for HCC in women [37]. Increased activation of androgen signaling pathways may increase the risk of hepatitis B virus (HBV)-related HCC in men [38]. During the last 2 decades there has been a rise in the number of cases in the United States from 1.4 per 100,000 between 1976 to 1980 to 2.4 per 100,000 between 1991 to 1995 [39]. Furthermore, the age-specific incidence of HCC has progressively shifted toward younger people (40 to 60 years old) [39]. This rise in incidence is linked to a rise in hepatitis C virus (HCV)-related liver disease and HBV infection. There are encouraging results from efforts to decrease hepatocellular cancer rates by vaccination to prevent transmission of hepatitis B infection [40].

1. Treatment of Hepatocellular Cancer

Despite a number of treatment modalities, the survival for HCC remains dismal, with less than 5% of patients alive at 5 years [41]. Even when resection of the tumor is an option, 70% of patients will have an intrahepatic recurrence. Orthotopic transplantation, the only complete cure, is also limited for HCC patients given limited donor availability. In highly selected patients with nonresectable HCC, chemoembolization improves survival when compared with supportive care alone [42]. Systemic chemotherapy has not been successful in improving survival in randomized trials, and patients should be encouraged to enter clinical trials of new therapeutic agents.

E. Biliary Duct and Gallbladder Cancer

Biliary duct and gallbladder cancer are uncommon malignancies, with an incidence of approximately 1 to 2 per 100,000 in the United States. Gallbladder cancer is exceptional among the upper GI malignancies because it occurs more frequently in women than in men, particularly in the age group younger than 65 years. Risk factors for biliary and gallbladder cancer include gallstones, sclerosing cholangitis, ulcerative colitis, and anatomic anomalies [43]. Reproductive history influences the risk of biliary cancers, possibly a consequence of the effect of endogenous estrogen and progesterone on the lithogenicity of bile. Younger age at menarche, early age at first pregnancy, increased number of pregnancies, and late menopause may enhance the risk of cancer of the biliary tract [44,45]. Multimodality therapies including surgery, chemotherapy, and radiation therapy have been used, but the best chance of cure remains complete surgical resection. Unfortunately only a small percentage of patients present early enough for this to be a viable therapeutic option.

II. Lower Gastrointestinal Malignancies

A. Colorectal Cancer

Colorectal cancer is the third most common cause of cancer-related mortality in the United States, accounting for approximately 60,000 deaths annually [3]. The incidence of colon cancer is marginally higher in women, whereas rectal cancer is slightly more common in men. Predisposing factors include smoking, diet, inflammatory bowel disease, and a family history of colon cancer. Women with a history of breast, ovarian, and endometrial cancer have an increased risk of developing colon cancer.

The role of diet in preventing colon cancer has been extensively examined in several large cohort studies [46]. The Nurses' Health Study has provided invaluable information with regard to the role of diet and exercise in prevention of colorectal cancer in women. Low-fat, specifically a low red meat, diet and moderate physical activity have been shown to decrease the incidence of colonic polyps and cancer in both men and women [47–49]. Only extended use of supplemental folic acid reduces the risk of colon cancer [50]. High-fiber diet likely provides no benefit against colon cancer but can be encouraged for its protective effect against cardiovascular disease [51,52].

The hereditary colon cancer syndromes have provided insight into the pathogenesis of sporadic colorectal cancer [53]. In familial adenomatous polyposis (FAP), mutations of the adenomatous polyposis coli (APC) protein results in deregulation of β-catenin and enhanced carcinogenesis. Mutations of the mismatch repair enzymes, manifesting as microsatellite instability (MSI), are responsible for the HNPCC syndromes. Both of these mechanisms are implicated in sporadic colon cancer. There are gender differences in the occurrence of MSI in colon tumors. Men are more likely then women to have MSI-negative tumors at a young age and women more likely to have MSI-positive tumors at an older age [54]. Exogenous estrogens appear to modify the risk of MSI-positive tumors and may account in some part for the reduced risk of colon cancer obtained from hormone replacement therapy [55]. Although meta-analyses of observational studies of hormone replacement therapy and the risk of colon cancer have been inconsistent in their results, reporting an insignificant 8% to a significant 33% reduction in the risk of colon cancer [56,57], the randomized Women's Health Initiative study of estrogen-progestin versus placebo in 16,608 healthy postmenopausal women confirmed an absolute risk reduction of six fewer cases of colorectal cancer per 10,000 woman-years [58]. However, an increased incidence of coronary heart disease (CHD), breast cancer, stroke, and pulmonary embolism prompted termination of this study and the recommendation that this combination of hormones not be prescribed.

1. Treatment of Colon Cancer

Although stage I colon cancer is effectively treated by surgical resection alone, there is an established role for 5-FU based chemotherapy in patients with stage III disease and in metastatic colon cancer [59,60]. Controversy remains regarding the overall benefit of adjuvant chemotherapy in stage II (Dukes B2) disease [61,62].

Patients with metastatic colon cancer treated with best supportive care have a median survival of 6 to 8 months. Currently available 5-FU based palliative chemotherapy significantly improves survival. Whether administered as a short infusion or continuously over 24 hours, 5-FU together with irinotecan and leucovorin (IFL) results in a median survival of 14 to 17 months, with overall 1-year survival of 20% [63,64]. Although outcome may be improved, the three-drug combination has increased toxicity and should be used cautiously in older patients with poor performance status, decreased albumin, and elevated lactate dehydrogenase (LDH). Data from a multi-institutional phase III trial comparing IFL with oxaliplatin and 5-FU show that the latter combination further improved survival (15 months vs 19.5 months) [65].

Patients with stage III colon cancer treated with surgery alone have a 5-year overall survival of approximately 50 to 60%. Six months of adjuvant 5-FU and leucovorin-based chemotherapy improves outcome by 15% [59,60]. Watanabe et al [66] reported that the 5-year survival rate for women is 10% higher than that for men receiving adjuvant chemotherapy for colon cancer. Conversely, a meta-analysis of five randomized trials shows that the 5-year survival in adjuvant (66% and 67%) and advanced disease (3% and 2%) is similar for women and men [67]. The results of adjuvant phase III trials comparing 5-FU/leucovorin with IFL and with oxaliplatin/5-FU are awaited with interest, because the recurrence rate in stage III patients remains distressingly high.

Several studies have sought to define the role of adjuvant chemotherapy in patients with stage II (Dukes B2) colon cancer. A meta-analysis of the NSABP colon cancer trials suggested a survival advantage for Dukes B2 patients receiving chemotherapy and recommended that all patients with Dukes B2 disease be offered treatment [61]. The IMPACT meta-analysis reported a small but not statistically significant survival benefit (3 to 8%) of adjuvant chemotherapy [62]. Stage II patients presenting with perforation, obstruction, or invasion of adjacent organs are at high risk of recurrence and should be offered adjuvant chemotherapy. Attempts to identify high-risk patients at the molecular level, which are currently still in development, may further define those patients who might benefit from this therapy and spare those who are unlikely to have recurrent disease [68].

Although newer chemotherapy agents such as irinotecan and oxaliplatin are improving outcome in patients with colon cancer, it is apparent that 5-FU remains an integral component of the adjuvant and metastatic disease chemotherapy regimens. Results from a number of trials suggest important differences in toxicity between men and women with colon cancer receiving 5-FU based regimens. A meta-analysis of data from seven clinical trials in which more than 1200 patients received either bolus or infusional 5-FU suggested that gender was a predictive factor for severe nonhematologic toxicities [69]. A small study of 23 men and 30 women treated with 5-FU based chemotherapy showed increased toxicity in women; the authors attributed this increased toxicity in women to deficiency of dihydropyrimidine dehydrogenase [70]. Further studies reported increased incidence of leukopenia and stomatitis but not diarrhea [71]. A recent meta-analysis of five North Central Cancer Treatment Group trials including more than 1400 patients treated with 5-FU in a 5-day bolus schedule confirmed that the incidence of stomatitis, alopecia, leukopenia, nausea, vomiting, and diarrhea was significantly greater in women than men. Furthermore, 53% of women as compared with 40% of men experienced severe toxicity. Severe nausea and vomiting, response to therapy, and survival were the same for both [67].

2. Treatment of Rectal Cancer

Combined modality therapy including radiation and chemotherapy is routinely used for the adjuvant treatment of localized rectal cancer. The initial National Surgical Adjuvant Breast and Bowel Project (NSABP) R-01 rectal cancer trial, comparing surgery alone to postoperative chemotherapy or radiation therapy, demonstrated a disease-free and overall survival advantage to chemotherapy with 5-FU, semustine, and vincristine (MOF) [72]. Inexplicably, the observed advantage was restricted to men. Radiation alone reduced local recurrence but did not affect survival. The subsequent NSABP R-02 trial of postoperative chemotherapy with or without radiation therapy confirmed a reduction in locoregional relapse for combined chemoradiation therapy [73]. The authors noted that men tolerated the 5-FU and leucovorin regimen better than women, with a lower incidence of grade 3 toxicities. The Intergroup 0114 trial studied various 5-FU based chemotherapy regimens in combination with radiotherapy following surgical resection in patients with T3/4 or node-positive rectal cancer [74]. Although there was no difference in disease-free survival or overall survival by regimen, there was a poorer overall survival rate for men than women. High-risk patients (T3N+ and T4) have lesser 5-year survival (55% vs 76%) and greater local recurrence (18% vs 9%) than low-risk (T1-2N+ or T3N0) patients. Toxicity was more severe in women, with 81% of women having ≥grade 3 toxicity compared with 69% of men.

Newer surgical techniques such as total mesorectal excision, in which the entire mesorectum is resected by sharp dissection, together with preoperative radiation reduces the risk of local recurrence [75]. Further prospective randomized trials are needed to answer many of the questions raised regarding treatment of rectal cancer, including the role of radiation therapy in low-risk patients, combination therapy with irinotecan and oxaliplatin, and the use of oral fluoropyrimidine such as capecitabine.

The data from trials of colon and rectal cancer provide confirmatory evidence of both increased incidence and severity of toxicity of 5-FU in women as compared with men. The mechanisms for this increase in toxicity are uncertain. Data on differences in levels of DPD or of the 5-FU target enzyme thymidylate synthase are inconsistent [68,76,77], and there is no evidence that the difference in some instances can be attributed to bias in reporting of subjective symptoms. Genetic polymorphisms of enzymes involved in the metabolism of chemotherapeutic agents may contribute to both toxicity and response to chemotherapy, and the role gender might play in their frequency awaits further elucidation [78–80].

B. Anal Cancer

Anal cancer is an uncommon malignancy, more frequent in women than in men, and accounts for approximately 2500 new cases of cancer per year. Smoking increases the risk of anal cancer up to 5-fold in premenopausal women [81]. As with cervical cancer, human papillomavirus type 16 has been implicated in the pathogenesis of anal intraepithelial neoplasia and invasive anal cancer [82]. The relative risk of anal cancer is 5-fold the expected rate in women with a history of cervical cancer. A number of epidemiologic studies have linked sexual practices and genital viral infections to the development of anal cancer. A case control study in women and heterosexual men demonstrated that the relative risk of anal cancer is highest in those with 10 or more sexual partners or a history of anal warts and sexually transmitted infections [83]. Receptive anal sex is a risk factor in both men and women. Whether human immunodeficiency virus (HIV) infection is directly involved in the pathogenesis of anal cancer remains unclear, but HIV infection predisposes to anal papillomavirus infection and an associated increased risk of anal cancer [84,85].

1. Treatment of Anal Cancer

The standard treatment of anal cancer includes radiation combined with 5-FU and mitomycin chemotherapy. Patients with persistent or recurrent disease can be salvaged by surgical resection or cisplatin-based chemotherapy [86,87]. Two randomized trials comparing radiation alone to radiation combined with chemotherapy confirm that multimodality therapy reduces local failure, colostomy rate, and recurrence and improves colostomy free–survival but not overall survival [88,89]. Multivariate analysis of the EORTC trial identified sex as a prognostic factor, with women having significantly better local control and survival [89].

III. The Management of Chemotherapy-related Emesis

There has been some progress in the ability to control chemotherapy-related nausea and vomiting. A better understanding of the pathogenesis of nausea and emesis, and the availability of new and more effective drugs to treat these problems has done much to improve patient quality of life [90]. Despite these advances, most patients still experience some degree of nausea and vomiting related to their therapy.

The three most frequent emetic problems encountered in patients receiving chemotherapy are anticipatory, acute, and delayed nausea and vomiting. Anticipatory emesis is a conditioned response in patients with prior poorly controlled nausea and vomiting, who experience nausea and vomiting before the administration of subsequent chemotherapy. Anticipatory nausea is a predictor of postchemotherapy nausea and vomiting. Acute emesis is emesis occurring within 24 hours, most frequently within the first 4 hours, of administration of chemotherapy. Factors predicting for chemotherapy-associated nausea and vomiting are apparent from numerous antiemetic studies and include younger age, no or minimal chronic alcohol consumption, lower performance status, and female gender [91–94]. Thus, younger women with no history of significant alcohol intake are at particularly high-risk for chemotherapy-related emesis. Delayed emesis is nausea or vomiting occurring greater than 24 hours after chemotherapy. The prevention of acute emesis is important, because occurrence of acute vomiting predicts for delayed emesis.

The emetogenicity of various chemotherapy agents and regimens have been established, with evidence-based guidelines provided for the prevention and treatment of acute, delayed, and anticipatory emesis [95,96]. For control of acute emesis when administering mildly emetogenic agents, prochlorperazine or metoclopramide are often adequate, whereas for moderately or highly emetogenic regimens, a combination of a serotonin antagonist and dexamethasone (20 mg) is recommended. For delayed emesis, dexamethasone with metoclopramide or a serotonin antagonist is effective [97]. Behavioral therapy and benzodiazepines may help control anticipatory emesis.

IV. Suggestions for Further Investigations

As has been outlined in this chapter, there are obvious gender disparities in tumors of the GI tract. Reasons for these differences are complex and results often are inconsistent. Future questions to be considered in research of the role gender plays in GI tumors include the following:

- How significant a role do sex hormones actually play in the pathogenesis of GI tumors, and how can we use this knowledge to develop safe targeted therapies for prevention?
- What role do genetic factors such as polymorphisms in catabolic enzymes and other proteins play in toxicity and the response to chemotherapy, and can this information be used to tailor patient therapy?
- Can we find and implement preventive strategies to decrease exposure to risk factors?

References

1. Parkin DM, Pisani P, Ferlay J. (1999). Global cancer statistics. *CA Cancer J Clin.* 49:33–64, 1.
2. Ries LAG, Eisner MP, Kosary CL *et al.* (2002). *SEER Cancer Statistics Review, 1973–1999.* Bethesda, MD: National Cancer Institute. http://seer.cancer.gov/csr/1973_1999/(2002)
3. Jemal A, Thomas A, Murray T, Thun M. (2002). Cancer statistics, 2002. *CA Cancer J Clin.* 52:23–47.
4. Gammon MD, Schoenberg JB, Ahsan H *et al.* (1997). Tobacco, alcohol, and socioeconomic status and adenocarcinomas of the esophagus and gastric cardia. *J Natl Cancer Inst.* 89:1277–1284.
5. Vaughan TL, Davis S, Kristal A, Thomas DB. (1995). Obesity, alcohol, and tobacco as risk factors for cancers of the esophagus and gastric cardia: Adenocarcinoma versus squamous cell carcinoma. *Cancer Epidemiol Biomarkers Prev.* 4(2):85–92.
6. Devesa SS, Blot WJ, Fraumeni JF Jr. (1998). Changing patterns in the incidence of esophageal and gastric carcinoma in the United States. *Cancer.* 83:2049–2053.
7. Campos GM, DeMeester SR, Peters JH *et al.* (2001). Predictive factors of Barrett esophagus: Multivariate analysis of 502 patients with gastroesophageal reflux disease. *Arch Surg.* 136:1267–1273.
8. Lagergren J, Bergstrom R, Lindgren A, Nyren O. (1999). Symptomatic gastroesophageal reflux as a risk factor for esophageal adenocarcinoma. *N Engl J Med.* 340:825–831.
9. Kelsen DP, Ginsberg R, Pajak TF *et al.* (1998). Chemotherapy followed by surgery compared with surgery alone for localized esophageal cancer. *N Engl J Med.* 339:1979–1984.
10. Cooper JS, Guo MD, Herskovic A *et al.* (1999). Chemoradiotherapy of locally advanced esophageal cancer: Long-term follow-up of a prospective randomized trial (RTOG 85-01). Radiation Therapy Oncology Group. *JAMA.* 281:1623–1627.
11. Ilson DH, Saltz L, Enzinger P *et al.* (1999). Phase II trial of weekly irinotecan plus cisplatin in advanced esophageal cancer. *J Clin Oncol.* 17:3270–3275.
12. Sun J, Misumi J, Shimaoka A *et al.* (2002). Stomach cancer-related mortality rate is higher in young Japanese women than in men. *Public Health.* 116:39–44.
13. Heuch I, Kvale G. (2001). Menstrual and reproductive factors and risk of gastric cancer: A Norwegian cohort study. *Cancer Causes Control.* 11:869–874.
14. La Vecchia C, D'Avanzo B, Franceschi S *et al.* (1994). Menstrual and reproductive factors and gastric-cancer risk in women. *Int J Cancer.* 59:761–764.
15. Inoue M, Ito LS, Tajima K *et al.* (2002). Height, weight, menstrual and reproductive factors and risk of gastric cancer among Japanese postmenopausal women: Analysis by subsite and histologic subtype. *Int J Cancer.* 97:833–838.
16. Uemura N, Okamoto S, Yamamoto S *et al.* (2001). Helicobacter pylori infection and the development of gastric cancer. *N Engl J Med.* 345:784–789.
17. Cuschieri A, Weeden S, Fielding J *et al.* (1999). Patient survival after D1 and D2 resections for gastric cancer: Long-term results of the MRC randomized surgical trial. Surgical Co-operative Group. *Br J Cancer.* 79:1522–1530.
18. Bonenkamp JJ, Hermans J, Sasako M, van de Velde CJ. (1999). Extended lymph-node dissection for gastric cancer. Dutch Gastric Cancer Group. *N Engl J Med.* 340:908–914.
19. Macdonald JS, Smalley SR, Benedetti J *et al.* (2001). Chemoradiotherapy after surgery compared with surgery alone for adenocarcinoma of the stomach or gastroesophageal junction. *N Engl J Med.* 345:725–730.
20. Vanhoefer U, Rougier P, Wilke H *et al.* (2000). Final results of a randomized phase III trial of sequential high-dose methotrexate, fluorouracil, and doxorubicin versus etoposide, leucovorin, and fluorouracil versus infusional fluorouracil and cisplatin in advanced gastric cancer: A trial of the European Organization for Research and Treatment of Cancer Gastrointestinal Tract Cancer Cooperative Group. *J Clin Oncol.* 18:2648–2657.
21. Silverman DT, Dunn JA, Hoover RN *et al.* (1994). Cigarette smoking and pancreas cancer: A case-control study based on direct interviews. *J Natl Cancer Inst.* 86:1510–1516.
22. Zheng W, McLaughlin JK, Gridley G *et al.* (1993). A cohort study of smoking, alcohol consumption, and dietary factors for pancreatic cancer (United States). *Cancer Causes Control.* 4:477–482.
23. Anderson KE, Johnson TW, Lazovich D, Folsom AR. (2002). Association between nonsteroidal anti-inflammatory drug use and the incidence of pancreatic cancer. *J Natl Cancer Inst.* 94:1168–1171.
24. Michaud DS, Giovannucci E, Willett WC *et al.* (2001). Physical activity, obesity, height, and the risk of pancreatic cancer. *JAMA.* 286:921–929.
25. Stolzenberg-Solomon RZ, Blaser MJ, Limburg PJ *et al.* (2001). Helicobacter pylori seropositivity as a risk factor for pancreatic cancer. *J Natl Cancer Inst.* 93:937–941.
26. Michaud DS, Giovannucci E, Willett WC *et al.* (2001). Coffee and alcohol consumption and the risk of pancreatic cancer in two prospective United States cohorts. *Cancer Epidemiol Biomarkers Prev.* 10:429–437.
27. Lynch HT, Smyrk T, Kern SE *et al.* (1996). Familial pancreatic cancer: A review. *Semin Oncol.* 23:251–275.
28. Goggins M, Schutte M, Lu J *et al.* (1996). Germline BRCA2 gene mutations in patients with apparently sporadic pancreatic carcinoma. *Cancer Res.* 56:5360–5364.
29. Gastrointestinal Tumor Study Group. (1987). Further evidence of effective adjuvant combined radiation and chemotherapy following curative resection of pancreatic cancer. *Cancer.* 59:2006–2010.
30. Neoptolemos JP, Dunn JA, Stocken DD *et al.* (2001). Adjuvant chemoradiotherapy and chemotherapy in resectable pancreatic cancer: A randomised controlled trial. *Lancet.* 358:1576–1585.
31. Moertel CG, Frytak S, Hahn RG *et al.* (1981). Therapy of locally unresectable pancreatic carcinoma: A randomized comparison of high dose (6000 rads) radiation alone, moderate dose radiation (4000 rads + 5-fluorouracil), and high dose radiation + 5-fluorouracil: The Gastrointestinal Tumor Study Group. *Cancer.* 48:1705–1710.
32. Burris HA 3rd, Moore MJ, Andersen J *et al.* (1997). Improvements in survival and clinical benefit with gemcitabine as first-line therapy for patients with advanced pancreas cancer: A randomized trial. *J Clin Oncol.* 15:2403–2413.
33. Colucci G, Giuliani F, Gebbia V *et al.* (2002). Gemcitabine alone or with cisplatin for the treatment of patients with locally advanced and/or metastatic pancreatic carcinoma: A prospective, randomized phase III study of the Gruppo Oncologia dell'Italia Meridionale. *Cancer.* 94:902–910.
34. Sherman WH, Fine RL. (2001). Combination gemcitabine and docetaxel therapy in advanced adenocarcinoma of the pancreas. *Oncology.* 60:316–321.
35. Kuper H, Tzonou A, Kaklamani E *et al.* (2000). Tobacco smoking, alcohol consumption and their interaction in the causation of hepatocellular carcinoma. *Int J Cancer.* 85:498–502.

36. Evans AA, Chen G, Ross EA *et al.* (2002). Eight-year follow-up of the 90,000-person Haimen City cohort: I. Hepatocellular carcinoma mortality, risk factors, and gender differences. *Cancer Epidemiol Biomarkers Prev.* 11: 369–376.

37. La Vecchia C, Negri E, Franceschi S, D'Avanzo B, (1992), Reproductive factors and the risk of hepatocellular carcinoma in women. *Int J Cancer.* 52: 351–354.

38. Yu MW, Cheng SW, Lin MW *et al.* (2000). Androgen-receptor gene CAG repeats, plasma testosterone levels, and risk of hepatitis B-related hepatocellular carcinoma. *J Natl Cancer Inst.* 92:2023–2028.

39. El-Serag HB, Mason AC. (1999). Rising incidence of hepatocellular carcinoma in the United States. *N Engl J Med.* 340:745–750.

40. Chang MH, Chen CJ, Lai MS *et al.* (1997). Universal hepatitis B vaccination in Taiwan and the incidence of hepatocellular carcinoma in children. Taiwan Childhood Hepatoma Study Group. *N Engl J Med.* 336:1855–1859.

41. Bruix J, Sherman M, Llovet JM *et al.* (2001). Clinical management of hepatocellular carcinoma. Conclusions of the Barcelona-2000 EASL conference. European Association for the Study of the Liver. *J Hepatol.* 35:421–430.

42. Llovet JM, Real MI, Montana X *et al.* (2002). Arterial embolisation or chemoembolisation versus symptomatic treatment in patients with unresectable hepatocellular carcinoma: A randomised controlled trial. *Lancet.* 359:1734–1739.

43. Sheth S, Bedford A, Chopra S. (2000). Primary gallbladder cancer: Recognition of risk factors and the role of prophylactic cholecystectomy. *Am J Gastroenterol.* 95:1402–1410.

44. Moerman CJ, Berns MP, Bueno de Mesquita HB, Runia S. (1994). Reproductive history and cancer of the biliary tract in women. *Int J Cancer.* 57:146–153.

45. Tavani A, Negri E, La Vecchia C. (1996). Menstrual and reproductive factors and biliary tract cancers. *Eur J Cancer Prev.* 5:241–247.

46. Willett WC. (2000). Diet and cancer. *Oncologist.* 5:393–404.

47. Giovannucci E, Rimm EB, Stampfer MJ *et al.* (1994). Intake of fat, meat, and fiber in relation to risk of colon cancer in men. *Cancer Res.* 54:2390–2397.

48. Colbert LH, Hartman TJ, Malila N *et al.* (2001). Physical activity in relation to cancer of the colon and rectum in a cohort of male smokers. *Cancer Epidemiol Biomarkers Prev.* 10:265–268.

49. Willett WC, Stampfer MJ, Colditz GA *et al.* (1990). Relation of meat, fat, and fiber intake to the risk of colon cancer in a prospective study among women. *N Engl J Med.* 323:1664–1672.

50. Giovannucci E, Stampfer MJ, Colditz GA *et al.* (1998). Multivitamin use, folate, and colon cancer in women in the Nurses' Health Study. *Ann Intern Med.* 129:517–524.

51. Fuchs CS, Giovannucci EL, Colditz GA *et al.* (1999). Dietary fiber and the risk of colorectal cancer and adenoma in women. *N Engl J Med.* 340:169–176.

52. Michels KB, Edward G, Joshipura KJ *et al.* (2000). Prospective study of fruit and vegetable consumption and incidence of colon and rectal cancers. *J Natl Cancer Inst.* 92:1740–1752.

53. Chung DC. (2000). The genetic basis of colorectal cancer: Insights into critical pathways of tumorigenesis. *Gastroenterology.* 119:854–865.

54. Malkhosyan SR, Yamamoto H, Piao Z, Perucho M. (2000). Late onset and high incidence of colon cancer of the mutator phenotype with hypermethylated hMLH1 gene in women. *Gastroenterology.* 119:598.

55. Slattery ML, Potter JD, Curtin K *et al.* (2001). Estrogens reduce and withdrawal of estrogens increase risk of microsatellite instability-positive colon cancer. *Cancer Res.* 61:126–130.

56. MacLennan SC, MacLennan AH, Ryan P. (1995). Colorectal cancer and oestrogen replacement therapy. A meta-analysis of epidemiological studies. *Med J Aust.* 162:491–493.

57. Nanda K, Bastian LA, Hasselblad V, Simel DL. (1999). Hormone replacement therapy and the risk of colorectal cancer: A meta-analysis. *Obstet Gynecol.* 93(5 Pt 2):880–888.

58. Writing Group for the Women's Health Initiative Investigators. (2002). Risks and benefits of estrogen plus progestin in healthy postmenopausal women: Principal results from the Women's Health Initiative randomized controlled trial. *JAMA.* 288:321–333.

59. Wolmark N, Rockette H, Mamounas E *et al.* (1999). Clinical trial to assess the relative efficacy of fluorouracil and leucovorin, fluorouracil and levamisole, and fluorouracil, leucovorin, and levamisole in patients with Dukes' B and C carcinoma of the colon: Results from National Surgical Adjuvant Breast and Bowel Project C-04. *J Clin Oncol.* 17:3553–3559.

60. International Multicentre Pooled Analysis of Colon Cancer Trials (IMPACT) investigators. (1995). Efficacy of adjuvant fluorouracil and folinic acid in colon cancer. *Lancet.* 345:939–944.

61. Mamounas E, Wieand S, Wolmark N *et al.* (1999). Comparative efficacy of adjuvant chemotherapy in patients with Dukes' B versus Dukes' C colon cancer: Results from four National Surgical Adjuvant Breast and Bowel Project adjuvant studies (C-01, C-02, C-03, and C-04). *J Clin Oncol.* 17:1349–1355.

62. International Multicentre Pooled Analysis of B2 Colon Cancer Trials (IMPACT B2) Investigators. (1999). Efficacy of adjuvant fluorouracil and folinic acid in B2 colon cancer. *J Clin Oncol.* 17:1356–1363.

63. Saltz LB, Cox JV, Blanke C *et al.* (2000). Irinotecan plus fluorouracil and leucovorin for metastatic colorectal cancer. Irinotecan Study Group. *N Engl J Med.* 343:905–914.

64. Douillard JY, Cunningham D, Roth AD *et al.* (2000). Irinotecan combined with fluorouracil compared with fluorouracil alone as first line treatment for metastatic colorectal cancer: A multicentre randomised trial. *Lancet.* 355: 1041–1047.

65. Goldberg RM, Sargent DJ, Morton RF *et al.* (2004). A randomized controlled trial of fluorouracil plus leucovorin, irinotecan, and oxaliplatin combinations in patients with previously untreated metastatic colorectal cancer. *J Clin Oncol.* 22:23–30.

66. Watanabe T, Wu TT, Catalano PJ *et al.* (2001). Molecular predictors of survival after adjuvant chemotherapy for colon cancer. *N Engl J Med.* 344:1196–1206.

67. Sloan JA, Goldberg RM, Sargent DJ *et al.* (2002). Women experience greater toxicity with fluorouracil-based chemotherapy for colorectal cancer. *J Clin Oncol.* 20:1491–1498.

68. Allegra CJ, Parr AL, Wold LE *et al.* (2002). Investigation of the prognostic and predictive value of thymidylate synthase, p53, and Ki-67 in patients with locally advanced colon cancer. *J Clin Oncol.* 20:1735–1743.

69. Meta-Analysis Group In Cancer. (1998). Toxicity of fluorouracil in patients with advanced colorectal cancer: Effect of administration schedule and prognostic factors. *J Clin Oncol.* 16:3537–3541.

70. Milano G, Etienne MC, Pierrefite V *et al.* (1999). Dihydropyrimidine dehydrogenase deficiency and fluorouracil-related toxicity. *Br J Cancer.* 79:627–630.

71. Cascinu S, Barni S, Labianca R *et al.* (1997). Evaluation of factors influencing 5-fluorouracil-induced diarrhea in colorectal cancer patients. An Italian Group for the Study of Digestive Tract Cancer (GISCAD) study. *Support Care Cancer.* 5:314–317.

72. Fisher B, Wolmark N, Rockette H *et al.* (1988). Postoperative adjuvant chemotherapy or radiation therapy for rectal cancer: Results from NSABP protocol R-01. *J Natl Cancer Inst.* 80:21–29.

73. Wolmark N, Wieand HS, Hyams DM *et al.* (2000). Randomized trial of postoperative adjuvant chemotherapy with or without radiotherapy for carcinoma of the rectum: National Surgical Adjuvant Breast and Bowel Project Protocol R-02. *J Natl Cancer Inst.* 92:388–396.

74. Tepper JE, O'Connell M, Niedzwiecki D *et al.* (2002). Adjuvant therapy in rectal cancer: Analysis of stage, sex, and local control–final report of intergroup 0114. *J Clin Oncol.* 20:1744–1750.

75. Kapiteijn E, Marijnen CA, Nagtegaal ID *et al.* (2001). Preoperative radiotherapy combined with total mesorectal excision for resectable rectal cancer. *N Engl J Med.* 345:638–646.

76. Cascinu S, Aschele C, Barni S *et al.* (1999). Thymidylate synthase protein expression in advanced colon cancer: Correlation with the site of metastasis and the clinical response to leucovorin-modulated bolus 5-fluorouracil. *Clin Cancer Res.* 5:1996–1999.

77. Diasio RB. (1998). The role of dihydropyrimidine dehydrogenase (DPD) modulation in 5-FU pharmacology. *Oncology (Huntingt).* 12(10 Suppl 7):23–27.

78. Stoehlmacher J, Park DJ, Zhang W *et al.* (2002). Association between glutathione S-transferase P1, T1, and M1 genetic polymorphism and survival of patients with metastatic colorectal cancer. *J Natl Cancer Inst.* 94:936–942.

79. Stoehlmacher J, Ghaderi V, Iobal S *et al.* (2001). A polymorphism of the XRCC1 gene predicts for response to platinum based treatment in advanced colorectal cancer. *Anticancer Res.* 21(4B):3075–3079.

80. Pullarkat ST, Stoehlmacher J, Ghaderi V *et al.* (2001). Thymidylate synthase gene polymorphism determines response and toxicity of 5-FU chemotherapy. *Pharmacogenomics J.* 1(1):65–70.

81. Frisch M, Glimelius B, Wohlfahrt J *et al.* (1999). Tobacco smoking as a risk factor in anal carcinoma: An antiestrogenic mechanism? *J Natl Cancer Inst.* 91:708–715.

82. Melbye M, Frisch M. (1998). The role of human papillomaviruses in anogenital cancers. *Semin Cancer Biol.* 8:307–313.

83. Frisch M, Glimelius B, van den Brule AJ *et al.* (1997). Sexually transmitted infection as a cause of anal cancer. *N Engl J Med.* 337:1350–1358.

84. Palefsky JM. (1998). Human papillomavirus infection and anogenital neoplasia in human immunodeficiency virus-positive men and women. *J Natl Cancer Inst Monogr.* 23:15–20.

85. Critchlow CW, Surawicz CM, Holmes KK *et al.* (1995). Prospective study of high grade anal squamous intraepithelial neoplasia in a cohort of homosexual men: Influence of HIV infection, immunosuppression and human papillomavirus infection. *AIDS.* 9:1255–1262.

86. Flam M, John M, Pajak TF *et al.* (1996). Role of mitomycin in combination with fluorouracil and radiotherapy, and of salvage chemoradiation in the definitive nonsurgical treatment of epidermoid carcinoma of the anal canal: Results of a phase III randomized intergroup study. *J Clin Oncol.* 14:2527–2539.

87. Doci R, Zucali R, La Monica G *et al.* (1996). Primary chemoradiation therapy with fluorouracil and cisplatin for cancer of the anus: Results in 35 consecutive patients. *J Clin Oncol.* 14:3121–3125.

88. UKCCCR Anal Cancer Trial Working Party. UK Co-ordinating Committee on Cancer Research. (1996). Epidermoid anal cancer: Results from the UKCCCR randomised trial of radiotherapy alone versus radiotherapy, 5-fluorouracil, and mitomycin. *Lancet.* 348:1049–1054.

89. Bartelink H, Roelofsen F, Eschwege F *et al.* (1997). Concomitant radiotherapy and chemotherapy is superior to radiotherapy alone in the treatment of locally advanced anal cancer: Results of a phase III randomized trial of the European Organization for Research and Treatment of Cancer Radiotherapy and Gastrointestinal Cooperative Groups. *J Clin Oncol.* 15:2040–2049.

90. Gralla RJ. (2002). New agents, new treatment, and antiemetic therapy. *Semin Oncol.* 29(1 Suppl 4):119–124.

91. Sullivan JR, Leyden MJ, Bell R. (1983). Decreased cisplatin-induced nausea and vomiting with chronic alcohol ingestion. *N Engl J Med.* 309:796.

92. Tsavaris N, Kosmas C, Mylonakis N *et al.* (2000). Parameters that influence the outcome of nausea and emesis in cisplatin based chemotherapy. *Anticancer Res.* 20(6C):4777–4783.

93. Osoba D, Zee B, Pater J *et al.* (1997). Determinants of postchemotherapy nausea and vomiting in patients with cancer. Quality of Life and Symptom Control Committees of the National Cancer Institute of Canada Clinical Trials Group. *J Clin Oncol.* 15:116–123.

94. Pollera CF, Giannarelli D. (1989). Prognostic factors influencing cisplatin-induced emesis. Definition and validation of a predictive logistic model. *Cancer.* 64:1117–1122.

95. Fauser AA, Fellhauer M, Hoffmann M *et al.* (1999). Guidelines for anti-emetic therapy: Acute emesis. *Eur J Cancer.* 35:361–370.

96. Gralla RJ, Osoba D, Kris MG *et al.* (1999). Recommendations for the use of antiemetics: Evidence-based, clinical practice guidelines. American Society of Clinical Oncology. *J Clin Oncol.* 17:2971–2994.

97. Kris MG, Gralla RJ, Tyson LB *et al.* (1989). Controlling delayed vomiting: Double-blind, randomized trial comparing placebo, dexamethasone alone, and metoclopramide plus dexamethasone in patients receiving cisplatin. *J Clin Oncol.* 7:108–114.

62

Gender Influences on the Development and Progression of Brain Tumors

CASILDA BALMACEDA, MD AND JENNIFER ROSSI, BA

The Neurological Institute, New York Presbyterian Hospital, New York, NY

I. Background

Gender may influence the development and progression of various types of brain tumors. Despite differences in the major tumor types, both children and adults exhibit the same gender trend: males have a greater overall incidence of brain tumors than females [1–6]. Skewed sex distributions are found across specific central nervous system (CNS) tumor subtypes: although males are twice as likely to develop a glioma, meningiomas are diagnosed twice as often in females [7,8]. Although the medical literature on this topic is scanty, several observations support the link between hormones and CNS cancers. Puberty, menstruation, pregnancy, and menopause—periods of relative hormonal excess—have all been observed to affect the incidence and outcomes of certain CNS tumors in women and men [9–15]. It has also been suggested that there is a link between the development of breast cancer, which is known to be hormonally influenced, and meningiomas.

Although the mechanism for this association is unclear, a growing body of work has identified and quantified certain steroid receptors, such as those for progesterone and estrogen, in primary brain tumors [16–26]. The lipophilic steroid hormones estrogen, progesterone, and testosterone can cross the blood-brain-barrier and penetrate neural cells. They exert action in the cell through binding with an intracellular hormone receptor, part of a family of transcription factors, which then binds DNA at promoter sites to affect gene transcription [27].

This chapter reviews the pertinent literature on the role of hormones in brain tumors from childhood through adulthood. We examine several areas: (1) childhood CNS cancers particularly gliomas, germ cell tumors, and meningiomas; (2) adult brain tumors with an emphasis on gliomas, acoustic neuromas, and meningiomas; and (3) changes in brain tumors through puberty, menstruation, menopause, and pregnancy. Lastly, we examine the therapeutic value of steroid hormones such as mifepristone and tamoxifen. We conclude that there is a growing body of evidence supporting pivotal roles of estrogen, progesterone, and androgens in a variety of primary brain cancer subtypes.

II. Childhood Brain Tumors

CNS cancers account for one fifth of all childhood malignancies [1]. Between 30,000 to 40,000 children are diagnosed with brain tumors annually worldwide, with rates increasing an average of 2% every year in the United States [1,28].

Gender differences in overall pediatric brain tumor incidence are present from birth and these gaps widen with age; boys are more prone to develop brain tumors than girls throughout childhood and adolescence (M/F ratio is 1.55, 0 to 14 years) [1,2,4,6,29]. The extent of male prevalence fluctuates because of the variable peak incidences of the various histologic tumor subtypes. The male-to-female ratios reported from several series are summarized in Table 62-1. Different types of childhood brain tumors are discussed in the following sections.

Major hormonal differences between the sexes arise during puberty—ovarian estrogen production begins in girls and testosterone production increases in boys. Such events may profoundly affect cells that lead to malignancy. Therefore, changing trends of brain tumor development during adolescence are of particular interest because they may reveal how gender, particularly sex hormones, can influence the development and progression of the malignancies.

Similar to the first decade of life, 10- to 14-year old boys have a larger number of tumors than their female counterparts; however, the gender gap is considerably wider at this time. In one study, girls had the lowest incidence rate during the pubertal years of any other pediatric age group [1,8]. As described in more detail later, diagnoses of several CNS cancer subtypes increase (germ cell tumors) or decrease (astrocytic tumors, primitive neuroectodermal tumor [PNET], medulloblastoma) throughout adolescence.

Interestingly, not only are boys more likely to develop CNS cancers, they are also more likely to have a poorer outcome than their female counterparts [30]. This could be because boys develop more malignant tumors; it could also be a reflection of a gender effect in tumor progression. These general observations yield two possible scenarios: (1) estrogen and progesterone may garner protection against certain malignancies, hence a lower tumor rate in girls and (2) testosterone could have harmful or tumor-promoting effects that contribute to the greater incidence and worse outcome in males. Possible hormonal roles in specific pediatric tumors are explored more fully in the following:

A. Glioma

The most common CNS tumors in childhood and adolescence are the astrocytomas; their overall prevalence is reported as 42 to 47% of pediatric brain tumors [5,29]. Mean age at diagnosis is 7.4 years [1]. As discussed later (see Section III.A), gliomas have a higher incidence in men than in women, but a different trend is observed in children. The incidence of astrocytomas is equal among girls and boys during the first 2 decades of life; however, there is a slight male predominance (1.1 M/F ratio after age four) [28]. The gender distribution

Table 62-1
Reported Gender Ratios in Childhood Central Nervous System Tumors

Author	Number of Patients	Pathology	M/F Ratio	Comments
Cho *et al* [1]	677	All CNS tumors	1.4:1	1959 to 2000
		Astrocytoma tumors	1.0	Patients <16 yr
		Pilocytic type	0.8	
		Excluding pilocytic	1.7	
		Anaplastic astrocytoma	1.4	
		GBM	0.8	
		Medulloblastoma	1.7	
		Craniopharyngioma	1.5	
		Germ cell tumors	1.7	
		ST-PNETs	1.8	
		Neuronal tumors	2.5	
		Oligodendroglial	0.8	
		Pituitary adenoma	0.6	
		Meningioma	2.3	
Rickert [4]	75	All CNS tumors (includes astrocytoma, ependymoma, PNET, medulloblastoma, teratoma, and others)	1.3	Patients <3 yr
Rickert and Paulus [5]	10,582	All CNS tumors	1.29	Meta-analysis patients <17 yr
Shah *et al* [6]	54	All CNS tumors	1.1	1995–1997
		Pilocytic astrocytoma	0.5	Patients <15 yr
		Medulloblastoma	9.0	
Gurney *et al* [28]	2578	All CNS tumors	1.2	Data from nine centers of the
		Astroglial	1.1	Surveillance, Epidemiology,
		PNET	1.5	and End Results Program of the
		Ependymoma	1.53	National Cancer 1974–1991
				Patients ≤14 yr

CNS, central nervous system; GBM, glioblastoma multiforme; PNET, primitive neuroectodermal tumors; ST-PNET, supratentorial primitive neuroectodermal tumors.
Gender ratios of selected histologic subtypes observed in each series are included.

becomes more skewed if only certain types of astrocytomas are considered. A study of 677 childhood CNS cancers reported the following M/F ratios among astrocytoma subtypes: astrocytoma excluding pilocytic type: 1.7, pilocytic astrocytoma: 0.8, anaplastic-astrocytoma: 1.4, and glioblastoma: 0.8 [1]. The changing gender ratios of these astrocytic tumors may indicate separate modes of development and progression in each.

One subtype of glioma—ependymomas—accounts for 8.5% of all pediatric CNS cancers [28] and 17.3% of those in children younger than age 3 years. The mean age at diagnosis is 5.1 years [1]. These tumors occur in the ventricles of the brain and often cause obstruction of the cerebrospinal fluid. They occur more often in males (M/F ratio = 1.5) (see Table 62-1) [28]. One report noted high estrogen receptor (ER) concentrations in both of two ependymomas taken from female patients [22]. The one tumor tested for progesterone receptor (PR) exhibited no binding. Therefore, estrogen, but not progesterone, action may contribute to the smaller incidence in females by retarding ependymoma growth, although the small sample size of this study necessitates that more conclusive research be conducted

Hormone receptor studies have focused primarily on adult tumors (Section III.A.2). One investigation that measured hormone receptors through a binding assay included four glial tumors (two astrocytomas, two ependymomas) from pediatric female patients [22]. One of two astrocytomas displayed significant estrogen binding. A progesterone binding assay was not performed on this tumor. Significant progesterone, but not estrogen, binding was detected in the other astrocytoma. Two of two ependymomas had significant estrogen binding.

B. Germ Cell Tumors

Intracranial germ cell tumors (GCTs) are a subset of extragonadal GCTs. These rare tumors most frequently arise in the pineal (49%) and suprasellar regions (34%) from primordial germ cells. Germ cell tumors can be divided into germinoma and nongerminomatous germ cell tumor (NGGCT). Elevated alpha-fetoproteins (AFPs) and beta human chorionic gonadotropins (βhCG) in the cerebrospinal fluid are suggestive of NGGCT, which is associated with a significantly shorter survival than germinomas (p < 0.0001) [31]. Germ cell tumors account for 0.4 to 3.4% of all CNS cancers in North American and 2.1 to 9.4% in Japan [31]. Although rarely occurring in the first few years of life, they account for almost one third of CNS cancers during the pubertal years (10- to 14-year age group) and 15% of pediatric intracranial tumors overall [29]. Peak age at diagnoses is between 10 to 12 years [1,31].

After age 9, a strong male predominance on the overall CNS GCT incidence appears: reported M/F ratios are 4.3 in the United States and 3.2 in Japan [31,32]. These ratios are even larger for nongerminomatous tumors. Gender influences the site of tumor development: 75% of female CNS GCTs are in the suprasellar region, whereas 67% of male GCTs are pineal [31]. Male-to-female ratios increase almost 3-fold when limited to the pineal region, whereas the M/F ratio of GCTs in the suprasellar location are approximately 1.0 [32]. The largest discrepancy between the sexes occurs from ages 20 to 24 in Japan and from ages 10 to 15 in Western countries [31,32].

The equal gender distribution in the first decade of life suggests against direct Y-linked effects. Male predominance, the rise of GCT incidence during periods of increased gonadotropin secretion (i.e., puberty), the association of gonadotropin (AFP and βhCG) secreting GCTs with a worse prognosis, and the location of most GCTs in close proximity to the pituitary all strongly suggest that sex hormones may trigger malignant development of primordial germ cells into CNS GCTs [31].

Further evidence for the hormonal influence of GCTs is the association between CNS GCT and Klinefelter's syndrome (males with XXY karyotype) [33]. Klinefelter's syndrome includes increased levels of serum and urinary gonadotropins, small testes with fibrosis and hyalinization of the seminiferous tubules, and impairment of function and clumping of Leydig cells. All four cases of XXY males with GCT reported in a recent series had an age of tumor onset between 12 and 20 years, which coincides with puberty [33].

Laboratory studies also support possible hormonal effects in GCT development. Some testicular GCTs display growth acceleration when exposed to andosterone in tissue culture, but this research has not yet been extended to include GCTs of the nervous system [31]. Both of two malignant teratomas examined in one series were found to have ERs and one also bound progesterone [22]. This supports a possible tumor-promoting role of testosterone and protective role of the female sex hormones estrogen and progesterone. More research on the exact roles of these hormones is necessary.

C. Primitive Neuroectodermal Tumors (PNETs)

Primitive neuroectodermal tumors are malignant small cell undifferentiated tumors that frequently develop in the cerebrum. In children, these tumors are most often diagnosed within the first 2 decades of life. Together with medulloblastomas they constitute 24.1% of tumors presenting in the first 3 years of life [4]. These tumors are diagnosed more frequently in boys than in girls, with a reported M/F ratio of 1.8 [1]. Medulloblastomas, like PNETs, are diagnosed more often in males (M/F ratio = 1.7) [1].

Hormone receptors in these tumors have not been extensively examined. A study of hormone binding in brain tumors found that neither of two PNETs exhibited ER binding [22]. One of two medulloblastomas exhibited estrogen binding, although conclusions cannot reliably be drawn from such a small sample size [22]. The four samples were not tested for PRs.

The reason for the male-skewed gender ratio has not been explored. Because these tumors peak before puberty, the cause of the greater male prevalence would provide information about gender differences that are not dependent on hormone levels (which do not differ dramatically until after age 10). Further research into this area is necessary.

D. Meningiomas

Meningiomas are uncommon in childhood and adolescence, accounting for only about 1.5% of brain tumors in patients younger than 15 years [1]. These tumors have a strong gender bias toward adult women (see Section III.C). This is in contrast with childhood patterns: one study of 29 pediatric meningiomas noted a clear male predominance (M/F ratio of 1.6) [34].

Sixty-two percent of childhood meningiomas occur between ages 10 and 15 years, during which the incidence of males is double that of females [1,34]. Shortly after puberty, meningioma incidences in women start to rise. The low rates in girls could result from reduced levels of female hormones progesterone and estrogen, which may not be sufficiently high to trigger meningioma development as in adult women. The stark difference between incidence of meningioma before and after puberty, as well as other observations noted in the discussion of adult meningiomas (Section III.C), strongly links meningioma incidence with hormonal effects.

III. Adult Brain Tumors

Adult tumors differ from childhood tumors in several important factors including histology and development but not in overall gender ratio: men, like boys, have an increased risk for developing a brain tumor than females of the same age. Every year in the United States, CNS cancers are diagnosed in 7.4 men and 5.3 women per 100,000 [3]. Only one study reported a higher age-adjusted incidence in women [8]. Gender preferences in several brain tumors types are summarized in Table 62-2.

A. Gliomas

1. Clinical Observations

Gliomas are the most prevalent type of brain tumor, accounting for 64 to 72% of all primary intracranial neoplasms [35]. They arise from glial cells; these include astrocytomas (low-grade astrocytoma; anaplastic astrocytoma; and glioblastoma multiforme [GBM], the most aggressive type of glioma), oligodendrogliomas, oligoastrocytomas (mixed glioma), and ependymomas. Gliomas develop more often in males than in females throughout adulthood, with the predominance increasing with age (M/F ratio of 1.59; p < 0.001) [16,35]. This trend contrasts with the almost equal gender ratios observed until puberty (see Section II.A), which indicates that glioma development is not governed by X- or Y-linked effects.

McKinley et al [36] performed a retrospective age- and sex-adjusted study on 11,204 glioblastomas (GBM) [36]. This study found an increasing risk of GBM with increasing age.

Table 62-2
Reported Gender Ratios in Adult Central Nervous System Tumors

Author	Number of Patients	Pathology	M/F Ratio	Comments
Kuratsu and Ushio [8]	1117	All CNS tumors	0.77	Japanese population
		Germ cell tumor	4.29	
		Neurinoma	1.32	
		Glioma	1.16	
		Pituitary adenoma	0.68	
		Meningioma	0.39	
Jukich et al [7]	16,078	All CNS tumors	0.92	Study population from state
		Glioblastoma	1.27	cancer registries in CT,
		Astrocytoma	1.17	DE, ID, MA, MO, UT
		Oligodendroglioma	1.27	Includes adult and pediatric
		Medulloblastoma/PNET	1.56	tumors
		Meningioma	0.41	
		Ependymoma	1.86	
Kasantikul et al [41]	103	Acoustic neuroma	0.72	
Fleury et al [35]	1376	All glioma	1.32	Patients from 6 French cancer
		Malignant astrocytoma	1.59	registries
		Low-grade astrocytoma	1.08	
		Oligodendroglioma	1.28	
		Unclassified	–	
		Without histologic confirmation	2.6	

CNS, central nervous system; PNET, primitive neuroectodermal tumor.

The risk in both genders was equal until the ages of 10 to 14 at which point girls begin to show a lower incidence than boys: their relative risk (RR) dropped from 1.02 to 0.78. As both gender populations aged, GBM incidence decreased in females relative to males until a maximum nadir at the age of 50 to 54 (start of menopause and stop of ovarian estrogen production) [36]. The female advantage begins to dissipate with age after menopause, although the RRs of the genders never become equal.

2. Animal and Laboratory Studies

Laboratory and animal studies reveal a physiologic basis for these observed incidences. Female rats with implanted U87 GBM tumor lines in their brains have a survival advantage over their male counterparts [37]. To investigate the cause of this observed advantage, suspected to be hormonal, nude rats received implanted GBM cells and were divided into several groups: males, females, females with ovariectomy, and sham ovariectomy. Two more groups undergoing ovariectomy were then given either benzoate or progesterone for 3 weeks. All implanted tumors appeared histologically similar. The female rats survived longer than their male counterparts (p = 0.02) [37]. Ovariectomy negated the survival advantage of females, but hormone replacement (estrogen) restored it subsequently. Progesterone had no effect on survival.

The higher levels of androgens, particularly testosterone, in males may contribute to their higher glioma incidence. Testosterone is suspected to alter the lipid composition of the cell membrane, which could have direct ramifications for cell signaling pathways and growth [38]. Neutral glycolipids (NGLs) of the cell membrane are promising diagnostic markers of human gliomas, and, although their biologic activity is still unknown, they have been reported to undergo compositional changes with growth, differentiation, and function in many disease processes including malignant transformation, which emphasizes their importance [38]. A greater abundance of NGL in males has been reported in some tissues, especially after puberty [38]. Ceramide dihexosides (CDHs) are a specific type of NGL known to increase in primary tumors of the CNS [38]. One recent study quantified the content of CDH in the cells of 181 human glial tumors: 45 oligodendrogliomas, 92 astrocytomas, 15 oligoastrocytomas, and 29 other primary brain tumors [38]. Of these tumors, 69 were from females and 112 from males [38]. The authors reported striking age- and sex-related difference in amount of CDH within these tumors; although CDH is equal in tumors of males and females until age 14, after puberty the median values of CDH in males increased to twice that of females. The CDH content of tumors from females does not increase until after age 50 (menopause), and gender differences in this age group are less pronounced. Female mice treated with testosterone displayed a greater content of NGL, especially CDH, which suggests that the observed sex differences are governed by sex hormones [38]. Notably, CDH levels were shown to correlate with the observed incidences of glioma in humans, for example, both the incidence and the CDH levels of human gliomas increase in postmenopausal women.

Studies on hormone receptors in gliomas are summarized in Table 62-3. Confounding the support for a role of estrogen in glial tumor development is that most glial tumors do not

Table 62-3
Hormone Receptors Reported on Gliomas

Author	Pathology	Percentage of Tumors Tested Positive for Hormone Receptor	Notes
Assimakopoulou et al [16]	90 astrocytomas (46 GBM, 20 anaplastic astrocytomas, 24 astrocytomas)	42% PR	GBM had statistically significant more PR than low-grade astrocytomas
Carroll et al [18]	Low-grade astrocytomas	100% AR 0% ER	PR detected more often in tumors of greater malignancy
Glick et al [22]	10 gliomas (5 malignant, 5 benign)	Malignant: 80% ER Benign: 20% ER	Difference between malignant and benign groups is significant (p<0.04) No significant sex-related preference for hormone binding

AR, androgen receptor; ER, estrogen receptor; GBM, glioblastoma multiforme; PR, progesterone receptor.

express ERs [16,19]. Progesterone receptors have been identified in a minority of astrocytic tumors. A study of 90 supratentorial astrocytic tumors (46 GBM, 20 anaplastic astrocytomas, 24 astrocytomas) found PRs in 38 (42%) of the tumors [16]. Of specific tumor types, glioblastomas have statistically significant more PR than benign astrocytomas: 59% of GBM, 45% of anaplastic astrocytomas, and only 8% of benign astrocytomas were PR positive. Age also appeared to influence PR expression: of the anaplastic astrocytoma group 55.5% of patients older than 50 tested positive for the receptor in comparison with 36% of those younger than 50 years, whereas of the glioblastoma group, 55% of patients older than 50 and 59% of patients younger than 50 had PR-positive tumors. There was no difference between mean PR score values in males and females.

Estrogen and progesterone levels in glial tumors differ from normal brain tissue: in tumors, estrogen concentrations are 10 to 30 times higher than normal, progesterone is about 10 times lower, and testosterone is not significantly different [39]. How estrogen may effect the cell without a receptor has not been explained; such high concentrations may build because the tumor cannot bind to the hormone [39]. The low concentrations of progesterone and the relative abundance of PR in tumors could indicate the rapid consumption of the hormone by the tumor [39]. Progesterone has been found to decrease the proliferation of glial cells of the CNS in vitro [40].

Together, these observations suggest that these tumors could be partly under hormonal influence, either because of a malignant effect of androgens (such as testosterone) or a protective effect of estrogen and/or progesterone. The lower female glioma incidence could correspond to a very basic hormonal suppression of estrogen [36,37]. The higher levels of estrogen and/or progesterone (or a metabolite) produced by women after menarche protect against GBM; the prohibitive effect then theoretically would diminish with the onset of menopause and the cessation of ovarian estrogen production [36]. However, the continuing female advantage past menopause indicates that estrogen is not the only factor that is responsible for the differing gender incidences. The presence of PRs on the tumors and the greater abundance of these receptors in astrocytic tumors of higher malignancy raise the additional possibility of progesterone influence, although

the presence of receptors does not guarantee that they are metabolically active—a normally suppressed gene could become derepressed in a malignant cell. Androgens in males may be a contributing factor to the development of such neoplasms.

B. Vestibular Schwannoma

1. Clinical Observations

Vestibular schwannomas (synonymous with acoustic neuroma and acoustic neuronoma) are benign neoplasms that represent nearly 6% of all intracranial tumors. The majority of these slow-growing tumors arise from the vestibular portion of the 8th cranial nerve within the internal ear canal. Most patients experience growth unilaterally. Common presentation includes balance change and hearing deficit, especially asymmetric. About 58% vestibular schwannomas occurred in women [41]. In addition, the tumors of women are likely to be larger and more vascularized than those found in males [41]. Vestibular schwannomas may undergo accelerated tumor growth during pregnancy and occur more frequently in women after menopause (discussed more fully in Sections IV.A and IV.B).

2. Laboratory and Animal Studies

The clinical observations discussed previously have led to investigations into the role of estrogen in the growth of vestibular schwannomas. One study examined the effect of estrogen on tumors in mice. Thirty-six nude mice with implanted human vestibular schwannomas were randomized to three treatment groups: controls, estrogen (17beta-estradiol), or estrogen and tamoxifen (an antiestrogen). Tumors in the mice treated with estrogen alone had statistically significant tumor growth when compared with either of the other groups. There was no difference between the controls and the group treated with estrogen and tamoxifen. These results support a correlation between estrogen and tumor growth in addition to tamoxifen's ability to block the effects of estrogen [42]. Not all published research supports such a conclusion. At odds with the previous study, Carroll et al [20] found that ER mRNA and protein were undetectable in vestibular schwannomas (Table 62-4).

Table 62-4
Hormone Receptors Reported on Acoustic Neuromas/Vestibular Schwannomas

Author	Pathology	Percentage of Tumors Tested Positive for Hormone Receptor	Notes
Carroll et al [20]	21 vestibular schwannomas	33% PR 9.5% AR 0% ER	Both tumors with PR were males PR detected in equal ratios of males and females
Glick et al [22]	8 vestibular schwannoma	50% ER	
Monsell and Wiet [43]	37 acoustic neuromas (21 males, 16 females)	19% ER 17% PR	No correlation of ER with gender
Siglock et al [26]	19 vestibular schwannomas (10 males, 9 females)	53% PR 0% ER 0% AR	Males and females exhibited a borderline difference in PR
Whittle et al [25]	7 acoustic neuromas	28% PR 0% ER	No correlation between gender and PR

AR, androgen receptor; ER, estrogen receptor; PR, progesterone receptor.

Vestibular schwannoma samples assayed for estrogen and progesterone binding ability reported that only a minority of tumors (19%) showed ER positivity and even less had PRs (17%) [43]. It is unclear how estrogen may affect growth in tumors that lack the necessary ERs. Further research in a human model is necessary for conclusive results.

Androgen receptor (AR) mRNA was reported in 2 males out of 21 tumors in one series [20] but was absent from all 19 vestibular schwannomas tested in another [26]; therefore, it is unlikely that testosterone affects tumor growth. Others report PRs in up to one third to one half of acoustic neuromas, with a preferential expression in women [20,26].

C. Meningiomas

1. Clinical Observations

Meningiomas arise from meningothelial cells found in the arachnoid villi of the meninges, which are the membranes covering the brain and spinal cord. They are most often benign and can be treated with surgical excision. Meningiomas account for one fifth of all primary intracranial and one fourth of all intraspinal neoplasms [19,21]. There are several lines of epidemiologic evidence that may link meningiomas with sex hormones: (1) meningioma incidence has a clear female predominance, occurring twice as often in women than in men; (2) they are diagnosed most often in the 5th and 6th decades with a decrease after menopause; and (3) there is a noted association between meningiomas and breast cancer [44–48]. Furthermore, pregnancy and menopause appear to influence tumor development, as discussed more fully in Sections IV.A and IV.B.

2. Laboratory and Animal Studies

A growing body of research has focused on the physiologic basis for hormonal influence in meningiomas, the mechanisms of which remain unclear. These studies concentrate on two areas: sex steroid receptor presence on meningiomas and the observed effects of hormones on meningioma cell growth both in vitro and in vivo.

Hormone receptors are present in a substantial proportion of meningiomas; therefore, these tumors may be hormone- and gender-dependent [16,17,19,21,23,25,44]. Table 62-5 summarizes the results of several studies that measured ERs, progesterone receptors (PRs), and/or ARs in meningiomas. The literature on the existence of ERs is inconsistent: ERs have been reported present in a majority [21,22] and none [23,25,44] of meningiomas tested. One study identified a trend toward increased estrogen binding by ERs in females [22], although most do not cite any gender differences in ER expressions. Estrogen receptors present in meningiomas are likely to be nonfunctional: no meningiomas tested with a nuclear binding assay, which only reveals activated receptors, were ER positive [49].

Data on PRs and ARs are more conclusive. Studies performed during the past 2 decades have demonstrated that meningiomas express abundant levels of PRs and ARs [17,19,23,25]. One study examined the mRNA expression of PRs, ERs and ARs in tumor samples collected intraoperatively from patients with meningioma [23]. Of nine meningiomas studies, AR mRNA transcripts and protein were detected in six of nine (55%) and PR mRNA transcripts and protein in eight of nine (88%) [23]. The authors did not find significant gender differences in hormone receptor expression. The presence of these receptors in the nucleus of meningioma cells [17] is strong evidence that they are likely functional and able to allow hormones to exert some degree of control over tumor growth and even malignant transformation.

A different study that focused on the expression of ARs in meningiomas found that 67% of 39 tumors expressed AR mRNA, of which more than two thirds were women and one third were men [19]. More than three fourths of the meningiomas negative for ARs were from men.

Meningioma cells have been subjected to hormonal influence in vitro. A medium with 17 beta-estradiol and progesterone caused 21 to 36% growth stimulation in tumor cells. The addition of

Table 62-5
Hormone Receptors Reported on Meningiomas

Author	Pathology	Percentage of Tumors Tested Positive for Hormone Receptor	Notes
Carroll et al [17]	33 meningiomas (11 male, 22 female)	64% PR (of these, 81% female and 19% male)	Women have statistically significant more tumors with PR
Carroll et al [19]	39 meningiomas (18 male, 21 female)	67% AR	Of positive tumors: 69% female, 31% male Of negative tumors: 23% female, 77% male
Carroll et al [21]	34 meningiomas (18 male, 16 female)	54–68% ER 64% PR	No correlation between ER and sex, age, or PR presence
Glick et al [22]	21 meningiomas	57% ER 75% PR	All 21 tumors tested for ER, 4 tested for PR Trend toward a sex-related preference for females (p > 0.13)
Maxwell et al [23]	9 meningiomas	88% PR 66% AR 0% ER	No correlation between gender and PR or AR
Salvati and Cervoni [44]	9 meningiomas	44% PR 0% ER	All 9 patients had breast cancer
Whittle et al [25]	29 meningiomas	55% PR 0% ER	No correlation between gender and PR

AR, androgen receptor; ER, estrogen receptor; PR, progesterone receptor.

tamoxifen, an estrogen antagonist, stimulated cell growth in one tumor by 35%, and it caused only transient stimulation or no effect in two others [50].

Patients with meningioma who underwent progesterone supplementation showed no positive response [51]. Of the nine patients who took 40 to 80 mg/day of megestrol acetate, three patients experienced rapid visual deterioration within the first 3 months. This result indicates a possible stimulatory effect of progesterone on meningioma growth. The positive results of several studies examining the efficacy of the antiprogesterone mifepristone (RU-486) also supports the contributing role of progesterone (Section V.B).

The exact mechanism of progesterone stimulation is still unclear. Recent investigations have focused on the response of cultured meningioma cells to epidermal growth factor (EGF) in the presence of progesterone [20,52]. Because EGF is present at all times and EGF receptors are expressed on human meningiomas, the interaction of sex hormones with EGF would appear as a direct effect of progesterone [20]. Cell suspensions of human meningioma tissue were prepared and grown in EGF either with 10 nM progesterone or without progesterone [52]. Four of five suspensions tested positive for PRs and all of these had EGF receptor. They found that the response to EGF was variable, but the sensitivity increased in the presence of progesterone. This supports the idea that sex steroids can increase the sensitivity of meningiomas to growth factors such as EGF, contributing to their proliferation.

3. Meningiomas and Breast Cancer

Several studies have reported a link between meningiomas and breast carcinoma [44–48]. Women may be diagnosed with breast cancer or meningioma first, and a few are diagnosed concurrently. A study of the Connecticut Tumor Registry observed eight cases of patients with meningioma and breast cancer, a larger number than the 3.7 cases the researchers expected to find [45]. A retrospective cohort analysis of the Western Washington State registry estimated that the risk of breast cancer after a diagnosis of meningioma was 1.54 with 95% confidence interval (CI) 0.77 to 2.75, and the risk of meningioma after the diagnosis of breast cancer was 1.40 with 95% CI 0.67 to 2.58 [47]. Although both CIs include 1.0, the risks for each cancer are elevated, especially in postmenopausal women. The small set of women who develop both cancers pose a difficulty to such studies and cause such large CIs.

Several explanations for this association have been proposed. One theory suggests that a malignant breast carcinoma cell metastasizes to a preexisting benign tumor, triggering a malignant meningioma development [48]. This is called a tumor collision. Others note that the bidirectional associations may be due to shared risk factors between the two cancers, such as female gender or similar responsiveness to hormones. At this time, the evidence that meningiomas respond to hormones in a similar way as breast malignancies is inconclusive. Breast cancer has been documented to be hormonally responsive; a link between breast cancers and meningiomas is strong support for an analogous influence of hormones in meningiomas as well. Interestingly, the two cancer types do not have the same hormone receptor profiles. Some meningiomas have PRs and rarely ERs, whereas receptor-positive breast cancers almost always have ER and only a minority has PR [44].

Although research on this topic is ongoing, neurosurgeons and oncologists should be aware of the association between the two. There are important clinical implications. Dural-enhancing lesions, in a patient with metastatic cancer, are not necessarily metastases (which may require irradiation), but may be meningiomas (potentially cured by surgical excision). If further evidence is found supporting the association, preventative measures against a second primary malignancy once a diagnosis of meningioma or breast carcinoma is established should be explored.

D. Other Central Nervous System Cancers

Data supporting gender associations in other CNS cancers is sparse.

1. Medulloblastomas

These highly aggressive tumors, although occurring primarily in children, also occur in adults. A retrospective review of 34 adult patients with cerebellar medulloblastoma showed that gender influenced the likelihood of a positive outcome [53]. The 5-year survival rates of patients with medulloblastoma were 92% for females and 40% for males.

2. Neurofibromas

These are benign tumors of the peripheral nerve sheath. Neurofibromatosis type I is a common genetic disorder that affects the nervous system and is associated with an increased risk for the development of benign and malignant tumors including neurofibromas. Like meningiomas, the incidence of these tumors corresponds with periods of increased hormone levels: they are rarely found before puberty and increase during pregnancy [24]. A majority of these tumors express PRs (75%) and only a small minority expresses ERs (5%) [24]. One author proposed that progesterone may play an important role in neurofibroma growth, similar to that of meningiomas, and suggested possible adjuvant therapy with antiprogesterones in treatment [24].

IV. Reproductive and Hormonal Associations

A. Menstrual Status and Brain Tumors

1. Menstruation

Neurologic symptoms of some patients with hemangiomas and meningiomas have been reported to worsen just before menstruation and recede during the week of menses, corresponding to the surge and subsequent fall of progesterone levels postovulation [9–11]. Although it is unclear whether the increased hormones directly affect the tumor or indirectly influence growth through the physiologic changes that they cause, such as increased water retention, these observations during the menstrual cycle further implicate that female hormones can influence brain tumor growth.

2. Menopause

Menopause has been associated with a change in the incidence rates of several brain tumors in women. A population-based case-control study of 127 females with brain tumors (60 meningiomas, 51 gliomas, 16 acoustic neuromas) revealed important trends associated with menopause [12]. Although the results of this study were not statistically significant because of a small sample size, after menopause, women were reported to have an increased RR for the development of gliomas and acoustic neuromas (RR = 1.31, 95% CI 0.51 to 2.07) and a greatly reduced risk for the development of meningiomas (RR = 0.58, 95% CI 0.18 to 1.90). Interestingly, there was a reduced risk for all three types of tumors in women with surgical induction of menopause, with the risk even lower for premenopausal women who underwent the bilateral oophorectomy more than 10 years before the brain tumor diagnosis. One study limitation was that hormonal replacement information was not attainable for all patients.

These observations suggest several possibilities regarding growth in each histologic tumor subtype in regards to hormonal levels. Two hormonal changes in menopause may contribute to the lower incidences of development in postmenopausal women: (1) the virtual cease in production of ovarian estrogen and (2) the slight increase in production of androgens and progesterone [12]. The effect of estrogen reduction is supported by the even lower risks observed in women who underwent bilateral oophorectomy, in whom the cessation of estrogen is immediate. The lower incidence in males, who have higher levels of androgens, supports the second hypothesis. In regards to the rise in incidence in glioma and acoustic neuroma after menopause, it is possible that estrogen slows tumor development and/or growth in the years before menopause. In addition, an increase in androgen levels, even if relative to other sex hormones, may contribute to the development of a glioma. This potential androgen effect can explain the increased risk for glioma development in menopausal women, who have increased androgen levels, and the overall male prevalence of this cancer (see Section III.A). Similarly, the reduced androgen levels that typically follow childbearing may account for the observed reduction in glioma risk in ever-parous women [54].

B. Pregnancy and Brain Tumors

Pregnancy is not a specific risk factor for brain tumor development because the relative frequency of CNS malignancies is equal in pregnant and nonpregnant women [11]. The incidence of brain neoplasms in pregnant patients is lower than calculated expected values in the normal population [55]. However, pregnancy can have a profound effect on the development of glioma, meningioma, vascular spinal tumors (hemangioma), and acoustic neuroma [10,11,14].

Several reports describe an exacerbation of symptoms in previously undiagnosed meningiomas during pregnancy [9–11]. These tumors most frequently arise in the 3rd trimester, and many patients experience a recession of symptoms with parturition [9–11]. Other types of tumors also experience growth increases during pregnancy. Gliomas tend to become symptomatic during the 1st trimester of pregnancy, whereas acoustic neuromas and vascular tumors such as hemangiomas manifest more commonly in the 3rd trimester [11,14].

There are two likely mechanisms of tumor exacerbation during pregnancy. First, the increased fluid retention and blood volume during pregnancy may cause tumor edema, especially in vascular tumors such as meningiomas and hemangiomas [11,14]. The fall of fluid levels could alleviate symptoms after pregnancy [10]. Second, sex steroid receptors have been reported in various amounts on these tumors (see Sections III.A to C, Table 62-3). The drastic changes in hormone levels during pregnancy—plasma concentrations of progesterone and estrogen increase six to seven times by the last 8 weeks of gestation—could trigger tumor growth via these receptors. *In vitro* studies have shown that estrogen and progesterone—hormones that increase during pregnancy—promote meningioma cell growth (see Section III.C.2) [50]. Progesterone is implicated in symptoms that arise during the luteal phase of menstruation or during pregnancy because its levels are elevated during these times. However, because symptoms typically evolve later in the course of pregnancy and progesterone levels remain relatively high for the duration of pregnancy, it is unlikely that only progesterone plays a role.

V. Hormone Therapies

Hormone therapies may prove to be useful adjuvant treatments for patients with brain tumors, especially against inoperable tumors and as salvage therapy when standard chemotherapy has failed. Investigations into such therapies have been promising, although inconclusive. We discuss tamoxifen, an estrogen antagonist, and mifepristone (RU-486), a progesterone antagonist.

A. Tamoxifen

Tamoxifen acts as an estrogen antagonist by inhibiting the protein kinase C (PKC) signal transduction pathway, which is used by many hormones to stimulate cell growth and migration [56]. As mentioned previously (Section III.B.2), tamoxifen blocks the growth stimulation of estrogen administration in human vestibular schwannomas grown in nude mice [42].

Malignant gliomas have increased PKC activity; this would be a potential target for tamoxifen therapy. Responses to tamoxifen (>50% reduction in tumor size) was observed radiographically via magnetic resonance imaging (MRI) and positron emission tomography (PET) and clinically in 3 of 11 adult patients (9 men, 2 women) with malignant glioma [56]. All three of the patients who responded were men; two had GBM, and one had progressive low-grade astrocytoma. One woman with GBM had stable disease. The other seven patients experienced progressive disease. In another study, two of three children with recurrent malignant gliomas had tumor reduction and clinical improvement after tamoxifen [57]. The third patient, a 5-year old girl with ependymoma, had stable disease for 17 months.

Another mechanism of tamoxifen action is its inhibition of the P-glycoprotein (Pgp) that serves as an efflux pump for some chemotherapy agents, thus increasing drug concentration in the area of the tumor [58]. It is feasible that new studies use tamoxifen not only for its PKC inhibition effects but also in conjunction with a chemotherapy regimen that would otherwise penetrate poorly across the blood-brain-barrier.

B. Mifepristone

Progesterone receptors are reported on meningiomas more than ERs [17,23]; therefore, hormone therapies have focused on antiprogesterone agents. The progesterone antagonist mifepristone (RU 486) inhibited meningioma growth in three of three human tumors supplanted into nude mice after 3 months

of treatment [59]. Patient trials reported promising results: the long-term administration of 200 to 400 mg/day of mifepristone to patients with unresectable meningiomas caused tumor regression or growth cessation in about one half of patients [60–62]. The most common side effect was fatigue and cessation of menses in premenopausal women. Most studies were unable to confirm the presence and quantity of PRs in all these tumors so it cannot be concluded whether the antiprogesterone treatment in nonresponsive patients failed because they lacked the needed receptor. Malignant meningioma cases and those with concurrent neurofibromatosis type 2 were more likely to see no improvement with mifepristone administration, indicating that this therapy is more effective in less-aggressive cases [60,61]. The long-term use of mifepristone or other steroidal hormones may be especially beneficial in patients with recurrent and unresectable meningioma.

Future studies may look at the status of the sex steroid receptors before administering hormone treatments in individual cases. Knowledge of receptors could enhance the selection of appropriate therapeutic interventions such as hormone therapies.

VI. Conclusions and Suggestions for Further Investigations

The hormonal effects of most CNS cancers are, at best, poorly understood. Awareness of gender influences on certain types of brain tumors, most notably gliomas, meningiomas, and GCTs, is still new. Although recognizing this association may allow earlier detection in certain groups of patients, the association has further implications. The detection of hormonal receptors in operative specimens may be used to study growth patterns, treatment sensitivity, and prognosis. Then therapeutic trials may be based on hormonal agents or hormonal manipulations with or without the addition of conventional chemotherapy. The following deserve future research:

- What are the mechanisms of hormonal action in the development and progression of brain tumors? What is the specific role of hormone receptors?
- Can hormones be targeted to antibodies to enhance tumor detection at diagnosis? Can treatment sensitivity and/or prognosis be determined via testing for the presence of hormone receptors on a tumor?
- How can hormonal therapy lead to tumor regression and/or stability?
- What is the exact nature of the link between breast cancer and meningiomas in women?
- Why do neurologic symptoms increase in only some pregnant women? Why do certain cancers manifest themselves at different times during pregnancy, for example, meningiomas most commonly in the third trimester and gliomas in the first trimester?

In this chapter, we report on possible gender associations in some brain tumors. This connection was first established through clinical observations. Many laboratory studies continue to explore the actions of the sex steroids on multiple CNS tumor subtypes. Although primary brain tumors are not classically hormone dependent, as described in this chapter, estrogen, progesterone, and testosterone have all been implicated in the development of certain brain tumors. They may protect against malignancy (e.g., estrogen against gliomas) or accelerate tumor growth (e.g., androgen in GCTs and estrogen in meningiomas). The exact mechanism by which hormones affect tumor growth is not known. Elucidating possible reasons for the development and progression of brain tumors may aid in the design of much needed novel treatment strategies.

Acknowledgments

We would like to thank our families and our patients for always being a source of inspiration. We would like to thank Ms. Dana Critchell for her literature searches. Dr. Balmaceda would like to thank her children, Cristián and Adrian, for their unfailing support.

References

1. Cho K, Wang K, Kim S *et al*. (2002). Pediatric brain tumors: Statistics of SNUH, Korea (1959–2000). *Child's Nerv Syst*. 18:30–37.

2. Gold EB, Gordis L. (1979). Patterns of incidence of brain tumors in children. *Ann Neurol*. 5:565–568.

3. Inskip PD, Linet MS, Heineman EF. (1995). Etiology of brain tumors in adults. *Epidemiol Rev*. 17:382–405.

4. Rickert CH. (1998). Epidemiological features of brain tumors in the first 3 years of life. *Child's Nerv Syst*. 14:547–550.

5. Rickert CH, Paulus W. (2001). Epidemiology of central nervous system tumors in childhood and adolescence based on the new WHO classification. *Child's Nerv Syst*. 17:503–511.

6. Shah HS, Soomro RN, Hussainy AS, Hassan SH. (1999). Clinicomorphological pattern of intracranial tumors in children. *J Pak Med Assoc*. 49:63–65.

7. Jukich PJ, McCarthy BJ, Surawicz TS *et al*. (2001). Trends in incidence of primary brain tumors in the United States, 1985–1994. *Neuro-Oncology*. 3:141–151.

8. Kuratsu J, Ushio Y. (1996). Epidemiological study of primary intracranial tumors: A regional survey in Kumamoto Prefecture in the southern part of Japan. *J Neurosurg*. 84:946–950.

9. Bickerstaff ER, Small JM, Guest IA. (1958). The relapsing course of certain meningiomas in relation to pregnancy and menstruation. *J Neurol Neurosurg Psychiatry*. 21:89–91.

10. Michelson JJ, New PFJ. (1969). Brain tumour and pregnancy. *J Neurol Neurosurg Psychiatry*. 32:305–307.

11. Roelvink NC, Kamphorst W, van Alphen AM, Rao BR. (1987). Pregnancy-related primary brain and spinal tumors. *Arch Neurol*. 44:209–215.

12. Schlehofer B, Blettner M, Wahrendorf J. (1992). Association between brain tumors and menopausal status. *J Natl Cancer Inst*. 84:1346–1349.

13. Custer BS, Koepsell TD, Mueller BA. (2002). The association between breast carcinoma and meningioma in women. *Cancer*. 94:1626–1635.

14. DeAngelis LM. (1994). Central Nervous System Neoplasms in Pregnancy. In *Neurological Complications of Pregnancy* (Devinsky O, Feldmann E, Hainline B, eds.). New York: Raven Press.

15. Simon RH. (1988). Brain tumors in pregnancy. *Semin Neurol*. 8:214–221.

16. Assimakopoulou M, Sotiropoulou-Bonikou G, Maraziotis T, Varakis J. (1998). Does sex steroid receptor status have any prognostic or predictive significance in brain astrocytic tumors? *Clin Neuropathol*. 17:27–34.

17. Carroll RS, Glowacka D, Dashner K, Black PM. (1993). Progesterone receptor expression in meningiomas. *Cancer Res*. 53:1312–1316.

18. Carroll RS, Zhang J, Dashner K *et al*. (1995). Steroid hormone receptors in astrocytic neoplasms. *Neurosurgery*. 37:496–504.

19. Carroll RS, Zhang J, Dashner K *et al*. (1995). Androgen receptor expression in meningiomas. *J Neurosurg*. 82:453–460.

20. Carroll RS, Zhang J, Black PM. (1997). Hormone receptors in vestibular schwannomas. *Acta Nurochir (Wien)*. 139:188–192.

21. Carroll RS, Zhang J, Black PM. (1999). Expression of estrogen receptors alpha and beta in human meningiomas. *J Neuro-Oncology*. 42:109–116.

22. Glick RP, Molteni A, Fors EM. (1983). Hormone binding in brain tumors. *Neurosurgery*. 13:513–519.

23. Maxwell M, Galanopoulos T, Neville-Golden J, Antoniades HN. (1993). Expression of androgen and progesterone receptors in primary human meningiomas. *J Neurosurg*. 78:456–462.

24. McLaughlin ME, Jacks T. (2003). Progesterone receptor expression in meningioma. *Cancer Res*. 63:752–755.

25. Whittle IR, Hawkins RA, Miller JD. (1987). Sex hormone receptors in intracranial tumors and normal brain. *Eur J Surg Oncol*. 13:303–307.

26. Siglock TJ, Rosenblatt SS, Finck F *et al*. (1990). Sex hormone receptors in acoustic neuromas. *Am J Otol*. 11:237–239.

27. Beato M. (1989). Gene regulation by steroid hormones. *Cell*. 56:335–344.

28. Gurney JG, Davis S, Severson RK *et al*. (1996). Trends in cancer incidence among children in the US. *Cancer*. 78:532–541.

29. Kuratsu J, Ushio Y. (1996). Epidemiological study of primary intracranial tumors in childhood. A population-based survey in Kumamoto Prefecture, Japan. *Pediatr Neurosurg*. 25:240–246.

30. Mostow EN, Byrne J, Connelly RR, Mulvihill JJ. (1991). Quality of life in long-term survivors of CNS tumors of childhood and adolescence. *J Clin Oncol*. 9:592–599.

31. Jennings MT, Gelman R, Hochberg F. (1985). Intracranial germ-cell tumors: Natural history and pathogenesis. *J Neurosurg*. 63:155–167.

32. Tada M. (1998). Epidemiology of CNS GCTs. In *Intracranial Germ Cell Tumors* (Sawamura Y, Shirato H, de Tribolet N, eds.), pp. 5–16. New York: Springer Wien.

33. Arens R, Marcus D, Engelberg S *et al*. (1988). Cerebral germinomas and Klinefelter syndrome. *Cancer*. 61:1228–1231.

34. Erdincler P, Lena G, Sarioglu AC *et al*. (1998). Intracranial meningiomas in children: Review of 29 cases. *Surg Neurol*. 49:136–140.

35. Fleury A, Menegoz F, Grosclaude P *et al*. (1997). Descriptive epidemiology of cerebral gliomas in France. *Cancer*. 79:1195–1202.

36. McKinley BP, Michalek AM, Fenstermaker RA, Plunkett RJ. (2000). The impact of age and sex on the incidence of glial tumors in New York state from 1976 to 1995. *J Neurosurg*. 93:932–939.

37. Plunkett RJ, Lis A, Barone TA *et al*. (1999). Hormonal effects on glioblastoma multiforme in the nude rat model. *J Neurosurg*. 90:1072–1077.

38. Yates AJ, Franklin TK, Scheithauer BW *et al*. (1999). Sex- and age-related differences in ceramide dihexosides of primary human brain tumors. *Lipids* 34:1–4.

39. von Schoultz E, Bixo M, Backstrom T *et al*. Sex steroids in human brain tumors and breast cancer. *Cancer*. 65:949–952.

40. Jung-Testas I, Schumacher M, Robel P, Baulieu EE. (1994). Actions of steroid hormones and growth factors on glial cells of the central and peripheral nervous system. *J Steroid Biochem Mol Biol*. 48:145–154.

41. Kasantikul V, Netsky MG, Glasscock ME 3rd, Hays JW. (1980). Acoustic neurilemmoma. Clinicoanatomical study of 103 patients. *J Neurosurg*. 52: 28–35.

42. Stidham KR, Roberson IB Jr. (1999). The effects of estrogen and tamoxifen on growth of human vestibular schwannoma in a nude mouse. *Otolaryngol Head Neck Surg*. 120:262–264.

43. Monsell EM, Wiet RJ. (1990). Estrogen and progesterone binding by acoustic neuroma tissue. *Otolaryngol Head Neck Surg*. 103:377–379.

44. Salvati M, Cervoni L. (1996). Association of breast carcinoma and meningioma: Report of 9 new cases and review of the literature. *Tumori*. 82:491–493.

45. Schoenberg BS, Christine BW, Whisnant JP. (1975). Nervous system neoplasms and primary malignancies of other sites. *Neurology*. 25:705–712.

46. Rubinstein AB, Schein M, Reichenthal E. (1989). The association of carcinoma of the breast with meningioma. *Surg Gynecol Obstet*. 169:334–336.

47. Custer BS, Koepsell TD, Mueller BA. (2002). The association between breast carcinoma and meningioma in women. *Cancer*. 94:1626–1635.

48. Miller RE. (1986). Breast cancer and meningioma. *J Surg Oncol*. 31:182–183.

49. Halper J, Colvard DS, Scheithauer BW *et al*. Estrogen and progesterone receptors in meningiomas: Comparison of nuclear binding, dextran-coated charcoal, and immunoperoxidase staining assays. *Neurosurgery*. 25:546–552.

50. Olson JJ, Beck DW, Schlechte JA, Loh PM. (1986). Hormonal manipulation of meningiomas *in vitro*. *J Neurosurg*. 65:99–107.

51. Grunberg SM, Weiss MH. (1990). Lack of efficacy of megestrol acetatein the treatment of unresectable meningioma. *J Neurooncol*. 8:61–65.

52. Koper JW, Lamberts SW. (1994). Meningiomas, epidermal growth factor and progesterone. *Hum Reprod*. 9(Suppl 1):190–194.

53. Le QT, Weil MD, Wara WM *et al*. (1997). Adult medulloblastoma: An analysis of survival and prognostic factors. *Cancer J Sci Am* 3:238–245.

54. Lambe M, Coogan P, Baron J. (1997). Reproductive factors and the risk of brain tumors: A population-based study in Sweden. *Int J Cancer*. 72:389–393.

55. Haas JF, Janisch W, Staneczek W. (1986). Newly diagnosed primary intracranial neoplasms in pregnant women: A population-based assessment. *J Neurol Neurosurg Psychiatry*. 49:874–880.

56. Couldwell WT, Weiss MH, DeGiorgio CM. (1993). Clinical and radiographic response in a minority of patients with recurrent malignant gliomas treated with high dose tamoxifen. *Neurosurgery*. 32:485–490.

57. Ben Arush MW, Postovsky S, Coldsher D *et al*. (1999). Clinical and radiographic response in three children with recurrent malignant cerebral tumors with high-dose tamoxifen. *Pediatr Hematol Oncol*. 16:245–250.

58. Rao US, Fine RL, Scarborough GA. (1994). Antiestrogens and steroid hormones: Substrates of the human P-glycoprotein. *Biochem Pharmacol*. 48:287–292.

59. Olson JJ, Beck DW, Schlechte JA, Loh PM. (1987). Effect of the antiprogesterone RU-38486 on meningioma implanted into nude mice. *J Neurosurg*. 66: 584–587.

60. Grunberg SM, Weiss MH, Spitz IM *et al*. (1991). Treatment of unresectable meningiomas with the antiprogesterone agent mifepristone. *J Neurosurg*. 74: 861–866.

61. Lamberts SW, Tanghe HL, Avezaat CJ *et al*. (1992). Mifepristone (RU 486) treatment of meningiomas. *J Neurol Neurosurg Psychiatry*. 55:486–490.

62. Haak HR, de Keizer RJ, Hagenouw-Taal JC *et al*. (1990). Successful mifepristone treatment of recurrent, inoperable meningioma. *Lancet*. 336: 124–125.

63

Gender Differences in Hereditary Cancer Syndromes: Risks, Management, and Testing for Inherited Predisposition to Cancer

DONNA RUSSO, MS AND WENDY K. CHUNG, MD, PhD

Columbia University Medical Center, New York, NY

I. Cancer Genetics Overview

The specific cause of cancer in most individuals is largely unknown but likely involves a combination of environmental and inherited genetic factors. For a minority of individuals, there is an inherited predisposition to cancer resulting from a (mono)genetic cancer predisposing mutation with high penetrance or likelihood that an individual will develop disease if he or she has inherited the genetic susceptibility. With advances in the field of human genetics, several of these genes that underlie cancer susceptibility have been identified and clinical diagnostic tests to identify mutations in these genes have been developed. These tests are available to physicians to be used in overall assessment of the risk of an individual's susceptibility to cancer so that an appropriate individualized management plan can be developed for each patient for prevention or early detection of cancer based on individual genetic predisposition. However, predictions for any one individual mutation carrier are limited because of the uncertainty of if, when, or in what organ a cancer may develop because predictions are based on population studies that cannot yet account for all individual variation. Furthermore, many of the hereditary cancers syndromes discussed in this chapter have different manifestations in men and women because they predispose to cancers of organs that are sex specific. In the future, additional genes and important gene environmental interactions will probably be identified to enable better strategies for cancer prevention.

Most individuals who develop cancer do not carry mutations in the inherited cancer genes that are discussed in this chapter. Individuals with mutations in highly penetrant genes can be clinically distinguished on the basis of their strong family history with multiple individuals in multiple generations affected with cancer, early age of onset of cancer, multiple primary cancers in a single individual, and clustering of particular types of cancer within either the individual or the family. In some cases, ethnicity also may be a predisposing factor. Although all ethnic groups have been found to carry mutations in these genes, certain ethnic groups may carry particular founder mutations at higher frequency. In addition to rare but highly penetrant monogenic (single gene) cancer susceptibility syndromes, another 5 to 30% of cancer is familial and likely represents the interaction of a small number of cancer susceptibility genes that in combination with each other and the environment increase the susceptibility to cancer. In families with familial rather than monogenic cancer susceptibility, the age of onset is often older and the number of affected family members is often fewer.

Most highly penetrant inherited cancer susceptibility genes are autosomal dominant. Autosomal dominant conditions are characterized by a 50% chance for both males and females to inherit a mutated gene from a carrier parent; they may pass it on to their children only if they are carriers. Although both males and females may carry a genetic mutation, this mutation may have different disease manifestations or expression in the two genders largely because of anatomic or hormonal differences between the sexes. This may give the appearance of "skipping a generation," if the gene is passed through an individual less likely to express disease (i.e., a male for a breast cancer gene). As discussed in further detail, the cancer spectrum differs by gender in cancer syndromes involving breast, prostate, ovarian, endometrial, and testicular cancer. Regardless of whether an individual manifests disease, individuals can still pass on this mutation to the next generation. This has important implications when taking a family history to assess risk of cancer because susceptibility is equally likely to be inherited through the paternal as the maternal side. For instance, when taking a family history for breast cancer, one should always ask about cases of breast cancer in paternal aunts, cousins, and grandmothers.

Although most cancer susceptibility genes are inherited in an autosomal dominant manner, they act recessively at a cellular level. Most cancer susceptibility genes are tumor suppressor genes that protect the cell from progression to uncontrolled growth. Although an individual has inherited a defect in one of these tumor suppressor genes, as long as the second copy of that gene functions normally, unregulated cell growth will still be suppressed. However, over time, the normal copy of the tumor suppressor gene may become somatically mutated. Such somatic mutations are not in the germline and are not passed down to the next generation, but these somatic mutations allow those somatic cells carrying two mutated genes to begin the process of tumor progression. The two hit hypothesis was originally described by Knudson for retinoblastoma [1], but it is equally relevant to most of the other cancer syndromes that are discussed in this chapter. In the two hit hypothesis, the first hit or mutation is inherited and the second hit is acquired somatically. Because a second somatic mutation must be acquired, an inherited mutation in a tumor suppressor gene greatly increases the likelihood of cancer but does not make it inevitable in many cases.

II. Breast Cancer

A. *Hereditary Breast Cancer Syndromes*

The hereditary breast cancer syndromes account for approximately 5 to 10% of all breast cancer and include a broad group of hereditary predisposition syndromes in which breast cancer is a component tumor. Among the hereditary breast cancers are hereditary breast-ovarian cancer (HBOC) syndrome, Cowden syndrome (CS), Li-Fraumeni syndrome (LFS), Peutz-Jeghers syndrome (PJS), and ataxia telangiectasia (ATM). The National Comprehensive Cancer Network (NCCN) Genetics/Familial High Risk Panel [2] has developed criteria for consideration of a hereditary breast cancer syndrome including (1) multiple cases of breast and/or ovarian cancer in the same individual or in close relatives; (2) clustering of breast cancer with male breast cancer, thyroid cancer, sarcoma, adrenocortical carcinoma, brain tumors, and/or leukemia and lymphoma in the same family; and (3) a member of a family with a known mutation in a breast cancer susceptibility gene. Although hereditary breast cancer syndromes primarily cause breast and ovarian cancer in women, men can be carriers of a cancer susceptibility gene and have increased risks for associated cancers.

1. Hereditary Breast-Ovarian Cancer Syndrome

Hereditary breast-ovarian cancer syndrome has variable expression and can present in families with breast cancer only, ovarian cancer only, or with both breast and ovarian cancers. One should consider HBOC when two or more first-degree relatives have breast and/or ovarian cancer, especially if the cancer onset is in young patients, if there is multifocal or bilateral disease, if breast and ovarian cancer occur in a single individual, and if a case of male breast cancer is present in the family. In addition, Ashkenazi ancestry is associated with a higher prevalence of breast and ovarian cancers resulting from HBOC.

There are two major HBOC cancer susceptibility genes, BRCA1 and BRCA2, both of which are tumor suppressor genes. Mutations in BRCA1 and BRCA2 are characterized by high lifetime risks for development of breast cancer (55 to 85%) and ovarian cancer (20 to 44%), as well as much lower risks of prostate cancer, colon cancer, pancreatic cancer, melanoma, male breast cancer, and other cancers [3,4]. More than 1600 distinct pathogenic mutations, polymorphisms, and variants of unknown significance have been identified in these two genes. There are founder mutations in certain populations, such as the Ashkenazim [5,6], Dutch [7,8], Icelandics [9], and French Canadians [10]. Importantly, one of the three founder mutations in Ashkenazi Jewish individuals, 185delAG and 5382insC in BRCA1 and 6174delT in BRCA2, account for 20 to 35% of early onset breast cancer and ovarian cancer at any age in Ashkenazi individuals [4] as compared with other populations in which germline BRC1/2 mutations were detected in only 5 to 10% of young patients with breast cancer or ovarian cancer [11,12].

DNA-based testing for BRCA1/2 cancer-predisposing mutations is available on a clinical basis for individuals identified by personal or family history to be at increased risk for having a germline BRCA1/2 mutation and for at-risk relatives of an individual with an identified BRCA1/2 mutation. At present, the available clinical testing includes direct sequence analysis of all coding exons and splice sites and analysis of common deletions. Current clinical testing is estimated to be at least 90% sensitive but could theoretically fail to detect intronic or promoter variants that would alter splicing or regulation. Furthermore, mutations of uncertain clinical significance may be identified, especially in minority populations with whom there is less experience to know which variants are benign polymorphisms segregating in the population without functional effects on BRCA1/2.

Given the substantially increased risk of breast, ovarian, and other cancers in HBOC, the management of individuals with BRCA1 or BRCA2 cancer-predisposing mutations includes discussion of enhanced cancer screening protocols, chemoprevention strategies, and options for prophylactic mastectomy and/or salpingo-oophorectomy. None of these strategies has been assessed by randomized clinical trials or case control studies in high-risk women, and current recommendations are made on the basis retrospective studies and clinical opinion.

Recommendations for cancer screening of individuals with a BRCA1 or BRCA2 mutation have been made by a task force convened by the Cancer Genetics Consortium (CGSC), an NIH-sponsored consortium of researchers assessing the ethical, legal, and social implications of genetic testing for cancer risk [13]. The CGSC recommendations for individuals with a BRCA1 or BRCA2 cancer-predisposing mutation are the following:

Breast Cancer Screening
Monthly breast self-examination starting in early adulthood
Semiannual clinical breast examination beginning at age 25 to 35 years
Annual mammography beginning at age 25 to 35 years

Men with BRCA2 cancer-predisposing mutations may also be at increased risk for breast cancer, and evaluation of any breast mass or change is advisable; however, there are insufficient data to recommend a formal program of surveillance.

Ovarian Cancer Screening
Annual or semiannual pelvic examination beginning at age 25 to 35 years
Annual or semiannual transvaginal ultrasound examination with color Doppler beginning at age 25 to 35 years
Annual serum CA-125 concentration beginning at age 25 to 35 years
Colon Cancer Screening
Annual stool occult blood testing beginning at age 50 years
Colonoscopy every 3 to 5 years beginning at age 50 years
Prostate Cancer Screening
Prostate specific antigen (PSA) serum screening
Clinical digital rectal examination usually starting at age 50

Chemoprevention strategies should be discussed with BRCA1/2 mutation carriers. The efficacy of tamoxifen for breast cancer risk reduction in women with BRCA1 or BRCA2 mutations is controversial. Although a randomized clinical trial of treatment with tamoxifen in women identified by the Gail model to have an increased breast cancer risk reported a 49% reduction in breast cancer in the treated group [14], tamoxifen reduced the incidence of breast cancers that were estrogen receptor positive but not estrogen receptor negative. Because breast cancers occurring in women with BRCA1 mutations are more likely to be estrogen receptor negative, it is difficult to estimate the benefit of tamoxifen prophylaxis in BRCA1 carriers. It is however possible that premalignant lesions in BRCA1 carrier are estrogen responsive and amenable to tamoxifen prophylaxis at least at some point during the premalignant phase.

The efficacy of oral contraceptives for ovarian cancer risk reduction in women with BRCA1/2 mutations is unclear. One case control study found a decreased risk of ovarian cancer in women with BRCA1 or BRCA2 carriers who took oral contraceptives for more than 3 years [15]. However, a more recent study did not confirm these findings and raised the concern that oral contraceptive use may increase the risk of breast cancer in women with BRCA1/2 cancer-predisposing mutations [16].

Because early detection does not prevent cancer, it is necessary to discuss the options of risk-reducing surgery including prophylactic mastectomy and prophylactic salpingo-oophorectomy. Tissue removed prophylactically should be carefully examined for malignancy, a finding that could alter medical management. Theoretical modeling and epidemiologic studies suggest that prophylactic surgeries do significantly decrease the risk of developing these cancers by greater than 90% but do not abolish it.

Cancer-predisposing mutations in BRCA1 and BRCA2 are inherited in an autosomal dominant manner; both men and women are equally likely to be mutation carriers. The most informative genetic result in a family is obtained by identifying the specific cancer-predisposing mutation in an affected family member before offering molecular genetic testing to asymptomatic at-risk family members. Without knowing if there is a BRCA1 or BRCA2 mutation segregating in the family, a negative genetic test result in an unaffected family member is ambiguous and cannot be easily interpreted. Therefore, genetic testing within a family should ideally begin with an individual with a history or breast and/or ovarian cancer. If there are multiple members in the family who are affected, the highest yield from the genetic testing is obtained by initially testing the youngest affected family member, an affected family member with breast and ovarian cancer, or an affected family member with bilateral breast cancer. First-degree relatives (parents, children, siblings) of individuals with a BRCA1 or BRCA2 mutations each have an independent 50% chance of inheriting the gene mutation.

2. Cowden Syndrome

Cowden syndrome is a rare cause of hereditary breast cancer characterized by multiple benign hamartomas including the pathognomonic trichilemmoma (a benign tumor of the infundibulum of the hair follicle), breast cancer, and thyroid cancer resulting from autosomal dominantly inherited mutations in the tumor suppressor gene phosphatase and tensin homolog deleted on chromosome ten (PTEN). Other clinical manifestations of CS include acral keratoses, verrucoid or papillomatous papules, goiter or thyroid adenoma, fibrocystic breasts, hamartomatous intestinal polyps, macrocephaly, and uterine leiomyomas. An increase in endometrial cancer has been reported. By age 40, most affected individuals develop the mucocutaneous features of CS. For carriers of PTEN mutations, there is a 3 to 10% lifetime risk of nonmedullary thyroid carcinoma, usually follicular [17,18]. Females with CS have a 67% risk of developing fibrocystic breast disease and a 25 to 50% lifetime risk of developing breast cancer [17,18]. The age of diagnosis of breast cancer approximately is 10 years earlier than average [17,19] but rarely before age 30. The estimated gene frequency for CS is 1 in a million [20], but it has been argued that this may be a gross underestimate resulting from underdiagnosis because of the variable and subtle clinical manifestations [21].

Clinical genetic testing of PTEN is available and can be useful in assessing risk to family members. The most specific clinical feature is trichilemmomas. Families with only thyroid and breast cancers without mucocutaneous lesions have only a 2% probability of having PTEN mutations [22]. PTEN mutations carriers should have annual physical examinations of the thyroid beginning in their late teens and annual breast examinations beginning in their mid 20s. Screening for endometrial cancer should begin at age 35. Annual mammograms and breast ultrasounds should be started at age 30 or 5 years before the earliest breast cancer in the family, whichever is younger.

3. Li-Fraumeni Syndrome

Li-Fraumeni syndrome is another rare cancer syndrome associated with a wide variety of pediatric and adult onset cancers. The clinical criteria for the diagnosis in an individual are bone or soft tissue sarcoma before the age of 45 with a family history significant for a first-degree relative with cancer before the age of 45 and a first- or second-degree relative with cancer before age 45 or sarcoma at any age. The most frequently associated cancers are soft tissue sarcomas and early onset breast cancer, often before the age of 30. Other less frequently occurring tumors include acute leukemias and brain, lung, pancreatic, skin, and adrenocortical tumors. Adrenocortical carcinoma is relatively specific to LFS, and as many as 50% of children with adrenocortical carcinoma even without a family history supportive of LFS have germline mutations in TP53 [23,24]. Three percent of children with osteosarcomas [25] and 9% of children with rhabdosarcomas [26] regardless of family history have inherited TP53 mutations with as many of 50% of those families not yet fulfilling clinical criteria for diagnosis. Cancer often develops in the parent of an affected child after the child has been diagnosed and emphasizes the need to constantly re-evaluate the dynamic family history over time. Affected individuals often have multiple primary cancers [27]. The relative risk of developing a second primary for TP53 carriers is 5.3 with a 57% chance of having a second primary in the 30-year period following diagnosis of the first cancer [27]. This cancer syndrome is autosomal dominantly inherited and is caused by missense mutations in the tumor suppressor gene TP53 that acts as a transcription factor to regulate expression of genes controlling cell growth. The mutation frequency is approximately 1 in 50,000 with a penetrance of 50% by age 30 and 90% by age 60 [28]. Age-specific penetrance is higher for females because of the association with breast cancer. The relative risk of mutation carriers in developing childhood cancer is 100 times the background. Somatic rather than inherited germline mutations of TP53 also commonly occur in a variety of cancers but are not associated with LFS.

Genetic testing for germline mutations in TP53 is available. However, it is currently unclear what effective therapeutic intervention options are available to mutations carriers. The cancers associated with LFS are difficult to cure with the exception of early stage breast cancer, childhood acute lymphoblastic leukemia, and germ cell tumors of the testis. The only effective intervention is increased and earlier surveillance for breast cancer in at-risk women [29]. For that reason, diagnostic genetic testing should be done only after careful genetic counseling to explore the impact of a genetic diagnosis on a given individual.

4. Peutz-Jeghers Syndrome

Peutz-Jeghers syndrome, a rare breast cancer syndrome, is characterized by mucocutaneous melanin pigmentation and intestinal hamartomatous polyposis [30] resulting from autosomal dominantly inherited inactivating mutations in the serine/threonine kinase LKB1. The melanotic pigmentation is seen in and around the mouth, on the hands and feet, and in the axilla. The pigmentation may be mild or even absent in some individuals. More specific are the hamartomatous polyps that have a core of smooth muscle cells with an arborizing pattern that extends to the lamina propria and that have overlying folded epithelium without evidence of neoplasia. Neoplastic changes can arise within these polyps. The numbers of polyps is usually small but can be as many as several dozen. The polyps are usually located in the small intestine and may present as a bowel obstruction. Unlike some of the other oncogenetic associations, the variety of neoplasms associated with PJS is large. Patients with this syndrome are predisposed to a variety of cancers including breast, cervical, ovarian, and gastrointestinal. Benign ovarian and testicular lesions such as granulosa cell tumors and Sertoli cell tumors, respectively, are also more common in patients with PJS [30]. The frequency of the syndrome itself is low (1 in 8300 to 1 in 29,000) [31], making accurate delineation of the clinical features difficult. The rate of de novo mutations is also relatively high, so that not all affected individuals have a significant family history [32]. The lifetime risk of all cancer in carriers is 18-fold higher in women and 6.2-fold higher in men [33].

Genetic testing for germline mutations in LKB1 can be useful in some families because the pigmentation findings are variable and not specific to PJS. There are no highly prevalent founder mutations, and most mutations are specific to the individual family. Once a mutation is identified within the family, other family members can then be genetically tested to stratify risk. At-risk individuals should then be monitored for gastrointestinal, breast, and gynecologic tumors.

5. Ataxia Telangiectasia

Ataxia telangiectasia is an autosomal recessive condition for which carriers may have a slightly higher risk of breast cancer. Ataxia telangiectasia is associated with progressive cerebellar ataxia, ocular apraxia, and telangiectasias in affected individuals. The gene ATM, encodes a large protein kinase and is thought to interact with proteins upstream of p53 in sensing DNA damage associated with double-stranded breaks. The incidence of ATM mutation is 1 in 40,000 live births and, therefore, has a heterozygote ATM mutation carrier frequency of ~1%. All ethnic groups are affected. Female ATM mutation carriers were initially reported to have a 5-fold increase in breast cancer [34,35]. However, subsequent studies have not replicated these initial findings [36–39]. The exact type of mutation, missense or nonsense, may be associated with different cellular phenotypes. It is possible that only missense mutations are associated with increased breast cancer susceptibility through a dominant negative effect [40]. It appears that ATM mutations account for a small proportion of inherited or familial breast cancer but may play a role in the more common apparently sporadic breast cancer that is due to the interaction of environmental factors with many low-penetrance genes.

III. Endometrial and Gastrointestinal Cancer

A. Hereditary Colon Cancer Syndromes

Most individuals with colorectal cancer have sporadic disease without a family history. However, in approximately 20% of individuals with colon cancer there is a definable genetic component [41,42]. Germline mutations conferring high lifetime risk of colorectal cancer account for 5 to 6% of all colorectal cancer cases. The two best defined colorectal cancer genetic syndromes are familial adenomatous polyposis (FAP) and hereditary non-polyposis colorectal cancer (HNPCC).

B. Familial Adenomatous Polyposis

Familial adenomatous polyposis is a colon cancer predisposition syndrome in which hundreds to thousands of precancerous colonic polyps develop, beginning at a mean age of 16 years (range 7 to 36 years) [43]. Seven percent of untreated patients with FAP develop colon cancer by age 21 years, 87% by 45 years, and 93% by 50 years with a mean age of colon cancer diagnosis of 39 years [44]. Associated extracolonic neoplasms include duodenal carcinomas, especially around the ampulla of Vater; follicular or papillary thyroid cancer; childhood hepato-blastoma; gastric carcinoma; and central nervous system tumors, predominantly medulloblastomas. Other benign manifestations include gastric and duodenal polyps, osteomas, dental anomalies, congenital hypertrophy of the retina pigment epithelium (CHRPE), and desmoid tumors [45]. Both sexes are equally affected.

Familial adenomatous polyposis is diagnosed clinically in individuals with greater than 100 colorectal adenomatous polyps or with fewer than 100 adenomatous polyps if there is a family history of FAP. Attenuated FAP is associated with fewer colonic adenomas than seen in classic FAP, and polyps are located predominantly in the proximal colon [46]. Colon cancer risk in attenuated FAP is usually delayed by approximately 12 years relative to classic FAP. Genetic testing is considered standard of care in families with FAP and should be performed in children by the age of 10 to determine if an individual is at risk and should begin screening.

Familial adenomatous polyposis is caused by inherited mutations in the APC gene [47], a tumor suppressor gene with more than 300 different disease-associated mutations [48]. Genetic testing of APC detects up to 95% of disease-causing mutations and is clinically available. Genetic testing is most often used to confirm the clinical diagnosis of FAP and to identify pre-symptomatic carriers in affected families. Protein truncating mutations in the extreme 5' or 3' end of the gene are associated with attenuated FAP [49,50]. Polymorphisms in APC have been identified and one specific missense mutation (Ile1307Lys), found exclusively in Ashkenazi Jewish individuals, results in a 2-fold relative risk of colonic adenomas and adenocarcinomas [51]. In contrast to classic FAP, this polymorphism does not predispose to the polyposis phenotype.

Familial adenomatous polyposis is autosomal dominantly inherited. Approximately 75 to 80% of individuals with FAP have an affected parent, and the mutation can be passed either from the maternal or paternal line. About 25% of cases present represent de novo mutations. Each child of an affected individual has a 50% chance of inheriting the familial mutation.

Early recognition of FAP and attenuated FAP allow for increased surveillance and surgical prophylaxis that improve survival. For this reason, FAP is one of the few cancer syndromes for which genetic testing is appropriate in children. Genetic testing for FAP should be offered to children at age 8 to 10 years before the commencement of colon cancer screening. For attenuated FAP, genetic testing is offered at age 18.

The American Gastroenterological Association [52] recommends surveillance of individuals with a known APC mutation or who are at 50% risk of FAP based on a family history. This surveillance includes the following:

- Annual screening for hepatoblastoma from birth to 5 years of age
- Sigmoidoscopy every 1 to 2 years beginning at age 10 to 12 years
- Colonoscopy once polyps are detected
- Upper endoscopy when colonic polyposis is detected or by age 25 and repeated every 1 to 3 years, the frequency of which is dependent on the severity of duodenal adenomas
- Small bowel x-ray when duodenal adenomas are detected or prior to colectomy, repeated every 1 to 3 years depending on findings and presence of symptoms
- Attention to extraintestinal manifestations
- Annual physical examination including palpation of the thyroid

The recommended surveillance of persons at risk for attenuated FAP includes the following:

- Colonoscopy every 2 to 3 years beginning at 18 to 20 years of age, depending on the number of polyps

Colectomy should be considered when polyps emerge with timing depending on the size and number of adenomatous polyps. For individuals with attenuated FAP, colectomy may ultimately be necessary but may be deferred until polyps become difficult to individually remove.

C. Hereditary Nonpolyposis Colon Cancer

Hereditary nonpolyposis colon cancer or Lynch syndrome is an autosomal dominantly inherited predisposition to colon carcinoma that is not associated with polyposis, unlike FAP.

Table 63-1

Amsterdam Criteria for Hereditary Nonpolyposis Colorectal Cancer

At least three affected relatives with colorectal cancer
At least one is a first-degree relative of the other two
Familial adenomatous polyposis has been excluded
At least two successive generations are affected
One colon cancer occurs before the age of 50

Several other types of cancer can also be associated including endometrial, small intestinal, ovarian, stomach, urinary tract, and brain cancer [53–55]. Lynch syndrome is genetically heterogeneous and involves inactivating mutations in one of several mismatch repair genes including MHS2, MLH1, MSH6, PMS1, and PMS2. Mutations in MSH2 and MLH1 account for 31% and 33% of families with HNPCC, whereas 32% of families have mutations in yet undefined genes [56]. Identification of the underlying genetic basis for HNPCC revealed a new mechanism of cancer progression with hypermutability leading to accumulation of changes in the DNA that ultimately lead to uncontrolled cell growth and division. This hypermutability can be detected in colonic polyps as acquired microsatellite instability (MSI), resulting from mutations of simple repetitive elements (usually dinucleotide repeats) called microsatellites. This hypermutability leaves cells susceptible to the accumulation of pathogenic mutations that ultimately lead to neoplasia. Clinical criteria to make the diagnosis of Lynch syndrome were developed in 1991 and are called the Amsterdam criteria [57] (Table 63-1). The diagnosis relies on an accurate and complete family history. However, these criteria were found to be too restrictive, and they decreased the sensitivity of identifying affected families. The criteria were, therefore, liberalized and these more inclusive criteria are called the Bethesda criteria (Table 63-2). A subset of HNPCC families have HNPCC-associated cancers and sebaceous gland tumors (adenomas, epitheliomas, and carcinomas) and keratoacanthomas and are called the Muir-Torre variant because of mutations in MSH2 [58,59]. Once a clinical diagnosis has been made, genetic testing can be used for risk assessment of unaffected members of the family.

Table 63-2

Betheseda Criteria for Hereditary Nonpolyposis Colorectal Cancer (HNPCC)

Families that meet Amsterdam criteria
Individuals with two HNPCC-related cancers including synchronous or metachronous colorectal cancer or extracolonic cancers including endometrial, ovarian, gastric, hepatobiliary, small bowel, or transitional cell carcinoma of the renal pelvis or ureter
Individuals with colorectal cancer and a first-degree relative with colorectal cancer and/or HNPCC-related extracolonic cancer and/or a colorectal adenoma; one of the cancers diagnosed at age younger than 45, the adenoma at age younger than 40
Individuals with colorectal cancer or endometrial cancer diagnosed at age younger than 45
Individuals with right-sided colorectal cancer with an undifferentiated pattern on histopathology diagnosed at age younger than 45
Individuals with signet ring cell type colorectal cancer diagnosed at age younger than 45
Individuals with adenomas diagnosed at age younger than 40

Expressivity of HNPCC is sex dependent. Men with HNPCC mutations are most likely to develop colon cancer, whereas women with HNPCC mutations are most likely to develop endometrial cancer. The lifetime risk of endometrial cancer has been estimated at 61% and 42% for MSH2 and MHL1 mutations, respectively [60] compared with the population risk of 3%. The median age of endometrial cancer diagnosis is 46 years [53]. The relative risk for other extracolonic HNPCC associated cancers is 4.1 to 4.4 for stomach, 6.4 to 8.0 for ovarian, 103 to 292 for small intestinal, and 75.3 for renal and ureteral [60]. The relative risk varies somewhat depending on the specific gene implicated. Identification of patients with HNPCC is important because of the high probability of a metachronous cancer after successful treatment of the first neoplasm. Surgical treatment of colon cancer should be total colon resection. Presymptomatic mutation carriers should follow a cancer surveillance protocol consisting of colorectal cancer surveillance and endometrial carcinoma screening starting at the age of 25 to 35. There is no consensus about the optimal method of endometrial carcinoma screening, but ultrasound and endometrial biopsy are usually done on an annual basis. Ovarian cancer screening consists of annual CA-125 and transvaginal ultrasound but is not associated with decreased mortality. Therefore, mutation carriers may consider prophylactic total hysterectomy to maximally reduce their cancer risk once childbearing is complete. Screening methods and frequency for other HNPCC-associated cancers has not yet been standardized.

IV. Testicular Cancer

Testicular cancer composes only 2% of all malignancies, but it is the most common type of cancer in men between the ages of 20 to 40 [61]. Several risk factors for testicular cancer have been identified including cryptorchidism, testicular dysgenesis, Klinefelter syndrome, prior history of a germ cell tumor, and a family history of an affected first-degree relative. There is a 6- to 10-fold relative risk of testicular cancer with an affected first-degree relative [62,63], and approximately 2% of all men with germ cell tumors have an affected family member [64]. The familial aggregation of testicular cancer is stronger with a history of an affected sibling rather than an affected father, which suggests that shared environmental contributions in addition to shared genetic factors are important. The International Testicular Cancer Linkage Consortium is working to identify genomic regions of linkage with testicular cancer, but the data to date have demonstrated only suggestive linkages with several chromosomal regions including Xq27–28, 18q22-qter, and 16p13 without clear identification of a major testicular cancer susceptibility locus [64]. Because no genes have been identified that confer high risk of testicular cancer, no clinical genetic testing is currently available for risk assessment.

V. Multiple Endocrine Neoplasia Type 2 (MEN 2)

Multiple endocrine neoplasia type 2 is a rare cancer syndrome associated with medullary thyroid cancer, pheochromocytomas, and parathyroid hyperplasia or adenomas affecting 1 in 30,000 individuals resulting from autosomal dominant inheritance of activating mutations in the oncogene rearranged in transfection (RET), a receptor tyrosine kinase. MEN2 families are characterized by

two or more of these endocrine tumors either in the same individual or in close relatives. Several subtypes of MEN2 have been identified including MEN2A with the clinical features described previously, which accounts for at least 65% of MEN2 families [65]. MEN2B is characterized by an earlier age of onset and more aggressive medullary thyroid cancer; pheochromocytomas; hyperplasia of the intestinal autonomic nerve plexuses; and disorganized growth of peripheral nerve axons in the lips, oral mucosa, and conjunctiva. MEN2B is also autosomal dominantly inherited resulting from mutations in RET. Familial medullary thyroid cancer is associated in some cases with pheochromocytoma and is also associated with mutations in the same RET gene. The location of mutations in RET tend to be specific to the phenotypes of MEN2A, MEN2B, or familial medullary thyroid cancer. The penetrance of MEN2A is approximately 70%, with an initial presentation usually of medullary thyroid cancer [66]. Approximately 50% of subjects with MEN1A develop pheochromocytoma and 5 to 10% develop hyperparathyroidism. MEN2B is characterized by an earlier mean age of onset of medullary thyroid cancer (18 years) and pheochromocytoma (24 years) [67].

Genetic testing of at-risk individuals is clinically available and considered the standard of care. It is imperative that at-risk individuals receive genetic testing before the age of 5 in MEN2A and before the age of 1 in MEN2B to prevent medullary thyroid cancer. Prophylactic total thyroidectomy is performed after the genetic diagnosis is made [68]. Presymptomatic mutation carriers are also followed by annual monitoring of blood pressure, urinary catecholamines, and serum metanephrine for pheochromocytomas and monitoring of serum calcium for evidence of hyperparathyroidism. In addition to testing those families with classic features of MEN2, some have advocated that all patients with medullary thyroid cancer regardless of family history be tested for inherited RET mutations because ~10% of these patients have RET mutations that would predispose them to pheochromocytomas or hyperparathyroidism.

VI. Prostate Cancer

Prostate cancer is the most common noncutaneous cancer and is the second leading cause of cancer death among men [69]. Evidence of an underlying genetic contribution to prostate cancer includes familial clustering and differing prevalence by ethnicity and country of origin [70]. Twenty-five percent of men with prostate cancer report a positive family history. The concordance rate of prostate cancer in monozygotic twins is 0.11 to 0.21 compared with dizygotic twins of only 0.03 to 0.06 [71–73], indicating that prostate cancer is likely a result of interactions of genetic and environmental factors. Prostate cancer is more common in African-American men, and among African-American men there is a higher proportion who present with metastases at diagnosis and a higher cancer-specific mortality [74]. Men with a single first-degree relative (father, brother, or son) with prostate cancer are twice as likely to develop prostate cancer as those without affected close relatives. As the number of affected relatives increases to two and three first-degree relatives, the risk of prostate cancer increases 5- and 11-fold, respectively [75]. Epidemiologic studies suggest that 5 to 10% of all prostate cancers are attributable to highly penetrant susceptibility genes [76].

Although there is clear evidence of a genetic contribution to prostate cancer, identifying those genes conferring increased susceptibility to prostate cancer has been difficult because of the multifactorial nature of the disease. Genetic models assuming a dominant mode of inheritance suggest that 9% of all prostate cancer and 43% of prostate cancer diagnosed before the age of 55 years could be attributable to a single gene with a mutant allele frequency of 0.36 to 1.67% [76,77]. There is evidence of locus heterogeneity for inherited factors with linkage of prostate cancer with several different chromosomal regions. The most significant of the prostate cancer loci identified is hereditary prostate cancer 1 (HPC1) on 1q24–q25 [78] identified as ribonuclease L (RNASEL). Several other susceptibility loci have been identified including on 20q13 [79], 1q42–q43 [80], Xq27–q28 [81], 16q23 [82], and 17p11 [83] leading to the identification ELAC2 as the gene responsible for the linkage on 17p11 [83].

Prostate cancer is seen at low frequency with some inherited cancer syndromes. Although BRCA1 and BRCA2 confer the majority of their cancer risk for breast and ovarian cancer, there have been reports of increased frequency of prostate cancer in men who carry mutations in either of these tumor suppressor genes [4,84,85] with an approximately 3-fold higher lifetime relative risk of developing prostate cancer in mutation-positive males [3] who have an earlier age of onset of prostate cancer. However, on a population-wide basis, the number of cases of prostate cancer attributable to mutations in either BRCA1 or BRCA2 is low. Currently, the only clinical genetic testing that is available for inherited prostate cancer is BRCA1 and BRCA2 testing, although this should change as additional genes are identified.

VII. Cancer Risk Assessment, Counseling, and Testing

With the recent identification of genes for a variety of hereditary cancer syndromes, risk assessment based on individual genetic test results is now feasible. When used appropriately, genetic testing for hereditary cancer facilitates the development of individualized surveillance and prevention strategies for at-risk individuals. However, care must be taken not to misinterpret negative test results to falsely reassure patients regarding risks for cancer in cases in which a familial mutation has not been identified. Currently, most research on the impact of testing for cancer predisposition has focused on hereditary breast/ovarian cancer (HBOC) families and hereditary non-polyposis colon cancer (HNPCC) families. The following section focuses on these two well-described cancer syndromes in relation to the process of genetic counseling. They serve as important models for understanding the medical, sociodemographic, psychologic, and family variables that arise in counseling individuals about increased cancer risks. Although limited research has been done on gender differences in genetic counseling for cancer-predisposing mutations, some preliminary information is available.

A. Genetic Counseling

Genetic counseling translates basic scientific advances into clinically practical and understandable information for patients. Accurate cancer risk assessment requires collection of accurate medical and family history and recognition of patterns of inheritance

and clinical characteristics of cancer syndromes. The National Society of Genetic Counselors has developed practice principles for genetic counseling including respect for autonomy and privacy of the individual, the need for confidentiality and informed consent, and the provision of information to the patient in a nondirective manner [86–88]. In oncogenetics, cancer prevention education is the central goal. Oncogenetic testing should include both pretest and post-test genetic counseling, informed consent, and careful interpretation and explanation of the results. Specialized programs have been developed to provide comprehensive services in cancer genetics (http://www.cancer.gov).

B. Importance of the Family History

The patient's personal history of cancer and a carefully ascertained three-generation family history of cancer remain the key components for identification of hereditary cancer syndromes. Based on this information, one can determine who in the family should be tested, which genes should be tested, and what the best surveillance and management strategy is. For all relatives it is important to document whether they have had any cancer, the primary cancer site(s), the age at diagnosis, the presence of bilaterality or multiple primary tumors, the tumor histology/stage, current age, history of chronic diseases that predispose to cancer (particularly Crohn's disease and ulcerative colitis for colon cancer risk), potential occupational and environmental exposures, age at and cause of death, and ethnic background. To accurately assess the family history often requires contacting multiple family members and obtaining medical records on deceased individuals. It is also important to note pieces of the family history that are unknown and to appreciate the limitations of self-reported family history. It is also important to consider other factors that may confound the pedigree interpretation, such as small family size, premature death because of trauma or war, prophylactic surgery that may mask the presence of a genetic susceptibility, and nonpaternity. Finally, family history is dynamic and changes over time and should be kept current.

The main features of a pedigree that suggest a hereditary cancer syndrome are the following:

- Autosomal dominant pattern of cancer
- A pattern of cancer types associated with a known cancer syndrome
- Early onset cancer
- Multiple relatives with the same or associated cancers
- Bilateral cancer or multiple primary cancers in the same individual
- Rare cancers, such as male breast cancer

In addition to assessing the family risk, the pedigree can also be important in identifying unaffected members who would benefit from enhanced cancer surveillance.

Before the advent of genetic testing, the diagnosis of a hereditary cancer syndrome was made on the basis of established clinical criteria and all at-risk relatives would be advised to have screening for the development of the cancers associated with the cancer syndrome. Now when a mutation is identified within a family, genetic testing allows accurate, relatively inexpensive risk stratification by differentiating presymptomatic genetic carriers from noncarriers who have no increased risk of cancer. It is important to note, however, that some families that meet the clinical criteria of a cancer syndrome may not have a detectable mutation because their cancer syndrome is caused by a mutation in an undiscovered gene or because the current testing method is not able to detect all mutations.

C. Genetic Testing

Several medical organizations have offered guidelines that support genetic testing for cancer risk. Some of these include the American Society of Clinical Oncology [89], the American College of Medical Genetics [90], the American Society of Human Genetics [90], and the American Gastroenterological Association [52]. Genetic testing offers many benefits, but, because of the inherent challenges, the following critical recommendations should be followed:

- Pretest genetic counseling and written informed consent should proceed genetic testing
- An *affected* individual should be the first in the family to be tested, whenever possible
- Genetic testing should be offered to families with a substantial pretest probability of carrying a mutation and used only when the results will influence the clinical management of the patient or family member
- The test must be interpretable

D. Informed Consent

The American Society of Clinical Oncology has identified essential elements to be discussed in conjunction with written informed consent for genetic testing [89]. First, information should be provided about the specific test being performed and the implications of a positive, a negative, and an uninformative result. Second, education about the medical aspects of the disorder, the mode of inheritance, cancer risks associated with a positive genetic test result, and the options and limitations of medical surveillance and screening should be provided. Third, the risks of genetic testing should be discussed, including short- and long-term psychologic effects of having a positive genetic test, the risk of insurance and employment discrimination, and patient confidentiality. Fourth, the technical accuracy of the test and the cost of genetic counseling and genetic testing should be explained. In addition, the Cancer Genetics Studies Consortium stresses that genetic professionals should assist patients in exploring their beliefs, values, and experiences with the disorder in the family.

E. Hereditary Breast-Ovarian Cancer Syndrome

Although it is clear that genetic testing for cancer risk has potential benefits for carefully selected and counseled patients and family members, it also has the potential to increase anxiety or depression and negatively affect family relationships [91]. Much of initial understanding of interest and use of predictive genetic testing comes from research studies that have offered BRCA1 and/or BRCA2 testing to persons in HBOC families. Studying HBOC families, Biesecker *et al* [49] reported that

55% of eligible relatives contacted by letter and telephone chose to participate in the education and counseling and to have BRCA1/2 testing. Most studies suggest that individuals seeking predictive genetic testing for BRCA1/2 are female and in their early to mid 40s [92,93].

In general, studies have shown that both unaffected women with a family history of breast or ovarian cancer and women affected with these cancers greatly overestimate their risk for breast cancer [94–96]. Young unaffected women experience more psychologic burden. Perception of personal breast cancer risk was nearly twice as high for unaffected women as compared with perceived risk before the diagnosis for the affected women (59% vs 31%), even with similar family histories [97]. Not surprisingly, a higher perception of risk is related to the expectation of being a gene carrier, which is overestimated before counseling. However, following genetic counseling the perception of cancer risk is markedly reduced [98]. Men usually seek genetic testing for HBOC for the sake of their children and are often referred by a family member, whereas females more often seek testing to manage their own clinical care and to reduce anxiety. Most men believe that they were at increased risk of development of cancer (prostate, breast, colorectal, and skin cancer), and, similar to their female counterparts, more than half (55%) had intrusive thoughts about their cancer risk [99].

F. Hereditary Nonpolyposis Colon Cancer

Analogous to benefits in families with BRCA1/2, the absence or presence of a HNPCC mutation is of considerable medical and psychologic significance. Importantly, patients with a predisposing mutation can benefit from a medical surveillance program that has been shown to reduce the risk of developing colorectal cancer and decrease the overall mortality by 65% [100,101]. In contrast to cancer risks in BRCA1/2 that predominantly affect female mutation carriers, HNPCC associated cancer risks affect both male and female mutation carriers. A recent study of 18 clinically ascertained HNPCC families (523 subjects) with identified mutations showed that slightly more women than men (62% vs 51%) sought genetic testing, which may reflect the additional risk for endometrial cancer in female mutation carriers [102].

G. Psychologic Issues

The potential adverse psychologic impact of genetic testing for hereditary cancer susceptibility is of great concern; however, there are scarce data to address this issue. Members of families with hereditary cancer syndromes often have been faced with close relatives who have died of cancer, sometimes at a young age. Knowledge of being at high risk of cancer has been associated with anxiety or depression [103] and the possibility of predisposition testing may add further psychologic burden. To date, studies performed worldwide on ethnically diverse populations show that genetic counseling and testing for BRCA1/2 gene mutations can be performed without a significant increase in anxiety and distress [96,104–108]. There were some initial concerns that genetic test results might negatively affect insurability, but there is now federal and state legislation in place to protect members of group health plans from having individually assessed health insurance rates or coverage determined on the basis of genetic predisposition.

VIII. Conclusion

During the last decade there have been major advances in clinical oncogenetics, and genetic testing for several hereditary cancer syndromes is now the standard of care. Recognizing the clues of hereditary cancer susceptibility can have lifesaving potential for the patient and at-risk relatives by developing an enhanced surveillance and/or preventive or therapeutic interventions based on the underlying genetic cancer predisposition. Additional cancer susceptibility genes including those that account for the less penetrant but more common familial cancer susceptibility are likely to be identified allowing for more accurate risk assessment and cancer prevention.

References

1. Hethcote HW, Knudson AG Jr. (1978). Model for the incidence of embryonal cancers: Application to retinoblastoma. *Proc Natl Acad Sci U S A.* 75:2453–2457.
2. Network NC. (1999). NCCN practice guidelines: Genetics. Familial high risk cancer. *Oncology.* 13:161–186.
3. Ford D, Easton DF, Bishop DT *et al.* (1994). Risks of cancer in BRCA1-mutation carriers. Breast Cancer Linkage Consortium. *Lancet.* 343:692–695.
4. Struewing JP, Hartge P, Wacholder S *et al.* (1997). The risk of cancer associated with specific mutations of BRCA1 and BRCA2 among Ashkenazi Jews. *N Engl J Med.* 336:1401–1408.
5. Roa BB, Boyd AA, Volcik K, Richards CS. (1996). Ashkenazi Jewish population frequencies for common mutations in BRCA1 and BRCA2. *Nat Genet.* 14:185–187.
6. Oddoux C, Struewing JP, Clayton CM *et al.* (1996). The carrier frequency of the BRCA2 6174delT mutation among Ashkenazi Jewish individuals is approximately 1%. *Nat Genet.* 14:188–190.
7. Petrij-Bosch A, Peelen T, van Vliet M *et al.* (1997). BRCA1 genomic deletions are major founder mutations in Dutch breast cancer patients. *Nat Genet.* 17:341–345.
8. Verhoog LC, Berns EM, Brekelmans CT *et al.* (2000). Prognostic significance of germline BRCA2 mutations in hereditary breast cancer patients. *J Clin Oncol.* 18(21 Suppl):119S–24S.
9. Thorlacius S, Olafsdottir G, Tryggvadottir L *et al.* (1996). A single BRCA2 mutation in male and female breast cancer families from Iceland with varied cancer phenotypes. *Nat Genet.* 13:117–119.
10. Tonin PN, Mes-Masson AM, Futreal PA *et al.* (1998). Founder BRCA1 and BRCA2 mutations in French Canadian breast and ovarian cancer families. *Am J Hum Genet.* 63:1341–1351.
11. Couch FJ, DeShano ML, Blackwood MA *et al.* (1997). BRCA1 mutations in women attending clinics that evaluate the risk of breast cancer. *N Engl J Med.* 336:1409–1415.
12. FitzGerald MG, MacDonald DJ, Krainer M *et al.* (1996). Germ-line BRCA1 mutations in Jewish and non-Jewish women with early-onset breast cancer. *N Engl J Med.* 334:143–149.
13. Burke W, Daly M, Garber J *et al.* (1997). Recommendations for follow-up care of individuals with an inherited predisposition to cancer. II. BRCA1 and BRCA2. Cancer Genetics Studies Consortium. *JAMA.* 277:997–1003.
14. Fisher B, Costantino JP, Wickerham DL *et al.* (1998). Tamoxifen for prevention of breast cancer: Report of the National Surgical Adjuvant Breast and Bowel Project P-1 Study. *J Natl Cancer Inst.* 90:1371–1388.
15. Narod SA, Risch H, Moslehi R *et al.* (1998). Oral contraceptives and the risk of hereditary ovarian cancer. Hereditary Ovarian Cancer Clinical Study Group. *N Engl J Med.* 339:424–428.
16. Modan B, Hartge P, Hirsh-Yechezkel G *et al.* (2001). Parity, oral contraceptives, and the risk of ovarian cancer among carriers and noncarriers of a BRCA1 or BRCA2 mutation. *N Engl J Med.* 345:235–240.
17. Starink TM, van der Veen JP, Arwert F *et al.* (1986). The Cowden syndrome: A clinical and genetic study in 21 patients. *Clin Genet.* 29:222–233.
18. Hanssen AM, Fryns JP. (1995). Cowden syndrome. *J Med Genet.* 32:117–119
19. Longy M, Lacombe D. (1996). Cowden disease. Report of a family and review. *Ann Genet.* 39:35–42.
20. Nelen MR, Padberg GW, Peeters EA *et al.* (1996). Localization of the gene for Cowden disease to chromosome 10q22–23. *Nat Genet.* 13:114–116.
21. Haibach H, Burns TW, Carlson HE *et al.* (1992). Multiple hamartoma syndrome (Cowden's disease) associated with renal cell carcinoma and primary neuroendocrine carcinoma of the skin (Merkel cell carcinoma). *Am J Clin Pathol.* 97:705–712.
22. Marsh DJ, Dahia PL, Caron S *et al.* (1998). Germline PTEN mutations in Cowden syndrome-like families. *J Med Genet.* 35:881–885.
23. Sameshima Y, Tsunematsu Y, Watanabe S *et al.* (1992). Detection of novel germ-line p53 mutations in diverse-cancer-prone families identified by selecting patients with childhood adrenocortical carcinoma. *J Natl Cancer Inst.* 84:703–707.
24. Wagner J, Portwine C, Rabin K *et al.* (1994). High frequency of germline p53 mutations in childhood adrenocortical cancer. *J Natl Cancer Inst.* 86:1707–1710.
25. McIntyre JF, Smith-Sorensen B, Friend SH *et al.* (1994). Germline mutations of the p53 tumor suppressor gene in children with osteosarcoma. *J Clin Oncol.* 12:925–930.
26. Diller L, Sexsmith E, Gottlieb A *et al.* (1995). Germline p53 mutations are frequently detected in young children with rhabdomyosarcoma. *J Clin Invest.* 95:1606–1611.
27. Draper GJ, Sanders BM, Kingston JE. (1986). Second primary neoplasms in patients with retinoblastoma. *Br J Cancer.* 53:661–671.
28. Williams WR, Strong LC. (1985). Genetic epidemiology of soft tissue sarcomas in children. In *Familial Cancer. First International Research Conference on Familial Cancer* (Muller H, Weber W, eds.). Basel, Karger.
29. Shapiro S. (1989). Determining the efficacy of breast cancer screening. *Cancer.* 63:1873–1880.
30. Phillips RS, Spigelman AD, Thompons JPS. (1994). *Familial Adenomatous Polyposis and Other Polyposis Syndromes.* London, Edward Arnold.
31. Finan MC, Ray MK. (1989). Gastrointestinal polyposis syndromes. *Dermatol Clin.* 7:419–434.
32. Westerman AM, Entius MM, Boor PP *et al.* (1999). Novel mutations in the LKB1/STK11 gene in Dutch Peutz-Jeghers families. *Hum Mutat.* 13:476–481.
33. Boardman LA, Thibodeau SN, Schaid DJ *et al.* (1998). Increased risk for cancer in patients with the Peutz-Jeghers syndrome. *Ann Intern Med.* 128: 896–899.
34. Swift M, Morrell D, Massey RB, Chase CL. (1991). Incidence of cancer in 161 families affected by ataxia-telangiectasia. *N Engl J Med.* 325:1831–1836.
35. Swift M, Reitnauer PJ, Morrell DJ, Chase CL. (1987). Breast and other cancers in families with ataxia-telangiectasia. *N Engl J Med.* 316:1289–1894.
36. Vorechovsky I, Rasio D, Luo L *et al.* (1996). The ATM gene and susceptibility to breast cancer: Analysis of 38 breast tumors reveals no evidence for mutation. *Cancer Res.* 56:2726–2732.
37. FitzGerald MG, Bean JM, Hegde SR *et al.* (1997). Heterozygous ATM mutations do not contribute to early onset of breast cancer. *Nat Genet.* 15:307–310.
38. Bay JO, Grancho M, Pernin D *et al.* (1998). No evidence for constitutional ATM mutation in breast/gastric cancer families. *Int J Oncol.* 12:1385–1390.
39. Chen J, Birkholtz GG, Lindblom P *et al.* (1998). The role of ataxia-telangiectasia heterozygotes in familial breast cancer. *Cancer Res.* 58: 1376–1379.
40. Gatti RA, Tward A, Concannon P. (1999). Cancer risk in ATM heterozygotes: A model of phenotypic and mechanistic differences between missense and truncating mutations. *Mol Genet Metab.* 68:419–423.
41. (2002). *Cancer Facts and Figures.* Atlanta, GA: American Cancer Society.
42. Burt RWPG. (1996). Familial Colorectal Cancer: Diagnosis and Management. In *Prevention of Early Colorectal Cancer* (Young CP, Rozen P, Levin B, eds.), pp. 171–194. London: WB Saunders.
43. Petersen GM, Slack J, Nakamura Y. (1991). Screening guidelines and premorbid diagnosis of familial adenomatous polyposis using linkage. *Gastroenterology.* 100:1658–1664.
44. Bussey H. (1975). *Familial Polyposis Coli. Family Studies, Histopathology, Differential Diagnosis and Results of Treatment.* Baltimore, Johns Hopkins University Press.
45. Burt RW. (2000). Colon cancer screening. *Gastroenterology.* 119:837–853.
46. Lynch HT, Smyrk TC, Watson P *et al.* (1992). Hereditary flat adenoma syndrome: A variant of familial adenomatous polyposis? *Dis Colon Rectum.* 35:411–421.
47. Kinzler KW, Nilbert MC, Su LK *et al.* (1991). Identification of FAP locus genes from chromosome 5q21. *Science.* 253:661–665.

48. Laurent-Puig P, Beroud C, Soussi T. (1998). APC gene: Database of germline and somatic mutations in human tumors and cell lines. *Nucleic Acids Res.* 26(1):269–270.

49. Biesecker BB, Ishibe N, Hadley DW *et al.* (2000). Psychosocial factors predicting BRCA1/BRCA2 testing decisions in members of hereditary breast and ovarian cancer families. *Am J Med Genet.* 93:257–263.

50. Giardiello FM, Brensinger JD, Luce MC *et al.* (1997). Phenotypic expression of disease in families that have mutations in the 5′ region of the adenomatous polyposis coli gene. *Ann Intern Med.* 126:514–519.

51. Laken SJ, Petersen GM, Gruber SB *et al.* (1997). Familial colorectal cancer in Ashkenazim due to a hypermutable tract in APC. *Nat Genet.* 17:79–83.

52. American Gastroenterological Association medical position statement: Hereditary colorectal cancer and genetic testing. (2001). *Gastroenterology.* 121:195–197.

53. Lynch HT, Lanspa S, Smyrk T *et al.* (1991). Hereditary nonpolyposis colorectal cancer (Lynch syndromes I & II). Genetics, pathology, natural history, and cancer control, Part I. *Cancer Genet Cytogenet.* 53:143–160.

54. Lynch HT, Ens J, Lynch JF, Watson P. (1988). Tumor variation in three extended Lynch syndrome II kindreds. *Am J Gastroenterol.* 83:741–747.

55. Vasen HF, Offerhaus GJ, den Hartog Jager FC *et al.* (1990). The tumour spectrum in hereditary non-polyposis colorectal cancer: A study of 24 kindreds in the Netherlands. *Int J Cancer.* 46:31–4.

56. Leach FS, Nicolaides NC, Papadopoulos N *et al.* (1993). Mutations of a mutS homolog in hereditary nonpolyposis colorectal cancer. *Cell.* 75:1215–1225.

57. Vasen HF, Mecklin J-P, Khan PM. (1991). The international collaborative group on hereditary non-polyposis colorectal cancer. *Dis Colon Rectum.* 34:424–428.

58. Honchel R, Halling KC, Schaid DJ *et al.* (1994). Microsatellite instability in Muir-Torre syndrome. *Cancer Res.* 54:1159–1163.

59. Kolodner RD, Hall NR, Lipford J *et al.* (1994). Structure of the human MSH2 locus and analysis of two Muir-Torre kindreds for msh2 mutations. *Genomics.* 24:516–526.

60. Vasen HF, Wijnen J, Menko F. (1996). Cancer risk in families with non-polyposis colorectal cancer diagnosed by mutation analysis. *Gastroenterology.* 110:1020–1028.

61. Schottenfeld DaWM. (1982). Testis. In *Cancer Epidemiology and Prevention* (Schalenfeld D, Fraumeni JF, eds.). London, WB Saunders, p. 947–957.

62. Forman D, Oliver RT, Brett AR *et al.* (1992). Familial testicular cancer: A report of the UK family register, estimation of risk and an HLA class 1 sib-pair analysis. *Br J Cancer.* 65:255–262.

63. Heimdal K, Lothe RA, Lystad S *et al.* (1993). No germline TP53 mutations detected in familial and bilateral testicular cancer. *Genes Chromosomes Cancer.* 6(2):92–97.

64. International Testicular Cancer Linkage Consortium. (1998). Candidate region for testicular cancer susceptibility genes. *Acta Pathol Microbiol Immunol Schand.* 106:64–72.

65. Eng C, Clayton D, Schuffenecker I *et al.* (1996). The relationship between specific RET proto-oncogene mutations and disease phenotype in multiple endocrine neoplasia type 2. International RET mutation consortium analysis. *JAMA.* 276:1575–1579.

66. Easton DF, Ponder MA, Cummings T *et al.* (1989). The clinical and screening age-at-onset distribution for the MEN-2 syndrome. *Am J Hum Genet.* 44:208–215.

67. Vasen HF, Nieuwenhuijzen Kruseman AC, Berkel H *et al.* (1987). Multiple endocrine neoplasia syndrome type 2: The value of screening and central registration. A study of 15 kindreds in The Netherlands. *Am J Med.* 83:847–852.

68. Gagel RF, Tashjian AH Jr, Cummings T *et al.* 1988. The clinical outcome of prospective screening for multiple endocrine neoplasia type 2a. An 18-year experience. *N Engl J Med.* 318:478–484.

69. Landis SH, Murray T, Bolden S, Wingo PA. (1999). Cancer statistics, 1999. *CA Cancer J Clin.* 49:8–31, 1.

70. Pienta KJ, Esper PS. (1993). Risk factors for prostate cancer. *Ann Intern Med.* 118:793–803.

71. Lichtenstein P, Holm NV, Verkasalo PK *et al.* (2000). Environmental and heritable factors in the causation of cancer—Analyses of cohorts of twins from Sweden, Denmark, and Finland. *N Engl J Med.* 343:78–85.

72. Ahlbom A, Lichtenstein P, Malmstrom H *et al.* (1997). Cancer in twins: Genetic and nongenetic familial risk factors. *J Natl Cancer Inst.* 89:287–293.

73. Verkasalo PK, Kaprio J, Koskenvuo M, Pukkala E. (1999). Genetic predisposition, environment and cancer incidence: A nationwide twin study in Finland, 1976–1995. *Int J Cancer.* 83:743–749.

74. Wingo PA, Bolden S, Tong T *et al.* (1996). Cancer statistics for African Americans, 1996. *CA Cancer J Clin.* 46:113–125.

75. Walsh PC, Partin AW. (1997). Family history facilitates the early diagnosis of prostate carcinoma. *Cancer.* 80:1871–1874.

76. Carter BS, Beaty TH, Steinberg GD *et al.* (1992). Mendelian inheritance of familial prostate cancer. *Proc Natl Acad Sci U S A.* 89:3367–3371.

77. Gronberg H, Damber L, Damber JE, Iselius L. (1997). Segregation analysis of prostate cancer in Sweden: Support for dominant inheritance. *Am J Epidemiol.* 146:552–557.

78. Smith JR, Freije D, Carpten JD *et al.* (1996). Major susceptibility locus for prostate cancer on chromosome 1 suggested by a genome-wide search. *Science.* 274:1371–1374.

79. Berry R, Schroeder JJ, French AJ *et al.* (2000). Evidence for a prostate cancer-susceptibility locus on chromosome 20. *Am J Hum Genet.* 67:82–91.

80. Berthon P, Valeri A, Cohen-Akenine A *et al.* (1998). Predisposing gene for early-onset prostate cancer, localized on chromosome 1q42.2–43. *Am J Hum Genet.* 62:1416–1424.

81. Xu J, Meyers D, Freije D *et al.* (1998). Evidence for a prostate cancer susceptibility locus on the X chromosome. *Nat Genet.* 20:175–179.

82. Suarez BK, Lin J, Burmester JK *et al.* (2000). A genome screen of multiplex sibships with prostate cancer. *Am J Hum Genet.* 66:933–944.

83. Tavtigian SV, Simard J, Teng DH *et al.* (2001). A candidate prostate cancer susceptibility gene at chromosome 17p. *Nat Genet.* 27:172–180.

84. Sigurdsson S, Thorlacius S, Tomasson J *et al.* (1997). BRCA2 mutation in Icelandic prostate cancer patients. *J Mol Med.* 75:758–761.

85. Easton DF, Steele L, Fields P *et al.* (1997). Cancer risks in two large breast cancer families linked to BRCA2 on chromosome 13q12–13. *Am J Hum Genet.* 61:120–128.

86. Kessler S. (1979). The Psychological Foundations of Genetic Counseling. In *Genetic Counseling: Psychological Dimensions.* Baltimore: Academic Press.

87. McKinnon WC, Baty BJ, Bennett RL *et al.* (1997). Predisposition genetic testing for late-onset disorders in adults. A position paper of the National Society of Genetic Counselors. *JAMA.* 278:1217–1220.

88. Fine B, Baker D, Fiddler MB. (1996). Practice-based competencies for accreditation of training in graduate programs in genetic counseling. *J Genet Counsel.* 5(3):113–122.

89. Statement of the American Society of Clinical Oncology: Genetic testing for cancer susceptibility. (1996). *J Clin Oncol.* 14(5):1730–1736.

90. Genetic testing for colon cancer: Joint statement of the American College of Medical Genetics and American Society of Human Genetics 2000. Joint Test and Technology Transfer Committee Working Group. (2000). *Genet Med.* 2(6):362–366.

91. Lerman C, Croyle R. (1994). Psychological issues in genetic testing for breast cancer susceptibility. *Arch Intern Med.* 154:609–616.

92. Lerman C, Schwartz MD, Lin TH *et al.* (1997). The influence of psychological distress on use of genetic testing for cancer risk. *J Consult Clin Psychol.* 65:414–420.

93. Reichelt JG, Dahl AA, Heimdal K, Moller P. (1999). Uptake of genetic testing and pre-test levels of mental distress in Norwegian families with known BRCA1 mutations. *Dis Markers.* 15(1–3):139–143.

94. Smith BL, Gadd MA, Lawler C *et al.* (1996). Perception of breast cancer risk among women in breast center and primary care settings: Correlation with age and family history of breast cancer. *Surgery.* 120:297–303.

95. Bluman LG, Rimer BK, Berry DA *et al.* (1999). Attitudes, knowledge, and risk perceptions of women with breast and/or ovarian cancer considering testing for BRCA1 and BRCA2. *J Clin Oncol.* 17:1040–1046.

96. Watson M, Lloyd S, Davidson J *et al.* (1999). The impact of genetic counselling on risk perception and mental health in women with a family history of breast cancer. *Br J Cancer.* 79:868–874.

97. MacDonald DJCJ, Ferrell B. (2000). Concerns of women presenting to a comprehensive cancer centre for genetic cancer risk assessment. *J Med Genet.* 39:526–530.

98. Bish A, Sutton S, Jacobs C *et al.* (2002). Changes in psychological distress after cancer genetic counselling: A comparison of affected and unaffected women. *Br J Cancer.* 86:43–50.

99. Liede A, Metcalfe K, Hanna D *et al.* (2000). Evaluation of the needs of male carriers of mutations in BRCA1 or BRCA2 who have undergone genetic counseling. *Am J Hum Genet.* 67:1494–1504.

100. Jarvinen HJ, Aarnio M, Mustonen H *et al.* (2000). Controlled 15-year trial on screening for colorectal cancer in families with hereditary nonpolyposis colorectal cancer. *Gastroenterology.* 118:829–834.

101. Renkonen-Sinisalo L, Aarnio M, Mecklin JP, Jarvinen HJ. (2000). Surveillance improves survival of colorectal cancer in patients with hereditary non-polyposis colorectal cancer. *Cancer Detect Prev.* 24:137–142.

102. Wagner A, Tops C, Wijnen JT *et al.* (2002). Genetic testing in hereditary non-polyposis colorectal cancer families with a MSH2, MLH1, or MSH6 mutation. *J Med Genet.* 39:833–837.

103. Lerman C, Daly M, Masny A, Balshem A. (1994). Attitudes about genetic testing for breast-ovarian cancer susceptibility. *J Clin Oncol.* 12:843–850.

104. Lerman C, Narod S, Schulman K *et al.* (1996). BRCA1 testing in families with hereditary breast-ovarian cancer. A prospective study of patient decision making and outcomes. *JAMA.* 275:1885–1892.

105. Croyle RT, Smith KR, Botkin JR *et al.* (1997). Psychological responses to BRCA1 mutation testing: Preliminary findings. *Health Psychol.* 16:63–72.

106. DudokdeWit AC, Tibben A, Frets PG *et al.* (1997). BRCA1 in the family: A case description of the psychological implications. *Am J Med Genet.* 71:63–71.

107. Wood ME, Mullineaux L, Rahm AK *et al.* (2000). Impact of BRCA1 testing on women with cancer: A pilot study. *Genet Test.* 4:265–272.

108. Broadstock M, Michie S, Marteau T. (2000). Psychological consequences of predictive genetic testing: A systematic review. *Eur J Hum Genet.* 8:731–738.

64
Cancer Screening

NASEEM ZOJWALLA, MD, DAVID FOGELMAN, MD, AND ALFRED I. NEUGUT, MD, PhD

Department of Medicine and the Herbert Irving Comprehensive Cancer Center, College of Physicians and Surgeons;
Department of Epidemiology, Mailman School of Public Health, Columbia University, New York, NY

I. Introduction

Cancer is the second leading cause of mortality in the United States after heart disease [1]. Prevention and early detection through screening can have a major impact on the fight against cancer. Cancer-screening guidelines are targeted toward both sex-specific and common cancers.

Gender differences in the screening guidelines of all cancers exist and can be explained by various factors. Female gender necessitates physician visits for certain nonmale issues, such as menstrual disorders, contraception, and pregnancy. Thus, women are more likely to see physicians, either for acute and chronic illnesses or for regular check-ups [2]. Because of this greater use of medical practitioners, cancer screening is easier to implement in the female population. Also, many of the cancer screening guidelines are geared toward female cancers—cervical, breast, and ovarian—whereas only prostate cancer screening is specifically directed toward the male population. Colorectal cancer screening is targeted toward both genders. However, women often encounter more barriers to health care, including access to care and gender discrimination [3]. This can affect adherence to screening practices.

The most important predictive factor in whether an individual has ever been screened is a recommendation from his or her health care provider. Studies have found that the sex of the physician influences recommendations for preventive care [4–7]. Lurie et al [8], in a large study of people enrolled in a Midwestern health plan, investigated differences between male and female physicians in the frequency of screening mammograms and Papanicolaou smears among their female patients. They found that women were more likely to undergo screening with Papanicolaou smears and mammograms if the women's physicians were female rather than male, particularly if the physicians were internists or family practitioners as opposed to obstetrician/ gynecologists.

Why do the female patients of female physicians have higher screening rates than the female patients of male physicians, or why do women have greater likelihood to get screened if they see a female physician? The same research group found that female physicians were more likely to inquire and implement preventive care and to promote mammography and reported more comfort in performing Papanicolaou smears and breast examinations [9]. Male physicians may be more uncomfortable with the examination of women's reproductive organs or with discussing issues related to sexuality and, therefore, more uneasy offering cancer-screening tests. They may also be concerned about accusations of sexual harassment and, thus,

less likely to perform Papanicolaou smears or clinical breast examinations.

Although male patients often prefer same-sex physicians [10], female patients tend to gravitate toward female physicians [11,12] because they are embarrassed to have male physicians perform screening tests such as Papanicolaou smears or clinical breast examinations [13]. These attitudes contribute to the higher screening rates by female physicians in female patients.

It is important for physicians of both genders to encourage all their patients to be screened regularly for cancer. Tools that have been shown to improve screening rates include flowsheets, chart reminders, computerized tracking, reminder systems, and aggressive follow-up [14–20]. Clinicians should remain up to date about the benefits and risks associated with various screening strategies so that they can provide patients with accurate and complete information to facilitate fully informed decision making.

II. Cancer Screening

In general, the appropriateness of any particular screening protocol is dependent on the natural history and biologic characteristics of a particular malignancy or its premalignant counterpart and on the efficacy of the test being used to screen for the cancer. Cancers that are ideally suited for screening are those with a recognizable presymptomatic latent stage that, if treated, favorably affects outcome and results in decreased mortality [21].

Although survival from the time of diagnosis of the disease is commonly reported in screening trials, this can be misleading because it is subject to lead-time bias, length-time bias, selection bias, and overdiagnosis bias. Lead-time bias occurs because the diagnosis of the disease is made earlier in the screened group, resulting in an apparent increase in survival time, although the time of death may not be affected. Length-time bias occurs because slower growing tumors have a longer potential detection period and are more likely to be detected when they are asymptomatic. As a result, a higher proportion of indolent tumors are usually found in the screened group, causing an apparent improvement in survival.

People who choose to participate in screening programs (volunteers) are likely to be different from the general population in that they are more likely to be health conscious than those who do not enter programs. Therefore, they are more likely to have a better outcome from their disease than the general population, resulting in selection bias. Overdiagnosis bias occurs when cancers are diagnosed in individuals who would not have presented with clinical symptoms during their lifetimes in the absence of screening [22].

Cancer screening should lead to effective treatment at the pre-clinical (asymptomatic) stage to reduce mortality in the screened group as compared with the unscreened group. The sensitivity, specificity, accessibility, cost, and associated morbidity of the screening tests must be reasonable and screening protocols should include tests that are cost-effective, sensitive, specific, and have acceptable positive and negative predictive values when applied to population-based screening (Table 64-1).

III. Cervical Cancer

Cervical cancer is the second most common cancer among women worldwide. In the United States, it is estimated that there will be 12,200 new cases of cervical cancer and 4100 deaths from cervical cancer in the year 2003 [23]. Risk factors for cervical cancer include early onset of sexual activity, multiple sexual partners, cigarette smoking, human immunodeficiency virus (HIV) infection, and infection with certain human papilloma-virus (HPV) strains.

Cervical cancer lends itself to screening because it has a long preinvasive stage that is easily detectable with a simple test [24]. Since the introduction of the Papanicolaou smear, a dramatic decrease has been observed in cervical cancer inci-dence and mortality in the United States. This is attributable to the ability of the Papanicolaou smear to identify precancerous changes and the availability of a number of effective local treatments.

The Papanicolaou test was introduced in the 1930's by Dr. George Papanicolaou. The Papanicolaou test is inexpensive, widely available, easily performed, and both specific and sensitive. The effectiveness of Papanicolaou screening has been demonstrated in case-control and cohort studies. A major study in Iceland reported declines in both the incidence and mortality of invasive cervical cancer after the introduction in 1964 of screening programs [25]. Case-control studies from Italy, Colombia, and Denmark all found decreases in invasive cervical cancer incidence, ranging from 60 to 90% [24]; Clarke and Anderson [26] in Toronto found a two-thirds decrease in incidence among women who had been screened with Papani-colaou smears compared with women who had not. Similarly, cervical cancer mortality in the United States decreased by 70% between 1947 and 1984, a change coincident with the introduc-tion of mass screening programs [27,28].

In 2000, the Behavioral Risk Factor Surveillance Survey found that 89% of women 18 to 44 years of age had received a Papanicolaou test within the past 3 years, and there was an 83% rate among women who were 45 years or older. These high rates reflect widespread acceptance of the Papanicolaou test among women and their health care providers and the convenience of testing [29].

Despite overall high rates of cervical cancer screening, certain minority groups continue to have lower screening rates compared with the general population. Although rates of screening in the African-American community are almost equiva-lent to rates among whites, American Indians/Alaska Native, Hispanic, and especially Asian American/Pacific Islander women

have lower Papanicolaou test-use rates [30]. Differences in use of cancer screening among racial and ethnic groups have been associated with various factors, including socioeconomic and cultural factors, lifestyle behaviors, education, access to health care, and physician recommendations.

Although screening rates in general in the United States are high, half of U.S. women in whom cervical cancer develops have never been screened [31], and efforts to encourage women to be screened can reduce the incidence and mortality of cervical cancer. Health care providers can help by offering screening to women who are being seen for other reasons. In one study of a large prepaid health plan with few barriers to access, most of the women with invasive cervical cancer had not had a Papanicolaou smear in the 3 years prior to their diagnosis, even though 75% of them had been seen in primary care outpatient clinics during that period [32].

Previously, the National Cancer Institute (NCI) and the American Cancer Society (ACS) recommended annual Papani-colaou tests for all women who have been sexually active or who have reached age 18. Less frequent screening was used when a low-risk woman had more than three consecutive, satis-factory, annual cytologic examinations with normal findings [33]. New guidelines for cervical cancer screening reflect a better understanding of the etiology of cervical neoplasia and incorporate new screening and diagnostic technologies. The ACS now recommends that screening for cervical cancer should begin three years after the onset of vaginal intercourse but no later than 21 years of age. Screening should be performed annually with cervical cytology smears or every two years with liquid-based cytology until the age of 30. After the age of 30, women who have had three consecutive negative cytology test results may continue screening every two to three years. Women who are age 70 years or older may discontinue cervical cancer screening if they previously have had 3 consecutive, sat-isfactory, negative cytology tests and have had no abnormal cytology tests wtihin a 10 year period prior to that time. There is no indication for cervical cancer screening in women who have had a total hysterectomy with cervix removal for benign gynecologic disease [34].

IV. Breast Cancer Screening

A. Epidemiology of Breast Cancer

Breast cancer remains the most commonly diagnosed cancer and the second most frequent cause of cancer death among women [23]. Of 1,334,100 estimated cancer cases in the United States in 2003, 211,300 cases of breast cancer, with 39,800 deaths, are expected [23]. Breast cancer mortality decreased by 1.6% annually from 1989 to 1995 and by 3.4% annually since 1995. Age at menarche and age at first pregnancy have been associated with breast cancer risk.

B. Trials of Screening

The New York State Health Insurance Plan (HIP) trial was the first to show a decrease in mortality from breast cancer [35,36]. It was a randomized trial in which 62,000 women, ages 40 to 64 years, were randomized to either a screening or control

Table 64-1
Cancer Screening Guidelines

	American Cancer Society*	American College of Obstetrics and Gynecologists**	U.S. Preventive Health Services Task Force†	National Cancer Institute's Physician Data Query (PDQ) System‡
Breast cancer	Women aged 40 and older should have a screening mammogram and a clinical breast examination (CBE) by a health care professional every year. The CBE should be scheduled close to and preferably before the scheduled mammogram.	Mammography should be performed every 1–2 years for women aged 40–49, and annually thereafter.	Routine screening every 1–2 years with mammography and clinical examination for women 50 and older. For women aged 40–49, the evidence that screening mammography reduces mortality from breast cancer is weaker, and the absolute benefit of mammography is smaller.	Screening by mammography, CBE, or both may decrease breast cancer mortality. The existence of benefit is uncertain because of the variable quality of the evidence and the inconsistency of results across studies.
Cervical cancer	Cervical cancer screening should begin 3 years after a woman begins having vaginal intercourse but no later than 21 years of age. Screening should be done every year with conventional Papanicolaou tests or every 2 years with liquid-based Papanicolaou tests. At or after age 30, women who have had 3 normal, consecutive test results may get screened every 2–3 years. Women 70 years of age or older who have had 3 or more normal Papanicolaou tests and no abnormal Papanicolaou tests in the last 10 years may choose to stop screening.	Papanicolaou test and pelvic examination yearly for all women who are, or have been, sexually active or who have reached 18. After three consecutive normal smears, Papanicolaou test less often at the discretion of physician.	Pap test every 1–3 years for all women who are sexually active and/or who have a cervix. No evidence to support an upper limit.	Evidence strongly suggests a decrease in mortality for regular screening with Papanicolaou tests in women who are sexually active or who have reached age 18. The upper limit at which such screening ceases to be effective is unknown.
Colorectal cancer	One of the following schedules for men and women age 50 and older: annual fecal occult blood testing (FOBT) and flexible sigmoidoscopy every 5 years; FOBT annually; colonoscopy every 10 years; double-contrast barium enema every 5 years, starting at age 50.	After the age of 50 years, one of three screening options: yearly fecal occult blood testing plus sigmoidoscopy every 5 years or colonoscopy every 10 years or double contrast barium enema (DCBE) every 5–10 years.	FOBT and/or sigmoidoscopy yearly at age 50 and older. A digital rectal exam should be performed at the time of each screening sigmoidoscopy, colonoscopy, or DCBE.	FOBT testing either annually or biennially using rehydrated or nonrehydrated stool specimens in people age 50 to 80 decreases mortality from colorectal cancer. Regular screening by sigmoidoscopy in people older than the age of 50 may decrease mortality from colorectal cancer. There is insufficient evidence to determine the optimal interval for such screening.

Continued

Table 64-1

(Continued)

	American Cancer Society*	American College of Obstetrics and Gynecologists**	U.S. Preventive Health Services Task Force†	National Cancer Institute's Physician Data Query (PDQ) System‡
Prostate cancer	Beginning at age 50, all men who have at least a 10-year life expectancy should be offered both the prostate-specific antigen (PSA) blood test and a digital rectal examination annually. Men in high-risk groups (African Americans, men with family history of prostate cancer) should begin testing at 45 years. Men should receive information regarding risks and benefits early. Men who ask their doctor to make the decision on their behalf should be tested. Men should not be discouraged from testing. Not offering the test is inappropriate.	N/A	Screening is not recommended.	There is insufficient evidence to establish whether a decrease in mortality from prostate cancer occurs with screening by digital rectal examination or serum PSA.

*Smith RA, Cokkinides V, Eyre HJ *et al*. (2003). American Cancer Society guidelines for the early detection of cancer. *CA Cancer J Clin*. 53:27–43 (available at www.cancer.org).

**ACOG Committee. "ACOG Committee Opinion. Routine cancer screening." (2003). 82:241–245.

†(2002, 2003). Guide to Clinical Preventive Services. Report of the U.S. Preventive Services Task Force, 3rd Edition. Washington DC: Department of Health and Human Services.

‡PDQ Screening and Prevention Editorial Board. (2003). PDQ Cancer Information Summaries: Screening/Detection National Cancer Institute. Bethesda, MD. www.cancer.gov/cancerinfo/pdq/screening.

group. The screening intervention consisted of a baseline mammogram and clinical breast examination, usually by a surgeon, followed by three additional annual evaluations. Of those women invited to undergo screening, 65% of the women accepted and went for a baseline examination; most (all but 12%) went for at least one additional examination.

After 9 years of follow-up, there were significantly fewer breast cancer deaths in the study group compared with the controls (91 vs 128, essentially a 30% reduction in breast cancer mortality). A separate analysis by Chu *et al* [37] in 1988 confirmed this improvement in breast cancer mortality. Importantly, there were fewer deaths among patients diagnosed with cancer (46.7 vs. 35.2 deaths per 100 cancer cases). Cancers detected by mammography had a case fatality rate of 33%, whereas those that were detected incidentally had a rate of 48%.

The investigators noted that there was no statistically significant difference in mortality between the screened and control populations in the 40- to 49-year age group and that the smaller number of deaths among the study group (39) compared with the control group (48) was attributable to the fewer deaths among cases after the women had progressed to the 50- to 54-year age group. Although this may suggest that screening was not efficacious in the 40- to 49-year age group, it may be that age at randomization, rather than age at diagnosis, is more important.

Other studies have confirmed the benefits of breast cancer screening. One such trial is the Swedish Two-County Trial [38,39], which randomized 133,000 women, ages 40 to 74 years, to mammography or to a control group. Breast cancer mortality was reduced by 32% among those women who were screened (22.3% among those screened vs 32.4% among controls). Screening saved one life per 4000 woman-years of screening, and there was one death per 7.4 cancers detected [40]. Another trial in Stockholm, Sweden, begun in 1981, enrolled 40,318 women [41]. This trial found a relative risk of death from breast cancer of 0.74 (95% confidence interval [CI] 0.5 to 1.1), although this was not statistically significant. The subgroup of women older than age 50 had a statistically significant mortality reduction of 38%. The UK Trial of Early Detection of Breast Cancer (TEDBC) [42] was started in 1979 and, after 16 years, found a 27% decrease in breast cancer mortality for screening.

Two Canadian trials evaluated the role of mammography; the first such study (Canadian National Breast Screening Study-1 [CNBSS-1]) [43] randomized 50,430 women aged 40 to 49 to receive a single clinical breast examination or to undergo annual mammography and physical examinations. More cancers were diagnosed initially in the mammography group in the first screen (3.89 vs 2.46 per 1000 subjects overall). Over the first 5 years of follow-up, more cancers were detected in the mammography group than the usual care group (72.7 per 1000 vs 59.3 per 1000). Despite the difference in detection, however, mortality from breast cancer proved higher in the mammography group (38 vs 28 cases). The authors concluded that screening this age group had no impact on mortality.

The second Canadian National Breast Screening Study evaluated the effect of mammography screening on breast cancer mortality in 39,405 women between the ages of 50 and 59 [44,45]. The women were randomized to either annual mammogram and clinical breast examination or to a clinical examination alone. The addition of mammography to physical examination detected more cancers (267 vs 148 cases on the initial screen). However, at 13 years of follow-up, there was no significant difference in the number of cancers detected by the two strategies (107 vs 105 deaths in the groups receiving physical examination with and without mammograms, respectively). The authors concluded that the addition of mammography to clinical examination did not reduce breast cancer mortality. Critics of the study have suggested that an effect of mammography would have been difficult to find in the presence of annual physical examination and have noted that the quality of the mammograms may have been poor [46].

C. A Recent Controversy

The trials cited previously on the efficacy of breast cancer screening were reviewed recently by Olsen and Gotzsche [47]. They classified the trials as high quality (none), medium quality (Malmo [48] and Canadian [45]), poor quality (Gothenburg [49], Stockholm [41], and Two-County [40]), and flawed (Edinburgh [50] and HIP [35]). The Swedish studies in particular were noted to have an imbalance in the ages of the women randomized, which suggested a poor trial methodology. For the two medium-quality trials alone, the relative risk of death from breast cancer after screening was 0.99 that of unscreened populations after 7 years and 1.00 after 13 years; the three poor-quality trials did not change the risk reduction (0.99 relative risk at 7 years). The authors noted that, although there was no benefit to be found in the medium-quality studies, there was a marked benefit at 7 and 13 years in the poor-quality trials (0.74 and 0.68 relative risk, respectively). These trials were carried out in women of all age groups; the authors concluded that screening women with mammography is not justified.

Gotzsche and Olsen also critiqued breast cancer mortality as an endpoint. Causes of death are difficult to assess in many cases and can be misleading. They argued that only all-cause mortality is a reliable indicator of mortality rather than cancer-specific mortality. Olsen and Gotzsche suggest that screening might result in a false-positive test in nearly half of women younger than the age of 50 after 10 years of annual screening and that 19% of these would undergo a biopsy. Furthermore, mastectomy would increase by 20% and surgery overall by 30%. Finally, they suggest that greater mortality might occur through the use of radiotherapy in otherwise low-risk patients [51].

This analysis generated a storm of controversy. One critique of the work is that excess stringency in rating the trials skewed the results unfairly toward the lower estimates of benefit [52]. Another critique lies in the defense of case fatality as a measure of screening effectiveness [53]. Despite varied reactions, the U.S. Preventive Service Task Force's (USPSTF's) reaffirmed their recommendations for mammography among 50-year-old women and added that women in their forties should undergo mammography [54].

D. Meta-analyses and Summary

The International Workshop On Screening For Breast Cancer examined the data from the various breast cancer screening trials in 1993. They noted that the randomized trials of breast cancer screening consistently showed a benefit in mortality in the 50 and older age groups. With respect to the 40- to 49-year age group, the working group found no benefit for screening at 5 to 7 years from study entry and an uncertain benefit at 10 to 12 years. The combined Swedish trials gave a non-statistically significant 13% decrease in mortality after 12 years of follow-up. A subsequent meta-analysis [55] of nine trials of screening mammography in this age group (40 to 49 years) also did not find a significantly lower risk.

Nystrom et al [56] conducted a recent meta-analysis of the Swedish screening studies. Published in response to the Danish criticism, the authors found that, over a median screening period of 16 years, there was a 21% decrease in breast cancer mortality achieved by mammography screening. This reduction was greatest in the 60- to 69-year age group, in whom a 33% decrease was found, although there was a smaller but significant decrease (24%) in the 55- to 59-age range as well. The authors found no significant mortality benefit for breast cancer screening in the 40- to 54-year age group, although there was a trend toward decreased mortality.

The USPSTF has laid out recommendations for screening women for breast cancer. Their second edition noted that

> Routine screening for breast cancer every 1–2 years, with mammography alone or mammography and annual clinical breast examination (CBE), is recommended for women aged 50–69. There is insufficient evidence to recommend for or against routine mammography or CBE for women aged 40–49 or aged 70 and older, although recommendations for high risk women aged 40–49 and healthy women aged 70 may be made on other grounds [57].

Recently, the USPSTF recommendations changed this advice for women in their forties. Released in February 2002 and revised (slightly) after the Nystrom report was published in March, their report now reads [54]:

> For women aged 40–49, the evidence that screening mammography reduces mortality from breast cancer is weaker, and the absolute benefit of mammography is smaller, than it is for older women. Most, but not all, studies indicate a mortality benefit for women undergoing mammography at ages 40–49, but the delay in observed benefit in women younger than 50 makes it difficult to determine the incremental benefit of beginning screening at age 40 rather than at age 50.

Other screening strategies have been suggested as well. One recommendation by Antman and Shea of Columbia University for the 40- to 49-year age group is to screen women who have specific risk factors, most notably family history, starting between 40 and 45 years. First-degree relatives of breast cancer patients might start mammography 10 years of age earlier than the first known case in their family. Those who are of average risk for breast cancer might start in the 45 to 49 age group [58].

E. Barriers to Screening

1. Effect of Race

The National Health Interview Survey (NHIS) reviews 49,000 households annually for knowledge and attitudes toward health. Results have shown that higher income, use of other kinds of screening, having a regular source of health care, living in the West or a metropolitan area, and having healthy lifestyle practices were associated with a higher likelihood of having regular mammograms among women aged 40 to 75 [59].

The NHIS found that the use of mammograms by the black population was lower than among whites in 1987 but also that blacks are closing the gap. In 1987, 14% of blacks were screened by mammography for breast cancer, whereas 18% of whites had the same test (p < 0.03). In 1990, however, 32% of both white and black respondents had mammograms.

Although Hispanic women have lower incidence and mortality rates from breast cancer than non-Hispanic white women, they are generally diagnosed at later stages and are more likely to die than non-Hispanic white women. The use of mammograms in Hispanics rose from 13 to 31% from 1987 to 1990 [59]. These findings are consistent with a review of the Colorado Mammography Project, which noted that non-White populations tended to return less frequently than whites for repeat mammograms, although this also correlated with education and insurance status [60].

2. Effect of Education and Income

Both education and income play a role in gaining access to screening. Stein-Merkin et al [61] noted that educational level, and to a lesser extent income, were associated with a lower stage at diagnosis. The odds ratio of developing advanced stage cancer in the lowest education quintile as compared with the highest was 1.84 (95% CI = 1.65 to 2.06). Notably, 55% of blacks were in the lowest quintile of education as compared with 30% of the white population. Also, 44% of black patients versus 11% of whites were in the lowest quintile of income.

To emphasize the barrier placed by financial impediments, Immonen-Raiha et al [62] documented the effect of instituting a $16 fee into what had been before 1997 a free screening system in Finland. Attendance dropped from 88 to 66% in the 40- to 49-year age group, and from 90 to 75% among the 60- to 69-year age group. This was irrespective of quintile of income, occupation, or employment status. In the 60- to 69-year-old group, however, the decrease in attendance was less among unmarried women.

In their review of the NHIS data, Breen et al [59] noted that nearly twice as many women whose family incomes were $20,000 or more reported having had a mammogram (22%) than those women whose family incomes were lower (11%) in 1987. By the time of the 1990 survey, these numbers were 39% and 24%, respectively.

The Hispanic EPESE study was a cohort study of 3050 Mexican Americans from Texas, Colorado, New Mexico, Arizona, and California. Field workers followed this population from 1993 to 1996, measured the use of cervical and breast cancer screening, and studied the association of screening with demographic, medical, and cultural factors. This population included 1625

women. This study found that women who were not married, had 5 years or less of education, or had no private insurance were significantly less likely to have had mammograms or Papanicolaou smears. Likewise, those women who had low levels of acculturation, as measured by the use of English in conversation with family, friends, and neighbors and the reading or viewing of English language literature, were less likely to have had cancer screening. However, with multivariate analysis, only age, insurance status, number of medical conditions, number of doctor visits, and having a history of a hysterectomy retained significant associations [63].

F. Attitudes toward Screening

Aro et al [64] published an analysis of the psychosocial factors that might influence a woman's decision to accept an invitation to breast cancer screening. They determined that socioeconomic predictors of participation in screening included marriage, working, low or middle level of education, and living in a rural setting. Notably, those with no serious illness and nonsmokers were more likely to be screened, as well as those who had not previously had a mammogram, those who infrequently performed breast self-examination, and those who saw a gynecologist regularly. The authors noted in a separate analysis that social isolation, anxiety, and depression were more prevalent in those who did not participate [65]. However, a recent mammogram was the strongest predictor of nonparticipation.

The effect of false-positive results on the psychologic well being of patients was studied by Olsson et al [66]. These authors noted that of women who were recalled for additional views on their mammograms, 54% coped well with no or mild distress. In this group, however, 30% had moderate or severe reactions that gradually resolved, and 15% had moderate or severe reactions that did not resolve after 6 months. Less educated women, those living in the most urban areas, and those with more children had significantly stronger reactions. Widows were noted to have better coping ability than others.

V. Prostate Cancer Screening

A. Burden of Disease

Prostate cancer remains the single most frequently diagnosed cancer in men. Its 220,900 cases constitute approximately 33% of cancers in men, and it is the second most frequent cause of cancer death among men. It is estimated that 85% of these cases are diagnosed at the local and regional stages, and, in these patients, 5-year survival rates approach 100%. The age-adjusted rate of prostate cancer is highest in African-American men, 275 per 100,000 men, compared with 173 per 100,000 among white men, 60.7 per 100,000 among Native Americans, 107 per 100,00 among Asian/Pacific Islanders, and 128 per 100,00 among Hispanics [23].

Despite the high incidence rate of prostate cancer in the older male population, screening for prostate cancer remains controversial; there is a lack of consensus regarding recommendations for prostate cancer screening. At this time, two randomized trials of prostate cancer screening are underway [67].

B. Methods of Screening

The three methods of screening for prostate cancer currently in use include digital rectal examination (DRE), prostate-specific antigen (PSA), and transrectal ultrasound. The first two of those are within the scope of primary care physicians and are discussed here.

DRE is an inexpensive test that has historically been part of routine health care. The true sensitivity and specificity of the test are unknown; studies of the test's accuracy have not included biopsy of normal appearing prostates. The positive predictive value (PPV) of the test seems to be approximately 15 to 30%.

PSA testing was begun in 1988; PSA levels greater than 4.0 ng/ml are usually considered suspicious. The PPV of PSA testing can be anywhere from 20 to 30% in men older than 50 years. PPV does vary with the magnitude of PSA elevation. Because many older men develop benign prostatic hyperplasia, which often elevates PSA levels, the specificity of the test declines with age. Serum levels of PSA can also be elevated after prostatitis, transrectal needle biopsy, acute urine retention, and prostate surgery [68]. Like the DRE, the actual sensitivity and specificity of the test are not well documented. One estimate comes from patients who were diagnosed with prostate cancer after participating in the Physicians' Health Study, who had serum drawn before their participation. The sensitivity of the test was only 46% among all patients diagnosed within 10 years, but was 53 to 87% among patients whose cancers were diagnosed within the subsequent 4 years. The lead time from such screening was determined to be approximately 5.5 years [69].

One study compared the utility of DRE and PSA among a group of 6630 male volunteers. PSA carried a PPV of 32 to 38% among all age groups, whereas the PPV of DRE alone rose with age, from 17% in the 50 to 59 age group to 38% in the 80+ age group [70]. Another analysis by the same group noted that of the 15% of men with an elevated PSA, 15% had a suspicious DRE, and 26% had abnormalities in one or both tests. PPV was higher for PSA (32%) than for DRE (21%). PSA alone detected 75% of organ-confined cancer, DRE 56%, and the two together 78% [71].

C. Risks and Benefits of Screening

Although no randomized trials of prostate cancer screening have been completed, two decision analysis models have been done to examine the effects of prostate cancer screening, and their results have conflicted. In one model, Krahn et al [72] found that screening men between the ages of 50 and 70 was found to increase longevity, particularly if transrectal ultrasound was combined with DRE and PSA. Using just the latter two tests, or just PSA alone, produced slightly smaller gains. DRE alone produced almost no increase in life expectancy. The model was sensitive to the increased perioperative mortality in older patients. In this model, the gains in life expectancy increased with advancing age.

Coley et al [73] came to a similar conclusion on the effects of screening on mortality in a separate decision analysis model. If aggressive screening is conducted using PSA and DRE, there will be a stage migration of detected cancers into earlier stages. If, in fact, men with organ-confined disease can be cured, one-time screening would result in an average increase of several weeks for each patient tested. For men who subsequently receive a diagnosis of cancer, aggressive treatment can potentially add up to 3 years of life.

Notably, however, Krahn's model predicted that quality of life would worsen with the use of screening, particularly at older ages. They concluded that although longevity would improve, quality-adjusted life-years would decrease with screening by 3 to 13 days. They further note that each life-year saved would cost from $113,000 to $729,000 (i.e., there would be no cost saving through prostate cancer screening).

Arguments against screening noted by the American College of Physicians (ACP) include observations that up to 40% of men who undergo screening require biopsy of their prostates. Of those men who are treated for clinically localized cancer, there is a 50% chance of sexual dysfunction, a 20 to 30% chance of impotence, and a 0.5% rate of perioperative death. Because the balance of good and harm resulting from early treatment with prostate cancer is unknown, the ACP has recommended that, rather than screening all men routinely, physicians should describe the risks and benefits of screening to patients and individualize the decision to screen. They further suggest that eligible men should participate in screening trials, when feasible. The ACP notes that men who are 50 to 69 years of age would enjoy the most benefit from screening, whereas older patients have less to gain.

Livingston et al [74] noted that 68% of the general population believed in prostate cancer screening, as compared with 55% of male physicians, and more patients than doctors had undergone screening (56% vs 45%, respectively). Likewise, 70% of a random sample of New York State residents wanted to be screened for early disease, and up to 77% of those surveyed had been screened [75]. However, in a cohort derived from the central Harlem section of New York City, only 25% of the community had undergone a PSA test. Of those who did have a PSA, 87% had also had a DRE. In the Harlem study, age, education, and a personal acquaintance having had prostate cancer were all shown to correlate with the frequency of prostate cancer screening [76]. The New York State sample differed from the Harlem study in that more of the population had some college education (42 to 54% vs 28%) and more had health insurance (94% vs 42%, excluding Medicare/Medicaid). Furthermore, the New York State sample was predominantly white (80%), whereas the Harlem study was geared toward African Americans.

In summary, there is no consensus yet on prostate cancer screening; the ACS [77] has recommended that DRE and PSA be offered to men older than 50 years and to high-risk patients, specifically African-Americans and first-degree relatives of cancer patients older than the age of 45. Conversely, the USP-STF has not recommended screening [54]. The Prostate, Lung, Colorectal and Ovarian Screening Trial now being conducted by the NCI may provide more evidence for or against the use of screening.

VI. Colorectal Cancer

Colorectal cancer is the third most common cancer in the United States among men and women, with an estimated 147,500 new cases and 57,100 deaths in 2003. More than half of the new cases and deaths will be in women [23]. Risk factors include age older than 50 years; a history of colorectal cancer or adenomas in a first-degree relative; a personal history of colorectal adenomas; and a previous diagnosis of endometrial, ovarian, or breast cancer. Colorectal cancer arises from adenomatous polyps, benign tumors that can be detected and removed by endoscopy. As a result, it is potentially appropriate for screening because there is a relatively long time from biologic onset to the development of the carcinoma, with a lengthy detectable preclinical phase.

Screening tests for colorectal cancer include the fecal occult blood testing (FOBT), sigmoidoscopy, and colonoscopy. FOBT has been assessed in two randomized controlled trials, as well as in case-control studies, and has been shown to reduce colorectal cancer-specific mortality rates [78–82]. One trial from the University of Minnesota demonstrated a nearly 40% reduction in the colorectal cancer mortality rate in the group undergoing FOBT compared with controls [81].

Cohort studies and case-control studies have demonstrated that flexible sigmoidoscopy screening decreases mortality from left-sided colorectal cancer by up to 85% [83,84]. Flexible sigmoidoscopy, however, cannot visualize the entire colon. Some studies have shown that the combination of sigmoidoscopy combined with FOBT improves sensitivity [85]. However, future recommendations for screening may favor colonoscopy over flexible sigmoidoscopy, because many physicians believe that flexible sigmoidoscopy fails to detect a substantial number of polyps or early invasive cancers because of their location proximal to the reach of the sigmoidoscope. In one recent study, asymptomatic patients were screened with only colonoscopy; the researchers found that a number of subjects had advanced proximal colonic lesions that presumably would not have been detected with flexible sigmoidoscopy [86].

Colorectal cancer screening rates among adults older than age 50 are low compared with other cancers, although these rates are improving. In 1997, only 18% of men and 21% of women older than 50 years reported an FOBT in the previous year, and 35% of men and 27% of women had a sigmoidoscopy in the previous 5 years [87]. These low rates in both genders contrast sharply with the high rates of cervical and breast cancer screening in women. Women are more likely to be screened with physician encouragement. The fact that age-adjusted colon cancer rates are higher in men than in women and that men are at higher risk for colorectal cancer than women may lead women to believe that colorectal cancer is a "man's disease" and, therefore, may result in underuse of screening procedures [88]. One study found that women were more likely to do home FOBT testing, whereas men were more likely to get a sigmoidoscopy or colonoscopy [89]. Another study compared the screening practices of men and women and found that a significantly smaller proportion of women underwent flexible sigmoidoscopy either for screening or diagnostic indications [90].

Among minority groups, screening rates vary; Hispanics and American Indians/Alaska Natives have lower rates than whites or African Americans. Cultural values or practices, access to health care, and knowledge concerning colorectal cancer and prevention affect screening [91]. Although differences in screening between genders and minority groups exist, it is important to encourage all groups to be screened for colon cancer through education and targeted interventions. Educational messages should encourage both women and men to be screened for colorectal cancer and in preventing cancer through early detection and removal of precancerous polyps through screening practices.

The ACS recommends one of the following schedules for men and women age 50 and older: annual FOBT and flexible sigmoidoscopy every 5 years, flexible sigmoidoscopy every 5 years, FOBT every year, colonoscopy every 10 years, or double-contrast barium enema every 5 years. Those with high risk for colorectal cancer should begin screening earlier and/or more frequently [77].

VII. Suggestions for Further Investigations

- Physicians should be informed of screening guidelines.
- Patients should be informed about the pros and cons of each screening method.
- Screening helps detect a number of cancers early, when treatment can be most effective.
- The patient and health care provider should share decision making.
- Community-based interventions should be developed to target minority and ethnically diverse communities to increase screening.
- Education should be used to promote screening.
- Access to health care should be facilitated.

References

1. Mirino AM, Smith BL. (2001). Deaths: Preliminary data for 2000. *Natl Vital Stat Rep.* 49(12):2–3.
2. Bertakis KD, Azari R, Helms LJ *et al.* (2000). Gender differences in the utilization of health care services. *J Fam Pract.* 49:147–152.
3. McKinlay JB. (1996). Some contributions from the social system to gender inequalities in heart disease. *J Health Soc Behav.* 37:1–26.
4. Hall JA, Palmer RH, Orav EJ *et al.* (1990). Performance quality, gender, and professional role: A study of physicians and nonphysicians in 16 ambulatory care practices. *Med Care.* 28:489–501.
5. Levy S, Dowling P, Boult L *et al.* (1992). The effect of physician and patient gender on preventive medicine practices in patients older than fifty. *Fam Med.* 24:58–61.
6. Osborn EH, Bird JA, McPhee SJ *et al.* (1991). Cancer screening by primary care physicians: Can we explain the differences? *J Fam Pract.* 32:465–471.
7. Henderson JT, Weisman CS. (2001). Physician gender effects on preventive screening and counseling: An analysis of male and female patients' health care experiences. *Med Care.* 39:1281–1292.
8. Lurie N, Slater J, McGovern P *et al.* (1993). Preventive care for women. Does the sex of the physician matter? *N Engl J Med.* 329:478–482.
9. Lurie N, Margolis K, McGovern PG *et al.* (1997). Why do patients of female physicians have higher rates of breast and cervical cancer screening? *J Gen Intern Med.* 12:34–43.
10. Kerssens JJ, Bensing JM, Andela MG. (1997). Patient preference for genders of health professionals. *Soc Sci Med.* 44:1531–1540.
11. Blake RL Jr. (1990). Gender concordance between family practice residents and their patients in an ambulatory-care setting. *Acad Med.* 65:702–703.
12. Kelly JM. (1980). Sex preference in patient selection of a family physician. *J Fam Pract.* 11:427–433.
13. Ahmad F, Stewart DE, Cameron JI, Hyman I. (2001). Rural physicians' perspectives on cervical and breast cancer screening: A gender-based analysis. *J Womens Health Gender Based Med.* 10:201–208.
14. Dietrich JJ, O'Conner GT, Keller A *et al.* (1992). Cancer: Improving early detection and prevention. A community practice randomized trial. *BMJ.* 304:91–95.

15. Dietrich JJ, Woodruff CB, Carney PA. (1994). Changing office routines to enhance preventive care. The preventive GAPS approach. *Arch Fam Med.* 3:176–183.

16. Gann P, Melville SK, Luckmann R. (1993). Characteristics of primary care office systems as predictors of mammography utilization. *Ann Intern Med.* 118:893–898.

17. Garr DR, Ornstein SM, Jenkins RG, Zemp LD. (1993). The effect of routine use of computer-generated preventive reminders in a clinical practice. *Am J Prev Med.* 9:55–61.

18. McPhee SJ, Bird JA, Jenkins CN, Fordham D. (1989). Promoting cancer screening. A randomized, controlled trial of three interventions. *Arch Intern Med.* 149:1866–1872.

19. McPhee SJ, Bird JA, Fordham D *et al.* (1991). Promoting cancer prevention activities by primary care physicians. Results of a randomized, controlled trial. *JAMA.* 266:538–544.

20. Engelstad LP, Stewart SL, Nguyen BH *et al.* (2001). Abnormal Pap smear follow-up in a high-risk population. *Cancer Epidemiol Biomarkers Prev.* 10.1015–1020.

21. Patz, EF, Goodman PC, Bepler G. (2000). Screening for lung cancer. *N Engl J Med.* 343:1627–1633.

22. Schottenfeld D, Fraumeni JF Jr, eds. (1996). *Cancer Epidemiology and Prevention,* 2nd Edition. New York: Oxford University Press.

23. Jemal A, Murray T, Samuels A, et al. (2003). Cancer statistics 2003. *CA Cancer J Clin.* 53:5–26.

24. Eddy DM. (1990). Screening for cervical cancer. *Ann Intern Med.* 113:214-226.

25. Johannesson G, Geirsson G, Day N. (1978). The effect of mass screening in Iceland, 1965–1974, on the incidence and mortality of cervical carcinoma. *Int J Cancer.* 21:418–425.

26. Clarke EA, Anderson TW. (1979). Does screening by "Pap" smears help prevent cervical cancer? A case-control study. *Lancet.* 2(8132):1–4.

27. Devesa SS, Silverman DT, Young JL Jr *et al.* (1987). Cancer incidence and mortality trends among whites in the United States, 1947–84. *J Natl Cancer Inst.* 79:701–770.

28. Koss LG. (1989). The Papanicolaou test for cervical cancer detection: a triumph and a tragedy. *JAMA.* 261:737–743.

29. Centers for Disease Control and Prevention (CDC). Behavioral Risk Factor Surveillance System Survey Data. Atlanta, Georgia: U.S. Department of Health and Human Services, Centers for Disease Control and Prevention, 2000.

30. National Center for Health Statistics. (2000). Data file documentation, National Health Interview Survey, 1998. National Center for Health Statistics. Hyattsville, Maryland.

31. (1996). Cervical cancer. NIH consensus statement, vol. 14, no. 1, pp. 1–38. Bethesda, MD: Office of Medical Applications of Research.

32. Kinney W, Sung HY, Keraney KA *et al.* (1998). Missed opportunities for cervical cancer screening of HMO members developing invasive cervical cancer. *Gynecol Oncol.* 71:428–430.

33. Smith RA, Cokkinides V, von Eschenbach *et al.* (2002). American Cancer Society guidelines for the early detection of cancer. *CA Cancer J Clin.* 52:8–22.

34. Saslow D, Runowicz CD, Solomon D, *et al.* (2002). American Cancer Society guidelines for the early detection of cervical neoplasia and cancer. *CA Cancer J Clin.* 52:342–362.

35. Shapiro S. (1977). Evidence on screening for breast cancer from a randomized trial. *Cancer.* 39:2772–2782.

36. Shapiro S, Venet W, Strax P, *et al.* (1982). Ten to fourteen year effect of screening on breast cancer mortality. *J Natl Cancer Inst.* 69:349–355.

37. Chu K, Smart C, Tarone R. (1988). Analysis of breast cancer mortality and stage distribution by age for the Health Insurance Plan Clinical Trial. *J Natl Cancer Inst.* 80:1125–1132.

38. Tabar L, Fagerberg CJ, Gad A, *et al.* (1985). Reduction in mortality from breast cancer after mass screening with mammography. *Lancet.* 1(8433):829–832.

39. Tabar L, Vitak B, Chen HH, *et al.* (2000). The Swedish Two-County Trial twenty years later. Updated mortality results and new insights from long-term follow-up. *Radiol Clin North Am.* 38:625–651.

40. Tabar L, Fagerberg G, Duffy S, Day N. (1989). The Swedish Two-County Trial of Mammographic Screening for breast cancer: Recent results and calculation of benefit. *J Epidemiol Community Health.* 43:107–114.

41. Frisell J, Lidbrink E, Hellstrom L, Rutqvist LE. (1997). Followup after 11 years–Update of mortality results in the Stockholm mammographic screening trial. *Breast Cancer Res Treat.* 45:263–270.

42. Moss S. (1999). 16-Year mortality from breast cancer in the UK Trial of Early Detection of Breast Cancer. *Lancet.* 353:1909–1914.

43. Miller A, Baines C, To T, Wall C. (1992). Canadian National Breast Screening Study: 1. Breast cancer detection and death rates among women aged 40 to 49 years. *Can Med Assoc J.* 147:1459–1476.

44. Miller A, Baines C, To T, Wall C. (1992). Canadian National Breast Screening Study: 2. Breast cancer detection and death rates among women aged 50 to 59 years. *Can Med Assoc J.* 147:1477–1488.

45. Miller A, To T, Baines J, Wall C. (2000). Canadian National Breast Screening Study-2: 13 Year results of a randomized trial in women aged 50–59 years. *J Natl Cancer Inst.* 92:1490–1499.

46. Gotzsche PC, Olsen O. (2000). Is screening for breast cancer with mammography justifiable? *Lancet.* 355:129–133.

47. Olsen O, Gotzsche PC. (2001). Screening for breast cancer with mammography (Cochrane Review). *Cochrane Database Syst Rev* 4:CD001877.

48. Garne JP, Aspergen K, Balldin G, Ranstam J. (1997). Increasing incidence of and declining mortality from breast carcinoma: Trends in Malmo, Sweden, 1961–1992, *Cancer.* 79:69–74.

49. Bjurstam N, Bjorneld L, Duffy SW *et al.* (1997). The Gothenburg Breast Screening Trial. *Cancer.* 80:2091–2099.

50. Alexander FE, Anderson TJ, Brown HK *et al.* (1999). 14 Years of follow-up from the Edinburgh randomized trial of breast cancer screening. *Lancet.* 353:1903–1908.

51. Olsen O, Gotzsche P. (2001). Cochrane review on screening for breast cancer with mammography. *Lancet.* 358:1340–1342.

52. McLellan F. (2002). Independent US panel fans debate on mammography. *Lancet.* 359:409.

53. Miettinen O, Henschke C, Pasmantier M *et al.* (2002). Mammographic screening: no reliable supporting evidence? *Lancet.* 359:404–406.

54. Guide to Clinical Preventive Services: Third Edition. (2002). U.S. Preventive Services Task Force. Washington DC: Department of Health and Human Services.

55. Kerlikowske K, Grady D, Rubin S *et al.* (1995). Efficacy of screening mammography: A meta-analysis. *JAMA.* 273:149–152.

56. Nystrom L, Andersson I, Bjurstam N *et al.* (2002). Long term effects of mammography screening: updated overview of the Swedish randomized trials. *Lancet.* 359:909–919.

57. Guide to Clinical Preventive Services: Second Edition. (1996). U.S. Preventive Services Task Force. Washington DC: Department of Health and Human Services.

58. Antman K, Shea S. (1999). Screening mammography under age 50. *JAMA.* 281:1470–1472.

59. Breen N, Kessler L. (1994). Changes in the use of screening mammography: Evidence from the 1987 and 1990 National Health Interview Surveys. *Am J Public Health.* 84:62–67.

60. Strzelczyk JJ, Dignan MB. (2002). Disparities in adherence to recommended follow-up on screening mammography: Interaction of sociodemographic factors. *Ethn Dis.* 12(1):77–86.

61. Stein Merkin S, Stevenson L, Powe N. (2002). Geographic socioeconomic status, race, and advanced-stage breast cancer in New York City. *Am J Public Health.* 92:64–70.

62. Immonen-Raiha P, Kauhava L, Parvinen I *et al.* (2001). Customer fee and participation in breast-cancer screening. *Lancet.* 358:1425.

63. Wu ZH, Black SA, Markides K. (2001). Prevalence and associated factors of cancer screening: Why are so many older Mexican American women never screened? *Prev Med.* 33:268–273.

64. Aro AR, de Koning HJ, Absetz P, Schreck M. (1999). Psychosocial predictors of first attendance for organised mammography screening. *J Med Screen.* 6:82–88.

65. Aro AR, de Koning HJ, Absetz P, Schreck M. (2001). Two distinct groups of non-attenders in an organized mammography screening program. *Breast Cancer Res Treat.* 70:145–153.

66. Olsson P, Armelius K, Nordahl G *et al.* (1999). Women with false positive screening mammograms: how do they cope? *J Med Screen.* 6:89–93.

67. Gohagan JK, Prorok PC, Kramer BS, Cornett JE. (1994). Prostate cancer screening in the prostate, lung, colorectal, and ovarian cancer screening trials of the National Cancer Institute. *J Urol.* 152:1905–1909.

68. Coley CM, Barry MJ, Mulley AG for the American College of Physicians. (1997). Screening for prostate cancer. *Ann Int Med.* 126:480–484.

69. Gann PH, Hennekens CH, Stampfer M. (1995). A prospective evaluation of plasma prostate-specific antigen for detection of prostate cancer. *JAMA.* 273:289–294.

70. Richie JP, Catalona WJ, Ahmann FR *et al*. (1993). Effect of patient age on early detection of prostate cancer with serum prostate-specific antigen and digital rectal examination. *Urology*. 42:365–374.

71. Catalona WJ, Richie JP, Ahmann FR *et al*. (1994). Comparison of digital rectal examination and serum prostate specific antigen in the early detection of prostate cancer: results of a multicenter clinical trial of 6,630 men. *J Urol*. 151:1283–1290.

72. Krahn MD, Mahoney JE, Eckman MH *et al*. (1994). Screening for prostate cancer. *JAMA*. 272:773–780.

73. Coley CM, Barry MJ, Fleming C, *et al*. (1997). Early detection of prostate cancer. Part II: Estimating the risks, benefits, and costs. *Ann Int Med*. 126:468–479.

74. Livingston P, Cohen P, Frydenberg M *et al*. (2002). Knowledge, attitudes, and experience associated with testing for prostate cancer: A comparison between male doctors and men in the community. *Int Med J*. 32:215–223.

75. McDavid K, Melnik T, Derderian H. (2000). Prostate cancer screening trends of New York State men at least 50 years of age, 1994 to 1997. *Prev Med*. 31:195–202.

76. Ashford, AR, Albert SM, Hoke G *et al*. (2001). Prostate carcinoma knowledge, attitudes, and screening behavior among African-American men in central Harlem, New York City. *Cancer*. 91:164–172.

77. Smith RA, Cokkinides V, Eyre HJ. (2003). American Cancer Society guidelines for the early detection of cancer, 2003. *CA Cancer J Clin*. 53:27–43.

78. Hardcastle JD, Camberlain JO, Robinson MH *et al*. (1996). Randomised controlled trial of faecal-occult-blood screening for colorectal cancer. *Lancet*. 348:1472–1477.

79. Kewenter J, Engaras B, Haglind E, Jensen J. (1990). Value of retesting subjects with a positive hemocult in screening for colorectal cancer. *Br J Surg*. 77:1349–1360.

80. Kronoborg O, Fenger C, Olsen J *et al*. (1996). Randomised study of screening for colorectal cancer with faecal-occult-blood test. *Lancet*. 348:1467–1471.

81. Mandel JS, Bond JH, Church TR *et al*. (1993). Reducing mortality from colorectal cancer by screening for fecal occult blood: Minnesota Colon Cancer Control Study. *N Engl J Med*. 328:1365–1371.

82. Winawer SJ, Flehinger BJ, Schottenfeld D, Miller DG. (1993). Screening for colorectal cancer with fecal occult blood testing and sigmoidoscopy. *J Natl Cancer Inst*. 85:1311–1318.

83. Newcomb PA, Norfleet RG, Storer BE *et al*. (1992). Screening sigmoidoscopy and colorectal cancer mortality. *J Natl Cancer Inst*. 84:1572–1575.

84. Selby JV, Friedman GD, Quesenberry CP Jr, Weiss NS. (1992). A case-control study of screening sigmoidoscopy and mortality from colorectal cancer. *N Engl J Med*. 326:653–657.

85. Berry DP, Clarke P, Hardcastle JD, Vellacott KD. (1997). Randomized trial of the addition of flexible sigmoidoscopy to faecal occult blood testing for colorectal neoplasia population screening. *Br J Surg*. 84:1274–1276.

86. Lieberman DA, Weiss DG, Bond JH *et al*. (2000). Use of colonoscopy to screen asymptomatic adults for colorectal cancer: Veterans Affairs Cooperative Study Group 380. *N Engl J Med*. 343:162–168.

87. Center for Disease Control and Prevention. (1999). Screening for colorectal cancer-United States, 1997. *MMWR Morb Mortal Wkly Rep*. 48:16.

88. Mandelson MT, Curry SJ, Anderson LA *et al*. (2000). Colorectal cancer screening participation by older women. *Am J Prev Med*. 19(3):149–154.

89. Shapiro JA, Seef LC, Nadel MR. (2001). Colorectal cancer-screening tests and associated health behaviors. *Am J Prev Med*. 21(2)132–137.

90. Herold AH, Riker AI, Warner EA *et al*. (1997). Evidence of gender bias in patients undergoing flexible sigmoidoscopy. *Cancer Detect Prev*. 21:141–147.

91. Bolen JC, Rhodes L, Powell-Griner EE *et al*. (2000). State-specific prevalence of selected health behaviors, by race and ethnicity—behavioral risk factor surveillance system, 1997. *MMWR Morb Mortal Wkly Rep*. 49(No. SS-02):1–60.

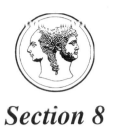

Section 8

NUTRITION

Ann M. Coulston, MS, RD

Nutrition Consultant, Stanford University School of Medicine, Stanford, CA

In this section we are faced with consideration of gender differences in nutrient requirements as well as gender considerations of nutrition-related disease conditions. The Institute of Medicine of The National Academies has completed a study of the Dietary Reference Intakes for most of the major nutrients and the macronutrients, carbohydrate, protein, fat, and energy. Leading nutrition scientists have reviewed published information about each specific nutrient and searched the world's literature to identify metabolic differences and needs and actions by age groupings as well as by gender. Publications are available on http://www.nap.edu. These reports include the commonly used Recommended Dietary Allowances (RDA) for those nutrients that had sufficient data for setting such individual guidelines and recommended Adequate Intakes (AI) for those nutrients without sufficient data. The reports for each nutrient are organized by gender and age groupings.

The Nutrition section covers a variety of physiologic areas and some have greater obvious gender differences than others. We have a considerably greater body of knowledge in energy requirements for men and women, and in the nutrient needs for athletic performance than areas like glucose metabolism, insulin resistance, and diabetes mellitus (DM), for example.

Some conditions, by nature of the body organs, pertain to only one gender such as prostate cancer, cervical, ovarian, and endometrial cancer. Most presentations of breast cancer will be in women, but it is not unknown in men, and information is needed to understand the natural history of the disease and the most appropriate treatment in men and women. Anorexia nervosa (AN) and related conditions have historically been conditions of women, however, reports of these conditions in young men are becoming more numerous.

Chapters in this section contain an excellent review of the literature of each topic, and where there is information, nutrient requirement, or utilization differences related to gender. As section editor, I am indebted to my colleagues for their thoughtful contributions and look forward to additional gender-specific, nutrition-related research stimulated by this publication.

65

Energy Requirements of Men and Women

SUSAN B. ROBERTS, PhD AND SAI KRUPA DAS, PhD

Jean Mayer USDA Human Nutrition Research Center on Aging at Tufts University, Boston, MA

I. Introduction

An individual's energy requirement is defined in the Dietary Reference Intakes (DRI) publication of the Food and Nutrition Board as "the dietary energy intake that is predicted to maintain energy balance in a healthy adult of a defined age, gender, weight, height, and level of physical activity consistent with good health" [1]. Thus, energy requirements are equal to total energy expenditure (TEE) in weight-maintaining individuals. As illustrated in Fig. 65-1, TEE is the sum of energy expended for different metabolic processes and activity, with three main components being typically defined.

Basal metabolic rate (BMR, sometimes termed resting metabolic rate [RMR] or resting energy expenditure [REE]) is the energy expended when a person is lying down completely at rest and represents the minimum energy needs of the body for such basic processes as respiration and circulation. In most adults this component of TEE represents about 60% of TEE.

Energy expenditure for physical activity and arousal (EEPA) is the second largest component of TEE, and is the energy expended for all movement whether strenuous or not as well as the state of being alert. This is the most variable component of TEE and typically represents about 30–40% of TEE.

Thermic effect of feeding (TEF) is the third component of TEE. This component, which contributes about 10% to the TEE, is the energy used to do the work of digesting, processing, and storing consumed food.

This chapter describes current methods for assessing usual energy needs, and summarizes national recommendations on energy intake using extracts from the DRI publication on energy and macronutrients [1].

A. *How Energy Requirements Are Determined*

Previous recommendations on energy needs [2] used the so-called "factorial method" for determination of TEE. The factorial method calculates 24h energy expenditure (EE) using information on the time devoted to different activities and the energy costs of each activity throughout a 24h period. The advantage of the factorial approach is that it allows theoretical estimation of 24h EE for defined activity patterns (using measured average costs of standard activities and activity durations). Thus, mean expected energy requirements for different levels of physical activity can be defined.

However, there are recognized theoretical problems with the factorial method. One problem is that there is a very wide range of activity types and levels of effort that are performed during normal life, and it is not feasible to measure the energy cost of each different activity. Even activities that were once thought to be equivalent to BMR (the minimum EE of a person who is awake and resting and measured at least 12 hours after consuming food), such as sleeping, have now been shown to have unique energy needs that require separate quantification [3]. Therefore the necessary generalizations about the energy costs of daily activities may result in substantial error. A further concern with the factorial method is that measurement of the energy costs of specific activities itself imposes constraints (due to embarrassment or awareness and the mechanical difficulties associated with performing an activity while wearing recording equipment) that could result in a change in effort level, thereby making the measured energy costs of different activities unrepresentative of the true costs of those activities. In addition, by definition and design, the factorial method only takes into account activities that can be specifically accounted for such as sleeping, walking, household work, occupational activity, and so on. However, 24h room calorimeter studies (which measure TEE) have shown that a significant amount of energy is expended in "non-accountable" activities (such as fidgeting) that can range from 100–800 kcal/day between individuals [4]. Thus, on theoretical grounds the factorial method has been suggested to underestimate

Components of Total Energy Expenditure

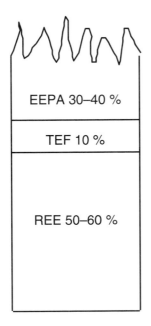

Fig. 65-1 Components of TEE, REE, TEF, and energy expenditure due to physical activity.

usual energy needs [5–11], and most [5,9–13] comparisons of the factorial approach with measurements of TEE have given significantly higher measured values for TEE than predicted from past recommended daily allowances (RDAs) [2].

The DRIs [1] adopted the alternative approach to estimating energy requirements of summarizing measurements of TEE determined using the doubly labeled water method for groups of individuals of normal body weight. Total energy expenditure includes all of the different subcomponents of EE previously summed in the factorial method, including RMR, EEPA, and TEF. For subjects in energy balance (i.e., who are neither gaining nor losing body fat), doubly labeled water measurements of TEE are equal to actual (rather than reported) energy intake, and so are equivalent to weight-maintenance energy needs.

As described elsewhere [14–16] the basis of the doubly labeled water method is that two stable isotopes of water ($H_2^{18}O$ and ^2H_2O) are administered and their disappearance rates from a body fluid such as urine or blood monitored for a period that is optimally equivalent to 1–3 half-lives for isotope disappearance (i.e., 7–21 days in most human subjects). The disappearance rate of ^2H_2O relates to water flux, whereas that of $H_2^{18}O$ reflects water flux plus carbon dioxide production rate through the rapid equilibration of the body water and bicarbonate pools resulting from the carbonic anhydrase reaction [17] (see Fig. 65-2). The difference between the two disappearance rates can therefore be used to calculate carbon dioxide production rate, from which TEE can be calculated.

Several validations of the doubly labeled water method have been conducted in which doubly labeled water-derived estimates of TEE were compared with measurements of EE in a whole-body calorimeter. Although validation studies conducted in whole-body calorimeters do not mimic normal life conditions, they do allow for an exact comparison of doubly labeled water with classic indirect calorimetry, which is considered a gold standard measurement of EE. As summarized elsewhere [18,19], there was a close agreement between means for CO_2 production rate determined by the two methods in all the validation studies. The precision of doubly labeled water measurements, as assessed by the variability of individual doubly labeled water measurements from the indirect calorimetry assessments, was 2–5% in the different studies. These validation studies show that the doubly labeled water method can provide an accurate assessment of carbon dioxide production rate and hence TEE in a wide range of human subjects.

One particular advantage of the doubly labeled water method for assessing energy requirements is that it provides a long-term index of TEE. Because 1–3 half-lives of isotope disappearance are needed for isotopic abundances to be measured accurately by mass spectrometry [20], optimal time periods for doubly labeled water measurements of TEE range from 1–3 weeks in most groups of human subjects. Thus, in contrast to other techniques such as the factorial method, doubly labeled water can provide EE estimations over biologically meaningful periods of time. Moreover, because doubly labeled water is noninvasive (requiring only that the subject drink the stable isotopes and provide 3+ urine samples over the study period), usual activity is not affected and measurements can be made in subjects leading their normal daily lives.

A critical mass of doubly labeled water data has now accumulated on a wide range of age groups and body sizes, and therefore, the new DRI [1] estimates of energy needs were based on doubly labeled water estimates of TEE (the complete dataset of individual results is given in the DRI publication).

II. Major Determinants of Energy Requirements

Equations for predicting the TEE (equal to energy requirements during weight-maintenance conditions) of women and men of healthy body weight (body mass index [BMI] 18.5–25 kg/m2) are given in Table 65-1. As summarized next, these equations were derived from the worldwide TEE database collected by the Food and Nutrition Board for determining DRIs [1]. Statistical modeling procedures were used to generate equations that fitted the data with allowance for four graded levels of EE for physical activity. Table 65-1 also shows equations for predicting RMR, the major component of TEE, from weight alone. The following sections of this chapter describe the effects of individual factors on TEE and RMR.

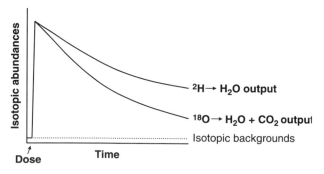

Fig. 65-2 Theoretical basis for the doubly labeled water method. Dose refers to the administration of the doubly labeled water $^2H_2^{18}O$, containing deuterium and oxygen 18. Carbon-dioxide, CO_2; Water, H_2O.

Table 65-1
Equations to Predict Total Energy Expenditure in Females and Males 19 and Older

For Females

TEE = 354.1−6.91 × Age [y] + PA × (9.36 × Weight [kg] + 726 × Height [m])
Where PA is the physical activity coefficient:
PA = 1.00 if PAL is estimated to be ≥1.0 <1.4 (Sedentary)
PA = 1.12 if PAL is estimated to be ≥1.4 <1.6 (Low Active)
PA = 1.27 if PAL is estimated to be ≥1.6 <1.9 (Active)
PA = 1.45 if PAL is estimated to be ≥1.9 <2.5 (Very Active)

For Males

TEE = 661.8−9.53 × Age [y] + PA × (15.91 × Weight [kg] + 539.6 × Height [m])
Where PA is the physical activity coefficient:
PA = 1.00 if PAL is estimated to be ≥1.0 <1.4 (Sedentary)
PA = 1.11 if PAL is estimated to be ≥1.4 <1.6 (Low Active)
PA = 1.25 if PAL is estimated to be ≥1.6 <1.9 (Active)
PA = 1.48 if PAL is estimated to be ≥1.9 <2.5 (Very Active)

Table 65-1
(Continued)
Equations to Predict Resting Metabolic Rate from Body Weight

Age Range	kcal/day	MJ/day
Females		
18–30	14.7 W + 496	0.0615 W + 2.08
30–60	8.7 W + 829	0.0364 W + 3.47
>60	10.5 W + 596	0.0439 W + 2.49
Males		
18–30	15.3 W + 679	0.0640 W + 2.84
30–60	11.6 W + 879	0.0485 W + 3.67
>60	13.5 W + 487	0.0565 W + 2.04

W, Body weight in kg.
(From Institute of Medicine of The National Academies. [2002]. *Dietary Reference Intakes: Energy, Carbohydrate, Fiber, Fat, Fatty Acids, Cholesterol, Protein, and Amino Acids.* Chapters 1–9. Washington, DC: The National Academy Press; National Academy of Sciences. [1989]. *Recommended Dietary Allowances.* 10th Edition. Washington, DC: The National Academy Press; and FAO, WHO, UNU. [1985]. Energy and protein requirements. Report of a joint FAO/WHO/UNU expert consultation. *Technical Report Series 724.* Geneva: World Health Organization.)

A. Body Size

Weight and height are important determinants of how much energy a person expends and therefore requires for body weight maintenance. Fig. 65-3 shows estimates of energy requirements (derived from Table 65-1 equations) for women of different heights and BMIs. It can be seen that for the same BMI, a woman of 1.73 m (5'8") will expend approximately 300 kcal/day more than a woman of 1.57 m (5'2") with the same level of physical activity. Both the additional height and the additional weight associated with that height contribute to the increased energy needs of the taller women. However, an increase in

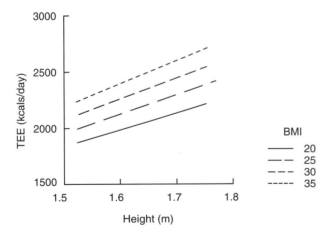

Fig. 65-3 Total energy expenditure in relation to height and BMI (predicted from the DRI equations for women). (From Institute of Medicine of The National Academies. [2002]. *Dietary Reference Intakes: Energy, Carbohydrate, Fiber, Fat, Fatty Acids, Cholesterol, Protein, and Amino Acids.* Chapters 1–9. Washington, DC: The National Academy Press.)

weight alone also causes TEE to increase. Contrary to the widespread belief that overweight women expend less energy to maintain weight than women of normal weight, the DRI database [1] of TEE measurements clearly indicates that heavier women have greater values for TEE than women of the same height but lower weight. For example, a woman with a BMI of 30 kg/m2 is predicted to have a greater TEE than a woman with a BMI of 25 kg/m2 in the same activity group by 200–240 kcal/day on average. In part this increase is due to increased RMR (as seen in the equations in Table 65-1, RMR is weight dependent; this is because additional body tissue has additional basal metabolic activity). Also, many of the daily activities, such as walking and running, are weight dependent and for the same workload heavier women will expend more energy. Even if activity is decreased in an overweight woman, TEE may still be high relative to that of a woman with normal BMI, because of the increase in energy needs associated with RMR.

It should be noted that the equations given in Table 65-1 for predicting energy requirements were developed from statistically modeling TEE data derived from women and men with values for BMI within the healthy range (18.5–25 kg/m2). However, as evaluated by the DRI group [1], inclusion of data from individuals >25 kg/m2 had very little effect on the parameter estimates, and thus the equations given are reasonably valid over a wide range of BMI values.

B. Gender

Much of the effect of gender on energy requirements can be traced to differences in body size between men and women. The reference woman weighs 13 kg less than the reference man, and is also 14 cm shorter. In consequence, size differences alone can exert a substantial impact on TEE and energy requirements. Fig. 65-4 shows calculated values for TEE based on the DRI equations for reference woman and men with different levels of activity. As seen, the TEE of women is consistently lower by 400 to 800 kcal/day.

There also appear to be cyclical changes in EE in women, especially for RMR, with most studies showing increased RMR in the luteal phase of the menstrual cycle compared with the follicular phase [21–25]. Two studies reported no increase in RMR in the luteal phase compared with the follicular phase [26,27] but in one of those studies both sleeping metabolic rate (SMR) and sedentary 24 h EE were significantly increased [26], suggesting that the lack of an increase in RMR may have been due to a methodologic problem.

Because of the weight of evidence indicating cyclical changes in RMR, and perhaps also sedentary 24 h EE in premenopausal adult women, studies examining whether women have lower energy requirements than men even after accounting for differences in body weight have usually adjusted or averaged for stage of the menstrual cycle. In such appropriately adjusted 24 h studies, two studies reported lower 24 h sedentary EE in women compared with men after adjusting for fat-free mass (FFM) and fat mass [28,29], although one study reported no significant gender effect in adjusted data [30]. The two studies showing lower 24 h EE are also consistent with the doubly labeled water TEE data of Carpenter *et al* [31] showing 16% lower TEE in women than men after controlling for the amount

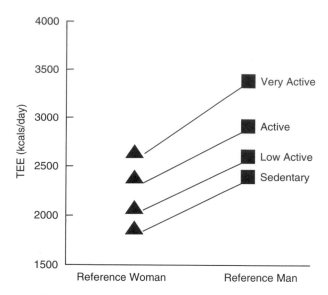

Fig. 65-4 Total energy expenditure in the reference woman vs reference man for different levels of activity (activity levels from the DRI). (From Institute of Medicine of The National Academies. [2002]. *Dietary Reference Intakes: Energy, Carbohydrate, Fiber, Fat, Fatty Acids, Cholesterol, Protein, and Amino Acids.* Chapters 1–9. Washington, DC: The National Academy Press.)

of lean tissue in the body, which was partly accounted for by lower RMR, and partly by other factors (presumably lower EEPA). Zurlo *et al* [32] also observed that spontaneous physical activity is correlated with subsequent weight change in men but not women, suggesting a tighter association between physical activity and body composition in men than women. Finally, menopause has also been associated with a further decrease in REE and decreased EEPA in association with increased body fat when no hormone replacement therapy is taken [33].

The question of whether the hormonal differences between premenopausal women and men are responsible for the observed differences in EE, or whether this is a secondary consequence to differences in body composition remains uncertain. Although most of the previously reviewed studies adjusted data for gender differences in the amount of lean tissue and fat mass, it was not possible to adjust for differences in the *quality* of FFM (i.e., the balance of different lean tissues). It is well recognized [34] that different body tissues have different metabolic rates, with brain and organ tissues having the highest values and muscle and adipose tissues having the lowest values. Therefore, it is possible that the lower RMR in women compared with men is due to a different balance of organ, brain, and skeletal muscle relative to men, rather than a lower EE per unit of individual tissues. Further studies are needed to address this issue.

C. Physical Activity

Energy expenditure for physical activity and arousal is the most variable component of TEE, and can vary from 400 to 3000 kcal/day between individuals. Exercise appears to have both immediate energy costs due to the work of the exercise, and longer-term effects on RMR.

The immediate energy cost of individual activities probably accounts for the majority of the effect of physical activity on energy requirements, and individuals who are more physically active tend to have a higher maximal oxygen consumption [35,36]. Table 65-2 shows average energy costs of a range of typical activities, with the values expressed as multiples of RMR, and Table 65-3 shows the absolute energy costs of these same activities expressed in terms of food equivalents.

In addition to the immediate energy cost of individual activities, physical activity also affects REE in the postexercise period by approximately +5% at least up to 24h after exercise [37]. The long-term effect of exercise in elevating REE is also seen in studies examining changes in RMR over several days in athletes who stop exercising [38,39].

There may also be chronic changes in EE associated with physical activity, resulting from changes in RMR due to alterations in body composition and alterations in the metabolic rate of muscle tissue, and changes in spontaneous physical activity associated with altered levels of fitness. However, the magnitude and direction of change in EE associated with these factors remains controversial. Concerning RMR, many studies have demonstrated that FFM is the major predictor of RMR [4,40] and therefore an increase in FFM due to increased physical activity would be expected to increase RMR. However, several studies do not support this relationship. In particular, three

Table 65-2
Energy Costs of Different Activities*

Activity	Energy Costs (Multiples of Basal Metabolism)
Sedentary Activities	
Sleeping	1.0
Sitting quietly	1.0
Sitting plus activity (e.g., sewing)	1.5
Walking	
Walking slowly (2 mph)	2.5
Walking at normal pace (3 mph)	3.3
Fast walking (4 mph)	4.5
Walking uphill at normal pace	6.9
Walking uphill at normal pace carrying 5 kg load	7.4
Home	
Household tasks, moderate effort	3.5
Gardening (no lifting)	4.4
Raking lawn	4.0
Lifting items	4.0
Recreational Sports	
Light activities (golf, bowling, sailing)	2.2–4.4
Moderate activities (dancing, cycling, tennis)	4.4–6.6
Heavy activities (skiing, jogging, rope skipping)	6.6+

*(From Institute of Medicine of The National Academies. [2002]. *Dietary Reference Intakes: Energy, Carbohydrate, Fiber, Fat, Fatty Acids, Cholesterol, Protein, and Amino Acids.* Chapters 1–9. Washington, DC: The National Academy Press.)

Table 65-3
Energy Costs of Different Activities Conducted for One Hour*

Activity	Energy Costs (calories above basal metabolism)	Food Equivalent
Sedentary Activities		
Sleeping	0	none
Sitting quietly	0	none
Sitting plus activity (e.g., sewing)	28	$\frac{1}{2}$ small cookie
Walking		
Walking slowly (2 mph)	83	$1\frac{1}{4}$ small cookies
Walking at normal pace (3 mph)	127	2 small cookies
Fast walking (4 mph)	193	3 small cookies
Walking uphill at normal pace	325	$5\frac{1}{2}$ small cookies
Walking uphill at normal pace carrying 5 kg load	353	6 small cookies
Household		
General household task, moderate effort	138	$2\frac{1}{4}$ small cookies
Gardening (no lifting)	188	3 small cookies
Raking lawn	166	$2\frac{3}{4}$ small cookie
Lifting items	166	$2\frac{3}{4}$ small cookie
Recreational Sports		
Light activities (golf, bowling, sailing)	66–188	1–3 small cookies
Moderate activities (dancing, cycling, tennis)	188–309	3–5 small cookies
Heavy activities (skiing, jogging, rope skipping)	309+	+5 small cookies

*Data recalculated for reference women of 57 kg with calculated BMR of 1325 kcal/d and assuming small cookie = 60 kcal.
(From Institute of Medicine of The National Academies. [2002]. *Dietary Reference Intakes: Energy, Carbohydrate, Fiber, Fat, Fatty Acids, Cholesterol, Protein, and Amino Acids*. Chapters 1–9. Washington, DC: The National Academy Press.)

studies [41–43], two of which hold energy intake constant [41,42] and promoted weight loss through dietary change, all reported no increase in RMR with increased physical activity. These data suggest that any potential increase in RMR with exercise training is easily negated by small opposing changes in energy balance.

The question of whether spontaneous nonexercise activity (sometimes loosely termed fidgeting) increases with intentional physical activity is also controversial. Spontaneous nonexercise activity has been reported to be quantitatively important, accounting for 100–800 kcal/day even in subjects residing in a whole body calorimeter chamber [4]. However, Shah *et al* [44] showed only a minimal (3%) increase in 24h EE, measured by whole-body calorimetry, with a 2-hour strenuous aerobic exercise program, presumably due to a corresponding decrease in EE at other times of the day. In another whole body calorimetry study, Van Etten *et al* [45] showed no significant increase in 24h EE with a standardized exercise program beyond that immediately associated with the energy cost of the exercise, whereas in contrast Blaak *et al* [46] reported a significant increase in spontaneous physical activity in obese boys enrolled in an exercise training program.

The question of whether different degrees of strenuousness may impact spontaneous nonexercise activity to different extents has also been addressed with mixed results. Shah *et al* [44] reported a bigger (5%) mean increase in 24h EE with a program of moderate exercise (walking) than with a strenuous aerobic training program conducted for an equivalent period (+3%),

suggesting that the subjects had lower levels of spontaneous movement after strenuous exercise because they were more tired. On the other hand, Schulz *et al* [47] reported no difference in sedentary 24h EE between aerobically fit and sedentary individuals, and Pacy *et al* [48] showed no differential effect of moderate vs strenuous activity on 24h EE after accounting for the energy costs of the exercise itself.

The combination of these different results indicate that the effects of planned physical activity on spontaneous activity at other times is highly variable (with overall effects on EE ranging from positive to negative), and probably depends on a number of factors including the nature of the exercise (strenuous vs moderate), the initial fitness of the subjects, and body composition and gender.

In contrast to the multiple potential effects of exercise, described previously, there appears to be minimal effects of age and gender on the energy costs of specific exercises [49] and no effect of exercise on TEF [50].

Quantification of the combined effects of physical activity on energy requirements is therefore clearly complex when a factorial approach is used to compute the separate effects of different aspects of physical activity. Therefore, studies have focused on using doubly labeled water to quantify the effects of physical activity on TEE. In cross-sectional studies, there is a substantial difference in physical activity level ([PAL] the ratio of TEE to REE) between long-term exercising women and sedentary women. For example, Withers *et al* [51] observed mean PAL values of 2.48 vs 1.87 in long-term active women reporting a mean 8.6 hr/week of aerobic exercise vs long-term nonexercisers. Concerning data from intervention studies, very intensive programs such as those training subjects to run a half marathon and requiring 8–10 hr/week of strenuous exercise, can also effect a substantial 15–50% increase in TEE in both adults and children [52–54]. However, more moderate exercise programs are reported to have a much smaller effect, with two studies (one with children and one with elderly individuals) reporting no significant increase in TEE [55,56]. This lack of TEE with a moderate increase in planned physical activity emphasizes the fact that intentional and spontaneous EE are interrelated and in some circumstances an increase in one component can be balanced by a decrease in the other component with the result that TEE can remain constant.

It is clear from the previous discussion of published data that although at a general level an increase in physical activity can be anticipated to increase TEE, this is not always the case. DRIs [1] provide for four different levels of physical activity (sedentary, low-active, active, very active) that are described in terms of walking equivalents (i.e., if all activity above the sedentary category was walking, how many miles would be walked daily?) as summarized in Table 65-4. Four activity categories were defined because at a general level the different categories can help to subdivide individuals with different energy requirements and PALs. However, it would be possible for an individual with a sedentary lifestyle who did little walking to expend energy that would classify her as active if she had high levels of spontaneous fidgeting and other unaccountable activity. For these reasons, further research is needed to provide methods for reliably placing individuals within their correct activity category, for the purpose of predicting energy requirements.

D. Age

As people get older, there is a tendency for all the major components of EE to decrease. Concerning RMR, there is an average decline in absolute RMR between young adult life and old age in both men and women [57], with a suggested breakpoint for more rapid decline apparently occurring around age 40 in men and 50 in women [58,59] (see Fig. 65-5). In the case of women, this may be due to an accelerated loss of FFM during menopause [60]. However, the change in absolute RMR with age also depends on weight change. Although RMR is generally

Table 65-4
Physical Activity Level Categories and Walking Equivalence

PAL Category*	PAL Range	Walking Equivalence** (miles/day at 2–4 mph)
Sedentary	1.0–1.39	0
Low Active	1.4–1.59	1.5–3.0
Active	1.6–1.89	3.0–7.5
Very Active	1.9–2.5	7.5–31.0

*PAL categories. (From Institute of Medicine of The National Academies. [2002]. *Dietary Reference Intakes: Energy, Carbohydrate, Fiber, Fat, Fatty Acids, Cholesterol, Protein, and Amino Acids*. Chapters 1–9. Washington, DC: The National Academy Press.)

**In addition to energy spent for generally unscheduled activities.

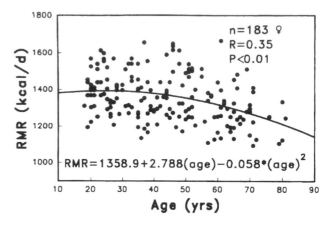

$$RMR = 1358.9 + 2.788(age) - 0.058*(age)^2$$

Fig. 65-5 Relationship between age and REE in women and men. (Adapted with permission from Poehlman ET. [1992]. Energy expenditure and requirements in aging humans. *J Nutr.* 122:2057–2065; and Poehlman ET, Berke EM, Joseph JR *et al.* [1992]. Influence of aerobic capacity, body composition and thyroid hormones on the age related decline in resting metabolic rate. *Metabolism.* 41:915–921.)

estimated to decline 1–2% per decade in individuals who maintain constant weight [57], this change must primarily be a consequence FFM loss and gain of less metabolically active fat associated with aging. In individuals who gain significant amounts of weight as they get older, RMR may actually increase due to gains of FFM and fat mass. In addition to FFM loss being a cause of age-associated decline in RMR, several [30,61–66] though not all [58,67] studies suggest that RMR adjusted for the change in FFM is decreased by about 5% in old adults compared to young ones. The reason for this change is not known, but may be due to loss of extremely metabolically active organ tissue and/or a decrease in metabolic rate per unit of specific lean tissues. There is also evidence suggesting that the RMR response to changes in energy balance may be attenuated in old vs young adults [68], which could be attributed to differences in FFM between young and old individuals. The equations for predicting RMR from body weight developed for the World Health Organization (WHO) (see Table 65-1) include an age effect. For example, a woman >60 is calculated to have a lower EE of approximately 11% than a woman of 18–30.

Concerning TEF, some studies report a decrease with aging [69–74], whereas other studies report no change or a nonsignificant increase [75–80]. Although this controversy cannot currently be resolved, a plausible explanation [80] is that TEF does not decline with aging per se, but that some studies may have included subjects with factors that decrease TEF independent of aging, such as obesity and digestive problems that limit nutrient absorption.

As seen in Fig. 65-6, which show cross-sectional differences in TEE between individuals of different ages, TEE declines substantially over the course of adult life. The regression equations predicting energy needs developed by the DRIs [1] (based on the data in Fig. 65-6) indicate that there is a progressive decline in TEE with age of 69 kcal/decade when there is no concomitant increase in body weight (which would tend to increase TEE, counterbalancing the effect of age) and no change in activity category. However, many individuals may also

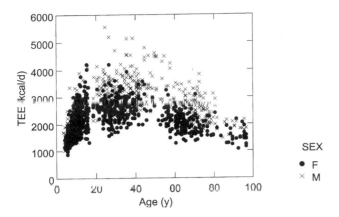

Fig. 65-6 Relationship between age and TEE in women and men. (From Institute of Medicine of The National Academies. [2002]. *Dietary Reference Intakes: Energy, Carbohydrate, Fiber, Fat, Fatty Acids, Cholesterol, Protein, and Amino Acids.* Chapters 1–9. Washington, DC: The National Academy Press.)

become much less active as they age, resulting in a greater decrease in TEE. These findings of decreased TEE with age based on doubly labeled water measurements are consistent with research based in whole body calorimeters showing that protocols with flexible activity result in lower 24h EE in elderly subjects compared to young ones [62].

The apparent decline in TEE and EE for physical activity in old age is also predicted by decreased reported strenuous physical activity in elderly men [81]. In addition, the decrease in TEE with age seen in the doubly labeled water and calorimeter studies closely parallels the increase in body fat mass [68], though the extent to which the increase in body fat mass with age is a consequence or a cause of the age-related decrease in EEPA is not known. In relation to this observation, it should be noted that some elderly individuals clearly are able to maintain very high levels of EE (for example, Withers *et al* [51] report PAL values of 2.48 among older women with routine exercise habits compared with 1.87 in nonexercising women). However, mean maximal oxygen consumption declines progressively with age at a similar rate in sedentary adults and professional athletes, suggesting that at least some parallel changes in fitness and EEPA with age are an inevitable consequence of the aging process rather than a cumulative consequence of long-term inactivity.

III. Other Determinants of Energy Requirements

A. Genetics and Racial Origin

Energy requirements vary substantially between individuals, primarily due to a combination of differences in body size and composition, gender, PAL, and age. Some of these differences may be mediated by the unique genetic inheritance of individuals, with transmissible and nontransmissible cultural factors contributing to variability also. Currently there is insufficient research data to predict the energy requirements of specific genetic and racial groups, but generalities can be made and as data accumulates more specific predictions may become possible.

The effects of genetic inheritance on body composition are well known, with most studies reporting that 25 to 50% of interindividual variability in body composition can be attributed to genetic factors [82–85]. Because FFM and fat mass are major determinants of both RMR and TEE [68], these genetic influences on FFM and FFM must translate into a strong effect on energy requirements secondary to a genetic effect on body composition.

In addition to these genetic influences on energy requirements mediated by genetic influences on body composition, there also appear to be genetic influences on EE independent of body composition. Bogardus *et al* reported a significant familial (i.e., intrafamily) influence on RMR independent of FFM, fat mass and sex [86]. In other words, for the same body size and composition, some families had higher or lower RMRs than others. Although the origin of this familial association is not currently known, it may potentially be due to differences in the relative sizes of FFM components (muscle, brain, organs) because work has suggested that organ size determined by magnetic resonance imaging (MRI) strongly predicts RMR [87]. In addition, Bouchard *et al* [88,89], reported that about 40% of the variance in RMR, TEF, and the energy costs of low- to moderate-intensity exercise is explained by inherited characteristics. The same group also reported [90] that there is a genetic component to the weight-gain response to 1000 kcal/day overfeeding, which must have been mediated by genetic influences on EE (because energy storage is equal to the difference between energy intake and EE).

The question of which specific genes underlie genetic differences in EE components is starting to be addressed, but few data are available as yet. Valve *et al* 1998 [91] reported that polymorphisms within the UCP1 gene had no effect on RMR, but a combination of polymorphisms in the UCP1 and beta 3-adrenergic receptor genes was associated with a significant 79 kcal/day decrease in RMR [91]. Klannemark *et al* 1998 [92] reported no association between polymorphisms in the UCP2 gene and RMR, whereas Astrup *et al* [93] reported significant associations of these polymorphisms with 24h EE determined in a whole body calorimeter and adjusted for FFM. The same group [93] also reported a small effect (6%) of circulating androstenedione and free T3 on 24h EE that may have had a genetic origin. The study of Astrup *et al* [93] suggesting an association of specific gene polymorphisms with sedentary EE is also consistent with the work of Heitmann *et al* [94] suggesting genetic influences on voluntary physical activity. Because EE for physical activity is the major variable component of TEE, it is likely that genetic influences on EEPA may contribute substantially to intraindividual variability in energy requirements, and further work in this area is needed.

In addition to the studies investigating general genetic influences in energy requirements, there have also been a number of studies investigating differences in energy requirements between specific racial groups. Most [31,95–100] but not all [102,103] studies comparing RMR or SMR between African-American and Caucasian adults have reported that RMR or SMR adjusted for differences in body composition are significantly lower in African-Americans by about 10%. Foster *et al*, 1999, [98] also reported that the decrease in RMR with weight loss adjusted for body composition change is greater in African-American women than Caucasian adults, even though weight loss of the African-American women in that study was less.

In addition, free-living EE for physical activity, measured using the doubly labeled water method, appears to be lower in African-American compared to Caucasian individuals by about 10% [31,101], whereas 24h sedentary EE measured by whole body calorimetry was not significantly different between African-American and Caucasian groups in two studies [100]. These studies suggest lower levels of intentional physical activities such as sports in African-Americans compared to white adults but no difference in spontaneous nonexercise EE, and as such are consistent with the separate reports of lower levels of reported physical activity in African-American vs Caucasian adults [103] and also lower maximal oxygen consumption (VO_2 max) [104]. The question of whether lower levels of physical activity in African-American vs Caucasian individuals reflect genetic or cultural differences between the groups is not known.

In addition to African-Americans, other minority races have been investigated for potential differences in energy requirements. Pima Indians, a racial group widely considered to have a form of genetic obesity, have no difference in RMR from Caucasians after adjustment for body composition [100,105], and similarly spontaneous physical activity was not different between Pima Indian and Caucasian children [105] although the same group observed that spontaneous physical activity is a familial trait [32]. Mohawk children were reported to have higher values for TEE than Caucasian children, due to high levels of EEPA [53]. Thus, although it is likely that there are racial differences in energy requirements, of either genetic or cultural origin, currently there is insufficient data to define specific differences in energy requirements between different racial groups and the equations of the DRIs [1] for predicting energy requirements are not specific for any particular race.

B. Climate

Mean outdoor daytime temperatures in the United States typically range from −20 to +40 C, with most values in the range −5 to +30 C. However, indoor temperatures are typically controlled within 20 to 25 C during winter by use of heaters, and are frequently controlled to within a similar range in summer with air conditioners. In addition, most individuals intentionally create a relatively consistent temperature microenvironment for themselves by using more insulating clothing in cold weather and lighter clothing in summer. Therefore, the question of whether normal variations in ambient temperature influence energy requirements is complex.

Potential effects of ambient temperature on energy requirements include effects on postprandial and postabsorptive metabolic rate (to include EE for shivering and nonshivering thermogenesis), the amount and types of voluntary and required physical activity, and the energy cost of that activity. Based on several studies involving measurement of TEE in climate-controlled whole-body calorimeters [106–111], the DRI report [1] concluded that there is a modest 2–5% increase in sedentary 24h EE at low-normal ambient temperatures compared to high-normal ambient temperatures. However, no specific allowance was made in the DRIs [1] for ambient temperature because the average

effects are included in the TEE database used to develop requirements and so and can be considered values averaged for all seasons of the year and all ambient temperatures.

IV. Summary and Conclusions

Equations developed from statistical modeling of measurements of TEE in healthy individuals now exist for predicting the energy requirements of groups and individuals from age, weight, height, and estimated level of physical activity. Other factors such as genetic inheritance, racial origin, and climate also exert some influence on energy requirements, but are probably quantitatively small relative to age, weight, height, and activity level. Use of the new equations should help improve estimates of energy needs required in clinical settings for both men and women.

V. Suggestions for Further Investigations

Issues that would add to the existing knowledge and further understanding of gender-based information on energy expenditure include:

- Research linking actual levels of physical activity to measurements of TEE.
- Studies identifying the underlying reasons for gender related differences in RMR.
- Studies examining the net effect of exercise regimens on TEE in women [112].

References

1. Institute of Medicine of The National Academies. (2002). *Dietary Reference Intakes: Energy, Carbohydrate, Fiber, Fat, Fatty Acids, Cholesterol, Protein, and Amino Acids.* Chapters 1–9. Washington, DC: The National Academy Press.
2. National Academy of Sciences. (1989). *Recommended Dietary Allowances.* 10th Edition. Washington, DC: The National Academy Press.
3. Garby L, Kurzer MS, Lammert O, Nielsen E. (1987). Energy expenditure during sleep in men and women: Evaporative and sensible heat losses. *Hum Nutr Clin Nutr.* 41:225–233.
4. Ravussin E, Lillioja S, Anderson TE, Christin L *et al.* (1996). Determinants of 24-hour energy expenditure in man, methods and results using a respiratory chamber. *J Clin Invest.* 78:1568–1578.
5. Roberts SB, Young VR, Fuss P *et al.* (1990). Energy expenditure and subsequent nutrient intakes in overfed young men. *Am J Physiol.* 259:R461–R469.
6. Durnin JVGA. (1990). Low energy expenditures in free-living populations. *Eur J Clin Nutr.* 44 95–102.
7. Durnin JVGA. (1990). Is satisfactory energy balance possible on low energy intakes? *Bull Nutr Found India.* 11:1–4.
8. Roberts SB, Heyman MB, Evans WJ *et al.* (1991). Dietary energy requirements of young adult men, determined by using the doubly labeled water method. *Am J Clin Nutr.* 54:499–505.
9. Roberts SB. (1993). Energy expenditure and the development of early obesity. *Ann NY Acad Sci.* 699:18–25.
10. Sawaya AL, Saltzman E, Young VR *et al.* (1995). Dietary energy requirements of young and older women determined by using the doubly labeled water method. *Am J Clin Nutr.* 62:338–344.
11. Jones PJ, Martin LJ, Su W, Boyd NF. (1997). Canadian recommended nutrient intakes underestimate true energy requirements in middle-aged women. *Can J Publ Health.* 88:314–319.
12. Haggarty P, McNeill G, Abu Manneh MK *et al.* (1994). The influence of exercise on the energy requirements of adult males in the UK. *Br J Nutr.* 72:799–813.
13. Leonard WR, Galloway VA, Ivakine E. (1997). Underestimation of daily energy expenditure with the factorial method: Implications for anthropological research. *Am J Phys Anthr.* 103:443–454.

14. Roberts SB, Leibel RL. (1998). Excess energy intake and low energy expenditure as predictors of obesity. *Int J Obesity*. 22:385–386.

15. Roberts SB. (1989). Use of the doubly labeled water method for measurement of energy expenditure, total body water, water intake, and metabolizable energy intake in humans and small animals. *Can J Physiol Pharm*. 67:1190–1198.

16. Schoeller DA. (1988). Measurement of energy expenditure in free-living humans by using doubly labeled water. *J Nutr*. 118:1278–1289.

17. Lifson N, Gordon GB, Visscher MB, Nier AO. (1949). The fate of utilized molecular oxygen and the source of oxygen of respiratory carbon dioxide, studied with the aid of heavy oxygen. *J Biol Chem*. 180:803–811.

18. Roberts SB, Coward WA, Schlingenseipen K-H *et al*. (1986). Comparison of the doubly labeled water (^{2}H2^{18}O) method with indirect calorimetry and a nutrient balance study for simultaneous determination of energy expenditure, water intake and metabolizable energy intake in preterm infants. *Am J Clin Nutr*. 44:315–322.

19. Schoeller DA, Webb P. Five-day comparison of the doubly labeled water method with respiratory gas exchange. *Am J Clin Nutr*. 1984; 40:153–158.

20. Schoeller DA. (1983). Energy expenditure from doubly labeled water: Some fundamental considerations in humans. *Am J Clin Nutr*. 38:999–1005.

21. Solomon SJ, Kurzer MS, Calloway DH. (1982). Menstrual cycle and basal metabolic rate in women. *Am J Clin Nutr*. 36:611–616.

22. Hessemer V, Bruch K. (1985). Influence of the menstrual cycle on thermoregulatory, metabolic, and heart rate responses to exercise at night. *J Appl Physio*. 59:1911–1917.

23. Bisdee JT, James WPT, Shaw MA. (1989). Changes in energy expenditure during the menstrual cycle. *Br J Nutr*. 61:187–199.

24. Meijer GAL, Westerterp KR, Saris WHM, ten Hoor F. (1992). Sleeping metabolic rate in relation to body composition and the menstrual cycle. *Am J Clin Nutr*. 55:637–640.

25. Melanson KJ, Saltzman E, Russell R, Roberts SB. (1996). Postabsorptive and postprandial energy expenditure and substrate oxidation do not change during the menstrual cycle in young women. *J Nutr*. 26:2531–2538.

26. Howe JC, Rumpler WV, Seale JL. (1993). Energy expenditure by indirect calorimetry in premenopausal women: Variation within one menstrual cycle. *J Nutr Biochem*. 4:268–273.

27. Piers LS, Diggavi SN, Rijskamp J *et al*. (1995). Resting metabolic rate and thermic effect of a meal in the follicular and luteal phases of the menstrual cycle in well-nourished Indian women. *Am J Clin Nutr*. 61:296–302.

28. Ferraro R, Lillioja S, Fontvielle AM *et al*. (1992). Lower sedentary metabolic rate in women compared with men. *J Clin Invest*. 90:780–784.

29. Dionne I, Despres JP, Bouchard C, Tremblay A. (1999). Gender difference in the effect of body composition on energy metabolism. *Int J Obes Relat Metab Disord*. 23(3):312–319.

30. Klausen B, Toubro S, Astrup A. (1997). Age and sex effects on energy expenditure. *Am J Clin Nutr*. 65:895–907.

31. Carpenter WH, Fonong T, Toth MJ *et al*. (1998). Total daily energy expenditure in free-living older African-Americans and Caucasians. *Am J Physiol*. 274:E96–E101.

32. Zurlo F, Ferraro RT, Fontvielle AM *et al*. (1992). Spontaneous physical activity and obesity: Cross-sectional and longitudinal studies in Pima Indians. *Am J Physiol*. 263:E296–300.

33. Poehlman ET, Toth MJ, Gardner AW. (1995). Changes in energy balance and body composition at menopause: A controlled longitudinal study. *Ann Int Med*. 123:673–675.

34. FAO, WHO, UNU. (1985). Energy and protein requirements. Report of a joint FAO/WHO/UNU expert consultation. *Technical Report Series 724*. Geneva: World Health Organization.

35. Berthouze SE, Pierre MM, Castells J *et al*. (1995). Relationship between mean habitual daily energy expenditure and maximal oxygen uptake. *Med Sci Sports Exerc*. 27:1170–1179.

36. Brochu M, Starling RD, Ades PA, Poehlman ET. (1999). Are aerobically fit older individuals more physically active in their free-living time? A doubly labeled water approach. *J Clin Endocrinol Metab*. 84(11):3872–3876.

37. Bielinski R, Schutz Y, Jequier E. (1985). Energy metabolism during the post-exercise recovery in man. *Am J Clin Nutr*. 42:69–82.

38. Tremblay A, Nadeau A, Fournier G, Bouchard C. (1988). Effect of a three-day interruption of exercise-training on resting metabolic rate and glucose-induced thermogenesis in trained individuals. *Int J Ob*. 12:163–168.

39. Herring JL, Mole PA, Meredith CN, Stern JS. (1992). Effect of suspending exercise training on resting metabolic rate in women. *Med Sci Sports Exerc*. 24:59–65.

40. Ravussin E, Bogardus C. (1989). Relationship of genetics, age, and physical fitness to daily energy expenditure and fuel utilization. *Am J Clin Nutr*. 49:968–975.

41. Tremblay A, Despres JP, Leblanc C *et al*. (1990). Effect of intensity of physical activity on body fatness and fat distribution. *Am J Clin Nutr*. 51:153–157.

42. Bingham SA, Goldberg GR, Coward WA *et al*. (1989). The effect of exercise and improved physical fitness on basal metabolic rate. *Br J Nutr*. 61:155–173.

43. Treuth M, Hunter G, Weinsier R, Kell S. (1995). Energy expenditure and substrate utilization in older women after strength training: 24-h calorimeter results. *J Appl Physiol*. 78:2140–2146.

44. Shah M, Geissler CA, Miller DS. (1988). Metabolic rate during and after aerobic exercise in post-obese and lean women. *Eur J Clin Nutr*. 42:455–464.

45. Van Etten LM, Westerterp KR, Verstappen FT *et al*. (1985). Racial differences in the energy cost of standardised activities. *Ann Nutr Metab*. 29:40–47.

46. Blaak EE, Westerterp KR, Bar-Or O *et al*. (1992). Total energy expenditure and spontaneous activity in relation to training in obese boys. *Am J Clin Nutr* 55:777–782.

47. Schulz S, Westerterp KR, Brück K. (1989). Comparison of energy expenditure by the doubly labeled water technique with energy intake, heart rate and activity recording in men. *Am J Clin Nutr*. 49:1146–1154.

48. Pacy PJ, Cox M, Khalouha M *et al*. (1996). Does moderate aerobic activity have a stimulatory effect on 24h resting energy expenditure: A direct calorimeter study. *Int J Food Sci Nutr*. 47.

49. Morio B, Beaufrere B, Montaurier C *et al*. (1997). Gender differences in energy expended during activities and in daily energy expenditure of elderly people. *Am J Physiol*. 273:E321–327.

50. Dallosso HM, James WPT. (1984). Whole-body calorimeter studies in adult men 1. The effect of fat over-feeding on 24h energy expenditure. *Br J Nutr*. 52:49–64.

51. Withers RT, Smith DA, Tucker RC *et al*. (1998). Energy metabolism in sedentary and active 49- to 70-yr-old women. *J Appl Physiol*. 84:1333–1340.

52. Westerterp KR, Meijer GA, Janssen EM *et al*. (1992). Long-term effect of physical activity on energy balance and body composition. *Br J Nutr*. 68:21–30.

53. Goran MI, Kashoun M, Johnson R *et al*. (1995). Energy expenditure and body fat distribution in Mohawk children. *Pediatrics*. 95:89–95.

54. Eliakim A, Barstow TJ, Brasel JA *et al*. (1996). Effect of exercise training on energy expenditure, muscle volume, and maximal oxygen uptake in female adolescents. *J Pediatr*. 129:537–543.

55. Goran MI, Poehlman ET. (1992). Total energy expenditure and energy requirements in healthy elderly persons. *Metabolism*. 41:744–753.

56. Treuth MS, Adolph AL, Butte NF. (1998). Energy expenditure in children predicted from heart rate and activity calibrated against respiration calorimetry. *Am J Physiol*. 275:E12–E18.

57. Keys A, Taylor HL, Grande F. (1973). Basal metabolism and age of adult man. *Metabolism*. 22:579–587.

58. Poehlman ET, Goran MJ, Gardner AW *et al*. (1993). Determinants of decline in resting metabolic rate in aging females. *Am J Physiol*. 264:E450–E455.

59. Poehlman ET. (1992). Energy expenditure and requirements in aging humans. *J Nutr*. 122:2057–2065.

60. Svendsen OL, Hassager C, Christiansen C. (1995). Age- and menopause-associated variations in body composition and fat distribution in healthy women as measured by dual-energy x-ray absorptiometry. *Metabolism*. 44:369–373.

61. Fukagawa NK, Bandini LG, Young JB. (1990). Effect of age on body composition and resting metabolic rate. *Am J Physiol*. 259:E233–E238.

62. Vaughan L, Zurlo F, Ravussin E. Aging and energy expenditure. *Am J Clin Nutr*. 1991; 53:821–825.

63. Poehlman ET, Melby CL, Bradylak SF. (1991). Relation of age and physical exercise status on metabolic rate in younger and older healthy men. *J Gerontol*. 46:B54–B58.

64. Visser M, de Groot LCPGM, Deurenberg P, van Staveren W. Dietary History Method Underestimates Energy Intake in a Group of Healthy Elderly Women. Second international conference on dietary assessment methods, Boston, MA, 1995.

65. Roberts SB. (1995). Influence of age on energy requirements. *Am J Clin Nutr*. 62(Suppl):1053A–1058A.

66. Pannemans DLE, Westerterp KR. (1995). Energy expenditure, physical activity and basal metabolic rate of elderly subjects. *Br J Nutr*. 73:571–581.

67. Tzankoff SP, Norris AH. (1977). Effect of muscle mass decrease on age-related BMR changes. *J Appl Physiol: Respirat Environ Exercise Physiol*. 43:1001–1006.

68. Roberts SB, Dallal GE. (1998). The effects of age on energy balance. *Am J Clin Nutr*. 68S:975S–979S.

69. Rolls BJ, Dimeo KA, Shide DJ. (1995). Age-related impairments in the regulation of food intake. *Am J Clin Nutr*. 62:923–931.

70. Steen B. (1988). Body composition and aging. *Nutr Rev*. 46:45–51.

71. Morley JE, Silver AJ. (1988). Anorexia in the elderly. *Neurobiology Aging*. 9:9–16.

72. Ferrannini E, Vichi S, Beck-Nielsen H *et al*. (1996). Insulin action and age. *Diabetes*. 45:947–953.

73. Marker JC, Cryer PE, Clutter WE. (1992). Attenuated glucose recovery from hypoglycemia. *Diabetes*. 41:671–678.

74. Meneilly GS, Cheung E, Tuokko H. (1994). Altered responses to hypoglycemia of healthy elderly people. *Clin Endocrinol Metab*. 78:1341–1348.

75. Meneilly GS, Cheung E, Tuokko H. (1994). Counterregulatory hormone responses to hypoglycemia in the elderly patient with diabetes. *Diabetes*. 43:403–410.

76. Brierley EJ, Broughton DL, James OFW, Alberti KGMM. (1995). Reduced awareness of hypoglycaemia in the elderly despite an intact counter-regulatory response. *QJ Med*. 88:439–445.

77. Minaker KL, Meneilly GS, Rowe JW. (1984). Endocrine systems. In *Handbook of the Biology of Aging*, (Finch C, Hayflick L, ed.), pp. 433–456. New York: Van Nostrand Reinhold.

78. Roth GS. (1979). Hormone action during aging: Alterations and mechanisms. *Mech Ageing Devel*. 9:497–514.

79. Committee on Statistics of the American Diabetes Association C. (1969). Standardization of the oral glucose tolerance test. *Diabetes*. 28:299–310.

80. Melanson KJ, Greenberg AS, Ludwig DS *et al*. (1998). Blood glucose and hormonal responses to small and large meals in healthy young and older women. *J Gerontol*. 53A:B299–B305.

81. Roberts SB. (1996). Energy requirements of older individuals. *Eur J Clin Nutr*. 50(Suppl 1):S112–S118.

82. Bouchard C, Savard R, Despres JP *et al*. (1985). Body composition in adopted and biological siblings. *Hum Biol*. 57:61–75.

83. Bouchard C, Perusse L. (1988). Heredity and body fat. *Ann Rev Nutr*. 8:259–277.

84. Bouchard C, Perusse L, Leblanc C. (1988). Inheritance of the amount and distribution of human body fat. *Int J Obesity*. 12:205.

85. Bouchard C, Perusse R, Tremblay L, Leblanc C. (1986). Inheritance of body composition and fat distribution. *Am J Phys Anthr*. 179:61–75.

86. Bogardus C, Lillioja S, Ravussin E *et al*. (1986). Familial dependence of the resting metabolic rate. *New Eng J Med*. 315:96–100.

87. Illner K, Brinkmann G, Heller M *et al*. (2000). Metabolically active components of fat free mass and resting energy expenditure in nonobese adults. *Am J Physiol*. 278:E308–E315.

88. Bouchard C, Despres J-P, Mauriege P. (1993). Genetic and nongenetic determinants of regional fat distribution. *Endocrine Rev*. 14:72–89.

89. Bouchard C, Tremblay A, Nadeau A *et al*. (1989). Genetic effects in resting and exercise metabolic rates. *Metab*. 4:364–370.

90. Bouchard C, Tremblay A, Despres J-P *et al*. (1990). The response to long-term overfeeding in identical twins. *New Eng J Med*. 322:1477–1482.

91. Valve R, Heikkinen S, Rissanen A *et al*. (1998). Synergistic effect of polymorphisms in uncoupling protein 1 and beta 3-adrenergic receptor genes on basal metabolic rate in obese Finns. *Diabetologia*. 41:357–361.

92. Klannemark M, Orho M, Groop L. (1998). No relationship between identified variants in the uncoupling protein 2 gene and energy expenditure. *Eur J Endocrinol*. 139:217–223.

93. Astrup A, Toubro S, Dalgaard LT *et al*. (1999). Impact of the v/v 55 polymorphism of the uncoupling protein 2 gene on 24-h energy expenditure and substrate oxidation. *Int J Obes Relat Metab Disord*. 23:1030–1034.

94. Heitmann BL, Kaprio J, Harris JR *et al*. (1997). Are genetic determinants of weight gain modified by leisure-time physical activity? A prospective study of Finnish twins. *Am J Clin Nutr*. 66:672–678.

95. Geissler CA, Aldouri MS. (1985). Racial Differences in the Energy Cost of Standardised Activities. *Ann Nutr Metab*. 29:40–47.

96. Albu J, Shur M, Curi M *et al*. (1997). Resting metabolic rate in obese, premenopausal black women. *Am J Clin Nutr*. 66:531–538.

97. Foster GD, Wadden TA, Vogt RA. (1997). Resting energy expenditure in obese African-American and Caucasian women. *Obes Res*. 5:1–8.

98. Foster GD, Wadden TA, Swain RM *et al*. (1999). Changes in resting energy expenditure after weight loss in obese African-American and white woman. *Am J Clin Nutr*. 69:13–17.

99. Jakicic JM, Wing RR. (1998). Differences in resting energy expenditure in African-American vs Caucasian overweight females. *Int J Obes Relat Metab Disord*. 22:236–242.

100. Weyer C, Snitker S, Bogardus C, Ravussin E. (1999). Energy metabolism in African-Americans: Potential risk factors for obesity. *Am J Clin Nutr*. 70:13–20.

101. Kushner RF, Racette SB, Neil K, Schoeller DA. (1995). Measurement of physical activity among black and white obese women. *Obes Res*. 3:261S–265S.

102. Nicklas BJ, Toth MJ, Goldberg AP, Poehlman ET. (1997). Racial differences in plasma leptin concentrations in obese postmenopausal women. *J Clin Endocrinol Metab*. 82:315–317.

103. Washburn RA, Kline G, Lackland DT, Wheeler FC. (1992). Leisure time physical activity: Are there black/white differences? *Prev Med*. 21:127–135.

104. Hunter GR, Weinsier RL, Darnell BE *et al*. (2000). Racial differences in energy expenditure and aerobic fitness in premenopausal women. *Am J Clin Nutr*. 71:500–506.

105. Fontvieille AM, Dwyer J, Ravussin E. (1992). Resting metabolic rate and body composition of Pima Indian and Caucasian children. *Int J Obes Relat Metab Disord*. 16:535–542.

106. Garby L, Lammert O, Nielsen E. (1990). Changes in energy expenditure of light physical activity during a 10 day period at 34 degrees Celsius environmental temperature. *Eur J Clin Nutr*. 44:241–244.

107. Blaza S, Garrow JS. (1983). Thermogenic response to temperature, exercise and food stimuli in lean and obese women, studied by 24h direct calorimetry. *Br J Nutr*. 49:171–180.

108. Warwick PM, Busby R. (1990). Influence of mild cold on 24h energy expenditure in 'normally' clothed adults. *Br J Nutr*. 63:481–488.

109. Buemann B, Astrup A, Christensen NJ, Madsen J. (1992). Effect of moderate cold exposure on 24-h energy expenditure: similar response in postobese and nonobese women. *Am J Physiol*. 263:E1040–E1045.

110. Nielsen E. (1987). Acute modest changes in relative humidity do not affect energy expenditure at rest in human subjects. *Hum Nutr Clin Nutr*. 41:485–488.

111. Valencia ME, McNeill G, Brockway JM, Smith JS. (1992). The effect of environmental temperature and humidity on 24h energy expenditure in men. *Br J Nutr*. 68:319–327.

112. Poehlman ET, Berke EM, Joseph JR *et al*. (1992). Influence of aerobic capacity, body composition and thyroid hormones on the age related decline in resting metabolic rate. *Metabolism*. 41:915–921.

66

Anorexia, Bulimia, Disordered Eating, and Obesity

DIANN M. ACKARD, PhD
Private Practice, Golden Valley, MN

The purpose of this chapter is to describe the impact of gender on eating and weight disorders. The prevalence of anorexia nervosa, bulimia nervosa, and disordered eating behaviors is greater among adolescent and adult females than among males by a factor of approximately 9:1. However, prevalence of binge eating disorder and obesity within community samples is comparable across gender. Prevalence rates of eating disorders among males may be too low, influenced by biases in diagnostic criteria, the assumption that these disorders are almost exclusively seen in females, and barriers to treatment accessibility for affected males. Specific characteristics associated with eating and weight disorders differ in males and among females. For example, males with eating disorders are more likely than females to report a homosexual orientation. Anorexic males have different reasons for losing weight than do anorexic females, and bulimic males are less likely to use extreme compensatory behaviors such as laxative use and vomiting than bulimic females. In addition, eating-disordered males are more likely to choose a realistic ideal body weight and report body satisfaction than their eating-disordered females of similar age, and are also more likely to report substance abuse than their eating-disordered female peers. Finally, obese women are more likely than obese men to report psychologic and social discrimination. Research on familial and genetic transmission of the disorder provides evidence of the heritability of eating disorders mainly among female relatives, although research among affected males is extremely limited. Prevention and treatment interventions need to be tailored to accommodate the rising awareness of eating disorders in both genders.

I. Introduction

Eating disorders are disturbances that are widely recognized among professionals and laypersons at present. However, early reports of anorexia nervosa and bulimia nervosa in males and females, although rare, appear as early as the 17th century [1]. One of the more striking findings regarding the etiology and epidemiology of eating disorders is that they are predominantly disorders afflicting women, and therefore, have been thought of as gender-specific. However, figures indicate that the rates of eating and weight disorders among males are increasing [2], a finding that brings to question whether these disorders are truly gender-specific, or whether the presence of eating and weight disorders among males has been under- or undetected?

Differences in male and female bodies are evident, and are first noticeable at birth because of the anatomic differences between boys' and girls' bodies. As early as toddler age, young boys and girls learn that their bodies are different from those of the opposite sex. During puberty, bodies of both boys and girls undergo tremendous changes. For example, girls' bodies change to a fuller figure by developing a greater percentage of adipose tissue typically concentrated at the breasts and lower extremities, whereas boys develop greater muscle mass, height, and lowered voice. Although these bodily changes may be challenging for both genders, these transitions have opposite effects with respect to the gender-specific cultural ideal. For boys, changes during puberty typically result in a body form that is closer to the current ideal. Among girls, the transition yields a body moving directly away from the current cultural ideal of prepubescent slenderness. These differences may explain why nearly twice as many girls as boys diet in grade school [3], despite similarities in body mass index (BMI) and obesity status.

There are also similarities in the ways that males and females experience their bodies. Regardless of gender, individuals who believe their bodies do not approximate the cultural ideal are at greater risk to utilize efforts, sometimes extreme, to transform the body into that which is more consistent with the ideal. Reports suggest that both genders are dissatisfied with their bodies, but in different ways [3]. Typically, females want to lose weight whereas males want to increase muscle mass. Females concentrate on losing "weight" or wanting to be a smaller size, whereas males focus on the shape of their body and pay less attention to weight. Females attempt to change their lower torso (legs, thighs, buttocks, abdomen), compared with males who target their upper torso (chest size, shoulders, biceps and triceps). And for both males and females, society plays a significant role in advertising the "ideal" body shape by gender. For females, this shape tends to be very thin and angular or with curves only at the bust, and for males it tends to be very muscular and lean.

There are also multiple similarities in the factors associated with eating disorders among both females and males. Individuals with eating disorders, when compared to those without a psychiatric diagnosis, are more likely to report symptoms of depression and anxiety, to struggle with body dissatisfaction, and to score lower on measures of self-esteem. The consequences of eating disorders, including medical, psychologic and social problems, do not know gender boundaries—both males and females seem to be equally affected.

In this chapter, eating and weight disorders (anorexia nervosa, bulimia nervosa, binge eating disorder, disordered eating, and obesity) are discussed with respect to gender, and within a multidimensional framework. Although there is limited research on the experiences of males with eating disorders, the available studies provide a foundation for what is known about gender differences and similarities in the field. Gaps in our current understanding of the gender differences serve to provide an excellent opportunity to raise questions for the future—what do

Table 66-1
Estimated Prevalence of Eating Disorders by Gender

Disorder	Males	Females
Anorexia Nervosa	0–0.2%	0.4–1.0%
Bulimia Nervosa	0–0.2%	1.1–6.0%
Binge Eating Disorder	0–5.3%	1.5–4.6%
Disordered Eating ("Dieting")	≤28%	≤47%
Obesity	≤20.2%	≤19.4%

we need to understand about females and males who have eating and weight disorders?

II. Anorexia Nervosa

A. Diagnostic Criteria

The term *anorexia* in medical terminology means "loss of appetite." However, it should not be assumed that individuals with anorexia nervosa do not experience appetite or hunger. According to the *Diagnostic and Statistical Manual of Mental Disorders*, 4th edition (DSM-IV) [4], the criteria for anorexia nervosa are:

1. Inability to maintain body weight at or above a minimally normal weight for age and height.
2. Intense fear of gaining weight or becoming fat, even though underweight.
3. Distorted sense of body, shape and size, undue influence of body weight on self-evaluation, or denial of the seriousness of the current low body weight.
4. In postmenarcheal females, amenorrhea (i.e., the absence of at least three consecutive menstrual cycles).

Obviously amenorrhea does not apply to diagnoses of males. To address changes in sexual functioning as a result of an eating disorder, the International Classification of Diseases, 10th revision (ICD-10) [5] includes loss of sexual interest and lack of potency as similar criteria for males. However, some clinicians choose to omit any criteria related to sexual interest or functioning when diagnosing males.

There are two classifications of anorexia nervosa: restricting type and binge-eating/purging type. Restricting type describes individuals who have not regularly engaged in binge-eating or purging behavior during the course of anorexia nervosa. Anorexia nervosa of the binge-eating/purging type classifies individuals who have regularly engaged in binge-eating or purging behaviors (self-induced vomiting, and/or the misuse of laxatives, diuretics, or enemas) during the episode of anorexia nervosa.

B. Prevalence Estimates

The prevalence of anorexia nervosa is estimated to range from 0.4% to 1.0% among females [4,6–7]. Prevalence rates for anorexia nervosa among males are limited [4], but are estimated to be between 0.0 and 0.2% [7,8]. Gender prevalence estimates for restricting type vs binge-eating/purging type are not known. The incidence rate of anorexia nervosa for females is approximately 18 cases, compared with two cases for males per 100,000 per year [6]. By gender, the ratio of community-based females to males with anorexia nervosa ranges from 6:1 to 20:1 [9], and among those who seek treatment (outpatient or inpatient) for anorexia nervosa is approximately 10:1 [10–13]. Although these rates illustrate that anorexia nervosa is not a common disorder, it has the highest mortality rate among all the psychiatric disorders [14].

C. Gender and Clinical Presentation

There exist similarities and differences between male and female anorexics in the presentation of the disorder. Several studies [15,16] found no significant differences by gender on the diagnostic features of the disorder, average age at onset of illness, age at first treatment and number of treatments, duration of illness, and sociodemographic characteristics such as familial mental illness, socioeconomic status, and birth order. However, these same studies do report several differences. Males were significantly more overweight (had a higher BMI) at the onset of weight loss prior to the development of anorexia nervosa, but were less likely to engage in the regular misuse of laxatives (such as would be characteristic of anorexia nervosa, binge-eating/purging type) than females. Furthermore, a greater percentage of males reported having a poor appetite in childhood than females.

According to Andersen *et al* [17], there are gender differences in the primary reasons for developing anorexia nervosa. Males are more likely than females to develop anorexia nervosa to avoid being teased for overweight, to enhance athletic performance (such as among wrestlers, jockeys, and ballet dancers), to avoid developing medical illnesses similar to a family member (most notably the father), and to improve a gay relationship [17]. In comparison, females often cite aesthetics related to body satisfaction and power/control as reasons for their weight loss.

There have been no systematic studies investigating the effectiveness of manual-based psychotherapy treatments for males as compared with females. Most of the information regarding treatment outcome for anorexic males is gleaned from inpatient and outpatient clinics that provide treatment to females and males, often with mixed-gender groups and interventions. Nonetheless, to date no gender differences in treatment outcome of anorexia nervosa have been found [18–19]; both males and females are likely to benefit from treatments proven to be effective. There is no current evidence to suggest that these treatments, when proven to be effective for females with anorexia nervosa, would not be comparably effective for males. However, separate groups for males may be one treatment difference worth consideration [9].

Medical complications to anorexia nervosa seem to be similar across genders (see Table 66-2 for a list of common medical complications associated with eating disorders). In addition to typical abnormalities in weight, dermatology, endocrinology, and cardiac systems, both males and females with anorexia nervosa have comparable bone mineral density deficiencies [20] and decreases in total brain volume and increases in ventricular volume [21]. One gender-specific laboratory finding is that males with anorexia nervosa often develop low testosterone levels and females with anorexia nervosa experience low estrogen levels, both attributed to low weight. In male patients, general physical evaluations should include initial and progressive assessments of serum testosterone levels [17]. Results from a testicular exam may indicate decreased size of testes in males with anorexia. In

Table 66-2
Common Medical Complaints and Possible Complications Associated with Eating Disorders

Medical System	Anorexia Nervosa	Bulimia Nervosa	Obesity
Cardiovascular			
Sinus bradycardia	✔		
Resting and orthostatic hypotension	✔	✔	
Hypertension			✔
Arrhythmia	✔		
EKG abnormalities (QT prolongation)	✔	✔	
Mitral valve prolapse	✔	✔	
Ipecac-related cardiomyopathy		✔	
Cardiovascular disease			✔
Stroke			✔
Dental and Oral			
Dental caries		✔	
Enamel erosion on lingual and occlusal surfaces		✔	
Frequent sore throats, esophagitis		✔	
Salivary gland hypotrophy (e.g., parotid glands)		✔	
Dermatology			
Hair loss, brittle nails, dry skin	✔	✔	
Calluses on knuckles (Russell's sign)	✔	✔	
Lanugo growth (fine, downy hair)	✔		
Skin rashes from skin rubbing together			✔
Endocrine			
"Euthyroid sick syndrome" (low T3, high rev. T3)	✔		
Fluid and Electrolyte			
Dehydration	✔	✔	
Hypokalemia		✔	
Hypochloremia		✔	
Metabolic alkalosis		✔	
Dyslipidemia	✔		✔
Hypercarotenemia	✔		
Gastrointestinal			
Nonfocal abdominal pain	✔	✔	✔
Constipation or diarrhea	✔	✔	✔
Gastroparesis (abdominal bloating)	✔	✔	✔
Delayed gastric and whole-gut emptying	✔	✔	
Gastric dilation, rupture	✔	✔	
Gastroesophageal reflux	✔	✔	
Esophageal burning, perforations and lacerations		✔	
Gallbladder disease			✔
Hematology			
Anemia	✔		
Leukopenia	✔		
Thrombocytopenia	✔		
Neurology			
EEG abnormalities	✔	✔	

Continued

Table 66-2
(Continued)

Medical System	Anorexia Nervosa	Bulimia Nervosa	Obesity
Orthopedic and Musculoskeletal			
Osteopenia, osteoporosis, bone fractures	✔		
Muscle weakness, loss of muscle mass	✔		
Arthritis			✔
Renal and Metabolic			
Hypokalemia	✔	✔	
Partial diabetes insipidus	✔		
Renal calculi	✔		
Hypoglycemia	✔	✔	✔
Diabetes mellitus (type 2, noninsulin dependent)			✔
Reproductive			
Amenorrhea	✔		
Low testosterone levels in males, sexual disinterest	✔		
Menstrual irregularity		✔	
Other Medical Complications			
Respiratory Disease			✔
Cancer			✔

the majority of cases, normal levels of testosterone and estrogen are established with weight gain. However testosterone replacement therapies for male patients should be considered as part of a treatment regimen until weight restoration and normal gonadal functioning has been achieved. For female patients, estrogen replacement therapy should be considered after weight has been restored if normal resumption of menses has not occurred [9].

D. Multidimensional Perspectives

Current understanding regarding the etiology of anorexia nervosa considers a range of factors including social, familial, cultural and genetic influences. Homosexual orientation seems to place males at greater risk than females for the development of eating disorders. Several studies have found that a higher percentage of males than females with anorexia nervosa are homosexual [22]; in fact, lesbian orientation among females has been cited as a protective factor against the development of an eating disorder [23]. Within gay culture, the ideal body type is more slender than that of heterosexual males; this difference may account for the increased likelihood that gay males want to lose or maintain a thin weight to approximate the ideal body type and appear more attractive to other males. Gay men are more likely than heterosexual men to report dissatisfaction with their body [24], and body dissatisfaction is a factor that is known to contribute significantly to dieting and the use of disordered eating behaviors. In comparison, lesbian females seem to accept a wider range of body shapes and sizes, thereby weakening the pressure to lose weight or be thin to be attractive to other lesbians.

The association between homosexual orientation among males and eating disorders is also supported by research on femininity and masculinity. Results from a meta-analysis of 22 studies indicate that there is a significant positive relationship between feminine characteristics (such as passivity, dependence, and need for others' approval) and disordered eating, meaning that the higher the rating of femininity, the greater the likelihood of disordered eating [25]. Findings also indicate the presence of an inverse relationship between masculine characteristics (assertiveness, independence) and eating problems [25] in that lower scores on a scale of masculinity were correlated with higher disordered eating symptoms. These results suggest that femininity is a risk factor, and masculinity is a protective factor, for the development of eating disorders. Although femininity and/or homosexual orientation among males is not a specific risk factor for the development of an eating disorder, research does suggest that it may place some individuals at heightened risk [26].

Involvement in certain athletics, most notably those with an association between weight and performance, has also been found to be a risk factor. For females, activities that are typically individually based and require a certain aesthetic appeal, such as dancing, gymnastics, modeling and acting, are considered high-risk [27,28] compared with team sports that promote strength and endurance such as basketball, field hockey, and soccer. For males, sports such as wrestling, running, jockeying, and ballet dancing may heighten risk [17,29,30]. These sports typically require maintenance of a strict range of body weight for peak performance or aesthetic appeal, or in the case of wrestling to be able to participate in a specific weight class.

There has been considerable attention to the contribution of family dynamics and familial psychiatric history on eating disorders. Unfortunately, there is a dearth of information on gender differences regarding familial experiences. For both males and females, keeping feelings and thoughts to oneself rather than expressing them openly has been found to be a risk factor for anorexia nervosa [31], and parental overprotection is associated with low body satisfaction.

Genetics research is a rapidly growing field and provides new information regarding the etiology of eating disorders. Some of the first studies to address familial transmission of eating disorders investigated the prevalence of eating disorders and eating disordered behaviors among first-degree relatives of afflicted individuals. In a study of female probands with anorexia nervosa, first-degree relatives were seven times as likely to have an eating disorder not otherwise specified and three times as likely to have any eating disorder, compared to first-degree relatives of noneating-disordered women [32]. An eating disorder "not otherwise specified" describes a constellation of behaviors that are similar in nature to either anorexia nervosa or bulimia nervosa, but do not meet full criteria for either disorder. By comparison, in a study of males with anorexia nervosa, no *male* relatives were affected [33]. However, the risk of developing anorexia nervosa in a first-degree *female* relative of a male proband was found to be 20 times greater than that for a first-degree female relative of a male who does not have anorexia nervosa. The risk for developing a subclinical level of anorexia nervosa was estimated to be 3 times as great for the female first-degree relative of a male proband than for a relative of an unaffected male [33].

Although family studies are important as a first step in assessing genetic factors, advances in identification of heritability using monozygotic twins have helped separate genetic effects from environmental influences. The range of heritability of liability estimates is broad, mainly due to differences in measurement and definition of the disorder. In an early study, heritability of anorexia nervosa was estimated to be about 70% [34], meaning that 70% of a person's liability to anorexia nervosa is genetic, and the remaining risk is due to environmental factors. In clinical cases of twin pairs where at least one twin has been diagnosed with anorexia nervosa in a clinical setting, heritability estimates are as high as 88% for additive genetic factors, 0% for the shared environment, and 12% for individual-specific environment effects [35]. One limitation of clinical twin-based studies is that the number of twins participating in the study is very small. Consequently, community-based samples often provide a better estimate of the heritability of a more diversity sample. In a population-based study of over 2000 female twins, anorexia nervosa was estimated to have a heritability of 58% [36]. There have been no systematic studies investigating the heritability of affected males due to the very small numbers of males, especially male twins, with anorexia nervosa.

III. Bulimia Nervosa

A. *Diagnostic Criteria*

The term *bulimia* means "ox hunger," a reference to the high consumption present during characteristic binge eating episodes. According to the DSM-IV [4], a diagnosis of bulimia nervosa is given to individuals who display the following behaviors and characteristics:

1. Recurrent episodes of binge eating (Binge eating is defined as eating within a discrete period an amount of food that is definitely larger than most people would eat during a similar period and under similar circumstances. Binge eating episodes are also characterized by a sense of lack of control over eating during the episode [a feeling that one cannot stop eating or control what or how much one is eating])
2. Recurrent inappropriate compensatory behavior to prevent weight gain, such as self-induced vomiting; misuse of laxatives, diuretics, enemas, or other medications; fasting; or excessive exercise.
3. The binge eating and inappropriate compensatory behaviors both occur, on average, at least twice a week for 3 months.
4. Self-esteem is unduly influenced by body shape and weight.
5. The disturbance does not occur exclusively during episodes of anorexia nervosa.

There are two classifications of bulimia nervosa: purging type and nonpurging type. Purging type is designated for individuals with bulimia nervosa who regularly engage in self-induced vomiting or the misuse of laxatives, diuretics, or enemas. Bulimia nervosa of the nonpurging type describes individuals who engage in binge eating, but who have used other compensatory behaviors such as fasting or excessive exercise to prevent weight gain, and have not regularly engaged in self-induced vomiting and/or the misuse of laxatives, diuretics, or enemas.

B. *Prevalence Estimates*

The prevalence of bulimia nervosa is estimated to range from 1.1% [7,37] to 6.0% [38] among girls and women. When broader diagnostic criteria are used, such as by lowering the minimum frequency of binge eating and purging to once per month, it is estimated that approximately 16.5% of girls engage in bulimic activities, but may not necessarily meet full diagnostic criteria [37,39–41]. Prevalence rates for bulimia nervosa among males range from 0.0 to 0.2% [7,38], and may be as high as 12.3% when assessing symptoms that are not as severe or frequent as those meeting criteria for the full disorder [37,39–41]. By gender, the ratio of females to males who seek treatment (outpatient or inpatient) for bulimia nervosa is approximately 20:1 [13] and in general in the community is 10:1–8:1 [2].

C. *Gender and Clinical Presentation*

There are several differences in the presentation between male and female bulimics. Onset age for bulimia is later among males than females [38]. This finding may be related to the earlier body dissatisfaction and pubertal changes among females that are likely to expedite the onset of bulimic behaviors for girls. Males are less likely than females to binge alone, and more likely to binge at mealtimes, and in public places. Other gender differences relate to the types of compensatory behaviors used to counteract binge eating. In a study of 15 bulimic men and 15 bulimic women matched on demographic variables and on factors related to symptom severity, findings suggest that males used fewer weight controls, such as vomiting or laxative use, than females [42]. These results were replicated by a larger study 10 years later [43]. Similar results have also been found among adolescents who binge and use compensatory behaviors, but who may not meet full diagnostic criteria for bulimia nervosa. Boys who binge eat and engage in compensatory behaviors were less likely than girls to skip meals (26.1% boys vs 78.4% girls), use diet pills (2.2% vs 26.3%), self-induce vomit (2.2% vs 35.2%) or use exercise (69.6% vs 94.6%) to lose or maintain weight [39]. These findings suggest that males may be more likely to fit diagnostic criteria for the nonpurging classification of bulimia nervosa than the purging type.

Further gender differences among individuals with bulimia nervosa relate to weight status, weight perception and body satisfaction. Affected males are more likely than females to perceive their ideal or desired weight as a more realistic weight for their height and age, and to report a higher current and past weight [38,42]. Females with full syndrome and subclinical bulimia are more likely than males to perceive themselves as too fat and to be actively dieting [39], and to be more concerned with weight control and obtaining what they believe to be their ideal weight [38,44].

It seems evident that females in general use bulimic behaviors as a means for weight control more than males, and as such are willing to use extreme measures to achieve weight loss or maintain control. This finding is supported by a longitudinal investigation of personality features among adolescent females and males with bulimia nervosa. Results indicate that females scored higher than males on a measure related to their intent to achieve thinness (drive for thinness). This raises the question of why males are engaging in these behaviors, if not primarily for weight control. In this same longitudinal study, bulimic males reported more traits of perfectionism and described greater interpersonal distrust than the bulimic females [45]. Other studies have found that bulimic men have more problems in their interpersonal relationships than do bulimic women. Affected males were less likely to be married or involved in romantic relationships, less likely to be sexually active, and more likely to report social isolation than females [42,44]. It is plausible that bulimic behaviors provide a different purpose, possibly related to relationships, for males than for females.

Common medical complications associated with bulimia nervosa can be found in Table 66-2 and are similar across affected males and females, with the exception of gonadal functioning. In low-weight patients, it is common to find males with low levels of testosterone and females with low levels of estrogen. These hormones should resume to normal levels with weight restoration, however replacement therapies may be considered as adjunct to conventional pharmacologic and psychotherapeutic treatments.

The extent of medical complications, notably cardiac problems, in individuals with bulimia nervosa is related to the frequency and severity of compensatory behaviors. Diuretic abuse is associated with the highest risk for cardiac abnormalities, enema and laxative abuse with moderate risk, and self-induced vomiting with milder risk [46]. However, the severity of cardiac risk is not the only factor to consider. A high frequency of a lower risk compensatory behavior, such as self-induced vomiting, could have equal or greater risk for cardiac complications if practiced regularly compared to a lesser-used compensatory behavior with higher risk. Other factors, such as exercise and "combining compensatory factors," (for example, regular use of several compensatory behaviors such as self-induced vomiting, excessive exercise, and laxative use) can also increase cardiac risk by placing strain on more systems of the body.

D. Multidimensional Perspectives

As cited earlier, homosexual orientation appears to be a risk factor for eating disorders among males, but a protective factor among females [26]. Research has demonstrated that a greater percentage of males than females with bulimia nervosa, in clinical and community samples, report a homosexual or bisexual orientation [47]. It is possible that the greater relationship problems that bulimic males experience compared with bulimic females may be related to homosexual orientation, although this hypothesis has not been thoroughly investigated.

Participation in high-risk athletics or other activities is also associated with bulimic behaviors. Dance, gymnastics, modeling and acting are considered high-risk activities for females [27,28], and wrestling, running, jockeying, and dancing are high-risk sports for males [17,29,30]. The bulimic behaviors may serve as a manner to maintain the aesthetic appeal (females), to enhance athletic performance (males), or in the case of wrestling, to meet criteria for competing in a particular weight class.

Males with bulimia nervosa are also more likely than females to have past and present problems with substance abuse. Among both adolescents [39] and adults [42], affected males reported more use of tobacco, alcohol, and other drugs than affected females. However, no significant differences on measures of depression and anxiety have been found by gender among individuals with bulimia.

Family studies provide evidence to suggest that bulimia nervosa can, at least in part, be genetically transmitted. First-degree female relatives of bulimic females, compared to female relatives of unaffected females, were found to be at 12 times greater risk of having an eating disorder not otherwise specified and 5 times greater risk of having either anorexia or bulimia nervosa [33]. Female relatives of female probands seem to be at risk for the development of an eating disorder; 43% of sisters and 26% of the mothers of bulimic probands had a lifetime diagnosis of an eating disorder, most notably an eating disorder not otherwise specified [48]. Male relatives of female probands were not affected. Unfortunately, family history studies of male probands have not been conducted due to the small percentage of affected males.

Genetics research also provides evidence of genetic transmission. An early study of bulimia nervosa among twin females indicated a heritability estimate of 10% [34]. Case studies involving twin pairs with at least one twin diagnosed with bulimia nervosa have indicated heritability as high as 47% for additive genetic factors, 30% for the shared environment, and 23% for individual-specific environment effects [35]. Studies of nonclinical bulimic females have provided similar results. Population-based studies of female twin pairs have reported estimates of genetic heritability of bulimia nervosa as high as 62% [49]. Subsequent studies have reported heritability estimates ranging from a low of 0% (no genetic contribution) [50] to a high of 83% [51] when bulimia is broadly defined by decreasing the minimum frequency of binge eating episodes. Most estimates of additive genetic factors among females range from 30% to 50% [35]. Due to the small number of male twin pairs with eating disorders, the heritability of bulimia nervosa among males has not yet been investigated.

IV. Binge Eating Disorder

A. Diagnostic Criteria

With the recognition that some individuals engage in binge eating but do not attempt to prevent weight gain by using inappropriate compensatory behaviors, researchers proposed criteria for a new eating disorder classification called binge eating disorder. The research criteria, which are provided in Appendix B of the DSM-IV [4] are:

1. Recurrent episodes of binge eating (Binge eating is defined as eating within a discrete period an amount of food that is definitely larger than most people would eat during a similar period and under similar circumstances. Binge eating episodes are also characterized by a sense of lack of control over eating during the episode [a feeling that one cannot stop eating or control what or how much one is eating].)

2. Binge eating episodes are associated with three or more of the following:

   - Eating much more rapidly than normal
   - Eating until feeling uncomfortably full
   - Eating large amounts of food when not feeling physically hungry
   - Eating alone because of being embarrassed by how much one is eating
   - Feeling disgusted with oneself, depressed, or very guilty after overeating

3. Marked distress regarding binge eating is present.
4. The binge eating occurs, on average, at least 2 days a week for 6 months.
5. The binge eating is not associated with the regular use of inappropriate compensatory behaviors (e.g., purging, fasting, excessive exercise) and does not occur exclusively during the course of anorexia nervosa or bulimia nervosa.

The diagnosis of binge eating disorder is relatively new. Consequently, there are gaps in our knowledge of the disorder and its association with anorexia and bulimia nervosa. One theory is that eating disorders are a continuum, with anorexia nervosa at one extreme point, obesity at the other, and with bulimia nervosa and binge eating disorder lying on points in between. Another theory is that there are distinct eating disorders mainly characterized by the presence or absence of binge eating, or the categorization of one's weight (underweight, normal weight, or overweight). These theoretic issues regarding eating disorder classification are currently unresolved. What we do know is that binge eating disorder is currently classified as a distinct eating disorder with specific criteria supported by research, descriptive statistics, and with distinct psychologic and medical consequences. Body weight patterns associated with binge eating are discussed later under the Obesity heading.

B. Prevalence Estimates

The prevalence of binge eating disorder is estimated to range from 1.5% to 3.1% among girls [7,52] and 1.8 to 4.6% among women [53]. Prevalence rates for binge eating disorder among males range from 0.0 to 0.9% for boys [7,52] and may be as high as 5.3% for men [54]. By gender, the ratio of females to males

who seek treatment (outpatient or inpatient) for binge eating disorder is approximately 10:1 [13], but in the community binge eating disorder is generally equal by gender [53].

Some researchers have hypothesized that infrequent binge eating behavior may be a precursor to more serious forms of eating disorders such as binge eating disorder and/or bulimia nervosa. Estimates of recurrent binge eating behavior are as high as 18.9% among girls and 17.5% among boys in a small study of school-age children [39], 25% of girls and 16% of boys in high schools [55], and 17.3% of girls and 7.8% of boys in population-based samples [52,56].

C. Gender and Clinical Presentation

Several features of the presentation of binge eating disorder vary by gender. Some researchers believe that binge eating is a more acceptable behavior for males than for females, a finding that has been replicated among samples of men [38] and boys [57]. Males are more likely than females to identify overeating, and sometimes binge eating, as normal behavior. Subsequently, males may consume a much larger quantity of food than females before they consider the eating episode to be a binge [58]. As a consequence, males are more likely to report gastrointestinal discomfort and complaints following an episode of binging, whereas females are more likely to report negative emotional states (feelings of guilt and upset about overeating, embarrassment, etc.) after eating a smaller amount of food [58]. Several reports indicate that males who binge are less likely than females to feel depressed or guilty about the eating episode [38,57].

In a community sample of obese adults, males and females diagnosed with binge eating disorder were similar in many ways. Both reported similar frequencies of prepubescent dieting and the number of times weight had been lost and regained, pounds for the largest amount of weight lost, levels regarding their perception of the importance of weight, and experiences of the extent of social pressures to lose weight [59]. However, females with binge eating disorder reported greater body dissatisfaction and demonstrated greater discrepancy between perceived current and ideal body figures than did males. Similar results have been found among adolescents; girls who engage in binge eating are more concerned than boys about their weight, and were more likely than boys to be trying to lose weight [39]. Women with binge eating disorder also reported a younger onset age of dieting than men [59].

Medical complications associated with binge eating disorder are often related to those for obesity (see Table 66-2). Binge eating can lead to weight gain, and can increase the risk for weight-related problems such as diabetes, cancer, and cardiac problems. Infrequent exercise can exacerbate medical complaints related to binge eating.

D. Multidimensional Perspectives

Aside from differences in the etiology and expression of symptoms, few differences by gender have been found regarding noneating disorder characteristics of those with binge eating disorder. There were no significant differences by gender on the abuse of substances such as alcohol, tobacco, marijuana, or other drugs [39] among adolescents, although results from an adult sample indicated that males with binge eating disorder were more likely than females to have had substance abuse problems [60]. No significant differences by gender were found on education level, household income, self-esteem, mood or anxiety disorders among an age-matched sample of males and females diagnosed with binge eating disorder [60].

Although no studies have investigated the heritability of binge eating disorder as a separate diagnosis, several studies have investigated heritability of binge eating behavior. One population-based study of female twins separated the symptoms of binge eating from vomiting. Estimates for binge eating behavior only were 46% for genetic effects, 0% for shared environmental effects, and 54% for individual-specific environment effects [61]. Another study of female twins sought to investigate the transition from binge eating to bulimia nervosa diagnosis [49]. These researchers found that heritability of binge eating behavior alone was estimated to be 44% for genetic effects, 0% for common environmental effects, and 56% for individual-specific environmental influence [49]. These results are similar to another study of female twin pairs that reported heritability of binge eating to be 50%, with the remaining variance attributable to individual-specific environment [51]. Estimates for heritability of binge eating behavior among males are not available.

V. Disordered Eating: Dieting and Unhealthy Weight-Control Behaviors

There are no criteria outlined in the DSM-IV [4] for dieting or disordered eating. Disordered eating describes a constellation of unhealthy eating and weight related behaviors and attitudes that do not meet criteria for a DSM-IV [4] eating disorder, but that have medical and/or psychologic consequences. Examples of disordered eating include, but are not limited to, infrequent use of or usage of low doses of compensatory behaviors such as laxative or diet pill use, self-induced vomiting, and a chaotic pattern of eating and fasting. Disordered eating differs from healthier approaches to dieting such as decreased consumption of fats and sugars, increased intake of fruits and vegetables, and adoption of a moderate exercise routine. Healthier dieting approaches can lead to improvement of overall health and fitness, whereas unhealthy eating approaches such as disordered eating can compromise psychologic and physical health.

If eating disorders lie on a continuum, then dieting and disordered eating may be one pathway by which an individual enters a more serious pattern of eating and weight-related behaviors. Many individuals report subclinical levels of an eating disorder prior to meeting full criteria [62]. Consequently, individuals who exhibit patterns of disordered eating should be routinely screened for later development of an eating disorder.

A. Prevalence Estimates

The prevalence of dieting is difficult to estimate due to the range of criteria used to assess these behaviors. In one study of youth, 4.7% of girls and 0.9% of boys described dieting as a "way to handle personal problems" [7]. In a large community-based sample of over 16,000 adolescents 14 or younger, 32% of girls and 20% of boys reported dieting; 2.4% of girls and 1.2% of boys reported chronic dieting [56]. The prevalence of dieting increases with age among adolescent females, but remains relatively stable for males. The percentage of girls trying to lose weight doubled from ages 9 (20%) to 14 (44%), whereas for boys, the percentages remained similar across ages (17% age 9 to 19% age 14, peaking at 23% age 12). Among public high school students, 47% of girls and 20% of boys reported trying to lose weight, and 28% girls and 10% boys have dieted in the past month [55]. Dieting behaviors are also prevalent among adults. Results from a telephone survey of over 60,000 adults indicated that approximately 38% of women and 24% of men were trying to lose weight, and 28% of women and 28% of men were trying to maintain their current weight [63].

Although many youth and adults engage in dieting practices, fewer report the use of disordered eating behaviors. Adolescents trying to lose weight reported the following prevalence rates of disordered eating behaviors: use of diet pills (6.2% girls and 4.8% boys); self-induced vomiting (5.5% girls and 3.1% boys); and skipping meals (72.1% girls and 56.7% boys) [64]. Various disordered eating behaviors have been used by adults to try to lose weight: taking diet pills (4% women and 2% men), taking special supplements (10% women and 7% men), fasting for a minimum of 24 hours (5% women and 5% men), and self-induced vomiting (0.3% women and 0.3% men) [63].

B. Gender and Clinical Presentation

There is a dearth of research comparing dieting and disordered eating and associated features by gender. The definition and measurement of disordered eating varies considerably across studies, thereby making identification of trends by gender essentially impossible. When assessing disordered eating behaviors, individuals should be asked questions about a range of behaviors, along with the frequency of (e.g., number of episodes per day, week, or month), severity of (e.g., number of pills taken and how many times per day, per week), and purpose behind the behavior (e.g., weight loss, body dissatisfaction, affect regulation).

Youth that report use of disordered eating behaviors are more likely to report other health-compromising behaviors when compared with youth who do not engage in disordered eating. Among those engaging in disordered eating behaviors, a greater percentage of girls than boys reported use of tobacco, to have attempted suicide, and to have had more than one sexual partner. Boys using disordered eating behaviors were more likely than girls to report use of alcohol, marijuana, to engage in delinquent behaviors (e.g., destruction of property, physical violence, stealing) [65].

Individuals who engage in disordered eating behaviors, but do not have full diagnosable eating disorders, may report medical complaints and complications typical of individuals with anorexia nervosa or bulimia nervosa (see Table 66-2). The majority of medical complications are exacerbated in relation to the frequency, severity, and length of use of the disordered eating behavior. Individuals who diet infrequently, or who use compensatory behaviors such as self-induced vomiting or laxative abuse on an irregular basis, may not experience any medical complaints. However, the risk for any of the medical complications associated with anorexia or bulimia increases with continued use of disordered eating behaviors.

C. Multidimensional Perspectives

There are factors related to disordered eating that demonstrate gender specificity with respect to disordered eating and weight-control behaviors. One of the identifiable risk factors toward the later development of disordered eating (and potentially toward the eventual diagnosis of an eating disorder) is participation in sports or occupations (such as flight attendants or actors/actresses) that require weight control for good or peak performance [2]. This includes involvement in sports such as wrestling and jockeying for males, and involvement in dancing, gymnastics, and swimming for girls.

Homosexual orientation is also associated with disordered eating for males but is a protective factor for females. Gay men scored higher than heterosexual men, and heterosexual women scored higher than lesbians, on measures of body dissatisfaction and dietary restraint. In addition, heterosexual women reported greater symptoms of bulimia and stronger drives for thinness than lesbians [66].

In a longitudinal study following over 1400 boys and girls over the course of 3 years, disordered eating at year 3 was significantly predicted by negative affect and attitudes at the first assessment [67]. This negativity was a better predictor for girls than for boys, but was a significant predictor for both genders.

Several studies have explored the contribution of genetics to the risk of developing disordered eating behaviors, and have hypothesized some interesting theories about the association between puberty and disordered eating onset. The studies were designed to evaluate heritability of problematic eating behaviors and attitudes (weight preoccupation). In the first study of female twins age 11 and age 17 from a population-based sample, results indicate no genetic influence among those age 11, but a heritability of 52 to 57% among those 17 [68]. The authors wondered whether the hormonal changes at puberty activate gene expression that subsequently increases heritability following puberty. To attempt to answer this question, they conducted a second study using the same population, but separating the 11-year-olds into prepubertal and pubertal groups [69]. Again, they found that there was no genetic influence among the prepubertal 11-year-olds. However, among the pubertal 11-year-olds, the heritability of problematic eating behaviors and attitudes was 26%. The authors concluded that the different heritability estimates of individuals who are the same age but who are of different pubertal status may provide evidence of a gene activation effect, most likely triggered by ovarian hormones [70]. Research would then need to investigate what triggers a similar activation process in males, if similar heritability trends are found.

VI. Obesity

A. Diagnostic Criteria

Obesity status can be identified using gender and age reference data for children, adolescents, and adults from the Center for Disease Control [71]. Typical weight status categories as defined by BMI (BMI: metric weight/height^2 as kg/m^2) are: underweight (BMI <15th percentile), average weight (BMI ≥15th percentile but <85th percentile), overweight (BMI ≥85th percentile but <95th percentile), and obese (BMI ≥95th percentile) [72]. Obesity status can also be defined by having a BMI ≥30 [72].

B. Prevalence Estimates

The percentage of individuals in the United States who are overweight or obese continues to increase. For both males and females, the greatest increase in the prevalence of overweight occurs between the ages of early 20 s to early 30 s. Statistics for the year 2000 indicate 20.2% of men and 19.4% of women are obese, a significant increase from 11.7% of men and 12.2% of women in 1991 [73]. In 1999 13% of youth age 6–11 and 14% of youth age 12–19 were categorized as obese; these results are also higher than those from the 1960s, which indicated that the prevalence of obesity among youth was 4% among those age 6–11 and 5% among those age 12–19 [74]. Sedentary lifestyle and changes in dietary intake and eating behaviors are the most likely causes of the steady increase of obesity among all demographic categories.

C. Gender and Clinical Presentation

There is limited information regarding differences in the ways males and females experience obesity. Obesity continues to be a stigmatized disorder; individuals struggling with obesity are less likely than nonobese to be accepted into prestigious colleges, to marry, and to be hired at an occupation, and are more likely to be discriminated against by health care professionals. Women who become obese in adolescence are more likely than men to remain obese in adulthood [75], and more likely than obese men to earn less, less likely to be married, and complete fewer years of school [76].

Obesity is associated with binge eating disorder, although not every obese person engages in binge eating behavior [77]. Binge eating certainly can contribute to increased weight and risk for obesity. However, other factors such as medications such as steroids or psychotropically active drugs, gender, genetics, and metabolic intake and energy expenditure also contribute to weight status.

Gender plays a significant role in fat distribution. Prior to puberty, both girls and boys have comparable percentages of body fat. However, during puberty girls increase the amount of adipose tissue on the body, most noticeably through the development of breasts and increased fat distribution to the buttocks and thighs. As a consequence of the complex changes that begin around puberty, women have a higher fat–lean tissue ratio than do men. Women also experience increases in fat distribution around childbirth and after menopause. Fat is more likely to be concentrated in the abdominal or torso area for men, compared with the buttocks and legs for women [78]. After menopause, however, women concentrate fat in the abdominal area.

The medical complications associated with obesity can affect both men and women (see Table 66-2). Carrying fat around the torso, typically seen among men who are overweight, is associated with greater risk for hypertension, dyslipidemia, and diabetes [79]. Obesity in general is associated with increased risk for diabetes, hypertension, stroke, dyslipidemia, cardiovascular disease, gallbladder disease, respiratory disease, cancer, arthritis, and gout. Obesity among women can lead to infertility problems [80].

D. Multidimensional Perspectives

Very little is known about gender-specific experiences of obesity with respect to social, cultural, and familial influences. One can assume that many of the differences associated with the eating disorders would apply. Body dissatisfaction is typically greater among females than among males, and is not necessarily associated with weight or obesity status. Females are more likely than males to be dissatisfied with their weight, and as a consequence, may engage in more frequent and possibly more extreme efforts to lose weight that may in fact have the undesirable consequence of weight gain.

However, body weight is a highly heritable condition [81]; approximately 70% of one's heritability of obesity is attributable to genetics. The remaining 30% of the variance can be accounted for by individual-specific environmental factors. This figure does suggest that although the risk for obesity is present among those individuals with a genetic predisposition, success at controlling one's environment through healthful eating and regular exercise may prevent the development of obesity.

E. Gender-Specific Prevention and Treatment Implications

Efforts to prevent the development of eating disorders among females have risen over the past decade. So has the prevalence of eating and weight disorders among both males and females. It is possible that the increased prevalence is associated with an increased willingness on behalf of affected persons to come forward, acknowledge the problem, and seek treatment. However, it is also possible that eating and weight disorders are becoming more prevalent due to factors related to society and cultural messages, genetics, poor nutrition and exercise regimens, and compromised psychologic health.

As exploration of the gender-specific aspects of the eating and weight disorders continues, attention to social and cultural factors that may place certain individuals at increased risk also needs to continue. Sociocultural factors related to increased risk for eating disorders among females include pressure to be thin, equating thinness with attractiveness and success, idealization of the thin body shape, and the normality of dieting behaviors [82]. Andersen suggests that obese boys be targeted for prevention [9]. Among both boys and girls involved in sports that are associated with higher risk for disordered eating, prevention programs should help coaches define appropriate weight standards to continue safe participation in a sport.

The monitoring and modification of media programming and advertising messages is critical toward developing an understanding of how the projection of a "body ideal" can be internalized. Pairing the body ideal with messages of happiness, success, and acceptance can have powerful and detrimental effects on the development of a positive and healthy self-esteem; one could believe that the only way to achieve happiness, success,

and acceptance is by attaining a certain body shape and size. The media impact on the body ideal has been widely recognized as a sociocultural pressure for women, as advertising campaigns have idealized thinness and promoted weight control methods and body shape alteration devices (e.g., girdles, push-up padded bras) for decades. There has been a rise in the weight- and shape-related advertising among men's magazines, although gender differences are still present. An investigation of popular magazines read by young adults reported higher rates of advertisements and articles promoting *weight loss* in women's magazines, but higher rates of advertisements and articles promoting *body shape changes* among men's magazines [83]. Prevention efforts are necessary for both genders, but the targeted message may be different. For females, acceptance of a wide range of body sizes and weights may be critical, whereas for men, education regarding body shape differences and reducing the association between masculinity and muscle mass may be more important.

Early intervention efforts need to be redesigned so that boys and men are not discriminated against in the diagnosis and treatment of eating disorders. The criterion of amenorrhea for the diagnosis of anorexia nervosa needs to be applied only to females [84], prevalence rates need to acknowledge the possibility of anorexia nervosa and bulimia nervosa in males, and these issues need to be clarified in future editions of the DSM-IV [4]. If eating disorders continue to be viewed as disorders that only affect young females, then older women and males of any age may not feel comfortable reporting their symptoms or seeking treatment. Acceptance of a wide range of symptomatology and of the idea that eating and weight disorders do not know boundaries by any demographic characteristic (gender, age, race, socioeconomic status, etc.) is imperative to providing accessible treatments.

Health care providers (e.g., physicians, nurses, school health staff) may be the first professionals that affected individuals turn to for assistance. Symptoms of an eating disorder may at first be "disguised" as fatigue, dizziness, weight changes, or cold intolerance. Some medical professionals may be less likely to acknowledge an eating disorder and more likely to seek medical explanation for weight loss among males [9]. It is critical to note the misconception that eating disorders are only disorders that affect females or gay males. Eating disorders are pervasive disorders across gender, ethnic, geographic, and economic borders. We need to be certain that we are training tomorrow's health care providers with today's knowledge.

To date, there have been no systematic investigations comparing the effectiveness of manual-based, proven treatments by gender. Treatments that have been found to be effective for treating anorexia nervosa and bulimia nervosa among females include cognitive-behavioral therapy, interpersonal therapy, family therapy, and pharmacologic interventions. These interventions focus on reestablishing normal dietary regimen, restoring weight as indicated, interrupting problematic behaviors such as binge-eating and purging, identifying situational and interpersonal factors that can trigger the behaviors, addressing distorted or erroneous beliefs that interfere with recovery, identifying interpersonal challenges that influence the behaviors, establishing a supportive environment among

Table 66-3
Summary of Predominant Differences in Eating and Weight Disorders by Gender

Disorder	Males	Females
Anorexia Nervosa	Low testosterone levels related to low weight Loss of sexual interest or lack of potency More overweight prior to weight loss History of poor childhood appetite problems Higher risk if wrestling, running, jockeying, dancing Higher risk if homosexual orientation, feminine Develop AN to avoid overweight teasing, to avoid medical illnesses, to improve gay relationship, to enhance athletic performance History of teasing for overweight	Amenorrhea More likely to engage in laxative misuse Moderate evidence for familial transmission Moderate evidence for genetic transmission Higher risk if dancing, gymnastics, modeling, acting. Develop AN for aesthetic reasons or for control
Bulimia Nervosa	Later age at onset of disorder More likely to binge at mealtimes or in public Higher risk if in wrestling, running, jockeying, dancing Greater interpersonal distrust, social isolation Ideal body type more realistic Greater perfectionism Higher risk if homosexual orientation Greater likelihood to abuse substances (past and present) Greater drive for thinness Greater body dissatisfaction, dieting	More likely to engage in vomiting or laxative use, skipping meals or fasting, diet pill use More likely to binge when alone Higher risk if dancing, gymnastics, modeling, acting Ideal body type less realistic, very slender Moderate evidence for familial transmission Moderate evidence for genetic transmission
Binge Eating Disorder	More likely to report gastrointestinal discomfort Greater likelihood to binge at mealtimes or in public More likely to perceive binge-eating as normal behavior Greater likelihood to abuse substances	More likely to relate binges to negative emotion Greater likelihood to binge when alone Greater body dissatisfaction Greater distortion of perceived body shape/size Younger age at onset of dieting Moderate heritability for binge behavior
Disordered Eating	Higher risk if wrestling, running, jockeying, dancing Homosexual orientation Greater likelihood to use alcohol, drugs May engage in delinquent behaviors More likely to have had >1 sexual partner Greater drive for thinness	Higher risk if dancing, gymnastics, modeling, acting Greater likelihood to smoke, use tobacco Greater risk for suicide attempts
Obesity	More likely to distribute fat in abdomen or torso, associated with greater risk for cardiovascular and endocrine problems	More likely to distribute in lower extremities Obese girls more likely to remain obese as women Greater body dissatisfaction

family and friends, assessing the need for pharmacologic treatments, treating co-morbid problems such as depression or substance use, and developing a relapse prevention plan. Cognitive-behavioral interventions are particularly effective for treating binge eating disorder among females. Effective treatments for disordered eating behaviors, although not systematically researched, are believed to be the same as those for the treatment of anorexia, bulimia, and binge eating disorder. There is reason to believe that these treatment interventions would be comparably effective for treating males with eating disorders.

Treatment of obesity among males and females typically includes a reduced-calorie dietary plan (typically increasing the intake of fruits and vegetables while decreasing the intake of fats and sweets), development of an exercise regimen, and identification and treatment of medical complications such as diabetes and thyroid disorders that may complicate weight loss or stabilization efforts. Medications to inhibit appetite and accelerate metabolism should be used with caution, as they may increase the risk for cardiovascular complications. Surgical treatments, such as gastric bypass, should be considered only for morbidly obese patients. Surgeries can be effective in the first year following the procedure, but a portion of the weight lost is often regained within 5 years of the surgery [80].

There are several caveats to standard treatment that should be explored. In many clinical settings across the country, males with eating disorders do not have the opportunity to participate in group psychotherapy solely devoted to affected males [85]. Separate male treatment groups should be offered when possible, and research should investigate whether the gender of the therapist matters in the effectiveness of single-gender groups. Females with eating disorders, as well as treating staff, may discriminate against affected males, and this behavior needs to be addressed in mixed-gender treatment milieus when present. It is important to address not only what it is like for an individual to have an eating disorder, but to address the concerns that are present when males are treated for eating disorders. Issues related to sexual orientation and functioning can be explored within the context of a safer environment if all male. For males who have experienced dramatic weight loss, testosterone replacement therapy is an important consideration during weight restoration to a normal weight. Andersen has suggested recommendations for testosterone replacement therapy [86].

Relapse prevention is essential. The effectiveness of most treatments is significantly influenced by appropriate attention to preventing a reoccurrence of symptoms and the disorder. Although differences by gender have not been studied on the effectiveness of relapse prevention or aftercare support groups, suggestions for leading support groups for males with eating disorders are available [87].

VII. Suggestions for Further Investigations

This chapter focused on biologic sex as it relates to the eating disorders and obesity. The field of eating disorders is generally viewed as young, and clearly research on males with eating disorders is in its infancy. To more fully understand the contribution of sex on the etiology, prevention, experience, and treatment of eating and weight disorders, we need to address the following questions.

- Studies indicate that weight status, body satisfaction, self-esteem, and psychologic health are essentially the same between boys and girls until they reach the middle of grade school (3rd–6th grade). Regarding prevention, what are some of the gender-specific factors that need to be addressed at this young age?
- What are the specific risk and protective factors influencing the development of eating disorders among males, and how are these factors similar to or different from those affecting the development of eating disorders among females?
- What is the heritability of anorexia nervosa, bulimia nervosa, binge eating disorder, disordered eating behaviors, and obesity among first-degree relatives of male probands and among male twin pairs?
- Treatment outcome studies need to include boys and men, both within current protocols as well as in protocols separate from females. Currently there are no studies that confirm that treatments typically effective for females, such as cognitive-behavioral therapy, family therapy, interpersonal therapy and pharmacotherapy, are equally effective for males. What are results of treatment outcome studies involving males with eating disorders?

References

1. Morton R. (1694). *Phthisidogica: Or a Treatise of Consumption*, London: Smith and Walford.
2. Braun DL, Sunday SR, Huang A, Halmi KA. (1999). More males seek treatment for eating disorders. *Int J Eating Disord.* 25:415–424.
3. Maloney M, McGuird J, Daniels S, Specker B. (1989). Dieting behavior and eating attitudes in children. *Pediatrics* 84:482–489.
4. American Psychiatric Association. (1994). *Diagnostic and Statistical Manual of Mental Disorders*, 4th Edition, Washington DC: American Psychiatric Association.
5. World Health Organization (WHO). (1992). *The ICD-10 classification of mental and behavioral disorders: Clinical descriptions and diagnostic guidelines.* Geneva: World Health Organization.
6. Pawluck DE, Gorey KM. (1998). Secular trends in the incidence of anorexia nervosa: Integrative review of population-based studies. *Int J Eating Disord.* 23:347–352.
7. Rosenvinge JH, Borgen JS, Borrensen R. (1999). The prevalence and psychological correlates of anorexia nervosa, bulimia nervosa, and binge eating among 15-year-old students: A controlled epidemiological study. *Eur Eating Disord Rev.* 7:382–391.
8. Pope HG, Katz DL, Hudson JI. (1993). Anorexia nervosa and "reverse anorexia" among 108 male body-builders. *Comp Psychiatry* 34:406–409.
9. Andersen AE. (1999). Gender-related aspects of eating disorders: A guide to practice. *J Gender Specific Med.* 2:47–54.
10. Rastam M, Gillberg C, Garton M. (1989). Anorexia nervosa in a Swedish urban region: A population-based study. *Br J Psychiatry.* 155:642–646.
11. Andersen A. (1992). Analysis of treatment experience and outcome from the Johns Hopkins Eating Disorders Program 1975–1990. In *Psychobiology and Treatment of Anorexia Nervosa and Bulimia Nervosa.* (Halmi KA, ed.), pp. 93–124. Washington DC: American Psychiatric Press, Inc.
12. Van Hoeken D, Lucas AR, Hoek HW. (1998). Epidemiology. In *Neurobiology in the Treatment of Eating Disorders*, (Hoek HW, Treasure JL, Katzman MA, ed.), pp. 97–126. New York: Wiley Press.
13. Striegel-Moore RH, Leslie D, Petrill SA *et al.* (2000). One-year use and cost of inpatient and outpatient services among female and male patients with an eating disorder: Evidence from a national database of health insurance claims. *Int J Eating Disord.* 27:381–389.
14. Sullivan PF. (1995). Mortality in anorexia nervosa. *Am J Psychiatry* 52:1073–1074.
15. Crisp AH, Burns T. (1983). The clinical presentation of anorexia nervosa in males. *Int J Eating Disord.* 2:5–10.
16. Crisp AH, Burns T, Bhat AV. (1986). Primary anorexia nervosa in the male and female: A comparison of clinical features and prognosis. *Br J Med Psychol.* 59:123–132.
17. Andersen A, Cohn L, Holbrook T. (2000). *Making Weight: Men's Conflicts with Food, Weight, Shape and Appearance.* Carlsbad: Gurze Books.
18. Burns T, Crisp A. (1990). Outcome of anorexia nervosa in males. In *Males with Eating Disorders.* (Andersen AE, ed.), pp. 163–186. New York: Brunner/Mazel.
19. Saccomani L, Savoini M, Cirrincione M *et al.* (1998). Long-term outcome of children and adolescents with anorexia nervosa: Study of comorbidity. *J Psychosom Res.* 44:565–571.
20. Andersen AE, Watson T, Schlechte J. (2000). Osteoporosis and osteopenia in men with eating disorders. *Lancet.* 355:1967–1968.
21. Swayze V, Andersen A, Arndt S *et al.* (1996). Reversibility in brain tissue loss in anorexia nervosa assessed with a computerized Talairach 3-D proportional grid. *Psychol Med.* 26:381–390.
22. Herzog D, Bradburn I, Newman K. (1990). Sexuality in males with eating disorders. In *Practica: Comprehensive Treatment of Anorexia Nervosa and Bulimia.* (Andersen AE, ed.), pp. 40–53. New York: Brunner/Mazel.
23. Siever MD. (1994). Sexual orientation and gender as factors in socio-culturally acquired vulnerability to body dissatisfaction and eating disorders. *J Consult Clin Psychol.* 62:252–260.
24. Russell CJ, Keel PK. (2002). Homosexuality as a specific risk factor for eating disorders in men. *Int J Eating Disord.* 31:300–306.
25. Murnen SK, Smolak L. (1997). Femininity, masculinity, and disordered eating: A meta-analytic review. *Int J Eating Disord.* 22:231–242.
26. Cantrell PJ, Ellis JB. (1991). Gender role and risk patterns for eating disorders in men and women. *J Clin Psychol.* 47:53–57.

27. Crago M, Yates A, Beutler LE, Arizmendi TG. (1985). Height-weight ratios among female athletes: Are collegiate athletics the precursor to an anorexic syndrome? *Int J Eating Disord.* 4:79–87.

28. Yates A, Leehy K, Shisslak LM. (1983). Running—An analogue of anorexia? *N Engl J Med.* 308:251–255.

29. Yates A. (1987). Eating disorders and long distance running. *Integrative Psychiatry.* 5:201–211.

30. King MB, Mezey G. (1987). Eating behaviour of male racing jockeys. *Psychol Med.* 17:249–253.

31. Felker KR, Stivers C. (1994). The relationship of gender and family environment to eating disorder risk in adolescents. *Adolesc.* 29:821–834.

32. Lilenfeld LR, Kaye WH, Greeno CG *et al.* (1998). A controlled family study of anorexia nervosa and bulimia nervosa: Psychiatric disorders in first-degree relatives and effects of proband comorbidity. *Arch Gen Psychiatry.* 55:603–610.

33. Strober M, Freeman R, Lampert C *et al.* (2001). Males with anorexia nervosa: A controlled study of eating disorders in first-degree relatives. *Int J Eating Disord.* 29:263–269.

34. Treasure J, Holland A. (1989). Genetic vulnerability to eating disorders: Evidence from twin and family studies. In *Child and Youth Psychiatry: European Perspectives.* (Remschmidt H, Schmidt MH, ed.), pp. 59–68. New York: Hogrefe and Huber.

35. Bulik CM, Sullivan PF, Wade TD, Kendler KS. (2000). Twin studies of eating disorders: A review. *Int J Eating Disord.* 27:1–20.

36. Wade TD, Bulik CM, Neale M, Kendler KS. (2000). Anorexia nervosa and major depression: Shared genetic and environmental risk factors. *Am J Psychiatry* 157:469–471.

37. Kaltiala-Heino R, Rissanen A, Rimpela M, Rantanen P. (1999). Bulimia and bulimic behaviour in middle adolescence: More common than thought? *Acta Psychiatrica Scandinavica* 100:33–39.

38. Carlat D, Camargo C. (1991). Review of bulimia nervosa in males. *Am J Psychiatry.* 148:831–843.

39. Ross HE, Ivis F. (1999). Binge eating and substance use among male and female adolescents. *Int J Eating Disord.* 26:245–260.

40. Gross J, Rosen JC. (1988). Bulimia in adolescents: Prevalence and psychosocial correlates. *Int J Eating Disord.* 7:51–61.

41. Ackard DM, Neumark-Sztainer D, Hannan PJ *et al.* (2001). Binge and purge behavior among adolescents: Associations with sexual and physical abuse in a nationally representative sample: the Commonwealth Fund survey. *Child Abuse Neglect.* 25:771–785.

42. Schneider JA, Agras WS. (1987). Bulimia in males: A matched comparison with females. *Int J Eating Disord.* 6:235–242.

43. Carlat DJ, Camargo CA, Herzog DB. (1997). Eating disorders in males: A report on 135 patients. *Am J Psychiatry.* 154:1127–1132.

44. Herzog DB, Norman DK, Gordon C, Pepose M. (1984). Sexual conflict and eating disorders in 27 males. *Am J Psychiatry.* 141:989–990.

45. Joiner TE, Katz J, Heatherton TF. (2000). Personality features differentiate late adolescent females and males with chronic bulimic symptoms. *Int J Eating Disord.* 27:191–197.

46. Powers PS. (1999). Eating disorders: Cardiovascular risks and management. In *Eating Disorders: A Guide To Medical Care And Complications.* (Mehler PS, Anderson AE, ed.), pp. 100–117. Baltimore: Johns Hopkins University Press.

47. Schneider JA, O'Leary A, Jenkins SR. (1995). Gender, sexual orientation, and disordered eating. *Psychol Health.* 10:113–128.

48. Stein D, Lilenfeld LR, Plotnicov K *et al.* (1999). Familial aggregation of eating disorders: Results from a controlled family study of bulimia nervosa. *Int J Eating Disord.* 26:211–215.

49. Wade TD, Bulik CM, Sullivan PF *et al.* (2000). The relation between risk factors for binge eating and bulimia nervosa: A population-based female twin study. *Health Psychol.* 19:115–123.

50. Hettema JM, Neale MC, Kendler KS. (1995). Physical similarity and the equal-environment assumption in twin studies of psychiatric disorders. *Behav Genetics.* 25:327–335.

51. Bulik CM, Sullivan PF, Kendler KS. (1998). Heritability of binge-eating and broadly defined bulimia nervosa. *Biol Psychiatry.* 44:1210–1218.

52. Ackard DM, Neumark-Sztainer D, Story M, Perry C. (2003). Overeating among adolescents: Prevalence and associations with weight-related characteristics and psychological health. *Pediatrics.* 111:67–74.

53. Castonguay LG, Eldredge KL, Agras WS. (1995). Binge eating disorder: Current state and future directions. *Clin Psychol Rev.* 15:865–890.

54. Taraldsen KW, Eriksen L, Goetestam KG. (1996). Prevalence of eating disorders among Norwegian women and men in a psychiatric outpatient unit. *Int J Eating Disord.* 20:185–190.

55. Field AE, Colditz GA, Peterson KE. (1997). Racial/ethnic and gender differences in concern with weight and in bulimic behaviors among adolescents. *Obes Res.* 5:447–454.

56. Field AE, Camargo CA, Taylor CB *et al.* (1999). Overweight, weight concerns, and bulimic behaviors among girls and boys. *J Am Acad Child Adolesc Psychiatry.* 38:754–760.

57. Snow J, Harris MB. (1989). Disordered eating in Southeastern Pueblo Indians and Hispanics. *J Adolesc.* 12:329–336.

58. LaPorte DL. (1997). Gender differences in perceptions and consequences of an eating binge. *Sex Roles.* 36:479–489.

59. Striegel-Moore RH, Wilson GT, Wilfley DE *et al.* (1998). Binge eating in an obese community sample. *Int J Eating Disord.* 23:27–37.

60. Tanofsky MB, Wilfley DE, Spurrell EB *et al.* (1997). Comparison of men and women with binge eating disorder. *Int J Eating Disord.* 21:49–54.

61. Sullivan PF, Bulik CM, Kendler KS. (1998). The genetic epidemiology of binging and vomiting. *Br J Psychiatry.* 173:75–79.

62. Whitaker AH. (1992). An epidemiological study of anorectic and bulimic symptoms in adolescent girls: Implications for pediatricians. *Pediatr Ann.* 21:752–759.

63. Serdula MK, Williamson DF, Anda RF *et al.* (1994). Weight control practices in adults: Results of a multistate telephone survey. *Am J Public Health.* 84:1821–1824.

64. Serdula MK, Collins E, Williamson DF *et al.* (1993). Weight control practices of U.S. adolescents and adults. *Ann Int Med.* 119:667–671.

65. Neumark-Sztainer D, Story M, French S. (1996). Covariations of unhealthy weight loss behaviors and other high-risk behaviors among adolescents. *Arch Pediatrics Adolesc Med.* 150:304–308.

66. Lakkis J, Ricciardelli LA, Williams R. (1999). Role of sexual orientation and gender-related traits in disordered eating. *Sex Roles.* 41:1–16.

67. Leon GR, Fulkerson JA, Perry CL *et al.* (1999). Three to four year prospective evaluation of personality and behavioral risk factors for later disordered eating in adolescent girls and boys. *J Youth Adolesc.* 28:181–196.

68. Klump KL, McGue M, Iacono WG. (2000). Age differences in genetic and environmental influences on eating attitudes and behaviors in preadolescent and adolescent twins. *J Abnormal Psychol.* 109:239–251.

69. Klump KL, McGue M, Iacono WG. (in press). Differential heritability of eating attitudes and behaviors in prepubertal versus postpubertal twins. *Int J Eating Disord.*

70. Klump KL, Kaye WH, Strober M. (2001). The evolving genetic foundations of eating disorders. *The Psychiatric Clinics of North America.* 24:215–225.

71. Center for Disease Control and Prevention National Center for Health Statistics. (2000). *CDC Growth Charts.* United States: Center for Disease Control and Prevention.

72. Must A, Dallal GE, Dietz WH. (1991). Reference data for obesity: 85th and 95th percentiles of body mass index (wt/ht^2) and triceps skinfold thickness. *Am J Clin Nutr.* 53:839–846.

73. Mokdad AH, Serdula MK, Dietz WH *et al.* (2000). The continuing epidemics of obesity in the United States. *JAMA.* 284:1650–1651.

74. Center for Disease Control and Prevention National Center for Health Statistics. (1999). *Prevalence of overweight among children and adolescents: United States 1999.* United States: Center for Disease Control and Prevention.

75. Gortmaker SL, Dietz WH, Sobol AM, Wehler CA. (1987). Increasing pediatric obesity in the United States. *Am J Diseases Childhood* 141:535–540.

76. Gortmaker SL, Must A, Perrin JM *et al.* (1993). Social and economic consequences of overweight in adolescence and young adulthood. *N Engl J Med.* 329:1008–1012.

77. Smith DE, Marcus MD, Lewis C *et al.* (1998). Prevalence of binge eating disorder, obesity, and depression in a biracial cohort of young adults. *Ann Behav Med.* 20:227–232.

78. Enzi G, Gaspar M, Biondetti PR *et al.* (1986). Subcutaneous and visceral fat distribution according to sex, age and overweight, evaluated by computed tomography. *Am J Clin Nutr.* 44:729–746.

79. Terry RB, Wood PD, Haskell WL *et al.* (1989). Regional adiposity patterns in relation to lipids, lipoprotein cholesterol and lipoprotein subfraction mass in men. *J Clin Endocrinol Metab.* 68:191–199.

80. Legato MJ. (1997). Gender-specific aspects of obesity. *Int J Fertil.* 42: 184–197.

81. Stunkard AJ, Harris JR, Pedersen NL, McClearn GE. (1990). The body-mass index of twins who have been reared apart. *N Engl J Med.* 322:1483–1487.

82. Rolls BJ, Fedoroff IC, Guthrie JF. (1991). Gender differences in eating behavior and body weight regulation. *Health Psychol.* 10:133–142.

83. Andersen AE, DiDomenico L. (1992). Diet vs shape content of popular male and female magazines: A dose response relationship to the incidence of eating disorders? *Int J Eating Disord.* 11:283–287.

84. Andersen AE, Holman JE. (1997). Males with eating disorders: Challenges for treatment and research. *Psychopharm Bull.* 33:391–397.

85. Woodside DB, Kennedy SH. (1995). Gender differences in eating disorders. In *Gender and Psychopathology*, (Violette M, ed.), pp. 253–268. Washington DC: American Psychiatric Press.

86. Andersen AE. (1999). Males with eating disorders: Medical considerations. In *Eating Disorders: A guide to medical care and complications*, (Mehler PS, Andersen AE, ed.), pp. 214–226. Baltimore: John Hopkins University Press.

87. Levine MP, Petrie TA, Gotthardt U, Sevig TD. (1990). A professionally-led support group for males with eating disorders. In *Males with Eating Disorders*, (Andersen AE, ed.), pp. 187–217. New York: Brunner/Mazel.

67

The Influence of Gender Differences in Metabolism upon Nutritional Recommendations for Athletes

MARK A. TARNOPOLSKY, MD, PhD

Department of Pediatrics and Medicine (Neurology and Rehabilitation), McMaster University, Hamilton, Ontario, Canada

I. Introduction

It has been assumed for years that men and women respond similarly to the metabolic stress of physical activity [1,2]. It is important to consider menstrual cycle phase, antecedent diet, habitual training status and aerobic capacity when conducting gender-comparative studies [1,3,4]. When training status and maximal aerobic capacity expressed relative to fat-free mass are controlled, there does not appear to be any gender difference in anaerobic threshold [5–7]. There is accumulating evidence that males and females differ in the metabolic response to endurance exercise, with females showing a higher relative lipid oxidation, and a lower protein and carbohydrate oxidation at submaximal exercise intensities [5,7–15]. Interestingly, the aerobic capacity adaptations to endurance exercise training also appear to be qualitatively and quantitatively similar between the genders [10,16,17]. In contrast, gender differences are apparent in the accumulation of muscle mass and strength following resistance exercise training; men show almost twice the response [18,19].

Sex hormones are likely a major contributor to these gender differences [20–23]. Testosterone has a potent anabolic effect on muscle growth and supraphysiologic doses clearly lead to significant strength and muscle mass gains, even in the absence of a resistance exercise-training program [20,24]. Estrogen itself has a mild anabolic effect and there is a decline in muscle mass in the early postmenopausal period that is attenuated with hormone replacement therapy (HRT) [25,26]. On the other hand, estrogen appears to have a significant effect on metabolic fuel selection during endurance exercise. Animal studies have shown an increase in carbohydrate oxidation and a lower lipid oxidation following ovariectomy, which is reversed with estrogen supplementation [27,28]. Male rats also show an increase in lipid oxidation and muscle glycogen "sparing" with estrogen supplementation [29–31]. For other hormones, the only consistent gender difference appears to be lower catecholamine response to endurance exercise in females as compared with males [8,12], although the growth hormone response shows an opposite gender pattern [6].

Whether these gender differences in metabolism have an impact on nutritional recommendations is unclear at this point; however, there are a few areas where some rational suggestions can be made. One area is protein requirement. The lower increase in amino acid oxidation seen in females during endurance exercise [5,15,16], suggests that any additional protein requirement for top sport female athletes would be lower than for their male counterparts. Also, females have an attenuated ability to increase muscle glycogen in response to an increase in the percentage of energy intake from dietary carbohydrate (carbohydrate loading)

[13]. However, this apparent inability of females to carbohydrate load is explained by a lower habitual energy (and resultant lower carbohydrate) intake. Increased energy intake and total carbohydrate intake for 4 days resulted in similar increases in muscle glycogen for female athletes [32]. Both men and women appear to show a similar muscle glycogen resynthesis response to the provision of early postexercise carbohydrate and carbohydrate-protein supplements when the carbohydrate intake is based upon body mass [33]. Finally, the administration of exogenous carbohydrate during endurance exercise can enhance exercise performance by a similar magnitude in males and females [34,35].

In the future it will be important to establish whether gender differences in metabolism exist across the menstrual cycle, that is, after menopause, and in the prepubertal state. Modern techniques such as proteomics and gene expression array analysis will help to understand the molecular basis for the gender differences and the influence of sex hormones. The implications of gender differences in metabolism upon nutritional recommendations is in its infancy and specific recommendations for recreational and top sport female athletes across the menstrual cycle will be an interesting practical area for future research.

II. Effect of 17-β-Estradiol on Substrate Metabolism During Endurance Exercise

Studies have found that 17 β-estradiol administration resulted in a decrease in glycogen utilization for both heart and skeletal muscle in male rats [30,31]. In addition, ovariectomy resulted in female rats showing a "male" metabolic pattern, with an increase in glycogen utilization and lower lipid utilization in both skeletal muscle and heart [27,28]. The "female" metabolic pattern of increased lipid and lower glycogen utilization was restored when the ovariectomized females were supplemented with 17 β-estradiol [27,28]. Although several of these studies used supraphysiologic doses of 17 β-estradiol [28–31], the metabolic effects were also seen with physiologically relevant doses [27], and performance improvements were apparent after only 3 days [31].

From a mechanistic standpoint, many of the effects on lipid metabolism appear to be occurring at the level of skeletal muscle. Addition of 17-β-estradiol increased intra-muscular triglyceride (IMTG) content in both heart and skeletal muscle [29]. These findings have now been extended to human muscle. Females show a higher IMTG content and a greater utilization rate during endurance exercise as compared with males [36]. 17 β-estradiol administration increased lipoprotein lipase (LPL) activity in skeletal muscle, and decreased it in adipocytes, which implied a "redirection" of lipid from the periphery towards skeletal muscle for storage and subsequent oxidation [29]. 17 β-estradiol supplementation also increased the maximal enzyme activities of carnitine palmitoyl transferase-1 (CPT-1) and β-3-OH-acyl-CoA-dehydrogenase in ovariectomized rats [37]. In contrast, there does not appear to be a significant gender difference in CPT-1 or total CPT activity between young men and women [2,38], and most [39,40], but not all [41], studies have not found gender differences in β-3-OH-acyl-CoA-dehydrogenase activity. Finally, there does appear to be a gender-related difference in one of the plasma membrane fatty acid transporters (FATP-1), which in females show twice the FATP-1 mRNA content as compared with males [42].

With respect to carbohydrate oxidation, there does not appear to be any effect of 17 β-estradiol on muscle glucose transporter 4 (GLUT-4) content, although the distribution of GLUT-4 was not determined in that study [43]. Another study found that ovariectomy resulted in a decrease in contraction stimulated glucose transport and an increase in glycogen utilization during exercise in rats [44]. The overexpression of GLUT-4 in a transgenic murine model resulted in an increase in the percentage of glucose disposal through glycolysis in male animals and an increase in that directed towards glycogen storage in female animals [45]. This latter finding may explain why muscle glycogen content is slightly higher in the luteal compared with follicular phase of the menstrual cycle in young females [46]. However, when comparing men and women directly, there does not appear to be a gender difference in basal muscle glycogen content at either phase of the female menstrual cycle [13,16,32,33,47]. There does not appear to be any gender difference in muscle glycogen breakdown during cycle ergometry in young subjects using the muscle biopsy technique [13,16]. In contrast, we have found lower glycogen utilization in females compared with males after a 15.5 km treadmill run [9]. Calculations of estimated glycogen breakdown during cycle ergometry exercise using stable isotope tracers have shown a lower glycogen utilization rate for females [7,8].

In addition to the effects of 17 β-estradiol on carbohydrate metabolism at the skeletal muscle level, 17 β-estradiol also has a major influence upon carbohydrate metabolism at the hepatic level [27,30,31,48,49]. The administration of 17 β-estradiol attenuated glycogen degradation during exercise in liver in rats [27,30,31]. Our group has found that short-term 17 β-estradiol administration to young men increased their plasma 17 β-estradiol concentration to midfollicular levels, yet did not affect muscle glycogen breakdown during endurance exercise [50]. In contrast, hepatic glucose production during endurance exercise was attenuated in both men [48], and women [49], following the administration of 17 β-estradiol. In support of the latter finding, several studies have found that glucose rate of appearance and disappearance [10] and glucose metabolic clearance rate [8] were lower for exercising females as compared with males. These latter findings imply that 17 β-estradiol reduces hepatic glucose production during exercise.

A very interesting study demonstrated the inter-relatedness of glucose and lipid oxidation and the relationship to 17 β-estradiol using a transgenic peripheral peroxisome activating receptor (PPARα$^{-/-}$) murine knockout model [51]. In this study, most of the male PPARα$^{-/-}$ mice died with severe hypoglycemia when an inhibitor of CPT activity (etoximir) was given, yet the majority of female mice survived [51]. Of further interest, the fatal effect of CPT-inhibition in this model in the males was prevented by 17 β-estradiol administration [51].

In summary, it appears that there are effects of 17 β-estradiol/gender on the expression of proteins in involved in FATP-1 and triglyceride hydrolysis (muscle LPL), that may be related to the higher IMTG content seen in females. There do not appear to be significant gender differences, but perhaps subtle effects from large differences in 17 β-estradiol concentration, upon the CPT system or the enzymes involved in β-oxidation. 17 β-estradiol does attenuate liver and muscle glycogen utilization in rodents, yet in humans the effect is consistently seen with estimates of liver glucose production, and inconsistently with muscle glycogen utilization. 17 β-estradiol confers protection from fatal hypoglycemia in a combined transgenic and CPT inhibitor model of human fatty acid oxidation defects.

III. Effect of Testosterone on Protein Turnover at Rest and During Resistance Exercise in Men

Testosterone is a steroid-based hormone produced by the testicular Leydig cells and the adrenal cortex. Testosterone is found in the plasma as a free molecule and bound to sex-hormone binding globulin. Plasma total testosterone concentrations are approximately 10-fold greater in males as compared with females. Anecdotally, the use of testosterone to enhance muscle mass accretion has been in use for decades, as evidenced by the abuse of anabolic steroids in the sporting arena.

More evidence has clearly shown that testosterone has a stimulatory effect on protein synthesis with a resultant increase in fat-free mass [20,24]. The administration of testosterone over 3 months resulted in a significant increase in lean body mass and mixed muscle protein synthetic rate in healthy sedentary males [24]. Similarly, another study found that 10 weeks of testosterone administration to healthy men resulted in a greater increase in strength and muscle size as compared with men receiving placebo [52]. As expected, the promotion of strength and muscle mass gains following testosterone supplementation is particularly robust in hypogonadal males [52,53]. Testosterone administration also potentiated the gains in fat-free mass, muscle size and strength consequent to a resistance exercise program in eugonadal young men [20]. Similar results were obtained in hypogonadal men with HIV wasting syndrome, where a testosterone supplement enhanced the muscle mass and strength gains following a resistance exercise program [52].

Earlier work had shown that testosterone administration did increase the fractional rate of mixed muscle protein synthesis [24]. Ferrando *et al* found that 5 days of testosterone enanthate administration resulted in a 2-fold increase in fractional protein synthetic rate with no change in fractional protein breakdown rate [23]. This group also showed that the protein synthetic stimulation effect was not mediated by an increase in amino acid transport but rather was due to an increase in the reutilization of intracellular amino acids [23].

It is clear that testosterone is a potent anabolic hormone and that its administration in supraphysiologic doses results in an increase in muscle mass in young men. At the skeletal muscle level, testosterone increases mixed protein synthesis rates by increasing the reutilization of intracellular amino acids. From a practical perspective, the current evidence does support that strength and power athletes would likely derive benefits from testosterone administration, and its place on doping lists appears to be legitimate. In the older adult male with sarcopenia or in the case of hypogonadism, the use of testosterone replacement is gaining increasing acceptance [22,54].

IV. Gender Differences in Metabolism During Endurance Exercise (Human Studies)

A. Carbohydrate Metabolism

To compare between genders, several major factors known to alter substrate oxidation rates must be controlled. Perhaps the most important variables that must be controlled in any comparison are training status and habitual and pre-exercise dietary intake. In addition, with gender-comparison studies, the menstrual cycle is known to alter substrate oxidation and must be specified in any comparison study [34,46]. We have previously suggested that one of the best ways to compare between the genders is to match men and women for training history and, given the higher percentage body fat content for females, by VO_{2peak} expressed relative to fat-free mass [55]. Another issue that is important to mention in the gender-difference literature is that studies should test males and females at the same time and not compare historical data. This issue is important. For example, one paper reported that there were no gender differences in substrate oxidation, yet the females appear to have been tested at least 6 years after the males [56]. This strategy will inherently increase the variance in the measurements, and any result could be related to a variety of factors including but not limited to a different metabolic cart, different calibration gas supply, a different person involved in the subject testing, etc.

Regardless of gender comparisons, there are two key factors that are important to accurately measure whole-body carbohydrate (and lipid) oxidation using indirect calorimetry during exercise. Accurate estimates of substrate oxidation require that the subjects be in steady state and exercising below the anaerobic threshold. Although the determination of anaerobic threshold is subject to more variability than the measurement of oxygen consumption, it is important that oxidation measurements are performed at exercise intensities that are lower than the anaerobic threshold. In untrained men and women, the anaerobic threshold may be as low as 66% of VO_{2peak} [6], and in the moderate-to well-trained athlete this may be as high as 80% of VO_{2peak} [5], with no gender difference. As a result, gender comparisons of substrate oxidation rates at higher exercise intensities may not be accurate. The majority of the gender-comparative studies that have been published have used exercise intensities that were appropriate for the subjects' training level [5,8–16,46,57–59].

When the aforementioned design issues are considered, there are a number of cross-sectional studies that have found that whole-body carbohydrate oxidation rates are lower for females as compared with males during endurance exercise at submaximal exercise intensities [5,8–11,13–16,57–59]. Although there are a few studies that have not found gender differences in whole-body carbohydrate oxidation [2,56,60], the majority of them violate one of the control parameters set forth previously [2,56]. Whole body respiratory exchange ratio (RER) values are lower for females as compared with males during endurance exercise even when every gender comparative study is combined into a "meta-analysis" (including those not showing an effect; Table 67-1). When substrate oxidation rates are calculated from the RER, there appears to be a lower carbohydrate oxidation rate for females as compared with males, which is evident in the meta-analytical calculations from the RER (Table 67-2).

One issue that further strengthens the observation of a gender difference in carbohydrate utilization is the fact that several gender comparative endurance exercise training studies have found these effects before and after the training program [8,10,14,16]. This approach removes the issue of matching for training status, because both the males and the females were exposed to exactly the same dose of training.

As discussed previously, the source of the reduction in carbohydrate oxidation for females is unclear, but likely involves an attenuation of predominantly hepatic and possibly muscle glycogen utilization. A study using the leg A-V balance method to examine substrate use across the leg in exercising men and women found no difference in carbohydrate utilization [60]. Confounding the interpretation of this study was the fact that 28% of oxygen consumption by the male leg remained unaccounted for by the sampling methods used [60]. Given that this study found that glucose rate of appearance was lower for the females [60], further support is provided that the sparing of carbohydrate oxidation must involve the liver to some extent. Further A-V balance studies are required with large numbers of men and women to identify the locus of the gender differences in metabolism.

B. Lipid Metabolism

As a corollary to the lower RER, indicating lower carbohydrate utilization for females during endurance exercise, this also indicates a greater lipid utilization for females [see Tables 67-1 and 67-2]. The finding of a higher lipid oxidation for females was confirmed using whole body calorimetry, where females were found to have higher rates of fat oxidation during waking hours and active periods of the day as compared with males [59]. Furthermore, this latter study found that females showed higher lipid oxidation during exercise at both 40 and 70% of VO_{2peak} as compared with males [59]. The source of the higher lipid use for the females during endurance exercise is likely to be a accounted by a greater use of IMTGs [36], and to a lesser extent, blood born free fatty acids (FFAs) [8,57].

Bente Kiens *et al* clearly demonstrated that the IMTG content was higher in females as compared with males and that only females showed a significant reduction with endurance exercise [36]. We have also found that females have a higher IMTG as compared with males using the same biochemic method and also with an electron microscopic method (Rennie *et al*, unpublished observations, 2002). The higher muscle LPL activity for females may direct the FFAs from blood derived chylomicrons and very low density lipoproteins towards a higher IMTG storage in females and a higher subsequent oxidation rate. In the paper by Kiens *et al*, the leg A-V balance data showed a 47% greater plasma FFA uptake for the females as compared with the males during endurance exercise, although this was not reported as being statistically significant [60]. Using

Table 67-1

Summary of Studies Where Whole Body Substrate Metabolism Was Reported in Males and Females

Reference	Subjects	Exercise	RER (mean)
Costill et al, 1979	12 F, T	60 min run @	F = 0.83
	12 M, T	70% VO$_{2max}$	M = 0.84
Froberg and Pederson, 1984	7 F, T	to exhaustion @	F = 0.93
	7 M, T	80 + 90% VO$_{2max}$	M = 0.97
Blatchford et al, 1985	6 F, T	90 min walk	F = 0.81
	6 M, T	@ 35% VO$_{2max}$	M = 0.85
Tarnopolsky et al, 1990	6 F, T	15.5 km run @	F = 0.876
	6 M, T	~ 65% VO$_{2max}$	M = 0.940
Phillips et al, 1993	6 F, T	90 min cycle @	F = 0.820
	6 M, T	65% VO$_{2max}$	M = 0.853
Tarnopolsky et al, 1995	8 F, T	60 min cycle @	F = 0.892
	7 M, T	75% VO$_{2max}$	M = 0.923
Tarnopolsky et al, 1997	8 F, T	90 min cycle @	F = 0.893
	8 M, T	65% VO$_{2max}$	M = 0.918
Horton et al, 1998	13 F, T + UT	120 min cycle @	F = 0.84
	14 M, T + UT	45% VO$_{2max}$	M = 0.86
Freidlander et al, 1998	17 F, UT→T	60 min cycle @	F = 0.885
	19 M, UT→T	45 & 65% VO$_{2max}$	M = 0.932
Romijn et al, 2000	8 F, T	20–30 min cycle @	F = 0.81
	5 M, T	65% VO$_{2max}$	M = 0.81
McKenzie et al, 2000	6 F, UT→T	90 min cycle @	F = 0.889
	6 M, UT→T	65% VO$_{2max}$	M = 0.914
Davis et al, 2000	8 F, UT	90 min cycle @	F = 0.92
	8 M, UT	50% VO$_{2max}$	M = 0.92
Goedecke et al, 2000	16 F, T	10 min @ 25,50,	F = 0.90
	45 M, T	and 75% VO$_{2max}$	M = 0.92
Rennie et al, 2000	6 F, UT→T	90 min cycle @	F = 0.893
	5, M, UT→T	60% VO$_{2max}$	M = 0.945
Carter et al, 2001	8 F, UT→T	90 min cycle @	F = 0.847
	8 M, UT→T	60% VO$_{2max}$	M = 0.900
Lamont et al, 2001	7 F, T + UT	60 min cycle @	F = 0.808
	7 M, T + UT	50% VO$_{2max}$	M = 0.868
Roepstorff et al, 2001	7 F, T	90 min cycle @	F = 0.886
	7 M, T58%	VO$_{2max}$	M = 0.905
Melanson et al, 2002*	8 F, T	400 kcal @40 +	F = 0.87
	8 M,T70%	VO$_{2max}$	M = 0.91
Mean	157 F		F = 0.867 (0.01)
	184 M		M = 0.899 (0.01)**

Values are mean (SD). A, active; F, females; M, males; T, trained; T + U, trained and untrained in same study; U, untrained; U→T, longitudinal training study: For longitudinal training studies, the pre/post-rides are all collapsed across time for each gender.

*The RER was a combination of those at both exercise intensities.

**Significant gender difference (P<0.001, 2-tailed independent t-test)

Table 67-2

Summary of Substrate Utilization in Several Studies (see Table 67-1) Directly Comparing Males and Females

Subjects	RER	CHO [%]	FAT [%]	PRO [%]*
N = 157 F	0.867 (0.01)	56 (10)	40 (9)	2 (2)
N = 184 M	0.899 (0.01)**	65 (9)†	29 (8)†	5 (3)†

Values are mean (SD).

*(From Tarnopolsky et al. [1989]; Phillips et al. [1993]; McKenzie et al. [2000]; Lamont et al. [2001].)

Gender difference (**P < 0.001; †P < 0.01).

CHO, carbohydrate; RER, respiratory exchange ratio.

glycerol tracers, we and others have found that females had a higher lipolytic rate as compared with males during endurance exercise, which supports the previous observation [8,57].

In summary, the balance of the data indicate that females have a higher lipid oxidation during endurance exercise that appears to be predominantly related to a higher IMTG content and possibly to a greater uptake of plasma FFAs.

C. Protein Metabolism

An attenuation of glucose utilization during endurance exercise would be expected to reduce amino acid oxidation [61]. Given the evidence for whole-body carbohydrate oxidation to be less for females as compared with males during endurance exercise, it would follow that amino acid oxidation would also be lower in females. During a 15.5 km treadmill run, we found a sparing of muscle glycogen in females with a corresponding lack of an increase in urinary urea nitrogen excretion on the exercise compared with control day [9]. Although indirect, these results implied that amino acid oxidation was lower during endurance exercise for females as compared with males [9].

To further address the question of gender differences in amino acid oxidation during endurance exercise we completed two trials using ^{13}C-leucine stable isotope methodology and training matched males and females [5,16]. During endurance exercise we found that leucine oxidation was lower for the females as compared with males [5]. Another study confirmed these findings by showing that females had a lower rate of leucine, but not lysine, oxidation during endurance exercise (60 min @ 50% of VO_{2peak}) as compared with males [15]. To examine the potential mechanism(s) behind this apparent gender difference in leucine oxidation, we studied six males and six females before and after a 31-day endurance exercise training program [16]. We measured ^{13}C-leucine oxidation at rest and during 90 min of exercise (60% VO_{2max}) and the active form of branched chain 2-oxo-acid dehydrogenase (BCOAD) in skeletal muscle. The females showed a lower leucine oxidation at rest and during exercise, yet we found identical BCOAD total activity levels and percentage activation before and after endurance training [16]. The lack of an effect of gender on the rate-limiting enzyme for muscle amino acid oxidation and a significantly lower leucine oxidation suggested that some of the sparing of amino acid oxidation may be occurring at the hepatic level. This would be in keeping with an attenuation of hepatic glycogen utilization during exercise for the females (see previous).

In addition to the lower leucine oxidation during exercise, both our study [16] and another by Volpi *et al* [62], found lower rates of basal leucine oxidation in females as compared with males. One final aspect of gender difference that needs to be considered in research studies is the effect of menstrual cycle phase on amino acid kinetics. One group used ^{13}C-leucine tracers to show that females had higher leucine oxidation during the luteal compared with follicular phase [63], and another study found that urinary urea nitrogen excretion was higher during the luteal compared with follicular phase of the menstrual cycle [64]. These findings suggest that there may be less of a gender difference in leucine oxidation during the luteal phase of the menstrual cycle (perhaps due to the testosterone-like properties of progesterone).

V. Protein Requirements for Athletes

Protein oxidation makes up a small proportion (0–6%) of the total energy demands of endurance exercise [5,16]. As a result, physical activity is not factored into most dietary protein requirements. Given the increase in leucine oxidation during endurance exercise [5,16], it would be predicted that dietary protein requirements could be affected if the exercise duration were sufficiently long or the intensity sufficiently high. Using nitrogen balance techniques, several researchers have found that the dietary protein requirements for top sport athletes is up to twice the national recommended intake levels in North

America. With modest intensity endurance exercise there does not appear to be an elevation of dietary protein requirements [65], and we have shown that BCOAD activation and leucine oxidation were lower at the same relative and absolute exercise intensity in both men and women after endurance exercise training [16]. The maximal BCOAD activity was greater after the training, which indicated that the capacity to oxidize amino acids was greater in the trained state [16].

There has only been one nitrogen balance study that has compared men and women directly [5]. This study found that even after a sufficient adaptation period, moderately trained, exercising men and women were both in negative nitrogen balance on a diet supplying protein just above the Canadian and U.S. government dietary protein requirements [5]. Even though the males were consuming marginally more dietary protein (0.94 g/kg/day) than the females (0.80 g/kg/day), the nitrogen balance was more negative for the males (−0.26 mg/kg/day) vs females (−16 mg/kg/day) [5]. These data suggest that any increase of dietary protein requirements in top sport female athletes will be somewhat less than for males (~ 25% lower). Clearly, longer-term and larger studies using several protein intakes will be required to clarify this issue.

VI. Carbohydrate Loading and Carbohydrate Dietary Manipulations for Endurance Activities

It has been known for decades that muscle glycogen stores are positively correlated with endurance exercise performance at intensities from 60–75% of maximal aerobic power [66,67]. Furthermore, dietary manipulations that lead to a higher carbohydrate intake can enhance endurance exercise performance at aforementioned intensities [68,69]. The dietary manipulation whereby an athlete increases carbohydrate intake and tapers their exercise training is termed carbohydrate loading and results in an increase in muscle glycogen store improvement and endurance exercise performance improvement [68,69].

The original studies that examined carbohydrate loading used exclusively or predominantly male subjects [68–71]. Based upon the aforementioned gender differences in carbohydrate metabolism, our group hypothesized that there may be gender differences in the ability to carbohydrate load [13]. Well-trained male and female athletes were given two dietary regimens providing 75% (LOAD) and 55% (HABITUAL) of total energy intake. They consumed each diet for 4 days before completing cycle ergometry for 60 min @ 75% VO_{2peak} followed by a performance ride to exhaustion at 85% VO_{2peak}. The males increased resting muscle glycogen content by 45%, which was correlated with a similar increase in performance, whereas the females showed neither an increase in glycogen content nor in exercise performance [13]. Subsequent work from Spreit *et al* supported these findings by showing that well-trained female athletes showed only minimal increases in muscle glycogen and exercise performance following carbohydrate loading and concluded that, "…the magnitude [of glycogen loading] was smaller than previously observed in men." [72].

Given that there do not appear to be any significant gender differences in hexokinase or GLUT-4 (see previous), we had hypothesized that one of the major factors responsible for the gender difference in the ability to carbohydrate load was the lower relative and absolute energy intake by the females which meant that females consumed less carbohydrate on a per kilogram body weight basis (<7 g/kg/day). In studies evaluating carbohydrate loading in men, the corresponding amount of dietary carbohydrate amounts to >8 g/kg/day [13,69,71]. Hence, if men and women are given dietary carbohydrate as a proportion of total energy intake, females are less likely to exceed a carbohydrate intake of 8 g/kg/day. Therefore, we completed a study where male and female athletes consumed three diets (habitual energy intake [55% CHO]; high carbohydrate intake [75% CHO]; and high carbohydrate + extra energy [75% CHO + 30% more energy than habitual intake] and muscle glycogen was measured) [32]. We found that increase in the percentage carbohydrate intake was insufficient for the females to increase muscle glycogen stores, yet when the additional energy was provided (hence greater CHO/kg body mass), there was a significant increase in muscle glycogen content [32]. These results were confirmed in a study where the ability to carbohydrate load in response to very high amounts of dietary carbohydrate (>12 g/kg fat-free mass/day) was evaluated in men and women (in both follicular and luteal phases of the menstrual cycle) [47]. This study found similar increases in muscle glycogen for both men and women in response to the load and between the menstrual cycle phases [47].

We have also compared the glycogen resynthesis rate in males and females following endurance exercise (90 min @ 65% of VO_{2peak}) with placebo, carbohydrate (1 g·kg^{-1} CHO) and carbohydrate/protein/fat (0.7 g/kg^{-1} CHO/0.1 g/kg^{-1} PRO/0.02 g/kg^{-1}·d^{-1} FAT) supplements given immediately and 1 hour after exercise. The rate of glycogen resynthesis in the first 4 hours was higher for the CHO and CHO/PRO/FAT as compared to placebo trials, yet was not significantly different between the genders [33]. These results confirmed that the glycogen resynthesis rates for men and women were similar in the postexercise period providing that the carbohydrate was expressed relative to body weight. Indirectly, these results provide some support for the aforementioned carbohydrate loading observations.

Many studies have found that the provision of exogenous carbohydrate during endurance exercise can delay the onset of fatigue and promote higher glucose oxidation rates in the latter stages of endurance exercise [73–77]. The majority of these studies had been completed with predominantly male subjects [73,76,77], and very few studies have examined the effect of exogenous carbohydrate intake on endurance exercise metabolism and performance in females [34,35]. One study found an 11–14% increase in exercise performance in young women during both the follicular and luteal phase of the menstrual cycle with a 6% glucose solution [35]. These findings have been extended by work showing greater improvement in performance from 6% glucose solution ingestion in both the follicular [19%] and luteal [26%] phase of the menstrual cycle [34]. We have extended these findings by showing that females oxidized a greater proportion of exogenous carbohydrate (8% carbohydrate solution) with a corresponding greater attenuation of endogenous glucose oxidation as compared with males during exercise [78].

In summary, it appears that the apparent inability for females to carbohydrate load was due to their low habitual energy intake which resulted in a relative carbohydrate intake of <8 g/kg/day. With additional energy and an increase in the proportion of carbohydrate, females can increase muscle glycogen content and performance. Similarly, in the immediate postexercise period, females and males show similar rates of glycogen resynthesis. Finally, males and females show similar responses to exogenous carbohydrate provision during exercise and both increase performance.

VII. Future Directions

The balance of the data is showing that there are gender differences in the metabolic fuel selection during endurance exercise. These differences consist of a higher lipid oxidation and a lower carbohydrate and protein oxidation for females as compared with males. It appears that much of the gender difference in carbohydrate metabolism is at the hepatic level and this may be related to the lower protein oxidation seen in females. A simple study would be to simultaneously measure both glucose and leucine turnover during endurance exercise in men and women in both phases of the menstrual cycle. Ideally transhepatic catheterization studies would answer the substrate balance question across the liver definitively, however, from a practical perspective, we will likely be limited to indirect evidence from animal studies.

The issue of gender differences in lipid utilization will require further characterization of IMTG use using magnetic resonance spectroscopy, biochemic measures and electron microscopic methods simultaneously with tracer turnover estimates. Furthermore, potential gender differences in the protein content and activity (where applicable) of the following proteins must be characterized at various stages of the menstrual cycle; each of the plasma membrane fatty acid binding proteins, cytosolic fatty acid binding protein, hormone sensitive lipase, CPT-2, PPAR, and each of the 10 different chain-length specific enzymes involved in β-oxidation. Two methods that must be employed to answer some of these questions are proteomics (proteome level) and gene expression arrays (transcriptome level).

Testosterone does appear to have potent effects on muscle mass accretion and protein turnover in women, however, the molecular basis behind these effects is not understood. Clearly, gene expression arrays looking at the interactive and independent effects of testosterone and resistance exercise will provide a great deal of insight.

The implications of gender differences in metabolism on nutritional recommendations are still in an embryonic level and even simple questions such as protein requirements for male and female athletes have not been characterized as yet. Future studies must also consider the issues of amenorrhea and menstrual cycle phase on nutritional recommendations for female athletes.

VIII. Suggestions for Further Investigations

Here is a list of research questions awaiting answers.

- What are the gender differences in muscle fatty acid storage, transport, and oxidation that explain the greater whole body lipid oxidation in women?
- Is the lower amino acid oxidation observed in females during exercise due to hepatic and/or muscle mediated factors?
- How does menstrual cycle phase affect the male–female gender comparison?
- What are effects of testosterone and 17 β-estradiol on skeletal muscle gene expression before and after exercise?
- Does the menstrual cycle phase alter gene expression in skeletal muscle?

- What are the protein requirements for female endurance and strength in athletes?
- Is 17 β-estradiol a potential treatment for inborn errors of metabolism in the fatty acid oxidation pathways?

Acknowledgement

Funding for the majority of our gender difference research has been from NSERC Canada.

References

1. Tarnopolsky MA. (2000). Gender differences in substrate metabolism during endurance exercise. Can J Appl Physiol. 25:312–327.
2. Costill DL, Fink WJ, Getchell LH et al. (1979). Lipid metabolism in skeletal muscle of endurance-trained males and females. J Appl Physiol. 47:787–791.
3. Cureton KJ. (1981). Matching of male and female subjects using VO2 max. Res Q Exerc Sport. 52:264–268.
4. Sparling, PB. (1980). A meta-analysis of studies comparing maximal oxygen uptake in men and women. Res Q Exerc Sport. 51:542–552.
5. Phillips SM, Atkinson SA, Tarnopolsky MA, MacDougall JD. (1993). Gender differences in leucine kinetics and nitrogen balance in endurance athletes. J Appl Physiol. 75:2134–2141.
6. Pritzlaff-Roy CJ, Widemen L, Weltman JY et al. (2002). Gender governs the relationship between exercise intensity and growth hormone release in young adults. J Appl Physiol. 92:2053–2060.
7. Ruby BC, Coggan AR, Zderic TW. (2002). Gender differences in glucose kinetics and substrate oxidation during exercise near the lactate threshold. J Appl Physiol. 92:1125–1132.
8. Carter SL, Rennie C, Tarnopolsky MA. (2001). Substrate utilization during endurance exercise in men and women after endurance training. Am J Physiol Endocrinol Metab. 280:E898–907.
9. Tarnopolsky LJ, MacDougall JD, Atkinson SA et al. (1990). Gender differences in substrate for endurance exercise. J Appl Physiol. 68:302–308.
10. Friedlander AL, Casazza GA, Horning MA et al. (1998). Training-induced alterations of carbohydrate metabolism in women: Women respond differently from men. J Appl Physiol. 85:1175–1186.
11. Horton TJ, Pagliassotti MJ, Hobbs K, Hill JO. (1998). Fuel metabolism in men and women during and after long-duration exercise. J Appl Physiol. 85:1823–1832.
12. Davis SN, Galassetti P, Wasserman DH, Tate D. (2000). Effects of gender on neuroendocrine and metabolic counterregulatory responses to exercise in normal man. J Clin Endocrinol Metab. 85:224–230.
13. Tarnopolsky MA, Atkinson SA, Phillips SM, MacDougall JD. (1995). Carbohydrate loading and metabolism during exercise in men and women. J Appl Physiol. 78:1360–1368.
14. Rennie CD, Brose AN, Carter SL, Tarnopolsky MA. (2000). Muscle enzyme changes following endurance exercise in males and females. [Abstract]. Med Sci Sports Exerc. 32:S363.
15. Lamont LS, McCullough AJ, Kalhan SC. (2001). Gender differences in leucine, but not lysine, kinetics. J Appl Physiol. 91:357–362.
16. McKenzie S, Phillips SM, Carter SL et al. (2000). Endurance exercise training attenuates leucine oxidation and BCOAD activation during exercise in humans. Am J Physiol Endocrinol Metab. 278:E580–E587.
17. Skinner JS, Jaskolski A, Jaskolska A, et al. (2001). Age, sex, race, initial fitness, and response to training: The HERITAGE Family Study. J Appl Physiol. 90:1770–1776.
18. Yarasheski KE, Pak-Loduca J, Hasten DL et al. (1999). Resistance exercise training increases mixed muscle protein synthesis rate in frail women and men >/=76 yr old. Am J Physiol. 277:E118–E125.
19. Tarnopolsky MA, Parise G, Yardley NJ et al. (2001). Creatine-dextrose and protein-dextrose induce similar strength gains during training. Med Sci Sports Exerc. 33:2044–2052.
20. Bhasin S, Storer TW, Berman N et al. (1996). The effects of supraphysiologic doses of testosterone on muscle size and strength in normal men. N Engl J Med. 335:1–7.
21. Ferrando, AA, Sheffield-Moore M, Yeckel CW et al. (2002). Testosterone administration to older men improves muscle function: Molecular and physiological mechanisms. Am J Physiol Endocrinol Metab. 282:E601–607.
22. Wolfe R, Ferrando A, Sheffield-Moore M, Urban R. (2000). Testosterone and muscle protein metabolism. Mayo Clin Proc. 75(Suppl):S55–60
23. Ferrando, AA, Tipton KD, Doyle D et al. (1998). Testosterone injection stimulates net protein synthesis but not tissue amino acid transport. Am J Physiol. 275:E864–871.
24. Griggs RC, Kingston W, Jozefowicz RF et al. (1989). Effect of testosterone on muscle mass and muscle protein synthesis. J Appl Physiol. 66:498–503.
25. Dionne IJ, Kinaman KA, Poehlman ET. (2000). Sarcopenia and muscle function during menopause and hormone-replacement therapy. J Nutr Health Aging. 4:156–161.
26. Phillips SK, Rook KM, Siddle NC et al. (1993). Muscle weakness in women occurs at an earlier age than in men, but strength is preserved by hormone replacement therapy. Clin Sci (Lond). 84:95–98.
27. Kendrick ZV, Steffen CA, Rumsey WL, DI Goldberg DI. (1987). Effect of estradiol on tissue glycogen metabolism in exercised oophorectomized rats. J Appl Physiol. 63:492–496.
28. Hatta H, Atomi Y, Shinohara S et al. (1988). The effects of ovarian hormones on glucose and fatty acid oxidation during exercise in female ovariectomized rats. Horm Metab Res. 20:609–611.
29. Ellis GS, Lanza-Jacoby S, Gow A, Kendrick ZV. (1994). Effects of estradiol on lipoprotein lipase activity and lipid availability in exercised male rats. J Appl Physiol. 77:209–215.
30. Rooney TP, Kendrick ZV, Carlson J et al. (1993). Effect of estradiol on the temporal pattern of exercise-induced tissue glycogen depletion in male rats. J Appl Physiol. 75:1502–1506.
31. Kendrick ZV, Ellis GS. (1991). Effect of estradiol on tissue glycogen metabolism and lipid availability in exercised male rats. J Appl Physiol. 71:1694–1699.
32. Tarnopolsky MA, Zawada C, Richmond LB et al. (2001). Gender differences in carbohydrate loading are related to energy intake. J Appl Physiol. 91:225–230.
33. Tarnopolsky MA, Bosman M, Macdonald JR et al. (1997). Postexercise protein-carbohydrate and carbohydrate supplements increase muscle glycogen in men and women. J Appl Physiol. 83:1877–1883.
34. Campbell SE, Angus DJ, Febbraio MA. (2001). Glucose kinetics and exercise performance during phases of the menstrual cycle: Effect of glucose ingestion. Am J Physiol Endocrinol Metab. 281:E817–E825.
35. Bailey SP, Zacher CM, Mittleman KD. (2000). Effect of menstrual cycle phase on carbohydrate supplementation during prolonged exercise to fatigue. J Appl Physiol. 88:690–697.
36. Steffensen, CH, Roepstorff C, Madsen M, Kiens B. (2002). Myocellular triacylglycerol breakdown in females but not in males during exercise. Am J Physiol Endocrinol Metab. 282:E634–E642.
37. Campbell SE, Febbraio MA. (2001). Effect of ovarian hormones on mitochondrial enzyme activity in the fat oxidation pathway of skeletal muscle. Am J Physiol Endocrinol Metab. 281:E803–E808.
38. Berthon, PM, Howlett RA, Heigenhauser GJ, Spriet LL. (1998). Human skeletal muscle carnitine palmitoyltransferase I activity determined in isolated intact mitochondria. J Appl Physiol. 85:148–153.
39. Carter SL, Rennie CD, Hamilton SJ, Tarnopolsky. (2001). Changes in skeletal muscle in males and females following endurance training. Can J Physiol Pharmacol. 79:386–392.
40. Gauthier JM, Theriault R, Theriault G et al. (1992). Electrical stimulation-induced changes in skeletal muscle enzymes of men and women. Med Sci Sports Exerc. 24:1252–1256.
41. Green HJ, Fraser IG, Ranney DA. (1984). Male and female differences in enzyme activities of energy metabolism in vastus lateralis muscle. J Neurol Sci. 65:323–331.
42. Binnert C, Koistinen HA, Martin G et al. (2000). Fatty acid transport protein-1 mRNA expression in skeletal muscle and in adipose tissue in humans. Am J Physiol Endocrinol Metab. 279:E1072–1079.
43. Hansen PA, McCarthy TJ, Pasia EN et al. (1996). Effects of ovariectomy and exercise training on muscle GLUT-4 content and glucose metabolism in rats. J Appl Physiol. 80:1605–1611.
44. Campbell SE, Febbraio MA. (2002). Effect of the ovarian hormones on GLUT4 expression and contraction-stimulated glucose uptake. Am J Physiol Endocrinol Metab. 282:E1139–E1146.
45. Tsao TS, Li J, Chang KS et al. (2001). Metabolic adaptations in skeletal muscle overexpressing GLUT4: Effects on muscle and physical activity. FASEB J. 15:958–969.
46. Nicklas BJ, Hackney AC, Sharp RL. (1989). The menstrual cycle and exercise: Performance, muscle glycogen, and substrate responses. Int J Sports Med. 10:264–269.

47. James, AP, Lorraine M, Cullen D *et al.* (2001). Muscle glycogen supercompensation: Absence of a gender-related difference. *Eur J Appl Physiol.* 85:533–538.

48. Carter S, McKenzie S, Mourtzakis M *et al.* (2001). Short-term 17beta-estradiol decreases glucose R(a) but not whole body metabolism during endurance exercise. *J Appl Physiol.* 90:139–146.

49. Ruby BC, Robergs RA, Waters DL *et al.* (1997). Effects of estradiol on substrate turnover during exercise in amenorrheic females. *Med Sci Sports Exerc.* 29:1160–1169.

50. Tarnopolsky MA, Roy BD, MacDonald JR *et al.* (2001). Short-term 17-beta-estradiol administration does not affect metabolism in young males. *Int J Sports Med.* 22:175–180.

51. Djouadi F, Weinheimer CJ, Saffitz JE *et al.* (1998). A gender-related defect in lipid metabolism and glucose homeostasis in peroxisome proliferator-activated receptor alpha-deficient mice. *J Clin Invest.* 102:1083–1091.

52. Bhasin S, Storer TW, Javanbakht M *et al.* (2000). Testosterone replacement and resistance exercise in HIV-infected men with weight loss and low testosterone levels. *JAMA.* 283:763–770.

53. Bhasin S, Storer TW, Berman N *et al.* (1997). Testosterone replacement increases fat-free mass and muscle size in hypogonadal men. *J Clin Endocrinol Metab.* 82:407–413.

54. Bhasin SL, Woodhouse R, Casaburi AB *et al.* (2001). Testosterone dose-response relationships in healthy young men. *Am J Physiol Endocrinol Metab.* 281:E1172–1181.

55. Tarnopolsky MA, Saris WH. (2001). Evaluation of gender differences in physiology: An introduction. *Curr Opin Clin Nutr Metab Care.* 4:489–492.

56. Romijn JA, Coyle EF, Sidossis LS *et al.* (2000). Substrate metabolism during different exercise intensities in endurance-trained women. *J Appl Physiol.* 88:1707–1714.

57. Friedlander AL, Casazza GA, Horning MA *et al.* (1998). Effects of exercise intensity and training on lipid metabolism in young women. *Am J Physiol.* 275:E853–E863.

58. Goedecke JH, St Clair A, Gibson L *et al.* (2000). Determinants of the variability in respiratory exchange ratio at rest and during exercise in trained athletes. *Am J Physiol Endocrinol Metab.* 279:E1325–E1334.

59. Melanson EL, Sharp TA, Seagle HA *et al.* (2002). Effect of exercise intensity on 24-h energy expenditure and nutrient oxidation. *J Appl Physiol.* 92:1045–1052.

60. Roepstorff C, Steffensen CH, Madsen M *et al.* (2002). Gender differences in substrate utilization during submaximal exercise in endurance-trained subjects. *Am J Physiol Endocrinol Metab.* 282:E435–E447.

61. Bowtell JL, Leese GP, Smith K *et al.* (2000). Effect of oral glucose on leucine turnover in human subjects at rest and during exercise at two levels of dietary protein. *J Physiol.* 525(Pt 1):271–281.

62. Volpi E, Lucidi P, Bolli GB *et al.* (1998). Gender differences in basal protein kinetics in young adults. *J Clin Endocrinol Metab.* 83:4363–4367.

63. Lariviere F, Moussalli R, Garrel DR. (1994). Increased leucine flux and leucine oxidation during the luteal phase of the menstrual cycle in women. *Am J Physiol.* 267:E422–E428.

64. Lamont LS, Lemon PW, Bruot BC. (1987). Menstrual cycle and exercise effects on protein catabolism. *Med Sci Sports Exerc.* 19:106–110.

65. Forslund AH, El-Khoury AE, Olsson RM *et al.* (1999). Effect of protein intake and physical activity on 24-h pattern and rate of macronutrient utilization. *Am J Physiol.* 276:E964–E976.

66. Hultman E. (1967). Studies on muscle metabolism of glycogen and active phosphate in man with special reference to exercise and diet. *Scand J Clin Lab Invest Suppl.* 94:1–63.

67. Bergstrom J, Hultman E. (1967). A study of the glycogen metabolism during exercise in man. *Scand J Clin Lab Invest.* 19:218–228.

68. Bergstrom J, Hermansen L, Hultman E, Saltin B. (1967). Diet, muscle glycogen and physical performance. *Acta Physiol Scand.* 71:140–150.

69. Sherman WM, Costill DL, Fink WJ, Miller JM. (1981). Effect of exercise-diet manipulation on muscle glycogen and its subsequent utilization during performance. *Int J Sports Med.* 2:114–118.

70. Hultman E, Bergstrom J. (1967). Muscle glycogen synthesis in relation to diet studied in normal subjects. *Acta Med Scand.* 182:109–117.

71. Karlsson J, Saltin B. (1971). Diet, muscle glycogen, and endurance performance. *J Appl Physiol.* 31:203–206.

72. Walker JL, Heigenhauser GJ, Hultman E, Spriet LL. (2000). Dietary carbohydrate, muscle glycogen content, and endurance performance in well-trained women. *J Appl Physiol.* 88:2151–2158.

73. Febbraio MA, Chiu A, Angus DJ *et al.* (2000). Effects of carbohydrate ingestion before and during exercise on glucose kinetics and performance. *J Appl Physiol.* 89:2220–2226.

74. Coggan AR, Swanson SC. (1992). Nutritional manipulations before and during endurance exercise: Effects on performance. *Med Sci Sports Exerc.* 24:S331–S335.

75. Coggan AR, Coyle EF. (1991). Carbohydrate ingestion during prolonged exercise: Effects on metabolism and performance. *Exerc Sport Sci Rev.* 19:1–40.

76. Coggan AR, Coyle EF. (1989). Metabolism and performance following carbohydrate ingestion late in exercise. *Med Sci Sports Exerc.* 21:59–65.

77. Burelle Y, Peronnet F, Charpentier S *et al.* (1999). Oxidation of an oral [13C] glucose load at rest and prolonged exercise in trained and sedentary subjects. *J Appl Physiol.* 86:52–60.

78. Riddell MC, Partington SL, Stupka N *et al.* (2002). Substrate utilization during exercise performed with and without glucose ingestion in female and male endurance-trained athletes. [Abstract]. *Int J Sport Nutr Metab.* (In review.)

68

Cardiovascular Disease, Genes, and Nutrition: Gender Matters

JOSE M. ORDOVAS, PhD* AND LI-MING LOH**

*Nutrition and Genomics Laboratory, JM-USDA-HNRCA at Tufts University, Boston, MA
**Department of Endocrinology, Singapore General Hospital, Singapore

I. Introduction

Cardiovascular disease (CVD), the leading cause of mortality in most industrialized countries, is a multifactorial disease that is associated with nonmodifiable risk factors, such as age, gender, and genetic background, and with modifiable risk factors, including elevated total and low-density lipoprotein cholesterol (LDL-C) levels, as well as reduced high-density lipoprotein cholesterol (HDL-C) levels. There is convincing evidence showing that lowering serum lipid levels will slow the progression or even induce regression in atherosclerotic lesions [1–3]. Based on this evidence, the National Heart, Lung, and Blood Institute's National Cholesterol Education Program (NCEP) has recommended that all adult Americans reduce their serum TC values to <5.18 mmol/L (200 mg/dL) and their LDL-C values to <3.37 mmol/L (130 mg/dL) and has put forward a set of guidelines for the prevention and management of high cholesterol in adults known as the Adult Treatment Panel III (ATPIII) [4].

The current ATPIII guidelines strengthen implementation of nutrition, physical activity, and weight control in the treatment of high blood cholesterol. These recommendations are now combined into what has been called therapeutic lifestyle change (TLC) treatment plan. The current dietary recommendations reflect the fact that during the last few years the intakes of both saturated fat (11–12% of total energy) and cholesterol (300–350 mg/day) are approaching the goals of previous NCEP recommendations of <10% of energy from saturated fat and <300 mg of dietary cholesterol, and sets more intensive guidelines aimed to achieve more efficiently the LDL-C goals. Another interesting addition is the recommendation of adding to the diet specifically formulated foods such as plant sterols-rich margarines and foods rich when soluble fiber if the dietary fat and cholesterol modifications are not enough to reach the optimal plasma LDL-C concentrations (see Table 68-1).

The ATPIII report is based on the evidence gathered from scores of studies that provide scientific support for the general recommendations shown in Table 68-1, and underscores the importance of nutrition on the primary and secondary prevention of CVD. According to the new cut points for plasma lipid and lipoprotein concentrations, the number of adults in the United States who need TLC is estimated at 65 million. However, these general recommendations do not take into account the well-known fact that individuals display a very wide range of responses to any therapeutic intervention, and it is not known how many individuals can achieve the recommended levels of serum lipids using the recommended approaches [4]. The major reason for this uncertainty is that although we have algorithms to predict plasma cholesterol response to changes in dietary fat and cholesterol in groups of individuals, we cannot predict at this time the individual's response.

The evidence for the Diet-Heart hypothesis began over 50 years ago, when several studies demonstrated that serum cholesterol could be modified by the composition of dietary fat [5,6]. Later on, studies by Keys *et al* [7] and Hegsted *et al* [8] provided the first quantitative estimates of the relative effects of the various classes of dietary fatty acids and amount of cholesterol on serum cholesterol changes. Other predictive algorithms have been developed, which include predictions of response for LDL-C and HDL-C [9–11]. As indicated previously, these relationships between dietary changes and serum lipid changes are well founded and predictable for groups; however, a striking variability in the response of serum cholesterol to diet between subjects was already reported as early as 1933 [12] and this variability has been the subject of multiple reports [11,13–16]. In some individuals, plasma total and LDL-C levels dramatically decrease following consumption of lipid-lowering diets, whereas they remain unchanged in others [11,13,14,17]. It has been shown already in studies in nonhuman primates that the serum lipoprotein response to dietary manipulation has a significant genetic component [18–20]. It is obvious that such genetic variability could have a significant impact on the success of public health policies and individual therapeutic interventions. In this regard, the Summary of a Scientific Conference on Preventive Nutrition: Pediatrics to Geriatrics convened by The Nutrition Committee of the American Heart Association (AHA), specifically states that

> *Theoretically, genetic differences can render a particular set of dietary conditions more harmful or beneficial in one ethnic group than in another. This is one explanation for why individuals of different ethnic groups who consume similar diets might have varying disease profiles.*

Moreover, the statement underscores the need to "*Identify specific genes and genetic variations that affect risk directly*

Table 68-1
Essential Components of Therapeutic Lifestyle Changes

Component	Recommendation
Saturated fats	<7% of total calories
Dietary cholesterol	<200 mg/day
Other alternatives for LDL lowering	
Plant stanols/sterols	2 g per day
Increased viscous (soluble) fiber	10–25 g per day

and indirectly by the way they interact with nutrients." [21] This message was also reflected in the latest revision of the AHA dietary guidelines [22].

The interest to elucidate the genetic factors responsible for the individual variability in response is highly worthy, and it will provide extremely important findings in terms of our understanding of basic metabolic regulation as well as public health recommendations; however, this excitement for genetic research has overshadowed the fact that gender may also affect the response to TLC.

Women were the "forgotten ones" when it came to CVD risk assessment and prevention. Cardiovascular disease was originally thought about as a male disease. Therefore, women were excluded or underrepresented from the major pharmacologic clinical trials that have defined the importance of lowering cholesterol to reduce CVD morbidity and mortality. Similarly, women have been absent or underrepresented in studies and trials involving dietary assessment or intervention. However, the current reality differs dramatically from the classic stereotype. Now we know that as many women as men die of CVD, although it happens about 8–10 years later. Moreover, women with disease have a worse prognosis than men. Therefore, we should make every effort to close this gap in our knowledge regarding the role of specific risk factors for CVD, as well as the proper therapeutic approaches to use in women. In this regard, it is worth noting the effort that the National Institutes of Health has placed on ensuring that women and minorities are properly represented in studies funded by the Institute.

In this chapter, we will examine how solid the evidence is for the current TLC recommendations, specifically those that relate to dietary modification, when it applies to women.

II. The Diet-Heart Hypothesis

A. Cross-Cultural Studies

The diet-heart hypothesis has been tested in long-term prospective observational studies, large-scale intervention studies and by scores of small dietary modification studies addressing different biochemic and/or clinical outcomes. Very strong initial evidence about the potential role of diet on the risk of coronary heart disease (CHD) came from cross-cultural studies. Probably the most influential of those original studies was the Seven Countries Study that began in 1958 [23–25]. This study consisted of 16 cohorts in seven countries: Finland, Greece, Italy, Japan, The Netherlands, United States, and Yugoslavia. The size of the study, 12,763 subjects, was impressive for that time, but in tune with the initial belief about CHD, only men were enrolled in this pivotal study. These subjects underwent physical examination, electrocardiograms were carried out and serum was collected to assess the classic biochemic risks at that time. Moreover, 7-day food records were collected in a random subset of the study participants. This study demonstrated that the average population intake of saturated fat was positively correlated with the 10- and 25-year CHD mortality rates and serum cholesterol was associated with 25-year population CHD mortality.

Another key cross-cultural study was the Nippon-Honolulu-San Francisco (Ni-Hon-San) [26–29]. This classical study was carried out between 1966 and 1970. Its specific goals were to: (1) precisely estimate the prevalence, incidence, and mortality of CHD and cerebrovascular disease among Japanese men (~8000, age 45–68 at baseline) in the three areas; (2) delineate the differences in the prevalence of established risk factors; and (3) determine the relations between risk factors and disease. California and Honolulu men were, on average, 8 kg heavier than their Japanese counterparts. Both American cohorts showed markedly higher serum cholesterol values than those in Japan (Japan: 176, Honolulu: 219, California: 228 at age 50–54). Blood pressure was distinctly higher in the California cohort. Serum glucose values determined 1 hour after an oral glucose load in Hawaii exceeded those in Japan at all ages. The mean value for total calories was only slightly lower in Japan than in Hawaii and California, but the fat intake in Japan was markedly lower than in America (15% vs 33% and 38% respectively).

These two studies are cited as landmarks supporting the importance of diet on determining CVD risk factors and the subsequent impact of disease morbidity and mortality. However, we should emphasize that in both instances, the populations examined were restricted to male subjects.

B. Intervention Studies

Several large diet intervention studies have been performed to assess the value of dietary modification on CVD risk. Unlike the clear evidence obtained from the cross-cultural studies regarding the modulating effect of diet over disease risk, the outcome of intervention studies has originated more controversy.

The cross-cultural studies referenced previously were long-term prospective observational studies looking at dietary patterns and subsequent CVD events. This approach provides information about associations between dietary factors and CVD risk. However, these studies are subjected to large numbers of confounding factors. Therefore, intervention studies, similar to those carried out for pharmacologic clinical trials are needed to provide solid evidence and to demonstrate cause (diet) and effect (CVD morbidity and/or mortality). This type of trial is essential in the current atmosphere of evidence-based medicine.

For the most part, dietary intervention studies have examined the effect of dietary modification on CHD risk factors (i.e., LDL-C, HDL-C) and the benefit of the observed changes are then extrapolated to a potential CHD benefit based on the impact of risk factor modification on disease risk. However, the final proof rests on demonstrating a direct effect of dietary intervention on clinical manifestation of disease.

A systematic review on the results of trials involving reduction or modification of dietary fat on the prevention of CVD has carefully compiled the data from 27 randomized trials including 40 intervention arms [30]. These trials included a total of 18,196 people, with even distribution among the control and the intervention groups. Assessment of the effects of dietary modification on CVD morbidity or mortality was the primary purpose of only nine of these trials. Whereas 13 of them were primarily designed to test intermediate CVD risk factors (i.e., plasma cholesterol or LDL-C levels), the remaining five had other pathologies as primary goals (i.e., breast cancer). Seven included only people at high CVD risk, six included subjects with moderate risk, and the remaining 14 incorporated low-risk individuals. Two of the 27 trials provided most of the nutritional needs to the participants over the duration of the study. Seventeen of the trials provided only dietary advice to decrease the amount or modify the type of fat. The remaining eight provided both dietary advice and supplementation. Dietary modification spanned from diets as low as 15% of energy as fat and as high as 45% replacing saturated by unsaturated fat. In addition, some of the protocols paid specific attention to other dietary components (i.e., reductions in dietary cholesterol or caloric intake, modification of the type of carbohydrates, and amounts of fiber, fruit and vegetables). Studies in which the major dietary intervention consisted of n-3 fatty acids were excluded because of their effects on other risk factors in addition to plasma lipid concentrations.

The fat interventions examined by these studies were low fat diets (usually isocaloric, with energy from fat being replaced with carbohydrate); modified fat diets (total fat remains constant, but saturated fat is replaced by unsaturated fats) and combinations of both. Those diets tend to have comparable effects on total serum cholesterol concentrations, but they may have different effects on CVD risk because of their effects on other CVD risk factors (i.e., HDL-C or triglycerides [Tgs]). For all studies combined, there was no significant effect of dietary modification for total mortality (relative risk [RR]: 0.98, 95% confidence interval [CI]: 0.86–1.12) and CVD mortality (RR: 0.91, 95% CI: 0.77–1.07).

Dietary change to reduce or modify dietary fat intake appears to reduce the incidence of combined cardiovascular events. This trend is statistically significant for all trials, but when a trial, which also increased omega-3 fat intake in the intervention group, is excluded, the results are no longer statistically significant. The protective effect is seen almost exclusively in those who continue to modify their diet over at least 2 years. The extent of this protection appears similar in both high- and low-risk populations, although the relationship does not achieve statistical significance in low-risk participants. Dietary advice to those at high risk of CVD (particularly where statins may not be available), and probably also to lower-risk population groups, should continue to include dietary fat modification, and it should be stressed that this is a permanent pattern of eating.

There was also a suggestion from these studies that dietary fat modification has a protective effect on total mortality and on cardiovascular mortality when the dietary modification is followed for at least 2 years, however, this trend is not statistically significant. It may be that not enough people were involved in long-term trials to show the protective effect of a change in dietary fat, or it may be that there is no such effect.

In terms of the specific topic of this review, the good news is that, overall, women made up 33% of all the participating subjects, but the bad news is that women represented 0% of the 3688 participants in trials including high-risk subjects. Thus, most of the CVD events of the reviewed trials occurred in men. Again, very little information has been gained from these studies regarding the impact of dietary modification on CVD risk in women.

Other sources of information regarding the potential effects of dietary modification on CVD risk factors come from the numerous small and, for the most part, short term dietary modification studies. The results from some of the early studies from the 1950s and 1960s were combined to determine how dietary fatty acids affect plasma cholesterol concentrations. Regression analyses reported in 1965 by Hegsted et al [8] and Keys et al [7] characterized the effects of dietary fat type and individual fatty acids on plasma total cholesterol (TC) concentrations, leading to the generation of the previously mentioned predictive equations that are still used today. However, as previously noted, the calculations used trials that included mostly men. The inclusion of women in dietary trials have shown that gender may affect plasma lipid responses to diets low in fat and cholesterol or with a high content of polyunsaturated fat. However, this is not a consistent finding and further research is needed.

The most systematic study aimed to identify differences between men and women on the response of serum cholesterol to dietary changes comes from an analysis by Weggemans et al [31] who studied sex differences in the response of serum cholesterol and lipoproteins to diet. They measured the responses of serum cholesterol to different types of intervention. Seven trials involving 126 men and 147 women involved a decrease in dietary saturated fat. Two trials (48 men and 57 women) consisted on a decrease in dietary trans fat. Eight trials (74 men and 70 women) examined a decrease in dietary cholesterol. They also measured responses to the coffee diterpene cafestol, which occurs in unfiltered coffee, in nine trials (72 men and 61 women). All subjects were lean and healthy. The response of TC to a decrease in the intake of saturated fat was greater in men (-0.62 mmol L-1) than in women (-0.48 mmol L-1; 95% CI: 0.04–0.23 mmol L-1). The response of TC to a decrease in the intake of cafestol was also larger in men (-1.01 mmol L-1) than in women (-0.80 mmol L-1; 95% CI: 0.04–0.39 mmol L-1). Responses to trans fat and to dietary cholesterol did not differ between men and women. The conclusions of this paper are in agreement with some previous studies suggesting that men have larger responses of total and LDL-C to saturated fat and cafestol than women do.

An article has reviewed the current status of our knowledge of lipoproteins, nutrition, and CHD [32]. Special emphasis was placed on dietary intervention studies. As described for the previous review, women were underrepresented in most of the studies covered in that article. Moreover, even in those cases in which women were part of the studies, the analyses were combined for both sexes.

C. Prospective Studies

Just like the cross cultural studies were essential to demonstrate the validity of the heart-diet hypothesis, large prospective studies are key components to gain understanding the effects of dietary factors on intermediate CVD risk factors and events in men and women.

In this regard several such studies have offered substantial information about diet, plasma lipids and CVD events in free-living populations in the USA. These are the Physicians' Health Study [33], the Nurses' Health Study [34], the Framingham Heart Study [35,36], and NHANES I and II [37,36].

The Physicians' Health Study is a randomized, double-blind, placebo-controlled trial of primary prevention initially designed to assess the effects of low-dose aspirin on CVD and of beta-carotene on risks of cancer. A total of 22,071 U.S. male physicians age 40 to 84 were randomized to one of four treatment groups: active aspirin and active beta-carotene, active aspirin and beta-carotene placebo, aspirin placebo and active beta-carotene, or both placebos. Data have been obtained related to a large number of variables, including demographics, personal medical history, family history, health habits, and diet. In the Health Professionals' Follow-up Study, diet was assessed in 1986 and 1990 by using food frequency questionnaires (FFQs) very similar to those in the 1984 Nurses' Health Study questionnaire.

In the Nurses' Health Study, dietary consumption and follow-up data from 84,688 female nurses, age 34 to 59 and free from CVD and cancer at baseline in 1980, were compared from validated questionnaires completed in 1980, 1984, 1986, 1990, and 1994. During 16 years of follow-up (1980–1996), there were 1513 incident cases of CHD (484 CHD deaths and 1029 nonfatal myocardial infarctions). The NHANES I Epidemiological Follow-up Study is a longitudinal cohort study of a national sample. Included in this analysis were 8825 white and black women and men age 25–74 who, when examined in 1971 through 1975, did not report a history of heart disease. Average follow-up for survivors of 18.8 years (maximum 22.1 years). The main outcomes measured were death (all causes, cardiovascular, noncardiovascular, cancer) and incidence of CHD.

Another source of information regarding the association between diet and disease in men but specially in women has been the Framingham Heart study. Dietary information has been collected using different dietary instruments at several time points during the long history of this study [38].

1. What Is the Evidence for the Benefit of Individual Nutrients and Dietary Patterns in Women Coming from Prospective Studies?

a. FATTY ACIDS. As previously discussed, there has been a lot of research evaluating the effects of varying amounts of total fat on risk factors for CVD and also for diabetes and overweight and obesity. The current evidence suggests that a diet moderate in total fat (25–35% energy) is probably advisable for the majority of individuals. However, we begin to realize the importance of individualizing dietary fat recommendations based on genetics, cultural diversity and specific pathologies. Thus, a diet higher in total fat (30–35% energy) may be more favorable for the lipid and lipoprotein risk profile than a lower-fat diet in individuals with diabetes, with the added benefit of better glycemic control.

It is not well known whether the effects of dietary fats on cardiovascular risk and risk factors are similar in men and women. In the Nurses' Health Study [39], each increase of 5% of energy intake from saturated fat, as compared with equivalent energy intake from carbohydrates, was associated with a borderline significant 17% increase in the risk of CHD (P = 0.10). As compared with equivalent energy from carbohydrates, the RR for a 2% increment in energy intake from transunsaturated fat was 1.93 (P<0.001); that for a 5% increment in energy from monounsaturated fat was 0.81 (P = 0.05); and that for a 5% increment in energy from polyunsaturated fat was 0.62 (P = 0.003). Total fat intake was not significantly related to the risk of CHD. For a 5% increase in energy from fat, the RR was 1.02 (P = 0.55).

The authors estimated that the replacement of 5% of energy from saturated fat with energy from unsaturated fats would reduce risk by 42% (P < 0.001) and that the replacement of 2% of energy from transfat with energy from unhydrogenated, unsaturated fats would reduce risk by 53% (P < 0.001). These findings suggest that replacing saturated and transunsaturated fats with unhydrogenated monounsaturated and polyunsaturated fats is more effective in preventing CHD in women than reducing overall fat. These results are in agreement with some previous dietary trials in men [40].

The relation between dietary fats and plasma lipids were also examined in a population-based sample of 695 premenopausal and 727 postmenopausal women participating in the Framingham Offspring Study. Multivariate regression analyses revealed that plasma Tgs were inversely related to polyunsaturated fat and directly related to saturated fat and oleic acid. A direct relationship between dietary fat and HDL cholesterol was limited to postmenopausal women. Plasma total and LDL-cholesterol levels were directly associated with consumption of saturated fat. In contrast, dietary cholesterol was not a predictor of plasma total or LDL cholesterol levels. Total cholesterol levels were also directly associated with total fat, oleic acid, and animal fat. Stepwise regressions with key nutrients indicated that saturated fat was consistently associated with total and LDL cholesterol levels in Framingham women [41,42].

The n-3 fatty acids deserve special attention. Evidence first reported 20 years ago from the Greenland Inuit population suggested that fatty fish and fish oils contained substances that reduced the incidence of ischemic heart disease (IHD) [43]. These substances, later determined to be omega-3 fatty acids, were found in early clinical trials to reduce platelet aggregation and to reduce hypertriglyceridemia by as much as 35%. More trials have found that omega-3 fatty acids also appear to reduce the risk of cardiac arrhythmia and sudden cardiac death and modestly reduce atherosclerotic plaque formation and hypertension. Some meta-analyses have provided further support to the cardioprotective protective properties of n-3 fatty acids from both fish and plant sources [44,45]. The accumulated consistent evidence was the basis for the AHA and the NCEP ATP III recommendations that fish be included as a part of a CHD risk reduction diet [22,4]. However, like for other nutrients, most of the studies have focused on men.

The potential benefits of fish and omega-3 fatty acids on cardiovascular risk in women has been examined in the Nurses' Health Study [46] and in the NHANES I [47] with different outcomes. In the Nurses' Health Study, compared women who rarely ate fish (<1 per month) to those with a higher intake of fish. The higher fish intake had a lower risk of CHD. After adjustment for age, smoking, and other CVD risk factors, the multivariable RR of CHD was 0.79 for fish consumption 1 to 3 times per month, 0.71 for once per week, 0.69 for 2 to 4 times per week, and 0.66 for 5 or more times per week (P for trend = .001). Similarly, women with a higher intake of omega-3 fatty acids had a lower risk of CHD, with multivariable RRs of 1.0, 0.93, 0.78, 0.68, and 0.67 (P<0.001 for trend) across quintiles of intake. For fish intake and omega-3 fatty acids, the inverse association appeared to be stronger for CHD deaths, multivariate RR for fish consumption 5 times per week was 0.55 for CHD deaths as compared with 0.73 for nonfatal myocardial infarction.

The conclusion from this study is that among women, higher consumption of fish and omega-3 fatty acids is associated with a lower risk of CHD, particularly CHD deaths. Consistent with this, a report from the Physicians' Health Study [48] found an inverse relationship between blood levels of eicosapentaenoic acid and docosahexaenoic acid and risk for sudden death in men, without a history of CVD. Compared with men whose blood levels were in the first quartile, RR for sudden death was significantly lower among men with levels in the third quartile (RR = 0.28) and the 4th quartile (RR = 0.19).

Conversely, in the NHANES I Epidemiologic Follow-up Study, [47] fish consumption at baseline was obtained from a 3-month FFQ. In this population, fish consumption (1 time/week or more) compared with no consumption was associated with lower mortality in white men age 25–74, but not in black men. This was primarily due to risk of noncardiovascular death. No consistent association of fish consumption and CHD incidence or mortality was seen. No significant findings were seen for white women and black women and men.

The reasons for these differences are not apparent. Both populations are United States-based with a similar follow-up period. The much larger sample size of the Nurses' Health Study may provide the required statistical power to detect minor effects and to adjust for other confounders.

b. DIETARY CHOLESTEROL. Reduction in egg consumption has been widely recommended to lower blood cholesterol levels and prevent CHD. The relationship between egg consumption and CHD was examined in the Nurses' Health Study. After adjustment for age, smoking, and other potential CHD risk factors, no evidence was found to support a significant association between egg consumption and risk of CHD or stroke in these women. The RRs of CHD across categories of intake (taking as baseline <1 per week) were: 1 per week (0.82), 2 to 4 per week (0.99), 5 to 6 per week (0.95), and ≥1 per day (0.82 [P for trend = .95]) [49]. Likewise, in the Framingham Heart Study, dietary cholesterol was not a predictor of plasma total or LDL-C levels [41,42]. In subgroup analyses from the Nurses' Health Study, higher egg consumption appeared to be associated with increased risk of CHD only among diabetic subjects (RR of CHD comparing >1 egg per day with <1 egg per week among diabetic women, 1.49 [P for trend = .008]. These findings suggest that consumption of up to 1 egg per day is unlikely to have substantial overall impact on the risk of CHD or stroke among healthy women. The apparent increased risk of CHD associated with higher egg consumption among diabetic women warrants further research.

c. FRUITS AND VEGETABLES. Many constituents of fruits and vegetables may reduce the risk for CHD. This concept has been supported by numerous epidemiologic studies, some of them focusing on women. Thus, in the Women's Health Study [50] when the lowest and highest quintiles of fruit and vegetable intake were compared, the multivariate adjusted RR for CVD risk and myocardial infarction as 0.45 (P=0.09) and 0.62 (P=0.07).

This association was also evaluated in the Nurses' Health Study [51]. Median total fruit and vegetable intake was 5.8 servings/day. With each one-serving/day increase in intake, the RR for CHD was 0.87. After additional adjustment for smoking,

the RR was 0.93. Further adjustment for additional risk factors produced a RR of 0.97. In this same report, the data from the Physicians' Follow-up Study shows very similar effects with RR values of 0.94; 0.96; and 0.93 respectively for the difference adjustments listed previously for women. All these effects were statistically significant in both men and women. For men and women combined, the RR for CHD was 0.80 when extreme quintiles of fruit and vegetable intake were compared. Moreover, the analytic model indicates a 4% lower risk for CHD for each 1 serving increase per day of fruits and vegetables.

A report about the health benefits of a high intake of fruits and vegetables comes from the NHANES study [52]. Over an average of 19 years, 888 strokes (218 fatal), 1786 IHD events (639 fatal), 1145 CVD deaths, and 2530 all-cause deaths were documented. Consuming fruit and vegetables ≥3 times/day compared with <1 time/day was associated with a 27% lower stroke incidence [RR: 0.73; P−0.01), a 42% lower stroke mortality (0.58; P=0.05), a 24% lower IHD mortality (0.76; P=0.07), a 27% lower CVD mortality (0.73; P=0.008), and a 15% lower all-cause mortality (0.85; P=0.02) after adjustment for established CVD risk factors.

These data support a protective effect of greater consumption of fruits and vegetables, in particular green leafy vegetables and vitamin C-rich fruits and vegetables, against risk for CHD. These results provide further support for recommendations to consume an abundance of fruits and vegetables also in women.

d. WHOLE GRAIN. Although current dietary guidelines for Americans recommend increased intake of grain products to prevent CHD, epidemiologic data relating whole-grain intake to the risk of CHD are sparse. The investigators of the Nurses' Health Study evaluated whether high whole-grain intake reduces risk of CHD in women. [53]. After adjustment for age and smoking, increased whole-grain intake was associated with decreased risk of CHD. For increasing quintiles of intake, the corresponding RRs were 1.0 (reference), 0.86, 0.82, 0.72, and 0.67 (95% CI comparing 2 extreme quintiles: 0.54, 0.84; P for trend <0.001). After additional adjustment for body mass index (BMI), postmenopausal hormone use, alcohol intake, multivitamin use, vitamin E supplement use, aspirin use, physical activity, and types of fat intake, these RRs were 1.0, 0.92, 0.93, 0.83, and 0.75 (95% CI: 0.59, 0.95; P for trend = 0.01). The inverse relation between whole-grain intake and CHD risk was even stronger in the subgroup of never smokers (RR = 0.49 for extreme quintiles; 95% CI: 0.30, 0.79; P for trend = 0.003). The lower risk associated with higher whole-grain intake was not fully explained by its contribution to intakes of dietary fiber, folate, vitamin B-6, and vitamin E. Therefore, increased intake of whole grains may protect against CHD in women. Moreover, this group has also shown a protective effect of whole grains in relation to ischemic stroke [54]. These findings are consistent with those from the Iowa Women's Health Study demonstrating a beneficial effect of whole grain [55] and fiber intakes on risk for IHD [56].

Because of the beneficial effects of whole grains, the AHA recommends 3 or more servings per day from whole grain breads and cereals [22]. Although whole grains are a good source of dietary fiber, it is now evident that their cardioprotective effects extend beyond dietary fiber, and include folate, vitamin

B_6, and vitamin E and likely numerous phytochemicals [53]. Nonetheless, whole grain foods are a source of soluble (viscous) fiber, which reduces LDL-cholesterol levels [5–10 g soluble (viscous) fiber reduces LDL-cholesterol by approximately 5%.

e. NUTS. There has been interest on the potential beneficial relationship between the intake of nuts and more specifically walnuts and the reduction and prevention of CHD. The health benefits of walnuts have been attributed to their specific fatty acid composition. Compared to most other nuts, which contain monounsaturated fatty acids (MUFAs), walnuts are unique because they are rich in n-6 (linoleate) and n-3 (linolenate) poly-unsaturated fatty acids (PUFAs). In addition, walnuts contain high levels of arginine, folate, fiber, tannins, and polyphenols. Several controlled, dietary walnut intervention trials have been carried out and they have consistently reported that walnuts as part of a heart-healthy diet, lower blood cholesterol concentrations. However, none of these studies were of extended duration that would be essential for evaluation of the sustainability of the observed outcomes. These results have been also supported by several large prospective observational studies in humans, demonstrating a dose response-related inverse association of the RR of CHD with the frequent daily consumption of small amounts of nuts, including walnuts.

The strongest initial evidence came from the Adventist Health Study, a prospective cohort investigation of 31,208 nonHispanic white California Seventh-Day Adventists. Extensive dietary information was obtained at baseline, along with the values of traditional coronary risk factors. These were related to risk of definite fatal CHD or definite nonfatal myocardial infarction. The data show that subjects who consumed nuts frequently (>4 times per week) experienced substantially fewer definite fatal CHD events (RR: 0.52) and definite nonfatal myocardial infarctions (RR: 0.49), when compared with those who consumed nuts <1 time per week. These findings persisted on covariate adjustment. This study also showed that subjects who usually consumed whole wheat bread experienced lower rates of definite nonfatal myocardial infarction (RR: 0.56) when compared with those who usually ate white bread. Men who ate beef at least 3 times each week had a higher risk of definite fatal CHD (RR: 2.31), but this effect was not seen in women or for the nonfatal myocardial infarction end point. [57]. The effects of nuts have also verified directly or indirectly in Iowa Women's Health Study [58,59].

The relation between nut consumption and risk of CHD was also examined in the Nurses' Health Study [60]. After adjusting for age, smoking, and other known risk factors for CHD, women who ate more than 5 units of nuts (1 unit equivalent = 1 oz of nuts) a week (frequent consumption) had a significantly lower risk of total CHD (RR: 0.65, P = 0.0009) than women who never ate nuts or who ate <1 unit a month (rare consumption). The magnitude of risk reduction was similar for both fatal CHD (0.61, P = 0.007) and non-fatal myocardial infarction (0.68, P = 0.04). Further adjustment for intakes of dietary fats, fiber, vegetables, and fruits did not alter these results. The inverse association persisted in subgroups stratified by levels of smoking, use of alcohol, use of multivitamin and vitamin E supplements, BMI, exercise, and intake of vegetables or fruits. In conclusion, frequent nut consumption was associated with a reduced risk of both fatal CHD and non-fatal myocardial infarction. These data, and those from other epidemiologic and clinical studies, support a role for nuts in reducing the risk of CHD.

Likewise, in the Physicians' Health Study, [61] dietary nut intake was associated with a significantly reduced risk of sudden cardiac death after controlling for known cardiac risk factors and other dietary habits (P = 0.01). Compared with men who rarely or never consumed nuts, those who consumed nuts 2 or more times per week had reduced risks of sudden cardiac death (RR: 0.53) and total CHD death (RR: 0.70).

Overall, the data indicate that consuming nuts >1 time (i.e., 1 oz serving) per week has similar protective effects for both men and women, with RR ranging from 0.49 to 0.82 for those who consumed nuts >5 times per week as compared with those who never consumed nuts.

f. PLANT STANOL/STEROL ESTER. The ATPIII [4] recommendations now include the use of plant stanols and sterol ester as part of the nutritional tools to reduce plasma LDL-C levels. In this case, and due to its commercialization as part of supplemented margarines, there is no epidemiologic evidence demonstrating a benefit over CHD risk. However, the evidence from clinical studies has shown that the consumption of 2–3 g/day of plant-derived stanol/sterol esters reduces LDL-cholesterol levels between 10% and 20%, without affecting HDL-cholesterol or Tgs [62,63]. These effects have been shown not only in men, but also in premenopausal and postmenopausal women.

g. OTHER FOODS WITH POTENTIALLY BENEFICIAL CARDIO-VASCULAR DISEASE EFFECTS. Although they may not be specifically listed in the ATPIII recommendations, several other commonly used foods have been shown and association with CVD risk factors and/or over the disease risk. The list is extensive and several of them have been reviewed [64]. We will present those, such as alcohol and legumes, for which there is evidence from the prospective studies discussed in this work.

a. ALCOHOL. It is quite well accepted that moderate alcohol consumption, that could be estimated as up to two drinks/day in men and one drink per day in women, is associated with lower CHD risk. For many years, there has been a heated discussion about whether the type of alcoholic beverage (wine, beer, spirits) has any influence over the reported associations [65–67]. The mechanisms by which alcohol drinking protects against CVD may be multiple. It is known that alcohol raises HDL-C. It has also been hypothesized that the antioxidants present in certain alcoholic beverages may protect against the development of atherosclerosis. Finally, alcohol drinking may also affect LDL-C levels. However, the data are very controversial in this regard. This may be due, as shown next, to the presence of significant gene-alcohol interactions. Moreover, this interaction may be gender dependent.

b. LEGUMES. Soybean protein and dietary fiber have been shown to reduce plasma cholesterol levels in intervention studies. Therefore, their consumption may be associated with lower CHD risk. This hypothesis has been demonstrated at the population level using data from the NHANES I [68]. These investigators demonstrated that legume consumption was inversely associated with risk for CHD and CVD. In that study, consumption of legumes 4 or more times per week vs <1 time per week was associated with a 22% lower (P=0.002), and 11% lower (P=0.02) CHD and CVD risk, respectively.

The legume that has raised more interest in terms of cardiovascular health is soybean, especially after a meta analyses including clinical trials concluded that a mean intake of 47 g/day soy protein was associated with a 13% reduction in LDL-cholesterol concentration [69]. This effect was even more significant among those subjects with higher baseline cholesterol concentrations. This hypocholesterolemic effect associated with soy products may be due to the estrogenic activities of soy isoflavones. However, this is a controversial issue. The initial studies demonstrated significant LDL-C effects in subjects with moderate hypercholesterolemia [70] and in certain phases of the menstrual cycle in women [71], other studies did not confirm such findings [72–75]. Despite these inconsistencies, the current evidence supports the notion that daily consumption of 25 g soy protein or more, directly or due to the presence of phytochemicals, can decrease LDL-C levels in moderately hypercholesterolemic individuals [76]. Therefore, these products are recommended as replacements for animal products rich in saturated fat and cholesterol.

D. Bringing All Together: Dietary Patterns

Although substantial information on individual nutrients or foods and risk of CHD is available, little is known about the role of overall eating pattern. This is an emerging concept and several mathematical models have been or are being developed to identify dietary patterns or clusters in different populations. Using dietary information from the Nurses' Health Study [77], two major dietary patterns—"prudent" and "Western"—were identified and factor scores were calculated of each pattern for individuals in the cohort. Logistic regression was used to examine prospectively the associations between dietary patterns and CHD risk. The prudent pattern was characterized by higher intakes of fruits, vegetables, legumes, fish, poultry, and whole grains, whereas the Western pattern was characterized by higher intakes of red and processed meats, sweets and desserts, French fries, and refined grains. After adjusting for coronary risk factors, the prudent diet score was associated with a RR of 0.76 (P=0.03) comparing the highest with lowest quintile. Extreme quintile comparison yielded an RR of 1.46 (P=0.02) for the Western pattern. Those who were jointly in the highest prudent diet quintile and lowest Western diet quintile had an RR of 0.64 (P<0.05) compared with those with the opposite pattern profile. These results support the concept that a diet high in fruits, vegetables, whole grains, legumes, poultry, and fish and low in refined grains, potatoes, and red and processed meats may lower risk of CHD in women.

The relation between dietary patterns and heart disease risk factors has also been examined in 1942 women age 18–76 participating in the Framingham Study. Ninety-four percent of the women were successfully assigned to one of the previously validated five dietary pattern clusters: Heart Healthy, Light Eating, Wine and Moderate Eating, High Fat, and Empty Calorie. Dietary patterns differed substantially in terms of individual nutrient intakes, overall dietary risk, heart disease risk factors, and predicted heart disease risk. Women in the Heart Healthy cluster had the most nutrient dense eating pattern, the lowest level of dietary risk, more favorable risk factor levels, and the lowest probability of developing heart disease. Those in the Empty Calorie cluster had a less nutritious dietary pattern, the greatest level of dietary risk, a heavier burden of heart disease risk factors, and a relatively higher probability of developing heart disease [78,79].

E. A Special Concern: Type 2 Diabetes Mellitus

A major risk factor for CVD, especially in women, is diabetes mellitus (DM). The prevalence of type 2 DM is increasing worldwide, in both industrialized and developing countries. Diabetes mellitus is another example of a complex disorder that results from gene-environment interaction. In this case, the environment consists of both behavioral factors, such as sedentary lifestyle and obesity, and also of dietary factors. Various studies involving ethnic groups at high risk of diabetes [80–82] have suggested that the adoption of a Western-type diet, as opposed to more traditional ones, have resulted in the worrying increases in prevalence seen. Interestingly, intervention studies targeting individuals most at risk of diabetes (i.e., those with impaired glucose tolerance), have shown dramatic reductions in the rate of developing diabetes when only lifestyle and diet are used [83–85]. These studies involved a good representation of both sexes.

1. Dietary Pattern

The role of dietary pattern in the development of diabetes was explored in the Health Professional Follow-up Study in 42,504 male professionals [86]. Two major dietary patterns were defined; the "prudent" pattern characterized by higher consumption of vegetables, fruit, fish, poultry, and whole grains and the Western pattern characterized by higher intakes of red meat, processed meat, French fries, high-fat dairy products, refined grains, sweets and desserts. In the 12-year follow-up, the prudent pattern was associated with a modestly lower risk, whereas the Western pattern with increased risk for type 2 diabetes (RR for extreme quintiles 0.84 [CI: 0.70–1.00] and 1.59 [CI: 1.32–1.93] respectively).

2. Dietary Fat Intake

The Nurses' Health Study studied the relation between dietary fat intake and the development of diabetes in women [87]. In the 14-year follow-up of 84,204 women, total fat intake was not found to be associated with the risk of diabetes. Neither was the intake of saturated fatty acids (SFAs) or MUFAs. The most significant finding of this study was that every 2% increase in energy from trans fatty acid was associated with a RR of 1.39 [CI: 1.15–1.67] whereas a 5% increase in energy from polyunsaturated fat related to a RR of 0.63 [0.53–0.76]. The authors proposed that by replacing 2% of energy from trans fatty acid isoenergetically with PUFA would result in a 40% lower risk of diabetes [0.48–0.75].

The similar finding was reported in older women, in the Iowa Women's Health Study [88], where 35,988 women age 55 to 69 were followed for 11 years using validated food-frequency questionnaires. Whereas no relationship was observed between the total fat intake, SFA, and MUFA and the risk of diabetes, the consumption of vegetable fat was inversely related, with a 22% reduction in the highest quintile (median 41.7 g/day). In contrast to the Nurses' Health Study, this study did not reveal an effect of trans fatty acid intake.

3. Dietary Fiber

In this same study, total grain, whole-grain, total dietary fiber, cereal fiber, and dietary magnesium intakes showed strong inverse associations with incidence of diabetes after adjustment for potential nondietary confounding variables [89]. Multivariate-adjusted RRs of diabetes were 1.0, 0.99, 0.98, 0.92, and 0.79 (P for trend: 0.0089) across quintiles of whole-grain intake; 1.0, 1.09, 1.00, 0.94, and 0.78 (P for trend: 0.005) across quintiles of total dietary fiber intake; and 1.0, 0.81, 0.82, 0.81, and 0.67 (P for trend: 0.0003) across quintiles of dietary magnesium intake. Intakes of total carbohydrates, refined grains, fruit and vegetables, and soluble fiber and the glycemic index were unrelated to diabetes risk.

Salmeron *et al* also showed that diets with highly refined grains with low fibre increased the risk of diabetes in both men [90] and women [91]. In contrast to the Iowa study, food high in glycemic load was positively associated with risk of diabetes.

III. Gender Differences in the Rates of Adherence to Dietary Interventions and Guidelines

Little information exists in the literature regarding gender differences in the adoption of healthful eating habits. The common knowledge suggests that women are more likely than men to report changing their diets and to be more compliant. This has been supported by some studies [92,93]. However, others have contradicted the prevailing sense by showing that gender differences are small, specifically among the elderly [94,95]. A survey documented that, in a nationally representative sample of the U.S. adult population, women gave more importance to good nutrition than did men [96]. Women also were more careful about selecting foods to achieve a healthful diet. The survey identified women age 35 to 54 and men age 25 to 34 as two subgroups of the population that may be most receptive to advice about improving dietary behaviors.

This issue has been tested in 2520 adult participants (1375 women and 1145 men) in the Framingham Offspring-Spouse Study surveyed between 1991 and 1995 using a cross-sectional analysis of nutrient intake estimated from 3-day food records [97]. These investigators examined gender differences in the proportions of persons who had intakes that met nutrient guidelines. The results show that population intake levels of certain key nutrients, including total and saturated fat, appear to be approaching recommended levels. High proportions of the Framingham population (70% or more) met current recommendations for intakes of protein, polyunsaturated and monounsaturated fat, cholesterol, alcohol, vitamins C and B-12, and folacin. About half or fewer met guidelines for carbohydrate; total and saturated fat; fiber; beta carotene; vitamins A, E, and B-6; calcium; and sodium. Important gender differences in the proportion of those meeting nutrient guidelines were observed

for 12 of the 18 nutrients examined, including carbohydrate; total, saturated, and monounsaturated fat; cholesterol; fiber; sodium; calcium; and several vitamins. Therefore, although progress has been made toward achieving population adherence to preventive nutrition recommendations, large proportions of adults fall short of guidelines for some key nutrients even in a population that has been exposed for a long time to the knowledge of CVD risk factors and the importance of nutrition as a preventive tool. Also very important are the differences in adherence rates between men and women that suggest areas for gender-specific, targeted nutrition messages and behavioral interventions. These investigators observed a number of significant (P < 0.01) gender differences in adherence to dietary recommendations in these subjects. Greater proportions of women than men met the recommendations for carbohydrate, total and saturated fat, cholesterol, vitamin A, beta carotene, and sodium, whereas more men than women met the guidelines for monounsaturated fat, dietary fiber, vitamin B-12, folacin, and calcium. These observations show men and women may have unique needs for nutrition information and interventions that are not adequately targeted by current global dietary recommendations. Preventive nutrition messages targeted to adult men need to emphasize reducing intakes of total and saturated fat, cholesterol, and sodium and increasing intakes of complex carbohydrates. In contrast, women appear to need messages that further emphasize adequate intakes of calcium, vitamin B-12, and folacin. Women also need specific nutrition messages that encourage the increased intake of foods higher in dietary fiber and lower in refined sugar. Recognition of differences in nutrient intake between men and women is important and may facilitate the improved formulation of behaviorally based, gender-specific nutrition messages and interventions.

Our knowledge about these issues will substantially increase as more information is made available from the Women's Health Initiative (WHI) Dietary Modification Trial. The WHI is examining the health of 161,855 postmenopausal women recruited and enrolled by 40 study sites throughout the United States. The WHI includes three randomized controlled clinical trials and one observational study. Women, age 50 to 79, will be followed for 7 to 12 years, depending on when they enrolled, with a mean follow-up of 8.5 years. Women randomly assigned to the intervention arm of the Dietary Modification study participate in a group-based low-fat intervention program. The Dietary Modification intervention arm includes 19,542 women. The program provides each participant with an individualized daily fat gram goal approximating 20% total energy from fat, common daily goals for fruit/vegetable and grain intakes (≥5 servings for fruit/vegetable, ≥6 servings for grain), methods for self-monitoring dietary intake, and a structured set of group sessions for learning and practicing dietary and behavior change skills. Nutritionists trained and certified by WHI facilitate the sessions. Group sessions started after randomization as soon as 8 to 12 women could be assigned to a specific time. The first 18 sessions, to be delivered within 12 months of the group start date, comprise the intensive phase of the intervention. During this first year, each participant meets individually with a nutritionist to discuss progress and address participant questions or concerns. Participants learn self-monitoring techniques and are assigned to turn in at least 1 fat gram score per session, starting with the third session. Each fat gram score represents the average daily fat gram intake during the number of days monitored. After the intensive first year of the study, quarterly annual maintenance sessions are held to reinforce self-monitoring skills. For study monitoring, food and nutrient intakes are assessed by a FFQ.

The objective of a publication from this study was to examine whether the effects of physical and emotional status on adherence to a low-fat (20% energy) dietary pattern are mediated by participation in an intervention program (attending sessions and self-monitoring). The data indicate that participating in the dietary intervention program reduced (mediated) the negative effect of poorer mental health on dietary adherence by 15%. Additional findings demonstrated a 10% increase in physical functioning that increased session attendance by 0.4% (P < .001) and a 10% increase in mental health predicted a decrease in percentage energy from fat of 0.3% (P < .001). Program participation had a marked effect on dietary adherence: A 10% increase in session attendance predicted a 1.2% decrease in percentage energy from fat (P < .001). In summary, this study concludes that understanding and using instruments to assess the physical and emotional status of a target population will help dietetic professionals promote healthful dietary change and maintenance [98].

Another publication based on the WHI explored some of the factors affecting dietary change for preventive purposes in older individuals [99]. The purpose of this study was to determine the major behavioral influences on older women's adherence to a dietary fat reduction intervention. The sample size for this exploratory study was small and consisted of a diverse sample of 92 women aged 55 to 80 recruited from two East Coast sites of the WHI. All the women participating in the dietary modification arm of WHI, had received the same dietary instruction, and were in the maintenance phase of the intervention. The women were classified by nutritionists as adherent or nonadherent to a diet limiting fat intake to <20% of total calories. Adherent women were more likely to report assertiveness, a lifelong commitment to reduced dietary fat, satisfaction with their lifestyle changes, and having applicable knowledge and skills. Nonadherent women reported more difficulty resisting negative emotions and prior food preferences and habits; they were also more concerned about negative responses from others. In conclusion, this study demonstrates that enhancing adherence of older women to a dietary fat reduction program will require shifting priorities away from conforming to social pressure and using high-fat foods for personal satisfaction, and moving toward enhancing motivation and commitment to long-term health.

IV. Gender, Genes, Diet and Cardiovascular Disease Risk

A. Apolipoprotein E

When it comes to the interplay between genetics, gender, environment and dislipidemias, the locus that has been more thoroughly examined is the apolipoprotein E gene *(apoE)*. Apolipoprotein E in serum is associated with chylomicrons, very-low-density lipoprotein (VLDL), and HDL, and serves as a ligand for the LDL receptor and the LDL receptor-related

protein (LRP) [100,101]. Genetic variation at the *apoE* locus results from three common alleles in the population, E4, E3, and E2, with frequencies in Caucasian populations of approximately 0.15, 0.77, 0.08 respectively [102]. Population studies have shown that plasma cholesterol, LDL cholesterol and *apoB* levels are highest in subjects carrying the *apoE*4 isoform, intermediate in those with the *apoE*3 isoform and lowest in those with the *apoE*2 isoform [103,104]. It has been suggested that *apoE* allelic variation may account for up to 7% of the variation in total and LDL cholesterol levels in the general population [102], with this effect being greater in women than in men. Therefore, variation at the *apoE* locus may determine the individual CVD risk. In this regard, the relation of *apoE* genotype to CVD was investigated in the Framingham Offspring Study [105]. Period prevalence of CVD between examinations one and five (1971–1994, [366 events]) was related to *apoE* genotype. Age adjusted period prevalence of CVD in men was 18.6% for Group E4, 18.2% for Group E2, and 12.7% for Group E3 (P = 0.004); whereas in women these rates were 9.9, 4.9, and 6.6%, respectively (P = 0.037). After adjustment for all CVD risk factors the relative odds in Group E2 men was 1.94 (P = 0.004) and in Group E4 men it was 1.51 (P = 0.0262). Therefore, the presence of the *apoE*2 or apo E4 alleles in men is associated with significantly greater CVD risk. In women, the *apoE*4 allele was also associated with increased CVD prevalence, but unlike men, the *apoE*2 allele was found to be protective.

These findings were supported also by another study that tested the hypothesis that risk of IHD differs as a function of *apoE* genotype in women and men [106]. These investigators genotyped 9241 white women and men from the general population and 940 white women and men with IHD. Their analyses suggested that *apoE* genotype may influence risk of IHD differently in women and men (p = 0.07). After age adjustment, the odds ratio (OR) for IHD for epsilon32 vs epsilon33 women was 0.57 (95% CI: 0.35–0.94) whereas epsilon43 and epsilon44 vs epsilon33 men had ORs of 1.16 (0.96–1.41) and 1.58 (1.01–2.45). After adjustment for age and other conventional cardiovascular risk factors, the equivalent ORs were for epsilon32 women 0.38 (0.18–0.79), for epsilon43 men 1.35 (1.02–1.78) and for epsilon44 men 1.58 (0.80–3.08). Equivalent ORs for epsilon43 and epsilon44 vs epsilon33 women and for epsilon32 vs epsilon33 men were all close to 1.0 and nonsignificant. Of the total risk of IHD relative to the epsilon33 genotype, the fraction attributed to epsilon32 in women was −9%, whereas the fractions attributed to epsilon43 and epsilon44 in men were +8% and +2%. Therefore, just like in the Framingham Study, the Copenhagen City Heart Study showed a gene-gender interaction in terms of the individual susceptibility to CVD and IHD, respectively.

In addition to the newly discovered gender effects, the *apoE*-related CVD risk varies from population to population, being relatively high in population with clustering of CVD risk factors (atherogenic diet, sedentary life style, obesity) and almost negligible in populations with low "metabolic stress." Many studies have been conducted to prove this hypothesis [2,107]. Some investigators reported greater plasma lipid responses in subjects carrying the *apoE*4 allele, whereas others failed to find significant associations between *apoE* genotype and plasma lipid response [108–110]. There are important differences among these studies that could account for some of the discrepancies observed. Thus, studies differed in gender, age and baseline lipid levels, and all these variables are known to play an important role in the variability of dietary response. Dreon *et al* [111] have shown that the *apoE*-dependent mechanism may be specific for large, buoyant LDL particles. Consequently, baseline LDL particle distribution will also play a significant role on the outcome of different studies and this variable should be controlled in future studies.

Overall, a significant diet by *apoE* gene interaction has been shown in studies with men alone. In those studies including men and women, significant effects were noted only in men, suggesting a significant gene-sex interaction. Another difference between the negative studies and those reporting significant *apoE* gene-diet interactions related to the baseline lipid levels of the subjects. Positive findings were frequently observed in those studies reporting significant associations included subjects who were moderately hypercholesterolemic and/or had significant differences in base TC and LDLC among the *apoE* genotype groups, suggesting that the significant gene by diet interaction is apparent only in subjects who are susceptible to hypercholesterolemia. Concerning differences in dietary interventions, significant interactions were more commonly observed among studies in which total dietary fat and cholesterol was modified. It is possible that dietary cholesterol may play a significant effect in this gene-diet interaction. It should also be noted that some reports have shown that cholesterol absorption is related to *apoE* genotype.

Several mechanisms have been proposed to explain these *apoE*-related differences in individual response to dietary therapy. Some studies have shown that intestinal cholesterol absorption is related to apo E phenotype, with *apoE*4 carriers absorbing more cholesterol than non-*apoE*4 carriers. Other mechanisms such as different distribution of *apoE* on the lipoprotein fractions, LDL apoB production, bile acid and cholesterol synthesis, and postprandial lipoprotein clearance may also be involved.

The focus of a report from the Framingham Offspring Study was on the interaction between alcohol drinking, and LDL-C concentrations [112]. In this study, men who reported to be non-drinkers did not show the traditional association between the *apoE* alleles and LDL-C concentrations (E2<E3<E4). Conversely, in those classified as drinkers, the *apoE*4 allele was associated with significantly elevated LDL-C concentrations, resulting in a significant *apoE*4-drinking-LDL-C interaction (p<0.001) after adjustment for age, BMI, smoking and diet. However, in women, no interaction was observed and in general, women who reported drinking alcohol had lower LDL-C concentrations, independently of *apoE* genotype. This interaction was also examined in another population in Spain. In that study the expected effect of the *apoE* genotype on LDL-C was observed in both men and women. However, an interaction was observed for women, with drinkers who carried either the E2 or the E4 alleles having lower LDL-C than non-drinkers. Djousse *et al* provided further information about this interaction [113]. These investigators examined the relation of *apoE*, cigarette smoking, alcohol drinking, and their interaction with carotid atherosclerosis on 544 individuals free of CHD in the NHLBI Family Heart Study (FHS). Carriers of E4 had lower blood pressure, lower HDL-C, and higher LDL-C. *apoE* alleles and alcohol drinking were not significantly associated with carotid atherosclerosis, but smoking was significantly associated. These investigators did not find evidence of an interaction between *apoE* and alcohol consumption. Therefore, in the FHS population, smoking but not alcohol consumption or *apoE* was associated with increased odds of carotid atherosclerosis, suggesting a synergistic effect between the E4 allele and smoking on carotid atherosclerosis.

Overall, the data suggest significant interactions between the *apoE* gene and behavioral factors; however, the fact that several of these factors have the potential to interact and that these may be differently distributed among populations, may result in one of the factors (i.e., alcohol drinking, smoking) having more weight in some populations and less in others. Along these lines, Lussier-Cacan *et al* have highlighted the importance of the context dependency of these interactions [114]. These authors examined data from a sample of about 1700 men and women participants in the Quebec Heart Health Survey. In this population, there was no evidence that the *apoE* gene effected the LDL-C and HDL-C association and alcohol after adjusting for age and BMI. However, in women carriers of the E4 allele, these authors found a significant alcohol by BMI interaction on TC, LDL-C, HDL-C, apoA-I, and apoB. Furthermore, smoking influenced this interaction. Their report highlights the complexity of these interactions and the context dependency of the influence of alcohol on lipid metabolism.

An "environmental" factor that has not received previous attention in the context of gene by environment interactions relates to pregnancy. It has been known for many years that pregnancy is associated with dramatic increases in both TC and Tg concentrations that peak towards the end of the second trimester and remain elevated until postpartum. These elevations are subjected to dramatic interindividual variability for which we don't have a good understanding. McGladdery *et al* [115] have examined the association between the pregnancy-related changes in plasma lipids and genetic factors including the *apoE* gene. The study included 250 unrelated women during their third trimester of their pregnancy. These authors found no significant differences in TG, HDL-C, LDL-C or TC in the E4 carriers as compared with the E3 homozygotes. Conversely, the E2 carriers had significantly lower TC and LDL-C but no significant differences in Tgs or HDL-C. Therefore, pregnancy did not increase the effects of the *apoE* gene on lipid levels, but rather eliminated the LDL-C raising effect associated with the E4 allele, while maintaining the lowering of LDL-C concentrations associated with the E2 allele. This study has been the first one to examine how genetic factors affect the lipid profile during pregnancy. This is potentially very important in light of the reported associations between fetal environment and future risk of disease [116].

Another behavioral factor that has been receiving increased and well-deserved attention relates to physical activity. Usually, it is very difficult to obtain reliable information about this variable in large population studies, especially when they have not been specifically designed to have physical activity as one of the major variables of the study. Despite those limitations, at least two studies have shown a reproducible interaction between *apoE* genotype and the effect of physical activity on

Table 68-2
Gene-Gender (Hormone) Interactions

Reference	Gene	Gender Interaction
[120]	ApoB/HincII; PvuII; XbaI; EcoRI	Less influence on quantitative trait variation in men than in women.
[120]	ApoA-I-CIII-AIV/BamHI; XmnI; TaqI, PstI, SstI, PvuII	Less influence on quantitative trait variation in men than in women.
[120]	CETP/TaqIA; TaqIB	TaqI-B(−) associated with quantitative variation in HDL-C in women but not in men.
[121]	apoA-I/-75(G/A)	The A allele associated with elevated HDL-C in men but not in women.
[122]	apoA-I/-75(G/A)	The A allele associated with elevated apoA-I in men but not in women.
[123]	LPL, Asp9Asn, and T(−93)—>G	The Asp9Asn substitution is in linkage disequilibrium with the T(−93)—>G mutation and that the double-heterozygous carrier status is associated with elevated plasma Tgs and an increased risk of IHD in men, but not so in women.
[124]	LPL, S447X	The S447X variant may confer significant protection against high Tg levels, low HDL-C, and premature CHD in men but not in women.
[125]	LPL, Asp9Asn and T(−93)—>G	The −93T—>G/D9N haplotype is associated with significantly higher levels of LDL-C and VLDL-C, and VLDL Tgs only in male carriers.
[126]	CETP, Ile405Val	Increased HDL-C levels caused by mutations in CETP are associated with an increased risk of IHD in white women. This effect was not observed in men.
[127]	CETP, TaqIB	In type 2 diabetic patients, Taq1b polymorphism seems to exert a modulating role in males only.
[128]	CETP, TaqIB	Variation at the CETP gene locus is a significant determinant of HDL-C levels, CETP activity, and lipoprotein size in men and women. Moreover, these effects appear to translate into a lower CHD risk among those men with the B2 allele, but this protection was not seen in women.

plasma lipid concentrations. The first one reported in a Spanish population that the association between HDL-C concentrations and physical activity (energy expenditure) is *apoE* dependent [117]. This interaction was confirmed and examined in more detail by Berstein *et al* [118]. These authors investigated this interaction in a population-based cross-sectional survey including 1708 men and women age 35 to 74. As described for alcohol, smoking and BMI, the findings are gender dependent. For men, increased physical activity had a greater protective effect in E4 carriers as compared with E3 homozygotes and E2 carriers in terms of HDL-C increases and TG decreases. In women, the protective effect of exercise on E4 carriers was limited to HDL-C and it was significant only for the difference vs carriers of the E2 allele. Along the same lines, there appears to be a significant interaction between exercise training and *apoE* genotype [119].

V. Gender and Genes: Other Loci

Previously *apoE* was used as an example of the multiple interactions that exist between genes and environmental factors, but also with gender. Table 68-2 contains a list of a few other examples showing that triple interaction between a particular polymorphism, a modifiable factor and gender. This is an ever-growing list, and this will be one of the challenges that genetic studies will have to address.

It is becoming obvious that the study of gene-environment interactions needs to seriously consider sex as another component of this complex picture. The question remains if there is a intrinsic effect of sex due to the hormonal differences, or, alternatively, as it has been proposed by others, sex should be considered part of the "environment" [129].

VI. Summary and Suggestions for Further Investigations

Cardiovascular disease, the leading cause of mortality in most industrialized countries, is a multifactorial disease that is associated with non modifiable risk factors, such as age, gender and genetic background, and with modifiable risk factors, including elevated total and LDL-C levels, as well as reduced HDL-C levels. The fact that these diseases were extremely rare just 100 years ago suggests that changes in the environment have been the major trigger for the current epidemic. Originally, this disease was thought to affect almost exclusively men and most of the initial efforts and many others that followed were devoted to studying CVD risk factors in men. Nowadays, we know that as many women as men die of CVD. However, most of the therapeutic approaches that are used for women are extrapolated from findings generated in men. This is especially true when it comes to dietary and behavioral interventions. It makes sense that a "prudent diet" will benefit both men and women. However, the final scientific proof is lacking for many of the recommendations. Reports from several prospective studies are showing the validity of such assumption and in the next few years we will be gaining specific information that should close the informational gender-gap that we currently have.

Several questions need to be addressed by current and future studies.

- Because much of the information coming from large population studies is obtained from dietary questionnaires, it remains to be determined whether the validity of self-reported data is similar for men and women. If one of the sexes provides less reliable information this would be an important confounder for the outcome of these studies.
- We don't have a firm understanding about gender-related differences in dietary compliance and in adherence to dietary recommendations. Again, some consensus is emerging about the need for gender-specific messages to increase the success of dietary modification programs.
- Some studies have suggested that, independent of potential differences in reporting and/or adherence to diets, there are intrinsic differences in dietary response. The current notion is that when it comes to changes in plasma lipid levels, women may respond less than men do to the same dietary intervention. However, this needs to be further examined.
- The interest in nutrigenomics is beginning to reveal interesting gene-diet interactions that could be of great interest for a more individualized and effective dietary therapy. As result from this emerging knowledge, we are beginning to uncover another layer of complexity involving the presence of three-way interactions. This would suggest that the differences in response associated with specific genetic mutations may affect differently men and women.
- If we assume that if we do the needed research we can definitively conclude that there are significant differences in the response of men and women to dietary modification and recommendations, more basic research will be needed to understand the molecular basis for such differences. Moreover, such differences would mandate the establishment of separate dietary guidelines and recommendations for men and women.
- Finally, we should keep in mind that women have different dietary needs at different life stages and that the final goal is healthier aging. Therefore, recommendations to decrease the risk of a specific age related disorder (i.e., CVD) should take into consideration the effects of those recommendations over the risk for other diseases (i.e., cancer, osteoporosis, and neurologic disorders). Studies like the WHI are addressing some of these issues, but again, we should keep in mind that by studying only one gender, we may miss the contrast and opportunity to examine the reasons for the differences.

Acknowledgement

Supported by NIH/NHLBI grant no. HL54776, NIH/NHLBI contract no. 1-38038, and contracts 53-K06-5-10 and 58-1950-9-001 from the U.S. Department of Agriculture Research Service.

References

1. Blankenhorn DH, Johnson RL, Mack WJ et al. (1990). The influence of diet on the appearance of new lesions in human coronary arteries [see comments]. JAMA. 263:1646–1652.
2. Scandinav Simvastatin Survival Study Group. (1994). Randomised trial of cholesterol lowering in 4444 patients with coronary heart disease: The Scandinavian Simvastatin Survival Study (4S). Lancet. 344:1383–1389.
3. Sacks FM, Pfeffer MA, Moye LA et al. (1996). The effect of pravastatin on coronary events after myocardial infarction in patients with average cholesterol levels. N Engl J Med. 335:1001–1009.
4. National Cholesterol Education Program. (2001.). Third Report of the Expert Panel on Detection, Evaluation, and Treatment of High Blood Cholesterol in Adults (Adult Treatment Panel III). Bethesda, MD: National Institutes of Health, National Heart, Lung and Blood Institute. NIH Publication No 01–3670.
5. Keys A, Anderson JT, and Grande F. (1957). "Essential" fatty acids, degree of unsaturation, and effect of corn oil on the serum cholesterol level in man. Lancet. 1:66–68.
6. Ahrens EH. (1957). Nutritional factors and serum lipid levels. Am J Med. 23:928–952.
7. Keys A, Anderson JT, Grande F. (1957). Prediction of serum cholesterol responses of man to changes in fats in the diet. Lancet. 2:959–966.
8. Hegsted DM, McGandy RB, Myers ML, Stare FJ. (1965). Quantitative effects of dietary fat on serum cholesterol in man. Am J Clin Nutr. 17:281–295.
9. Hegsted DM, Ausman LM, Johnson JA, Dallal GE. (1993). Dietary fat and serum lipids: An evaluation of the experimental data. Am J Clin Nutr. 57:875–883.
10. Mensink RP, Katan MB. (1992). Effect of dietary fatty acids on serum lipids and lipoproteins: A meta-analysis of 27 trials. Arterioscler Thromb. 12:911–919.
11. Cobb MM, Teitlebaum H. (1994). Determinants of plasma cholesterol responsiveness to diet. Br J Nutr. 71:271–282.
12. Okey R, Stewart D. (1933). Diet and blood cholesterol in normal women. J Biol Chem. 99:717–727.
13. Katan MB, Beynen AC, de Vries JH, Nobels A. (1986). Existence of consistent hypo- and hyperresponders to dietary cholesterol in man. American Journal of Epidemiology. 123:221–234.
14. Jacobs DR, Anderson JT, Hannan P et al. (1983). Variability in individual serum cholesterol response to change in diet. Arterio. 3:349–356.
15. Cobb MM, Risch N. (1993). Low-density lipoprotein cholesterol responsiveness to diet in normolipidemic subjects. Metabolism. 42:7–13.
16. O'Hanesian MA, Rosner B, Bishop LM, Sacks FM. (1996). Effects of inherent responsiveness to diet and day-to-day diet variation on plasma lipoprotein concentrations. Am J Clin Nutr. 64:53–59.
17. Schaefer EJ, Lichtenstein AH, Lamon-Fava S et al. (1995). Efficacy of a National Cholesterol Education Program Step 2 diet in normolipidemic and hypercholesterolemic middle-aged and elderly men and women. Arterioscler Thromb Vasc Biol. 15:1079–1085.
18. Rainwater DL. (1994). Genetic effects on dietary response of Lp(a) concentrations in baboons. Chem Phys Lipids. 67–68:199–205.
19. Singh ATK, Rainwater DL, Kammerer CM et al. (1996). Dietary and genetic effects an LDL size measures in baboons. Arterioscler Thromb Vasc Biol. 16:1448–1453.
20. McGill HC Jr, McMahan CA, Mott GE et al. (1988). Effects of selective breeding on the cholesterolemic responses to dietary saturated fat and cholesterol in baboons. Arterio. 8:33–39.
21. Deckelbaum RJ, Fisher EA, Winston M et al. (1999). Summary of a scientific conference on preventive nutrition: Pediatrics to geriatrics. Circ. 100:450–456.
22. Krauss RM, Eckel RH, Howard B et al. (2001). Revision 2000: A statement for healthcare professionals from the Nutrition Committee of the American Heart Association. J Nutr. 131:132–146.
23. Keys A, Menotti A, Karvonen MJ et al. (1986). The diet and 15-year death rate in the Seven Countries Study. Am J Epidemiol. 124:903–915.
24. Verschuren WMM, Jacobs DR, Bloemberg BPM et al. (1995). Serum total cholesterol and long-term coronary heart disease mortality in different cultures: Twenty-five-year follow-up of the seven countries study. JAMA. 274:131–136.
25. Menotti A, Blackburn H, Kromhout D et al. (2001). Cardiovascular risk factors as determinants of 25-year all-cause mortality in the seven countries study. Eur J Epidem. 17:337–346.
26. Takeya Y, Popper JS, Shimizu Y et al. (1984). Epidemiologic studies of coronary heart disease and stroke in Japanese men living in Japan, Hawaii and California: Incidence of stroke in Japan and Hawaii. Stroke. 15:15–23.
27. Syme SL, Marmot MG, Kagan H, Rhoads G. (1975). Epidemiological studies of coronary heart disease and stroke in Japanese men living in Japan, Hawaii and California: Introduction. Am J Epidemiol. 102:477–480.
28. Nichaman MZ, Hamilton HB, Kagan A et al. (1975). Epidemiological studies of coronary heart disease and stroke in Japanese men living in Japan, Hawaii

and California: Distribution of biochemical risk factors. *Am J Epidemiol.* 102:491–501.

29. Worth RM, Kato H, Rhoads GG *et al.* (1975). Epidemiologic studies of coronary heart disease and stroke in Japanese men living in Japan, Hawaii and California: mortality. *Am J Epidemiol.* 102:481–490.

30. Brunner EJ, Thorogood, M. (2002). Dietary interventions for reducing cardiovascular risk. *Cochrane Database of Systematic Reviews Cochrane Heart Group (2).*

31. Weggemans RM, Zock PL, Urgert R, Katan MB. (1999). Differences between men and women in the response of serum cholesterol to dietary changes. *Eur J Clin Invest.* 29:827–834.

32. Schaefer EJ. (2002). Lipoproteins, nutrition and heart disease. *Am J Clin Nutr.* 75:191–212.

33. Manson JE, Buring JE, Satterfield S, Hennekens CH. (1991). Baseline characteristics of participants in the Physicians' Health Study: A randomized trial of aspirin and beta-carotene in U.S. physicians. *Prev Med.* 7:150–154.

34. Belanger C, Hennekens CH, Rosner B, Speizer FE. (1978). The Nurses' Health Study. *Am J Nurs.* 78:1039–1040.

35. Dawber TR, Meadors GF, Moore R. (1951). Epidemiological approaches to heart disease: The Framingham Study. *Am J Public Health.* 41:279–286.

36. Gartside PS, Glueck CJ. (1995). The important role of modifiable dietary and behavioral characteristics in the causation and prevention of coronary heart disease hospitalization and mortality: The prospective NHANES I follow-up study. *J Am Coll Nutr.* 14:71–79.

37. Gartside PS, Glueck CJ. (1993). Relationship of dietary intake to hospital admission for coronary heart and vascular disease: The NHANES II national probability study. *J Am Coll Nutr.* 12:676–684.

38. Millen BE, Quatromoni PA. (2001). Nutritional research within the Framingham Heart Study. *J Nutr Health Aging.* 5:139–143.

39. Hu FB, Stampfer MJ, Manson JE *et al.* (1997). Dietary fat intake and the risk of coronary heart disease in women. *N Engl J Med.* 337:1491–1499.

40. Ascherio A, Rimm EB, Giovannucci EL *et al.* (1996). Dietary fat and risk of coronary heart disease in men: Cohort follow up study in the United States. *British Med J.* 313:84–90.

41. Millen BE, Franz M, Quatromoni PA *et al.* (1996). Diet and plasma lipid in women. I. Macronutrients and plasma total and LDL cholesterol in women. The Framingham Nutrition Studies. *Am J Epidemiol.* 49:657–653.

42. Sonnenberg LM, Quatromoni PA, Gagnon DR *et al.* (1996). Diet and plasma lipids in women. II. Macronutrients and plasma triglycerides, HDL and total to HDL cholesterol ratio in women. The Framingham Nutrition Studies. *Am J Epidemiol.* 49:665–672.

43. Kromhout D, Bosschieter EB, De Lezenne Coulander C. (1985). The inverse relation between fish consumption and 20-year mortality from coronary heart disease. *N Engl J Med.* 312:1205–1209.

44. Marckmann P, Gronaek M. (1999). Fish consumption and coronary heart disease mortality. A systematic review of prospective cohort studies. *Eur J Clin Nutr.* 53:585–590.

45. Bucher HC, Hengstler P, Schindler C, Meier G. (2002). N-3 polyunsaturated fatty acids in coronary heart disease: A meta-analysis of randomized controlled trials. *Am J Med.* 112:298–304.

46. Hu FB, Bronner L, Willett WC *et al.* (2002). Fish and omega-3 fatty acid intake and risk of coronary heart disease in women. *JAMA.* 287:1815–1821.

47. Gillum RF, Mussolino ME, Madans JH. (2000). The relation between fish consumption, death from all causes, and incidence of coronary heart disease. the NHANES I Epidemiologic Follow-up Study. *J Clin Epidemiol.* 53:237–244.

48. Albert CM, Campos H, Stampfer M *et al.* (2002). Blood levels of long-chain n-3 fatty acids and the risk of sudden death. *N Engl J Med.* 346:1113–1118.

49. Hu FB, Stampfer MJ, Rimm EB *et al.* (1999). A prospective study of egg consumption and risk of cardiovascular disease in men and women. *JAMA.* 281:1387–1394.

50. Liu S, Manson JE, Lee IM *et al.* (2000). Fruit and vegetable intake and risk of cardiovascular disease: The Women's Health Study. *Am J Clin Nutr.* 72:922–928.

51. Joshipura KJ, Hu FB, Manson JE *et al.* (2002). The effect of fruit and vegetable intake on risk for coronary heart disease. *Ann Intern Med.* 134:1106–1114.

52. Bazzano LA, He J, Ogden LG *et al.* (2002). Fruit and vegetable intake and risk of cardiovascular disease in U.S. adults: The first National Health and Nutrition Examination Survey Epidemiologic Follow-up Study. *Am J Clin Nutr.* 76:93–99.

53. Liu S, Stampfer MJ, Hu FB *et al.* (1999). Whole-grain consumption and risk of coronary heart disease: Results from the Nurses' Health Study. *Am J Clin Nutr.* 70:412–419.

54. Liu S, Manson JE, Stampfer MJ *et al.* (2000). Whole grain consumption and risk of ischemic stroke in women: A prospective study. *JAMA.* 284:1534–1540.

55. Jacobs DR, Meyer KA, Kushi LH, Folsom AR. (1998). Whole-grain intake may reduce the risk of ischemic heart disease death in postmenopausal women: The Iowa Women's Health Study. *Am J Clin Nutr.* 68:248–257.

56. Jacobs DR, Pereira MA, Meyer KA, Kushi LH. (2000). Fiber from whole grains, but not refined grains, is inversely associated with all-cause mortality in older women: The Iowa Women's Health Study. *J Am Coll Nutr.* 326S–330S.

57. Fraser GE, Sabate J, Beeson WL, Strahan TM. (1992). A possible protective effect of nut consumption on risk of coronary heart disease: The Adventist Health Study. *Arch Intern Med.* 152:1416–1424.

58. Prineas RJ, Kushi LH, Folsom AR *et al.* (1993). Walnuts and serum lipids. *N Engl J Med.* 329:359.

59. Kushi LH, Folsom AR, Prineas RJ *et al.* (1996). Dietary antioxidant vitamins and death from coronary heart disease in postmenopausal women. *N Engl J Med.* 334:1156–1162.

60. Hu FB, Stampfer MJ, Manson JE *et al.* (1998). Frequent nut consumption and risk of coronary heart disease in women: Prospective cohort study. *British Med J.* 317:1341–1345.

61. Albert CM, Gaziano JM, Willett WC, Manson JE. (2002). Nut consumption and decreased risk of sudden cardiac death in the Physicians' Health Study. *Arch Intern Med.* 162:1382–1387.

62. Cater NB. (2000). Plant stanol ester: Review of cholesterol-lowering efficacy and implication for coronary heart disease risk reduction. *Prev Cardiol.* 3:121–130.

63. Lichtenstein AH, Deckelbaum RJ. (2001). A statement for healthcare professionals from the Nutrition Committee of the Council on Nutrition, Physical Activity, and Metabolism of the American Heart Association. *Circ.* 103:1177–1179.

64. Kris-Etherton PM, Etherton TD, Carlson J, Gardner C. (2002). Recent discoveries in inclusive food-based approaches and dietary patterns for reduction in risk of cardiovascular disease. *Curr Opin Lipidol.* 13:397–407.

65. Rimm EB, Klatsky A, Grobbee D, Stampfer MJ. (1996). Review of moderate alcohol consumption and reduced risk of coronary heart disease: Is the effect due to beer, wine, or spirits. *British Med J.* 312:731–736.

66. Klatsky AL, Armstrong MA, Friedman GD. (1997). Red wine, white wine, liquor, beer, and risk for coronary artery disease hospitalization. *Am J Cardiol.* 80:416–420.

67. Gronbaek M, Deis A, Sorensen TI *et al.* (1995). Mortality associated with moderate intakes of wine, beer, or spirits. *British Med J.* 310:1165–1169.

68. Bazzano LA, He J, Ogden LG *et al.* (2001). Legume consumption and risk of coronary heart disease in U.S. men and women. NHANES I Epidemiologic Follow-Up Study. *Arch Intern Med.* 161:2573–2578.

69. Anderson JW, Johnstone BM, Cook-Newell ME. (1995). Meta-analysis of the effects of soy protein intake on serum lipids. *N Engl J Med.* 333:276–282.

70. Crouse JR III, Morgan T, Terry JG *et al.* (1999). A randomized trial comparing the effect of casein with that of soy protein containing varying amounts of isoflavones on plasma concentrations of lipids and lipoproteins. *Arch Intern Med.* 159:2070–2076.

71. Merz-Demlow BE, Duncan AM, Wangen KE *et al.* (2000). Soy isoflavones improve plasma lipids in normocholesterolemic, premenopausal women. *Am J Clin Nutr.* 71:1462–1469.

72. Gardner C, Newell K, Cherin R, Haskell W. (2001). The effect of soy protein with or without isoflavones relative to milk protein on plasma lipids in hypercholesterolemic postmenopausal women. *Am J Clin Nutr.* 73:728–735.

73. Baum JA, Teng H, Erdman JW *et al.* (1998). Long-term intake of soy protein improves blood lipid profiles and increases mononuclear cell low-density-lipoprotein receptor messenger RNA in hypercholesterolemic, postmenopausal women. *Am J Clin Nutr.* 68:545–551.

74. Nestel PJ, Yamashita T, Sasahara T *et al.* (1997). Soy isoflavones improve systemic arterial compliance but not plasma lipids in menopausal and perimenopausal women. *Arterioscler Thromb Vasc Biol.* 17:3392–3398.

75. Simons LA, Von Konigsmark M, Simons J, Celermajer DS. (2000). Phytoestrogens do not influence lipoprotein levels or endothelial function in healthy, postmenopausal women. *Am J Cardiol.* 85:1297–1301.

76. Erdman JW, Jr. (2000). Soy protein and cardiovascular disease. A statement for healthcare professionals from the Nutrition Committee of the AHA. *Circ.* 102:2555–2559.

77. Fung TT, Willett WC, Stampfer MJ *et al.* (2001). Dietary patterns and the risk of coronary heart disease in women. *Arch Intern Med.* 161:1857–1862.

78. Millen BE, Quatromoni PA, Copenhafer DL *et al.* (2001). Validation of a dietary pattern approach for evaluating nutritional risk: The Framingham Nutrition Studies. *J Am Dietet Assoc.* 101:187–194.

79. Quatromoni PA, Copenhafer DL, Demissie S *et al.* (2002). The internal validity of a dietary pattern analysis. The Framingham Nutrition Studies. *Journal of Epidemiology & Community Health.* 56:381–388.

80. Williams DE, Knowler WC, Smith CJ *et al.* (2001). The effect of Indian or Anglo dietary preference on the incidence of diabetes in Pima Indians. *Diabetes Care.* 24:811–816.

81. McMurry MP, Cerqueira MT, Connor SL, Connor WE. (1991). Changes in lipid and lipoprotein levels and body weight in Tarahumara Indians after consumption of an affluent diet. *N Engl J Med.* 325:1704–1708.

82. Swinburn BA, Boyce VL, Bergman RN *et al.* (1991). Deterioration in carbohydrate metabolism and lipoprotein changes induced by modern, high fat diet in Pima Indians and Caucasians. *J Clin Endocrinol Metab.* 73:156–165.

83. Pan XR, Li GW, Hu YH *et al.* (1997). Effects of diet and exercise in preventing NIDDM in people with impaired glucose tolerance—The Da Qing IGT and diabetes study. *Diabetes Care.* 20:537–544.

84. Tuomilehto J, Lindstrom J, Eriksson JG *et al.* (2001). Prevention of type 2 diabetes mellitus by changes in lifestyle among subjects with impaired glucose tolerance. *N Engl J Med.* 344:1343–1350.

85. Knowler WC, Barret-Connor E, Fowler SE *et al.* (2002). Reduction in the incidence of type 2 diabetes with lifestyle intervention or metformin. *N Engl J Med.* 346:393–403.

86. Van Dam RM, Willett WC, Rimm EB *et al.* (2002). Dietary patterns and risk for type 2 diabetes mellitus in U.S. men. *Ann Intern Med.* 136:201–209.

87. Salmerón J, Hu FB, Manson JE *et al.* (2001). Dietary fat intake and risk of type 2 diabetes in women. *Am J Clin Nutr.* 73:1019–1026.

88. Meyer KA, Kushi LH, Jacobs DR Jr, Folsom AR. (2001). Dietary fat and incidence of type 2 diabetes in older Iowa women. *Diabetes Care.* 24:1528–1535.

89. Meyer KA, Kushi LH, Jacobs DR *et al.* (2000). Carbohydrates, dietary fiber, and incident type 2 diabetes in older women. *Am J Clin Nutr.* 71:921–930.

90. Salmerón J, Ascherio A, Rimm EB *et al.* (1997). Dietary fiber, glycemic load, and risk of NIDDM in men. *Diabetes Care.* 20:545–550.

91. Salmerón J, Manson JE, Stampfer MJ *et al.* (1997). Dietary fiber, glycemic load, and risk of non-insulin-dependent diabetes mellitus in women. *JAMA.* 277:472–477.

92. Ferrini R, Edelstein S, Barret-Connor E. (1994). The association between health beliefs and health behavior change in older adults. *Prev Med.* 23:1–5.

93. Ferrini R, Edelstein SL, Barret-Connor E. (1994). Factors associated with health behavior change among residents 50 to 96 years of age in Rancho Bernardo, California. *American Journal of Preventive Medicine.* 10:26–30.

94. Popkin BM, Haines PS, Patterson RE. (1992). Dietary changes in older Americans. *Am J Clin Nutr.* 55:823–830.

95. Horwath CC. (1992). Dietary changes reported by a random sample of elderly people. *J Nutr Elderly.* 12:13–27.

96. Morreale S, Schwartz NE. (1995). Helping Americans eat right: Developing practical and actionable public nutrition education messages based on the ADA Survey of American Dietary Habits. *J Am Dietet Assoc.* 95:305–308.

97. Millen BE, Quatromoni PA, Franz MM *et al.* (1997). Population nutrient intake approaches dietary recommendations: 1991 to 1995 Framingham Nutrition Studies. *J Am Dietet Assoc.* 97:742–747.

98. Tinker LF, Perri MG, Patterson RH *et al.* (2002). The effects of physical and emotional status on adherence to a low-fat dietary pattern in the Women's Health Initiative. *J Am Dietet Assoc.* 102:789–794.

99. Kearney MH, Rosal MC, Ockene JK, Churchill LC. (2002). Influences on Older Women's Adherence to a Low-Fat Diet in the Women's Health Initiative. *Psychosom Med.* 64:450–457.

100. Beisiegel U, Weber W, Ihrke G *et al.* (1989). The LDL-receptor-related protein, LRP, is an apolipoprotein E-binding protein. *Nature.* 341:162–164.

101. Mahley RW. (1988). Apolipoprotein E: Cholesterol transport protein with expanding role in cell biology. *Science.* 240:622–630.

102. Davignon J, Gregg RE, Sing CF. (1988). Apolipoprotein E polymorphism and atherosclerosis. *Arterio.* 8:1–21.

103. Ordovas JM, Litwack-Klein L, Wilson PWF *et al.* (1987). Apolipoprotein E isoform phenotyping methodology and population frequency with identification of apoE1 and apoE5 isoforms. *J Lipid Res.* 28:371–380.

104. Schaefer EJ, Lamon-Fava S, Johnson S *et al.* (1994). Effects of gender and menopausal status on the association of apolipoprotein E phenotype with plasma lipoprotein levels: Results from the Framingham Offspring Study. *Arterioscler Thromb.* 14:1105–1113.

105. Lahoz C, Schaefer EJ, Cupples LA *et al.* (2001). Apolipoprotein E genotype and cardiovascular disease in the Framingham Heart Study. *Athero.* 154:529–537.

106. Frikke-Schmidt R, Tybjaerg-Hansen A, Steffensen R *et al.* (2000). Apolipoprotein E genotype: Epsilon32 women are protected while epsilon43 and epsilon44 men are susceptible to ischemic heart disease: The Copenhagen City Heart Study. *J Am Coll Cardiol.* 35:1192–1199.

107. Ordovas JM, Schaefer EJ. (1999). Genes, variation of cholesterol and fat intake and serum lipids. *Current Opinion in Lipidology.* 10:15–22.

108. Glatz JFC, Demacker PNM, Turner PR, Katan MB. (1991). Response of serum cholesterol to dietary cholesterol in relation to apolipoprotein E phenotype. *Nutr Metab Cardiovasc Dis.* 1:13–17.

109. Ginsberg HN, Karmally W, Siddiqui M *et al.* (1994). A dose-response study of the effects of dietary cholesterol on fasting and postprandial lipid and lipoprotein metabolism in healthy young men. *Arterioscler Thromb.* 14:576–586.

110. Friedlander Y, Berry EM, Eisenberg S *et al.* (1995). Plasma lipids and lipoproteins in response to a dietary challenge: Analysis of four candidate genes. *Clin Genet.* 47:1–12.

111. Dreon DM, Fernstrom HA, Miller B, Krauss RM. (1995). Apolipoprotein E isoform phenotype and LDL subclass response to a reduced-fat diet. *Arterioscler Thromb.* 15:105–111.

112. Corella D, Tucker K, Lahoz C *et al.* (2001). Alcohol drinking determines the effect of the *apoE* locus on LDL-cholesterol concentrations in men: The Framingham Offspring Study. *Am J Clin Nutr.* 73:736–745.

113. Djousse L, Myers RH, Province MA *et al.* (2002). Influence of apolipoprotein E, smoking, and alcohol intake on carotid atherosclerosis: National Heart, Lung, and Blood Institute Family Heart Study. *Stroke.* 33:1357–1361.

114. Lussier-Cacan S, Bolduc A, Xhignesse M *et al.* (2002). Impact of alcohol intake on measures of lipid metabolism depends on context defined by gender, body mass index, cigarette smoking, and apolipoprotein E genotype. *Arterioscler Thromb Vasc Biol.* 22:824–831.

115. McGladdery S, Frohlich JJ. (2001). Lipoprotein lipase and *apoE* polymorphisms: Relationship to hypertriglyceridemia during pregnancy. *J Lipid Res.* 42:1905–1912.

116. Hubinette A, Cnattingius S, Ekbom A *et al.* (2001). Birthweight, early environment, and genetics: A study of twins discordant for acute myocardial infarction. *Lancet.* 357:1997–2001.

117. Corella D, Guillen M, Saiz C *et al.* (2001). Environmental factors modulate the effect of the *apoE* genetic polymorphism on plasma lipid concentrations: Ecogenetic studies in a Mediterranean Spanish population. *Metabolism.* 50:936–944.

118. Bernstein MS, Costanza MC, James RW *et al.* (2002). Physical activity may modulate effects of *ApoE* genotype on lipid profile. *Arterioscler Thromb Vasc Biol.* 22:133–140.

119. Hagberg JM, Ferrell RE, Katzel LI *et al.* (1999). Apolipoprotein E genotype and exercise training-induced increases in plasma high-density lipoprotein (HDL)- and HDL2-cholesterol levels in overweight men. *Metabolism.* 48.

120. Kessling A, Ouellette S, Bouffard O *et al.* 1991). Patterns of association between genetic variability in apolipoprotein (apo) B, apo AI-CIII-AIV, and cholesterol ester transfer protein gene regions and quantitative variation in lipid and lipoprotein traits: Influence of gender and exogenous hormones. *Am J Hum Genet.* 50:92–106.

121. Sigurdsson G Jr, Gudnason V, Sigurdsson G, Humphries SE. (1992). Interaction between a polymorphism of the Apo A-I promoter region and smoking determines plasma levels of HDL and Apo A-I. *Arterioscler Thromb.* 12:1017–1022.

122. Saha N, Tay JSH, Low PS, Humphries SE. (1994). Guanidine to adenine (G/A) substitution in the promoter region of the apolipoprotein AI gene is associated with elevated serum apolipoprotein AI levels in Chinese non-smokers. *Genet Epidemiol.* 11:255–264.

123. Wittrup HH, Tybjaerg-Hansen A, Steffensen R *et al.* (1999). Mutations in the lipoprotein lipase gene associated with ischemic heart disease in men. The Copenhagen City Heart Study. *Arterioscler Thromb Vasc Biol.* 99:2901–2907.

124. Gagne SE, Larson MG, Pimstone SN *et al.* (1999). A common truncation variant of lipoprotein lipase (Ser447X) confers protection against coronary heart disease: The Framingham Offspring Study. *Clin Genet.* 55:450–454.

125. Hoffer MJ, Bredie SJ, Snieder H *et al.* (1998). Gender-related association between the −93T−>G/D9N haplotype of the lipoprotein lipase gene and elevated lipid levels in familial combined hyperlipidemia. *Athero.* 138:91–99.

126. Agerholm-Larsen B, Nordestgaard BG, Steffensen R *et al.* (2000). Elevated HDL cholesterol is a risk factor for ischemic heart disease in white women

when caused by a common mutation in the cholesteryl ester transfer protein gene. *Circ.* 101:1907–1912.

127. Durlach A, Clavel C, Girard-Globa A, Durlach V. (1999). Sex-dependent association of a genetic polymorphism of cholesteryl ester transfer protein with high-density lipoprotein cholesterol and macrovascular pathology in type II diabetic patients. *J Clin Endocr Metab.* 84: 3656–3659.

128. Ordovas JM, Cupples LA, Corella D *et al.* (2000). Association of cholesteryl ester transfer protein-TaqIB polymorphism with variations in lipoprotein subclasses and coronary heart disease risk: The Framingham study. *Arterioscler Thromb Vasc Biol.* 20:1323–1329.

129. Lawlor DA, Ebrahim S, Davey Smith G. (2001). Sex matters: Secular and geographical trends in sex differences in coronary heart disease mortality. *British Med J.* 323:541–545.

69

Insulin Resistance and Type 2 Diabetes Mellitus: Gender Differences and Similarities

ANN M. COULSTON, MS, RD

Nutrition Consultant, Stanford University School of Medicine, Stanford, CA

I. Introduction

As the incidence of type 2 diabetes increases so has interest in understanding the origins of the disease and disease management. In general, diabetes mellitus (DM) has not been diagnosed more often in men or women. Consequently, research on disease management and complications has not focused on men or women specifically, but most often studied mixed populations. The one exception is gestational diabetes. Obviously, this is a condition of women only and research on the management, medical and nutritional, of gestational diabetes is in its infancy. We are only beginning to understand the medical consequences of insulin resistance, which is at the root of both type 2 diabetes and gestational diabetes [1]. Consequently, information on nutritional considerations of this condition is scarce and especially so for potential gender differences. Over the last few years, insights have been gleaned from cohort epidemiology studies of women and men, but nutrition intervention studies comparing women and men, other than weight loss, are essentially nonexistent.

II. Description of Insulin Resistance and Type 2 Diabetes Mellitus

A. Insulin Resistance

Insulin resistance is a genetic predisposition in which the normal actions of insulin are impaired. It can be detected long before deterioration of glucose tolerance occurs. Insulin normally increases uptake, storage and oxidation of glucose in tissues. Only in the face of environmental stress of such factors as decreased physical activity or excess body weight, does this genetic trait present as an abnormal condition called the metabolic syndrome, or insulin resistance syndrome, or syndrome X. Under these conditions, insulin resistance increases the risk for developing DM and cardiovascular disease (CVD) [2,3]. This syndrome, with its many names, has insulin resistance as a common denominator. The insulin resistance syndrome or metabolic syndrome is a clustering of cardiovascular risk factors, namely, glucose intolerance, dyslipidemia (elevated plasma triglyceride [TG] concentration, decreased high-density lipoprotein cholesterol [HDL-C]), abdominal obesity, hypertension, and elevated coagulation factors (Table 69-1) [4,5].

Examination of the Third National Health and Nutrition Examination Survey (NHANES III) data reveals a 24% age-adjusted prevalence of the metabolic syndrome. Prevalence differed little among men (24%) and women (23.4%), but was higher among Mexican Americans (31.9%) and lowest among whites (23.8%). Among African Americans, women had about a 57% higher prevalence than men. Among Mexican Americans, women had about 26% higher prevalence than men [5].

When the World Health Organization (WHO) criteria for the metabolic syndrome (Table 69-1) were applied to the Botina study cohort [6], the prevalence in women and men respectively was 10% and 15% in subjects with normal glucose tolerance, 42% and 64% in those with impaired glucose tolerance and 78% and 84% in those with type 2 diabetes [3]. In women with normal glucose tolerance, the prevalence of insulin resistance increased from 19% in the age decade from 40–49 to 35% in the age decade of 60–69 [3].

Insulin resistance and its potential sequelae have now been widely accepted [1]. Disease progresses as insulin resistance worsens and frank diabetes appears when the beta cell of the pancreas can no longer compensate with increased insulin secretion. Women with insulin resistance are prone to develop gestational diabetes during pregnancy and both men and women who have insulin resistance can progress to type 2 diabetes primarily prompted by age, increased body weight, and decreased physical activity.

B. Type 2 Diabetes Mellitus

Approximately 16 million people in the United States have diabetes. Over 400,000 die each year, and nearly half of these deaths are directly related to diabetes or its complications. The NHANES III data (1988–1994) indicates that the prevalence of diabetes in the U.S. population is 5.9% [7]. The 1998 Behavior Risk Factor Surveillance System (BRFSS) indicated that about 13 million have diagnosed diabetes, including women with gestational diabetes. The prevalence of self-reported diagnosed diabetes among adults, including gestational diabetes, increased from 4.9% in 1990 to 6.5% in 1998 [8]. These estimates include all types of diabetes, but 90–95% of people over age 20 with diabetes have type 2 DM, and 7% of all pregnancies annually result in the development of gestational diabetes [9]. Gestational diabetes mellitus (GDM) describes glucose intolerance that is first detected during pregnancy. Women with known diabetes prior to conception are not part of this group. Ten to twenty years postpartum as many as 30–40% of women with gestational diabetes will develop impaired glucose tolerance or type 2 diabetes. Conversion of GDM to type 2 diabetes occurs most commonly within 5 years of delivery and most often among those with higher fasting plasma glucose levels [10]. Frequent blood glucose testing over this time period is recommended.

Table 69-1
Definition of the Metabolic Syndrome

	WHO*	ATP III**
Hypertension	>160/>90 mmHg	≥130/85 mmHg
Dyslipidemia: TG	>1.7 mmol/L	≥1.69 mmol/L (150 mg/dL)
HDL-C	<0.9 mmol/L men	≤1.04 mmol/L (40 mg/dL) men
	<1.0 mmol/L women	≤1.29 mmol/L (50 mg/dL) women
Fasting glucose	(see note below)	≥6.1 mmol/L (110 mg/dl)
BMI	≥30 kg/m^2	(none)
Waist–Hip ratio	>0.90 men	
	>0.85 women	
Abdominal obesity		>102 cm (>40 in) men
(waist circumference)		>88 cm (>35 in) women
Microalbuminuria (urinary albumin excretion rate)	>20 μg/min	

ATP III, Adult Treatment Panel III

*A person with type 2 diabetes or IFG/IGT must fulfill 2 of criteria, whereas person with NGT must also demonstrate insulin resistance. (From Isomaa B, Almgren P, Tuomi T *et al.* [2001]. Cardiovascular morbidity and mortality associated with the metabolic syndrome. *Diabetes Care.* 24:683–689.)

**A person with 3 or more for diagnosis of metabolic syndrome. (From Expert Panel on Detection, Evaluation, and Treatment of High Blood Cholesterol in Adults. [2001]. Executive summary of the third report of the National Cholesterol Education Program [NCEP] expert panel on detection, evaluation, and treatment of high blood cholesterol in adults [Adult Treatment Panel III]. *JAMA.* 285:2486–2497.)

Table 69-2
Prevalence of Type 2 Diabetes Among U.S.
Adults Age ≥20 by Body Weight Status (Percentage with Diabetes)

Weight Status	BMI (kg/m^2)	Women	Men
Underweight	<18.5	4.8	4.7
Normal weight	>18.5–24.9	2.4	2.0
Overweight	25.0–29.9	7.1	4.9
Obese class 1	30.0–34.9	7.2	10.1
Obese class 2	35.0–39.9	13.2	12.3
Obese class 3	>40.0	19.9	10.7

(Adapted from Must A, Spadano J, Coakley EH *et al.* [1999]. The disease burden associated with overweight and obesity. *JAMA.* 282:1523–1529.)

The latest group to develop type 2 diabetes is children and adolescents. Once thought to be a disease of adults, the incidence of type 2 diabetes in this population parallels the epidemic of childhood obesity. Because type 2 diabetes in children and adolescents is a relatively new phenomenon, accurate statistics regarding the number of cases have not been generated. However, reports indicate that 8–45% of children with newly diagnosed diabetes have type 2 diabetes (www.diabetes.org [as of 10/8/2002]). Previously, the prevalence was considered to be 2–4% among children and adolescents with type 2 diabetes.

Diabetes prevalence increases with age; nearly 19% of U.S. population over 65 has diabetes. Diabetes prevalence is similar for men and women up to age 65; however, above age 65, prevalence rates are higher for men than for women. Despite this statistic, in the adult population 45% of people with diabetes are male and 55% female. In the adult population, onset of type 2 diabetes is predominately after age 40–45, and about 50% of men and 70% of women are obese. Although prevalence rates are the same, about 55% of all people with diabetes are female. Differences in diabetes prevalence between men and women may reflect a number of factors including different distributions of risk factors, longer life expectancy for women, and racial and ethnic distribution [11].

Type 2 diabetes, presents with insulin resistance and relative insulin deficiency, and progress over time to a defect in insulin secretion and insulin resistance. Type 2 diabetes is characterized in most patients by insulin resistance with inadequate insulin response to maintain normal levels of blood glucose [12]. Because there is not an absolute absence of insulin in early disease, type 2 diabetes may have been undiagnosed for many years. Thus, people diagnosed with type 2 may have normal, depressed, or elevated insulin levels. High insulin levels, indicating insulin resistance, are most typical in the early phase. Insulin secretion decreases as the disease progresses. At the time of diagnosis of type 2 diabetes, about 50% of insulin secreting capacity is lost. Attention to maintaining glycosylated hemoglobin in the range of 6.5% delays further decline. People with type 2 diabetes do not depend on exogenous insulin for survival, but many require insulin therapy for adequate blood glucose control.

III. Obesity and Type 2 Diabetes Mellitus

Total body adiposity is an established risk factor for type 2 diabetes. Data from NHANES III indicate a 5-fold increased risk for type 2 diabetes for obese compared with normal weight individuals [13]. In addition, a longer duration of obesity increases risk for type 2 diabetes. Data from the Nurses' Health Study cohort found a 2–3-fold increased relative risk for diabetes in women who had experienced a 10–20 pound weight gain since age 18 [14]. However, not all overweight people develop diabetes and type 2 diabetes is also found in nonobese adults (see Table 69-2). In the United States, an individual who is either obese or has one parent with diabetes is twice as likely to develop diabetes as an individual with neither risk factor. Obese people with at least one parent with diabetes is four times as likely to develop diabetes as an individual with neither risk [15].

A related risk factor for diabetes is a sedentary lifestyle. Physical activity decreases the risk of type 2 diabetes: In the Nurses' Health Study cohort, an episode of physical activity once or more per week was associated with a 20% decrease in type 2 diabetes [16]. The Iowa women's study also showed an increase in diabetes in inactive postmenopausal women [17]. These observations are of particular interest in light of the Diabetes Prevention Program. This large, multicenter study enrolled over 3000 people with impaired glucose tolerance and observed them for almost 3 years. In the group of participants who were instructed to increase physical activity to 30 minutes per day and to lose weight, the incidence of new onset diabetes was 4.8 cases per 100 years, compared to 11.0 cases per 100 years in the placebo group. The lifestyle intervention consisted of 150 minutes of physical activity per week, body weight loss of 7%, and resulted in a decreased incidence of diabetes by 58% as compared to placebo [18]. Sixty-eight percent of those randomized to the lifestyle modification were women. The weight reduction plan was a regular food, low-calorie, low-fat diet. Physical activity was achieved by brisk walking.

Although there is a strong genetic predisposition for the development of type 2 diabetes, lifestyle and dietary factors, particularly those that promote obesity, are contributors [19]. Because about 90% of people with type 2 diabetes are obese, weight loss is essential in management. In one study, comparison of weight loss in patients with type 2 diabetes on diets that were 30% protein vs 15% protein resulted in the same amount of total weight loss (weight loss was independent of diet composition); however, women experienced significantly greater total fat and abdominal fat weight loss on the higher protein diet [20]. For men the differences in fat tissue loss was not different between the two diets. Triglyceride concentrations decreased equally in both men and women and HDL-C didn't change during weight loss. However, low-density lipoprotein cholesterol (LDL-C) and total cholesterol concentrations decreased, the impact was greater on the higher protein diet, but there was no gender difference.

Reduced calorie diets, aerobic exercise, and resistance exercise are all independent effect treatments for reducing metabolic risk factors in women [21–25]. These data suggest that a combination of diet and exercise would have a greater impact on metabolic risk factors than weight loss alone. However, when Janssen *et al* studied premenopausal women comparing diet alone to diet with aerobic exercise and diet with resistance training, significant reductions in total, visceral, and intermuscular fat were observed in each group following a 10% weight loss [26]. Glucose, insulin, and cholesterol concentrations also improved with no differences across treatment group. A report in obese men demonstrated a 2-fold greater improvement in insulin action in response to diet combined with aerobic or resistance exercise than with diet alone [27].

IV. Insulin Resistance, Type 2 Diabetes, and Lipid Metabolism

The most common pattern of dyslipidemia in insulin resistance and patients with type 2 diabetes is elevated TG levels and decreased HDL cholesterol levels. The concentration of LDL-C is usually not significantly different from nondiabetic individuals; however, people with insulin resistance and type 2 diabetes have a preponderance of smaller, denser LDL particles, which possibly accounts for the increase atherogenicity even when the absolute concentration of LDL-C is not significantly increased. For patients with type 2 disease, the LDL-C concentration target is <100 mg/dl because diabetes is considered a risk factor for CVD [28].

The prevalence of dyslipidemia and hypertension were both increased 2-fold in type 2 patients with diabetes as compared with normal glucose tolerance. Hypertension was associated with microalbuminuria and seen more often in men 22% as compared with 12% in women. Cardiovascular mortality was 12% in patients with the metabolic syndrome and 2.2% in those without it, thus confirming the steep rise in risk conferred by the association of these specific risk factors against a background of glucose intolerance or frank diabetes [3].

Diabetes is a major risk factor for CVD, especially in women. Diabetes increases the incidence of cardiovascular events in women more than in men, equalizing the age-adjusted rates [29]. The relative risk of mortality from myocardial infarction was 1.4 for men but 1.9 for women with diabetes [30]. Overall heart disease in women with diabetes increased 23% in a 10-year follow-up study despite a decline in men with and without diabetes [31]. The relative protection from CVD enjoyed by women is blunted with diabetes. The prevalence of type 2 DM is increasing worldwide, in both industrialized and developing countries and with it increased attention of the association of diabetes with CVD. Complication risk surveys conducted among patients with diabetes indicate that most patients know about the complications like blindness and amputation, but 68% failed to identify heart disease and stroke as a serious threat to their health. Studies have shown that, in general, people with diabetes are two to four times more likely to die from heart disease than people without diabetes. Heart disease is the leading cause of death accounting for about 40% of all deaths of people with diabetes. People with diabetes are four times as likely to have peripheral vascular disease and stroke is 2–4 times more common in people with diabetes [28].

Clinical manifestations of atherosclerosis occur primarily in the coronary arteries, lower extremities, and carotid arteries. To my knowledge, gender differences in plaque location have not been described for people with diabetes. Type 2 diabetes not only increases heart disease risk but also accelerates the clinical course 3–4-fold over normoglycemic people [32]. For example, in a population-based study, the incidence of first myocardial infarction or death for patients with diabetes was 20% and only 3.5% in nondiabetic patients [33].

V. Birth Weight and Type 2 Diabetes Risk

Birth weight has been shown to be inversely related to subsequent risk for insulin resistance or type 2 diabetes in men and women [34–36]. Low birth weight or small body size at birth as a result of reduced intrauterine growth is associated with increased rates of coronary heart disease and type 2 diabetes in adult life [37]. The association has been explained etiologically as representing long-term effects of nutritional deprivation *in utero* on fetal growth and the development of the endocrine pancreas, as a selective survival of small babies [38]. These findings support the "fetal origins" hypothesis—that susceptibility to these chronic adult conditions, including diabetes and insulin resistance, may be programmed *in utero*. The most popular hypothesis for explaining these observations is that inadequate nutrition permanently programs the endocrine system involved in nutritional homeostasis [39]. This has caused scientists to focus on lifestyle and nutrition factors, as well as maternal nutritional status before and during pregnancy. It has been observed that lower birth weight is associated with higher serum insulin concentrations in relation to their body size among Pima Indian children and young adults living in the United States [40]. They are more insulin resistant than those with normal birth weight, and this may explain their increased risk for type 2 diabetes. Maternal nutrition contributes to fetal development *in utero* and is one of the factors that determines birth weight [41].

As a result of these observations, it is clear that more research needs to be conducted investigating the relation between markers of a women's own growth *in utero* and her subsequent risk for gestational diabetes. An examination of a database maintained by the New York State Department of Health: The live birth registry and New York State hospital discharge records lends some interesting information [42]. Birth weight alone and adjusted for gestational age, showed a U-shaped relationship to risk for gestational diabetes. Risk of gestational diabetes rose with lower prepregnancy body mass index (BMI) and maternal diabetes. There is a strong inverse association of birth weight and risk for GDM. After adjusting for gestational age and prepregnancy weight, birth weight <2500 g was associated with a 2.3-fold increase in risk for GDM [42]. Nutrition, therefore, is a potential modifiable risk factor: It can modify maternal weight before and during pregnancy. This study is among the first to demonstrate a clear, dose-response relationship between relative fetal growth and adult risk for GDM, an important complication of pregnancy and a strong predictor of diabetes and other insulin resistance conditions. The genotype for insulin resistance and type 2 diabetes remains strong and passed through progeny.

VI. Observational Studies of Women and Type 2 Diabetes Mellitus

Diabetes mellitus is an example of a complex disorder that results from a gene-environment interaction. In this case, the environment consists of a sedentary lifestyle and obesity, as well as of dietary factors. Various observations of ethnic groups at high risk of diabetes [43–45] suggest that the adoption of a Western type diet, as opposed to more traditional ones, have resulted in the increases in prevalence seen.

The role of dietary patterns in the development of diabetes was explored in the Health Professional Follow-up Study in 42,504 male professionals [46]. Two major dietary patterns were defined; the "prudent" pattern characterized by higher consumption of vegetables, fruit, fish, poultry and whole grains and the "western" pattern characterized by higher intakes of red meat, processed meat, French fries, high-fat dairy products, refined grains, sweets and desserts. In the 12-year follow-up, the prudent pattern was associated with a modestly lower risk, whereas the western pattern with increased risk for type 2 diabetes.

The Nurses' Health Study studied the relationship between dietary fat intake and the development of diabetes in women [47]. In the 14-year follow-up of 84,204 women, total fat intake was not found to be associated with the risk of diabetes. Neither was the intake of saturated or monounsaturated fatty acids. The most significant finding of this study was that every 2% increase in energy from trans fatty acid was associated with a relative risk of 1.39, whereas a 5% increase in energy from polyunsaturated fat related to a relative risk of 0.63.

A similar finding was reported in older women, in the Iowa Women's Health Study [48] where 35,988 postmenopausal women were followed for 11 years dietary assessment was achieved with food-frequency questionnaires. No relationship was observed between the total fat intake, saturated and monounsaturated fatty acids, and the risk of diabetes; however, the consumption of vegetable fat was inversely related with a 22% disease incidence reduction.

The Iowa Women's study also reported that whole grain, total dietary fiber, cereal fiber, and dietary magnesium intakes showed strong inverse associations with incidence of diabetes after adjustment for potential confounding variables [49]. Intakes of total carbohydrates, refined grains, fruit and vegetables, and soluble fiber and the glycemic index were unrelated to diabetes risk.

Salmeron *et al* also showed that diets of highly refined grains with low fiber increased the risk of diabetes in both men [50] and women [51]. In contrast to the Iowa study, a diet pattern high in glycemic load (calculated as the total amount of carbohydrate multiplied by the glycemic index of the food) was positively associated with risk of diabetes.

VII. Evidence-Based Nutrition Guidelines

The American Diabetes Association (ADA) has published evidence-based nutrition principles and recommendations for the treatment and prevention of diabetes after a comprehensive review of the literature [52]. No gender-based recommendations were made apart from a section on pregnant and lactating women. The outcome goals for nutrition therapy include maintaining blood glucose in the normal or near normal range, a lipoprotein profile that reduces the risk of CVD, and blood pressure levels that reduce risk for stroke.

Because of the marked increased risk of CVD in both men and women with diabetes, attention to dietary fat modification aimed at reducing risk is a major dietary consideration. The primary goal is to reduce the intake of saturated fatty acids and dietary cholesterol. Compared to diabetic subjects, both men and women have a higher risk of CVD with higher intakes of dietary cholesterol [53]. In a meta-analysis of dietary intervention studies LDL-C was decreased by 12% with diets containing <10% calories from saturated fat and <300 mg cholesterol. When diets were further reduced to <7% saturated fat and <200 mg cholesterol, LDL was reduced by 16% [54].

Although there is universal agreement on this recommendation, the controversy focuses on whether to achieve the energy decrease by lowering saturated fat and cholesterol and substituting unsaturated fatty acids or dietary carbohydrate. In controlled intervention studies, diets that are increased in carbohydrate do not alter the fasting plasma glucose or insulin levels, but increase postprandial glucose and insulin concentrations, increase fasting and postprandial TG and decrease fasting HDL cholesterol concentrations [55]. When saturated fatty acids are replaced with unsaturated fats (monounsaturated and/or polyunsaturated) postprandial glucose and TG concentrations are not elevated and LDL-C levels fall. This has been demonstrated in patients with type 2 diabetes and patients with insulin resistance. However, proponents of lower total fat diets point out that observational studies indicate that higher fat diets are associated with insulin resistance [56,57]. As a result of the ongoing debate, no specific guidelines are recommended for how much of the caloric intake should come from carbohydrate and how much from unsaturated fatty acids. Rather the practitioner must follow the outcome measures of glycemic control using glycosylated hemoglobin and plasma lipid concentrations.

Because observational studies have associated glycemic load of the diet as a risk factor for diabetes [50,51], some nutritionists feel that the glycemic index of the diet should be lowered for patients with type 2 diabetes. However, intervention studies in much smaller groups of patients with type 2 diabetes have not convincingly demonstrated a beneficial effect of selecting low glycemic index foods [58,59]. Similar enthusiasm has been generated by the addition of fiber to the diet in hopes of modulating plasma glucose response and decreasing lipid concentrations. A study by Chandalia *et al* [60] that included 50 gm of fiber per day in the form of selected food choices demonstrated significant improvement in glycemic control. This study was done in men and the amount of fiber included is twice the general recommendation, which is already about double the amount consumed by the general population. Adding fiber to the diet to decrease LDL-C is more promising. A meta-analysis of controlled clinical trials supported improved lipid concentrations with diets high in soluble fiber [61]. Historically, the most widely held belief about nutrition and diabetes was that added sugars should be avoided. This concept was based on the notion that sucrose was more rapidly digested and absorbed than carbohydrates from more complex molecules like starch. Numerous studies have demonstrated no difference in glycemic control when sucrose is substituted for starch in the meal pattern of patients with diabetes [62]. Thus, the conclusion reached by the ADA review committee regarding dietary carbohydrate is that the total amount of carbohydrate in meals or snacks has a greater effect on blood glucose control than the source or type of carbohydrate [52].

Because diabetes may be a state of increased oxidative stress there has been increasing interest in the use of antioxidant vitamins and minerals for people with diabetes. Several large observational studies have looked at association of insulin resistance and type 2 diabetes with certain of the antioxidant nutrients with some promise [63–66]. However, the Institute of Medicine in its review of antioxidant vitamins and minerals [67] concluded that supplementation with any of these dietary antioxidants has not been demonstrated to protect against CVD, diabetes, or various forms of cancer [67].

Chromium is another nutrient frequently associated with insulin action in people with insulin resistance or type 2 diabetes. Two well-controlled studies conducted in Chinese diabetic subjects demonstrated improvement in glycemic control with chromium supplementation [68,69]. However, a closer examination of the subjects indicates that they had marginal baseline chromium status. In the United States, adequacy of chromium status appears not to be a problem, and studies that have supplemented chromium in patients with glucose intolerance [70] and women with gestational diabetes [71] have observed small improvements. Despite these findings, supplementation with chromium is not recommended by the ADA [52].

In summary, there are no specific nutritional management recommendations for men vs women with insulin resistance or type 2 diabetes. Rather, nutrition recommendations should be individualized around the general principles put forth by the ADA [52] with attention given to treatment goals, individual eating patterns, and desired plasma glucose, lipid, blood pressure, body weight goals, and disease complications.

VIII. Socioeconomic Status of Women with Diabetes

The socioeconomic status of women with diabetes affects health care delivery and access to food. Data from the BRFSS indicate that the socioeconomic status of women with diabetes is markedly lower than that of women without diabetes [72]. In this survey women were classified as having low socioeconomic status if they did not complete high school or resided in a household with an annual income of <$25,000. Of the women from this sample, 6.3% had diabetes, by self-report. These women were more likely than women without diabetes to be nonwhite; divorced, separated or widowed; living alone; retired; or unable to work.

Persons with low socioeconomic status have poorer health than others and are less likely to have adequate access to care or receive adequate clinical and preventive services [73]. Thus, it is apparent that the low socioeconomic status of many women with diabetes might compromise their ability to benefit from treatments that might reduce their risks for complications and premature death. Hence, programs designed to meet the needs of women with diabetes should take socioeconomic status into account. The Centers for Disease Control and Prevention have initiated a program entitled "Diabetes and Women's Health Across the Life Stages: A Public Health Perspective" which can be accessed online for additional information and action [72].

IX. Research Needs

Research in the area of gender differences and insulin resistance and type 2 diabetes is clearly in need of attention. As we have pointed out, not much work has been done in this area, partly because the incidence and prevalence of type 2 diabetes is not that different between men and women. However, the impact of diabetes as a risk factor for coronary artery disease on the two sexes is significantly different. In addition, we have only relatively recently had the research tools to tease out the differences in response to medical and nutritional therapies. Insulin resistance is truly a "new kid on the block" with regard to gender-based research. Although some clinical scientists have been interested in this topic for the past several decades, acceptance of the prevalence and health consequences have been recognized only in the past decade.

A. Suggestions for Further Investigations

* The recognition of diabetes as an independent risk factor for CVD will open pocketbooks to support prevention and therapeutic studies in this area. Because women carry a heavier burden than men in this area, research should lead to gender-based studies of diabetes and CVD.
* Interventional studies (with a special focus on nutrition) powered to determine gender differences are needed particularly on differences in metabolism, which may alter how fat and carbohydrate are handled in men and women.
* Nutritional intervention studies, which advance our understanding of nutrition *in utero*, will be important if we can ever hope to stem the rising tide of insulin resistance and type 2 diabetes.
* Finally, in the face of the recognized ability to prevent or delay the onset of diabetes through weight loss or prevention of further gain and regular physical activity, identifying effective strategies to increase the numbers of people choosing this life style are essential.

X. Conclusions

Insulin resistance and type 2 diabetes are complex conditions which carry with them major health risk of increased morbidity and mortality. This is one of the major chronic diseases for which nutrition therapy or altered food choices is a key component of medical management. Fortunately or unfortunately, the treatment is behavioral in nature. The nutrition component of behavioral change does not require expensive medications and treatments, but does require a commitment to appropriate food choices as well as the financial and cultural ability to access those choices. As health care providers we owe it to our patients to acknowledge the role of nutrition therapy in these conditions and provide them with the tools to achieve positive results.

References

1. Weyer C, Bogardus C, Mott DM, Pratley RE. (1999). The natural history of insulin secretory dysfunction and insulin resistance in the pathogenesis of type 2 diabetes mellitus. *J Clin Invest.* 104:787–794.
2. Haffner SM, Valdez RA, Hazuda HP *et al.* (1992). Prospective analysis of the insulin-resistance syndrome (syndrome X). *Diabetes.* 41:715–722.
3. Isomaa B, Almgren P, Tuomi T *et al.* (2001). Cardiovascular morbidity and mortality associated with the metabolic syndrome. *Diabetes Care.* 24:683–689.
4. Expert Panel on Detection, Evaluation, and Treatment of High Blood Cholesterol in Adults. (2001). Executive summary of the third report of the National Cholesterol Education Program (NCEP) expert panel on detection, evaluation, and treatment of high blood cholesterol in adults (Adult Treatment Panel III). *JAMA.* 285:2486–2497.
5. Ford ES, Giles WH, Dietz WH. (2002). Prevalence of the metabolic syndrome among U.S. adults: Findings from the third National Health and Nutrition Examination Survey. *JAMA.* 287:356–359.
6. Groop L, Forsblom C, Lehtovirta M *et al.* (1996). Metabolic consequences of a family history of NIDDM (the Botnia Study): Evidence for sex-specific parental effects. *Diabetes.* 45:1585–1593.
7. Harris MI, Flegal KM, Cowie CC *et al.* (1998). Prevalence of diabetes, impaired fasting glucose, and impaired glucose tolerance in U.S. adults. The third National Health and Nutrition Examination Survey, 1988–1994. *Diabetes Care.* 21:518–524.
8. Center for Disease Control. *Behavioral Risk Factor Surveillance System.* http://www.cdc.gov/brfss (Accessed August 2002).
9. American Diabetes Association. (2002). Gestational diabetes mellitus. *Diabetes Care.* 25:(Suppl 1):S94–S96.
10. Kim C, Newton, KM, Knopp RH. (2002). Gestational diabetes and the incidence of type 2 diabetes. *Diabetes Care.* 25:1862–1868.
11. American Diabetes Association. (2001). Diabetes statistics. In *Diabetes 2001: Vital Statistics*, pp. 13–27. Alexandria, VA: American Diabetes Association.
12. Kahn CR. (1994). Banting lecture: Insulin action, diabetogenes, and the cause of type 2 diabetes. *Diabetes.* 43:1066–1084.
13. Must A, Spadano J, Coakley EH *et al.* (1999). The disease burden associated with overweight and obesity. *JAMA.* 282:1523–1529.
14. Colditz GA, Willett WC, Rotnitzky A, Manson JE. (1995). Weight gain as a risk factor for clinical diabetes mellitus in women. *Ann Intern Med.* 122:481–486.
15. American Diabetes Association. (2001). Risk factors for diabetes. In *Diabetes 2001: Vital Statistics*, pp. 28–42. Alexandria, VA: American Diabetes Association.
16. Manson JE, Rimm EB, Stampfer MJ *et al.* (1991). Physical activity and incidence of non-insulin-dependent diabetes mellitus in women. *Lancet.* 338:774–778.
17. Folsom AR, Kushi LH, Hong CP. (2000). Physical activity and incident diabetes mellitus in postmenopausal women. *Am J Public Health.* 90:134–138.
18. Knowler WC, Barret-Connor E, Fowler SE *et al.* (2002). Reduction in the incidence of type 2 diabetes with lifestyle intervention or metformin. *N Engl J Med.* 346:393–403.
19. Haffner GM. (1998). Epidemiology of type 2 diabetes: Risk factors. *Diabetes Care.* 21(Suppl 3):S3–S6.
20. Parker B, Noakes M, Luscombe N, Clifton P. (2002). Effect of a high-protein, high-monounsaturated fat weight loss diet on glycemic control and lipid levels in type 2 diabetes. *Diabetes Care.* 25:425–430.
21. DeFronzo RA, Sherwin RS, Kraemer N. (1987). Effect of physical training on insulin action in obesity. *Diabetes.* 36:1379–1385.
22. Fujioka S, Matsuzawa Y, Tokunaga K *et al.* (1991). Improvements of glucose and lipid metabolism associated with selective reduction of intra-abdominal visceral fat in premenopausal women with visceral fat obesity. *Int J Obes.* 15:853–859.
23. Wing RR, Jeffery RW. (1995). Effect of modest weight loss on changes in cardiovascular risk factors: Are there differences between men and women or between weight loss and maintenance? *Int J Obes.* 19:67–73.
24. Henriksson J. (1995). Influence of exercise on insulin sensitivity. *J Cardiovasc Risk.* 2:303–309.
25. Ryan AS, Pratley RE, Goldberg AP, Elahi D. (1996). Resistive training increases insulin action in postmenopausal women. *J Gerontol.* 51A:M199–M205.
26. Janssen I, Fortier A, Hudson R, Ross R. (2002). Effects of an energy-restrictive diet with or without exercise on abdominal fat, intermuscular fat, and metabolic risk factors in obese women. *Diabetes Care.* 25:431–438.
27. Rice B, Janssen I, Hudson R, Ross R. (1999). Effects of exercise and/or diet on insulin, glucose and abdominal adipose tissue in obese men. *Diabetes Care.* 22:684–691.
28. Haffner SM. (1998). Management of dyslipidemia in adults with diabetes (Technical Review). *Diabetes Care.* 21:160–178.
29. Beckman JA, Creager MA, Libby P. (2002). Diabetes and atherosclerosis: Epidemiology, pathophysiology, and management. *JAMA.* 287:2570–2581.
30. Zuanetti G, Lantini R, Maggioni AP *et al.* (1993). Influence of diabetes on mortality in acute myocardial infarction. *J Am Coll Cardiol.* 22:1788–1794.
31. Gu K, Cowie CC, Harris MI. (1999). Diabetes and decline in heart disease mortality in U.S. adults. *JAMA.* 281:1291–1297.
32. Feskens EJ, Kromhout D. (1992). Glucose intolerance and the risk of cardiovascular disease: The Zutphen Study. *J Clin Epidemiol.* 45:1327–1334.
33. Haffner SM, Lehto S, Ronnemaa T *et al.* (1998). Mortality from coronary heart disease in subjects with type 2 diabetes and in nondiabetic subjects with and without prior myocardial infarction. *N Engl J Med.* 339:229–234.
34. Phipps K, Barker DJP, Hales CN *et al.* (1993). Fetal growth and impaired glucose tolerance in men and women. *Diabetologia.* 36:225–228.

35. Phillips DI. (1998). Birth weight and the future development of diabetes: A review of the evidence. *Diabetes Care*. 21(Suppl 2):B150–B155.

36. Rich-Edwards J, Colditz G, Stampfer M *et al*. (1999). Birth weight and risk for type 2 diabetes mellitus in adult women. *Ann Intern Med*. 130:278–284.

37. Barker DJ. (2000). *In utero* programming of cardiovascular disease. *Theriogenology*. 53:555–574.

38. McCance DR, Pettitt DJ, Hanson RL *et al*. (1994). Birth weight and non-insulin-dependent diabetes: Thrifty genotype, thrifty phenotype, or surviving small baby genotype? *BMJ*. 308:942–945.

39. Godfrey KM, Barker DJ (2000). Fetal nutrition and adult disease. *Am J Clin Nutr*. 71(Suppl):1344S–1352S.

40. Dabelea D, Pettitt DJ, Hanso RL *et al*. (1999). Birth weight, type 2 diabetes, and insulin resistance in Pima Indian children and young adults. *Diabetes Care*. 22:944–950.

41. King JC. (2002). Physiology of pregnancy and nutrient metabolism. *Am J Clin Nutr*. 71(Suppl):1218S–1225S.

42. Innes KE, Byers TE, Marshall JA *et al*. (2002). Association of a woman's own birth weight with subsequent risk for gestational diabetes. *JAMA*. 287:2534–2541.

43. Williams DE, Knowler WC, Smith CJ *et al*. (2001). The effect of Indian or Anglo dietary preference on the incidence of diabetes in Pima Indians. *Diabetes Care*. 24:811–816.

44. McMurry MP, Cerqueira MT, Connor SL, Connor WE. (1991). Changes in lipid and lipoprotein levels and body weight in Tarahumara Indians after consumption of an affluent diet. *N Engl J Med*. 325:1704–1708.

45. Swinburn BA, Boyce VL, Bergman RN *et al*. (1991). Deterioration in carbohydrate metabolism and lipoprotein changes induced by modern, high fat diet in Pima Indians and Caucasians. *J Clin Endocrinol Metab*. 73:156–165.

46. Van Dam RM, Willett WC, Rimm EB *et al*. (2002). Dietary patterns and risk for type 2 diabetes mellitus in U.S. men. *Ann Intern Med*. 136:201–209.

47. Salmerón J, Hu FB, Manson JE *et al*. (2001). Dietary fat intake and risk of type 2 diabetes in women. *Am J Clin Nutr*. 73:1019–1026.

48. Meyer KA, Kushi LH, Jacobs DR Jr, Folsom AR. (2001). Dietary fat and incidence of type 2 diabetes in older Iowa women. *Diabetes Care*. 24:1528–1535.

49. Meyer KA, Kushi LH, Jacobs DR *et al*. (2000). Carbohydrates, dietary fiber, and incident type 2 diabetes in older women. *Am J Clin Nutr*. 71:921–930.

50. Salmerón J, Ascherio A, Rimm EB *et al*. (1997). Dietary fiber, glycemic load, and risk of NIDDM in men. *Diabetes Care*. 20:545–550.

51. Salmerón J, Manson JE, Stampfer MJ *et al*. (1997). Dietary fiber, glycemic load, and risk of non-insulin-dependent diabetes mellitus in women. *JAMA*. 277:472–477.

52. Franz MJ, Bantle JP, Beebe CA *et al*. (2002). Technical review: Evidence-based nutrition principles and recommendations for the treatment and prevention of diabetes and related complications. *Diabetes Care*. 25:148–198.

53. Hu FB, Stampfer MJ, Rimm EB *et al*. (1999). A prospective study of egg consumption and risk of cardiovascular disease in men and women. *JAMA*. 281:1387–1394.

54. Yu-Poth S, Zhao G, Etherton T *et al*. (1999). Effects of the National Cholesterol Education Program's Step I and Step II dietary intervention programs of cardiovascular disease risk factors: A meta-analysis. *Am J Clin Nutr*. 69:632–646.

55. Garg A, Bantle JP, Henry RR *et al*. (1994). Effects of varying carbohydrate content of diet in patients with non-insulin-dependent diabetes mellitus. *JAMA*. 271:1421–1428.

56. Lovejoy JC, Windhauser MM, Rood JC, de la Bretonee JA. (1998). Effect of a controlled high-fat vs low-fat diet on insulin sensitivity and leptin levels in African-American and Caucasian women. *Metabolism*. 47:1520–1524.

57. Mayer-Davis EJ, Monaco JH, Hoen HM *et al*. (1997). Dietary fat and insulin sensitivity in a triethnic population: The role of obesity. The Insulin Resistance Atherosclerosis Study. *Am J Clin Nutr*. 65:79–87.

58. Jenkins DJA, Wolever TMS, Buckley G *et al*. (1988). Low glycemic index starchy food in the diabetic diet. *Am J Clin Nutr*. 48:248–254.

59. Luscombe ND, Noakes M, Clifton PM. (1999). Diets high and low in glycemic index versus high monounsaturated fat diets: Effects on glucose and lipid metabolism in NIDDM. *Eur J Clin Nutr*. 53:473–478.

60. Chandalia M, Garg A, Luthohann D *et al*. (2000). Beneficial effects of a high dietary fiber intake in patients with type 2 diabetes. *N Engl J Med*. 342:1392–1398.

61. Brown L, Rosner B, Willett WW, Sacks FM. (1999). Cholesterol-lowering effects of dietary fiber: A meta-analysis. *Am J Clin Nutr*. 69:30–42.

62. Bantle JP, Swanson JE, Thomas W, Laine DC. (1993). Metabolic effects of dietary sucrose in type II diabetes subjects. *Diabetes Care*. 16:1301–1305.

63. Will JC, Ford ES, Bowman BA. (1999). Serum vitamin C concentrations and diabetes: Findings from the Third National Health and Nutrition Examination Survey 1988–1994. Vit C in diabetes. NHANES III. *Am J Clin Nutr*. 70:49–52.

64. Mayer-Davis EJ, Bell KA, Reboussin BA *et al*. (1998). Antioxidant nutrient intake and diabetic retinopathy: The San Luis Valley Diabetes Study. *Ophthalmology*. 105:2264–2270.

65. Mayer-Davis EJ, Monaco JH, Marshall JA, Rushing J *et al*. (1997). Vitamin C intake and cardiovascular disease risk factors in persons with non-insulin-dependent diabetes mellitus: From the Insulin Resistance Atherosclerosis Study and the San Luis Valley Diabetes Study. *Prev Med*. 26:277–283.

66. Sanchez-Lugo L, Mayer-Davis EJ, Howard G *et al*. (1997). Insulin sensitivity and intake of vitamins E and C in African American, Hispanic, and non-Hispanic white men and women: The Insulin Resistance and Atherosclerosis Study (IRAS). *Am J Clin Nutr*. 66:1224–1231.

67. Food and Nutrition Board (FNB). (2000). Dietary Reference Intakes for vitamin C, vitamin E, selenium, and carotenoids. Washington, DC: National Academy of Press.

68. Anderson RA, Cheng N, Bryden NA *et al*. (1997). Beneficial effects of chromium for people with diabetes. *Diabetes*. 46:1786–1791.

69. Cheng N, Zhu X, Shi H *et al*. (1999). Follow-up survey of people in China with type 2 diabetes mellitus consuming supplemental chromium. *J Trace Elem Exp Med*. 12:55–60.

70. Cefalu WT, Bell-Farrow AD, Stegner J *et al*. (1999). Effect of chromium picolinate on insulin sensitivity *in vivo*. *J Trace Elem Exp Med*. 12:71–83.

71. Jovanovic L, Guiterrez M, Peterson CM. (1999). Chromium supplementation for women with gestational diabetes mellitus. *J Trace Elem Exp Med*. 12:91–97.

72. Beckles GLA, Thompson-Reid PE, ed. *Diabetes and Women's Health Across the Life Stages: A Public Health Perspective*. http://www.dkd.gov/diabetes/pubs/english.htm (Accessed August 2002).

73. Fiscella K, Franks P, Gold MR, Clancy CM. (2000). Inequality in quality: Addressing socioeconomic, racial, and ethnic disparities in health care. *JAMA*. 283:2579–2584.

70

The Role of Nutrition in the Modulation of Sex Steroids

ALISON M. DUNCAN, PhD, RD*, WILLIAM R. PHIPPS, MD**, AND MINDY S. KURZER, PhD†
*Department of Human Biology and Nutritional Sciences, University of Guelph, Guelph, Ontario, Canada
**Department of Obstetrics and Gynecology, University of Rochester, Rochester, NY
†Department of Food Science and Nutrition, University of Minnesota, St. Paul, MN

I. Introduction

There is an abundance of literature exploring the role of diet in modulating concentrations and metabolism of sex steroids. The research primarily stems from the hypothesis that such modulating effects may mediate the relationship of various nutrients to the risk of hormone-dependent diseases, including cancers of the breast, endometrium, and prostate, as well as cardiovascular disease. The flow of science supporting a role for nutrition in sex steroid modulation was initiated through results of ecologic studies comparing diets of populations at different risks for hormone-dependent diseases. These studies led to other epidemiologic studies comparing serum levels of sex steroids as well as risk of diseases related to sex steroids in individuals with differing diets, such as vegetarians and non-vegetarians. Human interventional studies closely followed, designed to evaluate whether a specific nutrient or combination of nutrients could influence concentration and/or metabolism of sex steroids.

This chapter will review the numerous nutrients and food components that have been linked to sex steroids, including dietary fiber, fat, carbohydrate, protein, micronutrients, alcohol and phytochemicals. In addition, the effect of obesity on sex steroids as well as studies comparing vegetarians to nonvegetarians will be discussed. Despite the desire to attribute changes in sex steroids to one specific nutrient, it should be recognized that it is often challenging to separate out the effects of various nutrients on sex steroid hormones. In addition, there are many studies that have evaluated a combination of nutrient manipulations on sex steroids, such as low-fat/high-fiber diets or a change in the protein–carbohydrate ratio. A discussion of the methodologic issues of importance when comparing multiple studies is included toward the end of this chapter.

II. Vegetarian Comparison Studies

A substantial amount of the evidence demonstrating an effect of nutrients on sex steroids originates from comparisons between vegetarians and nonvegetarians. One population often studied is that of Seventh-Day Adventists (SDAs), approximately 50% of whom consume a lacto-ovo vegetarian diet, with high intakes of fruits, vegetables, whole grains, and nuts [1]. SDAs also have a lower risk of hormone-dependent cancers; for example their incidence of breast cancer is 60–80% that of the general American population [2] and their mortality from prostate cancer is 30% that of males in the general California population [1]. Although the studies comparing vegetarians to nonvegetarians

provide valuable insight into how nutrition can affect sex steroids, it must be kept in mind that the study groups differ in their intakes of many nutrients, making it challenging to attribute hormone differences to one specific nutrient.

In a frequently cited study, Goldin *et al* measured estrogens in the plasma, urine and feces of 10 vegetarian and 10 nonvegetarian premenopausal women [3]. Vegetarians, who consumed less fat and more fiber, had significantly higher fecal weights, higher fecal estradiol, estriol, and total estrogens and lower urinary estriol, when compared with nonvegetarians [3]. In addition, the vegetarians had 17% lower concentrations of plasma estrone and estradiol than the nonvegetarians, and their plasma concentrations of these steroids correlated negatively with fecal estrogen. Finally, although the data were not statistically significant, vegetarians had lower fecal β-glucuronidase activity and lower estriol-3-glucuronide, a compound formed upon reabsorption of free-estriol from the intestine [3]. The authors concluded that increasing fiber and decreasing fat may reduce the intestinal deconjugation of steroids and in so doing, decrease their intestinal reabsorption, their plasma and urinary concentrations and increase their fecal excretion [4]. This hallmark study, showing strong statistical significance despite the small sample size, provided a clear indication that nutrients can affect estrogen metabolism.

Other cross-sectional studies comparing estrogens between premenopausal vegetarians and nonvegetarians have also reported lower serum concentrations of estrogen in vegetarians [5,6], although differences did not always reach statistical significance [6]. In a comparison of the urinary estrogen profile of 11 young Finnish vegetarians and 12 omnivores, Adlercreutz *et al* [7] found no significant differences, but did find that dietary intake of total and grain fiber were negatively associated with urinary excretion of 10 of the 13 estrogens measured. The relation of grain consumption to estrogens and possibly breast cancer risk was supported by another Finnish study showing that pre-menopausal breast cancer patients had significantly lower grain intake when compared with lacto-ovo vegetarians and omnivorous control groups [8]. A larger study that compared 640 premenopausal and 457 postmenopausal British meat eaters, vegetarians, and vegans, found slightly higher plasma sex hormone-binding globulin (SHBG) and lower plasma estradiol within the vegetarians and vegans, but these differences disappeared following adjustment for body mass index (BMI) [9]. This observation led the authors to argue that any association between a vegetarian diet and low-estrogen/high-SHBG concentrations may be due to a relatively low BMI among vegetarians.

Studies of postmenopausal vegetarian women provide convincing evidence of lower estrogen exposure in vegetarians.

Armstrong *et al* [10] reported significantly higher plasma SHBG and lower urinary total-estrogens and estriol in 43 SDA vegetarians, compared to 44 nonvegetarians. Similarly, Barbosa *et al* [11] reported significantly lower plasma estradiol in 12 SDA vegetarians compared to 12 nonvegetarians, as well as a significant negative relationship between dietary fiber and serum estradiol. Finally Adlercreutz *et al* [12] studied groups of postmenopausal omnivores, vegetarians, and breast cancer patients and reported that vegetarians had higher plasma SHBG and that a diet high in fat and protein and low in fiber and carbohydrate was associated with higher plasma levels of androstenedione, total and nonprotein-bound testosterone and lower plasma SHBG levels. Higher plasma SHBG and lower estradiol and testosterone levels have also been observed in postmenopausal women from rural areas in China (who usually consume more fiber and less fat), when compared with British women [13]. An increase in SHBG may increase the metabolic clearance of sex steroids and subsequently reduce their serum concentrations [14].

Given that there is a lower incidence of prostate cancer in men who consume vegetarian diets [15], there have been numerous studies comparing levels of serum sex hormones between male vegetarians and nonvegetarians. To address the potential relation between diet, hormones and prostate cancer, Hill *et al* showed that South African men, who have a low risk of prostate cancer and normally consume vegetarian diets, have significantly lower levels of urinary estrogens and androgens than their nonvegetarian North American counterparts [16,17]. Furthermore, when South African men were fed a Western diet, their urinary total androgens and estrogens increased, whereas when North American men were fed a vegetarian diet, their urinary total androgen and estrogens decreased [16,17]. In agreement with Hill's research, Howie *et al* [18] showed that plasma testosterone and estradiol correlated negatively with dietary fiber and were significantly lower in male SDA vegetarians, compared with SDA nonvegetarians. Other studies have reported significantly higher serum SHBG in male vegetarians [19,20]; however, they have not shown statistically significant differences in serum androgens [19,20] or estrogens [20,21]. A small study comparing 14 vegetarian to 15 omnivorous men observed a significantly decreased free androgen index (testosterone–SHBG ratio) in vegetarians, suggesting a decrease in the percentage of free testosterone [19]. However, a subsequent study comparing 51 male vegans and 57 controls observed no significant difference in free testosterone [20]. Results of two small interventional trials testing effects of lacto-ovo vegetarian diets showed significant reductions in serum total testosterone [22] and urinary dehydroepiandrosterone-sulfate (DHEA-S) [23]. Studies including males following strict vegan diets have reported higher serum concentrations of SHBG [24] and higher fecal estrone [21] in the vegans when compared to lacto-ovo vegetarians, however, there have also been results showing no significant differences in plasma estrogens [21] or androgens [24]. Interestingly, in a study comparing male SDA vegetarians to nonvegetarians, Pusateri *et al* [21] observed positive correlations between dietary fiber and fecal weight as well as fecal excretion of estrogen and testosterone. Although there were no significant correlations between the concentrations of fecal and plasma steroids (as was observed in premenopausal women [3]), the

data still provide support for the hypothesis that high-fiber diets can entrap hormones in the intestine, thereby increasing their fecal excretion [21].

III. Dietary Fat and Fiber

Although the serum sex steroid levels of vegetarians provide insight into the effects of diet on steroid hormones, interventional studies allow for more control and consequently have produced more consistent results. Following the observations from vegetarian studies, the hypothesis of these studies has been that a low-fat, high-fiber diet would be associated with reduced plasma and urinary estrogens and increased fecal estrogen excretion, and that these changes are beneficial for risk of hormone-dependent diseases.

In the first of a series of controlled interventional studies, 17 premenopausal women consumed a typical Western diet (12 g fiber/day, 40% of calories from fat) for 4 weeks followed by a low-fat (25%), high-fiber (40 g/day) diet for 2 menstrual cycles [25]. Results showed a significant decrease in serum levels of estrone-sulfate; however, there were no significant changes in any other serum estrogens or androgens. The authors speculate that due to the longer half-life and higher concentration of estrone-sulfate relative to estradiol or estrone, serum levels remain more constant during the menstrual cycle, making it easier to show a consistent change in short-term studies [25]. A significant decrease in serum estrone-sulfate, with no change in estrone or estradiol was also observed by Schaefer *et al* [26] in 22 premenopausal women who consumed a low-fat (16–18%), high-fiber (40 g/day) diet for 2 menstrual cycles, when compared to a baseline diet (40% fat, 12 g fiber/day) for 4 weeks. Other results included a significant reduction in androstenedione and no significant change in testosterone or SHBG [26].

Other studies in premenopausal women have detected significant decreases in other estrogens besides estrone-sulfate. When 13 premenopausal women consumed a diet containing 30% fat and 15–25 g fiber for 1 month followed by a diet containing 10% fat and 25–35 g fiber/day for 2 months, there were significant reductions in serum estrone and estradiol, however, there were no significant changes in serum estrone-sulfate or SHBG [27]. Furthermore, consuming a low-fat (20%), high-fiber (40 g/day) diet for 2 menstrual cycles significantly decreased serum estrone, estrone-sulfate and increased androstenedione in 18 African-American women, when compared to consuming a control diet (40% fat, 12 g fiber/day) for 3 weeks [28]. Finally, as part of an ongoing breast cancer prevention trial in Canada, Boyd *et al* [29] reported that 2 years of a low-fat (21.2%), high-carbohydrate (60.3%) diet significantly reduced serum estradiol, compared with a control diet (33.1% fat, 48.8% carbohydrate) in premenopausal women with high mammmographic densities.

To assess the independent effects of fat and fiber on serum estrogens, Goldin *et al* [30] studied 48 premenopausal women who lived on a metabolic ward and were randomized to a control diet or various isocaloric diets differing in their fat and fiber content for 2 menstrual cycles. Results showed that when dietary fat was lowered to 25–20% of calories and fiber was simultaneously increased to 40 g/day, there were statistically significant reductions in serum estrone, estrone-sulfate, testosterone, androstenedione and SHBG and marginally significant reductions in estradiol (p=0.07) and free estradiol (p=0.10) [30]. When the independent effects of fat and fiber were evaluated, results showed that the decrease in fat was found to be the major determinant of the decreases in serum estrone, free estradiol, testosterone, and androstenedione. The increase in fiber was the major determinant for the decreases in serum estradiol and SHBG, and both fat and fiber were equally important for the decrease in serum estrone-sulfate [30].

Effects of a low-fat, high-fiber diet have produced consistent results in postmenopausal women. Fowke *et al* [31] reported that a decrease in the dietary fat–fiber ratio was associated with an increase in the ratio of urinary 2/16α-hydroxyestrone in 37 postmenopausal women not using hormone replacement therapy (HRT). This finding is of particular relevance to breast cancer risk, given the reported carcinogenic properties of 16α-hydroxyestrone [32] and the inverse relation of the 2/16α-hydroxyestrone ratio to breast cancer risk [33]. Results from other interventional studies have shown a significant reduction in serum estradiol in 13 postmenopausal women not using HRT, who consumed a low-fat (<10%), high-fiber (34–45 g/1000 kcal/day) diet for 22 days [34] and a significant increase in serum SHBG in 22 postmenopausal women, regardless of HRT use, following 3 weeks of a low-fat (10%) high-fiber (35–40 g/1000 kcal/day) diet combined with exercise [35]. Finally, in a large study involving 312 postmenopausal women not using HRT, 4.5 months of a comprehensive dietary intervention combining low-fat, low saturated fat, and high complex carbohydrates and phytoestrogens, resulted in a significant increase in serum SHBG and a decrease in testosterone [36].

Studies of low-fat, high-fiber diets in men have shown effects on sex steroids that may be considered beneficial for reducing prostate cancer risk. Significant reductions in serum total and free testosterone were observed in 30 healthy men who consumed their customary diet (40% fat, 45% carbohydrate) for 2 weeks followed by a low-fat (25% kcal), higher polyunsaturated fatty acid (PUFA)–saturated fatty acid (SFA) ratio and high-fiber (57% carbohydrate) diet for 6 weeks [37]. Plasma SHBG-bound testosterone and urinary testosterone were also significantly reduced by a low-fat (18%), high-fiber (61.8 g/day) diet in 43 men, when compared with a high-fat (41%), low-fiber (26.4 g/day) diet [38]. The same study found that the low-fat, high-fiber diet significantly increased urinary estrogens and their 2-hydroxylated metabolites [38]. Interventions involving low-fat, high-fiber diets combined with exercise programs have also shown significant changes in sex steroids including increased serum SHBG following a 3-week intervention [39] and decreased serum estradiol, but no change in serum testosterone following a 26-day intervention [40], however neither of these studies included a control group.

IV. Dietary Fat

A number of studies have attempted to separate out the effects of dietary fat from those of dietary fiber. Whether a reduction in dietary fat is a preventive measure for cancer is an issue of great debate [41,42]. Nonetheless, there is epidemiologic evidence indicating that risk of hormone-dependent cancers, particularly breast and prostate may be related to a high consumption of fat [43,44]. Furthermore, it is thought that the relationship between fat and cancer may be mediated by high concentrations of sex steroids, particularly estrogen [45,46].

Cross-sectional studies have reported that fat intake relates positively to serum estrogens in pre- and postmenopausal women. In a comparison of Oriental and Caucasian pre- and postmenopausal women, it was found that Caucasians, who consume significantly more fat than their Oriental counterparts, had significantly greater plasma estrone and estradiol as well as plasma testosterone and androstenedione [47]. Other studies in Japanese premenopausal women have also reported positive correlations between fat intake and serum estrogens [48,49].

Interventional studies in women have not yielded consistent results. When 33 women (18 premenopausal and 15 postmenopausal) consumed a control diet (40% fat) or a low-fat (20%) diet for 2 months each in a randomized crossover design, results showed nonsignificant decreases in nonprotein bound estradiol (p=0.07) and testosterone (p=0.11) for all women, however there were no significant changes in serum concentrations of total estradiol, total testosterone, DHEA-S, or SHBG [50]. This is consistent with a nonrandomized study of 18 premenopausal and 19 postmenopausal women that observed no significant effects in total or free estradiol following a reduced-fat (23–24%) diet for 4 weeks [45].

In contrast, there are numerous studies that do support a positive relationship between dietary fat and serum estrogens. In a group of 16 premenopausal women with cystic breast disease, Rose *et al* [51] reduced the fat intake from 35 to 21% of calories for 3 months and showed significant reductions in serum concentrations of luteal phase total estrogens, estrone, and estradiol. Because there were no significant effects on luteinizing hormone or progesterone, the authors argued that effects could be attributed to alterations in the enterohepatic circulation of estrogen rather than the pituitary-ovarian axis [51]. Williams *et al* [52] also observed a significant reduction in luteal phase estradiol in 15 premenopausal women who consumed a low-fat (36 g/day) diet for 2 months. A smaller study in 6 healthy premenopausal women reported no significant effects of a low-fat (25%) diet for 2 months on serum follicular phase estradiol, but did observe a significant shift in estrogen metabolism, as reflected by significant reductions in follicular phase urinary 16α-hydroxyestrone and urinary estriol as well as an increase in urinary 2-hydroxylated estrogen metabolites [53].

Interventional studies in postmenopausal women have demonstrated more consistent decreases in serum estrogens following low-fat diets. Boyar *et al* [54] found a significant reduction in serum estradiol, following 5 months of a low-fat diet (20%) in 19 postmenopausal women with breast cancer, although there were no significant changes in estrone or total estrogens. A pilot study of the Women's Health Initiative reported that 73 postmenopausal women not taking HRT who reduced their dietary fat from 40 to 20% of calories for 10–22 weeks had significantly reduced serum estradiol as well as nonsignificantly reduced serum estrone-sulfate and SHBG [55]. Finally, Rose *et al* [56] showed that 6–12 months of a low-fat (20%) diet significantly reduced serum estradiol and SHBG in postmenopausal breast cancer patients not receiving tamoxifen, however there were no significant changes in estrone or estrone-sulfate. On the other hand, Holmes *et al* [57] reported an inverse association between dietary fat and serum estradiol in 381 postmenopausal women, results that are inconsistent with the hypothesis that fat intake increases breast cancer risk by increasing endogenous estrogen concentrations.

In an effort to consolidate the numerous dietary fat interventional studies, a meta-analysis of fat interventional studies by Wu *et al* [46] reported that a low-fat (10–25%) diet for 2–3 months resulted in an overall significant decrease of 13.4% in serum estradiol in pre- and postmenopausal women. It should be noted that the heterogeneity among studies was statistically significant and that some of the 13 studies included in the analysis also included manipulations in fiber intake [46].

Studies of a low-fat diet in men have shown both a decrease in serum testosterone and an increase in serum SHBG. Six weeks of a 25% fat diet significantly decreased serum total and free testosterone as well as androstenedione in 30 healthy men [58], whereas 2 weeks of a low-fat diet (<20 g/day) significantly increased SHBG and decreased free testosterone in six healthy men [59]. In contrast, an acute study showed that a high-fat (57%) meal significantly reduced free and total testosterone [60].

In addition to the quantity of dietary fat, the type of fat may also be important. Experimental studies have reported inverse correlations between the PUFA–SFA ratio and plasma estrogens in women [61] and androgens in men [38]. In addition, a study in Asian women showed that serum estradiol correlated positively with SFA (p=0.06), but not PUFA [47]. Omega-3 fatty acids may be particularly important, as suggested by an inverse correlation between intake of omega-3 fatty acids from fish and serum total testosterone in Japanese men [62]; however, the same study found no significant relationships with serum concentrations of free testosterone or estrogens [62]. A related 3-month interventional study in 26 premenopausal women showed no significant effects of a fish diet on serum sex hormones or SHBG, when compared to a meat or vegetarian diet [63]. Although there are not substantial data focusing on fat type, there is some evidence suggesting it may contribute toward serum hormones and as such, may also be contributing toward the inconsistent results observed in dietary fat interventional studies. Regardless, the observation that Eskimos who consume high amounts of high-fat fish have a low rate of breast cancer [64], warrants further investigation into the effect of fat type on sex steroids related to hormone-dependent cancers.

V. Dietary Fiber

Dietary fiber on its own is hypothesized to protect against breast cancer through effects on serum estrogens [65]. A New Zealand study involving 60 healthy premenopausal women reported that dietary fiber intakes >25 g/day were negatively correlated with plasma follicular and luteal phase estradiol [66]. Moreover, a significant reduction in serum luteal phase estrone and estradiol was observed in 62 premenopausal women who supplemented their diet with wheat bran to increase their fiber intake from 15 to 30 g/day for 2 months [67]. Interestingly, there were no significant effects of fiber from oat or corn bran [67]. The estrogen-lowering effect of wheat bran was confirmed in a follow-up study that showed a dose-dependent decrease in serum luteal phase estrone and estradiol following 1–2 months

of 10 or 20 grams of wheat bran per day in premenopausal women [68]. These effects were not, however, confirmed in an intervention with wheat bran in 17 African-American postmenopausal women that did not show any significant effects of wheat bran on serum estrogens, regardless of HRT use [69]. It is possible that the relatively lower concentrations of estrogens in postmenopausal women made it harder to detect any effect [69].

Studies focusing on the effect of fiber in men are less frequent and have shown fewer significant effects on sex steroids. A randomized crossover trial was performed in 14 men with dyslipidemia, who consumed diets high in soluble or insoluble fiber for 4 months each (25–30 g/1000 kcal/day), separated by a 2-month washout [70]. Results showed that the soluble fiber diet significantly lowered serum prostate-specific antigen, when compared with the insoluble fiber diet, however no treatment difference was observed in serum estradiol or free testosterone [70].

Overall, it appears that there is consistent evidence that fiber alone can decrease serum estrogens in premenopausal women. The observation that wheat bran is particularly effective supports the hypothesis that fiber, particularly insoluble fiber like wheat bran, may decrease estrogens by binding the intestinal steroids with subsequent interruption of steroid reabsorption and increased fecal excretion [47]. Data on the effects of fiber alone in postmenopausal women and in men are less convincing.

VI. Protein and Carbohydrate

The majority of studies evaluating the effect of dietary protein and/or carbohydrate on steroid hormones have involved a manipulation of the protein–carbohydrate ratio. In a cross-sectional study of Finnish women, Adlercreutz *et al* [8] reported a significant positive association between the protein–carbohydrate ratio and the urinary 2-hydroxyestrone–4-hydroxyestrone ratio. The interventional studies exploring protein and carbohydrate have been primarily done in males and have shown significant effects on the concentration and metabolism of sex steroids. In a nonrandomized study, it was demonstrated that 2 weeks of a high-protein, low-carbohydrate diet (44% protein, 35% carbohydrate, 21% fat) significantly decreased the 5α-reduction of testosterone and increased the 2-hydroxylation of estradiol, when compared to 2 weeks of a low-protein, high-carbohydrate diet (10% protein, 70% carbohydrate, 20% fat) in eight young males [71]. The effect on estrogen metabolism was confirmed in a subsequent study of identical design in which the high-protein, low-carbohydrate diet significantly increased 2-hydroxylation, but did not change 16α-hydroxylation of estrogens, when compared with the low-protein, high-carbohydrate diet [72]. A final study by the same group of investigators explored effects on plasma hormones and showed that a high-protein, low-carbohydrate diet (44% protein, 35% carbohydrate, 21% fat) significantly decreased plasma testosterone and SHBG, compared with a low-protein, high-carbohydrate diet (10% protein, 70% carbohydrate, 20% fat) in seven healthy men [73]. There were no significant changes in plasma DHEA, androstenedione, or estradiol in this study.

VII. Micronutrients

There has not been substantial research evaluating the effect of specific micronutrients on concentrations of sex steroids. In assessing the relation of numerous dietary variables to serum and/or urinary sex hormones, some epidemiologic studies have included selected micronutrients in their analyses.

In a cross-sectional study of 1241 middle-age American men, Field et al [74] observed that serum free and total testosterone were inversely associated with niacin intake, that serum SHBG was inversely associated with vitamin D intake and that serum DHEA-S was inversely associated with riboflavin intake. The authors did not make any conclusions about these findings due to the lack of prestudy hypotheses. Other cross-sectional studies have reported significant positive associations between serum sex hormones and various micronutrients including serum testosterone with phosphorus and zinc [75], as well as serum estradiol with retinol, vitamin E, vitamin C, and beta-carotene [75]. Retinol intake also showed significant positive correlations with urinary estradiol, estrone, and catechol estrogens in premenopausal women [8], and negative correlations with serum testosterone and estradiol in men [75]. Finally, plasma DHEA-S showed significant positive correlations with plasma retinol and inverse correlations with multivitamin intakes in a group of men from the Physician's Health Study [76].

Vitamin E has received considerable attention as a micronutrient that may affect sex steroids. Using baseline samples from the Alpha-Tocopherol Beta-Carotene Cancer Prevention (ATBC) study, Hartman et al [77] reported a significant inverse association between serum alpha-tocopherol and serum concentrations of testosterone, androstenedione, estrone, and SHBG in 204 men age 50 to 69. Results from the ATBC intervention revealed that supplementation with alpha-tocopherol significantly reduced serum testosterone and androstenedione [78]. These changes corresponded with significant reductions in the incidence and mortality of prostate cancer [79], providing indirect evidence that vitamin E supplementation may affect prostate cancer through modulation of sex hormones. To date, there have not been any studies to address specifically how alpha-tocopherol may affect sex hormones, although Hartman et al [78] suggest there are some data to suggest a prostaglandin-mediated mechanism [80,81].

Overall, there has been minimal research evaluating the effects of specific micronutrients on sex hormones. The findings that have emerged from epidemiologic studies may serve as a step for the generation of hypotheses and future studies.

VIII. Alcohol

Epidemiologic studies have reported that breast cancer risk is greater among women who consume alcohol, and it is thought that this risk may be mediated by increases in serum estrogen concentrations [82]. Cross-sectional [83] and acute experimental studies [84] in premenopausal women demonstrate that alcohol consumption is significantly associated with increased serum estradiol, however another study was unable to detect a significant relationship [85]. A 3-month interventional study in 34 premenopausal women found that moderate alcohol consumption (30 g/day) did result in significant increases in plasma and urinary estrogens within various menstrual cycle phases [86]. Other interventional studies have also found significant increases in plasma estradiol following moderate alcohol consumption, however only within oral contraceptive users [87,88]. Serum estrone has been unaffected by alcohol consumption in some

studies [85,87], leading to speculation that the alcohol-mediated decrease in the hepatic NAD–NADH ratio could result in reduced oxidation of estradiol to estrone [84,87]. Androgens are also increased in response to alcohol consumption in premenopausal women. Associational studies report positive relationships between alcohol and serum concentrations of androstenedione [85] and DHEA [86]. Moreover, interventional studies have consistently demonstrated significant increases in plasma testosterone following alcohol administration, regardless of oral contraceptive use [88–91].

In postmenopausal women, blood estrogens are consistently positively associated with moderate alcohol consumption [92–95] and are significantly elevated in patients with alcohol-induced cirrhosis [96–98]. Furthermore, acute alcohol interventions significantly increase serum estradiol, however this has only been observed in women taking estrogen replacement therapy (ERT) [99,100]. It is possible that alcohol enhances the effect of ERT by increasing estradiol absorption through the gut in the case of oral ERT [100] or increasing vasodilation of the skin in the case of transdermal ERT [99]. However, as pointed out by Ginsburg et al [100], it is unlikely to explain the full effect, because premenopausal women who do not take endogenous estrogens, experience consistent significant rises in estradiol following alcohol consumption [84,86]. A more likely explanation would be an alcohol-induced increase in the rate of androgen aromatization, a major source of estrogens in postmenopausal women. The observation of significantly increased estradiol–testosterone ratio in postmenopausal alcoholics supports this mechanism [97]. The overall estrogen-elevating effect of alcohol in postmenopausal women may help to explain its positive association with breast cancer risk [101] and negative association with cardiovascular disease risk [102].

Alcohol is also able to exert effects on sex steroids in males. Serum testosterone is significantly reduced in male alcoholics [103] and in healthy men administered alcohol, at least under certain experimental conditions [104–106]. Alcohol also appears to alter the metabolism of testosterone, as indicated by a significant decrease in its production rate [104], as well as significant increases in its metabolic clearance [104] and the activity of 5α-reductase [107] in 4-week interventional studies involving daily alcohol consumption in healthy men. The opposite effects of alcohol on serum testosterone in men vs premenopausal women suggest a gender-specific effect, as was confirmed in an acute alcohol study in adolescent males and females [108]. In contrast to its effects on androgens, alcohol has been shown to increase serum estrogens in men [109,110]. It is possible that increased estrogen concentrations could be due to increased peripheral aromatization of androgens [111], which could also help explain the decreased concentrations of testosterone observed.

IX. Obesity and Body Fatness

Effects of energy on sex steroids have been studied indirectly through the use of obesity (as defined by BMI >30 kg/m^2) as an independent variable. Increasing body weight and obesity have been associated with alterations in sex hormone concentrations and metabolism in both men and women [112]. Within women, the relationship between obesity and breast cancer risk is dependent on estrogen, however the effects depend upon menopausal status. In postmenopausal women, obesity increases breast cancer risk [113], likely in part due to increased estrogen exposure through increased peripheral aromatization of androgens to estrogens in adipose tissue [114]. In contrast, studies assessing obesity and breast cancer risk in premenopausal women have found either no association or a modest inverse association [115], possibly due to obesity-induced menstrual abnormalities leading to anovulation and lower overall estrogen exposure [116]. The most consistently observed hormonal effect of obesity within premenopausal women, postmenopausal women, and men is a significant inverse relationship between BMI and serum SHBG [74,117–121]. On average, SHBG is about twice as high in thin individuals (BMI $<20\,\text{kg/m}^2$) compared with obese individuals (BMI $>30\,\text{kg/m}^2$), an effect attributed largely to obesity-induced hyperinsulinemia [116].

In pre- and postmenopausal women, there is a clear significant increase in serum estrogens associated with obesity [122–124]. The peripheral conversion of androgens to estrogens also increases as a function of obesity [125,126], further contributing to higher serum estrogens. In addition, estrogen metabolism is affected by increasing body weight as has been demonstrated by increased urinary concentrations of the more estrogenic 16α-hydroxylated metabolites [127] and decreased concentrations of the less estrogenic 2-hydroxylated metabolites [127,128]. The opposite estrogenic properties of these metabolites further contribute to the hyper-estrogenic state of obese females and the subsequent implications for higher risk of hormone-dependent diseases such as breast cancer [129]. Androgen production rates and serum concentrations are elevated in pre- and postmenopausal obese women [123,130–133], however data is not as consistent as serum estrogens [134].

Obesity in men has been positively associated with serum estrogens [75,135,136], peripheral conversion of androgens to estrogens [135,137,138] and altered metabolism of estradiol toward decreased levels of 2-hydroxylated metabolites [128]. In contrast to effects in women, obesity in men is consistently negatively associated with serum androgens [74,75,135,139–141]. It is proposed that the decreased levels of SHBG found in obese men results in accelerated clearance and lowered serum androgen concentrations [134], although this does not appear to be the case in women.

In addition to body fat amount, body fat distribution is also known to affect sex steroids. Body fat distribution has been linked to gender, with upper body fat associated with maleness and lower body fat associated with femaleness [142]. This has led to the hypothesis that upper body obesity would be associated with more androgenic activity, when compared with lower body obesity [142]. This hypothesis is supported by cell culture research showing that adipose cells derived from abdominal fat have a lower estrone–androgens ratio, when compared to cells from the thigh-buttock area [143]. Furthermore, numerous human studies have associated upper body obesity with increased androgens [130,132,142], decreased SHBG [132,142,144,145], and increased free testosterone [132,142,145] in pre- and postmenopausal women.

X. Phytochemicals

Numerous phytochemicals have demonstrated potential to interact with sex steroids *in vitro* [146–151]; however, the majority of research has focused on phytoestrogens [152]. Phytoestrogens are naturally occurring plant chemicals, the two most relevant to sex steroids being isoflavones and lignans [152]. Isoflavones are found primarily in soybean products [153] whereas lignans are more widespread in plants but are exceptionally high in flaxseed [154]. Epidemiologic research reporting that consumption of phytoestrogens is linked to decreased risk of hormone-dependent diseases [155,156] has prompted evaluation of their effects on sex steroids in women and men.

Isoflavones are hypothesized to reduce serum estrogens and androgens in men and women, however the data have been inconsistent [157]. In premenopausal women, isoflavone-rich soy consumption has correlated negatively with serum estradiol [158], yet interventional studies have been inconsistent in their effects on concentrations of serum estrogens and androgens [157]. More consistency exists in the effect of soy isoflavone consumption on urinary estrogens, including significant decreases in urinary estradiol, estrone, estriol and total estrogens [159], as well as significant increases in the $2/16\alpha$-hydroxyestrone ratio [159,160]. Most interventional studies in postmenopausal women have been unable to detect significant effects of soy consumption on serum sex steroids [161–165]. Although some studies have observed statistically significant increases in plasma SHBG [166,167] and decreases in serum estrogens and androgens [167], the changes were of minimal physiologic significance. Interestingly, in agreement with results in premenopausal women [159], Xu *et al* [168] observed a significant increase in the urinary $2/16\alpha$-hydroxyestrone ratio when 18 postmenopausal women consumed isoflavone-rich soy, compared to soy-free baseline values. In men, soy intake has correlated negatively with serum estradiol as well as estrone, total and free testosterone, although the latter three relationships were of borderline significance [169]. Interventional studies in men have been unable to detect significant effects of soy on sex steroids [170–172], however there have been trends [p $=0.05$–0.07] toward decreased levels of estrone [170], the testosterone–estradiol ratio [171] and the free androgen index [171].

There are fewer human interventional studies evaluating the effect of lignans on sex steroids. In a randomized crossover study in 18 premenopausal women, consumption of lignan-rich flaxseed for 3 menstrual cycles resulted in significant increases in follicular phase testosterone and luteal phase progesterone–estradiol ratio [173], however no changes were observed in serum estrogens or SHBG. In another randomized crossover study in 28 postmenopausal women, 7 weeks of flaxseed consumption significantly reduced serum estradiol and estrone-sulfate [174], however no changes were observed in serum estrone, androgens or SHBG. Interestingly, the urinary $2/16\alpha$-hydroxyestrone ratio has been significantly reduced by flax consumption in both premenopausal [175] and postmenopausal [176] women. A small study in healthy men (n $=6$) reported no significant effects of 6 weeks of flax consumption on plasma SHBG, free or total testosterone [177]. In contrast, a larger study in 25 men recently diagnosed with prostate cancer reported that 34 days of flaxseed supplementation combined with a low-fat (20%) diet significantly reduced serum prostate specific antigen, testosterone and the free androgen index [178].

Another group of phytochemicals of particular interest with respect to sex steroids are the indole-3-carbinols, found primarily in *Brassica* vegetables such as brussels sprouts, broccoli, cabbage, cauliflower, kale, turnips, and collard [179]. Interventional studies have consistently reported significant increases in the urinary 2/16α-hydroxyestrone ratio in men and women who add *Brassica* vegetables [179,180] or concentrated pills containing indole-3-carbinol [181] to their daily diets. An increase in the urinary 2-hydroxyestrone–estriol ratio [182] as well as significant decreases in urinary estrogens [181] have also been observed in men and women following consumption of pills containing indole-3-carbinol.

XI. Methodologic Issues

It is important to consider methodologic issues when interpreting and comparing studies that explore nutrition and sex steroids. Arguably, the largest methodologic challenge is attributing an effect of sex steroids to a single nutrient. It takes substantial experimental control to ensure the treatment and control diets are similar in every way except the nutrient of interest. Without this, the introduction of confounding variables such as weight gain and changes in other nutrients can preclude clear and valid conclusions.

With regard to epidemiologic studies that relate diet to sex hormones, the validity and accuracy of the dietary assessment method should be noted. Another issue is the timing of the blood sample in terms of menstrual cycle day in premenopausal women and/or time of day in all populations in consideration of the cyclic and circadian rhythms of sex hormones. In addition, if the effect of diet on hormones is a substudy of a larger epidemiologic study, care should be exercised to make sure the data necessary for the comparison have been gathered in the appropriate manner to test the hypotheses.

With regards to interventional studies assessing the effect of diet on sex steroids, one of the most important issues is the existence of a control group. Many studies simply measure the dependent variables before and after an intervention, rather than including a control group arm or a control study period. Other methodologic issues include if and/or how compliance to the dietary intervention is assessed, whether the treatments were randomized or not, and sample size.

XII. Conclusions and Suggestions for Further Investigations

The link between sex steroids and hormone-dependent diseases has rationalized the substantial research effort into the effect of nutrients on sex steroids. Studies comparing vegetarians to nonvegetarians have suggested that low-fat, high-fiber diets are associated with lower serum estrogens, lower urinary estrogens, and higher fecal estrogens. Subsequent studies focusing on the effects of specific nutrients have revealed that metabolism and concentrations of sex steroids can be modulated by changes in amounts of many nutrients, including fiber, fat, carbohydrate and protein, alcohol, and phytochemicals. The significance of these changes have been linked to associations with increased or decreased risk of hormone-dependent diseases, primarily breast cancer, prostate cancer, and cardiovascular disease. It has also been consistently shown that obesity and body fatness contribute

to variation in sex steroids. The greatest challenge facing an overall consensus of the data is the difficulty of attributing effects to a single nutrient. In addition, the numerous methodologic issues facing investigators often makes it harder to detect statistically significant effects. In terms of future research, the following areas show potential:

- Some studies suggest that there may be gender-specific effects of nutrients on sex steroids. Future research could focus on this hypothesis by designing studies specifically to examine the effect of gender when exploring nutrition and sex steroids.
- The significance of the effects of nutrients on sex steroids relates to risk of hormone-dependent diseases. It would be interesting to have more research comparing the effect of nutrition on sex steroids in individuals with and without the relevant diseases.
- Apart from associational analyses, there has been very little done in the area of micronutrients and sex steroids. These associations can provide the basis for future hypotheses. In particular vitamin E shows promise as a potential contributor to variation in sex steroids and warrants more research.

References

1. Phillips RL. (1975). Role of life-style and dietary habits in risk of cancer among Seventh-Day Adventists. *Cancer Res.* 35:3513–3522.
2. Phillips RL, Garfinkel L, Kuzma JW *et al.* (1980). Mortality among California Seventh-Day Adventists for selected cancer sites. *J Natl Cancer Inst.* 65:1097–1107.
3. Goldin BR, Adlercreutz H, Gorbach SL *et al.* (1982). Estrogen excretion patterns and plasma levels in vegetarian and omnivorous women. *N Engl J Med.* 307:1542–1547.
4. Goldin BR, Gorbach SL. (1994). Hormone studies and the diet and breast cancer connection. *Adv Exp Med Biol.* 364:35–46.
5. Shultz TD, Leklem JE. (1983). Nutrient intake and hormonal status of premenopausal vegetarian Seventh-day Adventists and premenopausal non-vegetarians. *Nutr Cancer.* 4:247–259.
6. Gray GE, Williams P, Gerkins V *et al.* (1982). Diet and hormone levels in Seventh-Day Adventist teenage girls. *Prev Med.* 11:103–107.
7. Adlercreutz H, Fotsis T, Bannwart C *et al.* (1986). Urinary estrogen profile determination in young Finnish vegetarian and omnivorous women. *J Steroid Biochem.* 24:289–296.
8. Adlercreutz H, Fotsis T, Hockerstedt K *et al.* (1989). Diet and urinary estrogen profile in premenopausal omnivorous and vegetarian women and in premenopausal women with breast cancer. *J Steroid Biochem.* 34:527–530.
9. Thomas HV, Davey GK, Key TJ. (1999). Oestradiol and sex hormone-binding globulin in premenopausal and post-menopausal meat-eaters, vegetarians and vegans. *Br J Cancer.* 80:1470–1475.
10. Armstrong BK, Brown JB, Clarke HT *et al.* (1981). Diet and reproductive hormones: A study of vegetarian and nonvegetarian postmenopausal women. *J Natl Cancer Inst.* 67:761–767.
11. Barbosa JC, Shultz TD, Filley SJ, Nieman DC. (1990). The relationship among adiposity, diet, and hormone concentrations in vegetarian and nonvegetarian postmenopausal women. *Am J Clin Nutr.* 51:798–803.
12. Adlercreutz H, Hamalainen E, Gorbach SL *et al.* (1989). Diet and plasma androgens in postmenopausal vegetarian and omnivorous women and post-menopausal women with breast cancer. *Am J Clin Nutr.* 49:433–442.
13. Key TJ, Chen J, Wang DY *et al.* (1990). Sex hormones in women in rural China and in Britain. *Br J Cancer.* 62:631–636.
14. Anderson DC. (1974). Sex-hormone-binding globulin. *Clin Endocrinol [Oxf].* 3:69–96.
15. Isaacson C SG, Kaye V. (1978). Cancer in the urban black of South Africa. *Cancer Bulletin* 22:49–84.
16. Hill P, Wynder E, Garbaczewski L *et al.* (1980). Plasma hormones and lipids in men at different risk for coronary heart disease. *Am J Clin Nutr.* 33:1010–1018.

17. Hill P, Wynder EL, Garbaczewski L et al. (1979). Diet and urinary steroids in black and white North American men and black South African men. Cancer Res. 39:5101–5105.

18. Howie BJ, Shultz TD. (1985). Dietary and hormonal interrelationships among vegetarian Seventh-Day Adventists and nonvegetarian men. Am J Clin Nutr. 42:127–134.

19. Belanger A, Locong A, Noel C et al. (1989). Influence of diet on plasma steroids and sex hormone-binding globulin levels in adult men. J Steroid Biochem. 32:829–833.

20. Key TJ, Roe L, Thorogood M et al. (1990). Testosterone, sex hormone-binding globulin, calculated free testosterone, and oestradiol in male vegans and omnivores. Br J Nutr. 64:111–119.

21. Pusateri DJ, Roth WT, Ross JK, Shultz TD. (1990). Dietary and hormonal evaluation of men at different risks for prostate cancer: Plasma and fecal hormone-nutrient interrelationships. Am J Clin Nutr. 51:371–377.

22. Raben A, Kiens B, Richter EA et al. (1992). Serum sex hormones and endurance performance after a lacto-ovo vegetarian and a mixed diet. Med Sci Sports Exerc. 24:1290–1297.

23. Remer T, Pietrzik K, Manz F. (1998). Short-term impact of a lactovegetarian diet on adrenocortical activity and adrenal androgens. J Clin Endocrinol Metab. 83:2132–2137.

24. Allen NE, Appleby PN, Davey GK, Key TJ. (2000). Hormones and diet: Low insulin-like growth factor-I but normal bioavailable androgens in vegan men. Br J Cancer. 83:95–97.

25. Woods MN, Gorbach SL, Longcope C et al. (1989). Low-fat, high-fiber diet and serum estrone sulfate in premenopausal women. Am J Clin Nutr. 49:1179–1183.

26. Schaefer EJ, Lamon-Fava S, Spiegelman D et al. (1995). Changes in plasma lipoprotein concentrations and composition in response to a low-fat, high-fiber diet are associated with changes in serum estrogen concentrations in premenopausal women. Metabolism. 44:749–756.

27. Bagga D, Ashley JM, Geffrey SP et al. (1995). Effects of a very low fat, high fiber diet on serum hormones and menstrual function. Implications for breast cancer prevention. Cancer. 76:2491–2496.

28. Woods MN, Barnett JB, Spiegelman D et al. (1996). Hormone levels during dietary changes in premenopausal African-American women. J Natl Cancer Inst. 88:1369–1374.

29. Boyd NF, Lockwood GA, Greenberg CV et al. (1997). Effects of a low-fat high-carbohydrate diet on plasma sex hormones in premenopausal women: Results from a randomized controlled trial. Canadian Diet and Breast Cancer Prevention Study Group. Br J Cancer. 76:127–135.

30. Goldin BR, Woods MN, Spiegelman DL et al. (1994). The effect of dietary fat and fiber on serum estrogen concentrations in premenopausal women under controlled dietary conditions. Cancer. 74:1125–1131.

31. Fowke JH, Longcope C, Hebert JR. (2001). Macronutrient intake and estrogen metabolism in healthy postmenopausal women. Breast Cancer Res Treat. 65:1–10.

32. Fishman J, Osborne MP, Telang NT. (1995). The role of estrogen in mammary carcinogenesis. Ann NY Acad Sci. 768:91–100.

33. Muti P, Bradlow HL, Micheli A et al. (2000). Estrogen metabolism and risk of breast cancer: A prospective study of the 2:16 alpha-hydroxyestrone ratio in premenopausal and postmenopausal women. Epidemiology. 11:635–640.

34. Heber D, Ashley JM, Leaf DA, Barnard RJ. (1991). Reduction of serum estradiol in postmenopausal women given free access to low-fat high-carbohydrate diet. Nutrition. 7:137–139; discussion 139–140.

35. Tymchuk CN, Tessler SB, Barnard RJ. (2000). Changes in sex hormone-binding globulin, insulin, and serum lipids in postmenopausal women on a low-fat, high-fiber diet combined with exercise. Nutr Cancer. 38:158–162.

36. Berrino F, Bellati C, Secreto G et al. (2001). Reducing bioavailable sex hormones through a comprehensive change in diet: The diet and androgens [DIANA] randomized trial. Cancer Epidemiol Biomarkers Prev. 10:25–33.

37. Hamalainen EK, Adlercreutz H, Puska P, Pietinen P. (1983). Decrease of serum total and free testosterone during a low-fat high-fibre diet. J Steroid Biochem. 18:369–370.

38. Dorgan JF, Judd JT, Longcope C et al. (1996). Effects of dietary fat and fiber on plasma and urine androgens and estrogens in men: A controlled feeding study. Am J Clin Nutr. 64:850–855.

39. Tymchuk CN, Tessler SB, Aronson WJ, Barnard RJ. (1998). Effects of diet and exercise on insulin, sex hormone-binding globulin, and prostate-specific antigen. Nutr Cancer. 31:127–131.

40. Rosenthal MB, Barnard RJ, Rose DP et al. (1985). Effects of a high-complex-carbohydrate, low-fat, low-cholesterol diet on levels of serum lipids and estradiol. Am J Med. 78:23–27.

41. Greenwald P. (1999). Role of dietary fat in the causation of breast cancer: Point. Cancer Epidemiol Biomarkers Prev. 8:3–7.

42. Hunter DJ. (1999). Role of dietary fat in the causation of breast cancer: Counterpoint. Cancer Epidemiol Biomarkers Prev. 8:9–13.

43. Carroll KK. (1981). Influence of diet on mammary cancer. Nutr Cancer. 2:232–236.

44. Greenwald P, Sherwood K, McDonald SS. (1997). Fat, caloric intake, and obesity: Lifestyle risk factors for breast cancer. J Am Diet Assoc. 97:S24–S30.

45. Crighton IL, Dowsett M, Hunter M et al. (1992). The effect of a low-fat diet on hormone levels in healthy pre- and postmenopausal women: Relevance for breast cancer. Eur J Cancer. 28A:2024–2027.

46. Wu AH, Pike MC, Stram DO. (1999). Meta-analysis: Dietary fat intake, serum estrogen levels, and the risk of breast cancer. J Natl Cancer Inst. 91:529–534.

47. Goldin BR, Adlercreutz H, Gorbach SL et al. (1986). The relationship between estrogen levels and diets of Caucasian American and Oriental immigrant women. Am J Clin Nutr. 44:945–953.

48. Kaneda N, Nagata C, Kabuto M, Shimizu H. (1997). Fat and fiber intakes in relation to serum estrogen concentration in premenopausal Japanese women. Nutr Cancer. 27:279–283.

49. Nagata C, Takatsuka N, Kawakami N, Shimizu H. (2000). Total and monounsaturated fat intake and serum estrogen concentrations in premenopausal Japanese women. Nutr Cancer. 38:37–39.

50. Ingram DM, Bennett FC, Willcox D, de Klerk N. (1987). Effect of low-fat diet on female sex hormone levels. J Natl Cancer Inst. 79:1225–1229.

51. Rose DP, Boyar AP, Cohen C, Strong LE. (1987). Effect of a low-fat diet on hormone levels in women with cystic breast disease. I. Serum steroids and gonadotropins. J Natl Cancer Inst. 78:623–626.

52. Williams CM, Maunder K, Theale D. (1989). The effect of a low-fat diet on luteal-phase prolactin and oestradiol concentrations and erythrocyte phospholipids in normal premenopausal women. Br J Nutr. 61:651–661.

53. Longcope C, Gorbach S, Goldin B et al. (1987). The effect of a low fat diet on estrogen metabolism. J Clin Endocrinol Metab. 64:1246–1250.

54. Boyar AP, Rose DP, Loughridge JR et al. (1988). Response to a diet low in total fat in women with postmenopausal breast cancer: A pilot study. Nutr Cancer. 11:93–99.

55. Prentice R, Thompson D, Clifford C et al. (1990). Dietary fat reduction and plasma estradiol concentration in healthy postmenopausal women. The Women's Health Trial Study Group. J Natl Cancer Inst. 82:129–134.

56. Rose DP, Connolly JM, Chlebowski RT et al. (1993). The effects of a low-fat dietary intervention and tamoxifen adjuvant therapy on the serum estrogen and sex hormone-binding globulin concentrations of postmenopausal breast cancer patients. Breast Cancer Res Treat. 27:253–262.

57. Holmes MD, Spiegelman D, Willett WC et al. (2000). Dietary fat intake and endogenous sex steroid hormone levels in postmenopausal women. J Clin Oncol. 18:3668–3676.

58. Hamalainen E, Adlercreutz H, Puska P, Pietinen P. (1984). Diet and serum sex hormones in healthy men. J Steroid Biochem. 20:459–464.

59. Reed MJ, Cheng RW, Simmonds M et al. (1987). Dietary lipids: An additional regulator of plasma levels of sex hormone binding globulin. J Clin Endocrinol Metab. 64:1083–1085.

60. Meikle AW, Stringham JD, Woodward MG, McMurry MP. (1990). Effects of a fat-containing meal on sex hormones in men. Metabolism. 39:943–946.

61. Dorgan JF, Reichman ME, Judd JT et al. (1996). Relation of energy, fat, and fiber intakes to plasma concentrations of estrogens and androgens in premenopausal women. Am J Clin Nutr. 64:25–31.

62. Nagata C, Takatsuka N, Kawakami N, Shimizu H. (2000). Relationships between types of fat consumed and serum estrogen and androgen concentrations in Japanese men. Nutr Cancer. 38:163–167.

63. Bennett FC, Ingram DM. (1990). Diet and female sex hormone concentrations: An intervention study for the type of fat consumed. Am J Clin Nutr. 52:808–812.

64. Nielsen NH, Hansen JP. (1980). Breast cancer in Greenland—Selected epidemiological, clinical, and histological features. J Cancer Res Clin Oncol. 98:287–299.

65. Prentice RL. (2000). Future possibilities in the prevention of breast cancer: Fat and fiber and breast cancer research. Breast Cancer Res. 2:268–276.

66. Feng W, Marshall R, Lewis-Barned NJ, Goulding A. (1993). Low follicular oestrogen levels in New Zealand women consuming high fibre diets: A risk factor for osteopenia? NZ Med J. 106:419–422.

67. Rose DP, Goldman M, Connolly JM, Strong LE. (1991). High-fiber diet reduces serum estrogen concentrations in premenopausal women. Am J Clin Nutr. 54:520–525.

68. Rose DP, Lubin M, Connolly JM. (1997). Effects of diet supplementation with wheat bran on serum estrogen levels in the follicular and luteal phases of the menstrual cycle. *Nutrition.* 13:535–539.

69. Stark AH, Switzer BR, Atwood JR *et al.* (1998). Estrogen profiles in postmenopausal African-American women in a wheat bran fiber intervention study. *Nutr Cancer.* 31:138–142.

70. Tariq N, Jenkins DJ, Vidgen E *et al.* (2000). Effect of soluble and insoluble fiber diets on serum prostate specific antigen in men. *J Urol.* 163:114–118.

71. Kappas A, Anderson KE, Conney AH *et al.* (1983). Nutrition-endocrine interactions: Induction of reciprocal changes in the delta 4–5 alpha-reduction of testosterone and the cytochrome P-450-dependent oxidation of estradiol by dietary macronutrients in man. *Proc Natl Acad Sci USA.* 80:7646–7649.

72. Anderson KE, Kappas A, Conney AH *et al.* (1984). The influence of dietary protein and carbohydrate on the principal oxidative biotransformations of estradiol in normal subjects. *J Clin Endocrinol Metab.* 59:103–107.

73. Anderson KE, Rosner W, Khan MS *et al.* (1987). Diet-hormone interactions: Protein/carbohydrate ratio alters reciprocally the plasma levels of testosterone and cortisol and their respective binding globulins in man. *Life Sci.* 40:1761–1768.

74. Field AE, Colditz GA, Willett WC *et al.* (1994). The relation of smoking, age, relative weight, and dietary intake to serum adrenal steroids, sex hormones, and sex hormone-binding globulin in middle-aged men. *J Clin Endocrinol Metab.* 79:1310–1316.

75. Tamimi R, Mucci LA, Spanos E *et al.* (2001). Testosterone and oestradiol in relation to tobacco smoking, body mass index, energy consumption and nutrient intake among adult men. *Eur J Cancer Prev.* 10:275–280.

76. Salvini S, Stampfer MJ, Barbieri RL, Hennekens CH. (1992). Effects of age, smoking, and vitamins on plasma DHEAS levels: A cross-sectional study in men. *J Clin Endocrinol Metab.* 74:139–143.

77. Hartman TJ, Dorgan JF, Virtamo J *et al.* (1999). Association between serum alpha-tocopherol and serum androgens and estrogens in older men. *Nutr Cancer.* 35:10–15.

78. Hartman TJ, Dorgan JF, Woodson K *et al.* (2001). Effects of long-term alpha-tocopherol supplementation on serum hormones in older men. *Prostate.* 46:33–38.

79. Heinonen OP, Albanes D, Virtamo J *et al.* (1998). Prostate cancer and supplementation with alpha-tocopherol and beta-carotene: Incidence and mortality in a controlled trial. *J Natl Cancer Inst.* 90:440–446.

80. Sakamoto W, Fujie K, Nishihira J *et al.* (1991). Inhibition of PGE2 production in macrophages from vitamin E-treated rats. *Prostaglandins Leukot Essent Fatty Acids.* 44:89–92.

81. Ratner A, Wilson MC, Srivastava L, Peake GT. (1974). Stimulatory effects of prostaglandin e-1 on rat anterior pituitary cyclic AMP and luteinizing hormone release. *Prostaglandins.* 5:165–171.

82. Longnecker MP. (1994). Alcoholic beverage consumption in relation to risk of breast cancer: Meta-analysis and review. *Cancer Causes Control.* 5:73–82.

83. Muti P, Trevisan M, Micheli A *et al.* (1998). Alcohol consumption and total estradiol in premenopausal women. *Cancer Epidemiol Biomarkers Prev.* 7:189–193.

84. Mendelson JH, Lukas SE, Mello NK *et al.* (1988). Acute alcohol effects on plasma estradiol levels in women. *Psychopharmacology [Berl].* 94:464–467.

85. Dorgan JF, Reichman ME, Judd JT *et al.* (1994). The relation of reported alcohol ingestion to plasma levels of estrogens and androgens in premenopausal women [Maryland, United States]. *Cancer Causes Control.* 5:53–60.

86. Reichman ME, Judd JT, Longcope C *et al.* (1993). Effects of alcohol consumption on plasma and urinary hormone concentrations in premenopausal women. *J Natl Cancer Inst.* 85:722–727.

87. Sarkola T, Makisalo H, Fukunaga T, Eriksson CJ. (1999). Acute effect of alcohol on estradiol, estrone, progesterone, prolactin, cortisol, and luteinizing hormone in premenopausal women. *Alcohol Clin Exp Res.* 23:976–982.

88. Eriksson CJ, Fukunaga T, Lindman R. (1994). Sex hormone response to alcohol. *Nature.* 369:711.

89. Sarkola T, Fukunaga T, Makisalo H, Peter Eriksson CJ. (2000). Acute effect of alcohol on androgens in premenopausal women. *Alcohol Alcohol.* 35:84–90.

90. Sarkola T, Adlercreutz H, Heinonen S, Eriksson CJ. (2001). Alcohol intake, androgen and glucocorticoid steroids in premenopausal women using oral contraceptives: An interventional study. *J Steroid Biochem Mol Biol.* 78:157–165.

91. Sarkola T, Adlercreutz H, Heinonen S *et al.* (2001). The role of the liver in the acute effect of alcohol on androgens in women. *J Clin Endocrinol Metab.* 86:1981–1985.

92. Gavaler JS, Love K, Van Thiel D *et al.* (1991). An international study of the relationship between alcohol consumption and postmenopausal estradiol levels. *Alcohol Alcohol.* (Suppl 1):327–330.

93. Gavaler JS, Van Thiel DH. (1992). The association between moderate alcoholic beverage consumption and serum estradiol and testosterone levels in normal postmenopausal women: Relationship to the literature. *Alcohol Clin Exp Res.* 16:87–92.

94. Gavaler JS, Deal SR, Van Thiel DH *et al.* (1993). Alcohol and estrogen levels in postmenopausal women: The spectrum of effect. *Alcohol Clin Exp Res.* 17:786–790.

95. Hankinson SE, Willett WC, Manson JE *et al.* (1995). Alcohol, height, and adiposity in relation to estrogen and prolactin levels in postmenopausal women. *J Natl Cancer Inst.* 87:1297–1302.

96. Jasonni VM, Bulletti C, Bolelli GF *et al.* (1983). Estrone sulfate, estrone and estradiol concentrations in normal and cirrhotic postmenopausal women. *Steroids.* 41:569–573.

97. Gavaler JS, Van Thiel DH. (1992). Hormonal status of postmenopausal women with alcohol-induced cirrhosis: Further findings and a review of the literature. *Hepatology.* 16:312–319.

98. Gavaler JS. (1995). Alcohol effects on hormone levels in normal postmenopausal women and in postmenopausal women with alcohol-induced cirrhosis. *Recent Dev Alcohol.* 12:199–208.

99. Ginsburg ES, Walsh BW, Gao X *et al.* (1995). The effect of acute ethanol ingestion on estrogen levels in postmenopausal women using transdermal estradiol. *J Soc Gynecol Investig.* 2:26–29.

100. Ginsburg ES, Mello NK, Mendelson JH *et al.* (1996). Effects of alcohol ingestion on estrogens in postmenopausal women. *JAMA.* 276:1747–1751.

101. Feigelson HS, Calle EE, Robertson AS *et al.* (2001). Alcohol consumption increases the risk of fatal breast cancer [United States]. *Cancer Causes Control.* 12:895–902.

102. Stampfer MJ, Colditz GA, Willett WC *et al.* (1988). A prospective study of moderate alcohol consumption and the risk of coronary disease and stroke in women. *N Engl J Med.* 319:267–273.

103. Southren AL, Gordon GG, Olivo J *et al.* (1973). Androgen metabolism in cirrhosis of the liver. *Metabolism.* 22:695–701.

104. Gordon GG, Altman K, Southren AL *et al.* (1976). Effect of alcohol [ethanol] administration on sex-hormone metabolism in normal men. *N Engl J Med.* 295:793–797.

105. Mendelson JH, Mello NK, Ellingboe J. (1977). Effects of acute alcohol intake on pituitary-gonadal hormones in normal human males. *J Pharmacol Exp Ther.* 202:676–682.

106. Mendelson JH, Ellingboe J, Mello NK, Kuehnle J. (1978). Effects of alcohol on plasma testosterone and luteinizing hormone levels. *Alcohol Clin Exp Res.* 2:255–258.

107. Rubin E, Lieber CS, Altman K *et al.* (1976). Prolonged ethanol consumption increases testosterone metabolism in the liver. *Science.* 191:563–564.

108. Frias J, Rodriguez R, Torres JM *et al.* (2000). Effects of acute alcohol intoxication on pituitary-gonadal axis hormones, pituitary-adrenal axis hormones, beta-endorphin and prolactin in human adolescents of both sexes. *Life Sci.* 67:1081–1086.

109. Andersson SH, Cronholm T, Sjovall J. (1986). Effects of ethanol on the levels of unconjugated and conjugated androgens and estrogens in plasma of men. *J Steroid Biochem.* 24:1193–1198.

110. Andersson SH, Cronholm T, Sjovall J. (1987). Effects of ethanol on conjugated gonadal hormones in plasma of men. *Alcohol Alcohol.* (Suppl 1):529–531.

111. Purohit V. (2000). Can alcohol promote aromatization of androgens to estrogens? A review. *Alcohol.* 22:123–127.

112. Kirschner MA, Ertel N, Schneider G. (1981). Obesity, hormones, and cancer. *Cancer Res.* 41:3711–3717.

113. Key TJ, Verkasalo PK, Banks E. (2001). Epidemiology of breast cancer. *Lancet Oncol.* 2:133–140.

114. Longcope C, Baker R, Johnston CC, Jr. (1986). Androgen and estrogen metabolism: Relationship to obesity. *Metabolism.* 35:235–237.

115. Ursin G, Longnecker MP, Haile RW, Greenland S. (1995). A meta-analysis of body mass index and risk of premenopausal breast cancer. *Epidemiology.* 6:137–141.

116. Key TJ, Allen NE, Verkasalo PK, Banks E. (2001). Energy balance and cancer: The role of sex hormones. *Proc Nutr Soc.* 60:81–89.

117. Semmens JB, Rouse IL, Beilin LJ, Masarei JR. (1983). Relationships between age, body weight, physical fitness and sex-hormone-binding globulin capacity. *Clin Chim Acta.* 133:295–300.

118. Gates JR, Parpia B, Campbell TC, Junshi C. (1996). Association of dietary factors and selected plasma variables with sex hormone-binding globulin in rural Chinese women. *Am J Clin Nutr.* 63:22–31.

119. Longcope C, Feldman HA, McKinlay JB, Araujo AB. (2000). Diet and sex hormone-binding globulin. *J Clin Endocrinol Metab.* 85:293–296.

120. Ukkola O, Gagnon J, Rankinen T *et al.* (2001). Age, body mass index, race and other determinants of steroid hormone variability: The HERITAGE Family Study. *Eur J Endocrinol.* 145:1–9.

121. Verkasalo PK, Thomas HV, Appleby PN *et al.* (2001). Circulating levels of sex hormones and their relation to risk factors for breast cancer: A cross-sectional study in 1092 pre- and postmenopausal women [United Kingdom]. *Cancer Causes Control.* 12:47–59.

122. Vermeulen A, Verdonck L. (1978). Sex hormone concentrations in post-menopausal women. *Clin Endocrinol [Oxf].* 9:59–66.

123. Poortman J, Thijssen JH, de Waard F. (1981). Plasma oestrone, oestradiol and androstenedione levels in post-menopausal women: Relation to body weight and height. *Maturitas.* 3:65–71.

124. Cauley JA, Gutai JP, Kuller LH *et al.* (1989). The epidemiology of serum sex hormones in postmenopausal women. *Am J Epidemiol.* 129:1120–1131.

125. Edman CD, MacDonald PC. (1978). Effect of obesity on conversion of plasma androstenedione to estrone in ovulatory and anovulatory young women. *Am J Obstet Gynecol.* 130:456–461.

126. MacDonald PC, Edman CD, Hemsell DL *et al.* (1978). Effect of obesity on conversion of plasma androstenedione to estrone in postmenopausal women with and without endometrial cancer. *Am J Obstet Gynecol.* 130:448–455.

127. Fishman J, Boyar RM, Hellman L. (1975). Influence of body weight on estradiol metabolism in young women. *J Clin Endocrinol Metab.* 41:989–991.

128. Schneider J, Bradlow HL, Strain G *et al.* (1983). Effects of obesity on estradiol metabolism: Decreased formation of nonuterotropic metabolites. *J Clin Endocrinol Metab.* 56:973–978.

129. Hershcopf RJ, Bradlow HL. (1987). Obesity, diet, endogenous estrogens, and the risk of hormone-sensitive cancer. *Am J Clin Nutr.* 45:283–289.

130. Samojlik E, Kirschner MA, Silber D *et al.* (1984). Elevated production and metabolic clearance rates of androgens in morbidly obese women. *J Clin Endocrinol Metab.* 59:949–954.

131. Wajchenberg BL, Marcondes JA, Mathor MB *et al.* (1989). Free testosterone levels during the menstrual cycle in obese versus normal women. *Fertil Steril.* 51:535–537.

132. Kirschner MA, Samojlik E, Drejka M *et al.* (1990). Androgen-estrogen metabolism in women with upper body versus lower body obesity. *J Clin Endocrinol Metab.* 70:473–479.

133. Sowers M, Beebe J, McConnell D *et al.* (2001). Testosterone concentrations in women aged 25–50 years: Associations with lifestyle, body composition, and ovarian status. *Am J Epidemiol.* 153:256–264.

134. Kirschner MA, Schneider G, Ertel NH, Worton E. (1982). Obesity, androgens, estrogens, and cancer risk. *Cancer Res.* 42:3281s–3285s.

135. Schneider G, Kirschner MA, Berkowitz R, Ertel NH. (1979). Increased estrogen production in obese men. *J Clin Endocrinol Metab.* 48:633–638.

136. Brind J, Strain G, Miller L *et al.* (1990). Obese men have elevated plasma levels of estrone sulfate. *Int J Obes.* 14:483–486.

137. Kley HK, Deselaers T, Peerenboom H, Kruskemper HL. (1980). Enhanced conversion of androstenedione to estrogens in obese males. *J Clin Endocrinol Metab.* 51:1128–1132.

138. Kley HK, Edelmann P, Kruskemper HL. (1980). Relationship of plasma sex hormones to different parameters of obesity in male subjects. *Metabolism.* 29:1041–1045.

139. Glass AR, Swerdloff RS, Bray GA *et al.* (1977). Low serum testosterone and sex-hormone-binding-globulin in massively obese men. *J Clin Endocrinol Metab.* 45:1211–1219.

140. Zumoff B, Strain GW, Miller LK *et al.* (1990). Plasma free and non-sex-hormone-binding-globulin-bound testosterone are decreased in obese men in proportion to their degree of obesity. *J Clin Endocrinol Metab.* 71:929–931.

141. Vermeulen A. (1996). Decreased androgen levels and obesity in men. *Ann Med* 28:13–15.

142. Kirschner MA, Samojlik E. Sex hormone metabolism in upper and lower body obesity. *Int J Obes.* 15(Suppl 2):101–108.

143. Killinger DW, Perel E, Daniilescu D *et al.* (1987). The relationship between aromatase activity and body fat distribution. *Steroids.* 50:61–72.

144. Evans DJ, Hoffmann RG, Kalkhoff RK, Kissebah AH. (1983). Relationship of androgenic activity to body fat topography, fat cell morphology, and metabolic aberrations in premenopausal women. *J Clin Endocrinol Metab.* 57:304–310.

145. Kaye SA, Folsom AR, Soler JT *et al.* (1991). Associations of body mass and fat distribution with sex hormone concentrations in postmenopausal women. *Int J Epidemiol.* 20:151–156.

146. Dai R, Jacobson KA, Robinson RC, Friedman FK. (1997). Differential effects of flavonoids on testosterone-metabolizing cytochrome P450s. *Life Sci.* 61:PL75–PL80.

147. Baker ME. Flavonoids as hormones. (1998). A perspective from an analysis of molecular fossils. *Adv Exp Med Biol.* 439:249–267.

148. Collins-Burow BM, Burow ME, Duong BN, McLachlan JA. (2000). Estrogenic and antiestrogenic activities of flavonoid phytochemicals through estrogen receptor binding-dependent and -independent mechanisms. *Nutr Cancer.* 38:229–244.

149. Eng ET, Williams D, Mandava U, Kirma N *et al.* (2001). Suppression of aromatase [estrogen synthetase] by red wine phytochemicals. *Breast Cancer Res Treat.* 67:133–146.

150. Grube BJ, Eng ET, Kao YC *et al.* (2001). White button mushroom phytochemicals inhibit aromatase activity and breast cancer cell proliferation. *J Nutr.* 131:3288–3293.

151. Ikeda K, Arao Y, Otsuka H *et al.* (2002). Terpenoids found in the umbelliferae family act as agonists/antagonists for ER[alpha] and ERbeta: Differential transcription activity between ferutinine-liganded ER[alpha] and ERbeta. *Biochem Biophys Res Commun.* 291:354–360.

152. Setchell KD. (1998). Phytoestrogens: The biochemistry, physiology, and implications for human health of soy isoflavones. *Am J Clin Nutr.* 68:1333S–1346S.

153. Reinli K, Block G. (1996). Phytoestrogen content of foods—a compendium of literature values. *Nutr Cancer.* 26:123–148.

154. Axelson M, Sjovall J, Gustafsson BE, Setchell KD. (1982). Origin of lignans in mammals and identification of a precursor from plants. *Nature.* 298:659–660.

155. Adlercreutz CH, Goldin BR, Gorbach SL *et al.* (1995). Soybean phytoestrogen intake and cancer risk. *J Nutr.* 125:757S–770S.

156. Jacobsen BK, Knutsen SF, Fraser GE. (1998). Does high soy milk intake reduce prostate cancer incidence? The Adventist Health Study [United States]. *Cancer Causes Control.* 9:553–557.

157. Kurzer MS. (2002). Hormonal effects of soy in premenopausal women and men. *J Nutr.* 132:570S–573S.

158. Nagata C, Kabuto M, Kurisu Y, Shimizu H. (1997). Decreased serum estradiol concentration associated with high dietary intake of soy products in premenopausal Japanese women. *Nutr Cancer.* 29:228–233.

159. Xu X, Duncan AM, Merz BE, Kurzer MS. (1998). Effects of soy isoflavones on estrogen and phytoestrogen metabolism in premenopausal women. *Cancer Epidemiol Biomarkers Prev.* 7:1101–1108.

160. Lu LJ, Cree M, Josyula S, Nagamani M *et al.* (2000). Increased urinary excretion of 2-hydroxyestrone but not 16alpha-hydroxyestrone in premenopausal women during a soya diet containing isoflavones. *Cancer Res.* 60:1299–1305.

161. Brezezinski A AH, Shaoul R, Rosler A *et al.* (1997). Short-term effects of phytoestrogen-rich diet on postmenopausal women. *The Journal of the North American Menopause Society.* 4:89–94.

162. Petrakis NL, Barnes S, King EB *et al.* (1996). Stimulatory influence of soy protein isolate on breast secretion in pre- and postmenopausal women. *Cancer Epidemiol Biomarkers Prev.* 5:785–794.

163. Wilcox G, Wahlqvist ML, Burger HG, Medley G. (1990). Oestrogenic effects of plant foods in postmenopausal women. *BMJ.* 301:905–906.

164. Baird DD, Umbach DM, Lansdell L *et al.* (1995). Dietary intervention study to assess estrogenicity of dietary soy among postmenopausal women. *J Clin Endocrinol Metab.* 80:1685–1690.

165. Persky VW, Turyk ME, Wang L *et al.* (2002). Effect of soy protein on endogenous hormones in postmenopausal women. *Am J Clin Nutr.* 75:145–153.

166. Pino AM, Valladares LE, Palma MA *et al.* (2000). Dietary isoflavones affect sex hormone-binding globulin levels in postmenopausal women. *J Clin Endocrinol Metab.* 85:2797–2800.

167. Duncan AM, Underhill KE, Xu X *et al.* (1999). Modest hormonal effects of soy isoflavones in postmenopausal women. *J Clin Endocrinol Metab.* 84:3479–3484.

168. Xu X, Duncan AM, Wangen KE, Kurzer MS. (2000). Soy consumption alters endogenous estrogen metabolism in postmenopausal women. *Cancer Epidemiol Biomarkers Prev.* 9:781–786.

169. Nagata C, Inaba S, Kawakami N *et al.* (2000). Inverse association of soy product intake with serum androgen and estrogen concentrations in Japanese men. *Nutr Cancer.* 36:14–18.

170. Nagata C, Takatsuka N, Shimizu H *et al.* (2001). Effect of soymilk consumption on serum estrogen and androgen concentrations in Japanese men. *Cancer Epidemiol Biomarkers Prev.* 10:179–184.

171. Habito RC, Montalto J, Leslie E, Ball MJ. (2000). Effects of replacing meat with soyabean in the diet on sex hormone concentrations in healthy adult males. *Br J Nutr.* 84:557–563.

172. Mitchell JH, Cawood E, Kinniburgh D *et al.* (2001). Effect of a phytoestrogen food supplement on reproductive health in normal males. *Clin Sci [Lond].* 100:613–618.

173. Phipps WR, Martini MC, Lampe JW *et al.* (1993). Effect of flax seed ingestion on the menstrual cycle. *J Clin Endocrinol Metab.* 77:1215–1219.

174. Hutchins AM, Martini MC, Olson BA *et al.* (2001). Flaxseed consumption influences endogenous hormone concentrations in postmenopausal women. *Nutr Cancer.* 39:58–65.

175. Haggans CJ, Travelli EJ, Thomas W *et al.* (2000). The effect of flaxseed and wheat bran consumption on urinary estrogen metabolites in premenopausal women. *Cancer Epidemiol Biomarkers Prev.* 9:719–725.

176. Haggans CJ, Hutchins AM, Olson BA *et al.* (1999). Effect of flaxseed consumption on urinary estrogen metabolites in postmenopausal women. *Nutr Cancer.* 33:188–195.

177. Shultz TD, Bonorden WR, Seaman WR. (1991). Effect of short-term flax-seed consumption on lignan and sex hormone metabolism in men. *Nutrition Research.* 11:1089–1109.

178. Demark-Wahnefried W, Price DT, Polascik TJ *et al.* (2001). Pilot study of dietary fat restriction and flaxseed supplementation in men with prostate cancer before surgery: Exploring the effects on hormonal levels, prostate-specific antigen, and histopathologic features. *Urology.* 58:47–52.

179. Fowke JH, Longcope C, Hebert JR. (2000). Brassica vegetable consumption shifts estrogen metabolism in healthy postmenopausal women. *Cancer Epidemiol Biomarkers Prev.* 9:773–779.

180. Kall MA, Vang O, Clausen J. (1996). Effects of dietary broccoli on human *in vivo* drug metabolizing enzymes: Evaluation of caffeine, oestrone and chlorzoxazone metabolism. *Carcinogenesis.* 17:793–799.

181. Michnovicz JJ, Adlercreutz H, Bradlow HL. (1997). Changes in levels of urinary estrogen metabolites after oral indole-3-carbinol treatment in humans. *J Natl Cancer Inst.* 89:718–723.

182. Bradlow HL, Michnovicz JJ, Halper M *et al.* (1994). Long-term responses of women to indole-3-carbinol or a high fiber diet. *Cancer Epidemiol Biomarkers Prev.* 3:591–595.

71

Nutrition and Cancers of the Breast, Endometrium, and Ovary

CHERYL L. ROCK, PhD, RD* AND WENDY DEMARK-WAHNEFRIED, PhD, RD**

*Associate Professor, Department of Family and Preventive Medicine, University of California at San Diego, La Jolla, CA
**Department of Surgery, Duke University Medical Center, Durham, NC

I. Introduction

Carcinomas of the breast, endometrium, and ovary are hormone-related cancers that have biologic similarities. Among U.S. women, breast cancer is far more common than endometrial or ovarian cancers. In 2004, it is estimated that approximately 215,990 women will be diagnosed with breast cancer, thus comprising roughly 32% of the incident cancers among females [1]. In contrast, cancers of the endometrium (uterine corpus) and ovary are estimated to comprise approximately 6% and 4% of female cancers, respectively. Due to differential effectiveness of treatments, the mortality estimates for these cancers vary a great deal [1,2]. Breast cancer will be the cause of death for approximately 40,110 women during 2004 (approximately 15% of cancer-related deaths among U.S. females), whereas ovarian and endometrial cancers account for approximately 6% and 3% of cancer-related mortality among women, respectively.

Breast cancer occurs infrequently in men. In 2004 an estimated 1450 men will be diagnosed with breast cancer, and 470 men will die of this disease [1], accounting for <2% of all malignancies and only 0.2% of cancer deaths in men. Although male breast cancer is uncommon, men tend to have a less favorable outcome than women. Older age and advanced stage at diagnosis largely are responsible for these gender differences [3,4]. However, anatomic differences between male and female breasts also may contribute to the more aggressive clinical behavior of mammary carcinoma in men [3].

Estrogens are thought to play an important role in breast, endometrial and ovarian cancers [3,5]. Normal cell proliferation and differentiation in these tissues is highly responsive to estrogens and the other gonadal hormones, as well as cellular factors and mitogens that affect growth regulation and apoptosis and thus influence carcinogenesis in all cell types. In addition to the ovarian steroids, other growth factors and mitogens influenced by nutritional factors and dietary patterns also appear to play an important role in the initiation and promotion of breast cancer. Two factors that are currently of intense scientific interest are insulin and insulin-like growth factor I (IGF-I), and the interactions of these factors with adiposity and weight gain [6,7].

Inherited variations in other biochemic or metabolic pathways relevant to mammary, endometrial and ovarian cell biology, such as those involved in estrogen metabolism or the growth factor axis, are currently under study [8], and their contributions to genetic risk of hormone-related cancers are not yet known. Interactions between genetic and dietary factors also are likely to be among the determinants of risk for these cancers, and these interactions are currently the focus of intensive research [9,10].

Diet and/or nutritional status are presumed to play a major role in the risk and progression of the hormone-related cancers, either through influence on the hormonal milieu, gene expression or via direct effects. The incidence of these cancers varies widely by geographic location and with migration, so environmental factors appear to contribute substantially to risk. Over the past several decades, there has been a considerable amount of research exploring the possible relationships between various nutritional factors and breast cancer. Only a limited amount of effort has been focused specifically on nutritional factors and breast cancer in males. However, female and male breast cancer share several clinical and biologic features, and the available epidemiologic evidence is similar; thus, findings from studies focused on nutrition and breast cancer in women are presumed to be relevant to breast cancer in men. Compared to the amount of research on breast cancer, far fewer studies have examined the relationship between nutritional factors and risk and/or progression of endometrial and ovarian cancers. However, significant associations are suggested by the extant data.

This chapter reviews and summarizes evidence on the relationships between nutritional factors and breast, endometrial and ovarian cancers. The emphasis is on clinical and epidemiologic studies, with the goal of identifying clinically useful strategies for prevention and patient management, as well as describing future directions for research.

II. Nutritional Factors and Breast Cancer

A. Nutritional Factors and Primary Breast Cancer Risk

1. Height, Weight and Body Fat Distribution

Several studies have found positive associations between adult height and breast cancer [11–17]. This association appears significant and has been noted consistently for postmenopausal disease, whereas it is less clear for breast cancer occurring among younger women. In a pooled analysis of seven prospective cohort studies that was comprised of 337,819 women and 4385 incident invasive breast cancer cases, a per height increment of 5 cm was associated with a relative risk (RR) of 1.03 (95% confidence interval ([CI] 0.96, 1.10) in premenopausal women and a RR of 1.07 (95% CI 1.03, 1.12) in postmenopausal women [18]. It is hypothesized that growth factors that drive skeletal development also may stimulate the proliferation of mammary stem cells [12]. Although these growth factors may be more controlled by heredity than diet, recognition of height as a risk factor may enhance the identification of high-risk women who then could be targeted for interventions. Other skeletal indices, such as increased elbow breadth (a frame size marker), femur length and bone density also have been associated with increased risk [14,19].

A clear discrepancy exists with regard to adiposity and its ability to affect risk for pre- vs postmenopausal disease. Leanness is a risk factor for premenopausal breast cancer, whereas obesity serves as a risk factor for postmenopausal disease [11,20,21]. In the pooled analysis noted previously, women with a body mass index (BMI) of >31 kg/m² had an RR of 0.54 (95% C.I. 0.34, 0.85] for premenopausal breast cancer, whereas women whose BMI was >28 kg/m² had a RR of 1.26 (95% CI 1.09, 1.46) for postmenopausal disease [18]. Although it has been postulated that leanness may enhance early detection among younger women [12], a more prevalent view is that premenopausal breast cancer may be governed more by genetic predisposition and growth factors, whereas postmenopausal breast cancer may be influenced more by long-term exposure to the interacting effects of ovarian steroid hormones and lifestyle factors [22,23].

Two observational studies that focused specifically on male breast cancer indicate that the relationship between obesity and risk for breast cancer in men is similar to the relationship observed in postmenopausal breast cancer in women. In a case-control study of 178 men who died of breast cancer and 512 men who died of other causes, Hsing et al [24] found increased risk for men who were described by their next of kin as being very overweight (odds ratio [OR] 2.3, 95% CI 1.1, 5.0). Ewertz et al [25] found obesity 10 years before diagnosis associated with increased risk for breast cancer in men (OR 3.3, 95% CI 1.0, 4.5) in a population-based, case-control study of 156 incident cases of male breast cancer and 468 matched controls.

Because body weight fluctuates throughout life, it is conceivable that risk may be modified by body weight status at differing ages. Studies that have assessed weight prior to adulthood suggest that obesity during childhood and adolescence may be protective [26,27]. This relationship appears logical for premenopausal breast cancer, in which obesity is a protective factor. However, given the relationship between increased weight and early menarche, as well as increased weight and postmenopausal breast cancer, it is difficult to reason why early obesity would be protective for postmenopausal disease. Studies, however, indicate that obese girls have significantly fewer ovulatory cycles and thereby have lower circulating levels of both estrogen and progesterone—hormones associated with mammary proliferation [28,29].Upon attainment of adulthood, there appears to be a consistent finding of weight gain and increased body weight being highly associated with increased risk for postmenopausal cancer [11,13,18,20,30–32]. This increased risk may be largely explained by the fact that as women age, their circulating levels of estrogen become more influenced by estrogens produced by adipose tissue rather than those produced by the ovary [22,31]. Weight gain after age 40 also is more likely to be deposited in an android vs gynoid pattern, and hence may promote insulin resistance and the increased production of insulin and insulin-like growth factors that may act synergistically with estrogen to confer risk [11,20,30].

Previous research suggests that body fat distribution plays a significant role in predicting risk. A majority of studies suggest that central or visceral obesity (primarily assessed via waist–hip

ratio) as an additional risk factor [11,15,33,34]. Studies by Sellers et al [35] and London et al [36] suggest that risk conferred by either obesity or increased waist–hip ratio may be further exacerbated by a positive family history.

2. Dietary Composition

In ecologic studies, a 5-fold difference in breast cancer mortality rates has been observed across countries, and dietary patterns are a major aspect of the environmental exposures that differ across these countries [37,38]. Also, risk for breast cancer increases upon relocation from low-risk countries to high-risk countries, concurrent with the adoption of the dietary and lifestyle patterns of the new locale [38–41]. These findings from hypothesis-generating ecologic and migration studies have inspired much research effort aimed toward identifying the specific dietary factors that increase risk for breast cancer.

Most of the observational studies that have examined the link between dietary intake and breast cancer risk have relied on self-reported dietary intake data, and only a limited number of studies have utilized serologic biomarkers of diet. Self-reported dietary intakes should be interpreted as estimates that may allow ranking rather than producing absolute values, even when the best developed methodologies are used. Thus, a high risk for reporting bias and misclassification of subjects is inherent in this type of research.

The possible link between dietary fat intake and risk for breast cancer has historically received the most attention. Several comprehensive reviews and discussions of the evidence reported to date, and the challenges in interpreting these data, have been published [42–48]. A major issue in the interpretation of the data suggesting an adverse effect of dietary fat on breast cancer risk is that fat intake, total energy consumption, and adiposity are typically inextricably linked, therefore, demonstrating an independent effect of total dietary fat per se is a challenge.

Despite a strong and direct link between fat intake and breast cancer risk in ecologic studies, this relationship has generally not been as evident in observational studies conducted within populations, particularly in cohort studies. For example, in a pooled analysis of a U.S. cohort of 337,819 U.S. women with 4980 incident cases [49], the multivariate RR of breast cancer was 1.05 (95% CI 0.94, 1.16), when comparing women in the highest quintile of energy-adjusted total fat intake to women in the lowest quintile. Relative risks for intakes of saturated, mono-unsaturated, and polyunsaturated fat also were nonsignificant. In a single large cohort study of 88,795 women, of whom 2956 were diagnosed with breast cancer over a 14-year follow-up, those consuming 30–35% energy from fat had an RR of 1.15 (95% CI 0.73, 1.80) compared to women consuming ≤20% energy from fat [50]. In that study, specific types of fat also were not found to be associated with risk of breast cancer, although a small but significant increase in risk was associated with intake of omega-3 fatty acids from fish (RR 1.09, 95% CI 1.03, 1.16), and trans fatty acid intake had a slightly protective effect (RR 0.92, 95% CI 0.86, 0.98). Disparate findings on the association between fat intake and breast cancer risk in ecologic vs within-population cohort studies have been attributed to the limited range of fat intake that is typically reported by the homogeneous within-country populations and also to the underreporting of high-fat foods, which may limit the capability to detect an effect and also increases risk of classification errors [43].

Laboratory animal studies quite consistently demonstrate that except for a specific tumor-promoting effect of linoleic acid, the effects of dietary fat on tumor growth is attributable to the high energy content of a high-fat diet, rather than the content of fat [51]. In laboratory animal models, omega-6 fatty acids (i.e., linoleic acid) have been shown to promote tumor development, particularly in comparison to omega-3 fatty acid-rich diets [47,48,52], theoretically by influencing tumor eicosanoid production and possibly other cellular mechanisms (e.g., protein kinase C, membrane permeability). However, epidemiologic studies have not consistently revealed a protective pattern of specific fatty acids, so the issue remains unresolved.

Given that a reduction in fat intake has been hypothesized to influence breast cancer risk by reducing serum estrogen concentrations, various feeding studies and small diet intervention trials have examined the effect of dietary fat reduction on serum estrogen levels. Low-fat diets were associated with an average 13% reduction in serum estradiol concentration in a meta-analysis of several small feeding studies [53]. However, significant weight loss occurred in the majority of the studies in which serum estradiol was significantly reduced, and dietary fiber was concurrently increased in eight of the 13 studies included in the analysis. Thus, an energy deficit, weight loss, or increased fiber intake could be the more important factors promoting a reduction in hormone levels, and an independent effect of fat intake cannot be assumed to be the primary factor modulating serum estrogens.

Several epidemiologic studies have examined the association between vegetable and fruit intake and risk for primary breast cancer. Two large observational studies addressed this relationship using combined and pooled data. These pooled studies were based on combinations of published observational studies with different study designs, and they produced somewhat divergent results. In a meta-analysis of 26 studies (21 case-control and five cohort studies) published from 1982 to 1997, the relationships between risk for breast cancer and intakes of vegetables, fruit, beta-carotene and vitamin C were examined [54]. High (vs low) consumption of vegetables exhibited the strongest protective effect (RR 0.75, 95% CI 0.66, 0.85), whereas the relationship with fruit consumption was not significant (RR 0.94, 95% CI 0.74, 1.11) [54]. Data from 11 of these studies allowed analysis of beta-carotene intake, which was significantly inversely associated with risk (RR 0.82, 95% CI 0.76, 0.91 for approximately >7000 vs <1000 μg/day). Results from this meta-analysis are very similar to a summary based on 19 case-control and three cohort studies reported in 1997 [55], which found at least a 25% reduction in risk in the majority of the studies and greater consistency for vegetable compared with fruit intake. In a subsequent pooled analysis of 7377 incident breast cancer cases from women enrolled in eight prospective cohort studies, the protective effect of total fruit and vegetable intake was found to be small and nonsignificant (RR 0.93, 95% CI 0.86, 1.00 for highest vs lowest quintiles) [56]. Differences in the study designs and in the approaches used to estimate intake likely contribute to these inconsistent results. The pooled analysis that relied exclusively on data from cohort studies utilizes a better study design, because the dietary data were collected prior to diagnosis. However, the number of fruit and vegetable questions on the

various instruments used to collect the dietary data across these cohort studies varied over 4-fold, and combining widely disparate ranges of servings and types of vegetables and foods may have limited the capability of identifying a relationship with risk. To date, only one study has explored the association between intake of selected foods and male breast cancer [24]. In that study, nonsignificant protective effects were suggested for intake of vegetables (OR 0.5, 95% CI 0.2, 1.7, for 7+ times/week vs <1 time/week), and to a lesser extent, intake of fruit (OR 0.8, 95% CI 0.4, 1.3 for 7+ times/week vs <1 time/day). Point estimates of red meat consumption from that study also suggested a nonsignificant direct association with risk for breast cancer in these men (OR 1.8, 95% CI 0.6, 4.9, for 7+ servings per week vs <1 serving/week) [24].

Fewer studies in which tissue concentrations of carotenoids (a marker of vegetable and fruit intake) have been quantified and analyzed in relation to risk for breast cancer have been reported. These have often (but not always) suggested a protective effect of higher concentrations of these compounds, indicative of a diet high in vegetables and fruit [57–61]. In a prospective cohort study that examined this relationship [61], the OR for the lowest vs highest quartile of total serum carotenoids was 2.31 (95% CI 1.35, 3.96), with serum concentrations of beta-carotene (OR 2.21, 95% CI 1.29, 3.79), alpha-carotene (OR 1.99, 95% CI 1.18, 3.34), and lutein (OR 2.08, 95% CI 1.11, 3.90) inversely associated with risk.

Several biologically feasible mechanisms and supportive laboratory evidence for constituents of vegetables and fruits have been demonstrated in cell culture. For example, carotenoids have retinoid-like effects on cellular differentiation and also exhibit inhibitory effects on mammary cell growth [62–65]. Antioxidants, such as vitamin C, may reduce the risk for breast cancer by protecting against DNA damage and other free-radical-induced cellular changes associated with neoplasia. Vegetables of the Brassica genus, such as broccoli, may favorably alter estrogen metabolism via the induction of cytochromes P450 [66].

Alcohol intake has been consistently and positively associated with risk for breast cancer in epidemiologic studies. Pooled analysis of data from cohort studies (N = 22,647) indicates that alcohol intake exhibits a dose response relationship with risk for breast cancer, at least up to 60 g/day [67]. The multivariate adjusted RR for total alcohol intake of 30–60 g/day (approximately 2–5 drinks/day), compared with no alcohol, was 1.41 (95% CI 1.18, 1.69). The prevailing theory is that alcohol intake promotes increased serum estrogen levels, which would theoretically increase risk for breast cancer. This effect of alcohol has been observed in studies of premenopausal women and in postmenopausal women administered hormone replacement but not among postmenopausal women who do not use estrogen replacement therapy [68].

Although an association with intake of folate per se and breast cancer risk has not been consistently observed in epidemiologic studies, results from several cohort studies suggest that dietary folate intake may influence breast cancer risk through an interaction with alcohol [69–71]. Alcohol has well-known effects on folate status by interfering with folate metabolism. In a large prospective U.S. cohort study involving 88,818 women with 3483 incident breast cancer cases over a 16-year follow-up [69], folate intake ≥600 ug/day compared to 150–299 ug/day was associated with a multivariate adjusted RR of 0.55 (95% CI 0.39, 0.76, P=0.01 for trend) among women who consumed ≥15 g/day of alcohol. A similar relationship was identified in a cohort of 41,836 postmenopausal women, in whom the RR of breast cancer associated with low folate intake was 1.08 (95% CI 0.78, 1.49) among nondrinkers, 1.33 (95% CI 0.86, 2.05) among drinkers of ≤4 g alcohol/day, and 1.59 (95% CI 1.05, 2.41) among drinkers of >4 g alcohol/day [71].

As previously noted, dietary fiber also may exert a protective effect against breast cancer. Postulated mechanisms include the effect of fiber on circulating estrogens, as fiber has been shown to bind to estrogen in the enterohepatic circulation and hinder reabsorption [72]. However, case-control and cohort studies that have examined the relationship between fiber intake and risk for breast cancer have generally not found a significant protective effect [42,44].

Evidence from large U.S. cohort and other studies have generally not found significant associations between vitamin E intake and risk for breast cancer [42,73–78]. Similarly, caffeine has not been identified as influencing risk for either breast cancer or fibrocystic breast condition in women [79]. Observational studies that addressed the relationship between meat and/or protein consumption and breast cancer risk in women have produced inconsistent results and generally do not support this relationship [55,80].

Countries that consume greater amounts of soy and soy products, mainly native Japanese and Chinese populations, have historically exhibited the lowest breast cancer mortality rates, when compared to the United States and most European countries [81]. Soy is a rich source of phytoestrogens, and soy isoflavones have been shown to exert hormonal effects in cell culture systems and laboratory animal models [82,83]. Thus, a role in breast cancer prevention for soy and soy isoflavones, as well as other phytoestrogens, has been investigated in numerous laboratory and epidemiologic studies. However, phytoestrogens can act as estrogen agonists as well as antagonists, so it is possible that phytoestrogens could potentially promote mammary neoplasia. This would be most relevant for postmenopausal women, who do not have high levels of endogenous estrogens in the circulation that would compete for estrogen receptor (ER) binding sites. Results from several types of studies, including cell culture, clinical and laboratory animal studies, have produced evidence suggesting the possibility of an adverse effect of soy phytoestrogens on risk and progression of breast cancer, when amounts greater than that provided by the typical Asian diet are consumed [84].

Table 71-1 summarizes the nature of the evidence for a relationship with breast cancer and nutrients and other dietary constituents. A large ongoing clinical trial is currently testing whether diet intervention can modify risk for breast cancer. In the Women's Health Initiative, postmenopausal women age 50–79 are enrolled at 40 clinical centers nationwide into a clinical trial (N=64,000) or an observational study (N=100,000) [85]. One arm of the randomized clinical trial is testing whether a low-fat eating pattern (≤20% of energy from fat, ≥5 servings/day vegetables and fruits, ≥6 servings/day grain products) may help to prevent breast cancer, colorectal cancer and cardiovascular disease. The Canadian Diet and Breast Cancer Prevention Trial, a multicenter randomized controlled study, is testing whether a low-fat

(15% of energy), high-carbohydrate diet intervention can reduce the incidence of breast cancer over 10 years among women age 30–65 who have increased mammographic density [86].

B. Nutritional Factors and Recurrence, Progression and Survival

Breast cancer mortality has been declining, a trend that has been attributed to earlier diagnosis and improvements in initial treatments [87]. A majority of all breast cancers are now diagnosed at a localized stage, with 96% 5-year relative survival rates [88]. As a result, there are increasing numbers of women in the population who are breast cancer survivors and who are at risk for breast cancer recurrence. Recurrence is an important issue in the management of these patients, because the yearly rate of secondary cancer events, even for women who have been diagnosed with very early stage cancers, does not return to the level of similarly aged women who have not been diagnosed with breast cancer [89].

1. Obesity and Overweight

The nutritional factor associated most consistently with reduced likelihood of survival is increased weight at diagnosis. A critical review and analysis of 13 cohort studies and one case-control study on the association between obesity at diagnosis and poor prognosis, published in 1990, concluded that increased body weight exerts a negative, yet modest, prognostic effect [90]. Since that time 26 published studies have examined associations either between premorbid weight status or weight status at the time of diagnosis (estimated by relative weight for height or BMI) and breast cancer recurrence and/or survival. In 17 of the 26 studies, increased BMI and/or body weight significantly increased the risk of recurrent disease or disease progression [91–107], seven studies produced null findings [108–114], and two studies showed a significant inverse association between weight status and local recurrence or survival [115,116]. In those studies that found a significant association, women categorized in the higher (vs lower) levels of obesity typically exhibited a 30–54% increased risk of death. This relationship appears to be more pronounced among women who are diagnosed with early stage disease [91,106] and among those who have ER positive tumors [104]. Although BMI was not found to be a risk factor for increased breast cancer mortality in one study [116], android body fat distribution (higher suprailiac–thigh ratio) was found to be a significant prognostic indicator, with a hazard ratio of 2.6 (95% CI 1.63, 4.17).

Also, many women gain weight after the diagnosis of breast cancer, and weight gain is undesirable for several reasons. Weight gain may negatively affect quality of life, and previous studies indicate that a majority of patients with breast cancer find weight gain distressing and report it as a major concern [95,117–120]. Also, weight gain may predispose women to other chronic disorders, such as hypertension, cardiovascular disease, gallbladder disease, orthopedic disturbances, and diabetes mellitus [121,122]. Finally, although not conclusive, there is evidence to suggest that weight gain adversely affects disease-free survival. Camoriano et al [95] followed 646 patients with breast cancer for a median of 6.6 years and found that premenopausal patients

Table 71-1
Nutrients, Foods and Dietary Factors Suggested to be Associated with Risk for Breast Cancer

Strength of Current Evidence	Nutrient, Food, or Dietary Constituent	Proposed Direction of Association	Comments
Fairly consistent evidence from epidemiologic analytic research, and biologic mechanism(s) are plausible	Vegetable and fruit intake	Decreases risk	Several potential contributing mechanisms, attributable to numerous dietary constituents
	Alcohol intake	Increases risk	Possibly affects risk through hormonal effects, although clinical studies suggest a complicated relationship; possibly linked through effect on folate status
Inconsistent evidence from epidemiologic analytic research, but biologic mechanism(s) are plausible and/or demonstrable in laboratory studies	Dietary fiber intake	Decreases risk	Effects on hormonal factors demonstrable in biologic systems
	Folate intake	Decreases risk	May contribute to beneficial effects of vegetables and fruits; possibly interacts with alcohol intake
	Carotenoid and vitamin A intake	Decreases risk	May contribute to beneficial effects of vegetables and fruits; strongly supportive evidence from cell culture studies
Evidence from epidemiologic analytic research generally not supportive, but biologic mechanism(s) may be plausible or demonstrable	Dietary fat	Decreases risk	Possible effects on hormonal factors, but clinical studies are difficult to interpret due to confounding variables
	Specific fatty acids	Variable effects	Cell culture studies show differential effects of omega-6 and omega-3 fatty acids, but relevance to dietary patterns is not established or evident
	Vitamin E, vitamin C, and selenium	Decreases risk	Antioxidant effects possible, hypothesized to interact with genetic polymorphisms (e.g., glutathione-S-transferase)
Insufficient evidence from epidemiologic analytic research, but biologic mechanism(s) may be plausible or demonstrable	Well-done meat	Increases risk	Linked to carcinogens such as heterocyclic amines, hypothesized to interact with genetic polymorphisms (e.g., N-acctyl transferase)
	Soy and soy isoflavones, flaxseed	Variable effects	Although inverse associations suggested by ecologic studies, cull culture studies indicate possibility of adverse effects as well
Evidence from epidemiologic analytic research generally not supportive, and biologic mechanism(s) unknown or not demonstrable	Caffeine	—	No association with increased risk found consistently in case-control and cohort studies
	Protein	—	Associated in some case-control but not cohort studies, may be confounded by other characteristics of the diet

(Used with permission from Rock CL, Demark-Wahnefried W. [2001]. Nutrition and breast cancer. In *Nutrition in the Prevention and Treatment of Disease*, [Coulston AM, Rock CL, Monsen ER, ed.], San Diego, CA: Academic Press.)

who gained more than the median amount of weight (5.9 kg) were 1.5 times more likely to relapse and 1.6 times more likely to die of their breast cancer. Results from studies conducted by Chlebowski *et al* [123] and Goodwin *et al* [124] parallel these findings.

2. Dietary Composition

The relationship between dietary composition and survival or recurrence has been examined in 13 studies involving cohorts of women who had been diagnosed with breast cancer. In most cases, the dietary data were collected at the time of diagnosis or soon thereafter. All of these studies examined the effect of intake of dietary fat or selected high-fat foods. Results of the analysis of the relationship between fat intake and survival are generally inconsistent, with some studies finding inverse associations between survival and dietary fat intake at diagnosis, either adjusted [125–127] or unadjusted [93,128,129] for energy, whereas others [108,130–132] have not. One study (N=472) found stage- and age-adjusted risk for recurrence to be associated with intakes of butter, margarine and lard with a risk ratio of 1.30 (95% CI 1.03, 1.64) for each time these foods were consumed per day [100]. In a prospective study by Holmes *et al* (N=1982), in which dietary data were collected preceding and after diagnosis, no apparent association between energy-adjusted fat intake and mortality was observed [133]. However, protein intake, mainly linked to poultry, fish and dairy food sources, was found to exert a protective effect in that cohort (RR 0.65, 95% CI 0.47, 0.88, for highest vs lowest quintile).

Protective effects of vegetables and fruits and the micronutrients provided by these foods (e.g., vitamin C, carotenoids) have been observed in several of these follow-up cohort studies, with findings somewhat more consistent than those for dietary fat, although the strength of the association is modest. Of the eight studies that examined these dietary factors, three found a significant inverse association with risk of death [125,127,134], one found that risk of dying was nonsignificantly decreased in association with frequent vegetable consumption [131], and one found a significant inverse association in women with node negative disease, who comprised 62% of that cohort (but not in the total group that included women at all stages of invasive breast cancer) [133]. In the studies that found an inverse relationship with survival and intakes of vegetables, fruit and related nutrients (beta-carotene, vitamin C), the magnitude of the protective effect was a 20–90% reduction in risk for death.

Although alcohol intake has been identified as a risk factor for primary breast cancer, no significant relationships between alcohol intake and survival or recurrence were found in the eight studies that examined this relationship, although one of these studies reported that risk of dying was slightly (but not significantly) increased in association with frequent alcohol consumption [131]. In a study that examined specific foods [100], beer intake was directly related to risk for recurrence (but not survival), and wine and hard liquor intake were unrelated to risk for either outcome. Likewise, significant associations between dietary fiber intake and likelihood of survival have generally not been observed in these cohort studies.

Two multicenter, randomized, controlled trials are currently examining whether diet modification can influence the risk for recurrence and overall survival following the diagnosis of early stage breast cancer. In the Women's Intervention Nutrition Study (WINS), which involves 2437 women randomized within 12 months of primary surgery, the primary dietary goal is a reduction in dietary fat intake (≤15% energy from fat). Preliminary data indicate good adherence, with an average reduction from 33 to 20% energy from fat at 6 months into the study [135]. In the Women's Healthy Eating and Living (WHEL) Study, the target population consists of 3088 women who have been diagnosed with breast cancer within the preceding 4 years and who have completed initial therapies, prior to randomization. The primary emphasis of the WHEL Study diet intervention is on increased vegetable and fruit intake, with daily dietary goals of five vegetable servings, 16 ounces of vegetable juice, three fruit servings, 15–20% energy from fat, and 30 g dietary fiber. Feasibility study reports and preliminary trial data from this study also indicate excellent adherence [136–138]. In both of these studies, participants will be followed over 6 years; results are anticipated after 2006.

III. Endometrial Cancer

Cancer of the endometrium (uterine corpus) is the most common invasive gynecologic cancer [88]. Similar to breast and ovarian cancers, endometrial cancer is most common after menopause and is more prevalent among whites, although blacks have higher rates of mortality. Relative 5-year survival rates are 96%, 63%, and 26% for cancers diagnosed at local, regional and distant stages, respectively [88]. High cumulative exposure to estrogen is the major risk factor for endometrial cancer, whereas exposure to progesterone is protective [88,139–142]. Hence, early menarche, late menopause and nulliparity are risk factors for endometrial cancer, just as they are for breast and ovarian cancers [88,140]. However, unlike these cancers, risk factors for endometrial cancer also include tamoxifen use and factors associated with unopposed estrogens [139–141]. Given the key role that unopposed estrogens play in this disease, it is not surprising that obesity is one of the major nutrition related risk factors for this cancer.

The link between obesity and endometrial cancer is well established [142–145]. Bergstrom et al [32] conducted a review of 14 studies that were comprised of at least 100 incident cases (if a cohort study) and at least 200 cases (if a population-based, case-control study). A significantly positive association was found between excess weight and cancer of the endometrium in four of five of the cohort studies and in all of the case-control studies. In their meta-analysis (which included data from four studies), they found an RR of 1.10 (95% CI 1.07, 1.14) for each unit increase in BMI, equating to a relative risk for overweight ($25 \, kg/m^2$ <BMI <$30 \, kg/m^2$) of 1.59 and a relative risk for obesity (BMI >$30 \, kg/m^2$) of 2.52. When compared to parallel meta-analyses conducted for cancers at other sites (i.e., cancers of the colon, gallbladder, kidney, prostate, and postmenopausal breast), Bergstrom et al [32] concluded that the strongest association was between excess weight and cancer of the endometrium. Reports from the one cohort and six population-based, case-control studies conducted after those assembled for the aforementioned review all show positive associations between excess weight and endometrial cancer [141,146–151]. Some studies show that these associations are stronger for weight gained after adulthood [152,153], for metastatic disease [154], and for disease occurring in older women [152,155], as well as with upper body fat patterning [153,155,156–164]; however, these findings are either conflicting or there is a lack of data to confirm reported associations [144]. Given the strength and consistency of the evidence for a link between obesity and risk for endometrial cancer, more evidence would be useful to identify women at risk and to further define the mediating hormonal factors [165].

To date, 13 studies that have explored various dietary factors in relation to endometrial carcinoma have been reported. Six of these studies were hospital-based, case-control studies [166–171], three were population-based, case-control studies [148,172,173], and four were cohort studies [147,174–176]. The cohort studies found relatively few significant associations, with Terry et al [175] reporting a sole significant association of increased risk with very low intakes of vegetables and fruit. Fruit consumption was found to be a protective factor in three of the 13 studies [167,168,173]; and vegetable intake also was found to be protective in three of the studies [148,166,168]. Intake of beta-carotene, a constituent of vegetables and fruit, was associated with reduced risk in five of 12 studies [148,166–169], with ORs suggesting an average 40% risk reduction when intakes in the 4th vs the 1st quartiles are compared. Data largely show no associations for other plant constituents, such as dietary fiber or lycopene; however, these elements were either not analyzed in several studies (as in the case of lycopene) or analysis did not take into account various forms (as in the case of fiber). No consistent associations have been found with various types of vegetables or fruit [177].

Prior to 1995, dietary fat was associated with risk in a majority of studies of associations between dietary intake and risk for endometrial cancer. However, especially in the cohort studies in which ORs have been adjusted for BMI, total energy intake and other confounding factors, dietary fat intake is less often found to be an independent risk factor for endometrial cancer. A similar situation is true for energy intake, and it is unclear whether excess energy intake independently affects risk, or whether risk is conferred largely by obesity [178]. A host of other foods and nutrients have been explored, such as intakes of carbohydrate, protein, whole grains, dairy products, sugar, processed meat, and fatty fish [179]. However, the data lack consistency or confirmation for these factors.

In addition, most studies have found no association between risk for endometrial cancer and alcohol intake [144,156,167, 175,180–183]. Findings of Weiderpass et al [184], however, suggest that the effect of alcohol may be age-related and may serve as a risk factor among women below age 50, yet be protective among women who are older. This may explain nonsignificant associations and the discrepant findings of Parazzini et al [185], who found a positive association between alcohol intake and risk, and others who found evidence of a protective effect [186–187]. Certainly, more research is needed to confirm whether age-related associations exist.

Very little is known or reported regarding nutritional issues after the diagnosis of endometrial cancer. Although there are several studies that report increased prevalence of treatment-related complications among obese patients [188–191], a retrospective case series by Anderson et al [192] of 492 women with endometrial carcinoma found that BMI was inversely related to grade, invasion, and stage. Their data suggest that obese patients not only had better differentiated, less invasive tumors of lower stage with negative washings, but also showed that BMI was significantly inversely related to time to recurrence (P=0.0136). Given that this is the sole reported study in this area, more research is needed to confirm these findings, and outcomes that relate to overall health status, and not only to disease-related morbidity and mortality, are reported.

IV. Ovarian Cancer

Ovarian cancer is the most lethal of these cancers, being the fourth most common cause of cancer death among U.S. women despite having a relatively low incidence rate [1]. Women diagnosed with ovarian cancer typically present at an advanced disease stage, because the early stages are asymptomatic. The established risk factors for ovarian cancer are older age (≥50), low parity, no prior oral contraceptive (OCs) use, and a family history of breast or ovarian cancer [193,194]. Although the etiology is still a focus of intense investigation, a current theory is that increased ovulation or hormonal stimulation of ovarian epithelial cells plays a role in the development of ovarian cancer [195]. Current prevention strategies for women at high risk

include OC use, tubal ligation, and prophylactic oophorectomy [196]. Relatively few studies on the relationship between nutritional factors and risk for ovarian cancer have been reported, and there is a dearth of research that examines how these factors may influence progression or survival after the diagnosis of ovarian cancer.

Several case-control and three prospective studies have examined the relationship between adiposity and risk for ovarian cancer, and the results are mixed. In two case-control studies [197,198] and one prospective study [199], obesity was found to be significantly protective against ovarian cancer. Lukanova et al [199] found in their multicenter prospective study that women in the highest vs lowest quartile of BMI had a 54% lower risk of ovarian cancer (OR 0.23, 95% CI 0.23, 0.92). In contrast, one population-based, case-control study found women in the highest vs lowest category of BMI to have an increased risk with an OR of 1.7 (95% CI 1.1, 2.7) [200], and two case-control studies [201,202] and one prospective study [203] found no association between degree of obesity and risk for ovarian cancer. The relationship between body fat distribution and risk for ovarian cancer was examined in one prospective study involving postmenopausal women [204], in which a direct relationship between risk and waist–hip ratio was suggested (RRs for the upper three quintiles compared with the lowest quintile were 2.0, 1.6, and 2.3). Based on the mixed findings of these studies, it appears that the relationship between obesity and ovarian cancer risk clearly differs from the relationships observed between obesity and risk for either postmenopausal breast cancer or endometrial cancer.

Similar to the evidence for breast cancer, international comparisons of incidence of ovarian cancer indicate a strong inverse relationship with per capita dietary fat consumption [41], and the hypothesis that dietary fat intake increases circulating estrogen concentrations (discussed previously) has stimulated several observational studies of the relationship between dietary fat intake and risk for ovarian cancer. One meta-analysis pooled data from all available observational studies that examined the relationship between dietary fat intake and risk of invasive ovarian cancer [205]. In eight observational studies (one prospective and seven case-control studies) involving 6689 subjects, the RR for total fat intake was 1.24 (95% CI 1.07, 1.43) for higher vs lower intakes, suggesting that fat intake imparts a modestly increased risk [205]. For saturated fat, the RR was 1.20 (95% CI 1.04, 1.39) and for animal fat, the RR was 1.70 (95% CI 1.43, 2.03). However, the data on fat intake were energy-adjusted in only four of these eight studies, so whether fat intake exerts an independent effect on risk for ovarian cancer remains unresolved. In a few studies, food sources of fat also have been quantified for analysis. Saturated fatty acids or sources of these fatty acids (i.e., red meat) have been associated with increased risk in a few studies; for example, Bosetti et al [206] found an OR of 1.53 (95% CI 1.13, 2.05) for the highest compared with the lowest quintile of red meat consumption. Intakes of fish [206,207] and monounsaturated fatty acids [208] have been identified as being protective. However, the data to support relationships between risk and intakes of these fat subtypes are still limited, and replication in additional populations is needed.

Since 1987, 14 observational studies (two cohort and 12 case-control studies) have examined the relationships between intakes of antioxidant micronutrients, selected food sources, and risk for ovarian cancer. The most consistent relationship that has been observed is an inverse association between intake of vegetables and fruit and risk for ovarian cancer, which was found in seven of these studies [207,209–214], with intakes of green leafy vegetables, carrots, and tomato sauce, the vegetables specifically associated with reduced risk. Additionally, one of the cohort studies found that women who consumed at least 2.5 servings of vegetables and fruit per day as adolescents had a 46% reduction in risk for ovarian cancer [215], although adult vegetable and fruit intake was unrelated to risk in that study. Data on the relationship between risk and specific nutrients examined in these studies are inconsistent. For example, four case-control studies found a protective effect of carotenoids [211,216–218], whereas two case-control studies [208,210] and two prospective studies [213,215] did not find a protective effect of carotenoid intake. Dietary vitamin C intake was examined in five studies [198,208, 213,216,217] and was found to be inversely related to risk in two of these studies [208,217]. Vitamin E intake from food sources has not been found to relate to risk [198,213]. One study found vitamin C and vitamin E intake from dietary supplements, but not from food sources, to be associated with reduced risk of ovarian cancer [198]; however, there was no indication of a dose response effect in that study, and the lifestyle and behavioral characteristics of dietary supplement users are known to differ from those of nonusers. Results of analysis of relationships between ovarian cancer risk and intakes of other micronutrients and dietary constituents, such as vitamin A and alcohol, are similarly inconsistent.

One small prospective cohort study (35 cases, 37 controls), examined associations between serum concentrations of micronutrients and risk for ovarian cancer [219], using sera collected prior to diagnosis. They found no relationship between risk and serum retinol, beta carotene, lycopene, and lipid-adjusted alpha-tocopherol and gamma-tocopherol concentrations, but serum selenium concentration was inversely associated with risk of ovarian cancer among cases diagnosed 4 or more years after blood collections (P = 0.02 for trend) [219]. In contrast to these findings linking serum selenium to risk, another prospective study did not find an association between toenail selenium level and ovarian cancer risk [220]. Several earlier case-control studies compared serum nutrient concentrations of patients with ovarian cancer to those of matched controls, but when blood samples are collected following diagnosis, the effect of the diagnosis and treatment cannot be ruled out.

A possible role for intake of lactose (or more specifically, galactose, a unique monosaccharide constituent of lactose) in the development of ovarian cancer has been the focus of some research. It has been suggested that increased exposure to galactose, due to high intakes of dairy foods or altered galactose metabolism, might be associated with the development of ovarian cancer. This suggestion was based on animal studies showing that a diet very high in galactose is toxic to oocytes and evidence that the genetic disorder of galactosemia causes premature ovarian failure in women. Indeed, an early case-control study found intake of dairy foods to be directly associated with risk for ovarian cancer [221]. Since that time, however, several case-control and cohort studies have investigated this relationship, and these studies have not found significant associations between intakes of lactose or dairy foods and risk for ovarian cancer [211,213,222–224]. Thus, the majority of the evidence

suggests that adult consumption of galactose, lactose or dairy foods are not associated with increased risk for ovarian cancer. Findings from studies on the possible role for galactose in the development of ovarian cancer indicate that women with ovarian cancer may be more likely to have genetic polymorphisms that affect the metabolism of galactose at very high concentrations [222,224]. The effects of these genetic differences would be more relevant to fetal galactose, which is influenced by both maternal and fetal genotypes, than to intakes of lactose and dairy foods in adulthood [224], and the clinical importance of intrauterine galactose exposure to later ovarian cancer risk is unknown.

To date, one epidemiological study has examined the relationship between dietary intakes and survival following the diagnosis of ovarian cancer [225]. In a cohort of 609 women with invasive ovarian cancer, improved five-year survival was observed for women who reported a higher intake of vegetables (hazard ratio [HR] 0.75, 95% CI, 0.57–0.99 for highest versus lowest tertile). Cruciferous vegetables in particular were associated with greater likelihood of survival (HR 0.76, 95% CI 0.57–0.98 for highest versus lowest tertile).

V. Summary and Conclusions

Although a considerable amount of research has been devoted to understanding the effects of nutritional factors on the risk for breast cancer, much remains to be learned. More research on the relationships between these factors and risk for endometrial and ovarian cancers is sorely needed, and few studies to date have examined how these factors may influence overall survival in persons who have been diagnosed with hormone-related cancers. At this time, guidelines from the American Cancer Society [226,227] (summarized in Table 71-2) and the American Institute for Cancer Research [55] form the basis of current dietary recommendations, with encouragement toward more plant-based diets that promote healthy weight control serving as the underlying theme behind these recommendations.

The risk for morbidity and mortality from causes other than breast, endometrial and ovarian cancer also should be considered in dietary recommendations for women and men at risk for cancer and cancer survivors, especially those diagnosed with early stage cancers [228]. For example, even though evidence to support a link between fat intake and breast cancer risk and prognosis is inconsistent, limiting saturated fat intake is an established strategy to reduce risk for cardiovascular disease. Similarly, eating a diet with adequate dietary fiber has been associated with decreased risk of coronary heart disease and may contribute to overall health [229], irrespective of a specific link between fiber and hormone-related cancers. Diets that emphasize fruits, vegetables, whole grains, low-fat dairy foods, and lean meats and poultry have been associated with decreased risk of all-cause mortality [230].

VI. Suggestions for Further Investigations

Future directions of research in this area, in addition to the ongoing clinical trials described previously, include the following:

- Refinement in the methodologies used to measure intakes of vegetables, fruit and other plant foods, or their constituents,

Table 71-2

American Cancer Society Guidelines on Nutrition and Physical Activity for Cancer Prevention: American Cancer Society Recommendations for Individual Choices

1. Eat a variety of healthful foods, with an emphasis on plant sources.

    Eat five or more servings of a variety of vegetables and fruits each day.

    Choose whole grains in preference to processed (refined) grains and sugars.

    Limit consumption of red meats, especially those high in fat and processed.

    Choose foods that maintain a healthy weight.

2. Adopt a physically active lifestyle.

    Adults: Engage in at least moderate activity for 30 minutes or more 5 or more days/week; 45 minutes or more of moderate to vigorous activity 5 or more days/week may further enhance reductions in the risk of breast and colon cancer.

    Children and adolescents: Engage in at least 60 minutes/day of moderate-to-vigorous physical activity at least 5 days/week.

3. Maintain a healthful weight throughout life.

    Balance caloric intake with physical activity.

    Lose weight if currently overweight or obese.

4. If you drink alcoholic beverages, limit consumption.

(Used with permission from Byers T, Nestle M, McTiernan A *et al* and the American Cancer Society 2001 Nutrition and Physical Activity Guidelines Advisory Committee. [2002]. American Cancer Society Guidelines on Nutrition and Physical Activity for Cancer Prevention: Reducing the risk of cancer with healthy food choices and physical activity. *CA Cancer J Clin.* 52:92–119.)

as the potential importance of phytochemicals provided by these foods is increasingly evident, based on results from cell culture and laboratory animal studies.

- Increased utilization of biomarkers that provide corroborative evidence of dietary intakes and biologic activities of the various dietary constituents, in addition to use of surrogate biomarkers that are indicative of effects on the process of neoplasia.

- Identification of diet-gene interactions that likely influence response to exposure and are anticipated to be among the determinants of response to diet intervention efforts to reduce risk and progression of the hormone-related cancers.

- Development and testing of interventions that can facilitate healthy weight management in the target population of persons at risk for the hormone-related cancers and cancer survivors.

References

1. Jemal A, Tiwari RC, Murray T *et al.* (2004). Cancer Statistics, 2002. *CA Cancer J Clin.* 54:8–29.

2. Marsden DE, Friedlander M, Hacker NF. (2000). Current management of epithelial ovarian carcinoma: A review. *Sem Surg Oncol.* 19:11–19.

3. Ravandi-Kashani F, Hayes TG. (1998). Male breast cancer: A review of the literature. *Eur J Cancer.* 34:1341–1347.

4. Donegan WL, Redlich PN, Lang PJ, Gall MT. (1998). Carcinoma of the breast in males. *Cancer.* 83:498–509.

5. Snekeker SM, Diaugustine R. (1996). Hormonal and environmental factors affecting cell proliferation and neoplasia in the mammary gland. In *Cellular and Molecular Mechanisms of Hormonal Carcinogenesis: Environmental Influences,* (Huff J, Boyd J, Barrett JC, ed.), New York, NY: Wiley-Liss.

6. Kaaks R, Lukanova A. (2001). Energy balance and cancer: The role of insulin and insulin-like growth factor-1. *Proc Nutr Soc.* 60:91–106.

7. Del Giudice ME, Fantus IG, Ezzat S *et al.* (1998). Insulin and related factors in premenopausal breast cancer risk. *Breast Cancer Res Treat.* 47:111–120.

8. Clemons M, Goss P. (2001). Estrogen and the risk of breast cancer. *N Eng J Med.* 344:276–285.

9. Ambrosone CB, Coles BF, Freudenheim JL, Shields PG. (1999). Glutathione-S-transferase (GSTM1) genetic polymorphisms do not affect human breast cancer risk, regardless of dietary antioxidants. *J Nutr.* 129(Suppl):565S–568S.

10. Zheng W, Deitz AC, Campbell DR *et al.* (1999). N-acetyltransferase 1 genetic polymorphism, cigarette smoking, well-done meat intake, and breast cancer risk. *Cancer Epidemiol Biomarkers Prev.* 8:233–239.

11. Ballard-Barbash R. (1994). Anthropometry and breast cancer. Body size—a moving target. *Cancer.* 74:1090–1100.

12. Clinton SK. (1997). Diet, anthropometry and breast cancer: Integration of experimental and epidemiologic approaches. *J Nutr.* 127(Suppl):916S–920S.

13. Ziegler RG. (1997). Anthropometry and breast cancer. *J Nutr.* 127(Suppl): 924S–928S.

14. Brinton LA, Swanson CA. (1992). Height and weight at various ages and risk of breast cancer. *Ann Epidemiol.* 2:597–609.

15. Ng EH, Gao F, Ji CY *et al.* (1997). Risk factors for breast carcinoma in Singaporean Chinese women: The role of central obesity. *Cancer.* 80:725–731.

16. Swanson CA, Jones DY, Schatzkin A *et al.* (1988). Breast cancer risk assessed by anthropometry in the NHANES I epidemiological follow-up study. *Cancer Res.* 48:5363–5367.

17. de Waard F. (1975). Breast cancer incidence and nutritional status with particular reference to body weight and height. *Cancer Res.* 35:3351–3356.

18. van den Brandt PA, Spiegelman D, Yaun SS *et al.* (2000). Pooled analysis of prospective cohort studies on height, weight, and breast cancer risk. *Am J Epidemiol.* 152:514–527.

19. Mondina R, Borsellino G, Poma S *et al.* (1992). Breast carcinoma and skeletal formation. *Eur J Cancer.* 28A:1068–1070.

20. Carroll KK. (1998). Obesity as a risk factor for certain types of cancer. *Lipids.* 33:1055–1059.

21. Cleary MP, Maihle NJ. (1997). The role of body mass index in the relative risk of developing premenopausal versus postmenopausal breast cancer. *Proc Soc Exp Biol Med.* 216:28–43.

22. Vihko R, Apter D. (1989). Endogenous steroids in the pathophysiology of breast cancer. *Crit Rev Oncol Hematol.* 9:1–16.

23. Stoll BA. (2000). Adiposity as a risk determinant for postmenopausal breast cancer. *Int J Obes Relat Metab Disord.* 24:527–533.

24. Hsing AW, McLaughlin JK, Cocco P *et al.* (19). Risk factors for male breast cancer (United States). *Cancer Causes Control.* 9:269–275.

25. Ewertz M, Holmberg L, Tretli S *et al.* (2001). Risk factors for male breast cancer – a case-control study from Scandinavia. *Acta Oncol.* 40:467–471.

26. Le Marchand L, Kolonel LN, Earle ME, Mi MP. (1988). Body size at different periods of life and breast cancer risk. *Am J Epidemiol.* 128:137–152.

27. Radimer K, Siskind V, Bain C, Schofield F. (1993). Relation between anthropometric indicators and risk of breast cancer among Australian women. *Am J Epidemiol.* 138:77–89.

28. Apter D. (1996). Hormonal events during female puberty in relation to breast cancer risk. *Eur J Cancer Prev.* 5:476–482.

29. Stoll BA. (1997). Impaired ovulation and breast cancer risk. *Eur J Cancer.* 33:1532–1535.

30. Stoll BA. (1999). Western nutrition and the insulin resistance syndrome: A link to breast cancer. *Eur J Clin Nutr.* 53:83–87.

31. Kumar NB, Lyman GH, Allen K et al. (1995). Timing of weight gain and breast cancer risk. *Cancer.* 76:243–249.

32. Bergstrom A, Pisani P, Tenet V et al. (2001). Overweight as an avoidable cause of cancer in Europe. *Int J Cancer.* 91:421–30.

33. Schapira DV, Clark RA, Wolff PA et al. (1994). Visceral obesity and breast cancer risk. *Cancer.* 74:632–639.

34. Sonnenschein E, Toniolo P, Terry MB et al. (1999). Body fat distribution and obesity in pre- and postmenopausal breast cancer. *Int J Epidemiol.* 28:1026–1031.

35. Sellers TA, Drinkard C, Rich SS et al. (1994). Familial aggregation and heritability of waist-to-hip ratio in adult women: The Iowa Women's Health Study. *Int J Obes Relat Metab Disord.* 18:607–613.

36. London SJ, Colditz GA, Stampfer MJ et al. (1989). Prospective study of relative weight, height, and risk of breast cancer. *JAMA.* 262:2853–2858.

37. Harris JR, Lippman ME, Veronesi U, Willett W. (1992). Breast cancer (1). *N Engl J Med.* 327:319–328.

38. Kelsey JL, Horn-Ross PL. (1993). Breast cancer: Magnitude of the problem and descriptive epidemiology. *Epidemiol.* Rev 15:7–16.

39. McMichael AJ, Giles GG. (1988). Cancer in migrants to Australia: Extending the descriptive epidemiological data. *Cancer Res.* 48:751–756.

40. Ziegler RG, Hoover RN, Pike MC et al. (1993). Migration patterns and breast cancer risk in Asian-American women. *J Natl Cancer Inst.* 85:1819–27.

41. Armstrong B, Doll R. (1975). Environmental factors and cancer incidence and mortality in different countries, with special reference to dietary practices. *Int J Cancer.* 15:617–631.

42. Hunter DJ, Willett WC. (1996). Nutrition and breast cancer. *Cancer Causes Control.* 7:56–68.

43. Wynder EL, Cohen LA, Muscat JE et al. (1997). Breast cancer: Weighing the evidence for a promoting role of dietary fat. *J Natl Cancer Inst.* 89:766–775.

44. Clavel-Chapelon F, Niravong M, Joseph RR. (1997). Diet and breast cancer: Review of the epidemiologic literature. *Cancer Detect Prev.* 21:426–440.

45. Greenwald P. (1999). Role of dietary fat in the causation of breast cancer: Point. *Cancer Epidemiol Biomarkers Prev.* 8:3–7.

46. Hunter DJ. (1999). Role of dietary fat in the causation of breast cancer: Counterpoint. *Cancer Epidemiol Biomarkers Prev.* 8:9–13.

47. Rose DP. (1997). Dietary fatty acids and cancer. *Am J Clin Nutr.* 66:998S–1003S.

48. Guthrie N, Carroll KK. (1999). Specific versus nonspecific effects of dietary fat on carcinogenesis. *Prog Lipid Res.* 38:261–271.

49. Hunter DJ, Spiegelman D, Adami HO et al. (1996). Cohort studies of fat intake and the risk of breast cancer—a pooled analysis. *N Engl J Med.* 334:356–361.

50. Holmes MD, Hunter DJ, Colditz GA et al. (1999). Association of dietary intake of fat and fatty acids with risk of breast cancer. *JAMA.* 281:914–920.

51. Klurfeld DM, Welch CB, Davis MJ, Kirtchevsky DM. (1989). Determination of degree of energy restriction necessary to reduce DMBA-induced mammary tumorigenesis in rats during the promotion phase. *J Nutr.* 119:286–291.

52. Bartsch H, Nair J, Owen RW. (1999). Dietary polyunsaturated fatty acids and cancers of the breast and colorectum: Emerging evidence for their role as risk modifiers. *Carcinogenesis.* 20:2209–2218.

53. Wu AH, Pike MC, Stram DO. (1999). Meta-analysis: Dietary fat intake, serum estrogen levels, and the risk of breast cancer. *J Natl Cancer Inst.* 91:529–534.

54. Gandini S, Merzenich H, Robertson C, Boyle P. (2000). Meta-analysis of studies on breast cancer risk and diet: The role of fruit and vegetable consumption and the intake of associated micronutrients. *Eur J Cancer.* 36:636–646.

55. World Cancer Research Fund, American Institute for Cancer Research Expert Panel. (1997). Food, Nutrition and the Prevention of Cancer: A Global Perspective. Washington, DC: American Institute for Cancer Research.

56. Smith-Warner SA, Spiegelman D, Yaun SS et al. (2001). Intake of fruits and vegetables and risk of breast cancer: A pooled analysis of cohort studies. *JAMA.* 285:769–776.

57. Potischman N, McCulloch CE, Byers T et al. (1990). Breast cancer and dietary and plasma concentrations of carotenoids and vitamin A. *Am J Clin Nutr.* 52:909–915.

58. Zhang S, Tang G, Russell RM et al. (1997). Measurement of retinoids and carotenoids in breast adipose tissue and a comparison of concentrations in breast cancer cases and control subjects. *Am J Clin Nutr.* 66:626–632.

59. Yeum KJ, Ahn SH, Rupp de Paiva SA et al. (1998). Correlation between carotenoid concentrations in serum and normal breast adipose tissue of women with benign breast tumor or breast cancer. *J Nutr.* 128:1920–1926.

60. Ching S, Ingram D, Hahnel R et al. (2002). Serum levels of micronutrients, antioxidants and total antioxidant status predict risk of breast cancer in a case control study. *J Nutr.* 132:303–306.

61. Toniolo P, Van Kappel AL, Akhmedkhanov A et al. (2001). Serum carotenoids and breast cancer. *Am J Epidemiol.* 153;1142–1147.

62. Rock CL, Kusluski RA, Galvez MM, Ethier SP. (1995). Carotenoids induce morphological changes in human mammary epithelial cell cultures. *Nutr Cancer.* 23:319–333.

63. Prakash P, Krinsky NI, Russell RM. (2000). Retinoids, carotenoids, and human breast cancer cell cultures: A review of differential effects. *Nutr Rev.* 58:170–176.

64. Dawson MI, Chao WR, Pine P et al. (1995). Correlation of retinoid binding affinity to retinoic acid receptor alpha with retinoid inhibition of growth of estrogen receptor-positive MCF-7 mammary carcinoma cells. *Cancer Res.* 55;4446–4451.

65. Sumantran VN, Zhang R, Lee DS, Wicha MS. (2000). Differential regulation of apoptosis in normal versus transformed mammary epithelium by lutein and retinoic acid. *Cancer Epidemiol Biomarkers Prev.* 9:257–263.

66. Fowke JH, Longcope C, Hebert JR. (2000). Brassica vegetable consumption shifts estrogen metabolism in healthy postmenopausal women. *Cancer Epidemiol Biomarkers Prev.* 9:773–779.

67. Smith-Warner SA, Spiegelman D, Yaun SS et al. (1998). Alcohol and breast cancer in women: A pooled analysis of cohort studies. *JAMA.* 279:535–540.

68. Ginsburg ES. (1999). Estrogen, alcohol and breast cancer risk. *J Steroid Biochem Mol Biol.* 69:299–306.

69. Zhang S, Hunter DJ, Hankinson SE et al. (1999). A prospective study of folate intake and the risk of breast cancer. *JAMA.* 281:1632–1637.

70. Rohan TE, Jain MG, Howe GR, Miller AB. (2000). Dietary folate consumption and breast cancer risk. *J Natl Cancer Inst.* 92:266–269.

71. Sellers TA, Kushi LH, Cerhan JR et al. (2001). Dietary folate intake, alcohol, and risk of breast cancer in a prospective study of postmenopausal women. *Epidemiol.* 12:420–428.

72. Arts CJ, Govers CA, van den Berg H et al. (1991). *In vitro* binding of estrogens by dietary fiber and the *in vivo* apparent digestibility tested in pigs. *J Steroid Biochem Mol Biol.* 38:621–628.

73. Stoll BA. (1998). Breast cancer and the Western diet: Role of fatty acids and antioxidant vitamins. *Eur J Cancer.* 34:1852–1856.

74. van't Veer P, Strain JJ, Fernandez-Crehuet J et al. (1996). Tissue antioxidants and postmenopausal breast cancer: The European Community Multicentre Study on Antioxidants, Myocardial Infarction, and Cancer of the Breast (EURAMIC). *Cancer Epidemiol Biomarkers Prev.* 5:441–447.

75. Graham S, Zielezny M, Marshall J et al. (1992). Diet in the epidemiology of postmenopausal breast cancer in the New York State Cohort. *Am J Epidemiol.* 136:1327–1337.

76. Hunter DJ, Manson JE, Colditz GA et al. (1993). A prospective study of the intake of vitamins C, E, and A and the risk of breast cancer. *N Engl J Med.* 329:234–240.

77. Kushi LH, Fee RM, Sellers TA et al. (1996). Intake of vitamins A, C, and E and postmenopausal breast cancer. The Iowa Women's Health Study. *Am J Epidemiol.* 144:165–174.

78. Dorgan JF, Sowell A, Swanson CA et al. (1998). Relationships of serum carotenoids, retinol, alpha-tocopherol, and selenium with breast cancer risk: Results from a prospective study in Columbia, Missouri (United States). *Cancer Causes Control.* 9:89–97.

79. Horner NK, Lampe JW. (2000). Potential mechanisms of diet therapy for fibrocystic breast conditions show inadequate evidence of effectiveness. *J Am Diet Assoc.* 100:1368–1380.

80. Ambrosone CB, Freudenheim JL, Sinha R et al. (1998). Breast cancer risk, meat consumption and N-acetyltransferase (NAT2) genetic polymorphisms. *Int J Cancer.* 75:825–830.

81. Henderson BE, Bernstein L. (1991). The international variation in breast cancer rates: An epidemiological assessment. *Breast Cancer Res Treat.* 18(Suppl 1):S11–S17.

82. Kurzer MS. (2000). Hormonal effects of soy isoflavones: Studies in premenopausal and postmenopausal women. *J Nutr.* 130:660S–661S.

83. Herman C, Aldercreutz H, Goldin BR et al. (1995). Soybean phytoestrogen intake and cancer risk. J Nutr. 125(Suppl):757S–770S.

84. Messina MJ, Loprinzi CL. (2001). Soy for breast cancer survivors: A critical review of the literature. J Nutr. 131:3095S–3108S.

85. The Women's Health Initiative Study Group. (1998). Design of the Women's Health Initiative clinical trial and observational study. Control Clin Trials. 19:61–109.

86. Boyd NF, Fishell E, Jong R et al. (1995). Mammographic densities as a criterion for entry to a clinical trial of breast cancer prevention. Br J Cancer. 72:476–479.

87. Chu KC, Tarone RE, Kessler LG et al. (1996). Recent trends in U.S. breast cancer incidence, survival, and mortality rates. J Natl Cancer Inst. 88:1571–1579.

88. American Cancer Society. (2002). Cancer Facts & Figures 2002. Atlanta, GA: American Cancer Society.

89. Hayes DF, Kaplan W. (1996). Evaluation of patients after primary therapy. In Diseases of the Breast, (Harris JR, Lippman ME, Morrow M, Hellman S, ed.), Philadelphia, PA: Lippincott-Raven.

90. Goodwin PJ, Boyd NF. (1990). Body size and breast cancer prognosis: A critical review of the evidence. Breast Cancer Res Treat. 16:205–214.

91. Senie RT, Rosen PP, Rhodes P et al. (1992). Obesity at diagnosis of breast carcinoma influences duration of disease-free survival. Ann Intern Med. 116:26–32.

92. Bastarrachea J, Hortobagyi GN, Smith TL et al. (1994). Obesity as an adverse prognostic factor for patients receiving adjuvant chemotherapy for breast cancer. Ann Intern Med. 120:18–25.

93. Zhang S, Folsom AR, Sellers TA et al. (1995). Better breast cancer survival for postmenopausal women who are less overweight and eat less fat. The Iowa Women's Health Study. Cancer. 76:275–283.

94. Kyogoku S, Hirohata T, Takeshita S et al. (1990). Survival of breast-cancer patients and body size indicators. Int J Cancer. 46:824–831.

95. Camoriano JK, Loprinzi CL, Ingle JN et al. (1990). Weight change in women treated with adjuvant therapy or observed following mastectomy for node-positive breast cancer. J Clin Oncol. 8:1327–1334.

96. Coates RJ, Clark WS, Eley JW et al. (1990). Race, nutritional status, and survival from breast cancer. J Natl Cancer Inst. 82:1684–1692.

97. Daling JR, Malone KE, Doody DR et al. (2001). Relation of body mass index to tumor markers and survival among young women with invasive ductal breast carcinoma. Cancer. 92:720–729.

98. Gordon NH, Crowe JP, Blumberg DJ, Berger NA. (1992). Socioeconomic factors and race in breast cancer recurrence and survival. Am J Epidemiol. 135:609–618.

99. Haybittle J, Houghton J, Baum M. (1997). Social class and weight as prognostic factors in early breast cancer. Br J Cancer Res. 75:729–733.

100. Hebert JR, Hurley TG, Ma Y. (1998). The effect of dietary exposures on recurrence and mortality in early stage breast cancer. Breast Cancer Res Treat. 51:17–28.

101. Holmberg L, Lund E, Bergstrom R et al. (1994). Oral contraceptives and prognosis in breast cancer: Effects of duration, latency, recency, age at first use and relation to parity and body mass index in young women with breast cancer. Eur J Cancer. 30:351–354.

102. Kimura M. (1990). Obesity as prognostic factors in breast cancer. Diabetes Res Clin Pract. 10:S247–S251.

103. Goodwin PJ, Ennis M, Pritchard KI et al. (2002). Fasting insulin and outcome in early-stage breast cancer: Results of a prospective cohort study. J Clin Oncol. 20:42–51.

104. Mæhle BO, Tretli S. (1996). Premorbid body-mass-index in breast cancer: Reversed effect on survival in hormone receptor negative patients. Breast Cancer Res Treat. 41:123–130.

105. Tornberg S, Carstensen J. (1993). Serum beta-lipoprotein, serum cholesterol and Quetelet's Index as predictors for survival of breast cancer patients. Eur J Cancer. 29A:2025–2030.

106. Tretli S, Haldorsen T, Ottestad L. (1990). The effect of pre-morbid height and weight on the survival of breast cancer patients. Br J Cancer. 62:299–303.

107. Vatten LJ, Foss OP, Kvinnsland S. (1990). Overall survival of breast cancer patients in relation to preclinically determined total serum cholesterol, body mass index, height and cigarette smoking: A population-based study. Eur J Cancer. 27:641–646.

108. Saxe GA, Rock CL, Wicha MS, Schottenfeld D. (1999). Diet and risk for breast cancer recurrence and survival. Breast Cancer Res Treat. 53:241–253.

109. den Tonkelaar L, de Waard F, Seidell JC, Fracheboud J. (1995). Obesity and subcutaneous fat patterning in relation to survival of postmenopausal breast cancer patients participating in the DOM-project. Breast Cancer Res Treat. 34:129–137.

110. Galanis DJ, Kolonel LN, Lee J, LeMarchand L. (1998). Anthropometric predictors of breast cancer incidence and survival in multi-ethnic cohort of female residents of Hawaii, United States. Cancer Causes Control. 9:217–224.

111. Jain M, Miller AB. (1994). Pre-morbid body size and the prognosis of women with breast cancer. Int J Cancer. 86:1390–1397.

112. Jain M, Miller AB. (1997). Tumor characteristics and survival of breast cancer patients in relation to premorbid diet and body size. Breast Cancer Res Treat. 42:43–55.

113. Lethaby AE, Mason BH, Harvey VJ, Holdaway IM. (1996). Survival of women with node negative breast cancer in the Auckland region. NZ Med J. 109:330–333.

114. Obermair A, Kurz C, Hanzal E et al. (1995). The influence of obesity on the disease-free survival in primary breast cancer. Anticancer Res. 15:2265–2269.

115. Marret H, Perrotin F, Bougnoux P et al. (2001). Low body mass index is an independent predictive factor of local recurrence after conservative treatment for breast cancer. Breast Cancer Res Treat. 66:17–23.

116. Kumar NB, Cantor A, Allen K, Cox CE. (2000). Android obesity at diagnosis and breast carcinoma survival: Evaluation of the effects of anthropometric variables at diagnosis, including body composition and body fat distribution and weight gain during life span, and survival from breast carcinoma. Cancer. 88:2751–2757.

117. Monnin S, Schiller MR, Sachs L, Smith AM. (1993). Nutritional concerns of women with breast cancer. J Cancer Educ. 8:63–69.

118. Ganz PA, Schag CC, Polinsky ML. (1987). Rehabilitation needs and breast cancer: The first month after primary therapy. Breast Cancer Res Treat. 10:243–253.

119. Goodwin PJ, Ennis M, Pritchard KI et al. (1999). Adjuvant treatment and onset of menopause predict weight gain after breast cancer diagnosis. J Clin Oncol. 17:120–129.

120. Kornblith AB, Hollis DR, Zuckerman E et al. (1993). Effect of megestrol acetate on quality of life in a dose-response trial in women with advanced breast cancer. The Cancer and Leukemia Group B. J Clin Oncol. 11:2081–2089.

121. Li FP, Stovall EL. (1998). Long-term survivors of cancer. Cancer Epidemiol Biomarkers Prev. 7:269–270.

122. Brown BW, Brauner C, Minnotte MC. (1993). Noncancer deaths in white adult cancer patients. J Natl Cancer Inst. 85:979–987.

123. Chlebowski RT, Weiner JM, Reynolds R et al. (1986). Long-term survival following relapse after 5-FU but not CMF adjuvant breast cancer therapy. Breast Cancer Res Treat. 7:23–30.

124. Goodwin PJ, Panzarella T, Boyd NF. (1988). Weight gain in women with localized breast cancer—a descriptive study. Breast Cancer Res Treat. 11:59–66.

125. Jain M, Miller AB, To T. (1994). Premorbid diet and the prognosis of women with breast cancer. J Natl Cancer Inst. 86:1390–1397.

126. Holm LE, Nordevang E, Hjalmar ML et al. (1993). Treatment failure and dietary habits in women with breast cancer. J Natl Cancer Inst. 85:32–36.

127. Rohan TE, Hiller JE, McMichael AJ. (1993). Dietary factors and survival from breast cancer. Nutr Cancer. 20:167–177.

128. Nomura AM, Marchand LL, Kolonel LN, Hankin JH. (1991). The effect of dietary fat on breast cancer survival among Caucasian and Japanese women in Hawaii. Breast Cancer Res Treat. 18(Suppl 1):S135–141.

129. Gregorio DI, Emrich LJ, Graham S et al. (1985). Dietary fat consumption and survival among women with breast cancer. J Natl Cancer Inst. 75:37–41.

130. Kyogoku S, Hirohata T, Nomura Y et al. (1992). Diet and prognosis of breast cancer. Nutr Cancer. 17:271–277.

131. Ewertz M, Gillanders S, Meyer L, Zedeler K. (1991). Survival of breast cancer patients in relation to factors which affect the risk of developing breast cancer. Int J Cancer. 49:526–530.

132. Newman SC, Miller AB, Howe GR. (1986). A study of the effect of weight and dietary fat on breast cancer survival time. Am J Epidemiol. 123:767–774.

133. Holmes MD, Stampfer MJ, Colditz GA et al. (1999). Dietary factors and the survival of women with breast carcinoma. Cancer. 86:826–835.

134. Ingram D. (1994). Diet and subsequent survival in women with breast cancer. Br J Cancer. 69:592–595.

135. Chlebowski RT, Blackburn GL, Buzzard IM et al. (1993). Adherence to a dietary fat intake reduction program in postmenopausal women receiving therapy for early breast cancer. The Women's Intervention Nutrition Study. J Clin Oncol. 11:2072–2080.

136. Pierce JP, Faerber S, Wright FA et al. (1997). Feasibility of a randomized trial of a high-vegetable diet to prevent breast cancer recurrence. Nutr Cancer. 28:282–288.

137. Rock CL, Flatt SW, Wright FA et al. (1997). Responsiveness of carotenoids to a high vegetable diet intervention designed to prevent breast cancer recurrence. Cancer Epidemiol Biomarkers Prev. 6:617–623.

138. Rock CL, Thomson C, Caan BJ et al. (2001). Reduction in fat intake is not associated with weight loss in most women after breast cancer diagnosis. Cancer. 91:25–34.

139. Hale GE, Hughes CL, Cline JM. (2002). Endometrial cancer: Hormonal factors, the perimenopausal "window of risk," and isoflavones. J Clin Endocrinol Metab. 87:3–15.

140. Stoll BA. (1999). New metabolic-endocrine risk markers in endometrial cancer. Br J Obstet Gynaecol. 106:402–406.

141. Shields TS, Weiss NS, Voigt LF, Beresford SA. (1999). The additional risk of endometrial cancer associated with unopposed estrogen use in women with other risk factors. Epidemiol. 10:733–738.

142. Carroll KK. (1998). Obesity is a risk factor for certain types of cancer. Lipids. 33:1055–1059.

143. Persson I. (2000). Estrogens in the causation of breast, endometrial and ovarian cancers—evidence and hypotheses from epidemiological findings. J Steroid Biochem Molec Biol. 74:357–364.

144. Hill HA, Austin H. (1996). Nutrition and endometrial cancer. Cancer Causes Control. 7:19–32.

145. Schottenfeld D. (1995). Epidemiology of endometrial neoplasia. J Cell Biochem 23(Suppl):151–159.

146. Anderson KE, Anderson E, Mink PJ et al. (2001). Diabetes and endometrial cancer in the Iowa women's health study. Cancer Epidemiol Biomarkers Prev. 10:611–616.

147. Jain MG, Rohan TE, Howe GR, Miller AB. (2000). A cohort study of nutritional factors and endometrial cancer. Eur J Epidemiol. 16:899–905.

148. McCann SE, Freudenheim JL, Marshall JR et al. (2000). Diet in the epidemiology of endometrial cancer in Western New York (United States). Cancer Causes Control. 11:965–974.

149. Weiderpass E, Persson I, Adami HO et al. (2000). Body size in different periods of life, diabetes mellitus, hypertension, and risk of postmenopausal endometrial cancer (Sweden). Cancer Causes Control. 11:185–192.

150. Salazar-Martinez E, Lazcano-Ponce EC, Lira-Lira GG et al. (2000). Case-control study of diabetes, obesity, physical activity and risk of endometrial cancer among Mexican women. Cancer Causes Control. 11:707–711.

151. Shoff SM. Newcomb PA. (1998). Diabetes, body size, and risk of endometrial cancer. Am J Epidemiol. 148:234–240.

152. Levi F, La Vecchia C, Negri E, Parazzini F et al. (1992). Body mass at different ages and subsequent endometrial cancer risk. Int J Cancer. 50:567–571.

153. Le Marchand L, Wilkens LR, Mi MP. (1991). Early-age body size, adult weight gain and endometrial cancer risk. Int J Cancer. 48:807–811.

154. Tretli S, Magnus K. (1990). Height and weight in relation to uterine corpus cancer morbidity and mortality. A follow-up study of 570,000 women in Norway. Int J Cancer. 46:165–172.

155. Tornberg SA, Carstensen JM. (1994) Relationship between Quetelet's index and cancer of breast and female genital tract in 47,000 women followed for 25 years. Br J Cancer. 69:358–361.

156. Austin H, Drews C, Partridge EE. (1993). A case-control study of endometrial cancer in relation to cigarette smoking, serum estrogen levels, and alcohol use. Am J Obstet Gynecol. 169:1086–1091.

157. Elliott EA, Matanoski GM, Rosenshein NB et al. (1990). Body fat patterning in women with endometrial cancer. Gynecol Oncol. 39:253–258.

158. Folsom AR, Kaye SA, Potter JD, Prineas RJ. (1989). Association of incident carcinoma of the endometrium with body weight and fat distribution in older women: Early findings of the Iowa Women's Health Study. Cancer Res. 49:6828–6831.

159. Lapidus L, Helgesson O, Merck C, Bjorntorp P. (1998). Adipose tissue distribution and female carcinomas. A 12-year follow-up of participants in the population study of women in Gothenburg, Sweden. Int J Obesity. 12:361–368.

160. Shu XO, Brinton LA, Zheng W et al. (1992). Relation of obesity and body fat distribution to endometrial cancer in Shanghai, China. Cancer Res. 52:3865–3870.

161. Schapira DV, Kumar NB, Lyman GH et al. (1991). Upper-body fat distribution and endometrial cancer risk. JAMA. 266:1808–1811.

162. Swanson CA, Potischman N, Wilbanks GD et al. (1993). Relation of endometrial cancer risk to past and contemporary body size and body fat distribution. Cancer Epidemiol Biomarkers Prev. 2:321–327.

163. de Waard F, de Ridder CM, Baanders-van Halewyn EA, Slotboom BJ. (1996). Endometrial cancer in a cohort screened for breast cancer. Eur J Cancer Prev. 5:99–104.

164. Goodman MT, Hankin JH, Wilkens LR et al. (1997). Diet, body size, physical activity, and the risk of endometrial cancer. Cancer Res. 57:5077–5085.

165. Akhmedkhanov A, Zeleniuch-Jacquotte A, Toniolo P. (2001). Role of exogenous and endogenous hormones in endometrial cancer: Review of the evidence and research perspectives. Ann NY Acad Sci. 943:296–315.

166. Barbone F, Austin H, Partridge EE. (1993). Diet and endometrial cancer: A case-control study. Am J Epidemiol. 137:393–403.

167. La Vecchia C, Decarli A, Fasoli M, Gentile A. (1986). Nutrition and diet in the etiology of endometrial cancer. Cancer. 57:1248–1253.

168. Levi F, Franceschi S, Negri E, La Vecchia C. (1993). Dietary factors and the risk of endometrial cancer. Cancer. 71:3575–3581.

169. Negri E, La Vecchia C, Franceschi S et al. (1996). Intake of selected micronutrients and the risk of endometrial carcinoma. Cancer. 77:917–923.

170. Tzonou A, Lipworth L, Kalandidi A et al. (1996). Dietary factors and the risk of endometrial cancer: A case-control study in Greece. Br J Cancer. 73:1284–1290.

171. Villani C, Pucci G, Pietrangeli D et al. (1986). Role of diet in endometrial cancer patients. Eur J Gynaecol Oncol. 7:139–143.

172. Potischman N, Swanson CA, Brinton LA et al. (1993). Dietary associations in a case-control study of endometrial cancer. Cancer Causes Control. 4:239–250.

173. Shu XO, Zheng W, Potischman N et al. (1993). A population-based case-control study of dietary factors and endometrial cancer in Shanghai, People's Republic of China. Am J Epidemiol. 137:155–165.

174. Hirose K, Tajima K, Hamajima N et al. (1996). Subsite (cervix/endometrium)-specific risk and protective factors in uterus cancer. Japan J Cancer Res. 87:1001–1009.

175. Terry P, Baron JA, Weiderpass E et al. (1999). Lifestyle and endometrial cancer risk: A cohort study from the Swedish Twin Registry. Int J Cancer. 82:38–42.

176. Zheng W, Kushi LH, Potter JD et al. (1995). Dietary intake of energy and animal foods and endometrial cancer incidence. The Iowa Women's Health Study. Am J Epidemiol. 142:388–394.

177. Verhoeven DT, Goldbohm RA, van Poppel G et al. (1996). Epidemiological studies on Brassica vegetables and cancer risk. Cancer Epidemiol Biomarkers Prev. 5:733–748.

178. Boyle P, Maisonneuve P, Autier P. (2000). Update on cancer control in women. Int J Gynaecol Obstet. 70:263–303.

179. Terry P, Wolk A, Vainio H, Weiderpass E. (2002). Fatty fish consumption lowers the risk of endometrial cancer: A nationwide case-control study in Sweden. Cancer Epidemiol Biomarkers Prev. 11:143–145.

180. Newcomb PA, Trentham-Dietz A, Storer BE. (1997). Alcohol consumption in relation to endometrial cancer risk. Cancer Epidemiol Biomarkers Prev. 6:775–778.

181. Kalandidi A, Tzonou A, Lipworth L et al. (1996). A case-control study of endometrial cancer in relation to reproductive, somatometric, and lifestyle variables. Oncol. 53:354–359.

182. Gapstur SM, Potter JD, Sellers TA et al. (1993). Alcohol consumption and postmenopausal endometrial cancer: Results from the Iowa Women's Health Study. Cancer Causes Cont. 4:323–329.

183. Kato I, Tominaga S, Terao C. (1989). Alcohol consumption and cancers of hormone-related organs in females. Japan J Clin Oncol. 19:202–207.

184. Weiderpass E, Baron JA. (2001). Cigarette smoking, alcohol consumption, and endometrial cancer risk: A population-based study in Sweden. Cancer Causes Control. 12:239–247.

185. Parazzini F, La Vecchia C, D'Avanzo B et al. (1995). Alcohol and endometrial cancer risk: Findings from an Italian case-control study. Nutr Cancer. 23:55–62.

186. Swanson CA, Wilbanks GD, Twiggs LB et al. (1993). Moderate alcohol consumption and the risk of endometrial cancer. Epidemiol. 4:530–536.

187. Webster LA, Weiss NS. (1989). Alcoholic beverage consumption and the risk of endometrial cancer. Cancer and Steroid Hormone Study Group. Int J Epidemiol. 18:786–791.

188. Eltabbakh GH, Shamonki MI, Moody JM, Garafano LL. (2000). Hysterectomy for obese women with endometrial cancer: Laparoscopy or laparotomy? Gynecol Oncol. 78:329–735.

189. Thomadsen BR, Paliwal BR, Petereit DG, Ranallo FN. (2000). Radiation injury from x-ray exposure during brachytherapy localization. *Medical Physics.* 27:1681–1684.

190. Holub Z, Bartos P, Jabor A *et al.* (2000). Laparoscopic surgery in obese women with endometrial cancer. *J Am Assoc Gynecol Laparoscopists.* 7:83–88.

191. Scribner DR Jr, Walker JL, Johnson GA *et al.* (2002). Laparoscopic pelvic and paraaortic lymph node dissection in the obese. *Gynecol Oncol.* 84:426–430.

192. Anderson B, Connor JP, Andrews JI *et al.* (1996). Obesity and prognosis in endometrial cancer. *Am J Obstet Gynecol.* 174:1171–1178.

193. Runnebaum IB, Stickeler E. (2001). Epidemiological and molecular aspects of ovarian cancer risk. *J Cancer Res Clin Oncol.* 127:73–79.

194. Edmondson RJ, Monaghan JM. (2001). The epidemiology of ovarian cancer. *Intl J Gynecol Cancer.* 11:423–429.

195. Risch HA. (1998). Hormonal etiology of epithelial ovarian cancer, with a hypothesis concerning the role of androgens and progesterone. *J Natl Cancer Inst.* 90:1774–1786.

196. Narod SA, Boyd J. (2002). Current understanding of the epidemiology and clinical implications of BRCA1 and BRCA2 mutations for ovarian cancer. *Curr Opin Obstet Gynecol.* 14:19–26.

197. Parazzini F, Moroni S, La Vecchia C *et al.* (1997). Ovarian cancer risk and history of selected medical conditions linked with female hormones. *Eur J Cancer.* 33:1634–1637.

198. Fleischauer AT, Olson SH, Mignone L *et al.* (2001). Dietary antioxidants, supplements, and risk of epithelial ovarian cancer. *Nutr Cancer.* 40:92–98.

199. Lukanova A, Toniolo P, Lundin E *et al.* (2002). Body mass index in relation to ovarian cancer: A multi-centre nested case-control study. *Int J Cancer.* 99:603–608.

200. Farrow DC, Weiss NS, Lyon JL, Daling JR. (1989). Association of obesity and ovarian cancer in a case-control study. *Am J Epidemiol.* 129:1300–1304.

201. Hartge P, Schiffman MH, Hoover R *et al.* (1989). A case-control study of epithelial ovarian cancer. *Am J Obstet Gynecol.* 161:10–16.

202. Mori M, Nishida T, Sugiyama T *et al.* (1998). Anthropometric and other risk factors for ovarian cancer in a case-control study. *Japan J Cancer Res.* 89:246–253.

203. Tornberg SA, Carstensen JM. (1994). Relationship between Quetelet's index and cancer of the breast and female genital tract in 47,000 women followed for 25 years. *Br J Cancer.* 69:358–361.

204. Mink PJ, Folsom AR, Sellers TA, Kushi LH. (1996). Physical activity, waist-to-hip ratio, and other risk factors for ovarian cancer: A follow-up study of older women. *Epidemiol.* 7:38–45.

205. Huncharek M, Kupelnick B. (2001). Dietary fat intake and risk of epithelial ovarian cancer: A meta-analysis of 6689 subjects from 8 observational studies. *Nutr Cancer.* 40:87–91.

206. Bosetti C, Negri E, Franceschi S, Pelucchi C *et al.* (2001). Diet and ovarian cancer risk: A case-control study in Italy. *Int J Cancer.* 93:911–915.

207. Fernandez E, Chatenoud L, La Vecchia C *et al.* (1999). Fish consumption and cancer risk. *Am J Clin Nutr.* 70:85–90.

208. Tzonou A, Hsieh CC, Polychronopoulou A *et al.* (1993). Diet and ovarian cancer: A case-control study in Greece. *Int J Cancer.* 55:411–414.

209. La Vecchia C, Decarli A, Negri E *et al.* (1987). Dietary factors and risk of epithelial ovarian cancer. *J Natl Cancer Inst.* 79:663–669.

210. Shu XO, Gao YT, Yuan JM *et al.* (1989). Dietary factors and epithelial ovarian cancer. *Br J Cancer.* 59:92–96.

211. Engle A, Muscat JE, Harris RE. (1991). Nutritional risk factors and ovarian cancer. *Nutr Cancer.* 15:239–247.

212. Risch HA, Jain M, Marrett LD, Howe CR. (1994). Dietary fat intake and risk of epithelial ovarian cancer. *J Natl Cancer Inst.* 86:1409–1415.

213. Kushi LH, Mink PJ, Folson AR *et al.* (1999). Prospective study of diet and ovarian cancer. *Am J Epidemiol.* 149:21–31.

214. Parazzini F, Chatenoud L, Chiantera V *et al.* (2000). Population attributable risk for ovarian cancer. *Eur J Cancer.* 36:520–524.

215. Fairfield KM, Hankinson SE, Rosner BA *et al.* (2001). Risk of ovarian carcinoma and consumption of vitamins A, C, and E and specific carotenoids. *Cancer.* 92:2318–2326.

216. Byers T, Marshall J, Graham S *et al.* (1983). A case-control study of dietary and nondietary factors in ovarian cancer. *J Natl Cancer Inst.* 71:681–686.

217. Slattery ML, Schuman KL, West DW *et al.* (1989). Nutrient intake and ovarian cancer. *Am J Epidemiol.* 130:497–502.

218. Cramer DW, Kuper H, Harlow BL, Titus-Ernistoff L. (2001). Carotenoids, antioxidants, and ovarian cancer risk in pre- and postmenopausal women. *Int J Cancer.* 94:128–134.

219. Helzlsouer KJ, Albert GJ, Norkus EP, Morris JS *et al.* (1996). Prospective study of serum micronutrients and ovarian cancer. *J Natl Cancer Inst.* 88:32–37.

220. Garland M, Morris JS, Stampfer MJ *et al.* (1995). Prospective study of toenail selenium levels and cancer among women. *J Natl Cancer Inst.* 87:497–505.

221. Cramer DW, Welch AR, Hutchinson GB *et al.* (1984). Dietary animal fat in relation to ovarian cancer risk. *Obstet Gynaecol.* 63:833–838.

222. Webb PM, Bain CJ, Purdie DM *et al.* (1998). Milk consumption, galactose metabolism, and ovarian cancer (Australia). *Cancer Causes Control.* 9: 637–644.

223. Mettlin CJ, Piver MS. (1990). A case control study of milk-drinking and ovarian cancer risk. *Am J Epidemiol.* 132:871–876.

224. Cramer DW, Greenberg ER, Titus-Ernstoff L *et al.* (2000). A case-control study of galactose consumption and metabolism in relation to ovarian cancer. *Cancer Epidemiol Biomarkers Prev.* 9:95–101.

225. Runnebaum IB, Stickeler E. (2001). Epidemiological and molecular aspects of ovarian cancer risk. *J Cancer Res Clin Oncol.* 127:73–79.

226. Byers T, Nestle M, McTiernan A *et al.* and the American Cancer Society 2001 Nutrition and Physical Activity Guidelines Advisory Committee. (2002). American Cancer Society Guidelines on Nutrition and Physical Activity for Cancer Prevention: Reducing the risk of cancer with healthy food choices and physical activity. *CA Cancer J Clin.* 52:92–119.

227. Brown J, Byers T, Thompson K *et al.* (2002). Nutrition during and after cancer treatment: A guide for informed choices by cancer survivors. *CA Cancer J Clin.* 51:153–187.

228. Rock CL, Demark-Wahnefrield W. (In press). Nutrition and survival after the diagnosis of breast cancer: A review of the evidence. *J Clin Oncol.*

229. Wolk A, Manson JE, Stampfer MJ *et al.* (1999). Long-term intake of dietary fiber and decreased risk of coronary heart disease among women. *JAMA.* 281:1998–2004.

230. Kant AK, Schatzkin A, Graubard BI, Schairer C. (2000). A prospective study of diet quality and mortality in women. *JAMA.* 283:2109–2115.

72

Nutrition and the Etiology and Prevention of Prostate Cancer

LAURENCE N. KOLONEL, MD, PhD

Cancer Research Center, University of Hawaii, Honolulu, HI

I. Introduction

Because of its high incidence and apparent relation to endogenous sex hormones, prostate cancer is often considered a male counterpart to breast cancer in women. Both organs share a common embryologic origin in the urogenital sinus epithelium [1]. This chapter discusses the current status of epidemiologic evidence for a role of dietary factors in the development of prostate cancer. Some findings from animal and *in vitro* studies, as well as possible mechanisms for the carcinogenic effects of diet, are presented in support of the epidemiologic findings.

A. Normal Prostate Anatomy and Function

The normal adult prostate gland is a walnut-sized organ that surrounds the urethra and the neck of the bladder. The gland is composed of three distinct zones: peripheral, central, and transition. The peripheral zone is comprised of left and right lobes that can be palpated during digital rectal examination (DRE). The transition zone is the region that enlarges in benign prostatic hyperplasia (BPH), which is common in older men [1]. The prostate gland is a male secondary sex organ that secretes a fluid component of semen that is essential for male fertility. Normal growth and activity of the prostate gland is under the control of androgenic hormones. Circulating testosterone, produced primarily in the testes, diffuses into the prostate where it is irreversibly converted by the enzyme steroid 5alpha-reductase type II (SRD5A2) to dihydrotestosterone (DHT), a metabolically more active form of the hormone. Dihydrotestosterone binds to the androgen receptor (AR), and this complex then translocates to the cell nucleus where it activates selected genes [2].

B. Pathology and Diagnosis of Prostate Cancer

Almost all prostate tumors are classified as adenocarcinomas (i.e., they arise from the glandular epithelial cells), and occur most commonly in the peripheral zone of the gland. Accordingly, a physician can often feel them during DRE. A unique feature of human prostate cancer is the high frequency of small, latent tumors in older men. Autopsy reports have found such asymptomatic lesions in more than 80% of men in the United States over the age of 80 [1]. Although the relationship between these occult tumors and those that become clinically apparent has not been established, it is commonly assumed that clinical lesions evolve from these latent foci as a consequence of additional genetic mutations.

Generally, prostate cancer in its early stages is asymptomatic. Enlargement of the prostate gland (BPH) is common in men after age 45, and eventually leads to urinary tract symptoms (difficult and frequent urination). Many cases of prostate cancer are diagnosed incidentally as a result of visits to physicians for relief of these symptoms. The prostate-specific antigen (PSA) test has come into widespread use. Unfortunately, this test is not specific for prostate cancer, and produces elevated values with any increased tissue growth in the gland, such as occurs in BPH. The sensitivity of the PSA test can result in the diagnosis of very early, microscopic tumors, which are often removed surgically. Because surgical excision carries a risk of major complications (most notably incontinence and/or impotence), whereas only a proportion (unknown) of these occult lesions would ever progress to clinical disease, controversy exists regarding the proper use of PSA as a screening test for early prostate cancer [3].

II. Descriptive Epidemiology of Prostate Cancer

A. Incidence and Mortality Trends

Prostate cancer is a common cancer among men in many western countries, and is the leading male incident cancer (excluding nonmelanoma skin cancers) in the United States, where 189,000 new cases are projected for the year 2002 [4,5]. Incidence trends in the United States show a rather slow increase over most of the last 50 years, with a striking increase between 1989 and 1992 [6] (Fig. 72-1), attributable in large measure to the widespread adoption of the PSA screening test that first became available in the early 1980s [7]. Since 1992 the incidence has declined, reflecting an end to the surge in cases due to the introduction of this new screening procedure [8], as well as a more judicious use of PSA screening in medical practice. Moreover, mortality from prostate cancer is low relative to its incidence. This is because prostate cancer is generally well controlled by treatment (surgery, radiation, and androgen ablation) and occurs at relatively late ages, so that even men who are not cured of the disease often die from other causes. Interestingly, a parallel increase in prostate cancer mortality did not occur during the period 1989–1992, suggesting that most of the additional cases diagnosed would not otherwise have led to fatal outcomes.

B. Risk Factors for Prostate Cancer

Few risk factors for prostate cancer have been established (Table 72-1). Age is the strongest risk factor. Prostate cancer incidence increases more sharply with age than does any other cancer; more than 50% of cases in the United States are diagnosed in men >70 [4,9]. Race/ethnicity is a second risk

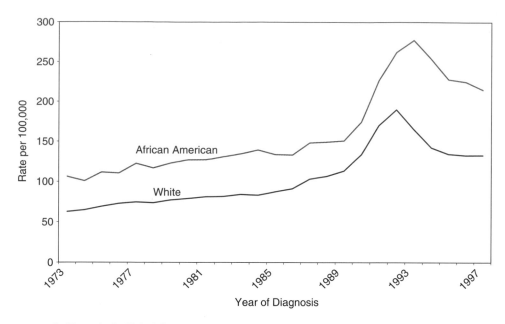

Fig. 72-1 Prostate cancer incidence in the United States, 1973–1997 (rates age-adjusted to the 1970 U.S. standard population. (From Ries LAG, Eisner MP, Kosary CL *et al*, ed. [2000]. SEER Cancer Statistics Review 1973–1997. NIH Pub No 00–2789 Bethesda, MD: National Cancer Institute.)

Table 72-1

Risk Factors for Prostate Cancer

Category	Characteristic or Exposure
Demographics	Age; ethnicity; geography
Genetics	Hereditary predisposing genes; polymorphisms in genes related to metabolism
Occupational Agents	Cadmium; metallic dusts and fluids; pesticides and other agricultural chemicals
Hormones/Growth Factors	Androgens (testosterone, DHT); insulin-like growth factors (IGF-I, IGF-binding proteins)
Lifestyle	Diet; alcohol; obesity; physical activity; sexually transmitted agents; smoking; vasectomy

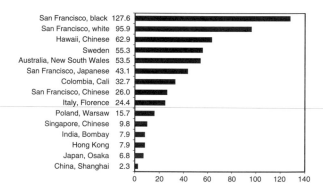

Fig. 72-2 Prostate cancer incidence in selected populations, 1988–1992 (rates age-adjusted to the world standard population). (From Parkin DM, Whelan SL, Ferlay J *et al*, ed. [1997]. *Cancer Incidence in Five Continents*. vol VII. IARC Sci Pub No 143. Lyon, France: IARC.)

factor for prostate cancer. In the United States, the lowest incidence rates are seen among Korean and Vietnamese men, both relatively recent immigrant groups from Asia; the rates are somewhat higher among Chinese, American Indian, Alaska Native, and Native Hawaiian men. Caucasian men have very high rates, but by far, the highest incidence of this cancer is among African-American men [10].

The incidence of prostate cancer varies more than 60-fold in populations around the world (Fig. 72-2). Indeed, of all common cancers, this site shows the widest variation between low- and high-risk countries or populations. High rates are seen in developed, especially western, countries, including the United States, Canada, parts of Europe, Australia, and New Zealand. Low rates tend to occur in Asia, particularly China [4,11]. The

highest reported rates in the world are among African-Americans, whereas the lowest reported rates are among Chinese men in Shanghai. Interestingly, Chinese men in more developed areas of Asia (Singapore and Hong Kong) and Chinese men in the United States (Hawaii and California) have much higher incidence rates than men in mainland China (see Fig. 72-2). Furthermore, immigrants from Japan to Brazil and the United States have higher rates than do men in Japan [9], suggesting the importance of the environment in determining prostate cancer risk. Although the incidence of prostate cancer in Japan increased about 3-fold between 1970 and 1990, which was similar to the rate of increase in the United States during the same period, the actual incidence in Japan remains very low (see Fig. 72-2).

Other than these risk factors, none of which by itself would be considered a causal agent, little is known about the etiology of prostate cancer. It is clear that men with a first-degree male relative who has had prostate cancer are at a 2- to 3-fold increased risk [12]. However, it is not clear whether this reflects a primary inherited predisposition for the disease or a shared environmental exposure among men growing up in the same household. The search for major predisposing genes for prostate cancer has identified some candidates, though none has yet been confirmed (see Section IV).

Several environmental (exogenous) etiologic agents have been proposed for prostate cancer: (1) occupational exposures (cadmium-containing products, such as paints and batteries; agriculture chemicals, especially pesticides; other metallic compounds) [13]; (2) diet, including alcohol consumption; (3) obesity; (4) physical activity; (5) sexually transmitted agents (cytomegalovirus, herpes simplex virus, human papillomavirus, and others) [14]; (6) smoking [15,16]; and (7) vasectomy [17]. However, the evidence is not yet convincing for any of these exposures.

Although it is suspected that most exogenous factors affecting prostate cancer risk exert their influence by altering endogenous androgen levels [18], epidemiologic studies have not yet clearly established the role of androgens in prostate cancer. Most studies of prediagnostic circulating levels of individual androgens have not shown a clear association with prostate cancer [19]. However, two studies showed weak positive relationships between the ratio of testosterone–DHT and prostate cancer [20,21]. A third study showed a strong positive association of plasma testosterone with prostate cancer only after adjustment for the sex hormone binding globulin (sHBG) level, suggesting that the level of free (unbound) testosterone is the critical factor [22].

The remainder of this chapter discusses evidence pertaining to diet (including alcohol), the most promising area of research into the etiology of prostate cancer. Because of the close association between diet, obesity and physical activity, the latter factors are also considered.

III. Studies of Diet in Relation to Prostate Cancer

A. Basis for the Diet-Prostate Cancer Hypothesis

Certain descriptive features of prostate cancer, especially the wide range in incidence for men of the same ethnic/racial group living in different geographic regions and the substantial changes in rates in migrant populations and their offspring [9], prompted a search for environmental risk factors in the etiology of this cancer. Diet became an important focus of this research for several reasons, including: (1) geographic variations in food and nutrient intakes are known to be large and could account for the observations in ethnic and migrant populations [11]; (2) ingested foods may contain carcinogenic compounds, either naturally occurring or produced during preservation or cooking [11]; (3) certain components of the diet can influence the levels of circulating androgens [23–25], which, as noted previously, are thought to play a role in prostate cancer risk. Many different dietary factors, including both foods and particular constituents of foods, have been studied. Some of these appear to increase risk, whereas others are possibly protective. These factors are listed in Table 72-2, and the supporting evidence is discussed in the following sections of this chapter.

Table 72-2
Possible Dietary Risk Factors for Prostate Cancer

Foods/Beverages	Food Constituents
Increase Risk	
Red meat	Total energy
Dairy products	Fat
Alcohol	Calcium
	Zinc/cadmium
Decrease Risk	
Vegetables	Vitamin D
Fruits	Vitamin E
Legumes	Carotenoids
Tea	Selenium
Fish	Other phytochemicals

B. Dietary Factors that Increase Risk

1. Foods and Drinks

a. RED MEAT.   Many epidemiologic investigations of different designs, including ecologic [26–28], case-control [29–35], and cohort [36–41] studies have reported positive associations between the consumption of meat, especially red meat, and prostate cancer. However, not all studies reproduced this finding [42–47].

Several alternative explanations for the association with meat are possible. Initially, the finding was thought to reflect a high exposure to dietary fat, especially saturated fat, because meat and dairy products are the major contributors to fat intake in the western diet. However, because the findings on dietary fat per se and prostate cancer are equivocal (see Section III.B.2.b), other explanations for the association need to be considered, including the following:

1. In the American diet, red meat is a major source of zinc, which is essential for testosterone synthesis and may have other effects in the prostate (see Section III.B.2.d).
2. Diets high in meat and other animal products may be relatively deficient in certain anticarcinogenic constituents found primarily in plant foods.
3. Many meats are cooked at high temperatures, such as by pan frying, grilling, or barbecuing.

Cooking meats at high temperatures can result in the formation of heterocyclic amines, which are potent carcinogens in animals, including the rat prostate [48]. Furthermore, when meats are cooked on charcoal grills, rendered fat is pyrolized by the coals, leading to the deposition of polycyclic aromatic hydrocarbons, which are also carcinogenic in animals, on the outer surface of the meat [49]. Few epidemiologic studies have been able to examine the relationship of such exposures to prostate cancer risk, as their levels in the diets of individuals cannot be easily and precisely assessed. One epidemiologic study that estimated heterocyclic amine intake from cooked meat and risk of prostate cancer did not lead to a clear result [50].

b. DAIRY PRODUCTS.   Several case-control [29,32,51,52] and cohort [33,36,39,40,53–55] studies found positive associations between the consumption of milk and other dairy products and the risk of prostate cancer. Nevertheless, some studies did not find this association [34,42,45,47,56,57]. One explanation for the positive association is an adverse effect of the high total and saturated fat content of dairy products. Another prominent constituent of these foods is calcium, which has also been proposed as a risk factor for prostate cancer (see Section III.B.2.c).

c. ALCOHOLIC BEVERAGES.   Although most case-control studies showed no association of prostate cancer with the intake of either total alcohol or specific alcoholic beverages [31,42, 43,58–61], some studies found positive associations with total alcohol [62] or specific types of alcoholic beverages, such as beer [63]. Similarly, several cohort studies found no association [36,39,58,64], whereas others saw an effect of total alcohol [65] or particular beverage types, including beer [47] and white (but not red) wine [66]. Thus, the data are quite inconsistent at present, and do not suggest an important relationship between alcoholic beverages and prostate cancer risk.

Some general mechanisms by which alcohol might enhance carcinogenesis have been proposed, including the activation of environmental nitrosamines, production of carcinogenic metabolites (acetaldehyde), immune suppression, and secondary nutritional deficiencies [58,62,66].

2. Nutrients and Other Food Constituents

a. ENERGY.   Total energy intake was not reported in early epidemiologic studies of diet and prostate cancer, because the dietary assessment methods used at the time were incomplete. However, several studies have examined this variable, particularly in relation to the effects of dietary fat intake. The findings have been very inconsistent. Some studies reported a positive association for energy intake and no independent association with dietary fat [67,68]. Others reported an effect of dietary fat, but no independent effect of energy [33,56,69,70]. One study reported a positive association with both total energy and total fat [34], and two studies found no association with either total energy or fat [43,71]. The conclusion that energy per se is unrelated to prostate cancer risk is supported by the finding that energy restriction in childhood and adolescence was not associated with a decrease in risk of prostate cancer in later life [72].

An experimental study in rodents (rats and mice) found that energy restriction reduced prostate tumor growth, possibly by inhibiting tumor angiogenesis [73].

b. FAT.   Dietary fat has been the most studied nutrient with regard to effects on prostate cancer risk. This topic has been the subject of reviews [74,75]. Total fat intake has been associated with the risk of prostate cancer in several case-control studies [31,33,56,59,76–78], although most found the association to be strongest for saturated or animal fat [30,33,69,76,77,79]. Of three cohort studies that examined total and saturated fat, one [71] found no evidence of an effect on prostate cancer, and two [38,80] found an elevated risk for total, but not saturated fat. When limited to studies that controlled for energy intake, however, the findings from both case-control and cohort studies are more equivocal, with many investigations showing no independent effect of fat [43,67,68,70,71]. In some studies, the

association with total and saturated fat was stronger for the advanced cases [33,38,69,78].

Some epidemiologic studies examined intakes of monounsaturated and polyunsaturated fat as well. The studies of monounsaturated fat are inconsistent, divided between those showing no association and those showing a positive association [75]. One case-control study [81] found an inverse association of prostate cancer with consumption of vegetable oils rich in monounsaturated fat, but not with total monounsaturated fat intake, suggesting that another component of these oils was responsible for the finding. For polyunsaturated fat, the findings are also equivocal, with some studies reporting no association and others a positive association [75].

Some investigators also examined specific fatty acids (including selected saturated, monounsaturated, omega-3 polyunsaturated, and omega-6 polyunsaturated fatty acids) based either on dietary intake data or biochemic measurements in blood or adipose tissue [75]. Although no clear associations have emerged, several studies reported positive associations of prostate cancer with alpha-linolenic acid, an omega-3 fatty acid found in vegetable oils and other terrestrial foods [38,41,79, 82,83]. In contrast, some studies found inverse associations with eicosapentaenoic acid (EPA) and/or docosahexaenoic acid (DHA), two long-chain omega-3 fatty acids found in fish oils [79,82,84]. The latter finding is supported by reports of an inverse association between fish consumption and prostate cancer (see Section III.C.1.e).

Some animal experiments have tested the fat-prostate cancer hypothesis. For example, a high fat diet increased prostate cancer incidence and shortened the latency period in Lobund Wistar rats treated with exogenous testosterone to induce the tumors [85]. Conversely, prostate tumor growth rate was reduced by a fat-free diet in Dunning rats [86] or by lowering dietary fat intake in athymic nude mice injected with LNCaP cells (a human prostate cancer cell line) [87]. With regard to specific types of fat, fish oils containing high levels of omega-3 fatty acids, such as EPA and DHA, generally suppressed prostate tumor growth in rodents, whereas other polyunsaturated fatty acids, including linoleic (omega-6) and alpha-linolenic (omega-3), promoted tumor growth [88,89]. Because most animal studies have been conducted in rodents, whose prostate glands differ anatomically from that of the human, extrapolation of these findings to humans is particularly tenuous.

A number of plausible mechanisms by which dietary fat could increase cancer risk have been proposed. These include, among others, the formation of lipid radicals and hydroperoxides that can produce DNA damage from oxidation of polyunsaturated fatty acids; increased circulating androgen levels from a high fat diet; decreased gap-junctional communication between cells from high polyunsaturated fat intake; altered activity of signal transduction molecules necessary for cellular growth control from high fat consumption; increased formation of eicosanoids that may influence prostate tumor cell growth from high intake of arachidonic acid; and decreased immune responsiveness from high intake of fatty acids [74].

c. CALCIUM.   As noted in Section III.B.1.b, a number of studies that examined the relationship of dairy product consumption to prostate cancer risk found a positive association. Dairy products could be a marker of exposure to calcium as well as saturated or animal fat, because this food group is a major source of both nutrients in the western diet. Data on calcium specifically are more limited, but one case-control study [52] and two cohort studies [54,55] reported statistically significant positive associations, especially with advanced or metastatic cancer. Furthermore, the data in these studies suggested that calcium, rather than dietary fat, was the relevant risk factor. However, a case-control study among U.S. whites and blacks [33], and a prospective analysis among men in Finland [57] did not show an independent effect of calcium on prostate cancer risk.

A mechanism for an adverse effect of calcium on prostate carcinogenesis has been proposed, based on the fact that a high intake of calcium decreases the levels of $1,25(OH)_2$ vitamin D which may inhibit cell proliferation and promote differentiation in prostatic tissue [90]. The role of vitamin D in prostatic carcinogenesis is discussed below.

d. ZINC AND CADMIUM. These trace elements are considered together because they act as antagonists in biologic systems. Few epidemiologic studies have examined dietary zinc or zinc supplement use in relationship to prostatic cancer. Most of the studies found no effect of zinc, especially after energy adjustment [43,56,67,78], although a positive association was suggested in two reports [77,91] and an inverse association in another [92]. The frequent association of prostate cancer risk with high intake of red meat (see Section III.B.1.a) could also be explained by a higher intake of zinc, rather than animal fat, because meat, especially red meat, is an important source of zinc in the American diet (other sources are shellfish, whole grain cereals, nuts and legumes) [93]. Reports based on zinc levels in serum or prostatic tissue of patients with cancer and controls have not been consistent [94,95], but such studies are unreliable, as the levels of zinc measured after diagnosis in the cases may reflect physiologic changes in the prostate as a result of the cancer.

As a major constituent of prostatic fluid [96,97], zinc is essential for normal prostate function. Zinc is also essential for normal testicular function, and high levels of zinc can increase the production of testosterone, leading to enhanced tissue growth in the prostate. Plasma levels of zinc have been positively correlated with testosterone and DHT levels in men [98,99]. Furthermore, in the rat prostate, zinc has been shown to increase 5α-reductase activity [100] and to potentiate AR binding [101]. Thus, one might speculate that higher intake of zinc could partially offset the normal decline in testosterone levels with age [102–104], thereby contributing to prostate cancer risk.

Epidemiologic evidence for cadmium as a risk factor for prostate cancer is also limited. Only two studies attempted to assess dietary exposure [105,106], and neither found very convincing evidence for an effect of diet alone, although both studies found some evidence for a positive association when the combined cadmium exposure from multiple sources (diet, cigarette smoking, occupation) was considered. Most studies of cadmium and prostate cancer have been among exposed workers in industries that utilize cadmium, and the findings of those investigations are only weakly suggestive of an adverse effect [107]. Cadmium is a competitive inhibitor of zinc in enzyme systems and accumulates in the body throughout life, because no mechanism exists for excreting it. Thus, the hypothesis that

cadmium may be carcinogenic for the prostate has biologic plausibility. This hypothesis is further supported by studies showing that cadmium is carcinogenic in animals, and that the effect can be blocked by simultaneous injection of zinc [108,109].

3. Obesity

Although obesity is not strictly a dietary risk factor, it is clearly related to diet. Unlike breast cancer in women, where the evidence for a positive association with obesity is strong, especially in postmenopausal patients, the evidence in support of an association between adult obesity and prostate cancer is limited. Although a few epidemiologic studies reported a significant positive association [29,42,53,80,110,111], most studies found no clear relationship of measures of obesity to prostate cancer risk [112]. Even when limited to prospective cohort investigations, the findings have been inconsistent [112]. The influence of obesity at younger ages is also unclear. One study suggested that childhood obesity may be protective against adult prostate cancer [113], but another study found that obesity at age 20 was associated with an increased risk [114].

The basis for an association between obesity and prostate cancer could involve endocrine factors, because adult obesity in men has been associated with decreased circulating levels of testosterone and sHBG, and increased levels of estrogen [115].

C. Dietary Factors that Decrease Risk

1. Foods and Drinks

a. VEGETABLES. Vegetables have been inversely associated with cancer risk at many sites. This has led to strong recommendations to consume significant quantities of these foods as part of a healthful diet. However, the evidence for a beneficial effect of vegetables on prostate cancer risk is not overwhelming. Although some case-control studies showed inverse associations with selected vegetables or vegetable groupings, including green and yellow vegetables, cruciferous vegetables, and carrots [31,34,116–119], others showed no significant associations [29,32,33,44,45,120,121]. The findings from prospective cohort studies have been mostly null [37,47,53,122–124]. The findings for legumes, a vegetable subgroup, are considered separately (Section IIIC.1.c. below), and the findings for tomatoes are included in the discussion of carotenoids (Section III.C.2.c).

Because vegetables contain numerous compounds that can act through a variety of mechanisms to inhibit carcinogenesis [125], an inverse association between vegetables and prostate cancer is plausible. For example, sulphoraphane, a major isothiocyanate found in cruciferous vegetables, was shown to induce phase 2 enzyme expression and activity in human prostate cancer cell lines [126]. Other mechanisms by which constituents of vegetables may protect against cancer of the prostate are discussed with respect to specific food constituents below.

b. FRUITS. The epidemiologic data on fruits and prostate cancer are also inconsistent, but interestingly, several studies, both case-control [44,77,116,117] and cohort [36,124], showed a direct (positive) association. Other case-control [32–34,45,56,

118,119] and cohort [37,47,53,122,123] studies showed either no association or a nonstatistically significant inverse relationship to prostate cancer risk. In one cohort [54], a statistically significant inverse association was found for fruit intake and advanced prostate cancer; this finding did not persist after adjustment for total fructose intake.

Why intake of fruits might have an adverse effect on the prostate is not clear. Fruits contain many of the same compounds with anticarcinogenic properties that are found in vegetables, such as various carotenoids and vitamin C [125]. Although this finding is not yet established firmly, it does appear that fruits have no particular benefit with regard to the risk of prostate cancer.

c. LEGUMES, INCLUDING SOY PRODUCTS.   Legumes, and particularly soy products, have become a focus of research on prostate cancer. Prostate cancer rates have traditionally been low in populations, such as those of Japan and China, where the intake of soy products is relatively high. A few case-control [43,44, 117,118] and cohort [36,37,124,127] studies have reported inverse associations between intake of legumes and prostate cancer, including soy foods specifically [36,44,118,127]. At present, the data are suggestive of a beneficial effect of legumes, but not soy products uniquely. Additional research may clarify this issue.

In the past, legumes were of interest in nutritional epidemiology primarily because of their important contribution to fiber intake. However, these foods also contain phytoestrogens, plant constituents that have mild estrogenic properties. Because estrogens may lower the risk of prostate cancer and are used in prostate cancer therapy, there is a good rationale for the hypothesis that phytoestrogen intake can protect against prostate cancer. Soybeans and many products made from soy, such as tofu, are rich in a class of bioactive phytoestrogens known as isoflavones (other classes of phytoestrogens include the coumestans and lignans). The main isoflavones found in soy include genistein, diadzein, and glycetein [128,129]. Although the mechanism for a protective effect of soy products on carcinogenesis in the prostate could entail the estrogenic effects of isoflavones, other actions of these compounds, such as inhibition of protein tyrosine phosphorylation, induction of apoptosis and suppression of angiogenesis have also been proposed [130]. Furthermore, legumes contain other bioactive microconstituents, including saponins, protease inhibitors, inositol hexaphosphate, γ-tocopherol, and phytosterols; mechanisms by which each of these compounds can inhibit carcinogenesis have been proposed [125,130,131–133].

Laboratory data based on human tissue as well as animal models offer support for the hypothesis that soy products may protect against prostate cancer [130]. Isoflavones added to the diet lowered plasma androgen levels in a rat model [134]. Lobund Wistar rats fed a diet in which soy protein isolate/ isoflavones replaced casein as a source of protein developed significantly fewer spontaneous prostate cancers than rats on the control diet [135]. In a transgenic mouse model, genistein in the diet reduced the incidence of poorly differentiated prostatic adenocarcinomas in a dose-dependent manner [136].

d. TEA.   Only a few studies have examined the relationship of tea consumption to prostate cancer risk, and the findings have been inconsistent. One cohort study in Hawaii and a case-control study in Canada showed an inverse relationship between daily tea consumption and prostate cancer risk [137,138], but other cohort [139,140] and case-control [43,44,141,142] studies did not reproduce this finding.

Tea contains polyphenols that are potentially anticarcinogenic because of their antioxidant properties, effects on signal transduction pathways, inhibition of cell proliferation, and other actions in the body [143].

e. FISH.   Only a few epidemiologic investigations have examined fish consumption in relation to prostate cancer risk. Although some studies reported inverse associations [35,144,145], other studies found no effect of fish [146,147]. The finding in a case-control study in New Zealand of an inverse association between the levels of two long-chain omega-3 fatty acids (EPA and DHA) in erythrocytes and prostate cancer risk supports this association [84]. In a study in Japan [25], the investigators found an inverse correlation between these long-chain fatty acids and total serum testosterone levels, suggesting one possible mechanism for a protective effect.

2. Nutrients and Other Food Constituents

a. VITAMIN D.   Evidence for a protective effect of vitamin D against prostate cancer is limited. In one cohort study [54], and two case-control studies [34,52], estimates of dietary vitamin D intake, whether from foods or supplements, were not associated with risk. Four cohort studies that examined the relationship of prediagnostic serum levels of 1,25-dihydroxyvitamin D ($1,25(OH)_2D$), the biologically active form of the vitamin, to subsequent development of prostate cancer produced discrepant results. One study found a clear inverse association [148], but the other three studies did not reproduce this finding [149–151].

Vitamin D reduces cell proliferation in the prostate (and other tissues) and enhances cell differentiation, both of which would be expected to lower the risk of cancer [90]. In mouse models and human prostatic cancer cell lines, $1,25(OH)_2D$ or vitamin D analogues were shown to inhibit tumor growth [152,153].

b. VITAMIN E.   The intake of vitamin E (alpha-tocopherol) is not adequately assessed with dietary histories, because much of the vitamin is obtained from fats and oils added during food preparation; estimating the amounts of added fats and oils is especially difficult. Nevertheless, a few epidemiologic studies attempted to determine vitamin E intake, with variable results. Several case-control studies [43,67,68,117] found no association with prostate cancer risk, whereas others [34,45] reported an inverse association with risk. Use of vitamin E supplements was not associated with prostate cancer risk overall in a cohort of U.S. men, although a reduced risk for advanced cancers was seen among current smokers and recent ex-smokers [154]. Some cohort studies reported on findings for vitamin E and prostate cancer based on prediagnostic serum levels. In one report, an inverse association was seen [155], whereas in three others, no association was found [156–158]. However, in an updated analysis [159] of one of these studies [157], an inverse association was found for vitamin E provided that levels of gamma-tocopherol (a related antioxidant consumed in the diet) were high. In an intervention trial among heavy smokers in Finland, an incidental finding was a reduced risk of prostate cancer associated with intake of vitamin E supplements (50 mg per day) [160,161]. Because the study was not specifically designed to test hypotheses related to prostate cancer, these results need confirmation. Furthermore, neither dietary nor serum vitamin E level at baseline was associated with subsequent development of prostate cancer in the nonvitamin E supplementation group [162].

Vitamin E inhibits the growth of human prostate tumors in nude mice [163]. Because vitamin E is a powerful antioxidant, one mechanism for a protective effect against carcinogenesis in the prostate would be inhibition of lipid peroxidation [164].

c. CAROTENOIDS (BETA-CAROTENE, LYCOPENE). The epidemiologic evidence related to carotenoids and prostate cancer is inconsistent. The results of case-control studies on dietary beta-carotene intake are mixed. Although some studies reported an inverse association [51,59,78,116], most offered no support for a protective effect of this nutrient [34,43,56,67,68,70,77, 119,121]. Furthermore, the findings often differed between younger and older men. Cohort studies have reported that dietary intake of beta-carotene decreased risk [47] or had no effect on risk [122,123], but, like the case-control studies, the findings sometimes differed between younger and older men [47]. A study showed that circulating levels of beta-carotene are significantly correlated with the levels in prostatic tissue [165]. However, studies of prostate cancer risk based on prediagnostic serum have reported both a positive [166] and no association [155,156,167] with elevated beta-carotene levels. Two intervention trials using beta-carotene have reported findings for prostate cancer. In a trial among physicians in the United States, beta-carotene supplementation (50 mg on alternate days) had no overall effect on prostate cancer incidence [168]; however, among men who had a low baseline serum beta-carotene, supplemenation was inversely associated with risk [169]. In an intervention trial among male smokers in Finland, beta-carotene supplementation was associated with a decreased risk of prostate cancer among nondrinkers of alcohol, but an increased risk among drinkers [160].

A carotenoid of particular interest with regard to prostate cancer is lycopene, found primarily in tomatoes and tomato products (other food sources include watermelon, grapefruit, and guava). Although a few case-control studies showed an inverse association between tomato consumption, particularly cooked tomatoes [33,45,117], most such studies found no association [43,44,118–121]. Of the case-control studies that estimated the intake of lycopene itself, none showed a clear inverse relationship to prostate cancer risk [34,43,117,121]. One study [33] found a weak inverse association with raw tomatoes but not cooked tomatoes, a surprising result, because the lycopene should be more bioavailable in the cooked tomatoes due to enhanced absorption as a result of heat processing and the presence of lipids [170]. Fewer analyses based on cohorts have been reported. Two such studies [37,123], including an updated analysis [171] of one of them [123] found significant inverse associations, although a third found no association [124]. Lycopene is unique among carotenoids in the diet, in that estimated intake

from fruits and vegetables is not a reliable predictor of blood levels [172]. However, the results of studies of prostate cancer based on prediagnostic circulating levels of lycopene are also inconsistent, two showing an inverse relationship [167,173] and one, no association [156].

Beta-carotene, lycopene, and other carotenoids are widely distributed in human tissues, including the prostate [165,174], where, as potent antioxidants, they help protect cell membranes, DNA, and other macromolecules from damage by reactive oxygen species [175]. Lycopene may also inhibit prostate carcinogenesis in humans by lowering insulin-like growth factor 1 (IGF-1) levels [176]. Other biologic activities of carotenoids, such as the upregulation of gap junctional communication [177] may also contribute to their anticarcinogenic effects. In three human prostate cancer cell lines (PC-3, DU 145 and LNCaP), beta-carotene significantly inhibited in vitro growth rates [178].

d. SELENIUM. Only a few epidemiologic studies have examined selenium and prostate cancer. Four case-control studies [43,56,78,117] found no association between estimated selenium intake and prostate cancer risk, and baseline selenium intake was not associated with subsequent development of prostate cancer in an intervention trial in Finland [162]. In addition, prediagnostic serum selenium was not related to prostate cancer in a prospective cohort in Finland [179], nor in a prospective analysis in the United States [180]. In contrast, prediagnostic selenium levels in toenails [159,181] and serum [182] were inversely associated with prostate cancer in three cohort studies; the findings from three other cohorts were suggestive of an inverse relationship [183–185]. Furthermore, in a selenium intervention trial to prevent skin cancer, an incidental finding was a reduced incidence of prostate cancer [186]. Because prostate cancer was not the primary end-point of the trial, this finding needs to be confirmed. A prostate cancer intervention trial using selenium as one of the interventions has begun (see Section V).

Selenium is a component of glutathione peroxidase, an important enzyme in certain antioxidative pathways. In an in vitro experiment, selenium was shown to inhibit the growth of human (DU-145) prostate carcinoma cells [187]. Selenium may exert its anticancer effects through any of several proposed mechanisms, such as antioxidation, enhanced immune function, inhibition of cell proliferation, and induction of apoptosis [188].

e. OTHER PHYTOCHEMICALS. The potential role of isoflavonoids in prostate carcinogenesis was discussed in the section on legumes (III.C.1.c). Similarly, the role of tea polyphenols and the isothiocyanate sulphoraphane was mentioned in the sections on tea (III.C.1.d), and vegetables (III.C.1.a).

3. Physical Activity

Physical activity, like obesity, is related to diet. Energy balance is only achieved when the combined caloric expenditure from basal metabolism and physical activity balance energy (caloric) intake. The role of physical activity in human prostate caricinogensis is at present quite unclear. Several epidemiologic studies have examined this relationship, but the findings have been highly inconsistent. Although several studies showed an inverse association, others showed no association, and some a positive association with prostate cancer risk [189,190]. These discrepancies may be resolved if future studies distinguish better between different types of physical activity, and can establish the time of life (e.g., young adulthood vs older ages) that may be most relevant.

Because exercise influences androgen levels in the body, an effect of physical activity on prostate cancer risk is biologically plausible. Exercise lowers testosterone in the blood, and also raises the level of sHBG, which reduces the circulating free testosterone levels, both of which would be expected to lower prostate cancer risk [191,192].

IV. Genetic Variation and Gene-Environment Interactions

As noted earlier, prostate cancer shows a familial association (i.e., men whose father or brothers have had prostate cancer are at a 2- to 3-fold higher risk of getting the disease than men without such a family history). The search for one or more highly penetrant genes that predispose to prostate cancer and that may explain at least part of this familial association has not yet been successful. Although candidate genes continue to be identified, attempts to reproduce the initial findings have led to inconsistent results [12,193].

However, genetic predisposition may have a more indirect relationship to prostate cancer. Androgenic hormones and various growth factors regulate cell growth and differentiation in the prostate. Several genes related to these cellular constituents, including the AR, SRD5A2, the vitamin D receptor (VDR), and insulin-like growth factor I (IGF-1), are polymorphic, and in some cases, variant forms of the gene have been shown to alter the activity of the gene product [194–200]. Several of these polymorphisms have been investigated in relation to prostate cancer risk [196–203], and although the findings are not yet entirely consistent, they indicate the potential of this new field of research.

A more complex and potentially useful area of investigation entails possible interactions between exogenous (environmental) exposures and such polymorphic genes. Because diet (as well as physical activity and other behaviors) can influence the levels of androgens, vitamin D, and IGF-1 in the body [204], there may be interactions between dietary exposures and inherited susceptibilities in determining actual risk for prostate cancer. Furthermore, many genes involved in the metabolism of dietary constituents (e.g., *CYP1A1* and *NAT2*, which encode specific cytochrome P450 and N-acetylating enzymes, respectively) are also polymorphic [205]. Thus, men whose diet is unhealthful and who also carry the high-risk variant of one or more of these genes may be at especially high risk for prostate cancer. Such gene-environment interactions offer considerable potential for elucidating the etiology of prostate cancer, and will no doubt be explored in future research.

V. Dietary Intervention Trials

A randomized intervention trial is the closest method to an experimental design that can be implemented in human subjects. Such a trial should be conducted only when there is considerable evidence for a beneficial effect, without apparent harm, based on observational studies and supported by animal

and *in vitro* studies. As the preceding review indicates, the data in support of most dietary factors and prostate cancer are either limited or inconsistent, and would not justify the expense and risks of an intervention trial. However, two randomized intervention trials that were conducted for other purposes have shown unexpected reductions in prostate cancer incidence in the intervention groups. One of these studies [186,206] was designed to test the potential of a daily selenium supplement (200 μg) to reduce the occurrence of basal and squamous cell skin cancers in men with a prior history of such lesions. The second trial [160,161] tested the effects of daily beta-carotene (20 mg) and/or vitamin E (50 mg *dl*-alpha-tocopherol acetate) on the risk of lung cancer in a group of male smokers. In both trials, the incidence of prostate cancer was significantly lower in the men who received the intervention compared with the placebo groups (in the lung cancer trial, the reduced incidence was in the men who received vitamin E rather than beta-carotene). However, because protection against prostate cancer was not a prespecified hypothesis in either trial, the results cannot be taken as definitive. Based on these findings, and the supportive evidence from other epidemiologic and laboratory research, a double-blind, randomized trial to test the potential benefit of supplemental selenium (200 μg) and vitamin E (400 mg), alone and in combination, is being conducted in the United States [207]. However, the results will not be available for several years.

VI. Role of Diet in Prostate Cancer Therapy

Currently, the primary treatment modalities for prostate cancer consist of surgery, radiation, and hormonal therapy. The fact that the findings for many dietary factors discussed previously were stronger in advanced or metastatic cases of prostate cancer (e.g., saturated fat, calcium) indicates that dietary effects can occur very late in the disease process. This suggests that dietary interventions have the potential not only to reduce the incidence but also to improve the survival rates of the disease.

Some early investigations offer support for this approach. A follow-up study of prostate cancer patients found significantly worse survival for men whose prediagnostic diet was high in saturated fat (>13.2% of calories) [208], whereas another study found that men with higher intake of monounsaturated fat prior to diagnosis had a better prostate cancer survival [209]. In a small intervention trial among prostate cancer patients prior to prostatectomy, the combination of fat restriction and supplementation with flaxseed (a rich source of the phytoestrogen lignan, as well as omega-3 fatty acids), significantly reduced total testosterone and free androgen (two possible biomarkers of prostate cancer risk) [210]. Finally, a very small intervention trial suggested that lycopene supplementation after diagnosis could have a beneficial effect on the progression of prostate cancer [211]. Although these results are preliminary, they support further research in this area as a complementary approach to the treatment of prostate cancer.

VII. Conclusions and Suggestions for Further Investigations

Considering the combined evidence from descriptive epidemiologic studies (especially the remarkable changes in migrant populations), analytic epidemiologic studies in widely varying populations, experimental studies in animals, and *in vitro* studies, the likelihood that certain dietary components or general patterns of eating influence the risk of prostate cancer remains high. However, at present, no specific relationships have been established conclusively. Continued research on this topic should be a high priority because diet is a modifiable risk factor and because prostate cancer incidence is extremely high in many populations. In addition, further research on genetic polymorphisms that affect susceptibility to prostate cancer should contribute to better identification of high risk groups of men who can be targeted for future preventive dietary interventions.

Among the many questions to be addressed in future research related to nutrition and prostate cancer are the following:

- When in the life cycle does diet exert its main effects on prostate carcinogenesis?
- What are the determinants of progression of latent tumors to clinically apparent disease? Can diet influence this process?
- Will the large-scale studies of interactions between dietary exposures and polymorphisms in genes related to food and hormonal metabolism clarify the specific effects of dietary constituents on carcinogenesis in the prostate?
- Are the risk factors for prostate cancer identical in men of all ethnicities? Are some populations, such as African-Americans, more susceptible to the effects of certain dietary exposures that increase prostate cancer risk?
- Can the identification of genes differentially expressed in malignant and normal prostate tissue [212] provide clues not only to prognosis but also to environmental exposures etiologically relevant to prostate cancer?

Based on current knowledge, highly specific dietary recommendations to prevent or treat prostate cancer are not possible. However, taken as a whole, the evidence offers reasonably strong support for a diet that emphasizes vegetables, including legumes, and is moderate or low in the consumption of meat, especially red meat, and dairy products.

References

1. Bostwick DG, Amin MB. (1996). Prostate and seminal vesicles. In *Anderson's Pathology*, 10th Edition, vol. 2. (Damjanov I, Linder J, ed.), pp. 2197–2230. St Louis, MO: Mosby.
2. Partin AW, Coffey DS. (1998). The molecular biology endocrinology and physiology of the prostate and seminal vesicles. In *Campbell's Urology*, 7th Edition, vol. 2, (Walsh PC, Retik AB, Vaughan ED Jr, Wein AJ, ed.), pp. 1381–1428. Philadelphia, PA: WB Saunders.
3. Barry MJ. (1998). PSA screening for prostate cancer: The current controversy–A viewpoint. Patient Outcomes Research Team for Prostatic Diseases. *Ann Oncol.* 9:1279–1282.
4. Parkin DM, Whelan SL, Ferlay J *et al*, ed. (1997). *Cancer Incidence In Five Continents.* vol VII. IARC Sci Pub No 143. Lyon France: IARC.
5. American Cancer Society. (2002). *Cancer Facts and Figures 2002.* Atlanta, GA: American Cancer Society.
6. Ries LAG, Eisner MP, Kosary CL *et al*, ed. (2000). SEER Cancer Statistics Review 1973–1997. NIH Pub No 00–2789. Bethesda, MD: National Cancer Institute.
7. Hankey BF, Feuer EJ, Clegg LX *et al*. (1999). Cancer surveillance series: Interpreting trends in prostate cancer–Part I: Evidence of the effects of screening in recent prostate cancer incidence mortality and survival rates. *J Natl Cancer Inst.* 91:1017–1024.

8. Legler JM, Feuer EJ, Potosky AL *et al*. (1998). The role of prostate-specific antigen (PSA) testing patterns in the recent prostate cancer incidence decline in the Unites States. *Cancer Causes Control.* 9:519–527.
9. Kolonel LN. (1997). Racial and geographic variations in prostate cancer and the effect of migration. In *Accomplishments in Cancer Research 1996*, (Fortner JG, Sharp PA, ed.), pp. 221–230. Philadelphia, PA: Lippincot-Raven.
10. Miller BA, Kolonel LN, Bernstein L *et al*, ed. (1996). *Racial/Ethnic Patterns of Cancer in the United States 1998–1992.* NIH Pub No 96–4104. Bethesda, MD: National Cancer Institute.
11. World Cancer Research Fund/American Institute for Cancer Research. (1997). *Food, Nutrition, and the Prevention of Cancer: A Global Perspective.* pp. 20–52, Washington, DC: American Institute for Cancer Research.
12. Stanford J, Ostrander E. (2001). Familial prostate cancer. *Epidemiol Rev.* 23:19–23.
13. Parent M-E, Siemiatycki J. (2001). Occupation and prostate cancer. *Epidemiol Rev.* 23:138–143.
14. Strickler H, Goedert J. (2001). Sexual behavior and evidence for an infectious cause of prostate cancer. *Epidemiol Rev.* 23:144–151.
15. Hickey K, Do K-A, Green A. (2001). Smoking and prostate cancer. *Epidemiol Rev.* 23:115–125.
16. Sharpe C, Siemiatycki J. (2001). Joint effects of smoking and body mass index on prostate cancer. *Epidemiol.* 12:546–551.
17. Giovannucci E. (2001). Medical history and etiology of prostate cancer. *Epidemiol Rev.* 23:159–162.
18. Wilding E. (1995). Endocrine control of prostate cancer. *Cancer Surveys.* 23:43–62.
19. Hsing A. (2001). Hormones and prostate cancer: What's next? *Epidemiol Rev.* 23:42–58.
20. Nomura A, Heilbrun LK, Stemmermann GN, Judd HL. (1988). Prediagnostic serum hormones and the risk of prostate cancer. *Cancer Res.* 48:3515–3517.
21. Hsing AW, Comstock GW. (1993). Serological precursors of cancer: Serum hormones and risk of subsequent prostate cancer. *Cancer Epidemiol Biomarkers Prev.* 2:27–32.
22. Gann PH, Hennekens CH, Ma J *et al*. (1996). Prospective study of sex hormone levels and risk of prostate cancer. *J Natl Cancer Inst.* 88:1118–1126.
23. Hamalainen E, Adlercreutz H, Puska P, Pietinen P. (1984). Diet and serum sex hormones in healthy men. *J Steroid Biochem.* 20:459–464.
24. Hill P, Wynder EL, Garbaczewski L *et al*. (1979). Diet and urinary steroids in black and white North American men and black South African men, *Cancer Res*, 39:5101–5105
25. Nagata C, Takatsuka N, Kawakami N, Shimizu H. (2000). Relationships between types of fat consumed and serum estrogen and androgen concentrations in Japanese men. *Nutr Cancer.* 38:163–167.
26. Howell MA. (1974). Factor analysis of international cancer mortality data and per capita food consumption. *Br J Cancer.* 29:328–336.
27. Armstrong B, Doll R. (1975). Environmental factors and cancer incidence and mortality in different countries with special reference to dietary practices. *Int J Cancer.* 15:617–631.
28. Koo LC, Mang OW, Ho JH. (1997). An ecological study of trends in cancer incidence and dietary changes in Hong Kong. *Nutr Cancer.* 28:289–301.
29. Talamini R, La Vecchia C, Decarli A *et al*. (1986). Nutrition social factors and prostatic cancer in a Northern Italian population. *Br J Cancer.* 53: 817–821.
30. Bravo MP, Castellanos E, del Rey Calero J. (1991). Dietary factors and prostatic cancer. *Urol Int.* 46:163–166.
31. Walker ARP, Walker BF, Tsotetsi NG *et al*. (1992). Case-control study of prostate cancer in black patients in Soweto South Africa. *Br J Cancer.* 65:438–441.
32. Talamini R, Franceschi S, La Vecchia *et al*. (1992). Diet and prostatic cancer: A case-control study in Northern Italy. *Nutr Cancer.* 113:277–286.
33. Hayes RB, Ziegler RG, Gridley G *et al*. (1999). Dietary factors and risks for prostate cancer among blacks and whites in the United States. *Cancer Epidemiol Biomarkers Prev.* 8:25–34.
34. Deneo-Pellegrini H, De Stefani E, Ronco A, Mendilaharsu M. (1999). Foods nutrients and prostate cancer: A case-control study in Uruguay. *Br J Cancer.* 80:591–597.
35. Ewings P, Bowie C. (1996). A case-control study of cancer of the prostate in Somerset and East Devon. *Br J Cancer.* 74:661–666.
36. Severson RK, Nomura AMY, Grove JS, Stemmermann GN. (1989). A prospective study of demographics diet and prostate cancer among men of Japanese ancestry in Hawaii. *Cancer Res.* 49:1857–1860.
37. Mills PK, Beeson WL, Phillips RL, Fraser GE. (1989). Cohort study of diet lifestyle and prostate cancer in Adventist men. *Cancer.* 64:598–604.

38. Giovannucci E, Rimm EB, Colditz GA *et al.* (1993). A prospective study of dietary fat and risk of prostate cancer. *J Natl Cancer Inst.* 85:1571–1579.
39. Le Marchand, L Kolonel LN, Wilkens LR *et al.* (1994). Animal fat consumption and prostate cancer: A prospective study in Hawaii. *Epidemiol.* 5:276–282.
40. Michaud D, Augustsson K, Rimm E *et al.* (2001). A prospective study on intake of animal products and risk of prostate cancer. *Cancer Causes Control.* 12:557–567.
41. Gann P, Hennekens CH, Sacks FM *et al.* (1994). Prospective study of plasma fatty acids and risk of prostate cancer. *J Natl Cancer Inst.* 86:281–286.
42. Gronberg H, Damber L, Damber JE. (1996). Total food consumption and body mass index in relation to prostate cancer risk: A case-control study in Sweden with prospectively collected exposure data. *J Urol.* 155:969–974.
43. Key TJ, Silcocks PB, Davey GK *et al.* (1997). A case-control study of diet and prostate cancer. *Br J Cancer.* 76:678–687.
44. Villeneuve PJ, Johnson KC, Kreiger N, Mao Y. (1999). The Canadian Cancer Registries Epidemiology Research Group Risk factors for prostate cancer: Results from the Canadian National Enhanced Cancer Surveillance System. *Cancer Causes Control.* 10:355–367.
45. Tzonou A, Signorello LB, Lagiou P *et al.* (1999). Diet and cancer of the prostate: A case-control study in Greece. *Int J Cancer.* 80:704–708.
46. Hirayama T. (1979). Epidemiology of prostate cancer with special reference to the role of diet. *Natl Cancer Inst Monogr.* 53:149–155.
47. Hsing AW, McLaughlin JK, Schuman LM *et al.* (1990). Diet tobacco use and fatal prostate cancer: Results from the Lutheran brotherhood cohort study. *Cancer Res.* 50:6836–6840.
48. Shirai T, Sano M, Tamano S *et al.* (1997). The prostate: A target for carcinogenicity of 2-amino-1 methyl-6-phenylimidazo[45-b]pyridine (PhIP) derived from cooked foods. *Cancer Res.* 57:195–198.
49. Lijinsky W, Shubik P. (1964). Benzo(a)pyrene and other polynuclear hydrocarbons in charcoal-broiled meat. *Science.* 145:53–55.
50. Norrish AE, Ferguson LR, Knize MG *et al.* (1999). Heterocyclic amine content of cooked meat and risk of prostate cancer. *J Natl Cancer Inst.* 91:2038–2044.
51. Mettlin C, Selenskas S, Natarajan N, Huben R. (1989). Beta-carotene and animal fats and their relationship to prostate cancer risk: A case-control study. *Cancer.* 64:605–612.
52. Chan JM, Giovannucci E, Andersson S-O *et al.* (1998). Dairy products calcium phosphorous vitamin D and risk of prostate cancer (Sweden). *Cancer Causes Control.* 9:559–566.
53. Snowdon AA, Phillips RL, Choi W. (1984). Diet obesity and risk of fatal prostate cancer. *Am J Epidemiol.* 120:244–250.
54. Giovannucci E, Rimm EB, Wolk A *et al.* (1998). Calcium and fructose intake in relation to risk of prostate cancer. *Cancer Res.* 58:442–447.
55. Chan J, Stampfer M, Ma J *et al.* (2001). Dairy products calcium and prostate cancer risk in the Physicians' Health Study. *Am J Clin Nutr.* 74:549–554.
56. Lee MM, Wang R-T, Hsing A *et al.* (1998). Case-control study of diet and prostate cancer in China. *Cancer Causes Control.* 9:545–552.
57. Chan JM, Pietinen P, Virtanen M *et al.* (2000). Diet and prostate cancer risk in a cohort of smokers with a specific focus on calcium and phosphorus (Finland). *Cancer Causes Control.* 11:859–867.
58. Dennis L, Hayes R. (2001). Alcohol and prostate cancer. *Epidemiol Rev.* 23:110–114.
59. Ross R, Shimizu H, Paganini-Hill A *et al.* (1987). Case-control studies of prostate cancer in blacks and whites in Southern California. *J Natl Cancer Inst.* 78:869–874.
60. Yu H, Harris RE, Wynder EL. (1988). Case-control study of prostate cancer and socioeconomic factors. *Prostate.* 13:317–325.
61. Tavani A, Negri E, Franceschi S *et al.* (1994). Alcohol consumption and risk of prostate cancer. *Nutr Cancer.* 21:25–31.
62. Hayes RB, Brown LM, Schoenberg JB *et al.* (1996). Alcohol use and prostate cancer risk in US blacks and whites. *Am J Epidemiol.* 143:692–697.
63. Sharpe C, Siemiatycki J. (2001). Case-control study of alcohol consumption and prostate cancer risk in Montreal Canada. *Cancer Causes Control.* 12: 589–598.
64. Hiatt RA, Armstrong MA, Klatsky AL, Sidney S. (1994). Alcohol consumption smoking and other risk factors and prostate cancer in a large health plan cohort in California (United States). *Cancer Causes and Control.* 5:66–72.
65. Hirayama T. (1992). Life-style and cancer: From epidemiological evidence to public behavior change to mortality reduction of target cancers. *Natl Cancer Inst Monogr.* 12:65–74.
66. Schuurman AG, Goldbohm RA, van den Brandt PA. (1999). A prospective cohort study on consumption of alcoholic beverages in relation to prostate cancer incidence (The Netherlands). *Cancer Causes Control.* 10:597–605.
67. Andersson SO, Wolk A, Bergstrom R *et al.* (1996). Energy nutrient intake and prostate cancer risk: A population-based case-control study in Sweden. *Int J Cancer.* 68:716–722.
68. Rohan TE, Howe GR, Burch JD, Jain M. (1995). Dietary factors and risk of prostate cancer: A case-control study in Ontario Canada. *Cancer Causes Control.* 6:145–154.
69. Whittemore AS, Kolonel LN, Wu AH *et al.* (1995). Prostate cancer in relation to diet, physical activity, and body size in blacks, whites, and Asians in the U.S. and Canada. *J Natl Cancer Inst.* 87:652–661.
70. Ghadiria P, Lacroix A, Maisonneuve P *et al.* (1996). Nutritional factors and prostate cancer: A case-control study of French Canadians in Montreal Canada. *Cancer Causes Control.* 7:428–436.
71. Schuurman AG, van den Brandt PA, Dorant E *et al.* (1999). Association of energy and fat intake with prostate carcinoma risk. *Cancer.* 86:1019–1027.
72. Dirx M, van den Brandt PA, Goldbohm RA, Lumey LH. (2001). Energy restriction in childhood and adolescence and risk of prostate cancer: Results from the Netherlands Cohort Study. *Am J Epidemiol.* 154:530–537.
73. Mukherjee P, Sotnikov AV, Mangian HJ *et al.* (1999). Energy intake and prostate tumor growth angiogenesis and vascular endothelial growth factor expression. *J Natl Cancer Inst.* 91:512–523.
74. Kolonel LN, Nomura AMY, Cooney B. (1999). Dietary fat and prostate cancer: Current status. *J Natl Cancer Inst.* 91:414–428.
75. Kolonel LN. (2001). Fat meat and prostate cancer. *Epidemiol Rev.* 23:72–81.
76. Graham S, Haughey B, Marshall J *et al.* (1983). Diet in the epidemiology of carcinoma of the prostate gland. *J Natl Cancer Inst.* 70:687–692.
77. Kolonel LN, Yoshizawa CN, Hankin JH. (1988). Diet and prostate cancer: A case-control study in Hawaii. *Am J Epidemiol.* 127:999–1012.
78. West DW, Slattery M, Robison LM *et al.* (1991). Adult dietary intake and prostate cancer risk in Utah: A case-control study with special reference to aggressive tumors. *Cancer Causes Control.* 2:85–94.
79. Harvei S, Bjerve KS, Tretli S *et al.* (1997). Prediagnostic level of fatty acids in serum phospholipids: ω-3 and ω-6 fatty acids and the risk of prostate cancer. *Int J Cancer.* 71:545–551.
80. Veierod M, Laake P, Thelle D. (1997). Dietary fat intake and risk of prostate cancer: A prospective study of 25,708 Norwegian men. *Int J Cancer.* 73: 634–638.
81. Norrish A, Jackson R, Sharpe S, Skeaff CM. (2000). Men who consume vegetable oils rich in monounsaturated fat: Their dietary patterns and risk of prostate cancer (New Zealand). *Cancer Causes Control.* 11:609–615.
82. Godley P, Campbell M, Gallagher P *et al.* (1996). Biomarkers of essential fatty acid consumption and risk of prostatic carcinoma. *Cancer Epidemiol Biomarkers Prev.* 5:889–895.
83. De Stefani E, Deneo-Pellegrini H, Boffetta P *et al.* (2000). Alpha-linolenic acid and risk of prostate cancer: A case-control study in Uruguay. *Cancer Epidemiol Biomarkers Prev.* 9:335–338.
84. Norrish AE, Skeaff CM, Arribas GLB *et al.* (1999). Prostate cancer risk and consumption of fish oils: A dietary biomarker-based case-control study. *Br J Cancer.* 81:1238–1242.
85. Pollard M, Luckert PH. (1986). Promotional effects of testosterone and high fat diet on the development of autochthonous prostate cancer in rats. *Cancer Lett.* 32:223–237.
86. Clinton SK, Palmer SS, Spriggs CE, Visek WJ. (1988). Growth of Dunning transplantable prostate adenocarcinoma in rats fed diets with various fat contents. *J Nutr.* 118:908–914.
87. Wang Y, Corr JG, Thaler HT *et al.* (1995). Decreased growth of established human prostate LNCaP tumors in nude mice fed a low-fat diet. *J Natl Cancer Inst.* 87:1456–1462.
88. Pandalai PK, Pilat MJ, Yamazaki K *et al.* (1996). The effects of omega-3 and omega-6 fatty acids on *in vitro* prostate cancer growth. *Anticancer Res.* 16:815–820.
89. Karmali RA, Reichel P, Cohen LA *et al.* (1987). The effects of dietary omega-3 fatty acids on the DU-145 transplantable human prostatic tumor. *Anticancer Res.* 7:1173–1179.
90. Feldman D, Zhao XY, Krishnan AV. (2000). Vitamin D and prostate cancer. *Endocrinology.* 141:5–9.
91. Schrauzer GN, White DA, Schneider CJ. (1977). Cancer mortality studies-III: Statistical associations with dietary selenium intakes. *Bioinorg Chem.* 7:23–34.
92. Kristal A, Stanford J, Cohen J *et al.* (1999). Vitamin and mineral supplement use is associated with reduced risk of prostate cancer. *Cancer Epidemiol Biomarkers Prev.* 8:887–892.
93. Shils ME, Olson JA, Shike M, ed. (1994). *Modern Nutrition in Health and Disease*, 8th Edition. Philadelphia PA: Lea & Febiger.

94. Feustel A, Wennrich R. (1986). Zinc and cadmium plasma and erythrocyte levels in prostatic carcinoma BPH urological malignancies and inflammations. *Prostate*. 8:75–79.

95. Whelan P, Walker BE, Kelleher J. (1983). Zinc vitamin A and prostatic cancer. *Br J Urol*. 55:525–528.

96. Tisell L-E, Fjelkegard B, Leissner K-H. (1982). Zinc concentration and content of the dorsal lateral and medial prostatic lobes and of periurethral adenomas in man. *J Urol*. 128:403–405.

97. Feustel A, Wennrich R. (1984). Determination of the distribution of zinc and cadmium in cellular fractions of BPH normal prostate and prostatic cancers of different histologies by atomic and laser absorption spectrometry in tissue slices. *Urol Res*. 12:253–256.

98. Habib F, Mason M, Smith P, Stitch S. (1979). Cancer of the prostate: Early diagnosis by zinc and hormone analysis. *Br J Cancer*. 39:700–704.

99. Hartoma T, Nahoul K, Netter A. (1977). Zinc plasma androgens and male sterility. *Lancet*. 2:1125–1126.

100. Om A-S, Chung K-W. (1996). Dietary zinc deficiency alters 5 alpha reduction and aromatization of testosterone and androgen and estrogen receptors in rat liver. *J Nutr*. 126:842–848.

101. Colvard DS, Wilson EM. (1984). Zinc potentiation of androgen receptor binding to nuclei *in vitro*. *Biochemistry*. 23:3471–3478.

102. Vermeulen A, Kautman JM, Giagulli VA. (1996). Influence of some biological indexes on sex hormone-binding globulin and androgen levels in aging or obese males. *J Clin Endocrinol Metab*. 81:1821–1826.

103. Wu AH, Whittemore AS, Kolonel LN *et al*. (1995). Serum androgens and sex hormone-binding globulins in relation to lifestyle factors in older African-American, white, and Asian men in the United States and Canada. *Cancer Epidemiol Biomarkers Prev*. 4:735–741.

104. Gray A, Feldman H, McKinlay J, Longcope C. (1991). Age disease and changing sex hormone levels in middle-age men: Results of the Massachusetts male aging study. *J Clin Endocrin Metab*. 73:1016–1025.

105. Kolonel LN, Winkelstein W Jr. (1977). Cadmium and prostatic carcinoma. *Lancet*. 2:566–567.

106. Abd Elghany N, Schumacher MC, Slattery ML *et al*. (1990). Occupation cadmium exposure and prostate cancer. *Epidemiology*. 1:107–115.

107. Nomura AMY, Kolonel LN. (1991). Prostate cancer: A current perspective. *Am J Epidemiol*. 13:200–227.

108. Haddow A, Roe FJC, Dukes CE, Mitchley BC. (1964). Cadmium neoplasia: Sarcomata at the site of injection of cadmium sulphate in rats and mice. *Br J Cancer*. 18:667–673.

109. Gunn SA, Gould TC, Anderson WAD. (1964). Effects of zinc on cancerogenesis by cadmium. *Proc Soc Exp Biol Med*. 115:653–657.

110. Andersson S-O, Wolk A, Bergstrom R *et al*. (1997). Body size and prostate cancer: A 20-yr follow-up study among 135,006 Swedish construction workers. *J Natl Cancer Inst*. 89:385–389.

111. Lew EA, Garfinkel L. (1979). Variations in mortality by weight among 750,000 men and women. *J Chron Dis*. 32:563–576.

112. Nomura AMY. (2001). Body size and prostate cancer. *Epidemiol Rev*. 23:126–131.

113. Giovannucci E, Rimm EB, Stampfer MJ *et al*. (1997). Height, body weight, and risk of prostate cancer. *Cancer Epidemiol Biomarkers Prev*. 6:557–563.

114. Schuurman AG, Goldbohm RA, Dorant E *et al*. (2000). Anthropometry in relation to prostate cancer risk in the Netherlands Cohort Study. *Am J Epidemiol*. 151:541–549.

115. Pasquali R, Casimirri F, Cantobelli S *et al*. (1991). Effect of obesity and body fat distribution on sex hormones and insulin in men. *Metabolism*. 40:101–104.

116. Ohno Y, Yoshida O, Oishi K *et al*. (1988). Dietary beta-carotene and cancer of the prostate: A case-control study in Kyoto Japan. *Cancer Res*. 48:1331–1336.

117. Jain MG, Hislop GT, Howe GR, Ghadirian P. (1999). Plant foods antioxidants and prostate cancer risk: Findings from case-control studies in Canada. *Nutr Cancer*. 34:173–184.

118. Kolonel LN, Hankin JH, Whittemore AS *et al*. (2000). Vegetables, fruits, legumes, and prostate cancer: A multiethnic case-control study. *Cancer Epidemiol Biomarkers Prev*. 9:795–804.

119. Cohen JH, Kristal AR, Stanford JL. (2000). Fruit and vegetable intakes and prostate cancer risk. *J Natl Cancer Inst*. 92:61–68.

120. Le Marchand L, Hankin JH, Kolonel LN, Wilkens LR. (1991). Vegetable and fruit consumption in relation to prostate cancer risk in Hawaii: A re-evaluation of the effect of dietary beta-carotene. *Am J Epidemiol*. 133:215–219.

121. Norrish AE, Jackson RT, Sharpe SJ, Skeaff CM. (2000). Prostate cancer and dietary carotenoids. *Am J Epidemiol*. 151:119–123.

122. Shibata A, Paganini-Hill A, Ross RK, Henderson BE. (1992). Intake of vegetables, fruits, beta-carotene, vitamin C, and vitamin supplements and cancer incidence among the elderly: A prospective study. *Br J Cancer*. 66:673–679.

123. Giovannucci E, Ascherio A, Rimm EB *et al*. (1995). Intake of carotenoids and retinol in relation to risk of prostate cancer. *J Natl Cancer Inst*. 87:1767–1776.

124. Schuurman AG, Goldbohm RA, Dorant E, van den Brandt PA. (1998). Vegetable and fruit consumption and prostate cancer risk: A cohort study in the Netherlands. *Cancer Epidemiol Biomarkers Prev*. 7:673–680.

125. Steinmetz KA, Potter JD. (1991). Vegetables, fruit, and cancer II mechanisms. *Cancer Causes Control*. 2:427–442.

126. Brooks JD, Paton VG, Vidanes G. (2001). Potent induction of phase 2 enzymes in human prostate cells by sulforaphane. *Cancer Epidemiol Biomarkers Prev*. 10:949–954.

127. Jacobsen BK, Knutsen SF, Fraser GE. (1998). Does high soymilk reduce prostate cancer incidence? The Adventist Health Study (United States). *Cancer Causes Control*. 9:553–557.

128. Wang H, Murphy PA. (1994). Isoflavone content in commercial soybean foods. *J Agric Food Chem*. 42:1666–1673.

129. Franke AA, Custer LJ, Wang W, Shi SJ. (1998). HPLC analysis of isoflavonoids and other phenolic agents from foods and from human fluids. *Proc Soc Exp Biol Med*. 211:163–173.

130. Fournier DB, Erdman Jr JW, Gordon GB. (1998). Soy, its components, and cancer prevention: A review of the *in vitro* animal and human data. *Cancer Epidemiol Biomarkers Prev*. 7:1055–1065.

131. Rao AV, Sung MK. (1995). Saponins as anticarcinogens. *J Nutr*. 125(Suppl 3): 717s–724s.

132. Kennedy AR. (1998). The Bowman-Birk inhibitor from soybeans as an anticarcinogenic agent. *Am J Clin Nutr*. (Suppl 68):1406s–1412s.

133. Wyatt CJ, Carballido SP, Mendez RO. (1998). Alpha- and γ-tocopherol content of selected foods in the Mexican diet: Effect of cooking losses. *J Agric Food Chem*. 46:4657–4661.

134. Weber KS, Setchell KD, Stocco DM, Lephart ED. (2001). Dietary soy-phytoestrogens decrease testosterone levels and prostate weight without altering LH prostate 5alpha-reductase or testicular steroidogenic acute regulatory peptide levels in adult male Sprague-Dawley rats. *J Endocrinol*. 170:591–599.

135. Pollard M, Wolter W. (2000). Prevention of spontaneous prostate-related cancer in Lobund-Wistar rats by a soy protein isolate/isoflavone diet. *Prostate*. 45:101–105.

136. Mentor-Marcel R, Lamartiniere CA, Eltoum I-E *et al*. (2001). Genistein in the diet reduces the incidences of poorly differentiated prostatic adenocarcinoma in transgenic mice (TRAMP). *Cancer Res*. 61:6777–6782.

137. Heilbrun LK, Nomura A, Stemmermann GN. (1986). Black tea consumption and cancer risk: A prospective study. *Br J Cancer*. 54:677–683.

138. Jain MG, Hislop GT, Howe GR *et al*. (1998). Alcohol and other beverage use and prostate cancer risk among Canadian men. *Int J Cancer*. 78:707–711.

139. Kinlen LJ, Willows AN, Goldblatt P, Yudkin J. (1988). Tea consumption and cancer. *Br J Cancer*. 58:397–401.

140. Ellison LF. (2000). Tea and other beverage consumption and prostate cancer risk: A Canadian retrospective cohort study. *Eur J Cancer Prev*. 9:125–130.

141. La Vecchia C, Negri E, Franceschi S *et al*. (1992). Tea consumption and cancer risk. *Nutr Cancer*. 17:27–31.

142. Slattery ML, West DW. (1993). Smoking, alcohol, coffee, tea, caffeine, and theobromine: risk of prostate cancer in Utah (United States). *Cancer Causes Control*. 4:559–563.

143. Yang CS, Chung JY, Yang G *et al*. (2000). Tea and tea polyphenols in cancer prevention. *J Nutr*. 130(Suppl 2S):472s–478s.

144. Terry P, Lichtenstein P, Feychting M *et al*. (2001). Fatty fish consumption and risk of prostate cancer. *Lancet*. 35:1764–1766.

145. Hebert JR, Hurley TG, Olendzki BC *et al*. (1998). Nutritional and socioeconomic factors in relation to prostate cancer mortality: a cross-national study. *J Natl Cancer Inst*. 90:1637–1647.

146. Schuurman AG, van den Brandt PA, Dorant E, Goldbohm RA. (1999). *Br J Cancer*. 80:1107–1113.

147. Hursting SD, Thornquist M, Henderson MM. (1990). Types of dietary fat and the incidence of cancer at five sites. *Prev Med*. 19:242–253.

148. Corder EH, Guess HA, Hulka BS *et al*. (1993). Vitamin D and prostate cancer: A prediagnostic study with stored sera. *Cancer Epidemiol Biomarkers Prev*. 2:467–472.

149. Gann PH, Ma J, Hennekens CH *et al*. (1996). Circulating vitamin D metabolites in relation to subsequent development of prostate cancer. *Cancer Epidemiol Biomarkers Prev*. 5:121–126.

150. Braun MM, Helzlsouer KJ, Hollis BW, Comstock GW. (1995). Prostate cancer and prediagnostic levels of serum vitamin D metabolites. *Cancer Causes Control*. 5:235–239.

151. Nomura AM, Stemmermann GN, Lee J *et al*. (1998). Serum vitamin D metabolite levels and the subsequent development of prostate cancer. *Cancer Causes Control*. 9:425–432.

152. Schwartz GG, Hill CC, Oeler TA *et al*. (1995). 125-Dihydroxy-16-ene-23-yne-vitamin D3 and prostate cancer cell proliferation *in vivo*. *Urology*. 46:365–369.

153. Miller GJ, Stapleton GE, Hedlund TE, Moffat KA. (1995). Vitamin D receptor expression 24-hydroxylase activity and inhibition of growth by 1-alpha25-dihydroxyvitamin D3 in seven human prostatic carcinoma cell lines. *Clin Cancer Res*. 1:997–1003.

154. Chan JM, Stampfer MJ, Ma J *et al*. (1999). Supplemental vitamin E intake and prostate cancer risk in a large cohort of men in the United States. *Cancer Epidemiol Biomarkers Prev*. 8:893–899.

155. Eichholzer M, Stahelin HB, Gey FK *et al*. (1996). Prediction of male cancer mortality by plasma level of interacting vitamins: 17-year follow-up of the Basel Study. *Int J Cancer*. 55:145–150.

156. Nomura AMY, Stemmermann GN, Lee J, Craft NE. (1997). Serum micronutrients and prostate cancer in Japanese Americans in Hawaii. *Cancer Epidemiol Biomarkers Prev*. 6:487–492.

157. Comstock GW, Bush TL, Helzlsouer K. (1992). Serum retinol beta-carotene vitamin E and selenium as related to subsequent cancer of specific sites. *Am J Epidemiol*. 135:115–121.

158. Knekt P, Aromaa A, Maatela J *et al*. (1988). Serum vitamin E and risk of cancer among Finnish men during a 10-year follow-up. *Am J Epidemiol*. 127:28–41.

159. Helzlsouer KJ, Huang H-Y, Alberg AJ *et al*. (2000). Association between alpha-tocopherol, selenium, and subsequent prostate cancer. *J Natl Cancer Inst*. 92:2018–2023.

160. Heinonen OP, Albanes D, Virtamo J *et al*. (1998). Prostate cancer and supplementation with alpha-tocopherol and alpha-carotene: Incidence and mortality in a controlled trial. *J Natl Cancer Inst*. 90:440–446.

161. The Alpha-Tocopherol Beta Carotene Cancer Prevention Study Group. (1994). The effect of vitamin E and beta-carotene on the incidence of lung cancer and other cancers in male smokers. *N Eng J Med*. 330:1029–1035.

162. Hartman TJ, Albanes D, Pietinen P *et al*. (1998). The association between baseline vitamin E selenium and prostate cancer in the Alpha-Tocopherol Beta-Carotene Cancer Prevention study. *Cancer Epidemiol Biomarkers Prev*. 7:335–340.

163. Fleshner N, Fir WR, Huryk R, Heston WD. (1999). Vitamin E inhibits the high-fat diet promoted growth of established human prostate LNCaP tumors in nude mice. *J Urol*. 161:1651–1654.

164. Burton GW, Ingold KU. (1981). Autooxidation of biological molecules 1. The antioxidant activity of vitamin E and related chain-breaking phenolic antioxidants *in vivo*. *J Am Chem Soc*. 103:6472–6477.

165. Freeman VL, Meydani M, Yong S *et al*. (2000). Prostatic levels of tocopherols carotenoids and retinol in relation to plasma levels and self-reported usual dietary intake. *Am J Epidemiol*. 151:109–118.

166. Knekt P, Aromaa A, Maatela J *et al*. (1990). Serum vitamin A and subsequent risk of cancer: Cancer incidence follow-up of the Finnish Mobile Clinic Health Examination Survey. *Am J Epidemiol*. 132:857–870.

167. Hsing AW, Comstock GW, Abbey H, Polk BF. (1990). Serologic precursors of cancer. Retinol carotenoids and tocopherol and risk of prostate cancer. *J Natl Cancer Inst*. 82:941–946.

168. Hennekens CH, Buring JE, Manson JE *et al*. (1996). Lack of effect of long-term supplementation with beta-carotene on the incidence of malignant and cardiovascular disease. *N Eng J Med*. 334:1145–1149.

169. Cook NR, Stampfer MJ, Ma J, Manson JE *et al*. (1999). Beta-carotene supplementation for patients with low baseline levels and decreased risks of total and prostate carcinoma. *Am Cancer Soc*. 86:1783–1792.

170. Sies H, Stahl W. (1998). Lycopene: Antioxidant and biological effects and its bioavailability in the human. *Proc Soc Exp Biol Med*. 218:121–124.

171. Giovannucci E, Rimm EB, Liu Y *et al*. (2002). A prospective study of tomato products, lycopene, and prostate cancer risk. *J Natl Cancer Inst*. 94:391–398.

172. Campbell DR, Gross MD, Martini MC *et al*. (1994). Plasma carotenoids as biomarkers of vegetable and fruit intake. *Cancer Epidemiol Biomarkers Prev*. 3:493–500.

173. Gann PH, Ma J, Giovannucci E *et al*. (1999). Lower prostate cancer risk in men with elevated plasma lycopene levels: Results of a prospective analysis. *Cancer Res*. 59:1225–1230.

174. Clinton SK, Emenhiser C, Schwartz SJ *et al*. (1996). Cis-trans lycopene isomers carotenoids and retinol in the human prostate. *Cancer Epidemiol Biomarkers Prev*. 5:823–833.

175. Chen L, Stacewicz-Sapuntzakis M, Duncan C *et al*. (2001). Oxidative DNA damage in prostate cancer patients consuming tomato sauce-based entrees as a whole-food intervention. *J Natl Cancer Inst*. 93:1872–1879.

176. Mucci LA, Tamimi R, Lagiou P *et al*. (2001). Are dietary influences on the risk of prostate cancer mediated through the insulin-like growth factor system? *B J U Int*. 87:814–820.

177. Bertram JS. (1999). Carotenoids and gene regulation. *Nutr Rev*. 57:182–191.

178. Williams AW, Boileau TW, Zhou JR *et al*. (2000). Beta-carotene modulates human prostate cancer cell growth and may undergo intracellular metabolism to retinal. *J Nutr*. 130:728–732.

179. Knekt P, Aromaa A, Maatela J *et al*. (1990). Serum selenium and subsequent risk of cancer among Finnish men and women. *J Natl Cancer Inst*. 32:864–868.

180. Goodman GE, Schaffer S, Bankson DD *et al* and the Carotene and Retinol Efficacy Trial (CARET) Co-Investigators. (2001). Predictors of serum selenium in cigarette smokers and the lack of association with lung and prostate cancer risk. *Cancer Epidemiol Biomarkers Prev*. 10:1069–1076.

181. Yoshizawa K, Willett WC, Morris SJ *et al*. (1998). Study of prediagnostic selenium levels in toenails and the risk of advanced prostate cancer. *J Natl Cancer Inst*. 90:1219–1224.

182. Nomura AMY, Lee J, Stemmermann GN, Combs GF Jr. (2000). Serum selenium and subsequent risk of prostate cancer. *Cancer Epidemiol Biomarkers Prev*. 9:883–887.

183. Criqui MH, Bangdiwala S, Goodman DS *et al*. (1991). Selenium retinol retinol-binding protein and uric acid associations with cancer mortality in a population-based prospective case-control study. *Ann Epidemiol*. 1:385–393.

184. Willett WC, Polk BF, Morris JS *et al*. (1983). Prediagnostic serum selenium and risk of cancer. *Lancet*. 2:130–134.

185. Coates RJ, Weiss NS, Daling JR *et al*. (1988). Serum levels of selenium and retinol and the subsequent risk of cancer. *Am J Epidemiol*. 128:515–523.

186. Clark LC, Combs GF, Turnbull BW *et al*. (1996). Effects of selenium supplementation for cancer prevention in patients with carcinoma of the skin. A randomized controlled trial. *JAMA*. 276:1957–1963.

187. Webber MM, Perez-Ripoll EA, James GT. (1985). Inhibitory effects of selenium on the growth of DU-145 human prostate carcinoma cells *in vitro*. *Biochem Biophys Res Commun*. 130:603–609.

188. Medina D. (1986). Mechanisms of selenium inhibition of tumorigenesis. *Adv Exp Med Biol*. 206:465–472.

189. Lee I-M, Sesso H-D, Chen J-J, Paffenbarger RS Jr. (2001). Does physical activity play a role in the prevention of prostate cancer. *Epidemiol Rev*. 23:132–137.

190. Bairati I, Larouche R, Meyer F *et al*. (2000). Lifetime occupational physical activity and incidental prostate cancer (Canada). *Cancer Causes Control*. 11:759–764.

191. McTiernan A, Ulrich C, Slate S, Potter J. (1998). Physical activity and cancer etiology: Associations and mechanisms. *Cancer Causes Control*. 9:487–509.

192. Hackney AC, Fahrner CL, Gulledge TP. (1998). Basal reproductive hormonal profiles are altered in endurance-trained men. *J Sports Med Phys Fitness*. 38:138–141.

193. Wang L, McDonnell SK, Elkins DA *et al*. (2001). Role of HPC2/ELAC2 in hereditary prostate cancer. *Cancer Res*. 61:6494–6499.

194. Ross RK, Pike MC, Coetzee GA *et al*. (1998). Androgen metabolism and prostate cancer: Establishing a model of genetic susceptibility. *Cancer Res*. 58:4497–4504.

195. Makridakis NM, Ross RK, Pike MC *et al*. (1999). Association of mis-sense substitution in SRD5A2 gene with prostate cancer in African-American and Hispanic men in Los Angeles U.S.A. *Lancet*. 354:975–978.

196. Platz EA, Giovannucci E, Dahl DM *et al*. (1998). The androgen receptor gene GGN microsatellite and prostate cancer risk. *Cancer Epidemiol Biomarkers Prev*. 7:379–384.

197. Stanford JL, Just JJ, Gibs M *et al*. (1997). Polymorphic repeats in the androgen receptor gene: Molecular markers of prostate cancer risk. *Cancer Res*. 57:1194–1198.

198. Habuchi T, Suzuki T, Sasaki R *et al*. (2000). Association of vitamin D receptor gene polymorphism with prostate cancer and benign prostatic hyperplasia in a Japanese population. *Cancer Res*. 60:305–308.

199. Ingles SA, Ross RK, Yu MC *et al.* (1997). Association of prostate cancer risk with genetic polymorphisms in vitamin D receptor and androgen receptor. *J Natl Cancer Inst.* 89:166–170.

200. Takacs I, Koller DL, Peacock M *et al.* (1999). Sibling pair linkage and association studies between bone mineral density and the insulin-like growth factor I gene locus. *J Clin Endocrinol Metab.* 84:4467–4471.

201. Hsing AW, Chokkalingam AP, Gao Y-T *et al.* (2002). Polymorphic CAG/CAA repeat length in the AIB1/SRC-3 gene and prostate cancer risk: A population-based case control study. *Cancer Epidemiol Biomarkers Prev.* 11:337–341.

202. Hsing AW, Chen C, Chokkalingam AP *et al.* (2001). Polymorphic markers in the SRD5A2 gene and prostate cancer risk: A population-based case-control study. *Cancer Epidemiol Biomarkers Prev.* 10:1077–1082.

203. Stanford JL, Noonan EA, Iwasaki LI *et al.* (2002). A polymorphism in the CYP17 gene and risk of prostate cancer. *Cancer Epidemiol Biomarkers Prev.* 11:243–247.

204. Tymchuk CN, Tonnler SB, Aronson WJ, Barnard RI (1998). Effects of diet and exercise on insulin sex hormone-binding globulin and prostate-specific antigen. *Nutr Cancer.* 31:127–131.

205. Chen C. (2001). Risk of prostate cancer in relation to polymorphisms of metabolic genes. *Epidemiol Rev.* 23:30–35.

206. Clark LC, Dalkin B, Krongrad A *et al.* (1998). Decreased incidence of prostate cancer with selenium supplementation: Results of a double-blind cancer prevention trial. *Br J Urol.* 81:730–734.

207. Klein EA, Thompson IM, Lippman SM *et al.* (2000). SELECT: The selenium and vitamin E cancer prevention trial–rationale and design. *Prostate Cancer Prostat Dis.* 3:145–151.

208. Meyer F, Bairati I, Shadmani R *et al.* (1999). Dietary fat and prostate cancer survival. *Cancer Causes Control.* 10:245–251.

209. Kim DJ, Gallagher RP, Hislop TG *et al.* (2000). Premorbid diet in relation to survival from prostate cancer (Canada). *Cancer Causes Control.* 11:65–77.

210. Denmark-Wahnefried W, Price DT, Polascik TJ *et al.* (2001). Pilot study of dietary fat restriction and flaxseed supplementation in men with prostate cancer before surgery: Exploring the effects on hormonal levels prostate-specific antigen and histopathologic features. *Urology.* 58:47–52.

211. Kucuk O, Sarkar FH, Sakr W *et al.* (2001). Phase II randomized clinical trial of lycopene supplementation before radical prostatectomy. *Cancer Epidemiol Biomarkers Prev.* 10:861–868.

212. Welsh JB, Sapinoso LM, Su AI *et al.* (2001). Analysis of gene expression identifies candidate markers and pharmacological targets in prostate cancer. *Cancer Res.* 61:5974–5978.

73

Human Papillomavirus Infection in Men and Women: The Impact of Nutrition on Cervical Cancer

MACK T. RUFFIN IV, MD, MPH* AND CHERYL L. ROCK, PhD, RD**

*Associate Professor, Department of Family Medicine, University of Michigan, Ann Arbor, MI

**Associate Professor, Department of Family and Preventive Medicine, University of California at San Diego, La Jolla, CA

I. Introduction

Cervical carcinoma and genital infections with human papillomavirus (HPV) are significant health problems worldwide. There has been little success in controlling either except with cervical cytology or Pap smear surveillance, which is not easily supported or afforded in developing countries. One variable often overlooked in these two diseases is the role of nutrition as a risk reduction strategy or a treatment method for early disease. The objectives of this chapter are to review the epidemiology of HPV and cervical cancer, explore the possible cofactors that contribute to the development of diseases, and review the data related to nutrition.

II. Description of the Continuum of Cervical Cancer

To bring order to the diagnostic confusion previously associated with Pap smear classifications, the Bethesda System was introduced in the United States [1–3]. This system combines clinically similar intraepithelial diagnosis into broad categories, specifically, low-grade squamous intraepithelial lesion (LGSIL) and high-grade squamous intraepithelial lesion (HGSIL). The Bethesda system was updated and revised [4]. This system was designed for use in cytologic screening. It remains technically more correct to use the detailed cervical intraepithelial neoplasia (CIN) scale for discussing cervical histopathology [5].

The progression of normal cervical epithelium through pre-invasive cervical lesions (LGSIL [HPV infection, CIN I], HGSIL [CIN II, CIN III, carcinoma *in situ*]) to invasive cancer is widely accepted as the continuum of cervical carcinoma. Squamous cell carcinoma usually arises from the squamo-columnar junction of the cervix and is preceded by, and thought to result from the progression of, cervical dysplasia and carcinoma *in situ* [6,7]. Rates of progression to carcinoma *in situ*, have ranged from 11 to 33% with a mean time of progression from CIN I to carcinoma of 86 months [6,8–10].

Several observations support the assertion of Kiviat *et al* [11] that only CIN II and III are the true precursor lesions. First, the anatomic distribution of CIN I is different (peripheral cervical lesions) from CIN II-III (central cervical lesions) [12]. Second, the mean age of women with CIN I and CIN II-III is comparable in incident case analysis [13] as distinguished from prevalent case analyses [14]. Third, 61% of women with CIN II-III never had a Pap smear showing CIN I [15]. Fourth, 50 to 90% of those CIN lesions most likely to regress are caused by HPV types other than "high-risk" types, whereas lesions most likely to progress to invasive carcinoma are caused by these high-risk HPV types [16]. Finally, *in vitro* infection of human keratinocytes

with HPV-16 produces a lesion that resembles CIN II-III, whereas infection with HPV-6 results in a lesion resembling CIN I [17].

A substantial proportion of CIN spontaneously regresses [9]. CIN I regresses more frequently than CIN II or III. The relative frequency of spontaneous regression varies widely from 11 to 44% [18–20]. In treatment protocols, the placebo response has ranged from 3 to 66% depending on population and mix of disease status [21–28]. The phase II study by Meyskens *et al* [26] is useful as it documented a placebo response rate of 27% in CIN II and 25% in CIN III.

Current treatment options for women with CIN II/III are still primarily ablation of the involved tissue. Newer techniques (e.g., loop electrosurgical excision procedure [LEEP]) still involve removal of tissue but have relatively few complications [29–38], yet retain similar treatment effectiveness compared to older procedures [39–42]. New modalities for prevention and treatment are under investigation.

A. Epidemiology

Cervical carcinoma is a significant health problem worldwide, being the second most common cancer among women, ranking first in many developing countries [43]. The worldwide incidence of cervical cancer is about 440,000 cases per year. The highest rates of cervical cancer have been reported from Cali, Colombia (42 per 100,000 person years) and Costa Rico (26 per 100,000 person years) [44]. In the United States, 12,900 new cases of invasive cervical cancer were predicted in 2001 with 4400 deaths attributable to this disease (1.8% of all cancer-related deaths in women) [45]. There have been increases in incidence and mortality rates among young women in countries with very low incidence rates. These countries include certain populations in the United States [46], Canada [47], Great Britain [48], Belgium [49], New Zealand [50], and Australia [51]. Yet, cervical carcinoma only represents a small portion of the burden created by cervical HPV infection. Annually in the United States, an estimated 3,550,000 women have cervical abnormalities noted on their Pap smear as highlighted in Fig. 73-1 [52]. These abnormalities create a great deal of anxiety and fear along with the burden of expensive and painful diagnostic colposcopic procedures.

B. Risk Factors

The epidemiologic association between HPV infection and cervical carcinoma fulfills all of the established epidemiologic

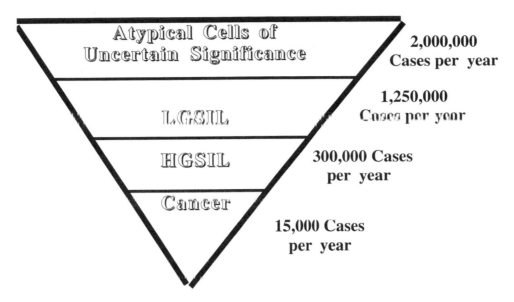

Fig. 73-1 Annual estimates of cervical cytologic abnormalities in the United States.

criteria for causality [16,53]. Genital HPV infection is the most common sexually transmitted infection (STI) in the United States [54]. At any one time, an estimated 20 million people in the United States have genital HPV infection that can be transmitted to others. Every year, about 5.5 million people acquire a genital HPV infection [54]. The prevalence of HPV infection in young women has been estimated to range from 20 to 46% in various countries, but results from studies in the United States suggest that 60% of college-aged women are infected with HPV at some time [55]. Persistent genital HPV infection among women represents a significant risk for the development of CIN [56,57] or persistent CIN [58].

III. Human Papillomavirus Mechanism of Action

The mere presence of HPV DNA at the cervix does not necessarily establish a clinical manifestation of squamous intraepithelial lesion (SIL) [59,60]. The natural history of a genital HPV infection, which can be characterized by changes in DNA positivity, HPV types, and number of HPV genomes over time, may influence the risk of developing squamous intraepithelial lesion of invasive cervical carcinoma. Some have argued that genital HPV infection is mainly transient, but this conclusion was based on small numbers and limited assessment points in time [61–65]. Cervical infection with HPV requires some type of cofactor before progression to significant disease. Some of these cofactors are viral persistence, viral load, viral integration, immune response to HPV and cervical carcinogenesis, which are reviewed in the next sections.

A. Viral Persistence

Few studies have examined prospectively the issues of persistent HPV cervical infections. Ho *et al* [58] examined the factors related to persistent SIL among 70 women followed every 3 months for 15 months. The risk of persistent SIL was

associated with persistent cervical-type specific HPV infection with an odds ratio (OR) of 3.9 (95% CI 1.58–9.65). In this study HPV persistence was defined as consecutive assessments positive for HPV. The Ho *et al* [55] study of 608 college women followed every 6 months for 3 years noted a cumulative 36-month incidence of HPV infection of 43%. The median duration of new infections was 8 months (95% CI 7–10 months), but the accuracy of this estimate was limited by the every-6-months assessment. The risk of developing an abnormal Pap smear increased with persistent HPV infection, particularly with high-risk types (relative risk [RR] 37.2, 95% CI 14.6 94.8) [55].

A number of studies have examined HPV persistence. In Table 73-1 is a selective summary of these studies highlighting techniques used for HPV detection, sample size, study population age, interval tested and follow-up length, and HPV outcome. It is difficult to draw conclusions given the different detection techniques used, unique study populations, various sampling methods, highly variable sampling intervals, and different lengths of observation. Most importantly, each study created a unique definition for persistence of genital HPV. In general, one can conclude that persistent genital HPV increases a woman's risk of developing an abnormal Pap smear. There are some other issues that are important to highlight from these studies. Koutsky *et al* noted a 2-year cumulative incidence of CIN II/III from first positive HPV as 28% [15]. In addition, this group noted no new cases of CIN II/III after 24 months regardless of HPV status [15]. Thus, women with HPV for 24 months are extremely unlikely to develop significant cervical abnormalities. Some would interpret the work of Moscicki *et al* [56,57] as a rationale for not treating genital HPV infections, because most women with HPV will clear it in 24 months. However, this same group also reported an RR of 14.1 (95% CI 2.3–84.5) for developing HGSIL, with at least three tests positive for high-risk HPV [56]. One of their studies found the RR for developing LGSIL as 7.4 for HPV 1 year, 10.3 for HPV for 1–2 years, and 6.11 for HPV 2–3 years [57]. Again, they confirmed the risk of persistent genital HPV infection.

Table 73-1
Summary of Studies Reporting Human Papillomavirus Persistence

Author/Technique	Sample Size	Age Years	Interval Tested	HPV Outcome
Rosenfeld [255] Southern Blot Tech	51	13–21 range	6–36 mos mean 13.3 mos	Base 39.2% follow-up 25.5%
Syrjanen [256] PCR	1,289	22 mean	Annual for 12 yrs	Base 3% follow-up 7% Annual incidence 7%
Koutsky [15] PCR	241	26.7 mean	Average 3 mos followed 25 mos	Base 18% 1st follow-up 7% 2nd follow-up 20%
DeVillers [257] Southern Blot	11,667	?	Over 5 yrs	Base 11.1% follow-up 11%
Moscicki [258] PCR	300	17.8 mean	Mean visits 6 over a mean of 27 mos	55% HPV + 33% consistently + 40% new HPV at follow-up
Hildesheim [63] PCR	393	26 mean 16–68 range	Median 14.9 mos	Base 26% follow-up 26%
Evander [259] PCR	276	Age cohorts of 19, 21, 23, 25	Median 24 mos (11–37)	Base 21% follow-up 8.3%
Hinchliffe [62] PCR	366	18–35 range	4 menstrual cycles apart	Base 7.4% follow-up 6.8%
Wheeler [260] PCR	72	<35 range	10 weekly visits	Base 36% weekly % HPV + range 20–47%
Moscicki [56] PCR	618	13–22 range	Q4 mos total 24 mos	All started as HPV + 70% HPV—at 24 mos
Moscicki [57] PCR	897	13–21 range	Q4 mos median 60 mos	496 prevalent HPV 105 negative 54 incident HPV

B. Viral Load

The viral load of HPV at the cervix could presumably be a marker of women with a greater chance of developing CIN or cervical cancer. Various measures of viral load have been explored. Early approaches assumed that HPV detected by Southern Blot techniques represents a high viral load compared to detection only by polymerase chain reaction (PCR) as low viral load [66]. Others have used more accurate measures of viral load under the name of copy number or number of HPV DNA per cells present [67–69]. The commonly used technique is quantitative, PCR-based fluorescent assays. Studies have questioned the utility of copy number given the large range of values (over 7 logs within a single disease category with a median copy number of 10^7 for normal and LGSIL disease and 10^9 for HGSIL), even after adjusting for HPV type and cervical disease status [69].

High viral load of oncogenic HPV DNA is considered a risk factor for potentially evolving LGSIL and HGSIL [70]. Average HPV-16 DNA copy number increases significantly with increasing epithelial abnormality, suggesting an association between HPV-16 DNA load and neoplastic progression [69]. In one study, women in the highest quintile for amount of HPV-16 DNA were at a 60-fold higher risk of developing cervical carcinoma in situ when compared with women negative for HPV-16 [71]. The data to date suggest an association between viral load of HPV-16 and the risk of more advanced cervical lesions. However, the influence of viral load on the natural history of HPV-16, especially among women with atypical squamous cells of uncertain significance (ASCUS) and LGSIL, remains uncertain.

C. Viral Integration

Integration of the viral genome into host cellular DNA can have implications in the initial stages of cell transformation, in the perpetuation of the transformed phenotype as well as in tumor progression. However, the direct effects on human genome integrity and gene function are largely unknown. Although it has been assumed that sites of integration of HPV are random, fluorescent in situ hybridization (FISH) data from a number of laboratories has shown an association between sites of HPV integration and chromosomal fragile sites [72,73]. It is possible that DNA strand breaks at fragile sites provide targets for viral integration.

FRA3B is the most common fragile site on normal human chromosomes and maps on the short arm of chromosome 3 (3p14.2). Cytologically, it is similar to the well known fragile X site associated with X-linked mental retardation. It differs in that it is present on chromosomes from all individuals and does not appear to be caused by a CCG trinucleotide repeat expansion. Like other fragile sites, it is a site of nonrandom chromosome breakage or instability seen following perturbation of DNA replication by folate deficiency or such drugs as FUdR or aphidicolin. FRA3B is the most "fragile" site in the human genome under these conditions [74]. It displays a number of interesting characteristics associated with site-specific chromosome breakage. Following induction in vitro, it acts as a site for production of translocations [75] and sister-chromatid exchanges [76] at a high rate, and is a preferred target of integration of transfected pSV2neo plasmid DNA [77]. Its location in the genome has been of interest in relation to carcinogenesis. It is indistinguishable cytogenetically from the t(3;8) breakpoint seen in a family with hereditary renal cell carcinoma [76], and lies in a region of 3p frequently deleted in a number of solid tumors such as lung, cervical, and renal [78–80], leading to the suggestions that the fragile site may play a mechanistic role in some of these deletion events.

The cloning of the fragile histidine triad (FHIT) gene was reported [81] in the FRA3B region. The search for the gene was based on the known existence of one or more putative tumor suppressor genes in 3p and on findings of homozygous deletions in 3p14.2 in gastrointestinal carcinoma cell lines [82]. The FHIT gene codes for a hydrolase involved in the catalysis of diadenosine tri- or tetra-phosphates. The gene and its transcripts exhibit very unusual behavior in a variety of tumors and tumor cell lines, including lung, esophageal, gastric and breast [81–84]. Multiple altered or "aberrant" transcripts, deleted for some of the FHIT coding exons, were seen in tumor tissue and tumor cell lines. The aberrant transcripts were shown in tumor cell lines to be caused by genomic deletions, often homozygous, within the FHIT gene. The origin of aberrant transcripts in fresh tumor specimens is less clear, and alternative splicing has been suggested to account for some findings [85]. Based on the hallmark characteristic of intragenic homozygous deletions, the FHIT gene has been suggested to be a tumor suppressor gene [81,83,84]. In addition, integration of HPV DNA has been identified at FRA3B within the FHIT gene in cervical cancer [86].

D. Immune Response to Human Papillomavirus

Papillomaviruses, with few exceptions, are exclusively intraepithelial pathogens, and it is presumed that the major route of presentation of viral antigens to the immune system is via the skin or mucous membranes. The viruses are not cytolytic and no inflammation accompanies infection and replication, a phenomenae that may retard initiation or even prevent an effective immune response. However, evidence from immunosuppressed individuals suggests strongly that the immune system is important in the pathogenesis of HPV-induced disease and malignant progression.

1. Humoral Response

Advances in the understanding of the humoral immune have lagged behind other areas of virology research for a number of reasons. These include difficulties in obtaining adequate quantities of virons and lack of appropriate animal models. The foremost reason is that the highest level of HPV gene expression occurs in the extreme outer layers of the epithelium with no detectable viremic stage. However, studies using enzyme-linked immunosorbent assay with HPV capsids or using in vitro translated early proteins has led many to believe that the humoral response to HPV has many important aspects.

The infected host responds to cutaneous papillomavirus infection by eliciting antibodies to structural viral proteins, which protects against reinfection [87]. Studies have focused on immune reactivity to nonstructural or capsid protein using synthetic peptides or expressed proteins as the test antigen. Serologic studies have used virus-like particles (VLP) produced from the expression of the L1 major capsid gene in vaccinia or baculovirus-expression systems. The L1 capsid protein self-

assembles to form 50 nm particles that resemble papillomavirus virions [88]. Virus-like particles for HPV-16 were used to test seropositivity in women that had HPV-16 DNA sequences in cervical scrapes. Sixty-seven percent of women with high HPV-16 DNA concentrations were seropositive, and only 37% of women with low DNA concentrations were positive. This contrasts to only 6% of women with no HPV-16 DNA being seropositive. In addition, women with CIN ranged from 45 to 75% seropositive [88]. HPV-16 VLP antibodies were detected in 73% and 81% of women with CIN III in Spain and Colombia, respectively. However, 46% of the Colombians were seropositive, whereas only 10% of the Spanish controls were positive. In addition, 59% of Spanish women with HPV-16 containing cervical cancers were seropositive and 51% of Colombian women had antibodies. Controls for Colombia showed 23% seropositivity, whereas only 3% of Spanish controls were positive [89]. Humoral response to virus capsid protein is slow. The mean time for development of antibodies from the detection of virus DNA is 350 days [90]. This likely is a reflection of the intraepithelial nature of the infection with relatively low amounts of virus capsid being made over a long period.

Fusion proteins are, in general, insoluble and need to be denatured and used in Western blot assays that provide only linear epitopes. Antibodies to HPV types 6, 16, or 18 early- and late-fusion proteins have been detected in up to 70% in children and asymptomatic adults [91,92]. Correlation has been found between the presence of HPV lesions or HPV DNA detection and seropositivity [93,94]. However, other studies have failed to reveal associations between antibody status and HPV infection [92,95]. Antibodies to HPV-16 E7 fusion protein are strongly associated with cervical cancer as are E6 antibodies. Antibodies to HPV-18 E6 and E7 in cervical cancer patients have also been reported [91,96–100]. There was no elevation in antibodies of patients with CIN. Some of the studies showed the strongest association to be with late stage cervical cancers suggesting antibodies to E6 and E7 develop after long-term exposure to antigens.

Antibody responses to numerous synthetic peptide epitopes have been defined for early and late open reading frames (ORFs) for HPV-16 and a few for HPV-18 [101]. Some of the epitopes have low sensitivity, whereas others show no apparent disease associations. For cervix cancer patients, response to the three HPV-16 epitopes range from 17 to 45% with the frequency being statistically significant over controls. Immunoglobulin G (IgG) antibodies to one epitope in E2 (peptide 245) is elevated among patients with cervix cancer and CIN and titers drop after treatment of CIN. An L2 epitope has been described to which an immunoglobulin A (IgA) response is preferentially found among patients with HPV-16 positive CIN. Titers to this epitope disappear upon spontaneous regression of the lesion.

2. Cell-Mediated Response

The cell-mediated reactions responding to HPV infections include: (1) production of cytokines with antiviral, antitumor, and immunoregulatory properties, (2) triggering of specific immune reactions, (3) recruitment of immunocompetent cells to the site of infection, and (4) cell-mediated cytotoxicity reactions against virus-infected cells.

a. CYTOKINES.   The main source of cytokines in mucosa are keratinocytes, epithelial cells, and infiltrating monocytes. Their role in anti-HPV reaction may include inhibition of HPV gene expression, modulation of HPV-infected cell growth, stimulation of leukocyte infiltrates, facilitating the death of HPV-infected cells, and control of angiogenic and metastatic potential of HPV-associated tumors. The primary cytokines that may be able to inhibit the expression of HPV genes and growth of HPV infected cells include tumor necrosis factor a (TNF-α), interleukin 1 (IL-1), transforming factor b (TGF-β), and interferons [102] The mechanism of down-regulation of HPV expression may involve activation of some transcription factors. Inhibition of growth of HPV infected cells may be related to the down-regulation of some cellular regulatory genes such as c-myc [103,104].

b. ANTIGEN PRESENTATION.   Immune response to HPV antigens may contribute to disease progression suggesting that particular human leukocyte antigen (HLA) class II genes are associated with persistence or progression of virally induced lesions. Han et al [105], using the cottontail rabbit papillomavirus system, demonstrated that papilloma regression and progression to carcinoma was linked to HLA class II alleles determined by restriction fragment length polymorphisms of the rabbit homologues of the DRA and DQA genes. Regression was associated with a given DRA allele and progression to a particular DQA allele. Cervical cancer risk in man is also linked to HLA class II genes. Wank et al [106] showed that German women with cervical cancer have a 7-fold increase in RR for cervical cancer if they are HLA-DQ3 antigen-positive as determined by serotyping. This has been confirmed in other populations using other techniques [107–111]. On the other hand, the presence of HLA-DR6 conferred a 12.7-fold decrease in the RR for cervical cancer. Other studies, however, have failed to detect a statistically significant association between DQB1*03 and increased risk for cervical cancer in English patients [112,113]. Hispanic women also failed to show a statistically significant association for increased risk of developing cervical cancer for DQB*03 alone; however, combinations of HLA class II alleles (the DRB1*0407/DQB1*0302 and DRB1*1501/DQB1*0602 haplotypes) were increased in patients with HPV-16-positive cancers [114].

Considering the premalignant stages of cervical cancer, associations have been found between CIN and DQB1*03 in Belgian women [115] and DQB1*0301, DRB1*0401 and English women [116,117]. HPV-16 seropositive Swedish women showed increased frequency of DQB1*0602, DQA1*0102, and DRB1*1501 compared with seronegative women [118]. The DRB1*1501/DQB1*0602 haplotype that is found in Hispanic cervical cancer patients is also found in Hispanics with HPV-16-containing CIN [119]. Less is known about HLA class I associations with cervical cancer. Wank et al [106] were unable to find differences in the frequencies of class I alleles in German cervical cancer patients. Human leukocyte antigen B7 and HLA A26 were more frequent in cervical cancer patients in England, but the differences were not statistically significant [113,120]. However, cervical cancer patients with HLA B7 had a significantly reduced survival time compared with patients without the allele [120].

Indirect evidence that regression of HPV-induced lesions is a cell-mediated event is reflected by the fact that renal allograft recipients have a 10-fold increase in RR for developing cervical neoplasia [121,122]. Spontaneous rejection of flat skin warts is characterized by a cellular infiltrate composed mainly of T lymphocytes and macrophages resembling a delayed type hypersensitivity (DTH) response [123,124]. In vitro studies have shown that proliferating keratinocytes from wart explants are destroyed by migration of T cells from the explants [125]. Immunohistologic studies reveal that regression of these warts is accompanied by an intense mononuclear dermal infiltrate of CD4+ lymphocytes and HLA-DR+ dendritic cells [126,127].

Normal cervical epithelial cells do not express HLA class II antigens. Human papillomavirus-infected cervical epithelial cells, however, do express class I and class II antigens but in varying amounts. These cells should, therefore, be able to present antigen to both CD4+ and CD8+ lymphocytes, both of which infiltrate cervical cancers [112,128,129]. T-cell clones obtained from tumor-infiltrating lymphocytes have varying levels of cytolytic activity to autologous or other tumor cells. The fact that a proportion of cervical cancer patients, patients with CIN and asymptomatic women are seropositive for HPV antigens [91,95] indicates specific T-helper cell function. Cervical epithelial cells lack expression of the accessory molecules B7.1 and B7.2 for correct antigen presentation that may lead to T-cell anergy or a biased T-helper response [130,131].

Human leukocyte antigen class I antigens are down-regulated in a variety of cancers, including cervical [132]. Complete loss of class I expression ranges from 5 to 48% with down-regulation of one or more class I alleles in 30 to 78% of cervical cancers and loss of expression of common alleles in 17 to 71% of cancers. Down-regulation of class I molecules may be important in the persistence of CIN associated with high risk HPVs. However, there are conflicting reports on down-regulation of class I molecules in CIN.

T-cell determinants have been mapped for HPV early proteins. Strang et al [133] established interleukin 2 (IL-2)-dependent human T-cell lines and clones from asymptomatic donors that responded to HPV-16 E6 synthetic peptides in an HLA-DR-restricted fashion. Studies in rodent systems using E7-expressing tumor cells have shown that E7 is a tumor rejection antigen and can elicit a DTH response [134–136]. CD4+ cytotoxic human T lymphocyte lines and T-cell clones have been established from peripheral blood mononuclear cells of asymptomatic HPV-16 seropositive donors responding to E7 synthetic peptides [137].

The apparent association of HLA class II molecules with increased risk for cervical cancer indicates the inability to immunologically respond to high-risk HPV. Functions of T lymphocytes depend upon interactions with other cells resulting in generation of cytotoxic T cells and T-helper cells that induce the proliferation and differentiation of antibody-secreting B-lymphocytes. Human leukocyte antigen molecules direct T-cell responses to the cell surface where foreign antigens are recognized as part of a complex with HLA products. Assuming this holds true for HPV antigens, then a number of possibilities exist to explain an impaired immune response to HPV. For example, DQB1*03 may be a surrogate marker for cervical cancer risk related to a nearby locus such as the polymorphic

DQA1 gene. This is a possibility, because different DQA1 alleles can be linked to one DQB1 allele resulting in DQ dimers differ in antigen presentation [138].

Human leukocyte antigen class II-antigen complexes may stimulate suppressor T cells to dampen the immune response. Sasazuki *et al* have found HLA DQ-restricted suppressor cells [139–141]. There are low responders to natural antigens such as tetanus toxoid, staphylococcal cell wall and hepatitis B surface antigen in the human population. Depletion of CD8+ T cells from low-responder T cells restores the response and the CD8+ T cells of low responders suppress the immune response of isolated CD4+ T cells from high responders [141]. The effect is linked to HLA-DQ, because anti-HLA-DQ monoclonal antibody restores the immune response in some low responders and there is a statistically significant association between low immune response and HLA-DQ [142]. Furthermore, antigen specific CD4+ T cells from nonresponders are restricted by DQA1*0102 or DQA1*0103 [143]. These results taken together suggest that HLA-DQ may down-regulate the immune response through induction of CD8+ suppressor T cells. Perhaps HLA-DQ presents antigens to HLA-DQ-restricted CD4+ suppressor/inducer T cells that in turn activate CD8+ T-suppressor cells [143].

The TCR is a heterodimeric glycoprotein expressed on the surface of T cells. This molecule confers immunity by the specific recognition of foreign antigen peptides in the context of HLA molecules. Heterogeneity of TCR molecules, which is needed to cope with the number of potential foreign antigens, occurs through somatic recombination of variable (V), diversity (D) and junctional (J) elements by mechanisms similar to immunoglobulin gene rearrangements. The epithelium of human skin, the gastrointestinal tract and the uterine cervix are populated predominately by T cells bearing the αβ receptor and contain a minority of γδT cells [144–146]. When compared to TCR β-chain variable region (Vβ)-expression in PBL, TCR αβ+ gastrointestinal epithelial T cells express a limited number of Vβ that varies, to some extent, among individuals [147]. In normal skin given Vβ families are absent when compared to peripheral blood lymphocytes (PBL), whereas other Vβ families are overrepresented [148]. It is likely that differences exist in TCR Vβ usage in cervical epithelium as compared with PBL. One could hypothesize, therefore, that in the case of cervical cancer, CIN progression to cancer may, in part, be due to expression of a limited T cell β repertoire in cervical epithelium capable of recognizing HLA-HPV antigen complexes.

E. Cervical Carcinogenesis

Epidemiologic studies have shown the high-risk HPVs (HPV-16 and HPV-18) to be the central etiologic factor for invasive cervical cancer and its precursor lesions [149]. However, HPV infection constitutes only one step in cervical carcinogenesis, because only a small percentage of women infected with high risk HPVs ever develop cervical cancer [150]. The putative target cell in the cervix for HPV infection is squamous metaplastic epithelium, because most CIN and cervical cancers occur within the transformation zone of the cervix [151]. The infection can become latent before or after a lesion develops. This transition may be regulated by the immune system, because lesions frequently develop during pregnancy and then spontaneously resolve, and women under immunosuppressive therapy have a high incidence of cervical neoplasia [151]. Experimentally, HPV sequences are frequently detected in cervical scrapes from asymptomatic women [152,153].

In all cell lines examined and in most cervical cancers, the viral genome is integrated, which is not true in CIN [154–156]. This integration preserves, at a minimum, the long control region, which contains numerous transcription factor binding sites, enhancer elements, the early region promoter, and the E6 and E7 ORFs [155–160]. This results in loss of the tight transcriptional regulation of E6 and E7 from downstream ORF products. Continued expression of these proteins is critical for maintenance of the malignant phenotype of cervical cancer cells [161]. In tissue culture, HPV-16 and HPV-18 E6 and E7 can profoundly influence growth and differentiation of human keratinocytes. Transfection of primary human keratinocytes with virus DNA results in immortalization of nontumorigenic cells [162,163]. Immortalization depends on continued expression of E6 and E7 [164]. Transfection of these cells with the activated ras oncogene converts the cells to a tumorigenic phenotype [165]. Therefore, additional mutational events are required for tumorigenicity. This is supported by the rare conversion of HPV-18-immortalized keratinocytes to tumorigenicity after prolonged passage [166].

Human papillomaviruses associated with cervical cancer efficiently immortalize primary human keratinocytes, whereas viruses not frequently detected in cervical cancer (HPV-6 and HPV-11) do not [167]. Insights into the biochemic basis of cell transformation have come from the demonstration that HPV-16 and HPV-18 E6 binds to and promotes the degradation of the tumor suppressor gene product p53 via the ubiquitin protease pathway [168–170], whereas low-risk virus E6 binds only weakly [171]. A nuclear protein, p53 regulates genes involved in apoptosis, cell cycle progression, and DNA damage and is frequently mutated in cancers. However, p53 is usually intact in HPV-positive cervical cancers and cell lines [172]. It is a potent activator of transcription through activation of promoters containing a p53 binding site. Cell cycle regulation by p53 is mediated through up-regulation of WAF-1 (CIP-1, p21) expression [173]. WAF-1 complexes with proliferating cell nuclear antigen (PCNA), which is required for stimulation of DNA polymerase [174]. WAF-1 is also a cdk inhibitor and blocks cells in G1 by inhibiting phosphorylation of the retinoblastoma tumor suppressor gene product (pRB) by cdc2 [175]. Phosphorylation of pRB releases the E2F transcription factor, which stimulates transcription of growth promoting genes. In response to DNA damage, p53 also stimulates transcription of GADD45 [176]. GADD45 stimulates excision repair and inhibits DNA replication presumably by forming a complex with PCNA. If cells cannot repair the DNA damage or there are conflicting signals to proliferate from an activated oncogene and growth suppression from wild type p53, apoptosis may ensue [177]; however, cells expressing E6 are resistant to radiation-induced apoptosis.

The E7 protein from these viruses, which is the most abundant viral protein in cervical cancer cells [178,179], binds to the hypophosphorylated forms of the pRB family of tumor suppressors [180] but E7 from low-risk viruses binds weakly [181].

Hypophosphorylated pRB interacts with the transcription factor E2F, and the complex acts as a transcriptional repressor. The binding of hypophosphorylated pRB by E7 functionally inhibits the sequestering of E2F and allows free forms of E2F to transcriptionally activate genes whose products are required for the G1/S transition. Overexpression of E2F induces apoptosis in cells with an intact p53 pathway [182] and may explain why HPV needs to target both cell cycle regulatory pathways. E7 has also been shown to inhibit WAF-1 function by binding to the carboxy-terminal end of the protein that overlaps with the PCNA binding site and the second cyclin binding motif [183].

IV. Nutrition and Cervical Cancer

Numerous epidemiologic studies have examined the associations between dietary factors and risk for cervical cancer. Based on current knowledge of the etiology of cervical cancer, interpretation of results from the early studies is constrained because accurate information on HPV status was generally not available to consider in the analysis. In more recent studies, HPV status is generally considered as a contributing or adjustment factor in the analysis, although this is arguably not an appropriate strategy because HPV status is in the causal pathway. Studies also have examined whether diet influences risk for persistence of HPV infection, which more specifically tests whether nutrient status or dietary intake is a determinant of the cellular and biologic response to HPV exposure and infection.

Various mechanisms have been proposed to explain the effects of nutrient status and dietary constituents on the process of cervical carcinogenesis, and in some cases, the proposed cellular mechanisms are demonstrable in cell culture models. In these cases, the effect on risk for malignancy or progression may be direct (for example, facilitating normal gene expression or promoting apoptosis in HPV-infected cells), and the specificity of the effect would thus be determined by the biologic functions and activities of the nutrient or dietary constituent. However, overall nutritional status and several micronutrients and dietary constituents are known to influence the immune response on several levels of the defense system. For example, both protein-energy malnutrition and obesity are associated with immunodeficiencies, and adequate energy and amino acid intakes are necessary to provide energy and substrates to enable the synthesis of cellular constituents and activities of the immune system [184]. Marginal and frank deficiencies of several essential minerals and vitamins are associated with impaired immune response, with vitamin A having probably the most well-established role in the immune response. In vitamin A deficiency, the immune response is depressed, the secretion of mucus (which provides a barrier function) is impaired, and the activity of T-helper cells is affected [185]. As another example, administration of vitamin E to persons who do not exhibit evidence of poor status or inadequate intake has been shown to improve *in vivo* immune response [186]. In addition to effects of energy, amino acids, and micronutrients, manipulations of lipids in the diet also have been demonstrated in clinical studies to have effects on the immune system [187,188].

In the majority of the epidemiologic studies of the relationship between nutritional factors and cervical cancer risk, the focus has been on risk for CIN or SIL rather than risk for invasive cervical cancer, because the disease is usually detected at the preneoplastic stages in women in developed countries. Similarly, the nutrition intervention studies conducted to date all have focused on increasing the regression rate of CIN, rather than on primary prevention or altering the response to HPV exposure. An important issue in this area of study is that the stage at which nutritional factors may influence the risk and progression of cervical cancer is unknown, and results from cell culture studies suggest that there may be stages at which the cell growth abnormalities cannot be reversed [189].

A critical and comprehensive review of the available evidence on nutrition and cervical neoplasia from clinical and analytic epidemiologic studies and intervention trials was conducted in 1996 by Potischman *et al* [190], which serves as a benchmark. Since that report, 17 analytic epidemiologic studies on this topic have been reported, with the majority (14 of 17) being case-control studies or comparisons across subgroups of women in clinical populations. Three prospective studies have been reported: two addressed the relationship between nutritional factors and risk for cervical cancer [191,192], and one addressed the relationship between dietary intakes and risk for SIL in HPV-positive women [193]. In addition to increased emphasis on assessment of HPV status (and adjustment for this crucial determinant of disease and disease progression in the analysis), an evident trend in this area of research is the increased utilization of serologic data and dietary biomarkers in these epidemiologic studies, rather than reliance on dietary intake data alone. Although not without limitations, serologic data generally provide a more objective and definitive assessment of intake and status, when compared with the reporting bias and classification error that is inherent in self-reported dietary data, which presents a problem even when the most well-developed dietary assessment methodologies are used. Also, several clinical trials that were in progress at the time of the 1996 review have been completed.

A. Vitamin A and Carotenoids

Vitamin A and the carotenoids have overlapping biologic activities, because approximately 10% of the carotenoids can function as vitamin A or retinoic acid precursors. However, the food sources for these compounds are distinctly different. Vegetables and fruit provide the overwhelming majority of carotenoids in the diet, and animal products (e.g., dairy foods, liver) are the major dietary sources of preformed vitamin A. Also, an important biologic difference that is relevant to interpreting the literature on nutrition and cervical neoplasia is that ingested preformed vitamin A is highly regulated in the human biologic system, so peripheral tissue levels of vitamin A-active compounds generally do not have a linear relationship with the levels of dietary intake, at least across the range typically consumed in the United States. Circulating vitamin A (retinol) concentration declines in response to low intake only in adults who have consumed low amounts of vitamin A or precursors over some period of time. In contrast, carotenoids are unregulated, with amounts in the circulation and in the peripheral tissue reflective of dietary intake of these compounds (and intakes of vegetables and fruit) in a linear manner, although responsiveness is attenuated somewhat by nondietary determinants such as smoking status (due to increased oxidation of the carotenoids) and increased body mass or adiposity (due to an increase in the size of the body compartments or pools). Also, the carotenoids have been shown to be metabolized *in vivo* to retinoic acid-like metabolic products that have unknown biologic activities, and other nonvitamin A activities, such as antioxidant activity, have been demonstrated *in vitro* [194].

In the earlier review, it was concluded that the majority of epidemiologic data did not suggest a relationship between cervical cancer risk and the levels of dietary preformed vitamin A or plasma or serum retinol concentrations [190]. Since that time, serologic vitamin A data have been examined in seven epidemiologic studies (including one prospective study), and three studies examined the relationship between dietary vitamin A and risk for cervical dysplasia or cancer. Of the seven studies involving serum or plasma vitamin A data, a significant inverse relationship between retinol concentration and risk was observed in three of these studies [195–197], and the point estimates were suggestive (although not significant, in association with very small sample sizes) in two of the studies [192,198]. Conversely, two studies that were both case-control studies focused on risk of CIN or SIL did not observe a relationship between serum retinol concentration and risk [199,200]. Notably, two of the studies that found a protective effect targeted minority groups that likely included a relatively large proportion of economically disadvantaged women (Native Americans in the Southwestern United States and nonHispanic African-American women) [195,198]. In the study by French *et al* [196], 1314 women with known human immunodeficiency virus infection were examined, and risk for SIL was found to be associated with retinol concentrations <1.05 umol/L (multivariate OR 1.62, 95% confidence interval [CI] 1.02, 2.58). In women already diagnosed with cervical dysplasia, Nagata *et al* [192] found the rate of progression to carcinoma *in situ* or invasive cervical cancer to be 4.5 times higher in those with lower serum retinol levels (P = 0.08).

Dietary vitamin A intake was not linked with risk for CIN or cervical cancer in the three studies [192,193,198]. In the study by Wideroff *et al* [193], the analysis was prospective and was focused solely on dietary data, but similar to the others, a relationship between intake and risk for SIL was not observed.

It is notable that a number of studies in which HPV status has been considered in the analysis have identified an adverse effect of poor vitamin A status (reflected in low serum retinol concentration) on risk for cervical dysplasia or cancer. The findings are somewhat supportive of a relationship when the focus is on plasma retinol concentration as the indicator of status but not when the focus is on self-reported intake. This suggests that poor vitamin A status may indeed be a risk factor for cervical cancer for some women and some subgroups, even in developed countries.

A relevant finding is that topical retinoic acid has been demonstrated in a controlled clinical trial to increase the regression rate of CIN II [26]. However, amounts of retinoic acid in peripheral tissues, such as the cervix, are generally not modifiable by ingested preformed vitamin A across the range of vitamin A

intake in the U.S. diet, and serum retinol in that study was not related to response or regression rate.

Since the earlier review [190], six observational epidemiologic studies have examined the relationship between serologic data on carotenoids and cervical neoplasia (including one cross-sectional study that focused on risk for HPV persistence), three studies incorporated an analysis of the relationship between estimated carotenoid intakes and risk for CIN or SIL, and two studies examined intakes of relevant foods (vegetables, fruit) and risk for CIN. Four of the six studies that conducted an analysis of risk based on serum or plasma carotenoids found a significant protective effect [197,200–202] and another one reported point estimates that suggest a nonsignificant protective effect [198]. Only one study that examined the relationship between serologic data on carotenoids and risk for CIN, adjusted for HPV status and other potential influencing factors, did not find a relationship [199]. In the studies in which an association between carotenoids and risk was observed, various carotenoids were identified as being protective against CIN, SIL, cervical cancer or HPV persistence, including α-carotene [201], β-carotene [202], β-cryptoxanthin [197,200–202], lutein/zeaxanthin [197,201,202], and lycopene [197,198]. In the studies that identified a protective effect, the risk for CIN or disease progression was typically reduced by 60%. In an observational study of 123 Hispanic women, Giuliano *et al* [202] found adjusted mean concentrations of serum β-carotene, β-cryptoxanthin, and lutein to be 24% lower (P<0.05) among women with persistent HPV infection (defined as HPV positive at both of two examinations, 3 months apart) compared with women without persistent HPV infection.

Of the three studies that examined the association between estimated carotenoid intakes and risk for CIN or SIL, one found a significant inverse relationship with risk for β-carotene intake [203], one found no relationship between carotenoid intake and risk [198], and one found a nonsignificant protective association (OR 0.6 for highest vs lowest quartile) between risk and β-carotene intake [193]. Because vegetables and fruit are the predominant food sources of carotenoids, analysis of associations between intakes of these foods and risk for cervical neoplasia are highly relevant to the potential role of carotenoids. These associations have been addressed in two studies. One case-control study did not find vegetable intake to be significantly related to risk of CIN [204], although the analysis revealed a marginally significant protective effect (adjusted OR 0.6 for highest vs lowest quartile, P = 0.09 for trend), whereas another found both vegetables and fruit to be consumed less frequently by women with HPV-associated cervical dysplasia compared to controls (P<0.05) [203].

Similar to the results of the earlier studies on carotenoids and cervical cancer risk [190], these observational epidemiologic studies indicate fairly consistent support for a protective effect. These findings and the earlier studies contributed to the rationale for the β-carotene supplement trials that have been conducted (discussed next); however, it is notable that the epidemiologic studies have linked the reduction in risk to several carotenoids and not just to β-carotene.

Both vitamin A metabolites (retinoids) and carotenoids have been shown to act on cell growth regulation and apoptosis [189,205]. At physiologic levels, retinoic acid suppresses

HPV-16-mediated transformation of human keratinocytes and inhibits the expression of the HPV-16 oncogenes [205]. Similarly, carotenoids such as β-carotene and astaxanthin induce significant growth retardation in HPV-16-infected cervical dysplasia cell lines, associated with chromatin condensations indicative of apoptosis [189]. In the case of vitamin A and the carotenoids, *in vitro* laboratory evidence for possible mechanisms of action in cervical carcinogenesis has been reported.

B. Vitamin C

Few studies involving serologic assessment of vitamin C status were available for review in 1996, but a majority of the case-control studies focused on dietary vitamin C intake that were available for review at that time indicated an inverse association with risk for cervical neoplasia [190]. Since that time, four observational epidemiologic studies involving analysis of vitamin C measurements in blood samples, including one study of the relationship with HPV persistence, have been reported. Two of these studies, both case-control studies focused on risk for CIN, found plasma vitamin C to be protective [199,200]. Although marginally significant across the entire population (OR 0.34, 95% CI 0.13, 1.00 per unit increase adjusted for HPV status and other influencing factors), plasma vitamin C was associated with reduced risk of CIN in HPV-positive individuals at a high level (≥0.803 mg/dL) (OR = 0.46, 95% CI 0.19, 0.89) in one of these studies [199]. Conversely, the other two studies in which serum vitamin C concentration was the focus of analysis did not find an association with risk or HPV persistence [195,202]. Of the three studies in which the association between vitamin C intake and risk for CIN was examined, two did not find a significant relationship [193,204] and one found a protective effect [203]. Because vegetables and fruit are the primary food sources of vitamin C (as well as the carotenoids), the somewhat favorable findings from the two studies that examined the associations between intake of these foods (discussed previously) and risk for cervical dysplasia provide findings that also are relevant to vitamin C intake and cervical neoplasia.

These newer findings on vitamin C from epidemiologic studies have been inconsistent, with outcomes that are evenly divided in the suggested effects on risk. Vitamin C exhibits biologic activity as a water-soluble antioxidant, which theoretically could reduce oxidative damage to DNA and thus, attenuate oxidative stress-related molecular changes associated with cervical carcinogenesis. Also, vitamin C has been shown to have several effects on immune system factors *in vivo* [194], so beneficial effects on the immune response to HPV exposure also are feasible.

C. Vitamin E

Early evidence from epidemiologic studies relating vitamin E intake to cervical cancer risk was less consistent than that for dietary carotenoid and vitamin C [190]. However, vitamin E has been shown to enhance cell-mediated immune response and phagocyte-derived functions in laboratory animal and human studies [186], so the possibility of a beneficial effect on risk for

cervical cancer, mediated by enhanced immune responsiveness, is an attractive theory. Several studies that have examined the relationship between serum vitamin E concentration or dietary intake and cervical neoplasia have been reported the past few years.

Of the six observational epidemiologic studies (including one observational study on HPV persistence) relating serologic vitamin E data to cervical neoplasia that have been reported since the earlier review, four found a significant protective effect for serum α-tocopherol concentration [197,199,200,202]. As an illustration of the magnitude of the effect observed in these studies, Ho *et al* [199] found a 52% reduction in risk for CIN associated with higher plasma α-tocopherol concentration (OR 0.48 for highest vs lowest quintile, P = 0.024 for trend), adjusted for HPV positivity and other possible influencing factors. Another case-control study reported a suggestive but nonsignificant point estimate for risk of CIN (OR 2.0 for low serum α-tocopherol) [195]. However, one case-control study did not report a relationship between serum α-tocopherol and risk for CIN [198].

In contrast with the reasonable consistency of a beneficial effect of plasma α-tocopherol (and sometimes gamma-tocopherol) concentration on risk or progression of disease, none of the three studies that examined associations between tocopherol intake and risk for CIN found a significant association [193,198,203]. However, vitamin E intakes are assumed to reflect a greater degree of underreporting than intakes of other micronutrients, because the richest sources of this vitamin are generally the high-fat foods that are known to be underreported in research studies and nutrition surveys [206]. Inaccuracies in dietary intake data provide one explanation for the disparity between findings based on serologic vs dietary data in these epidemiologic studies on vitamin E and cervical neoplasia.

D. Folate

Morphologic similarities between the cytologic features of megaloblastosis due to folate deficiency and the changes associated with cervical dysplasia have historically suggested a role for folate in cervical cancer risk. Also, folate functions in a key role in one-carbon metabolism and thus, plays a crucial role in DNA methylation and gene expression [207]. A few other nutrients that are involved in the one-carbon metabolic pathway (thus linked to DNA methylation and normal DNA synthesis and repair), especially vitamin B12, have also been examined in several studies related to the role of folate in cervical neoplasia. Homocysteine is a sensitive indicator of folate intake that provides some insight about folate status, because increased homocysteine concentration occurs with suboptimal folate status. Thus, homocysteine and cysteine (a related metabolite) have been examined in some of the studies on folate and cervical neoplasia [208,209].

Based on the earlier evidence, Potischman *et al* [190] concluded that dietary folate seemed to be generally associated with risk for early CIN rather than for carcinoma *in situ* or invasive cancer. Since that review, six observational epidemiologic studies have examined associations between risk for CIN, SIL, cervical cancer or HPV persistence, and serum or erythrocyte folate concentration, and many of these studies also collected and analyzed data on related nutrients and metabolites (e.g., vitamin B12, vitamin B6, homocysteine, cysteine). Two of these studies did not identify a relationship between erythrocyte or serum folate concentration and risk for CIN [195,198], but the results from four of these studies suggest a nonsignificant protective effect in association with higher folate or vitamin B12, or lower homocysteine or cysteine, concentrations [191,200,210,211]. For example, Weinstein et al [211] found a 64% increase in risk for invasive cervical cancer associated with lower erythrocyte folate concentration, adjusted for HPV status and other influencing factors (OR 1.64 for lowest vs highest quartile, P = 0.09 for trend). In a cross-sectional study of HPV persistence, Sedjo et al [210] found higher serum vitamin B12 (but not folate) concentration to be associated with a reduction in risk.

Further support for a role in the etiology of cervical cancer for one-carbon metabolism, and the nutrients associated with the metabolic pathways relevant to those biochemic activities, is suggested by results of a study that examined a diet-gene interaction. Polymorphisms in the gene for the enzyme methylenetetrahydrofolate reductase (MTHFR) are associated with an increased requirement for folate and elevated plasma homocysteine concentration [212]. In a case-control study focused on risk for SIL, Goodman et al [213] found that low folate intake in the presence of the most common MTHFR polymorphism was associated with significantly increased risk (OR 5.0, 95% CI 2.0, 12.2 for below vs above the median folate intake). Of the six studies (five observational and one prospective) that included an analysis of folate intake and risk for CIN, SIL or HPV infection that have been reported since the earlier review [193,198,203,204,210], only the study by Goodman et al [213] found dietary intakes of folate, vitamin B6, and vitamin B12 to be inversely related to the ORs for cervical SIL after adjustment for HPV and other influencing factors.

Thus, results from these findings have not ruled out a role for folate and other nutrients involved in one-carbon metabolism, and instead seem to suggest that some relationship exists, although it may be complicated by genetic factors. A relationship between circulating and cervical tissue folate concentrations and degree of DNA hypomethylation in biopsied cervical tissue has been reported [214,215], which provides some in vivo evidence to support the hypothesized relationship between one-carbon metabolism, related nutrients, and cervical neoplasia.

E. Intervention Trials with Supplements and Diet Modification

On the basis of the earlier epidemiologic evidence, intervention studies involving supplemental folate, β-carotene, and vitamin C were initiated several years ago to test the effect on regression of dysplasia. Three controlled studies of the effect of folic acid supplementation on regression of CIN have been conducted and reported. Following a preliminary trial that found beneficial results in 47 women with CIN [216], Butterworth et al [24] randomized 235 women with CIN I and II to receive 10 mg folate or placebo daily for 6 months. No differences in HPV or CIN status between the treatment and placebo groups were observed. The third trial was a multicenter study in which 331 women with atypia and CIN I and II were randomly assigned to receive 5 mg folate or placebo daily for 6 months, and again, no significant differences were found between the two study groups in terms of rate or degree of improvement [217].

Based on the strength and consistency of the earlier observational studies on β-carotene and risk for CIN or cervical cancer, five randomized, controlled trials testing whether β-carotene supplements could increase the rate of regression of cervical dysplasia were initiated, and all have been completed [21,28,218–220]. In one of these studies [219], the β-carotene supplementation was administered with or without supplemental vitamin C (500 mg/day). Details about these studies are summarized in Table 73-2. None of these studies found a beneficial effect of β-carotene supplementation compared with placebo. Two clinical trials using dietary supplements reported plasma retinol concentrations were associated with better outcomes regardless of study group assignment [24,220].

An alternative approach is to modify the diet to resemble the pattern suggested by the observational studies of nutrients associated with protection against persistent HPV infection, progression of cervical dysplasia, and development of cervical cancer. Specifically, epidemiologic studies have suggested that dietary intakes of carotenoids, vitamin C, and folate are negatively correlated with risk for cervical dysplasia and cancer, and vegetables and fruits have been the primary sources of these nutrients in the U.S. diet [194,221]. A controlled study testing the effect of diet modification on rate of regression of CIN I and II was initiated in 1996, and preliminary data from the study indicate good adherence to the high-vegetable and fruit diet intervention [222]. In this study, 150 women with

Table 73-2

Randomized Controlled Trials of β-Carotene Supplements and Regression of Cervical Intraepithelial Neoplasia (CIN)

Investigators	Number of Subjects	Targeted Group	Amount of β-Carotene	Length of Follow-up	Results
De Vet et al [218]	278	CIN I, II, and III	10 mg/day	3 mos	Same response as placebo
Fairley et al [21]	111	Atypia, HPV, CIN I and II	30 mg/day	12 mos	Same response as placebo
Romney et al [28]	69	CIN I, II, and III	30 mg/day	9 mos	Same response as placebo
Mackerras et al [219]	141	Atypia, CIN I	30 mg/day ± 500 mg/day vitamin C	2 yrs	Same response as placebo
Keefe et al [220]	103	CIN II and III	30 mg/day	2 yrs	Same response as placebo

cervical dysplasia (63% CIN I, 37% CIN II) were enrolled and randomized to the diet intervention arm or control arm and followed for 1 year. When the study ended, preliminary intent to treat analysis indicated no statistically significant difference in response rate observed across the two study groups. However, analysis of response after adjustment for HPV status and other factors associated with regression of dysplasia in these women, and other secondary analysis, is currently underway.

A limitation of the intervention trials conducted to date is that all of these studies have been focused on increasing the regression rate of established CIN, and nutritional factors may have a more meaningful clinical effect earlier in the HPV exposure and infection process. Also, most of the intervention studies conducted to date have been constrained by limited statistical power, so that interpretation of results is severely constrained. It is notable that the spontaneous regression rate for CIN typically falls in the range at which the number of subjects needed to detect a treatment effect is very high, so implementing a study focused on regression of CIN is operationally challenging. Screening, confirmation of histopathologic status, and the availability of ablative treatments substantially reduce the pool of subjects who are eligible and willing to participate in clinical trials of this type.

Future directions of research are moving beyond the focus on CIN and instead are exploring the feasibility of primary prevention. Clinically, evaluating the overall nutritional status and adequacy of the diet of the woman at risk for cervical cancer may provide some insight that will help her improve her diet and thus, improve the immune response.

V. The Role of Men in Human Papillomavirus and Cervical Cancer

Although HPV is a highly prevalent STI, the majority of research has focused on female cohorts due to specific sequelae of SIL and cervical cancer as noted. However, the risk of HPV in women is directly linked to male issues [13,223–225]. Male HPV infections and diseases are very common in sexually active men, manifesting in many forms ranging from clinically inapparent to warts and anogenital malignancies. Condylomata are common in male partners of women with CIN, but the lesions are frequently not apparent unless magnification and acetic acid are used [226]. However, the evidence is not consistent for a causal role of HPV in immuno-competent men with respect to penile, bladder, prostate, or rectal cancer. Human papillomavirus DNA is found commonly in all grades of penile intraepithelial neoplasia [227] but does not influence the prognosis of invasive penile cancer, a very rare cancer in the United States [228]. Among 57 transitional cell bladder carcinoma specimens, none had evidence of HPV DNA [229]. The involvement of HPV in the pathogenesis of prostate cancer remains controversial. Early studies suggested a link between HPV and prostate cancer [230–232]. However, the data suggest no link [233–235].

The reservoir for HPV in men remains unclear. At one time it was believed to be urethral epithelium, but this has not been proven [236]. Human papillomavirus has been detected in semen in several studies [237–240]. These results conflict with the early work of Nieminen [241], which claimed that HPV was not transmitted by semen, because semen of the sexual partners of 17 women positive for HPV were uninfected. The other likely reservoir in men for transmission of HPV is the prostate [242–246]. Limitations of these studies include inadequate study population sample size, limited anatomic sampling, and laboratory detection methods. The role of the foreskin as a reservoir has been brought back to our attention, as circumcision was noted to reduce the risk of penile HPV infection and cervical cancer among their current female partners after adjusting for history of multiple partners and other potential confounders [247]. However, this study also failed to sample multiple anatomic sites.

Information on the concordance of HPV infection between men and their sexual partners has been limited by the number of subjects studied, the accuracy of HPV detection methods used [248], and the anatomic site sampled [249]. The introduction of colposcopy and acetic acid application for detection of genital lesions in both genders has revealed that 53 to 80% of male partners of women with various forms of cervical diseases have evidence of HPV-associated genital lesions [236,250–252]. However, the utility of these results are limited by the determination of HPV infection based upon clinical manifestation of genital warts, which is not accurate. The use of cytology from penile warts or penile biopsy does not improve the accuracy of determining a man's HPV status [236,248]. The actual detection of HPV DNA in men is the best detection method available to define a man's HPV status. A few early studies have used Southern blot techniques [236,238,248] followed by studies using polymerase chain reaction (PCR) techniques [236,237, 253,254]. From these studies, it is clear that the standard method to detect the presence of HPV DNA in men is PCR. However, this technique has not been applied to multiple anatomic samples from a population-based sample of men to establish the ideal anatomic site to sample.

Any current effort to develop a public health strategy to reduce the burden of HPV lacks critical information. The missing information includes the prevalence of HPV among sexually active healthy men. This information cannot be collected until one can determine the best anatomic site to sample men to determine their HPV status. Once this information is available, then several hypotheses that may provide an explanation for the different impact of HPV in the men and women can be started.

VI. Conclusion

Cervical carcinoma and genital infections with HPV are significant health problems worldwide. There has been little success in controlling either except with cervical cytology or Pap smear surveillance, which is not easily supported or afforded in developing countries. A variety of variables contribute to a woman's exposure to HPV and development of diseases. These variables include male factors, HPV type, viral load, viral persistence, immune response, and nutrition. Other than sexual behavior, only nutrition is a modifiable factor that could contribute to prevention and/or treatment of disease. The studies of nutrition as an intervention method have been limited by the focus on a single or combination of micronutrients in women with evidence of cytologic or pathologic disease. This reductionist approach is far too focused and does not reflect the observation epidemiologic data, which suggest that a diet high in fruit and vegetables reduces the risk of HPV and preinvasive cervical disease. Future directions of research are moving beyond the focus on CIN and instead are exploring the feasibility of primary prevention. Clinically, evaluating the overall nutritional status and adequacy of the diet of the woman at risk for cervical cancer may provide some insight that will help her improve her diet and thus, improve the immune response.

VII. Suggestions for Further Investigations

- Studies of diet interventions to reduce the persistence of cervical HPV.
- Exploration of molecular, protein, and immune markers related to persistence of cervical HPV and progression to cervical disease.
- Examination of the immune response (cervical and systemic) to cervical HPV infection.
- Studies of heterosexually active men to determine the anatomical site of HPV infection and predictors of spreading the infection.

References

1. NCI Workshop. (1989). The 1988 Bethesda system for reporting cervical/vaginal cytological diagnoses. *JAMA*. 262(7):931–933.
2. Shepherd JC, Fried RA. (1995). Preventing cervical cancer: The role of the Bethesda System. *Am Fam Phys*. 51:434–440.
3. Bethesda System Committee. (1992). The Bethesda System for reporting cervical and vaginal cytologic diagnoses: Report of the 1991 Bethesda Workshop. *J Fam Pract*. 35(1):98–101.
4. Solomon D, Davey D, Kurman R *et al.* (2002). The 2001 Bethesda System: Terminology for reporting results of cervical cytology. *JAMA*. 287:2114–2119.
5. Schiffman MH, Brinton LA, Devesa SS, Fraumeni JF. (1996). Cervical cancer. In *Cancer Epidemiology and Prevention*, (Schottenfeld D, Fraumeni JF, ed.), pp. 1090–1116. New York: Oxford University Press.
6. Peterson O. (1956). Spontaneous course of cervical pre-cancerous conditions. *Am J Obstet Gynecol*. 72:1063.
7. Richard R. (1967). Natural history of cervical intraepithelial neoplasm. *Clin Obstet Gynecol*. 10:883.
8. Hall JE, Walton L. (1968). Dysplasia of the cervix: A prospective study of 206 cases. *Am J Obstet Gynecol*. 100:662–671.
9. Richart RM, Barron BA. (1969). A follow-up study of patients with cervical dysplasia. *Am J Obstet Gynecol*. 105:386–393.
10. Richart RM, Townsend DE, Crisp W *et al.* (1980). An analysis of "long-term" follow-up results in patients with cervical intraepithelial neoplasia treated by cryotherapy. *Am J Obstet Gynecol*. 137:823–826.
11. Kiviat NB, Koutsky LA. (1993). Specific human papillomavirus types as the causal agents of most cervical intraepithelial neoplasia: Implications for current views and treatment. *J Natl Cancer Inst*. 85:934–935.
12. Burghardt E, Ostor AG. (1983). Site and origin of squamous cervical cancer: A histomorphologic study. *Obstet Gynecol*. 62:117–127.
13. Wright VC, Riopelle MA. (1982). Age at time of first intercourse v. chronologic age as a basis for Pap smear screening. *Can Med Assoc J*. 127:127–131.
14. Koss L. (1979). *Diagnostic Cytopathology*. Philadelphia: JB Lippincott.
15. Koutsky LA, Holmes KK, Critchlow CW *et al.* (1992). A cohort study of the risk of cervical intraepithelial neoplasia grade 2 or 3 in relation to papillomavirus infection. *N Engl J Med*. 327:1272–1278.
16. Schiffman MH, Bauer HM, Hoover RN *et al.* (1993). Epidemiologic evidence showing that Human Papillomavirus infection causes most cervical intraepithelial neoplasia. *J Natl Cancer Inst*. 85(12):958–964.
17. Merrick DT, Blanton RA, Gown AM, McDougall JK. (1992). Altered expression of proliferation and differentiation markers in human papillomavirus 16 and 18 immortalized epithelial cells grown in organotypic culture *Am J Pathol*. 140:167–177.
18. Kinlen LJ, Spriggs AI. (1978). Women with positive cervical smears but without surgical intervention. A follow-up study. *Lancet*. 2:463–465.
19. Campion MJ, McCance DJ, Cuzick J, Singer A. (1986). Progressive potential of mild cervical atypia: Prospective cytological, colposcopic, and virological study. *Lancet*. 2:237–240.
20. Carmichael JA, Maskens PD. (1989). Cervical dysplasia and human papillomavirus. *Am J Obstet Gynecol*. 160:916–918.
21. Fairley C, Tabrizi S, Chen S *et al.* (1996). A randomized clinical trial of beta-carotene vs placebo for the treatment of cervical HPV infection. *Int J Gynecol Cancer*. 6:225–230.
22. Greenberg ER, Baron JA, Stukel TA *et al.* (1990). A clinical trial of beta-carotene to prevent basal-cell and squamous-cell cancers of the skin. The Skin Cancer Prevention Study Group. *N Engl J Med*. 323:789–795.
23. Romney SL, Palan PR, Duttagupta C *et al.* (1981). Retinoids and the prevention of cervical dysplasias. *Am J Obstet Gynecol*. 141:890–894.
24. Butterworth CE Jr, Hatch KD, Soong SJ *et al.* (1992). Oral folic acid supplementation for cervical dysplasia: A clinical intervention trial. *Am J Obstet Gynecol*. 166:803–809.
25. Childers JM, Chu J, Voigt LF *et al.* Chemoprevention of cervical cancer with folic acid: A phase III Southwest Oncology Group Intergroup study. *Cancer Epidemiol Biomarkers Prev*. 4:155–159.
26. Meyskens FL Jr, Surwit E, Moon TE *et al.* (1994). Enhancement of regression of cervical intraepithelial neoplasia II (moderate dysplasia) with topically applied all-trans-retinoic acid: A randomized trial. *J Natl Cancer Inst*. 86:539–543.
27. Meyskens F, Surwit E, Childers J *et al.* (1993). Phase III randomized trial of trans-retinoic acid to prevent progression of cervical intraepithelial neoplasia (CIN): would new biomarkers have helped along the way? *CCPC-93: Second International Cancer Chemo Prevention Conference*. 45.
28. Romney S, Ho G, Palan P *et al.* (1997). Effects of beta-carotene and other factors on outcome of cervical dysplasia and human papillomavirus infection. *Gynecol Oncol*. 65:484–492.
29. Ferenczy A, Choukroun D, Arseneau J. (1996). Loop electrosurgical excision procedure for squamous intraepithelial lesions of the cervix: Advantages and potential pitfalls. *Obstet Gynecol*. 87:332–337.
30. Biel MA. (1996). Photodynamic therapy and the treatment of head and neck cancers. *J Clin Laser Med Surg*. 14:239–244.
31. Dougherty TJ. (1996). A brief history of clinical photodynamic therapy development at Roswell Park Cancer Institute. *J Clin Laser Med Surg*. 14:219–221.
32. Fritsch C, Stege H, Saalmann G *et al.* (1997). Green light is effective and less painful than red light in photodynamic therapy of facial solar keratoses. *Photodermatol Photoimmunol Photomed*. 13:181–185.
33. Gossner L, Stolte M, Sroka R *et al.* (1998). Photodynamic ablation of high-grade dysplasia and early cancer in Barrett's esophagus by means of 5-aminolevulinic acid. Comment in: *Gastroenterology*, 1998, 114(3):604–606. *Gastroenterology*. 114:448–455.
34. Kato H, Okunaka T, Shimatani H. (1996). Photodynamic therapy for early stage bronchogenic carcinoma. *J Clin Laser Med Surg*. 14:235–238.
35. Kato H. (1998). Photodynamic therapy for lung cancer—a review of 19 years' experience. *J Photochem Photobiol B*. 42:96–99.
36. Kennedy JC, Marcus SL, Pottier RH. (1996). Photodynamic therapy (PDT) and photodiagnosis (PD) using endogenous photosensitization induced by 5-aminolevulinic acid (ALA): Mechanisms and clinical results. *J Clin Laser Med Surg*. 14:289–304.
37. Kick G, Messer G, Plewig G. (1996). Historical development of photodynamic therapy. *Hautarzt*. 47:644–649.
38. Kingsbury JS, Cecere W, Mang TS, Liebow C. (1997). Photodynamic therapy for premalignant lesions in DMBA-treated hamsters: A preliminary study. *J Oral Maxillofac Surg*. 55:376–381.
39. Mitchell MF, Tortolero-Luna G, Cook E *et al.* (1998). A randomized clinical trial of cryotherapy, laser vaporization, and loop electrosurgical excision for treatment of squamous intraepithelial lesions of the cervix. *Obstet Gynecol*. 92:737–744.
40. Ljubojevic N, Babic S, Audy-Jurkovic S *et al.* (1998). Loop excision of the transformation zone (LETZ) as an outpatient method of management for women with cervical intraepithelial neoplasia: Our experience. *Collegium Antropologicum*. 22:533–543.
41. Duggan BD, Felix JC, Muderspach LI *et al.* (1999). Cold-knife conization versus conization by the loop electrosurgical excision procedure: A randomized, prospective study. *Am J Obstet Gynecol*. 180:276–282.
42. Huang LW, Hwang JL. (1999). A comparison between loop electrosurgical excision procedure and cold knife conization for treatment of cervical dysplasia:

Residual disease in a subsequent hysterectomy specimen. *Gynecol Oncol.* 73:12–15.

43. Parkin D, Pisani P, Frelay J. (1993). Estimates of the worldwide frequency of eighteen major cancers in 1985. *Int J Cancer.* 1993:594–606.

44. Parkin D, Muir C, Whelan S. (1992). *Cancer Incidence in Five Continents, vol VI.* Lyon: IARC.

45. Greenlee R, Hill-Harmon M, Murray T, Thun M. (2001). Cancer Statistics 2001. *CA Cancer J Clin.* 51:15–56.

46. Beral V, Hermon C, Munoz N, Devesa SS. (1994). Cervical cancer. In *Cancer Surveys Volume 19/20: Trends in Cancer Incidence and Mortality,* vol. 19/20, (Doll R, Fraumeni JJ, Muir C, ed.), pp. 265–285. Cold Spring Harbor, NY: Cold Spring Harbor Laboratory Press.

47. Carmichael J, Clarke D, Moher D *et al.* (1986). Cervical carcinoma in women aged 34 and younger. *Am J Obstet Gynecol.* 154:264–269.

48. Parkin D, Nguyen-dinh X, Day N. (1985). The impact of screening on the incidence of cervical cancer in England and Wales. *Br J Obstet Gynaecol.* 92:150–157.

49. Vyslouzilova S, Arbyn M, Van Oyen H *et al.* (1997). Cervical cancer mortality in Belgium, 1955–1989, a descriptive study. *Eur J Cancer.* 33:1841–1845.

50. Green G. (1979). Rising cervical cancer mortality in young New Zealand women. *NZ Med J.* 89:89–91.

51. Holman C, Armstrong B. (1987). Cervical cancer mortality trends in Australia—an update. *Med J Aust.* 146:410–412.

52. Rock CL, Michael CW, Reynolds RK, Ruffin MT. (2000). Prevention of cervix cancer. *Crit Rev Oncol Hematol.* 33:169–185.

53. Hill A. (1965). Environment and disease: Association or causation? *Proc R Soc Med.* 58:295–300.

54. Cates W, Jr. (1999). Estimates of the incidence and prevalence of sexually transmitted diseases in the United States. American Social Health Association Panel. *Sex Transm Dis.* 26:S2–S7.

55. Ho GY, Bierman R, Beardsley L *et al.* (1998). Natural history of cervicovaginal papillomavirus infection in young women. *N Engl J Med.* 338:423–428.

56. Moscicki AB, Shiboski S, Broering J *et al.* (1998). The natural history of human papillomavirus infection as measured by repeated DNA testing in adolescent and young women. *J Pediatr.* 132:277–284.

57. Moscicki AB, Hills N, Shiboski S *et al.* (2001). Risks for incident human papillomavirus infection and low-grade squamous intraepithelial lesion development in young females. *JAMA.* 285:2995–3002.

58. Ho GY, Burk RD, Klein S *et al.* (1995). Persistent genital human papillomavirus infection as a risk factor for persistent cervical dysplasia. *J Natl Cancer Inst.* 87:1365–1371.

59. Morrison EA. (1994). Natural history of cervical infection with human papillomaviruses. *Clin Infect Dis.* 18:172–180.

60. Bauer HM, Ting Y, Greer CE *et al.* (1991). Genital human papillomavirus infection in female university students as determined by a PCR-based method. *JAMA.* 265(4):472–477.

61. Brisson J, Bairati I, Morin C *et al.* (1996). Determinants of persistent detection of human papillomavirus DNA in the uterine cervix. *J Infect Dis.* 173:794–799.

62. Hinchliffe SA, van Velzen D, Korporaal H *et al.* (1995). Transience of cervical HPV infection in sexually active, young women with normal cervicovaginal cytology. *Br J Cancer.* 72:943–945.

63. Hildesheim A, Schiffman MH, Gravitt PE *et al.* (1994). Persistence of type-specific human papillomavirus infection among cytologically normal women. *J Infect Dis.* 169:235–240.

64. Moscicki AB, Palefsky JM, Gonzales J *et al.* (1992). Colposcopic and histologic findings and human papillomavirus (HPV) DNA test variability in young women positive for HPV DNA. *J Infect Dis.* 166:951–957.

65. Rosenfeld WD, Rose E, Vermund SH *et al.* (1992). Follow-up evaluation of cervicovaginal human papillomavirus infection in adolescents. *J Pediatr.* 121:307–311.

66. Morrison EA, Ho GY, Vermund SH *et al.* (1991). Human papillomavirus infection and other risk factors for cervical neoplasia: A case-control study. *Int J Cancer.* 49:6–13.

67. Berumen J, Casas L, Segura E *et al.* (1994). Genome amplification of human papillomavirus types 16 and 18 in cervical carcinomas is related to the retention of E1/E2 genes. *Int J Cancer.* 56:640–645.

68. Berumen J, Unger ER, Casas L, Figueroa P. (1995). Amplification of human papillomavirus types 16 and 18 in invasive cervical cancer. *Hum Pathol.* 26:676–681.

69. Swan DC, Tucker RA, Tortolero-Luna G *et al.* (1999). Human papillomavirus (HPV) DNA copy number is dependent on grade of cervical disease and HPV type. *J Clin Microbiol.* 37:1030–1034.

70. Clavel C, Masure M, Putaud I *et al.* (1998). Hybrid capture II, a new sensitive test for human papillomavirus detection. Comparison with hybrid capture I and PCR results in cervical lesions. *J Clin Pathol.* 51:737–740.

71. Josefsson AM, Magnusson PK, Ylitalo N *et al.* (2000). Viral load of human papilloma virus 16 as a determinant for development of cervical carcinoma in situ: A nested case-control study. *Lancet.* 355:2189–2193.

72. Smith P, Friedman C, Bryant E, McDougall J. (1992). Viral integration and fragile sites in human papillomavirus-immortalized human keratinocyte cell lines. *Genes Chrom Cancer.* 5:150–157.

73. Popescu N, DiPaolo J. (1989). Preferential sites for viral integration on mammalian genome. *Cancer Genet Cytogenet.* 42:157–171.

74. Glover TW, Berger C, Coyle J, Echo B. (1984). DNA polymerase alpha inhibition by aphidicolin induces gaps and breaks at common fragile sites in human chromosomes. *Hum Genet.* 67:136–142.

75. Glover TW, Stein CK. (1988). Chromosome breakage and recombination at fragile sites. *Am J Hum Genet.* 43:265–273.

76. Glover TW, Stein CK. (1987). Induction of sister chromatid exchanges at common fragile sites. *Am J Hum Genet.* 41:882–890.

77. Rassool FV, McKeithan TW, Neilly ME *et al.* (1991). Preferential integration of marker DNA into the chromosomal fragile site at 3p14: An approach to cloning fragile sites. *Proceedings of the National Academy of Sciences of the United States of America* 88:6657–6661.

78. Chung GT, Huang DP, Lo KW *et al.* (1992). Genetic lesion in the carcinogenesis of cervical cancer. *AntiCancer Res.* 12:1485–1490.

79. Hibi K, Takahashi T, Yamakawa K *et al.* (1992). Three distinct regions involved in 3p deletion in human lung cancer. *Oncogene.* 7:445–449.

80. Sanchez Y, el-Naggar A, Pathak S, Killary Am. (1994). A tumor suppressor locus within 3p14-p12 mediates rapid cell death of renal cell carcinoma in vivo. *Proceedings of the National Academy of Sciences of the United States of America* 91:3383–3387.

81. Ohta M, Inoue H, Cotticelli MG *et al.* (1996). The FHIT gene, spanning the chromosome 3p14.2 fragile site and renal carcinoma-associated t(3;8) breakpoint, is abnormal in digestive tract cancers. *Cell.* 84:587–597.

82. Kastury K, Baffa R, Druck T *et al.* (1996). Potential gastrointestinal tumor suppressor locus at the 3p14.2 FRA3B site identified by homozygous deletions in tumor cell lines. *Cancer Res.* 56:978–983.

83. Negrini M, Monaco C, Vorechovsky I *et al.* (1996). The FHIT gene at 3p14.2 is abnormal in breast carcinomas. *Cancer Res.* 56:3173–3179.

84. Sozzi G, Veronese Ml, Negrini M *et al.* (1996). The FHIT gene 3p14.2 is abnormal in lung cancer. *Cell.* 85:17–26.

85. Thiagalingam S, Lisitsyn NA, Hamaguchi M *et al.* (1996). Evaluation of the FHIT gene in colorectal cancers. *Cancer Res.* 56:2936–2939.

86. Wilke C, Hall BK, Hoge A *et al.* (1996). FRA3B extends over a broad region and contains a spontaneous HPV16 integration site: Direct evidence for the coincidence of viral integration sites and fragile sites. *Hum Mol Genet.* 5:187–195.

87. Kirchner H. (1986). Immunobiology of human papillomavirus. *Prog Med Virology.* 33:1–41.

88. Kirnbauer R, Booy F, Cheng N *et al.* (1992). Papillomavirus L1 major capsid protein self-assembles into virus-like particles that are highly immunogenic. *Proceedings of the National Academic Science USA.* 89:12180–12184.

89. Nonnenmacher B, Hubbert NL, Kirnbauer R *et al.* (1995) Serologic response to human papillomavirus type 16 virus-like particles in HPV-16 DNA-positive invasive cervical cancer and cervical intraepithelial neoplasia grade III patients and controls from Colombia and Spain. *J Infect Dis.* 172:19–24.

90. Carter JJ, Koutsky LA, Wipf GC *et al.* (1996). The natural history of human papillomavirus type 16 capsid antibodies among a cohort of university women. *J Infect Dis.* 174:927–936.

91. Jochumus-Kudielka I, Schneider A, Braun R *et al.* (1989). Antibodies against human papillomavirus type 16 early proteins in huma sera: Anti-E7 reactivity correlates with cervical cancer. *J Natl Cancer Inst.* 81:1698–1704.

92. Jenison SA, Yu XP, Valentine JM *et al.* (1990). Evidence of prevalent genital type human papillomavirus infections in adults and children. *J Infect Dis.* 162:60–69.

93. Wikstrom A, van Doornum GJ, Quint WG *et al.* (1995). Identification of human papillomavirus seroconversions. *J Gen Virol* 76:529–539.

94. van Doornum GJ, Prins M, Pronk L *et al.* (1994). A prospective study of antibody responses to defined epitopes of human papillomavirus (HPV) type 16

in relationship to genital and anorectal presence of HPV DNA. *Clin Diagn Lab Immunol.* 1:633–639.

95. Kochel HG, Sievert K, Monazahian M *et al.* (1991). Antibodies to human papillomavirus type-16 in human sera as revealed by the use of prokaryotically expressed viral gene products. *Virology.* 182:644–654.

96. Mann VM, de Lao SL, Brenes M *et al.* (1990). Occurrence of IgA and IgG antibodies to select peptides representing human papillomavirus type 16 among cervical cancer cases and controls. *Cancer Res.* 50:7815–7819.

97. Hamsikova E, Novak J, Hofmannova V *et al.* (1994). Presence of antibodies to seven human papillomavirus type 16-derived peptides in cervical cancer patients and healthy controls. *J Infect Dis.* 170:1424–1431.

98. Mandelson MT, Jenison SA, Sherman KJ *et al.* (1992). The association of human papillomavirus antibodies with cervical cancer risk. *Cancer Epidemiol Biomarkers Prev.* 1:281–286.

99. Muller M, Viscidi RP, Sun Y *et al.* (1992). Antibodies to HPV-16 E6 and E7 proteins as markers for HPV-16-associated invasive cervical cancer. *Virology.* 187:508–514.

100. Sun Y, Eluf-Neto J, Bosch FX *et al.* (1994). Human papillomavirus-related serological markers of invasive cervical carcinoma in Brazil. *Cancer Epidemiol Biomarkers Prev.* 3:341–347.

101. Dillner J. (1996). *Antibody Responses to Defined HPV Epitopes in Cervical Neoplasia,* (Lacey C, ed.), pp. 121–130. Leeds, UK: Leeds University Press.

102. Majewski S, Marczak M, Szmurlo A *et al.* (1996). Interleukin-12 inhibits angiogenesis induced by human tumor cell lines *in vivo. J Invest Dermatol.* 106:1114–1118.

103. Woodworth CD, Notario V, DiPaolo JA. (1990). Transforming growth factors beta 1 and 2 transcriptionally regulate human papillomavirus (HPV) type 16 early gene expression in HPV-immortalized human genital epithelial cells. *J Virol.* 64:4767–4775.

104. Yarden A, Kimchi A. (1986). Tumor necrosis factor reduces c-myc expression and cooperates with interferon-gamma in HeLa cells. *Science.* 234:1419–1421.

105. Han R, Breitburd F, Marche PN, Orth G. (1992). Linkage of regression and malignant conversion of rabbit viral papillomas to MHC class II genes. *Nature.* 356:66–68.

106. Wank R, Thomassen C. (1991). High risk of squamous cell carcinoma of the cervix for women with HLA-DQw3. *Nature.* 352:723–725.

107. Helland A, Borresen AL, Kaern J *et al.* (1992). Scientific correspondence–HLA antigens and cervical carcinoma. *Nature.* 356:23.

108. Sastre-Garau X, Loste MN, Vincent-Salomon A *et al.* (1996). Decreased frequency of HPV DRB1*13 alleles in Frenchwomen with HPV-positive carcinoma of the cervix. *Int J Cancer.* 69:159–164.

109. Nawa A, Nishiyama Y, Kobayashi T *et al.* (1995). Association of human leukocyte antigen-B1*03 with cervical cancer in Japanese women aged 35 years and younger. *Cancer.* 75:518–521.

110. Wank R, ter Meulen J, Luande Eberhardt HC, Pawlita M. (1993). Cervical intraepithelial neoplasia, cervical carcinoma, and risk for patients with HLA-DQB1*0602, *0301, *0303 alleles. *Lancet.* 341:1215.

111. Gregoire L, Lawrence WD, Kukuruga D *et al.* (1994). Association between HLA-DQB1 and increased risk for cervical cancer in African-American women. *Int J Cancer.* 57:504–507.

112. Glew SS, Duggan-Keen M, Cabrera T, Stern PL. (1992). HLA class II antigen expression in human papillomavirus-associated cervical carcinoma. *Cancer Res.* 52:4009–4016.

113. Glew SS, Duggan-Keen M, Ghosh AK *et al.* (1993). Lack of association of HLA polymorphisms with human papillomavirus-related cervical cancer. *Hum Immunol.* 37:157–164.

114. Apple RJ, Erlich HA, Klitz W *et al.* (1994). HLA DR-DQ associations with cervical carcinomas show papillomavirus-type specificity. *Nat Genet.* 6:157–162.

115. Vandenvelde C, De Foor M, Van Beers D. (1993). HLA DQB1*03 and cervical intraepithelial neoplasia grades I-III. *Lancet.* 341:442–443.

116. Odunsi K, Terry G, Ho L *et al.* (1996). Susceptibility to human papillomavirus-associated cervical intraepithelial neoplasia is determined by specific HLA DR-DQ alleles. *Int J Cancer.* 67:595–602.

117. Odunsi K, Terry G, Ho L *et al.* (1995). Associations between HLA DQB1*03 and cervical intraepithelial neoplasia. *Mol Med.* 1:161–171.

118. Sanjeevi CB, Hjelmstrom P, Hallmans G *et al.* (1996). Different HLA-DR-DQ haplotypes are associated with cervical intraepithelial neoplasia among human papillomavirus type-16 seropositive and seronegative Swedish women. *Int J Cancer.* 68:409–414.

119. Apple RJ, Becker TM, Wheeler CM, Erlich HA. (1995). Comparison of human leukocyte antigen DR-DQ disease associations found with cervical dysplasia and invasive carcinoma. *J Natl Cancer Inst.* 87:427–436.

120. Duggan-Keen MF, Keating PJ *et al.* (1996). Immunogenetic factors in HPV-associated cervical cancer: Influence on disease progression. *Eur J Immunogenet.* 23:275–284.

121. Morison WL. (1975). Viral warts, herpes simplex and herpes zoster in patients with secondary immunodeficiencies and neoplasms. *Br J Dermatol.* 92:625.

122. Porreco R, Penn I, Droegenmuller W *et al.* (1975). Gynecological malignancies in immunosuppressed organ homograft recipients. *J Obstet Gynecol.* 45:359–367.

123. Berman A, Winklemann RK. (1977). Flat warts undergoing involution: Histopathologic findings. *Arch Dermatol.* 113:1219–1221.

124. Iwatuski K, Tagami H, Takigawa M, Yamada M. (1986). Plane warts under spontaneous regression: Immunopathologic study of cellular constituents leading to the inflammatory reaction. *Arch Dermatol.* 122:655–659.

125. Tagami H, Oku T, Iwatsuki K. (1985). Primary tissue culture of spontaneously regressing flat warts. *In vitro* attack by mononuclear cells against wart-derived epidermal cells. *Cancer.* 55:2437–2441.

126. Aiba S, Rokego M, Tagaini H. (1986). Immunohistological analysis of the phenomenon of spontaneous regression of numerous flat warts. *Cancer.* 58:1246–1251.

127. Chardonnes Y, Viac J, Staquet MJ, Thivolet J. (1985). Cell-mediated immunity to human papillomavirus. *Clin Dermatol.* 3:156–162.

128. Torres LM, Cabrera T, Concha A *et al.* (1993). HLA class I expression and HPV-16 sequences in premalignant and malignant lesions of the cervix. *Tissue Antigens.* 41:65–71.

129. Ghosh AK, Moore M. (1992). Tumor-infiltrating lymphocytes in cervical carcinoma. *Eur J Cancer.* J28A:1910–1916.

130. Leung HT, Linsley PS. (1994). The CD28 costimulatory pathway. *Ther Immunol.* 1:217–218.

131. Clark EA, Ledbetter JA. (1994). How B and T cells talk to each other. *Nature.* 367:425–428.

132. Bretiburd F, Ramoz N, Salmon J, Orth G. (1996). HLA control in the progression of human papillomavirus infections. *Semin Cancer Biol.* 7:359–371.

133. Strang G, Hickling JK, McIndoe GA *et al.* (1990). Human T cell responses to human papillomavirus type 16 L1 and E6 synthetic peptides: Identification of T cell determinants, HLA-DR restriction and virus type specificity. *J Gen Virol.* 71:423–431.

134. Meneguzzi G, Cerni C, Kieny MP, Lathe P. (1991). Immunization against human papillomavirus type 16 tumor cells with recombinant vaccinia viruses expressing E6 and E7. *Virology.* 181:62–69.

135. Chen TEK, Hu SL, Hellstrom I, Hellstrom KE. (1991). Human papillomavirus type 16 nucleoprotein E7 is a tumor rejection antigen. *Proceedings of the National Academic Science USA.* 88:110–114.

136. McLean CS, Sterling JS, Mowat J *et al.* (1993). Delayed-type hypersensitivity response to the human papillomavirus type 16 E7 protein in a mouse model. *J Gen Virol.* 74:239–245.

137. Altmann A, Jochmus-Kudielka I, Frank R *et al.* (1992). Definition of immunogenic determinants of the human papillomavirus type 16 nucleoprotein E7. *Eur J Cancer.* 28:326–333.

138. Kwok WW, Mickelson E, Masewicz S *et al.* (1990). Polymorphic DQ alpha and DQ beta interactions dictate HLA class II determinants of allorecognition. *J Exp Med.* 171:85–95.

139. Sasazuki T, Kohno Y, Iwamoto I *et al.* (1978). Association between an HLA haplotype and low responsiveness to tetanus toxoid in man. *Nature.* 272:359–361.

140. Sasazuki T, Kaneoka H, Nishimura Y *et al.* (1980). An HLA-linked immune suppression gene in man. *J Exp Med.* 152:297–313.

141. Watanbe H, Matsushita S, Kamikawaji N *et al.* (1988). Immune suppression gene on HLA-Bw54-DR4-DRw53 haplotype controls nonresponsiveness in humans to hepatitis B surface antigen via CD8+ suppressor T cells. *Hum Immunol.* 22:9–17.

142. Kamikawaji N, Fujisawa K, Yoshizume H *et al.* (1991). HLADQ-restricted CD4+ T cells specific to streptococcal antigen present in low but not high responders. *J Immunol.* 146:2560–2567.

143. Nishimura Y, Kamikawaji N, Fujisawa K *et al.* (1991). Genetic control of immune response and disease susceptibility by the HLA-DQ gene. *Res Immunol.* 142:459–466.

144. Foster CA, Yokozeki H, Rappersberger K *et al.* (1990). Human epidermal T cells predominately belong to the lineage expressing alpha/beta T cell receptor. *J Exp Med.* 171:997–1013.

145. Groh V, Fabbi M, Hochstenbach F, Maziarz RT. (1989). Double negative (CD8-CD4) lymphocytes bearing T cell receptor alpha and beta chains in normal human skin. *Proceedings of the National Academic Science USA.* 86:5059–5063.

146. Rosini S, Colasante A, Aiello FB *et al.* (1991). Intraepithelial immune cells in normal uterine cervix and HPV-associated disease. *J Immunol Res.* 3:155–162.

147. Van Kerckhove C, Russell GJ, Deusch K *et al.* (1992). Oligoclonality of human intestinal intraepithelial cells. *J Exp Med.* 175:57–63.

148. Dunn DA, Gadenne AS, Simha S *et al.* (1993). T-cell receptor V beta expression in normal human skin. *Proceedings of the National Academic Science USA.* 90:1267–1271.

149. Brinton LA. (1992). Epidemiology of cervical cancer—overview. In *The Epidemiology of Cervical Cancer and Human Papillomaviruses,* (Munoz N, Bosch FX, Shah KV, Meheus A, ed.), pp. 3–23. Lyon: IARC.

150. zur Hausen H, Schneider A. (1987). The role of papillomaviruses in human anogenital cancer. In *The Papovaviridae: The Papillomaviruses,* vol. 2, (Salzman NP, Howley PM, ed.), pp. 245–263. New York: Plenum Press.

151. Jenson AB, Lancaster WD. (1990). Association of HPV with benign, premalignant and malignant anogenital lesions. In *Papillomaviruses and Human Cancer.* (Pfister H, ed.), pp. 11–44. Boca Raton: CRC Press.

152. Lorincz AT, Temple GF, Patterson JA *et al.* (1986). Correlation of cellular atypia and human papillomavirus DNA sequences in exfoliated cells of the uterine cervix. *Obstet Gynecol.* 68:508–512.

153. Fuchs P, Girardi G, Pfister H. (1988). Human papillomavirus DNA in normal, metaplastic, preneoplastic and neoplastic epithelia of the cervix uteri. *Int J Cancer.* 41:41.

154. Crum CP, Ikenberg H, Richart RM, Gissmann L. (1984). Human papillomavirus type 16 and early cervical neoplasia. *N Engl J Med.* 310:880–883.

155. Durst M, Kleinheinz A, Hotz Mgissmann L. (1985). The physical state of human papillomavirus type 16 DNA in benign and malignant genital tumors. *J Gen Virol.* 66:1515–1522.

156. Cullen, AP, Reid R, Campion M, Lorincz AT. (1991). Analysis of the physical state of different human papillomavirus DNAs in intraepithelial and invasive cervical neoplasm. *J Virol.* 65:606–612.

157. Schwarz E, Freese UK, Gissmann L *et al.* (1985). Structure and transcription of human papillomavirus sequences in cervical carcinoma cells. *Nature.* 314:111–114.

158. Schneider-Gadicke A, Schwarz E. (1986). Different human cervical carcinoma cell lines show similar transcription patterns of human papillomavirus type 18 early genes. *EMBO J.* 5:2285–2292.

159. Wilczynski SP, Pearlman L, Walker J. (1988). Identification of HPV 16 early genes retained in cervical carcinomas. *Virology.* 166:624–627.

160. Matsukura T, Koi S, Sugase M. (1989). Both episomal and integrated forms of human papillomavirus type 16 are involved in invasive cervical cancers. *Virology.* 172:63–72.

161. DiMaio D. (1991). Transforming activity of bovine and human papillomaviruses in cultured cells. *Adv Cancer Res.* 56:133–159.

162. Durst M, Dzarlieva-Petrusevska RT, Boukamp P *et al.* (1987). Molecular and cytogenetic analysis of immortalized human primary keratinocytes obtained after transfection with human papillomavirus type 16 DNA. *Oncogene.* 1:251–256.

163. Pirisi L, Yasumoto S, Feller M *et al.* (1987). Transformation of human fibroblasts and keratinocytes with human papillomavirus type 16 DNA. *J Virol.* 61:1061–1066.

164. Munger K, Phelps WC, Bubb V *et al.* (1989). The E6 and E7 genes of the human papillomavirus type 16 together are necessary and sufficient for transformation of primary human keratinocytes. *J Virol.* 63:4417–4421.

165. DiPaolo J, Woodworth CD, Popescu N *et al.* (1989). Induction of human squamous cell carcinoma by sequential transfection with human papillomavirus 16 DNA and viral Harvey ras. *Oncogene.* 4:395–399.

166. Hurlin PJ, Kaur P, Smith PP *et al.* (1991). Progression of human papillomavirus type 18-immortalized human keratinocytes to a malignant phenotype. *Proceedings of the National Academic Science USA.* 88:570–574.

167. Storey A, Pim D, Murray A *et al.* (1988). Comparison of the *in vitro* transforming activities of human papillomavirus types. *EMBO J.* 7:1815–1820.

168. Werness BA, Levine AJ, Howley PA. (1990). Association of human papillomavirus types 16 and 18 E6 proteins with p53. *Science.* 248:76–79.

169. Scheffner M, Werness BA, Huibregtse JM *et al.* (1990). The E6 oncoprotein encoded by human papillomavirus types 16 and 18 promotes the degradation of p53. *Cell.* 63:1129–1136.

170. Crook T, Tidy JA, Vousden KH. (1991). Degradation of p53 can be targeted by HPV E6 sequences distinct from those required for p53 binding and trans-activation. *Cell.* 67:547–556.

171. Huibregtse JM, Beaudenon SL. (1996). Mechanism of HPV E6 proteins in cellular transformation. *Semin Cancer Biol.* 7:317–326.

172. Crook T, Wrede D, Tidy JA *et al.* (1992). Clonal p53 mutation in primary cervical cancer: Association with human-papillomavirus-negative tumors. *Lancet.* 339:1070–1073.

173. El-Deiry WS, Tokino T, Velculescu VE *et al.* (1993). WAF1 a potential mediator of p53 tumor suppression. *Cell.* 75:817–825.

174. Waga S, Hannon GJ, Beach D, Stillman B. (1994). The p21 inhibitor of cyclin-dependent kinases controls DNA replication by interaction with PCNA. *Nature.* 369:574–578.

175. Riley DJ, Lee E-H, Lee WH. (1994). The retinoblastoma protein: More than a tumor suppressor. *Ann Rev Cell Biol.* 10:1–29.

176. Kastan MB, Zhan Q, El-Deiry WS *et al.* (1992). A mammalian cell cycle checkpoint pathway utilizing p53 and GADD45 is defective in ataxia-telangiectasia. *Cell.* 71:587–597.

177. Debbas M, White E. (1993). Wild-type p53 mediates apoptosis by E1A which is inhibited by E1B. *Genes Dev.* 7:546–554.

178. Smotkin D, Wettstein FO. (1986). Transcription of human papillomavirus-type 16 early genes in a cervical cancer and a cancer-derived cell line and identification of the E7 protein. *Proceedings of the National Academic Science USA.* 83:4680–4684.

179. Crook T, Morgenstern J, Crawford L, Banks L. (1990). Continued expression of HPV16 E7 protein is required for maintenance of the transformed phenotype of cells contransformed by HPV16 and EJ-ras. *EMBO J.* 8:513–519.

180. Munger K, Werness BA, Dyson N *et al.* (1989). Complex formation of 5 human papillomavirus E7 proteins with the retinoblastoma tumor suppressor gene product. *EMBO J.* 8:4099–4105.

181. Heck DV, Yee CL, Howley PM, Munger K. (1992). Efficiency of binding the retinoblastoma protein correlates with the transforming capacity of the E7 oncoproteins of the human papillomaviruses. *Proceedings of the National Academic Science USA.* 89:4442–4446.

182. Hiebert SW, Packham G, Strom DK *et al.* (1995). E2F-1:DP-1 induces p53 and overrides survival factors to trigger apoptosis. *Mol Cell Biol.* 15:6864–6874.

183. Funk JO, Waga S, Harry JB *et al.* (1997). Inhibition of CDK activity and PCNA-dependent DNA replication by p21 is blocked by interaction with the HPV 16 E7 oncoprotein. *Genes Dev.* 11:2090–2100.

184. Yoshida SH, Keen CL, Ansari AA, Gershwin ME. (1999). Nutrition and the immune system. In *Modern Nutrition in Health and Disease,* (Shils ME, Olson JA, Shike M, Ross AC, ed.), pp. 725–750. Baltimore: Williams & Wilkins.

185. Olson JA. (1994). Hypovitaminosis A: Contemporary scientific issues. *J Nutr.* 124:1461S–1466S.

186. Meydani SN, Meydani M, Blumberg JB *et al.* (1997). Vitamin E supplementation and *in vivo* immune response in healthy elderly subjects. A randomized controlled trial. *JAMA.* 277:1380–1386.

187. Calder P, Yagoob P, Thies F *et al.* (2002). Fatty acids and lymphocyte functions. *Br J Nutr.* 87(Suppl):S31–S48.

188. de Pablo MA, Alvarez de Cienfuegos G. (2000). Modulatory effects of dietary lipids on immune system functions. *Immunol Cell Biol.* 78:31–39.

189. Muto Y, Fujii J, Shidoji Y *et al.* (1995). Growth retardation in human cervical dysplasia-derived cell lines by beta-carotene through down-regulation of epidermal growth factor receptor. *Am J Clin Nutr.* 62:1535S–1540S.

190. Potischman N, Brinton LA. (1996). Nutrition and cervical neoplasia. *Cancer Causes Control.* 7:113–126.

191. Alberg AJ, Selhub J, Shah KV *et al.* (2000). The risk of cervical cancer in relation to serum concentrations of folate, vitamin B12, and homocysteine. *Cancer Epidemiol Biomarkers Prev.* 9:761–764.

192. Nagata C, Shimizu H, Higashiiwai H *et al.* (1999). Serum retinol level and risk of subsequent cervical cancer in cases with cervical dysplasia. *Cancer Invest.* 17:253–258.

193. Wideroff L, Potischman N, Glass AG *et al.* (1998). A nested case-control study of dietary factors and the risk of incident cytological abnormalities of the cervix. *Nutr Cancer.* 30:130–136.

194. Rock CL, Jacob RA, Bowen PE. (1996). Update on the biological characteristics of the antioxidant micronutrients: Vitamin C, vitamin E, and the carotenoids. *J Am Diet Assoc.* 96:693–702.

195. Yeo AS, Schiff MA, Montoya G *et al.* (2000). Serum micronutrients and cervical dysplasia in Southwestern American Indian women. *Nutr Cancer.* 38:141–150.

196. French AL, Kirstein LM, Massad LS *et al.* (2000). Association of Vitamin A Deficiency with Cervical Squamous Intraepithelial Lesions in Human Immunodeficiency Virus-Infected Women. *J Infect Dis.* 182:1084–1089.

197. Peng YM, Peng YS, Childers JM *et al.* (1998). Concentrations of carotenoids, tocopherols, and retinol in paired plasma and cervical tissue of patients with cervical cancer, precancer, and noncancerous diseases. *Cancer Epidemiol Biomarkers Prev.* 7:347–350.

198. Kanetsky PA, Gammon MD, Mandelblatt J *et al.* (1998). Dietary intake and blood levels of lycopene: Association with cervical dysplasia among non-Hispanic, black women. *Nutr Cancer.* 31:31–40.

199. Ho GY, Palan PR, Basu J *et al.* (1998). Viral characteristics of human papillomavirus infection and antioxidant levels as risk factors for cervical dysplasia. *Int J Cancer.* 78:594–599.

200. Goodman MT, Kiviat N, McDuffie K *et al.* (1998). The association of plasma micronutrients with the risk of cervical dysplasia in Hawaii. *Cancer Epidemiol Biomarkers Prev.* 7:537–544.

201. Schiff MA, Patterson RE, Baumgartner RN *et al.* (2001). Serum carotenoids and risk of cervical intraepithelial neoplasia in Southwestern American Indian women. *Cancer Epidemiol Biomarkers Prev.* 10:1219–1222.

202. Giuliano AR, Papenfuss M, Nour M *et al.* (1997). Antioxidant nutrients: Associations with persistent human papillomavirus infection. *Cancer Epidemiol Biomarkers Prev.* 6:917–923.

203. Kwasniewska A, Charzewska J, Tukendorf A, Semczuk M. (1998). Dietary factors in women with dysplasia colli uteri associated with human papillomavirus infection. *Nutr Cancer.* 30:39–45.

204. Kjellberg L, Hallmans G, Ahren AM *et al.* (2000). Smoking, diet, pregnancy and oral contraceptive use as risk factors for cervical intra-epithelial neoplasia in relation to human papillomavirus infection. *Br J Cancer.* 82:1332–1338.

205. Creek KE, Jenkins GR, Khan MA *et al.* (1994). Retinoic acid suppresses human papillomavirus type 16 (HPV16)-mediated transformation of human keratinocytes and inhibits the expression of the HPV16 oncogenes. *Adv Exp Med Biol.* 354:19–35.

206. Board FAN. (2000). Reference intakes for Vitamin C, Vitamin E, selenium, and carotenoids. Institute of Medicine: Washington, DC.

207. Kim Y, Pogribny I, Basnakian A *et al.* (1997). Folate deficiency in rats induces DNA strand breaks and hypomethylation within the p53 tumor suppressor gene. *Am J Clin Nutr.* 65:46–52.

208. Goodman MT, McDuffie K, Hernandez B *et al.* (2000). Case-control study of plasma folate, homocysteine, vitamin B(12), and cysteine as markers of cervical dysplasia. *Cancer.* 89:376–382.

209. Thomson SW, Heimburger DC, Cornwell PE *et al.* (2000). Correlates of total plasma homocysteine: Folic acid, copper, and cervical dysplasia. *Nutrition.* 16:411–416.

210. Sedjo R, Inserra P, Abrahamsen M *et al.* (2002). Human papillomavirus persistence and nutrients involved in the methylation pathway among a cohort of young women. *Cancer Epidemiol Biomarkers Prev.* 11:353–359.

211. Weinstein SJ, Ziegler RG, Frongillo EA *et al.* (2001). Low serum and red blood cell folate are moderately, but nonsignificantly associated with increased risk of invasive cervical cancer in U.S. women. *J Nutr.* 131:2040–2048.

212. Bailey LB, Gregory JF 3rd. (1999). Polymorphisms of methylenetetrahydrofolate reductase and other enzymes: Metabolic significance, risks and impact on folate requirement. *J Nutr.* 129:919–922.

213. Goodman MT, McDuffie K, Hernandez B *et al.* (2001). Association of methylenetetrahydrofolate reductase polymorphism C677T and dietary folate with the risk of cervical dysplasia. *Cancer Epidemiol Biomarkers Prev.* 10:1275–1280.

214. Kim YI, Giuliano A, Hatch KD *et al.* (1994). Global DNA hypomethylation increases progressively in cervical dysplasia and carcinoma. *Cancer.* 74:893–899.

215. Fowler BM, Giuliano AR, Piyathilake C *et al.* (1998). Hypomethylation in cervical tissue: Is there a correlation with folate status? *Cancer Epidemiol Biomarkers Prev.* 7:901–906.

216. Butterworth CE Jr, Hatch KD, Gore H *et al.* (1982). Improvement in cervical dysplasia associated with folic acid therapy in users of oral contraceptives. *Am J Clin Nutr.* 35:73–82.

217. Childers J, Chu J, Voigt L *et al.* (1995). Chemoprevention of cervical cancer with folic acid: A phase III Southwest Oncology Group Intergroup study. *Cancer Epidemiol Biomarkers Prev.* 4:155–159.

218. de Vet HC, Knipschild PG, Willebrand D *et al.* (1991). The effect of beta-carotene on the regression and progression of cervical dysplasia: A clinical experiment. *J Clin Epidemiol.* 44:273–283.

219. Mackerras D, Irwig L, Simpson JM *et al.* (1999). Randomized double-blind trial of beta-carotene and vitamin C in women with minor cervical abnormalities. *Br J Cancer.* 79:1448–1453.

220. Keefe KA, Schell MJ, Brewer C *et al.* (2001). A randomized, double blind, Phase III trial using oral beta-carotene supplementation for women with high grade cervical intraepithelial neoplasia. *Cancer Epidemiol Biomarkers Prev.* 10:1029–1035.

221. Tucker KL, Selhub J, Wilson PW, Rosenberg IH. (1996). Dietary intake pattern relates to plasma folate and homocysteine concentrations in the Framingham Heart Study. *J Nutr.* 126:3025–3031.

222. Rock CL, Moskowitz A, Huizar B *et al.* (2001). High vegetable and fruit diet intervention in premenopausal women with cervical intraepithelial neoplasia. *J Am Diet Assoc.* 101:1167–1174.

223. Hulka BS. (1982). Risk factors for cervical cancer. *J Chronic Dis* 35:3–11.

224. Miller AB, Barclay TH, Choi NW *et al.* (1980). A study of cancer, parity and age at first pregnancy. *J Chronic Dis.* 33:595–605.

225. Peters RK, Thomas D, Hagan DG *et al.* (1986). Risk factors for invasive cervical cancer among Latinas and non-Latinas in Los Angeles County. *J Natl Cancer Inst.* 77:1063–1077.

226. Krebs HB, Schneider V. (1987). Human papillomavirus-associated lesions of the penis: Colposcopy, cytology, and histology. *Obstet Gynecol.* 70:299–304.

227. Aynaud O, Ionesco M, Barrasso R. (1994). Penile intraepithelial neoplasia. Specific clinical features correlate with histologic and virologic findings. *Cancer.* 74:1762–1767.

228. Bezerra AL, Lopes A, Santiago GH *et al.* (2001). Human papillomavirus as a prognostic factor in carcinoma of the penis: Analysis of 82 patients treated with amputation and bilateral lymphadenectomy. *Cancer.* 91:2315–2321.

229. Aynaud O, Tranbaloc P, Orth G. (1998). Lack of evidence for a role of human papillomaviruses in transitional cell carcinoma of the bladder. *J Urol.* 159:86–89;discussion 90.

230. McNicol PJ, Dodd JG. (1990). Detection of papillomavirus DNA in human prostatic tissue by Southern blot analysis. *Can J Microbiol.* 36:359–362.

231. McNicol PJ, Dodd JG. (1990). Detection of human papillomavirus DNA in prostate gland tissue by using the polymerase chain reaction amplification assay. *J Clin Microbiol.* 28:409–412.

232. McNicol PJ, Dodd JG. (1991). High prevalence of human papillomavirus in prostate tissues. *J Urol.* 145:850–853.

233. Cuzick J. (1995). Human papillomavirus infection of the prostate. *Cancer Surv.* 23:91–95.

234. Noda T, Sasagawa T, Dong Y *et al.* (1998). Detection of human papillomavirus (HPV) DNA in archival specimens of benign prostatic hyperplasia and prostatic cancer using a highly sensitive nested PCR method. *Urol Res.* 26:165–169.

235. Strickler HD, Burk R, Shah K *et al.* (1998). A multifaceted study of human papillomavirus and prostate carcinoma. *Cancer.* 82:1118–1125.

236. Barrasso R. (1992). HPV-related genital lesions in men. In *The Epidemiology of Cervical Cancer and Human Papillomavirus.* (Munoz N, Bosch F, Shah K, Meheus A, ed.), pp. 85–92. Lyon: International Agency for Research on Cancer.

237. Green J, Monteiro E, Bolton VN *et al.* (1991). Detection of human papillomavirus DNA by PCR in semen from patients with and without penile warts. *Genitourin Med.* 67:207–210.

238. Green J, Monteiro E, Gibson P. (1989). Detection of human papillomavirus DNA in semen from patients with intrameatal penile warts. *Genitourin Med.* 65:357–360.

239. Kyo S, Inoue M, Koyama M *et al.* (1994). Detection of high-risk human papillomavirus in the cervix and semen of sex partners. *J Infect Dis.* 170:682–685.

240. Lai YM, Yang FP, Pao CC. (1996). Human papillomavirus deoxyribonucleic acid and ribonucleic acid in seminal plasma and sperm cells. *Fertil Steril.* 65:1026–1030.

241. Nieminen P, Koskimies AI, Paavonen J. (1991). Human papillomavirus DNA is not transmitted by semen. *Int J of STD & AIDS.* 2:207–208.

242. Anderson M, Handley J, Hopwood L *et al.* (1997). Analysis of prostate tissue DNA for the presence of human papillomavirus by polymerase chain reaction, cloning, and automated sequencing. *J Med Virol.* 52:8–13.

243. Dodd JG, Paraskevas M, McNicol PJ. (1993). Detection of human papillomavirus 16 transcription in human prostate tissue. *J Urol.* 149:400–402.

244. Sarkar FH, Sakr WA, Li YW *et al.* (1993). Detection of human papillomavirus (HPV) DNA in human prostatic tissues by polymerase chain reaction (PCR). *Prostate.* 22:171–180.

245. Tu H, Jacobs SC, Mergner WJ, Kyprianou N. (1994). Rare incidence of human papillomavirus types 16 and 18 in primary and metastatic human prostate cancer. *Urology.* 44:726–731.

246. Wideroff L, Schottenfeld D, Carey TE *et al.* (1996). Human papillomavirus DNA in malignant and hyperplastic prostate tissue of black and white males. *Prostate.* 28:117–123.

247. Castellsague X, Bosch FX, Munoz N *et al.* (2002). Male circumcision, penile human papillomavirus infection, and cervical cancer in female partners. *N Engl J Med.* 346:1105–1112.

248. Nuovo GJ, Hochman HA, Eliezri YD *et al.* (1990). Detection of human papillomavirus DNA in penile lesions histologically negative for condylomata. Analysis by *in situ* hybridization and the polymerase chain reaction. *Am J Surg Pathol.* 14:829–836.

249. Schneider A, Sawada E, Gissmann L, Shah K. (1987). Human papillomaviruses in women with a history of abnormal Papanicolaou smears and in their male partners. *Obstet Gynecol.* 69:554–562.

250. Levine RU, Crum CP, Herman E *et al.* (1984). Cervical papillomavirus infection and intraepithelial neoplasia: A study of male sexual partners. *Obstet Gynecol.* 61(1):16–20.

251. Sedlacek TV, Cunnane M, Carpiniello V. (1986). Colposcopy in the diagnosis of penile condyloma. *Am J Obstet Gynecol.* 154(3):494–496.

252. Sand PK, Bowen LW, Blischke SO, Ostergard DR. (1986). Evaluation of male consorts of women with genital human papilloma virus infection. *Obstet Gynecol.* 68:679–681.

253. Wikstrom A, Popescu C, Forslund O. (2000). Asymptomatic penile HPV infection: A prospective study. *Int J STD & AIDS.* 11:80–84.

254. Lazcano-Ponce E, Herrero R, Munoz N *et al.* (2001). High prevalence of human papillomavirus infection in Mexican males: Comparative study of penile-urethral swabs and urine samples. *Sex Transm Dis.* 28:277–280.

255. Rosenfeld W, Rose E, Vermund S *et al.* (1992). Follow-up evaluation of cervicovaginal human papillomavirus infection in adolescents. *J Pediatr.* 121:307–311.

256. Syrjanen K, Hakama M, Saarikoski S *et al.* (1990). Prevalence, incidence, and estimated lifetime risk of cervical human papillomavirus infections in a nonselected Finnish female population. *Sex Transm Dis.* 17:15–19.

257. De Villiers E, Wagner D, Schneider A *et al.* (1992). Human papillomavirus DNA in women without and with cytological abnormalities: Results of a 5-year follow-up study. *Gynecol Oncol.* 44:33–39.

258. Moscicki AB, Palefsky J, Smith G *et al.* (1993). Variability of human papillomavirus DNA testing in a longitudinal cohort of young women. *Obstet Gynecol.* 82:578–585.

259. Evander M, Edlund K, Gustafsson A *et al.* (1995). Human papillomavirus infection is transient in young women: A population-based cohort study. *J Infect Dis.* 171:1026–1030.

260. Wheeler CM, Greer CE, Becker TM *et al.* (1996). Short-term fluctuations in the detection of cervical human papillomavirus DNA. *Obstet Gynecol.* 88:261–268.

74

Nutritional Antioxidants, Vitamins, Cognition, and Neurodegenerative Disease

ANTONIO MARTIN, MD, PhD*, MARK A. SMITH, PhD**, GEORGE PERRY, PhD**,
AND JAMES JOSEPH, PhD†

*Nutrition and Neurocognition Laboratory at the Jean Mayer USDA Human Nutrition Research Center on Aging
at Tufts University, Boston, MA
**Institute of Pathology, Case Western Reserve University, Cleveland, OH
†Neuroscience Laboratory at the Jean Mayer USDA Human Nutrition Research Center on Aging at Tufts University, Boston, MA

Abstract

More than 4 million Americans have Alzheimer's disease AD and other dementias. The prevalence of these disorders will increase markedly with the aging of the population. There is tremendous interest in the prevention and treatment of AD, particularly through nutrition and dietary supplements. Cross-sectional and prospective studies in humans show that higher intakes of B vitamins and antioxidants decrease the risk of AD, other dementias, and cognitive impairment. Antioxidant vitamins, such as vitamins E and C, are receiving a great deal of attention because several studies have shown that higher intake of these nutrients is associated with a decreased risk of cognitive impairment and dementia. In addition, studies have shown new evidence on the potential role that these nutrients may have in reducing the risk of cancer. Vitamin E is a fat-soluble vitamin that exists in eight different forms. Each form has its own biologic activity. The most active form of vitamin E in humans is α-tocopherol, a powerful biologic antioxidant.

Vitamin C has an essential role in human nutrition. In addition to its role in collagen formation and other life-sustaining functions, this nutrient serves as a key immune system nutrient and a potent free radical fighter. Antioxidants such as vitamins E and C and flavonoids present in fruits and vegetables act to protect cells in the body against the effects of free radicals, which are potentially damaging by-products of the body's metabolism. In addition, these nutrients have other roles at the molecular level by participating in biochemic processes relevant to cell function and body homeostasis.

I. Introduction

Elders suffer from multiple co-occurring chronic conditions, including cognitive decline and dementia, with incidence and prevalence sharply increasing as people age. With increasing numbers of elderly people in the population, the number of patients with dementia is growing rapidly. Cognitive impairment and dementia are major causes of disability in our nation, and their financial impact and long-term care costs, are enormous. The major cause of dementia is Alzheimer's disease. Aging clearly results in declines in brain size, weight, and function [1–3]. However, to date the cellular and morphologic substrates underlying these changes remain poorly characterized. Although long-held dogma suggested that aging is associated with a significant loss of neurons in the brain, careful studies have uncovered modest, if any, change in cell number and size in a variety of brain regions with aging, including the neocortex and hippocampus [4–7]. A lack of evident morphologic changes associated with neurodegeneration in the entorhinal cortex with aging further supports the concept that there are fundamental differences between the type of changes that occur in normal "healthy" aging and the pathologic changes that occur in age-related neurodegenerative processes, such as AD.

Among the clear functional changes that occur in the brain with aging are declines in various aspects of cognition and memory. In particular, short-term memory [8], memory acquisition and early retrieval [2], working memory [9], recognition memory [10,11], reasoning [12], and processing speed [13,14] are affected with aging. In fact, a great deal of research has shown, in both humans and animal models, the occurrence of numerous neuronal and behavioral deficits during aging in the absence of neurodegenerative disease. These changes may include decrements in receptor sensitivity, most notably: (a) adrenergic [15]; (b) dopaminergic [16,17]; (c) muscarinic [18,19] and (d) opioid [20]. These decrements and those involving neuronal signaling [21] and decreases in neurogenesis [22] can be expressed, ultimately, as alterations in both motor [23,24] and cognitive behaviors [25]. The alterations in motor function may include decreases in balance, muscle strength and coordination [23], whereas cognitive deficits are seen primarily with respect to spatial learning and memory [26,27]. Indeed, these characterizations have been supported by a great deal of research both in animals [25–27] and humans [28]. Age-related deficits in motor performance are thought to be the result of alterations either in the striatal dopamine (DA) system (as the striatum shows marked structural and functional changes with age and in Parkinson's disease [PD]) or in the cerebellum, which also shows age-related alterations [29,30].

Memory alterations appear to occur primarily in secondary memory systems and are reflected in the storage of newly acquired information [19,31]. It is thought that the hippocampus mediates allocentric spatial navigation (i.e., place learning), and that the prefrontal cortex is critical to acquiring the rules that govern performance in particular tasks (i.e., procedural knowledge), whereas the dorsomedial striatum mediates egocentric spatial orientation (i.e., response and cue learning) [32–35]. More importantly, data from a variety of experiments suggest that the contributing factors to the behavioral decrements seen in aging involve oxidative stress (OS) [36] and inflammation [37,38].

A. *Gender Differences in Dementia*

Epidemiologic observations and evidence of gender-related differences in cognition and behavior suggest that there may be important genetic and/or biologic factors related to gender that are operating in the pathogenesis of neurologic disease, and particularly in AD. Clinicians who diagnose and treat patients with AD recognize that there is heterogeneity in its cognitive and behavioral manifestations. Research suggests that gender may be an important modifying factor in AD's development and expression. One of the most intriguing aspects concerning the epidemiology of AD is that the prevalence rate in women is roughly twice that in men and this skewed sex ratio is specific for AD, but not for other dementias. Age is the most important risk factor associated with dementia. Males tend to have shorter life spans than females and even though the life-span gap narrows as men live longer, still at the age of 75 and older, there are significantly more women with AD than men. American women enjoy an average life expectancy of 79.10 years, whereas males are expected to live 74.1 years.

Long-term effects of the metabolic and hormonal differences among men and women may play a relevant role on the age-associated cognitive impairment and behavioral changes observed in the elderly. Some studies have considered cerebral glucose metabolic differences between men and women as an important factor in cognitive decline. Studies have only shown a decreased parietal activity in early-onset dementia of AD, independent of a gender effect [39]. Another aspect regarding differences in prevalence of AD among men and women focused on the roles of estrogen and testosterone in disease pathogenesis, and there are a number of lines of evidence suggesting that estrogen deficiency, following menopause, may contribute to the etiology of AD in women [40,41]. The decreased incidence [42] and a delay in the onset [43] of AD among women on hormone replacement therapy following menopause [44] has also contributed to believe that these agents may play a relevant role in brain function and cognitive decline associated with aging [45]. However, a decline in estrogen or testosterone does not explain why males with Down's syndrome are at significantly higher risk of developing AD-type changes and at an earlier age than their female counterparts [46]. Indeed, the concentration of estrogen and testosterone in both sexes is similar in patients with Down's syndrome to those in the general population. Studies have cast doubt on estrogen-replacement therapy as being protective against AD [47–50].

There are a number of other hormones involved in the hypothalamic-pituitary-gonadal axis that regulates reproductive function and, importantly, receptors for these other hormones are expressed in many nonreproductive tissues including the brain. Supporting evidence indicates that other hormones of the hypothalamic-pituitary-gonadal axis may be playing a central role in the pathogenesis of AD [51].

Several studies of gender differences in cognition have pointed to greater language deficits in women with AD as compared with men [52,53]. However, studies have reported absence of gender-related language differences or other measures of cognition, including memory and perception in AD [54,55].

The most prominent change noted in patients with AD, are changes in cognition. However, behavioral disturbances also frequently occur. Interestingly, although, several reports have suggested that increased behavioral disturbance in AD is related to dementia severity across gender, qualitative differences between men and women in the manifestation of the disturbances also have been reported. Female patients with AD exhibited tendencies to be more reclusive and emotionally labile. In comparison, men with AD showed more psychomotor and vegetative changes and aggressive behaviors [56]. Male patients exhibit greater problems than female patients in wandering, abusiveness, and social impropriety, particularly in the more advanced stages of the disorder. In addition, male patients with AD have increased physical, verbal, and sexual aggression than women [57–59]. Depression, on the other hand, does appear to be more prevalent in female than in male patients with AD [60]. Thus, several observations suggest that there may be important genetic factors related to gender that are operative in the pathogenesis of AD. However, it remains controversial whether men and women differ in the incidence of AD and whether there are clearly recognizable sex disparities operating in the cognition and behavior changes among those afflicted.

B. *Oxidative Stress in Aging*

The central nervous system (CNS) appears to be especially vulnerable to OS effects, partially as a result of additional factors such as increases in the ratio of oxidized to total glutathione [61], significant lipofuscin accumulation [62] with bcl-2 gene increases [63], increases in membrane lipid peroxidation [64], reduced glutamine synthetase [65], reductions in redox active iron [62], and alterations in membrane lipids [66]. Importantly, in addition to these considerations, it has been shown that not only is the CNS particularly vulnerable to OS, but this vulnerability increases during aging [67,68]. Research has also shown that besides the factors discussed previously, OS vulnerability in aging may be the result of three additional factors: (a) alterations in the membrane microenvironment, (b) alterations in calcium buffering ability, and (c) differential vulnerability of neurotransmitter receptors. The latter of these will be discussed in more detail in a later section, but in the case of membranes and aging, indications are that age-related changes in the neuronal plasma membrane molecular structure and physical properties (e.g., increased rigidity) may increase vulnerability to OS and inflammation [68,69].

In addition, various reports have shown increased reactive carbonyls in association with OS in AD [70]. These changes have been identified in senile plaques [71,72], neurofibrillary tangles (NFT) [72,73], and the primary component of the latter, tau protein (τ) [73,74]. The significance of these findings was initially questioned by suggestions that the lesions of AD, such as those that occur in vessel walls [75,76], accumulate damage through low protein turnover [77]. What was missing from this criticism was not the accumulative nature of carbonyl modification but that the products first identified, advanced glycation end products (AGE), are "active-modifications", by which we mean they are the result of metal-catalyzed redox chemistry and are continuing sites of redox chemistry [78]. Also, we have demonstrated that the lesions not only are sites of AGE accumulation but also continuing sites of glycation, because the initial Amadori product is closely associated with NFT [79].

Early reports of oxidative modifications were followed in close succession by the identification in NFT of reactive carbonyls [80,81] and protein adducts of the lipid peroxidation product, hydroxynonenal [82,83]. What was remarkable in using these different markers either resulting from carbonyl adduction or, in the case of reactive carbonyls, from direct protein oxidation, is that although highly stable modifications involving cross-linked proteins are predominantly associated with the lesions, metastable modifications are more commonly associated with the neuronal cytoplasm. Specifically, populations of neurons involved in AD, and not others, show this change, suggesting that the most active site of oxidative damage is the neuronal cytoplasm.

Studies analyzing certain physical properties of the oxidized proteins forming cross-linking compounds, specifically, those properties which make these biologic molecules refractory to light, have shown the presence of modified proteins in the brain of AD patients [84]. In addition, oxidation of the modified proteins not only renders the modified protein more resistant to degradation but also appears to competitively inhibit the proteosome [84]. These changes may underlie the accumulation of ubiquitin conjugates observed in neurons in AD [85]. Protein nitration is a noncross-link-related oxidative modification of protein resulting from either peroxynitrite attack or peroxidative nitration. In investigating the distribution of nitrotyrosine in AD, we found that the major site of nitrotyrosine was in the cytoplasm of nonNFT-containing neurons [86] and that neurons containing NFT actually showed lower levels of nitrotyrosine than similar neurons lacking NFT. These relationships were confirmed when we examined RNA, a cellular component with a relatively rapid turnover rate. A major oxidation product of RNA, 8-hydroxyguanosine (8OHG), has a distribution similar to nitrotyrosine, except that it is absent from NFT and reduced in the surrounding cytoplasm [87], even though NFT contain associated RNA [88]. The concurrence of RNA and protein damage suggests that the major site of oxidative damage in AD is localized predominantly in the neuronal cytoplasm.

1. Source of Reactive Oxygen Species

Both location and type of damage are important to understand the source of oxidative damage. First, the location of damage, which involves every category of biomacromolecules, appears to be restricted to neurons. Classically, nitrotyrosine is considered the product of peroxynitrite attack of tyrosine, and 8OHG is considered the product of •OH attack of guanosine. However, the separation is not simple; nitrotyrosine can be formed from peroxidative nitration by nitrite and H_2O_2, and peroxynitrite is produced by the reaction of nitric oxide (NO^-) with superoxide (O_2^-). In the case of peroxidative nitration, treating tissue sections with nitrite and H_2O_2 yields increased nitrotyrosine of the same distribution found during the disease in AD, but not control, cases [89]. An issue with peroxynitrite is diffusibility, being the result of the fusion of nitric oxide (NO) and O_2^-; it can diffuse several cell diameters from its source to attack vulnerable target proteins [90]. In AD, one of the most striking findings is the

restriction of damage to the cell bodies of vulnerable neurons. Although amyloid-β deposits and NFT contain redox-active iron, like oxidative damage, the most conspicuous changes in iron are within the cytoplasm of vulnerable neurons [91,92]. Significantly, cytoplasmic redox-active iron is barely detectable in controls. Redox-active iron is the critical element for Fenton chemistry generation of •OH from H_2O_2. Ultrastructural localization of iron shows it is diffusely associated with the cytoplasm, primarily in the endoplasmic reticulum, but also in granules identified as lipofuscin as well as their associated vacuoles.

Lipofuscin is thought to represent the terminal phase of autophagic lysosomes that involve iron-rich mitochondria [93]. Therefore, the increased redox-active iron in such lysosomes in AD lends credence to the notion of mitochondrial abnormalities in AD. To examine this issue further, we performed *in situ* hybridization for mitochondrial DNA (mtDNA). Mitochondrial DNA, as well as the protein cytochrome oxidase-1, was increased several-fold in vulnerable neurons in AD. Ultrastructural examination showed, although both markers were in mitochondria, in AD the increased levels were in the cytoplasm and, in the case of mtDNA, in vacuoles associated with lipofuscin, the same sites showing increased redox-active iron. It is tempting to consider that electron-dense lipofuscin may play a role in modulating metal release from mitochondrial turnover. Ultrastructural examination of the site of oxidative damage points to mitochondria. We note that the majority of iron is in the endoplasmic reticulum suggesting that a role for mitochondria is probably not to directly supply •OH but instead to supply its precursors, H_2O_2 and redox-active metals. Although the proposed mechanism is distinct from nonmetal-catalyzed peroxynitrite formation, it does not discount an important role for NO. Neurons in AD show activation of NO synthetase as well as its modulator, dimethylargininase [94]. Nitric oxide has strong antioxidant activity (see next) as well as inhibitor activity for cytochromes. The latter could play a role in the hypometabolism consistently found in AD [95] as well as the altered mitochondrial dynamics noted here.

2. Relationship to Lesions

In AD, the putative source of the reactive oxygen species was supposed to be the lesions. Amyloid-β by itself was proposed to generate reactive oxygen species [96]. This mechanism has fallen into question for both chemical and biologic issues [97]. Nevertheless, amyloid-β, under some circumstances, can bind iron and promote catalytic redox cycling, yielding reactive oxygen [98]. Therefore, it was a surprise when we noted *in vivo* that oxidative damage is inversely correlated to amyloid-β load, indicating that rather than being a source of the reactive oxygen, amyloid-β may be a modulator that can either increase or decrease reactive oxygen production [69,99,100]. Further, the relative paucity of short-lived oxidative changes surrounding amyloid-β deposits [87], rather than those that accumulate in long-lived proteins [72], also puts into question the idea that reactive oxygen resulting from inflammation is an important mechanism for oxidative damage. In fact, although the notion of inflammation in AD is well established [101], this appears to be a secondary response to the underlying pathologic changes. Alternatively, NO resulting from microglia may be playing an antioxidant role [94].

3. Inflammation

A large body of evidence indicates that inflammatory events in the CNS play an important role in functional changes associated with aging, and especially in the pathogenesis of neurodegenerative processes, like AD [102–107]. For example, by middle age there is an increased glial fibrillary acid protein expression [108] that later, in the elderly, even occurs in the absence of an inflammatory stimulus [109,110]. In conjunction with this observation, it has also been reported that tumor necrosis factor a (TNFα) is produced in higher amounts during cytotoxic reactions in the elderly [111] and that neuronal inhibition of glial activities may be lost during aging [111]. Other studies have reported increases in TNFα and interleukin-6 (IL-6) in the sera of aged mice and humans [112,113]. In fact, it has been suggested that the up-regulation of C-reactive protein represents a relevant marker associated with the risk of age-related neurodegenerative diseases, and predisposes patients to poor prognoses and to death [114].

Relevant to the inflammatory processes is the potential association between expression of proinflammatory cytokines and generation of ROS. For example, ROS-independent activation of NF-kappaB by IL-1ß in epithelial cells appears to involve the acidic sphingomyelinase/ceramide-transduction pathway [115]. There is also evidence for flavoenzyme-generated ROS in the induction of c-*fos*, and collagenase expression by IL-1 in chondrocytes [116]. In fact, most growth factors and cytokines appear to generate ROS at or near the plasma membrane.

Also paralleling the results seen with respect to OS are increases in sensitivity to inflammatory mediators with aging. For example, studies [117,118] showed that old rats were more sensitive to kainate-induced excitotoxic brain injuries and enhanced 5-lipoxygenase expression in limbic structures. The results of such increases in inflammatory reactions involving such factors as cytokines, complement proteins, and adhesion molecules may represent extracellular signals that act in concert with OS to initiate decrements in neuronal function or glial-neuronal interactions [119–122]. Thus, it appears that the increases in sensitivity that are seen with respect to OS and inflammation in senescence may play a role in mediating the deficits in behavior that have been observed in aging.

4. Age–Alzheimer Disease Parallels

As discussed previously there are increases in oxidative and inflammatory stressors as a function of age that appear to be involved in the decrements seen in both cognitive and motor behaviors. If this is the case, then it might be postulated that neurodegenerative diseases, which are age-dependent would be superimposed upon an environment already vulnerable to these insults. Indeed, OS plays a major role in the cascade of effects associated with AD (e.g., damage to DNA, protein oxidation, lipid peroxidation; see Joseph *et al*, 2001, for review [69]), and abnormal sequestration of metals [123–125], that may be independent of amyloid beta deposition. Thus, the free radical perturbations would have an even greater effect in an aged organism, because as pointed out previously, there is increased vulnerability to OS in senescence.

In addition to these OS considerations there are also indications of increased inflammation in AD. These inflammatory mediators are prominent in the AD brain and as pointed out previously, they also have been observed in lower concentrations in non-demented (ND) brains from aged individuals. Multiple endogenous sources including microglia, astrocytes (HA), and brain endothelial cells can produce these inflammatory mediators in AD [126–129]. Glial cells play important roles in supporting survival of neurons [130–133] and are extraordinarily sensitive to changes in the brain microenvironment. Brain astrocytes (HA) in particular show reactive gliosis to several forms of CNS lesions [134,135]. Additionally, gliosis, which can lead to brain damage by several mechanisms [136], is a feature common to virtually every neurodegenerative disease (e.g., multiple sclerosis, AD, tumor, HIV encephalitis, or prion disease) [137–141].

5. Antioxidant Vitamins

Given that people age 65 or over represent over 50% of all those who have ever attained this age throughout all of human history, and that in all probability the incidence of AD will rise exponentially in the ensuing years, then it is critical to find ways to reduce the vulnerability of the aged brain to OS and inflammation. A failure to do so will significantly increase the health care costs in the coming years. One method that has been employed to reverse or forestall the deleterious effects of brain aging on behavior in our laboratory has been to utilize nutritional supplementation. Diets supplemented with micronutrients like vitamins E and C, and fruits or vegetables high in vitamin C and polyphenolic compounds have multiple effects involving antioxidant levels and anti-inflammatory properties [142–145]. In this review, we will discuss the efficacy of these various treatments to date in reversing or forestalling the deleterious effects of aging and neurodegenerative disease.

For more than half a century after its discovery, vitamin E remained an enigma. However, cell, animal, and epidemiologic studies have heralded the benefits of both vitamin E and vitamin C. These antioxidant nutrients, in addition to being necessary for normal brain function, prevent cognitive declines and reduce the risk of dementia. Vitamin E has been reported to be significantly lower in patients with vascular dementia (VaD) in comparison to patients with AD and controls [146]. They also have other important roles in health including the improvement of immune function, and protection against heart disease, cancer, aging, diabetic damage, exercise fatigue, and environmental toxins. Several studies have reported that vitamin E helped reduce the risk for diabetes [147], high blood pressure [148,149], and cancer [150]. Additionally, work from our laboratory and others discussed next has shown that foods high in antioxidant and anti-inflammatory activity (e.g., blueberries) may forestall or prevent the deleterious effects of aging on neuronal function and behavior [143,151]. Results support the hypothesis that long-duration, generous intake of antioxidant vitamins E and C may reduce the risks for declines in cognitive and physical functioning, and chronic disease, including cancer.

6. Vitamin E

The lipid-soluble antioxidant vitamin E is localized in the cell membrane and has received the most attention with respect to atherosclerosis and vascular function. A decreased concentration of antioxidants including vitamin E in the presence of a stimuli such as infection, bacterial colonization, exposure to various toxins, and/or metabolic changes such as increased sugar levels could increase free radical concentrations and alter normal brain vascular function. Various studies have assessed the effects of vitamin E intake on vitamin E concentration in different brain regions and its influence on neurologic function. We have previously assessed the effect of a graded dietary vitamin E intake on brain levels and brain function following a 2-month feeding of diets supplemented with 5, 30, 60, 250, or 500 mg α-tocopherol-acetate/kg diet [152]. Animals on this diet exhibited a significant increase of vitamin E concentration in the brain and peripheral tissues. Interestingly, the CNS increased its vitamin E concentration in a dose-response manner only when the diet was supplemented with certain concentrations (i.e., 5, 30, or 60 mg E/kg diet). Vitamin E in food plus 60 mg vitamin E as a supplement = 80 mg E/kg diet was the optimum intake for the CNS tissue to become maximally enriched. Compared to the low vitamin E groups, rats on diets supplemented with the 60 mg E/kg diet showed a significant enhancement on brain function as assessed by dopamine release from striatum, and this finding supports previous work where vitamin E supplementation prevented cognitive behavioral deficits in aged rats. Therefore, although the brain has a limited capacity to incorporate vitamin E, the optimal intake of this nutrient may provide long-term significant benefits on brain performance.

Evidence linking vitamin E deficiency and neurologic sequelae in humans is now firmly established. Several neuropathologic observations are associated with vitamin E deficiency in humans, indicating the importance of this nutrient in the CNS. Studies have shown that increased vitamin E intake slows the progression of dementia in AD, enhances vasculature performance, and improves CNS function [145,153–156].

The reported effects of nutrients such as vitamin E and the drug selegiline in prolonging time to institutionalize patients or in significantly decreasing the disease process, are examples of the feasibility of this approach. Several prospective studies, including the U.S. Nurses' Health Study and the U.S. Health Professionals Follow-up Study, found a significant reduction (about 40%) in the risk of having a cardiac event for those taking vitamin E supplements [157,158]. The Iowa Women's Health Study found a 47% reduction in cardiac mortality [158,159]. This is highly relevant because cardiovascular disease (CVD) is one of the leading causes of morbidity and mortality among the elderly. However, results of randomized, controlled clinical trials have not been consistent with the previous studies. Although the Cambridge Heart Antioxidant Study observed a 47% reduction in fatal and nonfatal myocardial infarction in patients who received 400 or 800 IU of vitamin E/day, no effect on mortality was detected [160]. Although several epidemiologic studies have suggested that inadequate antioxidant status is related to the development of vascular disease, particularly CVD, results from intervention trials have been contradictory [161]. One trial did not find cardiovascular protection with vitamin E supplements at a dose of 400 IU/day in high-risk patients. However, vitamin E has shown some promise in the treatment of AD and CVD. Although strong data suggest the potential benefit of vitamin E on vascular function [162], no clear consensus has been reached for primary prevention of CVD. Animal studies have provided further evidence for the benefits of vitamin E by suggesting that free radical-mediated sublethal changes and inflammatory processes in endothelial cells may promote thrombosis, directly damage vascular cells, and interfere with vasomotor regulation [145,163,164]. A common complication of diabetes is the accelerated atherosclerosis or hardening of the arteries, which interferes with normal blood flow and increases the risk of heart attacks and strokes [165]. One of the reasons for decreased circulation is the abnormal function of the endothelium. Thus, a generous intake of this nutrient could play a beneficial role in human health, and may contribute to the prevention or delay of neuropathologic processes. Interestingly, the Food and Nutrition Board, in addition to increasing its recommended dietary allowances by 50%, has set an upper limit for this nutrient of 1000 mg/day. Therefore, vitamin E, through dietary supplementation alone or in combination with anti-inflammatory drugs, may provide valuable protection against the vascular diseases and neurodegenerative changes associated with cognitive impairment.

Interestingly, population-based studies of antioxidants suggest that a diet rich in foods containing vitamin E may help protect some people against AD [155,156]. These reports are part of a series of existing reports on vitamin E and dementia. The new findings heighten interest in the outcome of clinical trials now underway to test the effectiveness of vitamin E and other antioxidants in preventing or postponing cognitive decline and AD. These studies and a number of other important population studies have suggested that vitamin E may work as a protective molecule against oxidative damage or other mechanisms associated with cognitive decline and dementia. Clinical studies and trials now underway will generate, in the near future, critical information to test these hypotheses, helping us to better understand the role of antioxidants in cognitive function and to determine whether vitamin E in food or in supplements, or taken together, can prevent or slow down the development of mild cognitive impairment or AD.

7. Vitamin C

Vitamin C, a water-soluble vitamin, participates in a large number of cell functions. All animal species appear to require vitamin C, but for humans, guinea pigs, monkeys, bats, certain fish, and perhaps certain reptiles, it is a dietary requirement. These species lack the enzyme L-gulonolactone oxidase, which is necessary for vitamin C synthesis from 6-carbon sugars. Vitamin C is rapidly absorbed into the circulatory system in the upper part of the small intestine. About 80–95% is absorbed when the intake is about 100 mg a day, and the absorption decreases with larger intake being only about 50% when the total intake is 1500 mg. In addition to the antioxidant-protective role in cell injury [166–169], vitamin C accelerates the degradation of intra- and extracellular proteins targeted to the lysosomal lumen by autophagic and heterophagic pathways, relevant for the removal of abnormal proteins that accumulate with aging [151]. Vitamin C also has specific and well-defined roles in the activation of two enzyme classes, the copper-containing hydroxylases (e.g., dopamine-hydroxylase and peptide glycine hydroxylase) and the iron-containing hydroxylases (e.g., procollagen proline 4-hydroxylase involved in collagen synthesis; aspartate-hydroxylase, precursor of protein C and involved in the clotting cascade; and carnitine synthase used by mitochondria for electron transfer in ATP synthesis). In addition, over the years, other enzymes, including tryptophan dioxygenase and tyrosine hydroxylase, have been found to be ascorbate-dependent.

The average body pool of vitamin C in adults is about 1500 mg with a fractional turnover rate of 3–4% daily, suggesting a need for about 60 mg/day for replacement. However, considering the absorption variability factor, food-viability, and that its catabolism rate varies with the intake, a reference intake of 80–100 mg/day has been recommended. Based on the RDA, 75 mg of vitamin C/day (before 2000 the RDA was 60 mg), a substantial number of people (20–30%) in the United States ingest vitamin C at or below the RDA recommendations. Researchers estimate that our paleolithic ancestors ingested several grams of vitamin C/day [170]. Although optimal vitamin C requirements are unknown, Levine *et al* estimated that they should be about 200 mg/day, based on concentrations in plasma and tissues, optimal vitamin C intake, and epidemiologic observations [171]. Some researchers believe that human requirements for vitamin C are considerably higher than those previously discussed, scaling up to 1–3 g/day.

During times of chemical, emotional, psychological, or psychologic stress, the urinary system excretes vitamin C at a significantly increased rate, thereby elevating the body's need for vitamin C during these times. Examples of chemical stressors include cigarette smoke, pollutants, and allergens. Extra intake of vitamin C in the form of supplementation or by drinking or eating foods with a high content of vitamin C is often recommended to keep the immune system working properly during times of stress. In certain instances, vitamin C supplementation is the only way to meet the concentrations needed for many health conditions. For example, cancer patients should supplement their diet with additional vitamin C and consume foods containing high levels of vitamin C, particularly vegetable juices because they are also a rich source of carotenes and flavonoids.

Vitamin C is highly concentrated in the brain, estimated at between 100–500 mmol/L. Although it is known that within the brain, vitamin C concentration changes rapidly in response to neural activity, its physiologic functions are not well understood. Vitamin C has been shown to significantly improve endothelium-dependent vasodilation in diabetics, perhaps by reducing excess superoxide production and thereby decreasing levels of NO inactivation. Higher vitamin C plasma concentrations have been significantly associated with better memory performance in patients with dementia [146,172–175]. Cognitive performance in normal older people as well as cognitive decline in patients with AD appears to be positively associated with vitamin C intake. Interestingly, the Food and Nutrition Board modified the dietary reference (April 2000) [175a], and, in addition to increasing its recommended dietary allowances by 25–50%, has set an upper limit for this nutrient of 2000 mg/day. Vitamin C treatment, through dietary supplementation alone or in combination with anti-inflammatory drugs and/or other antioxidants, may provide valuable protection against the neurodegenerative changes associated with cognitive impairment. High intakes of vitamin C, of which no toxic effects have been found, may cause diarrhea and abdominal bloating for some people, and should not be recommended to patients who are iron-overloaded, have hemochromatosis, thalasemia major, sideroblastic anemia, or other diseases requiring multiple red blood cell transfusions. It is not known whether ascorbate induces iron overabsorption in healthy people.

8. Roles of Vitamin E and C in Brain

Nutrient intake evaluation in a study regarding cognitive function was evaluated in all 921 trial subjects with ages varying from 65 to >85. Of all nutritional factors evaluated, the vitamin C intake was shown to have the strongest influence on the cognitive functioning [176]. This observation increases in importance with the fact that a low consumption of vitamin C as well as a low plasma level of this nutrient was associated with a greater risk of cognitive disorders. Interestingly, 20 years later, when 842 individuals had died, it could be calculated that the death risk of persons with a low cognitive score was 2-fold higher than those with a normal score [176]. This higher mortality in people suffering from cognitive impairment involved, in particular, a higher risk of dying from a stroke. The relation between cognitive function and risk of death from stroke suggests that cerebrovascular disease may be an important contributor of declining cognitive function. Vitamin C status may be a determinant of cognitive function in elderly people by acting in both the vasculature [177], and directly in brain, improving degradation of modified proteins [144,151]. Although vitamin C is the most popular vitamin supplement in the United States, in many respects it is the most controversial. In general, the literature strongly supports the notion that high vitamin C intake may protect against both cognitive impairment and cerebrovascular disease.

9. Fruit and Vegetable Polyphenolic Supplementation

There have been numerous studies in which antioxidants have been examined with respect to reducing the deleterious effects of brain aging, with mixed results (following). However, our research (following) suggests that the combinations of antioxidant/anti-inflammatory polyphenolics found in fruits and vegetables may show efficacy in aging. Plants, including food plants (fruits and vegetables), synthesize a vast array of chemical compounds that are not involved in their primary metabolism. These 'secondary compounds' instead serve a variety of ecologic functions, ultimately, to enhance the plant's survivability. Interestingly, these compounds also may be responsible for the multitude of beneficial effects of fruits and vegetables on an array of health-related bioactivities; two of the most important may be their antioxidant and anti-inflammatory properties. Because OS appears to be involved in the signaling and behavioral losses seen in senescence, an important question becomes whether increasing antioxidant intake would forestall or prevent these changes, and the literature is replete with studies in which a large variety of dietary agents have been employed to alter behavioral and neuronal deficits with aging. These studies have included such nutritional supplements as vitamins C or E, garlic [178], herbals (e.g., ginseng, ginkgo biloba, Ding lang see [142]), and dietary fatty acids [179].

As indicated previously, we believed that given the considerable antioxidant/anti-inflammatory potential of the fruits and vegetables, they might show considerable efficacy in reducing the deleterious effects of aging [144]. In our first study we utilized fruits and vegetables identified as being high in antioxidant activity via the Oxygen Radical Absorbance Capacity Assay (ORAC) [180–182], and showed that long-term (from age 6 to 15 months; F344 rats) feeding with a supplemented American Institute of Nutrition (AIN)-93 diet (strawberry extract or spinach extract [1–2% of the diet] or vitamin E [500 IU]), retarded age-related decrements in cognitive or neuronal function. Results indicated that the supplemented diets could prevent the onset of age-related deficits in several indices (e.g., cognitive behavior, Morris water-maze performance) [143].

In a subsequent experiment [183] we found that dietary supplementation (for 8 weeks) with spinach, strawberry or blueberry (BB) extracts in an AIN-93 diet was effective in reversing age-related deficits in neuronal and behavioral (cognitive) function in aged (19 mo) F344 rats. However, only the BB-supplemented group exhibited improved performance on tests of motor function. Specifically, the BB-supplemented group displayed improved performance on two motor tests that rely on balance and coordination, rod walking, and the accelerating rotarod, whereas none of the other supplemented groups differed from control on these tasks. (Note that the beneficial effects of BB on motor function seen in rodents have also been observed in aged humans [mean age 65]. Preliminary results from a study in which reaction speed was examined to a stimulus indicated that as the daily intake of blueberries was increased from 0 to 2 cups/day over 12 weeks, subjects showed a significant 6% increase in reaction speed per Joseph *et al*, in preparation [184].)

In the Joseph *et al* study [183] the rodents in all diet groups, but not the control group, showed improved working memory (short-term memory) performance in the Morris water maze, demonstrated as one-trial learning following the 10 minute retention interval. We also observed significant increases in several indices of neuronal signaling (e.g., MAChR sensitivity), and found that BB diet reversed age-related "dysregulation" in Ca^{45} buffering capacity. Examinations of reactive oxygen species production (ROS) in the brain tissue obtained from animals in the various diet groups indicated that the striata obtained from all of the supplemented groups exhibited significantly lower ROS levels (by assaying DCF;$2',7'$-dichlorofluorescein diacetate) than the controls. A subsequent study using a BB-supplemented NIH-31 diet replicated the previous findings [185]. However, it was clear from these supplementation studies [183,185] that the significant effects of BBs on both motor and cognitive behavior were due to a multiplicity of actions, in addition to those involving antioxidant and anti-inflammatory activity. We also have shown that BB-supplemented senescent animals show increased neurogenesis [186].

With respect to AD, we have shown in a study [184] that BB-supplemented (from age 1 to 12 mo) mice transgenic for amyloid precursor protein and presenilin-1 mutations (which show the formation of numerous plaques in the brain, similar to those seen in AD) do not show behavioral deficits in Y-maze performance as seen by those given a control diet. The supplemented mice also showed enhancements in several signaling molecules associated with cognitive function (e.g., extracellular signal-regulated kinase activity). The findings suggest that it is possible to delay and/or prevent cognitive dysfunction despite the pathologic changes in this model, and further suggest that the inclusion of fruits high in antioxidant activity may help prevent the deleterious effects of this disease later in life.

Vegetables (especially broccoli, peppers, potatoes, and brussels sprouts) also contain high levels of vitamin C, even though most people think of citrus fruits as the best source of this nutrient. However, exposure to air destroys vitamin C, so it is important to eat fresh foods as quickly as possible. Although a salad from a salad bar is a healthy choice, the vitamin C content of the fruits and vegetables from a salad bar is only a fraction of what it would be in a fresh salad. Other nutrients previously described appear to be more stable; however, further studies need to be performed to evaluate this perception. For example, freshly sliced vegetables, if left standing, lose about 50% of their vitamin C content within the first 3 hours, and about 35% in the refrigerator in <24 hours.

II. Conclusions

From the previous sections, it should be clear that there are a number of sources of OS and inflammation and that these insults are superimposed upon an increasingly vulnerable environment in aging. Moreover, in genetic aberrations in conditions such as AD or PD this vulnerability increases even further. Because this is the case, it is critical that methods be explored to reduce this vulnerability. What we have tried to show in this review is that one method of accomplishing this may be through diets containing antioxidants. An abundance of epidemiologic data indicates that diets rich in antioxidants may play a pivotal role in maintaining human health [187–189].

It is evident that these antioxidants should include Vitamin E and C. These vitamins can help to protect cells and intracellular organelles, and prevent their decline in function with aging. A deficiency of vitamin E can cause breakdown of red blood cells, especially in infants, resulting in anemia. Vitamin E is also necessary for the maintenance of the immune system and nervous tissue. Deficiency of vitamin E can result in neurologic disorders affecting the spinal cord and retina. Plant oils are rich in vitamin E as are margarine and some fruits and vegetables. Grains such as oatmeal and wheat germ, and nuts, are also good sources. In individuals with fat malabsorption, 200–400 IU/day for adults are usually prescribed to supplement the diet.

In addition to vitamins E and C, it is also important for the diets to contain fruits and vegetables, and this appears to be especially true in aging and possibly in AD. We have reviewed studies that have shown reversals in age-related cognitive and motor behaviors with fruit or vegetable supplementation [183] and have increased signaling and prevented cognitive decline in APP/PS1 mice [184]. In the case of AD, there is an inverse correlation between the intake of wine flavonoids [190] or fruit and vegetable intake [191], and the development of dementia. Thus, these studies, as well as those reviewed previously, suggest a positive role for dietary antioxidants in both the prevention and delay of the deleterious effects of aging and AD. Finally, it should be pointed out that studies in cell models indicate that green tea extracts may also be of some benefit in reducing the neurotoxicity associated with PD [192–194]. Given these considerations, it is evident that antioxidants may be critical elements in a diet to maintain motor and cognitive health throughout the lifespan and should increase the likelihood of achieving successful aging.

III. Suggestions for Further Investigations

- To assess the existing gaps in the role that oxidative stress and inflammation may play in the etiology of neurodegenerative disease associated with aging.
- To investigate to what extent nutritional intervention, with a generous intake of fruits and vegetables, is critical on maintaining cognitive function and prevention of AD.

Acknowledgement

The authors would like to thank Dr. Donna Bielinski for her editing comments on the preparation of this manuscript.

References

1. Cabeza R, Grady CL, Nyberg L *et al.* (1997). Age-related differences in neural activity during memory encoding and retrieval: A positron emission tomography study. *J Neurosci.* 17:391–400.
2. Small SA, Stern Y, Tang M, Mayeux R. (1999). Selective decline in memory function among healthy elderly. *Neurology.* 52:1392–1396.
3. Murphy DG, DeCarli C, Schapiro MB *et al.* (1992). Age-related differences in volumes of subcortical nuclei, brain matter, and cerebrospinal fluid in healthy men as measured with magnetic resonance imaging. *Arch Neurol.* 49:839–845.
4. Morrison JH, Hof PR. (1997). Life and death of neurons in the aging brain. *Science.* 278:412–419.
5. West MJ. (1993). Regionally specific loss of neurons in the aging human hippocampus. *Neurobiol Aging.* 14:287–293.
6. Ball MJ, West MJ. (1998). Aging in the human brain: A clarion call to stay the course. *Neurobiol Aging.* 19:1.
7. Peters A, Morrison JH, Rosene DL, Hyman BT. (1998). Feature article: Are neurons lost from the primate cerebral cortex during normal aging? *Cereb Cortex.* 8:295–300.
8. Bartus RT, Fleming D, Johnson HR. (1978). Aging in the rhesus monkey: Debilitating effects on short-term memory. *J Gerontol.* 33:858–871.
9. Grady CL, McIntosh AR, Bookstein F *et al.* (1998). Age-related changes in regional cerebral blood flow during working memory for faces. *Neuroimage.* 8:409–425.
10. Moss MB, Killiany RJ, Lai ZC *et al.* (1997). Recognition memory span in rhesus monkeys of advanced age. *Neurobiol Aging.* 18:13–19.
11. Rapp PR, Amaral DG. (1991). Recognition memory deficits in a subpopulation of aged monkeys resemble the effects of medial temporal lobe damage. *Neurobiol Aging.* 12:481–486.
12. Gilinsky AS, Judd BB. (1994). Working memory and bias in reasoning across the life span. Psychol Aging 9:356–371.
13. Kail R, Salthouse TA. (1994). Processing speed as a mental capacity. *Acta Psychol (Amst).* 86:199–225.
14. Robbins TW, James M, Owen AM *et al.* (1994). Cambridge Neuropsychological Test Automated Battery (CANTAB): A factor analytic study of a large sample of normal elderly volunteers. *Dementia.* 5:266–281.
15. Gould TJ, Chadman K, Bickford PC. (1998). Antioxidant protection of cerebellar beta-adrenergic receptor function in aged F344 rats. *Neurosci Lett.* 250:165–168.
16. Joseph JA, Berger RE, Engel BT, Roth GS. (1978). Age-related changes in the nigrostriatum: A behavioral and biochemical analysis. *J Gerontology.* 33:643–649.
17. Cepeda C, Colwell CS, Itri JN *et al.* (1998). Dopaminergic modulation of NMDA-induced whole cell currents in neostriatal neurons in slices: Contribution of calcium conductances. *J Neurophysiol.* 79:82–94.
18. Egashira T. (2000). Effects of breeding conditions on neurochemical cholinergic and monoaminergic markers in aged rat brain. *Nippon Ronen Igakkai Zasshi.* 37:233–238.
19. Joseph JA. (1992). The putative role of free radicals in the loss of neuronal functioning in senescence. *Integr Physiol Behav Sci.* 27:216–227.
20. Kornhuber J, Schoppmeyer K, Bendig C, Riederer P. (1996). Characterization of [3H]pentazocine binding sites in postmortem human frontal cortex. *J Neural Transm.* 103:45–53.
21. Galli RL, Shukitt-Hale B, Youdim KA, Joseph JA. (2002). Fruit polyphenolics and brain aging: Nutritional interventions targeting age-related neuronal and behavioral deficits. *Ann N Y Acad Sci.* 959:128–132.
22. Kuhn HG, Dickinson-Anson H, Gage FH. (1996). Neurogenesis in the dentate gyrus of the adult rat: Age-related decrease of neuronal progenitor proliferation. *J Neurosci.* 16:2027–2033.
23. Joseph JA, Bartus RT, Clody D *et al.* (1983). Psychomotor performance in the senescent rodent: Reduction of deficits via striatal dopamine receptor up-regulation. *Neurobiol Aging.* 4:313–319.
24. Kluger A, Gianutsos JG, Golomb J *et al.* (1997). Motor/psychomotor dysfunction in normal aging, mild cognitive decline, and early Alzheimer's disease: Diagnostic and differential diagnostic features. *Int Psychogeriatr.* 9(Suppl 1):307–316; discussion 317–321.
25. Bartus RT. (1990). Drugs to treat age-related neurodegenerative problems. The final frontier of medical science? *J Am Geriatr Soc.* 38:680–695.
26. Ingram DK, Spangler EL, Iijima S *et al.* (1994). New pharmacological strategies for cognitive enhancement using a rat model of age-related memory impairment. *Ann N Y Acad Sci.* 717:16–32.
27. Shukitt-Hale B, Mouzakis G, Joseph JA. (1998). Psychomotor and spatial memory performance in aging male Fischer 344 rats. *Exp Gerontol.* 33:615–624.
28. Muir JL. (1997). Acetylcholine, aging, and Alzheimer's disease. *Pharmacol Biochem Behav.* 56:687–696.
29. Bickford P, Heron C, Young DA *et al.* (1992). Impaired acquisition of novel locomotor tasks in aged and norepinephrine-depleted F344 rats. *Neurobiol Aging.* 13:475–481.
30. Bickford P. (1993). Motor learning deficits in aged rats are correlated with loss of cerebellar noradrenergic function. *Brain Res.* 620:133–138.
31. Bartus RT, Dean RL, Beer B. (1982). Neuropeptide effects on memory in aged monkeys. *Neurobiol Aging.* 3:61–68.
32. Devan BD, Goad EH, Petri HL. (1996). Dissociation of hippocampal and striatal contributions to spatial navigation in the water maze. *Neurobiol Learn Mem.* 66:305–323.
33. McDonald RJ, White NM. (1994). Parallel information processing in the water maze: Evidence for independent memory systems involving dorsal striatum and hippocampus. *Behav Neural Biol.* 61:260–270.
34. Oliveira MG, Bueno OF, Pomarico AC, Gugliano EB. (1997). Strategies used by hippocampal- and caudateputamen-lesioned rats in a learning task. *Neurobiol Learn Mem.* 68:32–41.
35. Zyzak DR, Otto T, Eichenbaum H, Gallagher M. (1995). Cognitive decline associated with normal aging in rats: A neuropsychological approach. *Learn Mem.* 2:1–16.
36. Shukitt-Hale B, Smith DE, Meydani M, Joseph JA. (1999). The effects of dietary antioxidants on psychomotor performance in aged mice. *Exp Gerontol.* 34:797–808.
37. Hauss-Wegrzyniak B, Willard LB, Del Soldato P *et al.* (1999). Peripheral administration of novel anti-inflammatories can attenuate the effects of chronic inflammation within the CNS. *Brain Res.* 815:36–43.
38. Hauss-Wegrzyniak B, Vannucchi MG, Wenk GL. (2000). Behavioral and ultrastructural changes induced by chronic neuroinflammation in young rats. *Brain Res.* 859:157–166.
39. Small GW, Kuhl DE, Riege WH *et al.* (1989). Cerebral glucose metabolic patterns in Alzheimer's disease. Effect of gender and age at dementia onset. *Arch Gen Psychiatry.* 46:527–532.
40. Jorm AF, Korten AE, Henderson AS. (1987). The prevalence of dementia: A quantitative integration of the literature. *Acta Psychiatr Scand.* 76:465–479.
41. McGonigal G, Thomas B, McQuade C *et al.* (1993). Epidemiology of Alzheimer's presenile dementia in Scotland, 1974–88. *BMJ.* 306:680–683.
42. Henderson VW, Paganini-Hill A, Emanuel CK *et al.* (1994). Estrogen replacement therapy in older women. Comparisons between Alzheimer's disease cases and nondemented control subjects. *Arch Neurol.* 51:896–900.
43. Tang MX, Jacobs D, Stern Y *et al.* (1996). Effect of oestrogen during menopause on risk and age at onset of Alzheimer's disease. *Lancet.* 348:429–432.
44. Kawas C, Resnick S, Morrison A *et al.* (1997). A prospective study of estrogen replacement therapy and the risk of developing Alzheimer's disease: The Baltimore Longitudinal Study of Aging. *Neurology.* 48:1517–1521.
45. Stam FC, Wigboldus JM, Smeulders AW. (1986). Age incidence of senile brain amyloidosis. *Pathol Res Pract.* 181:558–562.
46. Schupf N, Kapell D, Nightingale B *et al.* (1998). Earlier onset of Alzheimer's disease in men with Down syndrome. *Neurology.* 50:991–995.
47. Mulnard RA. (2000). Estrogen as a treatment for Alzheimer's disease. *JAMA.* 284:307–308.

48. Mulnard RA, Cotman CW, Kawas C et al. (2000). Estrogen replacement therapy for treatment of mild to moderate Alzheimer disease: A randomized controlled trial. Alzheimer's Disease Cooperative Study. *JAMA*. 283:1007–1015.

49. Wang PN, Liao SQ, Liu RS et al. (2000). Effects of estrogen on cognition, mood, and cerebral blood flow in AD: A controlled study. *Neurology*. 54: 2061–2066.

50. Seshadri S, Zornberg GL, Derby LE et al. (2001). Postmenopausal estrogen replacement therapy and the risk of Alzheimer disease. *Arch Neurol*. 58:435–440.

51. Genazzani AR, Castaldi M, Didzinska D et al. (1992). The brain as a target organ of gonadal steroids. *Psychoneuroendocrinology*. 17:385–390.

52. Ripich DN, Petrill SA, Whitehouse PJ, Ziol EW. (1995). Gender differences in language of AD patients: A longitudinal study. *Neurology*. 45:299–302.

53. Buckwalter JG, Sobel E, Dunn ME et al. (1993). Gender differences on a brief measure of cognitive functioning in Alzheimer's disease. *Arch Neurol*. 50:757–760.

54. Hebert LE, Wilson RS, Gilley DW et al. (2000). Decline of language among women and men with Alzheimer's disease. *J Gerontol B Psychol Sci Soc Sci*. 55:P354–360.

55. Bayles KA, Azuma T, Cruz RF et al. (1999). Gender differences in language of Alzheimer disease patients revisited. *Alzheimer Dis Assoc Disord*. 13:138–146.

56. Ott BR, Tate CA, Gordon NM, Heindel WC. (1996). Gender differences in the behavioral manifestations of Alzheimer's disease. *J Am Geriatr Soc*. 44:583–587.

57. Drachman DA, Swearer JM, O'Donnell BF et al. (1992). The Caretaker Obstreperous-Behavior Rating Assessment (COBRA) Scale. *J Am Geriatr Soc*. 40:463–470.

58. Lyketsos CG, Steele C, Galik E et al. (1999). Physical aggression in dementia patients and its relationship to depression. *Am J Psychiatry*. 156:66–71.

59. Lyketsos CG, Chen LS, Anthony JC. (1999). Cognitive decline in adulthood: An 11.5-year follow-up of the Baltimore Epidemiologic Catchment Area Study. *Am J Psychiatry*. 156:58–65.

60. Cohen D, Eisdorfer C, Gorelick P et al. (1993). Sex differences in the psychiatric manifestations of Alzheimer's disease. *J Am Geriatr Soc*. 41:229–232.

61. Olanow CW. (1992). An introduction to the free radical hypothesis in Parkinson's disease. *Ann Neurol*. 32 Suppl:S2–9.

62. Gilissen EP, Jacobs RE, McGuinness ER, Allman JM. (1999). Topographical localization of lipofuscin pigment in the brain of the aged fat-tailed dwarf lemur (Cheirogaleus medius) and grey lesser mouse lemur (Microcebus murinus): Comparison to iron localization. *Am J Primatol*. 49:183–193.

63. Sadoul R. (1998). Bcl-2 family members in the development and degenerative pathologies of the nervous system. *Cell Death Differ*. 5:805–815.

64. Yu BP, Suescun EA, Yang SY. (1992). Effect of age-related lipid peroxidation on membrane fluidity and phospholipase A2: Modulation by dietary restriction. *Mech Ageing Dev*. 65:17–33.

65. Carney JM, Smith CD, Carney AM, Butterfield DA. (1994). Aging- and oxygen-induced modifications in brain biochemistry and behavior. *Ann N Y Acad Sci*. 738:44–53.

66. Denisova NA, Erat SA, Kelly JF, Roth GS. (1998). Differential effect of aging on cholesterol modulation of carbachol-stimulated low-K(m) GTPase in striatal synaptosomes. *Exp Gerontol*. 33:249–265.

67. Joseph J, Dalton T, Hunt W. (1988a). Age-related decrements in the muscarinic enhancement of K+-evoked release of endogenous striatal dopamine: An indicator of altered cholinergic-dopaminergic reciprocal inhibitory control in senescence. *Brain Res*. 454:140–148.

68. Joseph J, Dalton T, Roth G, Hunt W. (1988b). Alterations in muscarinic control of striatal dopamine autoreceptors in senescence: A deficit at the ligand-muscarinic receptor interface? *Brain Res*. 454:149–155.

69. Joseph J, Shukitt-Hale B, Denisova NA et al. (2001). Copernicus revisited: Amyloid beta in Alzheimer's disease. *Neurobiol Aging*. 22:131–146.

70. Smith CD, Carney JM, Tatsumo T et al. (1992). Protein oxidation in aging brain. *Ann N Y Acad Sci*. 663:110–119.

71. Vitek MP, Bhattacharya K, Glendening JM et al. (1994). Advanced glycation end products contribute to amyloidosis in Alzheimer disease. *Proc Natl Acad Sci USA*. 91:4766–4770.

72. Smith MA, Taneda S, Richey PL et al. (1994). Advanced Maillard reaction end products are associated with Alzheimer disease pathology. *Proc Natl Acad Sci USA*. 91:5710–5714.

73. Yan SD, Chen X, Schmidt AM et al. (1994). Glycated tau protein in Alzheimer disease: A mechanism for induction of oxidant stress. *Proc Natl Acad Sci USA*. 91:7787–7791.

74. Ledesma MD, Bonay P, Colaco C, Avila J. (1994). Analysis of microtubule-associated protein tau glycation in paired helical filaments. *J Biol Chem*. 269:21614–21619.

75. Salomon RG, Subbanagounder G, O'Neil J et al. (1997). Levuglandin E2-protein adducts in human plasma and vasculature. *Chem Res Toxicol*. 10:536–545.

76. Sayre LM, Perry G, Smith MA. (1999). *In situ* methods for detection and localization of markers of oxidative stress: Application in neurodegenerative disorders. *Methods Enzymol*. 309:133–152.

77. Mattson MP, Carney JW, Butterfield DA. (1995). A tombstone in Alzheimer's? *Nature*. 373:481.

78. Smith MA, Sayre LM, Vitek MP et al. (1995). Early AGEing and Alzheimer's. *Nature*. 374:316.

79. Castellani RJ, Harris PL, Sayre LM et al. (2001). Active glycation in neurofibrillary pathology of Alzheimer disease: N(epsilon)-(carboxymethyl) lysine and hexitol-lysine. *Free Radic Biol Med*. 31:175–180.

80. Smith MA, Perry G, Richey PL et al. (1996). Oxidative damage in Alzheimer's. *Nature*. 382:120–121.

81. Smith MA, Sayre LM, Anderson VE et al. (1998). Cytochemical demonstration of oxidative damage in Alzheimer disease by immunochemical enhancement of the carbonyl reaction with 2,4-dinitrophenylhydrazine. *J Histochem Cytochem*. 46:731–735.

82. Montine TJ, Amarnath V, Martin ME et al. (1996). E-4-hydroxy-2-nonenal is cytotoxic and cross links cytoskeletal proteins in P19 neuroglial cultures. *Am J Pathol*. 148:89–93.

83. Sayre LM, Zelasko DA, Harris PL et al. (1997). 4-Hydroxynonenal-derived advanced lipid peroxidation end products are increased in Alzheimer's disease. *J Neurochem*. 68:2092–2097.

84. Friguet B, Stadtman ER, Szweda LI. (1994). Modification of glucose-6-phosphate dehydrogenase by 4-hydroxy-2-nonenal. Formation of cross-linked protein that inhibits the multicatalytic protease. *J Biol Chem*. 269:21639–21643.

85. Mori H, Kondo J, Ihara Y. (1987). Ubiquitin is a component of paired helical filaments in Alzheimer's disease. *Science*. 235:1641–1644.

86. Smith MA, Richey Harris PL, Sayre LM et al. (1997). Widespread peroxynitrite-mediated damage in Alzheimer's disease. *J Neurosci*. 17:2653–2657.

87. Nunomura A, Perry G, Pappolla MA et al. (1999). RNA oxidation is a prominent feature of vulnerable neurons in Alzheimer's disease. *J Neurosci*. 19:1959–1964.

88. Ginsberg SD, Crino PB, Lee VM et al. (1997). Sequestration of RNA in Alzheimer's disease neurofibrillary tangles and senile plaques. *Ann Neurol*. 41:200–209.

89. Nunomura A, Perry G, Aliev G et al. (2001). Oxidative damage is the earliest event in Alzheimer disease. *J Neuropathol Exp Neurol*. 60:759–767.

90. Sampson JB, Ye Y, Rosen H, Beckman JS. (1998). Myeloperoxidase and horseradish peroxidase catalyze tyrosine nitration in proteins from nitrite and hydrogen peroxide. *Arch Biochem Biophys*. 356:207–213.

91. Smith MA, Harris PL, Sayre LM, Perry G. (1997). Iron accumulation in Alzheimer disease is a source of redox-generated free radicals. *Proc Natl Acad Sci USA*. 94:9866–9868.

92. Sayre LM, Perry G, Harris PL et al. (2000). *In situ* oxidative catalysis by neurofibrillary tangles and senile plaques in Alzheimer's disease: A central role for bound transition metals. *J Neurochem*. 74:270–279.

93. Brunk UT, Jones CB, Sohal RS. (1992). A novel hypothesis of lipofuscinogenesis and cellular aging based on interactions between oxidative stress and autophagocytosis. *Mutat Res*. 275:395–403.

94. Smith MA, Vasak M, Knipp M et al. (1998). Dimethylargininase, a nitric oxide regulatory protein, in Alzheimer disease. *Free Radic Biol Med*. 25:898–902.

95. Small GW, Mazziotta JC, Collins MT et al. (1995). Apolipoprotein E type 4 allele and cerebral glucose metabolism in relatives at risk for familial Alzheimer disease. *JAMA*. 273:942–947.

96. Hensley K, Carney JM, Mattson MP et al. (1994). A model for beta-amyloid aggregation and neurotoxicity based on free radical generation by the peptide: Relevance to Alzheimer disease. *Proc Natl Acad Sci USA*. 91:3270–3274.

97. Sayre LM, Zagorski MG, Surewicz WK et al. (1997). Mechanisms of neurotoxicity associated with amyloid beta deposition and the role of free radicals in the pathogenesis of Alzheimer's disease: A critical appraisal. *Chem Res Toxicol*. 10:518–526.

98. Rottkamp CA, Raina AK, Zhu X et al. (2001). Redox-active iron mediates amyloid-beta toxicity. *Free Radic Biol Med*. 30:447–450.

99. Perry G, Nunomura A, Raina AK, Smith MA. (2000). Amyloid-beta junkies. *Lancet*. 355:757.

100. Smith MA, Joseph JA, Perry G. (2000). Arson. Tracking the culprit in Alzheimer's disease. *Ann N Y Acad Sci*. 924:35–38.

101. Lukiw WJ, Bazan NG. (2000). Neuroinflammatory signaling upregulation in Alzheimer's disease. *Neurochem Res.* 25:1173–1184.

102. Townsend KP, Obregon D, Quadros A *et al.* (2002). Proinflammatory and vasoactive effects of Abeta in the cerebrovasculature. *Ann N Y Acad Sci.* 977:65–76.

103. Lue LF, Walker DG. (2002). Modeling Alzheimer's disease immune therapy mechanisms: Interactions of human postmortem microglia with antibody-opsonized amyloid beta peptide. *J Neurosci. Res* 70:599–610.

104. Butterfield DA, Griffin S, Munch G, Pasinetti GM. (2002). Amyloid beta-peptide and amyloid pathology are central to the oxidative stress and inflammatory cascades under which Alzheimer's disease brain exists. *J Alzheimers Dis.* 4:193–201.

105. Rostagno A, Revesz T, Lashley T *et al.* (2002). Complement activation in chromosome 13 dementias. Similarities with Alzheimer's disease. *J Biol Chem.* 277:49782–49790.

106. Russo C, Venezia V, Salis S *et al.* (2002). Molecular aspects of neurodegeneration in Alzheimer's disease. *Funct Neurol.* 17:65–70.

107. Bamberger ME, Landreth GE. (2002). Inflammation, apoptosis, and Alzheimer's disease. *Neuroscientist.* 8:276–283.

108. Rozovsky I, Finch CE, Morgan TE. (1998). Age-related activation of microglia and astrocytes: *In vitro* studies show persistent phenotypes of aging, increased proliferation, and resistance to down-regulation. *Neurobiol Aging.* 19:97–103.

109. McGeer PL, McGeer EG. (1995). The inflammatory response system of brain: Implications for therapy of Alzheimer and other neurodegenerative diseases. *Brain Res.* Rev. 21(2):195–218.

110. McGeer P, McGeer E. (1995). The inflammatory response system of brain: Implications for therapy of Alzheimer and other neurodegenerative diseases. *Brain Res.* Rev. 21:195–218.

111. Chang HN, Wang SR, Chiang SC *et al.* (1996). The relationship of aging to endotoxin shock and to production of TNF-α. *J Gerontology.* 51: M220–M222.

112. Spaulding CC, Walford RL, Effros RB. (1997). Calorie restriction inhibits the age-related dysregulation of the cytokines TNF-alpha and IL-6 in C3B10RF1 mice. *Mech Ageing Dev.* 93:87–94.

113. Volpato S, Guralnik JM, Ferrucci L *et al.* (2001). Cardiovascular disease, interleukin-6, and risk of mortality in older women: The Women's Health and Aging Study. *Circulation.* 103:947–953.

114. Kushner I. (2001). C-reactive protein elevation can be caused by conditions other than inflammation and may reflect biologic aging. *Cleve Clin J Med.* 68:535–537.

115. Bonizzi G, Piette J, Merville MP, Bours V. (1997). Distinct signal transduction pathways mediate nuclear factor-kappaB induction by IL-1beta in epithelial and lymphoid cells. *J Immunol.* 159:5264–5272.

116. Lo YY, Conquer JA, Grinstein S, Cruz TF. (1998). Interleukin-1 beta induction of c-*fos* and collagenase expression in articular chondrocytes: Involvement of reactive oxygen species. *J Cell Biochem.* 69:19–29.

117. Tueting P, Costa E, Dwivedi Y *et al.* (1999). The phenotypic characteristics of heterozygous reeler mouse. *Neuroreport.* 10:1329–1334.

118. Manev H, Uz T. (1999). Primary cultures of rat cerebellar granule cells as a model to study neuronal 5-lipoxygenase and FLAP gene expression. *Ann N Y Acad Sci.* 890:183–190.

119. Woodroofe MN. (1995). Cytokine production in the central nervous system. *Neurol.* 45 (6 Suppl 6):S6–S10.

120. Steffen B, Breier G, Butcher E *et al.* (1996). ICAM-1, VCAM-1, and MAd-CAM-1 are expressed on choroid plexus epithelium but not endothelium and mediate binding of lymphocytes *in vitro. Am J Pathol.* 148:1819–1838.

121. Schipper H. (1996). Astrocytes, brain aging, and neurodegeneration. *Neurob Aging.* 17:467–480.

122. Rosenman SJ, Shrikant P, Dubb L *et al.* (1995). Cytokine-induced expression of vascular cell adhesion molecule-1 (VCAM-1) by astrocytes and astrocytoma cell lines. *J Immunol.* 154(4):1888–1899.

123. Christen Y. (2000). Oxidative stress and Alzheimer disease. *Am J Clin Nutr.* 71:621S–629S.

124. Markesbery WR, Carney JM. (1999). Oxidative alterations in Alzheimer's disease. *Brain Pathol.* 9:133–146.

125. Ham D, Schipper HM. (2000). Heme oxygenase-1 induction and mitochondrial iron sequestration in astroglia exposed to amyloid peptides. *Cell Mol Biol (Noisy-le-grand).* 46:587–596.

126. Agrimi U, Di Guardo G. (1993). Amyloid, amyloid-inducers, cytokines and heavy metals in scrapie and other human and animal subacute spongiform encephalopathies: Some hypotheses. *Med Hypotheses.* 40:113–116.

127. Paris D, Townsend KP, Obregon DF *et al.* (2002). Pro-inflammatory effect of freshly solubilized beta-amyloid peptides in the brain. *Prostaglandins Other Lipid Mediat.* 70:1–12.

128. Meda L, Baron P, Scarlato G. (2001). Glial activation in Alzheimer's disease: The role of Abeta and its associated proteins. *Neurobiol Aging.* 22:885–893.

129. McGeer E, McGeer P. (1998). The importance of inflammatory mechanisms in Alzheimer disease. *Exp Gerontol.* 33:371–378.

130. Yoshida M, Saito H, Katsuki H. (1995). Neurotrophic effects of conditioned media of astrocytes isolated from different brain regions on hippocampal and cortical neurons. *Experientia.* 51:133–136.

131. Wiese S, Metzger F, Holtmann B, Sendtner M. (1999). Mechanical and excitotoxic lesion of motoneurons: Effects of neurotrophins and ciliary neurotrophic factor on survival and regeneration. *Acta Neurochir Suppl (Wien).* 73:31–39.

132. Paratcha G, Ledda F, Baars L *et al.* (2001). Released GFRalpha1 potentiates downstream signaling, neuronal survival, and differentiation via a novel mechanism of recruitment of c-Ret to lipid rafts. *Neuron.* 29:171–184.

133. Rakowicz WP, Staples CS, Milbrandt J *et al.* (2002). Glial cell line-derived neurotrophic factor promotes the survival of early postnatal spinal motor neurons in the lateral and medial motor columns in slice culture. *J Neurosci.* 22:3953–3962.

134. Garcia-Ovejero D, Veiga S, Garcia-Segura LM, Doncarlos LL. (2002). Glial expression of estrogen and androgen receptors after rat brain injury. *J Comp Neurol.* 450:256–271.

135. Malhotra SK, Shnitka TK, Elbrink J. (1990). Reactive astrocytes: A review. *Cytobios.* 61:133–160.

136. McGraw J, Hiebert GW, Steeves JD. (2001). Modulating astrogliosis after neurotrauma. *J Neurosci. Res* 63:109–115.

137. Brown DR. (2001). Microglia and prion disease. *Microsc Res Tech.* 54:71–80.

138. Persidsky Y, Limoges J, Rasmussen J *et al.* (2001). Reduction in glial immunity and neuropathology by a PAF antagonist and an MMP and TNFalpha inhibitor in SCID mice with HIV-1 encephalitis. *J Neuroimmunol.* 114:57–68.

139. Gendron FP, Neary JT, Theiss PM *et al.* (2003). Mechanisms of P2X7 receptor-mediated ERK1/2 phosphorylation in human astrocytoma cells. *Am J Physiol Cell Physiol.* 284:C571–581.

140. Irizarry MC, Hyman BT. (2001). Alzheimer disease therapeutics. *J Neuropathol Exp Neurol.* 60:923–928.

141. Kobayashi K, Hayashi M, Nakano H *et al.* (2002). Apoptosis of astrocytes with enhanced lysosomal activity and oligodendrocytes in white matter lesions in Alzheimer's disease. *Neuropathol Appl Neurobiol.* 28:238–251.

142. Cantuti-Castelvetri I, Shukitt-Hale B, Joseph JA. (2000). Neurobehavioral aspects of antioxidants in aging. *Int J Dev Neurosci.* 18:367–381.

143. Joseph J, Shukitt-Hale B, Denisova N *et al.* (1998). Long-term dietary strawberry, spinach, or vitamin E supplementation retards the onset of age-related neuronal signal-transduction and cognitive behavioral deficits. *J Neurosience.* 18:8047–8055.

144. Martin A, Cherubini A, Andres-Lacueva C *et al.* (2002). Effects of fruits and vegetables on levels of vitamins E and C in the brain and their association with cognitive performance. *J Nutr Health Aging.* 6:392–404.

145. Martin A, Youdim K, Szprengiel A *et al.* (2002). Roles of vitamins E and C on neurodegenerative diseases and cognitive performance. *Nutr Rev.* 60:308–326.

146. Ryglewicz D, Rodo M, Kunicki PK *et al.* (2002). Plasma antioxidant activity and vascular dementia. *J Neurol Sci.* 203–204:195–197.

147. Mayer-Davis EJ, Costacou T, King I *et al.* (2002). Plasma and dietary vitamin E in relation to incidence of type 2 diabetes: The Insulin Resistance and Atherosclerosis Study (IRAS). *Diabetes Care.* 25:2172–2177.

148. Boshtam M, Rafiei M, Sadeghi K, Sarraf-Zadegan N. (2002). Vitamin E can reduce blood pressure in mild hypertensives. *Int J Vitam Nutr Res.* 72:309–314.

149. Chen J, He J, Hamm L *et al.* (2002). Serum antioxidant vitamins and blood pressure in the United States population. *Hypertension.* 40:810–816.

150. Jacobs EJ, Henion AK, Briggs PJ *et al.* (2002). Vitamin C and vitamin E supplement use and bladder cancer mortality in a large cohort of US men and women. *Am J Epidemiol.* 156:1002–1010.

151. Martin A, Joseph JA, Cuervo AM. (2002). Stimulatory effect of vitamin C on autophagy in glial cells. *J Neurochem.* 82:538–549.

152. Martin A, Janigian D, Shikitt-Hale B *et al.* (1999). Effect of vitamin E intake on levels of vitamin E and C in the central nervous system and peripheral tissues: Implications for health recommendations. *Brain Res.* 845:50–59.

153. Sano M, Ernesto C, Thomas RG et al. (1997). A controlled trial of sele-giline, alpha-tocopherol, or both as treatment for Alzheimer's disease. The Alzheimer's Disease Cooperative Study [see comments]. *New England Journal of Medicine*. 336:1216–1222.

154. Meydani M. (2001). Nutrition interventions in aging and age-associated disease. *Ann N Y Acad Sci*. 928:226–235.

155. Morris M, Evans D, Bienias J et al. (2002). Dietary intake of antioxidant nutrients and the risk of incident Alzheimer disease in a biracial community study. *JAMA*. 287:3230–3237.

156. Engelhart M, Ruitenberg A, van Swieten J et al. (2002). Dietary intake of antioxidants and risk of Alzheimer disease. *JAMA*. 287:3223–3229.

157. Gaziano JM. (1994). Antioxidant vitamins and coronary artery disease risk. *Am J Med*. 97:18S–21S; discussion 22S–28S.

158. Manson JE, Gaziano JM, Spelsberg A et al. (1995). A secondary prevention trial of antioxidant vitamins and cardiovascular disease in women. Rationale, design, and methods. The WACS Research Group [see comments]. *Annals of Epidemiology*. 5:261–269.

159. Manson JE, Gaziano JM, Jonas MA, Hennekens CH. (1993). Antioxidants and cardiovascular disease: A review. *J Am Coll Nutr*. 12:426–432.

160. Emmert DH, Kirchner JT. (1999). The role of vitamin E in the prevention of heart disease. *Arch Fam Med*. 8:537–542.

161. Duthie GG, Bellizzi MC. (1999). Effects of antioxidants on vascular health. *Br Med Bull*. 55:568–577.

162. Stampfer MJ, Hennekens CH, Manson JE et al. (1993). Vitamin E consumption and the risk of coronary disease in women [see comments]. *N Engl J Med*. 328:1444–1449.

163. Ames BM, Shigena MK, Hagen TM. (1993). Oxidants, antioxidants and the degenerative diseases of aging. *Proc Natl Acad Sci USA*. 90:7915–7922.

164. Martin A, Foxall T, Blumberg JB, Meydani M. (1997). Vitamin E (α-T) decreases intracellular adhesion molecule (ICAM-1) expression and mono-cyte adhesion to human aortic endothelial cells. *Arterioscl Thromb Vasc Bio*. 17:429–436.

165. Skyrme-Jones RA, O'Brien RC, Berry KL, Meredith IT. (2000). Vitamin E supplementation improves endothelial function in type I diabetes mellitus: A randomized, placebo-controlled study. *J Am Coll Cardiol*. 36:94–102.

166. Majewska MD, Bell JA. (1990). Ascorbic acid protects neurons from injury induced by glutamate and NMDA. *Neuroreport*. 1:194–196.

167. Blasiak J, Kowalik J. (2001). Protective action of vitamin C against DNA damage induced by selenium-cisplatin conjugate. *Acta Biochim Pol*. 48:233–240.

168. Martin A, Frei B. (1997). Both intracellular and Extracellular vitamin C inhibit atherogenic modification of LDL by human vascular endothelial cells. *Arterioscler Thromb Vasc Biol*. 17:1583–1590.

169. Fennessy FM, Moneley DS, Wang JH et al. (2003). Taurine and vitamin C modify monocyte and endothelial dysfunction in young smokers. *Circulation*. 107:410–415.

170. Eaton SB, Konner M. (1985). Paleolithic nutrition. A consideration of its nature and current implications. *N Engl J Med*. 312:283–289.

171. Levine M, Dhariwal KR, Welch RW et al. (1995). Determination of optimal vitamin C requirements in humans. *Am J Clin Nutr*. 62:1347S–1356S.

172. Foy C, Passmore A, Vahidassr M, Young I, Lawson J. (1999). Plasma chain-braking antioxidants in Alzheimer's disease, vascular dementia and Parkinson's disease. *QJM*. 92:39–45.

173. Perrig WJ, Perrig P, Stahelin HB. (1997). The relation between antioxidants and memory performance in the old and very old. *J Am Geriatr Soc*. 45:718–724.

174. Paleologos M, Cumming RG, Lazarus R. (1998). Cohort study of vitamin C intake and cognitive impairment. *American Journal of Epidemiology*. 148:45–50.

175. Bonnefoy M, Drai J, Kostka T. (2002). Antioxidants to slow aging, facts and perspectives. *Presse Med*. 31:1174–1184.

175a. National Academy of Sciences, Institute of Medicine, Food and Nutrition Board. (2000). Dietary Reference Intakes for Vitamin C, Vitamin E, Selenium, and Carotenoides. Washington, DC: National Academies Press.

176. Gale CR, Martyn CN, Cooper C. (1996). Cognitive impairment and mortality in a cohort of elderly people. *BMJ*. 312:608–611.

177. d'Uscio LV, Milstien S, Richardson D et al. (2003). Long-term vitamin C treatment increases vascular tetrahydrobiopterin levels and nitric oxide synthase activity. *Circ Res*. 92:88–95.

178. Youdim KA, Joseph JA. (2001). A possible emerging role of phytochemicals in improving age-related neurological dysfunctions: A multiplicity of effects. *Free Radic Biol Med*. 30:583–594.

179. Youdim KA, Martin A, Joseph J. (2000). Essential fatty acids and the brain: Possible health implications. *Inter J Develop Neuroscience*. 18:383–399.

180. Cao G, Giovanoni M, Prior RL. (1996). Antioxidant capacity in different tissues of young and old rats. *Proc Soc Exp Biol Med*. 211:359–365.

181. Prior RL, Cao G. (1999). Antioxidant capacity and polyphenolic components of teas: Implications for altering *in vivo* antioxidant status. *Proc Soc Exp Biol Med*. 220:255–261.

182. Wang SY, Lin HS. (2000). Antioxidant activity in fruits and leaves of black-berry, raspberry, and strawberry varies with cultivar and developmental stage. *J Agric Food Chem*. 48:140–146.

183. Joseph J, Shukitt Hale B, Denisova N et al. (1999). Reversals of age-related declines in neuronal signal-transduction, cognitive, and motor behavioral deficits with blueberry, spinach, or strawberry dietary supplementation. *J Neuroscience*. 19:8114–8121.

184. Joseph JA, Denisova NA, Arendash G et al. (2003). Blueberry supplementa-tion enhances signaling and prevents behavioral deficits in Alzheimer's disease model. *Nutritional Neurosci*. 6:153–162.

185. Youdim KA, Shukitt-Hale B, MacKinnon S et al. (2000). Polyphenolics enhance red blood cell resistance to oxidative stress: *In vitro* and *in vivo*. *Biochim Biophys Acta*. 1523:117–122.

186. Casadesus G, Stellwagen H, Szprengiel A et al. (2002). Modulation of hippocampal neurogenesis and cognitive performance in the aged rat: The blueberry effect. *Soc Neurosci Abs*. 28:294.

187. Miquel J. (2001). Nutrition and ageing. *Public Health Nutr*. 4:1385–1388.

188. Kris-Etherton PM, Keen CL. (2002). Evidence that the antioxidant flavo-noids in tea and cocoa are beneficial for cardiovascular health. *Curr Opin Lipidol*. 13:41–49.

189. Kris-Etherton PM, Hecker KD, Bonanome A et al. (2002). Bioactive com-pounds in foods: Their role in the prevention of cardiovascular disease and cancer. *Am J Med*. 113(Suppl 9B):71S–88S.

190. Commenges D, Scotet V, Renaud S et al. (2000). Intake of flavonoids and risk of dementia. *Eur J Epidemiol*. 16:357–363.

191. Grant WB, Campbell A, Itzhaki RF, Savory J. (2002). The significance of environmental factors in the etiology of Alzheimer's disease. *J Alzheimers Dis*. 4:179–189.

192. Levites Y, Amit T, Youdim MB, Mandel S. (2002). Involvement of protein kinase C activation and cell survival/cell cycle genes in green tea polyphenol-epigallocatechin 3-gallate neuroprotective action. *J Biol Chem*. 277: 30574–30580.

193. Levites Y, Weinreb O, Maor G et al. (2001). Green tea polyphenol-epigal-locatechin-3-gallate prevents N-methyl-4-phenyl-1,2,3,6-tetrahydropyridine-induced dopaminergic neurodegeneration. *J Neurochem*. 78:1073–1082.

194. Levites Y, Youdim MB, Maor G, Mandel S. (2002). Attenuation of 6-hydroxydopamine (6-OHDA)-induced nuclear factor-kappaB (NF-kappaB) activation and cell death by tea extracts in neuronal cultures. *Biochem Pharmacol*. 63:21–29.

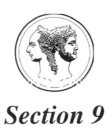

Section 9

DRUG METABOLISM

Janice B. Schwartz, MD

Institute on Aging and Jewish Home of San Francisco, University of California, San Francisco, CA

I. Introduction

Women make up more than half of the population of the world and of the United States; however, information regarding diseases of women and the treatment of common diseases in women fills far less than half the medical or scientific literature. We all recognize that men and women are different; however, we are only now acknowledging that our approach to the treatment of men and women may need to take gender into consideration. Most therapeutic interventions are pharmacologic, making appropriate drug selection and dosing regimens important. Despite the under-representation of women in clinical drug studies [1–3], there is mounting evidence that the physiologic differences between men and women can result in different responses to drugs in women compared with men.

Clinical pharmacology is often defined as the study of drugs in humans. In the following chapters, the clinical pharmacology of oral contraceptives and hormone replacement strategies in women and the approach to pharmacologic agents during pregnancy are reviewed as are the treatment of pain, depression and obesity, and the female patient requiring anticoagulation. In these chapters, leading experts in the area summarize the known information and highlight areas of uncertainly regarding gender differences. Finally, experience related to gender-specific information during the evaluation of new pharmacologic agents is presented by experts from the Center on Drug Evaluation of the Food and Drug Administration.

On reading these chapters, one cannot help but acknowledge the existence of gender differences in the prevalence of diseases, manifestations of diseases, and differences in responses to therapies for some but not all disorders. A common observation is also the relative paucity of data and the need for further investigations of gender differences and the underlying mechanisms. Although much remains to be learned, perhaps one area that has been studied more than most others relates to drug metabolism.

II. Pharmacokinetic Differences Between the Genders

Pharmacokinetics is a term that defines the processes of drug absorption, distribution, and clearance from the body. Extensive reviews of pharmacokinetic differences between the sexes have been published [2,4], but a few key points warrant presentation here (and are summarized in Table 1).

A. Size and Distribution Volumes

Size does matter. On average, men are heavier and have greater body water, intravascular volumes, and muscle mass compared with women. As a matter of scientific principle, many studies investigate drug clearance and report the results in amount of drug cleared per unit of measure. This tests whether pound for pound or gram for gram, the metabolic enzyme works at the same rate. This is scientifically sound, but perhaps not the best way to impart concepts that facilitate optimal dosing for patients because medications are not currently universally dosed based on size. A conclusion from an investigation that there are no differences in drug clearance between men and women – (when analyzed on an mg/kg basis) may not be translated into doses that differ by weight. In fact, many clinical guidelines mention optimal doses that are for a condition and do not consider either sex or weight. However, for

Table 1
Overview of Gender Differences in Pharmacokinetic Parameters

	Men > Women	Men = Women	Women > Men
Bioavailability			
Oral			X
Transdermal		X	
Bronchial	X		
Distribution volume*			
Water soluble, nonlipophilic	X		
Lipophilic			X
Protein binding			
Albumin		X	
Alpha-1-acidglycoprotein	X		
Renal drug clearance			
Glomerular filtration	X		
Tubular reabsorption	X		
Tubular secretion	X		
Hepatic Drug Clearance			
Phase I			
CYP1A, 2D6, 2E1	X		
CYP 2C9, 2C19		X	
CYP3A			X
Phase II (conjugation, glucuronidation, catechol-O-methyltransferase, thiopurine methyltransferase)	X		

*In general, total volumes are greater in men because of greater body size.

therapeutic drugs with known target concentrations or concentrations directly related to toxicity, the most important factor in adjusting medication dosages between men and women may be to incorporate an adjustment for body size [2,5]. The need for body size adjustment is most obvious for loading doses of medications in chemotherapeutic regimens or when administering initial or loading doses of drugs with a narrow therapeutic to toxic ratio (anticoagulants, aminoglycoside antibiotics, thrombolytics, antiarrhythmic drugs, sedative/hypnotics). The smaller size of women compared with men with the resultant lower distribution volume for alcohol is the major reason for greater initial concentrations and increased effects for a given amount of alcohol consumed [6]. Widespread applicability of this finding is demonstrated by materials developed to prevent drunk driving. Separate tables are provided for men compared with women that show that women reach legal driving limits for blood alcohol after fewer drinks per unit time compared with men.

Women are not only smaller than men but they also tend to have more body fat compared with men, with differences decreasing at older ages [7]. Higher body fat may increase distribution volumes for lipophilic drugs such as benzodiazepines leading to increased durations of sedation in women compared with men [8–12]. For most drugs, body fat usually produces only small effects on the pharmacokinetic profile.

B. Clearance Differences Between the Genders

There are also differences in drug pharmacokinetics that persist after weight differences are taken into account. The most consistent of these are gender differences in renal drug elimination by glomerular filtration.

1. Glomerular Filtration

Glomerular filtration is consistently, on average, higher in men than in women. Although directly proportional to body weight [13], there may also be a weight-independent sex difference in glomerular filtration rate (GFR) [14]. Glomerular filtration rate is often estimated by use of creatinine clearance rates because creatinine is eliminated by glomerular filtration. Because men produce more creatinine than women resulting from greater muscle mass, formulas to estimate creatinine clearance often include sex and weight [15] or sex and race [16,17]. The effects of sex on renal secretion and renal reabsorption are less clear.

2. Nonrenal Drug Clearance

The data on gender differences in hepatic (and intestinal) drug clearance are large and do not all reach the same conclusion. Most data converge on several points [2,5,18–20]. First, that phase II hepatic drug metabolism (conjugative: glucuronidation, sulfation, acetylation, methylation, glutathione conjugation) is generally faster in men compared with women, and second, that oxidative pathways (cytochrome P450 [CYP]) show variable differences between the sexes.

a. PHASE II HEPATIC METABOLISM. Phase II metabolism sex differences have clinical significance. A classic example relates to thiopurine methyltransferases (TPMTs). Greater bone marrow toxicity is seen in patients with low activity after chemotherapeutic agents metabolized by this pathway are administered [21,22]. Human liver biopsies have shown higher TPMT levels in men compared with women [23,24] and higher erythrocyte TPMT activity is seen in men compared with women [23]. Higher doses of 6-mercaptopurine are needed for equivalent therapeutic efficacy in boys compared with girls with leukemia [22,25,26]. 5-Fluorouracil clearance is dramatically lower in women than in men [27–29], and toxicity is higher in women compared with men even after dosages adjusted for body size [30,31]. Drugs such as temazepam and oxazepam that are metabolized solely by conjugation are, in general, cleared faster by men than by women [32,33]. A sex difference is also seen for the enzyme catechol-O-methyltransferase (COMT) that metabolizes the neurotransmitters norepinephrine, epinephrine and dopamine, and levo-dopamine. Concentrations of COMT are reported to be about 25% higher in men compared with women [34–37]. Oral contraceptives are another important influence on glucuronidation rates in women and have been reported to increase glucuronidation rates [38,39].

b. PHASE I HEPATIC METABOLISM. Phase I metabolism (oxidation, reduction, and hydrolysis) appears to demonstrate pathway specific gender differences. CYP3A is the human enzyme involved in the metabolism of the largest number of currently available medications. Faster clearance of a number of CYP3A substrates (alfentanil, cyclosporine, diazepam, erythromycin, methylprednisolone, midazolam, nifedipine, tirilazad, verapamil), has been reported in women compared with men [12,40–56]. Not all investigations detected sex differences with putative CYP3A substrates [9,57–61]. Nonetheless, the bulk of data suggest sex differences in CYP3A-mediated hepatic and intestinal clearance that is of mild to modest size and is influenced by concomitant medications and alternative routes of drug metabolism. Data on other CYP pathways follow.

For CYP1A, greater clearance is seen in men compared with women [62–65]. Hormone replacement therapy or oral contraceptive administration may eliminate sex differences in clearance of the CYP1A2 substrate paracetamol [38], but estrogen or oral contraceptive administration has more commonly been reported to impair clearance of CYP1A2 substrates such as caffeine [62] and ropinirole [66]. For CYP2D6, either no gender differences exist or higher clearance of substrates is seen in healthy men compared with healthy women matched for metabolizer phenotype [63,67–73]. Data from clinical populations receiving CYP2D6 substrates are limited; however, clomipramine and nortriptyline concentrations have been reported to be higher in women compared with men [74,75]. Potential sex differences of CYP2C19 have been less well studied, but the data suggest no sex difference in clearance of CYP2C19 substrates in the most prevalent phenotype (extensive metabolizer) [76,77]. Observed differences have been seen in some studies that have been attributed to the inhibitory effects of oral contraceptives or lack of correction of parameters for weight [76–79]. CYP2C9 appears not to display sex differences [80–83]. Sex differences have been found For CYP2E1 with higher clearance of chlorzoxazone (about 30%) in healthy men compared with healthy women [84–86].

c. MIXED HEPATIC METABOLISM. A number of drugs are metabolized by combined oxidative and conjugative processes or mixed hepatic processes. Methadone is one such drug. A steady-state methadone pharmacokinetic study in opiate addicts found longer methadone elimination times in women compared with men that could not be explained on the basis of body weight, comedications or other variables [87]. Clearance of labetalol (cleared by combined processes) is also reported to be higher in male hypertensive patients compared with female patients [88].

C. Absorption

Absorption of most orally administered drugs occurs in the intestine where metabolism and active transport back into the gut lumen can affect the amount of drug that reaches the circulation. Investigations using probes of drug metabolizing enzymes found in the intestine (CYP3A) suggest more drug appears in the body of women compared with men for some CYP3A substrates and greater increases in drug concentration are seen in women compared with men if this enzyme is inhibited [43,52,89]. Sex differences in the P-glycoprotein (Pgp) transporter that pumps drugs (that are also CYP3A substrates for the most part) back into the gut have been hypothesized based on reported differences in hepatic content [90]. However, investigations in humans using the Pgp substrate, fexofenadine, found no sex differences in plasma concentration time profiles [91]. The impact of sex differences in dietary content on drug absorption is not known.

Drugs are also administered by nonoral routes. Data are limited, but it appears that neither transdermal drug delivery or inhalation routes of delivery appear to be significantly affected by gender.

D. Sex-specific Influences on Pharmacokinetics (PK) in Women (Also See Chapter 79)

1. The Menstrual Cycle

Most data suggest little clinically relevant effect of the menstrual cycle on drug pharmacokinetics. This topic has also been recently reviewed [2,92].

2. Oral Contraceptives

Estrogens and progestins undergo intestinal absorption and metabolism, hepatic metabolism, and enterohepatic recycling. Hepatic metabolism is via oxidation by the CYP enzymes including CYP3A. Intestinal metabolism by CYP3A may also occur. Data suggest that oral contraceptives can increase or decrease concentrations of coadministered medications, and coadministered medications can reduce the efficacy of contraceptives leading to contraceptive failure. The inducers of hepatic metabolism that have been reported to reduce contraceptive efficacy or concentrations include the anticonvulsant drugs phenytoin, primidone, and carbamazepine and the anti-infectious agents rifampin, penicillin, ampicillin, tetracycline, and the cephalosporins. Oral contraceptives may decrease the effects or concentrations of the benzodiazepines lorazepam, temazepam, and oxazepam; clofibric acid; cyclosporin; phenytoin; rifampicin; and warfarin when added to their administration. Increased drug effect or concentrations of the antidepressants imipramine and amitriptyline, caffeine, the corticosteroids prednisone and prednisolone, selegiline, or theophylline may be seen with the addition of oral contraceptives to their administration.

3. Hormone Replacement Therapy

In studies to date, no effect of estrogen has been seen on clearance of coadministered CYP3A substrates, and neither estradiol nor estriol affect GFR or tubular reabsorption. Combined estrogen and progesterone hormone replacement is prescribed less frequently and has been less well investigated. Data from oral contraceptive interaction studies suggest that progesterone may be more likely to interact with concomitantly administered drugs that are metabolized by CYP3A than estrogen.

III. Conclusion

There is mounting evidence that clinically important differences between the sexes exist in the pharmacokinetic processes that determine drug concentrations and in the pharmacodynamic processes that determine physiologic responses to pharmacologic agents. This leads to the logical conclusion that sex should be considered during the selection of medications and dosages of medications. However, the information base to make such adjustments is woefully inadequate. Optimal care for women will require further investigation of medications for women and of therapies for disorders that are common in women. I hope that the following chapters contribute to an understanding of what we currently know about modifications of pharmacologic therapies for women and point us in the directions needed to obtain further information.

References

1. Schmucker D, Vesell E. (1993). Underrepresentation of women in clinical drug trials. *Clin Pharmacol Ther.* 54:11–15.
2. Wizeman T, Pardue M-L, eds. (2001). *Exploring the Biological Contributions to Human Health. Does Sex Matter?* Washington DC: Institute of Medicine, Report No.: ASBN 0–309–07281–6.
3. Harris D, Douglas P. (2000). Enrollment of women in cardiovascular clinical trials funded by the National Heart, Lung, and Blood Institute. *N Engl J Med.* 343:475–480.
4. Schwartz J. (2003). The influence of sex on pharmacokinetics. *Clin Pharmacokinet.* 42:4–10.
5. Beierle I, Meibohm B, Derendorf H. (1999). Gender differences in pharmacokinetics and pharmacodynamics. *Int J Clin Pharmacol Ther.* 37:529–547.
6. Wedel M, Pieters J, Pikaar N, Ockhuizen T. (1991). Application of a three-compartment model to a study of the effects of sex, alcohol dose and concentration, exercise and food consumption on the pharmacokinetics of ethanol in healthy volunteers. *Alcohol Alcohol.* 26:329–336.
7. Vahl N, Moller N, Lauritzen T *et al.* (1998). Metabolic effects and pharmacokinetics of a growth hormone pulse in healthy adults: Relation to age, sex, and body composition. *J Clin Endocrinol Metab.* 82:3612–3618.
8. Greenblatt D, Wright C. (1993). Clinical pharmacokinetics of alprazolam: Therapeutic implications. *Clin Pharmacokinet.* 24:453–471.
9. Kirkwood C, Moore A, Hayes P *et al.* (1991). Influence of menstrual cycle and gender on alprazolam pharmacokinetics. *Clin Pharmacol Ther.* 50:404–409.
10. Kristjansson F. (1991). Disposition of alprazolam in human volunteers. Differences between genders. *Acta Pharm Nord.* 3:249–250.
11. Ochs H, Greenblatt D, Divoll M *et al.* (1981). Diazepam kinetics in relation to age and sex. *Pharmacology.* 23:24–30.
12. Greenblatt D, Allen M, Harmatz J, Shader R. (1980). Diazepam disposition determinants. *Clin Pharmacol Ther.* 27:301–312.
13. Rowland M, Tozer T. (1995). *Clinical Pharmacokinetics: Concepts and Applications*, 3rd Edition. Philadelphia: Williams & Wilkins.
14. Gross J, Friedman R, Azevedo M *et al.* (1992). Effects of age and sex on glomerular filtration rate measured by 51 Cr-EDTA. *Braz J Med Biol Res.* 25:129–134.
15. Cockcroft DW, Gault MH. (1976). Prediction of creatinine clearance from serum creatinine. *Nephron.* 16:31–41.
16. Manjunath G, Sarnak M, Levey A. (2001). Prediction equations to estimate glomerular filtration rate: An update. *Curr Opin Nephrol Hypertens.* 10:785–792.
17. Levey A, Bosch J, Lewis J *et al.* (1999). A more accurate method to estimate glomerular filtration rate from serum creatinine: A new prediction equation. *Ann Intern Med.* 130:461–470.
18. Harris R, Benet L, Schwartz J. (1995). Gender effects in pharmacokinetics and pharmacodynamics. *Drugs.* 50:222–239.
19. Tanaka E. (1999). Gender-related differences in pharmacokinetics and their clinical significance. *J Clin Pharm Ther.* 24:339–346.
20. Fletcher C, Acosta E, Strykowski J. (1994). Gender differences in human pharmacokinetics and pharmacodynamics. *J Adolesc Health.* 15:619–629.
21. Lennard L, Van Loon J, Lilleyman J, Weinshilboum R. (1987). Thiopurine pharmacogenetics in leukemia: Correlation of erythrocyte thiopurine methyltransferase activity and 6-thioguanine nucleotide concentrations. *Clin Pharmacol Ther.* 41:18–25.
22. Lennard L, Lilleyman J, Van Loon J, Weinshilboum R. (1990). Genetic variation in response to 6-mercaptopurine for childhood acute lymphoblastic leukaemia. *Lancet.* 336:225–229.
23. Szumlanski C, Honchel R, Scott M, Weinshilboum R. (1992). Human liver thiopurine methyltransferase pharmacogenetics: Biochemical properties, liver-erythrocyte correlation and presence of isozymes. *Pharmacogenetics.* 2:148–159.
24. Klemetsdal B, Tollefsen E, Loennechen T *et al.* (1992). Interethnic differences in thiopurine methyltransferase activity. *Clin Pharmacol Ther.* 51:24–31.
25. Chessells J, Richards S, Bailey C *et al.* (1995). Gender and treatment outcome in childhood lymphoblastic leukaemia: Report from the MRC UKALL trials. *Br J Haematol.* 89:364–372.
26. Lennard L, Welch J, Lilleyman J. (1997). Thiopurine drugs in the treatment of childhood leukaemia: The influence of inherited thiopurine methyltransferase activity on drug metabolism and cytotoxicity. *Br J Clin Pharmacol.* 44:455–461.
27. Milano G, Cassuto-Viguier E, Thyss A *et al.* (1992). Influence of sex and age on fluorouracil clearance. *J Clin Oncol.* 10:1171–1175.
28. Port R, Daniel B, Ding R, Herrmann R. (1991). Relative importance of dose, body surface area, sex, and age for 5-fluorouracil clearance. *Oncology.* 48:277–281.
29. Zalcberg J, Kerr D, Seymour L, Palmer M. (1998). Haematological and non-haematological toxicity after 5-fluorouracil and leucovorin in patients with advanced colorectal cancer is significantly associated with gender, increasing age and cycle number. *Eur J Cancer.* 34:1871–1875.
30. Sloan J, Loprinzi C, Novotny P *et al.* (2000). Sex differences in fluorouracil-induced stomatitis. *J Clin Oncol.* 18:412–420.
31. Sloan J, Goldberg R, Sargent D *et al.* (2002). Women experience greater toxicity with 5-Fu based chemotherapy for colorectal cancer. *J Clin Oncol.* 20:1491–1498.
32. Divoll M, Greenblatt D, Harmatz J, Shader R. (1981). Effect of age and gender on disposition of temazepam. *J Pharm Sci.* 70:1104–1107.
33. Greenblatt D, Divoll M, Harmatz J, Shader R. (1980). Oxazepam kinetics: Effects of age and sex. *J Pharmacol Exp Ther.* 215:86–91.
34. Boudikova B, Szumlanski C, Maidak B, Weinshilboum R. (1990). Human liver catechol-O-methyltransferase pharmacogenetics. *Clin Pharmacol Ther.* 48:381–389.
35. Fahndrich E, Coper H, Christ W *et al.* (1980). Erythrocyte COMT activity in patients with affective disorders. *Acta Psychiatr.* 61:427–437.
36. Floderus Y, Ross S, Wetterberg L. (1981). Erythrocyte catechol-O-methyltransferase activity in a Swedish population. *Clin Genet.* 19:389–392.
37. Halbreich U, Vital-Herne J, Goldstein S, Zander K. (1984). Sex differences in biological factors putatively related to depression. *J Affect Disord.* 7:223–233.
38. Miners J, Attwood J, Birkett D. (1983). Influence of sex and oral contraceptive steroids on paracetamol metabolism. *Br J Clin Pharmacol.* 16:503–509.
39. Macdonald J, Herman R, Verbeeck R. (1990). Sex-difference and the effects of smoking and oral contraceptive steroids on the kinetics of diflunisal. *Eur J Clin Pharmacol.* 38:175–179.
40. Watkins PB, Murray SA, Winkelman LG *et al.* (1989). Erythromycin breath test as an assay of glucocorticoid-inducible liver cytochromes P-450. *J Clin Invest.* 83:688–697.
41. Thummel KE, O'Shea D, Paine MF *et al.* (1996). Oral first-pass elimination of midazolam involves both gastrointestinal and hepatic CYP3A-mediated metabolism. *Clin Pharmacol Ther.* 59:491–502.
42. Hunt C, Westerkam W, Stave G. (1992). Effect of age and gender on the activity of human hepatic CYP3A. *Biochem Pharmacol.* 44:275–283.
43. Greenblatt D, Abernethy D, Locniskar A *et al.* (1984). Effect of age, gender, and obesity on midazolam kinetics. *Anesthesiology.* 61:27–35.

44. Lew K, Ludwig E, Milad M et al. (1993). Gender-based effects on methyl-prednisolone pharmacokinetics and pharmacodynamics. Clin Pharmacol Ther. 54:402–414.

45. Krecic-Shepard M, Barnas C, Slimko J et al. (2000). Gender-specific effects on verapamil pharmacokinetics and pharmacodynamics in humans. J Clin Pharmacol. 40:219–230.

46. Krecic-Shepard M, Park K, Barnas C et al. (2000). Race and sex influence clearance of nifedipine: Results of a population study. Clin Pharmacol Ther. 68:130–142.

47. Krecic-Shepard M, Barnas C, Slimko J et al. (1999). In vivo comparison of putative probes of CYP3A4/5 activity: Erythromycin, dextromethorphan, and verapamil. Clin Pharmacol Ther. 66:40–50.

48. Schwartz J, Capili H, Daugherty J. (1994). Aging of women alters S-verapamil pharmacokinetics and pharmacodynamics. Clin Pharmacol Ther. 55:509–517.

49. Hunt C, Strater S, Stave G. (1990). Effect of normal aging on the activity of human hepatic cytochrome P450IIE1. Biochem Pharmacol. 40:1666–1669.

50. Krivoruk Y, Kinirons M, Wood A, Wood M. (1994). Metabolism of cytochrome P4503A substrates in vivo administered by the same route: Lack of correlation between alfentanil clearance and erythromycin breath test. Clin Pharmacol Ther. 56:608–614.

51. Hulst L, Fleishaker J, Peters G et al. (1994). Effect of age and gender on tirilazad pharmacokinetics in humans. Clin Pharmacol Ther. 55:378–384.

52. Gorski J, Jones D, Haehner-Daniels B et al. (1998). The contribution of intestinal and hepatic CYP3A to the interaction between midazolam and clarithromycin. Clin Pharmacol Ther. 64:133–143.

53. Kahan B, Kramer W, Wideman C et al. (1986). Demographic factors affecting the pharmacokinetics of cyclosporine estimated by radioimmunoassay. Transplantation. 41:459–464.

54. Kinirons M, O'Shea D, Kim R et al. (1999). Failure of erythromycin breath test to correlate with midazolam clearance as a probe of cytochrome P4503A. Clin Pharmacol Ther. 66:224–231.

55. Fleishaker JC, Pearson PG, Wienkers LC et al. (1996). Biotransformation of tirilazad in human: 2. Effect of ketoconazole on tirilazad clearance and oral bioavailability. J Pharmacol Exp Ther. 277:991–998.

56. Fleishaker J, Fiedler-Kelly J, Grasela T. (1999). Population pharmacokinetics of tirilazad: Effects of weight, gender, concomitant phenytoin, and subarachnoid hemorrhage. Pharm Res. 16:575–583.

57. Yee G, Kennedy M, Storb R, Thomas E. (1984). Effect of hepatic dysfunction on oral cyclosporine pharmacokinetics in marrow transplant patients. Blood. 64:1277–1279.

58. Holazo A, Winkler M, Patel I. (1988). Effects of age, gender and oral contraceptives on intramuscular midazolam pharmacokinetics. J Clin Pharmacol. 28:1040–1045.

59. Gupta S, Atkinson L, Tu T, Longstreth J. (1995). Age and gender related changes in stereoselective pharmacokinetics and pharmacodynamics of verapamil and norverapamil. Br J Clin Pharmacol. 40:325–331.

60. Fleishaker J, Peters G. (1996). Pharmacokinetics of tirilazad and U-89678 in ischemic stroke patients receiving a loading regimen and maintenance regimen of 10 mg/kg/day of tirilazad. J Clin Pharmacol. 36:809–813.

61. Fleishaker J, Pearson L, Pearson P et al. (1999). Hormonal effects on tirilazad clearance in women: Assessment of the role of CYP3A. J Clin Pharmacol. 39:260–267.

62. Kalow W, Tang B. (1991). Use of caffeine metabolite ratios to explore CYP1A2 and xanthine oxidase ratios. Clin Pharmacol Ther. 50:508–519.

63. Bock K, Schrenk D, Forster A et al. (1994). The influence of environmental and genetic factors on CYP2D6, CYP1A2 and UDP-glucuronosyltransferases in man using sparteine, caffeine, and paracetamol as probes. Pharmacogenetics. 4(4):209–218.

64. Relling M, Lin J, Ayers G, Evans W. (1992). Racial and gender differences in N-acetyltransferase, xanthine oxidase, and CYP1A2 activities. Clin Pharmacol Ther. 52:643–658.

65. Ou-Yang D-S, Huang S-L, Wang W et al. (2000). Phenotypic polymorphism and gender-related differences of CYP1A2 activity in a Chinese population. Br J Clin Pharmacol. 49:141–151.

66. Kaye C, Nicholls B. (2000). Clinical pharmacokinetics of ropinirole. Clin Pharmacokinet. 39:243–254.

67. May DG, Porter J, Wilkinson G, Branch R. (1994). Frequency distribution of dapsone N-hydroxylase, a putative probe for P4503A4 activity, in a white population. Clin Pharmacol Ther. 55:492–500.

68. Pollock B, Altieri L, Kirshner M et al. (1992). Debrisoquine hydroxylation phenotyping in geriatric psychopharmacology. Psychopharmacol Bull. 28:163–168.

69. Labbe L, Sirois C, Pilote S et al. (2000). Effect of gender, sex hormones, time variables, and physiological urinary pH on apparent CYP2D6 activity as assessed by metabolic ratios of marker substrates. Pharmacogenetics. 10:425–438.

70. Timmer C, Sitsen J, Delbressine L. (2000). Clinical pharmacokinetics of mirtazapine. Clin Pharmacokinet. 38:461–474.

71. Gilmore D, Gal J, Gerber J, Nies A. (1992). Age and gender influence the stereoselective pharmacokinetics of propranolol. J Pharmacol Exp Ther. 261:1181–1186.

72. Walle T, Byington R, Furberg C et al. (1985). Biologic determinants of propranolol disposition. Results from 1308 patients in the beta-blocker heart attack trial. Clin Pharmacol Ther. 38:509–518.

73. Hong-Guang X, Xiu C. (1995). Sex differences in pharmacokinetics of oral propranolol in healthy Chinese volunteers. Acta Pharmacologica Sinica. 16:468–470.

74. Gex-Fabry M, Balant-Gorgia A, Balant L et al. (1990). Clomipramine metabolism: Model-based analysis of variability factors from drug monitoring data. Clin Pharmacokinet. 19:241–255.

75. Dahl M, Bertilsson L, Nordin C. (1996). Steady-state plasma levels of nortriptyline and its 10-hydroxy metabolite: Relationship to the CYP2D6 genotype. Psychopharmacology. 123:315–319.

76. Tamminga A, Wemer J, Oosterhuis B et al. (1999). CYP2D6 and CYP2C19 activity in a large population of Dutch healthy volunteers: Indications for oral contraceptive-related gender differences. Eur J Clin Pharmacol. 55:177–184.

77. Hooper WD, Qing M-S. (1990). The influence of age and gender on the stereoselective metabolism and pharmacokinetics of mephobarbital in humans. Clin Pharmacol Ther. 48:633–640.

78. Laine K, Tybring G, Bertilsson L. (2000). No sex-related differences but significant inhibition by oral contraceptives of CYP2C19 activity as measured by the probe drugs mephenytoin and omeprazole in healthy Swedish white subjects. Clin Pharmacol Ther. 68:151–159.

79. Karin Z, Noveck R, McMahon F et al. (1997). Oxaprozin and piroxicam, nonsteroidal antiinflammatory drugs with long half-lives: Effect of protein-binding differences on steady-state pharmacokinetics. J Clin Pharmacol. 37:267–278.

80. Jokubaitis L. (1996). Development and pharmacology of fluvastatin. Br J Clin Pract Suppl. 77A:11–15.

81. Scripture C, Pieper J. (2001). Clinical pharmacokinetics of fluvastatin. Clin Pharmacokinet. 40:263–281.

82. Vachharajani N, Shyu W, Smith R, Greene D. (1998). The effects of age and gender on the pharmacokinetics of irbesartan. Br J Clin Pharmacol. 46:611–613.

83. Houghton G, Richens A, Leighton M. (1975). Effect of age, height, weight and sex on serum phenytoin concentration in epileptic patients. Br J Clin Pharmacol. 2(3):251–256.

84. Lucas D, Menez C, Girre C et al. (1995). Cytochrome P450 2E1 genotype and chlorzoxazone metabolism in healthy and alcoholic Caucasian subjects. Pharmacogenetics. 5:298–304.

85. Kim R, O'Shea D, Wilkinson G. (1995). Interindividual variability of chlorzoxazone 6-hydroxylation in men and women and its relationship to CYP2E1 genetic polymorphisms. Clin Pharmacol Ther. 57:645–655.

86. O-Shea D, Davis S, Kim R, Wilkinson G. (1994). Effect of fasting and obesity in humans on the 6-hydroxylation of chlorzoxazone: A putative probe of CYP2E1 activity. Clin Pharmacol Ther. 56:359–367.

87. de Vos JW, Geerlings P, van den Brink W et al. (1995). Pharmacokinetics of methadone and its primary metabolite in 20 opiate addicts. Eur J Clin Pharmacol. 48:361–366.

88. Johnson J, Akers W, Herring V et al. (2000). Gender differences in labetalol kinetics: Importance of determining stereoisomer kinetics for racemic drugs. Pharmacotherapy. 20:622–628.

89. Kates R, Keefe D, Schwartz J et al. (1981). Verapamil disposition kinetics in chronic atrial fibrillation. Clin Pharmacol Ther. 30:44–51.

90. Schuetz E, Furuya K, Schuetz J. (1995). Interindividual variation in expression of P-glycoprotein in normal human liver and secondary hepatic neoplasms. J Pharmacol Exp Ther. 275:1011–1018.

91. Kim R, Leake B, Choo E et al. (2001). Identification of functionally variant MDR1 alleles among European Americans and African Americans. Clin Pharmacol Ther. 70:189–199.

92. Kashuba A, Nafziger A. (1998). Physiological changes during the menstrual cycle and their effects on the pharmacokinetics and pharmacodynamics of drugs. Clin Pharmacokinet. 34:203–218.

75

Anticoagulants/Antithrombotic Therapy

STEVEN R. KAYSER, PHARMD

Professor of Clinical Pharmacy, Department of Clinical Pharmacy, School of Pharmacy,
University of California, San Francisco, CA

Abstract

The development of newer and more effective antithrombotic strategies has lead to the routine use of combination approaches to the treatment of both venous and arterial thromboembolic disease. Because of the increased potential and risk for adverse events, efforts have increased to tailor therapy for individual groups of patients and for individual patients. There is general consensus that women do benefit from antithrombotic therapy but that some differences in response do exist, both from a therapeutic and an adverse reaction perspective. Pharmacologic agents available to influence coagulation include antiplatelet inhibitors, thrombolytics, and indirect and direct inhibitors of thrombin.

I. Introduction

The application of antithrombotic therapy in the management of cardiovascular and cerebrovascular disease has increased dramatically in the last 30 years. The development of newer and more effective strategies has lead to the routine use of combination antithrombotic approaches in an effort to further improve clinical outcomes. Because of the increased potential and risk for adverse events, efforts have increased to tailor therapy for individual groups of patients and for individual patients. It is well recognized that women have been under-represented in most of the large-scale clinical trials involving antithrombotic agents. Despite this, there is general consensus that women do benefit from antithrombotic therapy but that some differences in response do exist, both from a therapeutic and an adverse reaction perspective. A recognition of these differences and of the factors influencing dosing is important in ensuring their rational application.

Sex-related characteristics, other than differences in body size and weight, in the ability to metabolize drugs has increasingly been postulated as a potential explanation for observations from some clinical trials. Some differences do exist in drug disposition among men and women. Women for example appear to have lower activity for the drug transporter, P-glycoprotein, but to have the same activity for certain drug metabolizing enzymes, CYP2C19 and CYP3A. For certain drugs, gender-specific differences in pharmacologic effect have been observed; however, the clinical significance of these differences has been debated because in many cases what determines the dose is usually a therapeutic outcome or surrogate endpoint (e.g., blood pressure, heart rate, or the influence on a laboratory test) [1]. No gender-related differences in antithrombotic drug metabolism have been confirmed for the currently available antithrombotic drugs. Despite the lack of difference in overall metabolism, lighter body weight and older age at time of presentation for therapy may predispose women to increased sensitivity to antithrombotic drugs.

II. Monitoring of Antithrombotic Therapy (See Table 75-1)

It is important to confirm the integrity of the coagulation system before initiating antithrombotic therapy. Baseline tests should include a platelet count, prothrombin time/international normalized ratio (PT/INR), and an activated partial thromboplastin time (APTT). The PT is particularly sensitive to factor VII and evaluates the extrinsic and common clotting pathway. The APTT is particularly sensitive to factor II but also is prolonged in the presence of abnormalities of factor IX and X. It evaluates the integrity of the intrinsic and common clotting pathway. In addition to measures of coagulation, a baseline complete blood count (CBC), urinalysis (UA), and fecal test for occult blood should be obtained to provide a basis for evaluating the presence or significance of any suspected bleeding.

A. Antiplatelet Therapy

No reliable laboratory test is yet available to monitor the therapeutic effect of antiplatelet agents. Thromboelastography represents the most promising way to evaluate the influence of the platelet GPIIbIIIa receptor antagonists; however, it has not become accepted as a standard in the clinical management of these agents [2]. Aspirin and the thienopyridines may influence the bleeding time, but this is not a useful test to evaluate their efficacy [2].

B. Thrombolytics

Thrombolytic therapy significantly influences global tests of coagulation, and although the thrombin time and APTT have been used historically to evaluate their influence on clotting, these have not proven to be useful tools for dosage adjustment. Most if not all doses are either standardized or weight based and are not adjusted on the basis of alterations in clotting tests. It is particularly important to pay attention to dosing in women because lighter body weight and older age are predictors of bleeding following thrombolytic therapy [2a].

C. Heparin and Low-Molecular-Weight Heparins

Standard unfractionated heparin (UFH) is monitored by the APTT or the activated clotting time (ACT). The APTT is the

Table 75-1
Monitoring of Antithrombotic Drug Therapy

Medication	Laboratory Monitoring	Therapeutic Goal
Antiplatelet agents: aspirin, thienopyridine antagonists (clopidogrel), glycoprotein IIb/IIIa platelet antagonists (abciximab, eptifibatide, tirofiban)	Laboratory monitoring is not required for dosage determination. Currently there is no routine test available to monitor their effectiveness. Thromboelastography may prove to be useful in the future	Not applicable
Unfractionated heparin (UFH)	Activated partial thromboplastin time (APTT) Note: High doses of heparin may interfere with prothrombin time (PT) measurements and result in prolonged PTs and international normalized ratios (INRs)	Institution-specific heparin dosing algorithms should be established with therapeutic ranges corresponding to heparin levels of 0.2–0.4 U/mL by protamine titration or 0.3–0.7 U/mL by antifactor Xa assay
Low-molecular-weight heparins: dalteparin (Fragmin), enoxaparin (Lovenox)	Anti-Xa levels	Levels for prophylaxis=0.3–0.5 U/mL Levels for therapy=0.5–1.0 U/mL
Warfarin	PT and INR $INR=(patient\ PT/\ PT\ control)^{ISI}$ ISI=international sensitivity index	Therapeutic INRs are within the range of 2.0–3.5. For most clinical indications an INR of 2.0–3.0 is adequate. An INR of 2.5–3.5 is indicated for patients with mechanical valve replacements in the mitral position, for patients with mechanical valves and additional risk factors, and for patients with recurrent thromboembolism (see also ref. 4)
Direct thrombin inhibitors: argatroban, bivalirudin, lepirudin	Activated clotting time (ACT), APTT, PT may be influenced by therapy with these agents. The ecarin clotting time (ECT) may prove to be a useful monitoring test in the future (see text for discussion). See also Table 75-4	
Thrombolytic agents: alteplase (tPA), reteplase, tenecteplase (TNK-tPA)	May influence all tests of coagulation	Not useful in determining dose. See text for discussion

Baseline laboratory tests should be obtained before initiation of any antithrombotic therapy (see text for discussion).

most commonly used test for monitoring and standards for its interpretation and targets for therapeutic ranges have been established [3]. The ACT is a whole blood test and is used commonly in the catheterization laboratory and surgical amphitheater for the management of heparin and direct thrombin inhibitors (DTIs) in patients undergoing percutaneous coronary interventions (PCIs) or extracorporeal bypass. Low-molecular-weight heparins (LMWHs) have certain advantages over UFH (see section IVA), one of which is the lack of need for routine laboratory monitoring in the absence of creatinine clearances less than 30 mL/min or morbid obesity or very small size where dosing can be difficult. Low-molecular-weight heparins are cleared by the kidneys, and accumulation may occur with standard doses. In this case, monitoring with an anti-factor Xa level may be useful. Similarly, patients who are obese (>40% ideal body weight [IBW]) may have an altered volume of distribution for these drugs, and anti-factor Xa monitoring may be useful to ensure that not only a therapeutic effect is achieved but that adverse effects are prevented.

D. Warfarin

The PT responds to a reduction in concentration of three of the four vitamin K dependent clotting factors (VII, X, and II) and has historically been the preferred test to evaluate the response to coumarin anticoagulants of which warfarin (Coumadin) is

the most widely prescribed one in the United States. The PT relies on a reference thromboplastin standard for its performance, and, because this may differ among commercial sources and laboratories, the INR was developed to overcome the differences that may exist from laboratory to laboratory. The INR is the ratio of the patients PT to the laboratory standard PT, raised to the power of the sensitivity of the thromboplastin reagent (international sensitivity index [ISI]) [4]. Target INRs for numerous therapeutic indications have been established and are the same for both men and women [4].

E. Direct Thrombin Inhibitors

The newest class of antithrombotic agents are the DTIs, argatroban (Argatroban), bivalirudin (Angiomax), and lepirudin (Refludan). These agents are used primarily in the management of heparin-induced thrombocytopenia (HIT), although they are finding increased utility in the management of acute coronary syndromes (ACSs) and in patients undergoing PCI. They can be managed with the APTT, ACT, or the ecarin clotting time (ECT). The ECT has not yet become widely available but shows promise in specifically monitoring these new agents [5]. This test is performed by adding ecarin, a purified snake venom that acts to generate thrombin in the patient's plasma sample. In the presence of a DTI most of the generated thrombin is neutralized; however, the excess free thrombin will proceed to stimulate the conversion of fibrinogen to fibrin. The prolongation of the ECT thus reflects the concentration of the drug (i.e., the greater the drug concentration, the less free thrombin and subsequently the less fibrin generation and subsequently a greater prolongation of the ECT) [5].

III. Pharmacologic Agents Influencing Platelet Activity

A. General Efficacy

Early approaches to the management of thrombosis with antiplatelet agents were limited by the availability of aspirin alone. In the management of stable angina, aspirin has been shown to result in a decrease in risk of approximately 33% in both men and women [6]. The efficacy of aspirin in ACSs has similarly been established [7]. With the advent of newer antiplatelet agents (e.g., the thienopyridine derivatives ticlopidine [Ticlid] and clopidogrel [Plavix]) and the inhibitors of platelet glycoprotein IIbIIIa receptors (abciximab [Reopro], eptifibatide [Integrilin], and tirofiban [Aggrastat]), similar questions of differences in efficacy have arisen. Initial reports from trials with the platelet glycoprotein inhibitors suggested a treatment benefit only in men. The Enhanced Suppression of the Platelet IIb/IIIa Receptor with Integrilin Therapy (ESPRIT) trial initially reported a lack of treatment benefit in women [7]. Meta-analyses have subsequently confirmed the efficacy of these agents in women not routinely scheduled for early revascularization when they were risk stratified for the presence of elevated serum troponins [7]. Women undergoing PCI have also been shown to favorably benefit from abciximab [9], eptifibatide, and tirofiban [9–11].

The thienopyridine derivative clopidogrel inhibits platelet activity primarily by inhibiting adenosine diphosphate (ADP), resulting in a decrease in platelet glycoprotein IIbIIIa activity indirectly. Ticlopidine has previously been used but it was associated with several adverse effects, neutropenia and thrombotic thrombocytopenic purpura (TTP), that have not been observed as frequently with clopidogrel. As a result, clopidogrel has become more widely used for the management of non-ST segment elevation myocardial infarction (MI) and in patients following PCI. Its efficacy has been established as a result of the Clopidogrel vs Aspirin in Patients at Risk of Ischemic Events (CAPRIE) and the Clopidogrel in Unstable Angina to Prevent Recurrent Ischemic Events (CURE) trials [12–14].

B. Dosing

To maximally inhibit platelet activity and to provide long-term protection for recurrence of symptoms, antiplatelet drugs are usually prescribed in combination not only with each other but with other antithrombotic agents. Heparin, either UFH or LMWHs, are usually also administered, and the efficacy of platelet inhibitors is increased in their presence. For patients presenting with ACS, immediate aspirin is mandatory in the absence of an aspirin allergy. For high-risk patients with ACSs, intravenous inhibitors of glycoprotein IIb/IIIa receptors (either tirofiban or eptifibatide) are indicated and should be administered concomitantly with aspirin and heparin. If the patient is to undergo PCI, either abciximab, eptifibatide, or tirofiban may

be considered, although this decision is often delayed until the patient is in the catheterization laboratory. Clopidogrel 300 mg orally is administered before the procedure, although caution is advised if there is a chance that the patient may require emergent coronary artery bypass grafting (CABG) because of the risk of perioperative and postoperative bleeding. The similar risk exists for the use of the intravenous inhibitors of glycoprotein IIb/IIIa. There are differences in the characteristics of the platelet glycoprotein inhibitors (Table 75-2), which should also be considered when dosing. Based on experience from CAPRIE and CURE, there does not appear to be a need to adjust the initial or maintenance dose of clopidogrel or to expect a difference in response for women as compared with men. Clopidogrel is usually administered for ACS at an initial loading dose of 300 mg followed by 75 mg daily for up to a year following non-ST elevation MI (NSTEMI) or PCI. For the treatment of peripheral arterial disease, dosing is initiated with a maintenance dose of 75 mg daily.

C. Risks and Adverse Effects

Hemorrhagic complications are the most frequently seen risks of antiplatelet therapy. Women appear to be at increased overall risk for bleeding; however, when adjusted for weight, age, and hypertension, the difference between men and women became nonsignificant in at least one report with the use of eptifibatide [8]. Bleeding does appear to be higher in patients undergoing PCI whether they receive abciximab or other platelet glycoprotein inhibitors or not. Thrombocytopenia has been reported with all of the agents used to inhibit platelet function, although the incidence is highest with the glycoprotein IIb/IIIa receptor antagonist abciximab. Clopidogrel was not initially thought to be associated with the same complications as ticlopidine; however, recent reports have demonstrated a real but lesser incidence of TTP and neutropenia. Abciximab has been associated with an immune mediated thrombocytopenia that may occur on subsequent readministration, although there have been successful cases of readministration without adverse effect. Because of the long duration of the platelet inhibition seen with abciximab (3 to 5 days), thrombocytopenia may be particularly troublesome. Thrombocytopenia secondary to eptifibatide and tirofiban occurs rarely. The shorter half-lives of these agents, approximately 2 to 2.5 hours, allows for more rapid recovery of normal platelet counts and function (see Table 75-2).

IV. Thrombolytic Agents

A. General Efficacy

The availability of thrombolytic agents to rapidly recanalize occluded coronary arteries provides a mechanism to preserve myocardium in jeopardy of infarction and to reduce mortality in women and men. For various reasons well described in the literature, women receive therapy with thrombolytic agents and with other therapies and interventions less often than men [15]. The results of numerous clinical trials have demonstrated the ability to achieve similar infarct related artery patency regardless of sex; however, the mortality benefit is less in women [16–18]. The clinical response to thrombolytics may be influenced in

Table 75-2
Platelet GP IIb/IIIa Receptor Antagonists

	Tirofiban (Aggrastat)	Eptifibatide (Integrilin)	Abciximab (Reopro)
Source	Nonpeptide	Peptide	Monoclonal antibody
Specificity for GP IIb/IIIa receptor without interference with other receptors	Yes	Yes	No
Antigenicity	No	No	Yes
Reversibility–return of normal platelet function	Fast	Fast	Slow
Half-life	~2 hr	~2.5 hr	~0.5 hr
Route of elimination	Renal, requires dose reduction with reduced renal function, decrease dose by 50% with CrCl <30 mL/min	Renal, requires dose reduction with serum Scr >2 mg/dL, avoid if Scr >4 mg/dL	Unknown, no dosage reduction required with increased Scr
Dose for acute coronary syndrome (ACS)*	0.4 µg/kg/min for 30 minutes, then 0.1 µg/kg/min for 48–108 hours	180 µg/kg bolus, then 2 µg/kg/min for up to 72 hours Max dosing weight 120 kg	0.25 mg/kg bolus, then 0.125 µg/kg/min (up to 10 µg/min) for 18–24 hours
Dose for percutaneous coronary intervention (PCI) without ACS	10 µg/kg over 3 minutes, then 0.15 µg/kg/min for 18–24 hours (RESTORE dose) *Not currently FDA approved	180 µg/kg bolus × 2, 10 minutes apart, 2 µg/kg/min × 18 hours ESPRIT	0.25 mg/kg bolus 10–60 min before procedure, then 0.125 µg/kg/min (max 10 µg/min) for 12 hours after
Adverse effects	Hemorrhage, thrombocytopenia	Hemorrhage, thrombocytopenia	Hemorrhage, immune-mediated thrombocytopenia

(From Lincoff AM, Califf RM, Topol EJ. (2000). Platelet glycoprotein IIb/IIIa receptor blockade in coronary artery disease. *J Am Coll Cardiol*. 35:1103–1115; and Kleiman NS. (1999). Pharmacokinetics and pharmacodynamics of glycoprotein IIb-IIIa inhibitors. *Am Heart J*. 138:S263–S275. CrCl, creatinine clearance; Scr, serum creatinine.)

Table 75-3
Thrombolytic Agents

Characteristic	Alteplase (Activase)	Reteplase (Retevase)	Tenecteplase (TNKase)
Antigenicity	No	No	No
Plasminogen activation	Direct	Direct	Direct
Fibrin specificity	++	+	+++
Plasma half-life	4–6 min	18 min	20 min
Dose	For patients >67 kg, 15 mg bolus followed by 50 mg over 30 minutes, then 35 mg over 60 minutes, not to exceed total dose of 100 mg. For patients <67 kg, 15 mg bolus, followed by 0.75 mg/kg over the next 30 minutes, not to exceed 50 mg and then 0.5 mg/kg over the next 60 minutes not to exceed 35 mg	10 unit bolus followed by a second 10 unit bolus intravenous (IV) 30 minutes later	0.5 mg/kg to a maximum total dose of 50 mg by bolus injection
Metabolism	Hepatic	Renal	Hepatic

women who are postmenopausal or on estrogen replacement therapy. Evidence suggests that the activity of plasminogen activator inhibitor [PAI-(1)] is increased in women following menopause and decreased in women taking estrogens [19]. Despite their efficacy, thrombolytic agents are associated with an increased incidence of adverse events (see later discussion) in women, especially older women, and this coupled with other issues have in some cases limited their application. Thrombolytic agents although used less frequently in the treatment of pulmonary embolism in general have shown similar benefits in women and men with a similar risk for hemorrhage in this population [20].

B. Dosing

Some currently available thrombolytic agents are adjusted for weight (Table 75-3); however, none are specifically adjusted for gender.

C. Adverse Effects and Risks

Intracranial hemorrhage occurs with increased frequency in women [21]. The exact mechanism for this observation is unknown, but it does increase in frequency particularly in association with advanced age. In at least one study there was a decrease in the incidence of intracranial hemorrhage with the use of weight-adjusted dosing of tenecteplase compared with alteplase [22,23]. Cardiac rupture has been reported to account for up to 10 to 15% of in-hospital deaths following MI [24]. Review of data from TIMI 9A and 9B of patients receiving thrombolytic therapy (weight-adjusted rtPA or 1.5 MU streptokinase), aspirin, and either heparin or hirudin demonstrated that female gender was associated with an odds ratio of 2.87, (95% confidence interval [CI] 2.53 to 5.35) for death. The association of cardiac rupture was independent of the type or intensity of thrombin inhibition with heparin or hirudin. Other factors observed by multivariate analysis to be predictive included age older than 70 years and prior angina. Beta-blocker and angiotensin converting enzyme inhibitor therapy were negatively associated with the occurrence of rupture, although the nonrandom distribution of their use limits interpretation of this observation. Female gender and the risk for cardiac rupture has also been observed in the Gruppo Italiano per lo Studio della Sterptochinasi nell'Infarcto Miocardico-2 (GISSI-2) trial [25,26]. The exact mechanism for the increase in cardiac rupture is unknown, but it has been proposed to be linked to the increase in plasmin generation and its possible adverse influence on promoting collagen degradation. Although most women presenting with MI are postmenopausal, there are occasional circumstances when thrombolytic therapy may be indicated in a woman who is menstruating. It is more likely that the indication will be acute stroke. Limited information is available that suggests, despite the usual contraindication to their use during menstruation, that they may be used with relative safety [27].

V. Heparin

A. General Efficacy and Use

The efficacy of heparin in the management of venous and arterial thrombotic disorders is well established for both men and women. Heparins act by binding to antithrombin III (ATIII). This induces a conformational change in the ATIII-heparin complex and facilitates the inactivation of primarily factors Xa and IIa with lesser influence on factor IXa. The half-life of UFH is usually 60 to 90 minutes, although it increases with increased dose. It is eliminated by the reticuloendothelial system and is not influenced by renal function. The inactivation of factor IIa (thrombin) results in prolongation of the APTT, which is the usual clinical marker of anticoagulation used to monitor the effect of UFH. Because of its larger size and higher molecular weight, UFH is more likely to be bound to endothelial cells and macrophages, which limits its systemic availability. This leads to changes in dose response based on the clinical situation. For example, patients with venous thromboembolic disease generally have a higher dose requirement than do patients with coronary artery disease [28] presumably because of a larger clot burden observed with venous disease. Low-molecular-weight heparins lack the ability to bind to factor IIa (thrombin) and subsequently

do not result in significant prolongation of the APTT. Because of their selective binding to factor Xa, monitoring of LMWHs is accomplished by measuring anti-Xa levels. Low-molecular-weight heparins have a number of potential advantages over UFH including more predictable dose response because of their smaller size and subsequently less binding to endothelial cells and macrophages, linear pharmacokinetics, higher bioavailability, lack of need for routine monitoring, lack of significant influence on the APTT and INR, rapid onset of action and longer half-life (~4 hours) that allows twice daily (q 12 h or even q24 h) dosing, reduced inhibitory effects on platelet aggregation or binding of fibrinogen to platelets, and possibly a tendency for fewer bleeding complications. Low-molecular-weight heparins are eliminated primarily by the kidneys. They may accumulate in patients with a creatinine clearance less than 30 mL/min, and it is in these patients that anti-Xa monitoring may be useful. This may be especially pertinent to the care of women older than the age of 70 for whom creatinine clearance estimates should be calculated to avoid missing the presence of significant asymptomatic decreased renal function that can be present in a small, older woman with a normal creatinine. For patients with decreased renal function, UFH may be preferable because its effect may be monitored with the APTT. Dosing of LMWHs in patients with obesity may also be problematic. They are usually dosed according to total body weight up to a maximum of 150 kg.

B. Dosing

Multiple factors may influence the dosing of heparin. As discussed previously, the dose may be influenced by the indication and dosing algorithms have been established to account for these differences (Fig. 75-1). Because the source of laboratory thromboplastin may vary among laboratories, institutional ranges need to be established that correlate the APTT in seconds with heparin levels. The desired (therapeutic) heparin levels determined by protamine titration are 0.2 to 0.4 U/mL. The desired anti-Xa levels are 0.3 to 0.7 U/mL [3]. Administration of standardized doses of UFH based on the indication, generally results in higher heparin levels and greater prolongation of the APTT in women compared with men. Similarly, LMWHs dosed in women result in higher anti-Xa levels [29,30]. These differences observed between men and women remain when age, body weight, and the presence of smoking are considered. Because the response to UFH is monitored frequently with the APTT, the presence of a greater than expected response usually results in a dosage reduction promptly and subsequently should limit the time that a patient is at a level associated with increased risk for bleeding. Because LMWHs are not routinely monitored the possibility that women could be at risk for higher anti-Xa levels and subsequently at greater risk for bleeding when these agents are used may occur. This has been observed in some studies but not all [31]. The therapeutic range for anti-Xa levels is quite broad, 0.5 to 1.0 U/mL, and there has not been a good correlation between bleeding and levels. It is thus likely that other factors and risks for bleeding may be as likely to result in bleeding as the higher than anticipated anti-Xa levels. Tailoring of dosing regimens on the basis of multiple factors including gender may result in safer and more efficacious regimens [31].

Intended for patients who will receive full doses of unfractionated heparin (UFH).

DATE		TIME	
ALLERGIES			

LABS Required PRIOR to initiation of heparin	☑ aPTT	☑ PT/INR	☑ Platelets	☑ Urinalysis	☑ Stool guaiac

INDICATION		DOSE SELECTION (For all doses round to nearest 100 units)
☐	Suspected or confirmed PE & <u>low bleeding risk</u>	LD: 100 units/kg (Min 5,000 units, Max 10,000 units) CI: 22 units/kg/hr
☐	DVT --or-- Suspected/confirmed PE with <u>high bleeding risk</u> -or- other (see below)	LD: 80 units/kg (Min 5,000 units, Max 10,000 units) CI: 18 units/kg/hr
☐	Acute Coronary syndromes (Unstable angina, AMI)	Use ANTITHROMBOTIC ORDER FORM-ACS
☐	Neurologic disorders (e.g. stroke,neurovascular disease)	LD: NONE CI: 15 units/kg/hr

TOTAL BODY WEIGHT(TBW):	WEIGHT:	_____	Kg
LOADING DOSE:	DOSE:	_____	Units
INITIAL CONTINUOUS INFUSION:	DOSE:	_____	Units/hr

☐   Follow ALGORITHM below   -- or -   ☐   DO NOT follow ALGORITHM below. Will re-write separate orders.

- **Other indications:** Atrial fibrillation, mechanical heart valve, or other conditions with thrombosis
- **See reverse side** for abbreviations & risk factors.
- **No IM injections** are to be administered during therapeutic heparin administration
- If long-term anticoagulation is desired, warfarin may be initiated on day 1 of heparin. **Warfarin dose must be ordered daily.**

ALGORITHM

☑   Obtain **first aPTT** <u>6 hrs</u> after initiation of heparin therapy

  1. Neurologic disorder ⇨ Follow TABLE below

  2. All other indications (after giving the initial bolus dose) if aPTT is:
        <55 sec ⇨ Follow TABLE below   **≥55 sec** ⇨ Do NOT Change Rate
                                                              • **Recheck aPTT** in <u>4 hrs</u> after previous blood draw
                                                              • Dose adjust rate according to the TABLE below

☑   Obtain **aPTT's** <u>Q6 hrs</u> until therapeutic or after a dose change and adjust rate using TABLE below*
☑   Obtain <u>daily</u> **aPTT** after aPTT is stable*
☑   Obtain <u>daily</u> **CBC & platelets**
☑   Obtain **stool guaiac** <u>every other day</u>

aPTT (seconds)	Re-bolus (units)	Hold drip (minutes)	Change drip (units/hr)	Repeat aPTT (After dose adjustment)
<40	Neuro Pt: None Others: 70 units/kg	0	+200	6 hrs
40-47	0	0	+200	6 hrs
48-54	0	0	+100	6 hrs
55-80 THERAPEUTIC RANGE	**0**	**0**	**0**	**Q6hrs** until stable* Once stabilized, then **QAM**
81-90	0	0	-100	6 hrs
91-100	0	30	-200	6 hrs
>100	0	60	-300	6 hrs

*Stable = 2 consecutive aPTT values within therapeutic range [aPTT 55-80])

Fig. 75-1   Intravenous heparin order form for adults.

Anticoagulation in Adults
General Information

---

1. **Risk factors** for bleeding on heparin:
   a. Surgery, trauma, or stroke within the previous 14 days.
   b. History of peptic ulcer disease, GI bleeding or GU bleeding.
   c. Platelet count < 150,000.
   d. Miscellaneous factors such as hepatic failure, uremia, or brain metastases or presence of underlying coagulopathy.
   e. Age > 70 years.
   f. Concomitant antithrombotic therapy (e.g. thrombolytics, antiplatelet therapy)
   g. Recent or anticipated central or arterial catheterization.

2. **Duration of heparin**: For patients who require concomitant heparin and warfarin therapy, a *minimum of 5 days overlap is required.*

3. For dosing of the **low molecular weight heparins** [e.g., enoxaparin (Lovenox®)], especially in the setting of renal compromise, contact the anticoagulation service.

4. **Warfarin (Coumadin®) dosing algorithm:**

Day	INR	Dosage
1	≤1.1	5 mg
2	<1.5	5 mg
	1.5-1.9	2.5 mg
	2.0 -2.5	1 - 2.5 mg
	>2.5	0 mg
3	<1.5	5 - 10 mg
	1.5-1.9	2.5 - 5 mg
	2.0-3.0	0 - 2.5 mg
	>3.0	0 mg
4	<1.5	10 mg
	1.5-1.9	5 - 7.5 mg
	2.0-3.0	0 - 5 mg
	>3.0	0
5	<1.5	10 mg
	1.5-1.9	7.5 - 10 mg
	2.0-3.0	0 - 5 mg
	>3.0	0 mg

For additional dosing recommendations please contact the anticoagulation service

NOTE: These guidelines are recommendations. They are not intended to replace an individual clinician's judgment.

5. Considerations for oral anticoagulation with warfarin:
   a. Many drugs may interfere with the anticoagulant effect of warfarin.
      - The addition or deletion of any medication(s) may alter this effect.
      - For a listing of interfering medications, contact anticoagulation service.
   b. Additional factors that may influence warfarin response include coagulopathy caused by disorders such as CHF, hepatic disease, nutritional vitamin K deficiency, and febrile illnesses.
   c. Warfarin should **not** be administered during *pregnancy*.
   d. PT/INR should be ordered daily.
   e. Any increase in INR of greater than 0.3-0.4 units per day should result in a dose reduction.
   f. Therapeutic range for warfarin:
      a. INR 2.5-3.5 for most mechanical prosthetic valves or recurrent systemic embolism
      b. INR 2.0-3.0 for most other indications.
   g. **Follow-up** appointments can be scheduled by calling...
   h. For patients being treated for unstable angina, NSTEMI or STEMI, please use **ANTITHROMBOTIC ORDER FORM**.
   i. Educational tools below are available:
      - Warfarin education booklets
      - Enoxaparin discharge teaching kits
      - For information regarding temporary interruption of therapy: **Recommendations for Perioperative Management of Patients on Long-Term Anticoagulation Therapy**
      - VTE risk assessment recommendations

ABBREVIATIONS
PE = Pulmonary embolism
DVT = Deep Vein Thrombosis
LD = Loading dose
CI = Continuous infusion
VTE = Venous thromboembolism

Fig. 75-1   *(Continued)*

C. Risks and Adverse Effects

1. Hemorrhage

Gender has been observed to be a strong predictor for hemorrhagic events from both UFH and LMWHs although there is not universal agreement from all investigators [32]. Antithrombotic therapy has become much more complicated in the last few years and the use of multiple antithrombotic agents (e.g., aspirin, heparin, glycoprotein IIb/IIIa inhibitors, or thrombolytics) could account for these observations. However, despite these concerns, gender does still predict likelihood for more frequent bleeding [32].

2. Thrombocytopenia

Thrombocytopenia secondary to heparin may occur with both UFH and LMWHs; however, the incidence is greater with UFH. There does not appear to be a greater frequency in women [33]. Heparin-induced thrombocytopenia may be of two types, type I is associated with a generally benign course and occurs early after the start of therapy (1 to 2 days) with a platelet nadir of approximately 100,000. Type II HIT is antibody mediated, occurs usually 5 to 7 days after initiation of heparin, may be associated with a much more precipitous drop in the platelet count, and is occasionally associated with a thrombosis syndrome. The onset may be earlier if the patient has previously been exposed and is antibody positive. With HIT type II, heparin must be immediately discontinued and if continued antithrombotic therapy is indicated, DTIs (lepirudin, bivalirudin, or argatroban) are indicated. Low-molecular-weight heparins should not be administered to patients with HIT. Although they are associated with a lower incidence of HIT, it may occur and there is significant (>87%) cross-reactivity [34]. A newly released synthetic pentasaccharide, a specific factor-Xa inhibitor, fondaparinux does not cross react with either UFH or LMWH and may prove to be another alternative when greater clinical experience is available [35].

3. Osteoporosis

Administration of UFH for greater than 1 month, but usually for 3 to 6 months, may result in decreased bone density and osteoporosis in up to a third of women [36,37]. Fracture occurs less frequently and has been observed in approximately 2 to 3% of patients. The use of LMWHs may be associated with a decreased incidence of bone loss [38].

4. Use in Pregnancy

Management of thrombotic conditions during pregnancy is usually accomplished with heparin because of the potential for fetal abnormalities with warfarin. Both UFH and LMWHs have been studied, and evidence suggests that they are safe for the development of the fetus [39,40]. Fetal and maternal hemorrhage are still possible complications of heparins and require close monitoring. There are little pharmacokinetic data available on the most appropriate way to dose LMWHs during pregnancy; nonetheless, there are several factors that are known to influence dosing. Total body weight increases during pregnancy and the renal clearance of enoxaparin increases [40a]. Both of these conditions may lead to an increased dose requirement. In selecting patients in whom to use LMWHs, it is recommended that the availability of anti-Xa levels be determined and that occasional anti-Xa monitoring be performed, particularly as the time course of the pregnancy advances and the mother's weight increases. Therapeutic anti-Xa levels are in the range of 0.5 to 1.0 IU/mL. If possible, the LMWH should be discontinued before delivery and substituted with UFH, because its longer half-life may result in more bleeding complications. Heparins do not cross into the breast milk.

VI. Warfarin

A. General Efficacy

Warfarin has been used for the management of antithrombotic disease for more than 50 years and is presently the only orally active drug available. The indications for warfarin have been well described elsewhere [4]. Warfarin acts at a postribosomal step in inhibiting the activation of precursor, vitamin K dependent clotting factors, II, VII, IX, and X. Vitamin K promotes the carboxylation of the glutamic acid residues on these precursor proteins and in this process confers calcium-binding affinity required for coagulation. This process requires the availability of active vitamin K, which is oxidized to vitamin K epoxide and is inactivated during this process. In the absence of warfarin, vitamin K epoxide is converted (reduced) back to the active form and subsequently participates in the further activation of additional new active clotting factors. In the presence of warfarin this reduction is inhibited and there is a buildup of inactive forms of vitamin K and subsequently an inhibition of the formation of clotting factors and hopefully a decrease in clot formation. In addition to the procoagulant vitamin K dependent factors, warfarin may also influence protein C and protein S, which are vitamin-K dependent, naturally occurring anticoagulants. With initiation of warfarin therapy there may subsequently be a reduction in these protective vitamin K dependent factors and it is during this time that coverage with heparin, which is immediate acting, is essential. The use of warfarin in the United States is increasing as the population ages and the incidence of cardiovascular and cerebrovascular diseases increases. The efficacy of warfarin has been clearly established for both men and women.

B. Dosing

Warfarin is subject to the influence of many different factors, and prediction of dose may be difficult [4]. Because warfarin acts indirectly to inhibit the coagulation factors there is a delay in the onset of its effect. Clotting factors that are present in the patients circulation are not influenced by warfarin and their elimination must rely on natural degradation. The half-lives of the vitamin K dependent clotting factors vary; factor VII is the shortest with a half life of approximately 7 hours, whereas factors IX and X are 20 to 40 hours and prothrombin (II) is the longest at around 60 hours. Thus, administration of larger doses of warfarin do not result in a more rapid response and only predispose the patient to a greater chance of bleeding because of the rapid decline in factor VII concentration. Therefore, the usual starting dose of warfarin is 5 mg [42,43]. Many other factors have been identified that influence the response to warfarin, including the presence of other drugs, diet, and acute (e.g., fever, diarrhea) and chronic illnesses (e.g., congestive heart failure [CHF], liver disease, thyroid dysfunction) [44]. Body size and age have been suggested to influence warfarin dose requirements but are inconsistently observed [45]. Gender does not predict warfarin dose requirements when controlled for age and weight. Because women generally live longer than men and may be of smaller body size, there may be a disproportionate observation of a decrease in warfarin dose requirements in women. Drugs may interfere with warfarin by a number of different mechanisms. There may be pharmacokinetic interactions as a result primarily of alterations in absorption, metabolism (either inhibition or induction), and possibly protein displacement. In addition there may be pharmacodynamic interactions as a result of influences on vitamin K availability and disposition or the combination of therapeutic agents that further inhibit blood clotting via inhibition of platelet function or fibrinolytic activity or stimulate blood clotting such as with the use of estrogens. Lists of drugs reported to interact with warfarin are available from a number of different sources and should be consulted whenever warfarin is being initiated and whenever a drug is being added to or deleted from a patient's medication regimen. Today it is also particularly important to consider the role of over-the-counter medications and herbal medications because of their popularity and availability [46]. Dietary influences on warfarin dose requirements are most often transient, and the content of vitamin K containing foods does not require alteration in patients taking warfarin. Maintaining a balance in the ingestion of vitamin K rich foods is more important. Patients who suffer an acute febrile illness may have an exaggerated response to warfarin because of the increased turnover of vitamin K. The presence of acute diarrheal illnesses may also lead to an increased sensitivity to warfarin because of the malabsorption of vitamin K and a decreased intake because the major source of physiologically active vitamin K is dietary [47]. The laboratory response to warfarin is based on measurement of the INR. When initiating therapy in patients on warfarin, in addition to the factors discussed, the race of the patient should be considered. Review of 440 patients attending the University of California, San Francisco Anticoagulation Clinic revealed that when drugs, comorbid conditions, indications for therapy, age, weight, and sex are controlled for, Asians have a significantly lower dose requirement. To achieve an INR of 2 to 3, Asians of all backgrounds required on the average 3.5 mg/day, Caucasians 5.2 mg/day, and African Americans 6.2 mg/day. The most likely explanation for this is a genetically determined polymorphism in cytochrome P450, 2C9 enzyme. Further study is necessary to confirm this and is ongoing [48–50].

C. Risks and Adverse Effects

1. Hemorrhage

Hemorrhage is the most common and serious adverse reaction to warfarin. Predictors of bleeding most commonly associated with warfarin include the intensity of effect as measured by the INR, individual patient characteristics, drug interactions, and duration of therapy. One of the major advances in the use of warfarin over the last few years has been the use of less intense

therapy. Accumulating evidence supports the efficacy of less intense therapy, and there is an effort to maintain an INR of 2 to 3 for most indications. The exception is the use of warfarin in patients with mechanical heart valves in the mitral position, patients with a previous history of systemic embolism, or patients with multiple risk factors for thrombosis (e.g., prosthetic valve with atrial fibrillation). In these patients an INR of 2.5 to 3.5 is the goal [1]. Increased bleeding has been reported in some studies to be higher in women, but this has been an inconsistent finding and other studies have not reported this observation [51]. If there is a difference, it may reflect the higher incidence of certain disease states in women (e.g., arthritis) and the use of drugs that may interact with warfarin [52]. There are several possible approaches to the management of elevated INRs. In the absence of bleeding, temporary discontinuation may be all that is required. The INR usually declines over 2 to 5 days, and then a decision can be made regarding what dose to resume. If a more rapid decrease is desired, which may be desirable in a patient at increased risk for bleeding, a low dose of oral vitamin K (e.g., 2.5 mg) can be administered and experience has demonstrated that the INR can be safely and more rapidly decreased toward the therapeutic range without normalization of the INR, which would be undesirable [53,54]. It appears that the oral route is more rapid, predictable, and effective than the subcutaneous route. If the patient is bleeding, further evaluation is recommended, and therapeutic approaches may require infusion of appropriate intravenous agents including fresh frozen plasma or specific factors (e.g., VII or IX).

2. Use in Pregnancy

Warfarin should be avoided during pregnancy especially between the 6th and 12th week because it is during this time that the fetus is most likely susceptible to the warfarin-induced embryopathy [38]. Because there is a risk at any time during pregnancy from either the embryopathy or fetal bleeding, warfarin should be avoided. Women of childbearing age should be counseled to use appropriate contraceptive methods to prevent the difficult decision of whether to terminate the pregnancy should they become pregnant while taking warfarin. For women who wish to become pregnant, warfarin should be discontinued and heparin started before the attempts at conception.

3. Osteoporosis

The long-term use of warfarin (12 months or more) has been associated with an increased risk of fractures in women, particularly an increase in vertebral and rib fractures. Most observations are retrospective in nature and the mechanism of osteoporosis has not been clearly elucidated. For women requiring long-term warfarin therapy, appropriate attention should be made to ensure that measures to prevent osteoporosis are made [55,56].

VII. Direct Thrombin Inhibitors

A. General Efficacy

A new class of antithrombotic agents, the DTIs, have recently become available. These agents are specific, direct

Table 75-4
Comparison of Direct Thrombin Inhibitors (DTIs)

	Bivalirudin (Angiomax)	Lepirudin (Refludan)	Argatroban	Melagatran (Active) Ximelagatran Is Prodrug (Investigational)
Approved indication(s)	Patients with UA undergoing PTCA	Patients with HIT	Prophylaxis or treatment in patients with HIT	DVT/PE-Rx+prevention Prevention of stroke in AF
Source	Synthetic	Derived from yeast cells	Synthetic	Synthetic
Binding to thrombin	Specific and direct reversible binding to catalytic and exosite 1	Specific, direct, and irreversible binding at both catalytic and exosite 1	Direct reversible binding near catalytic site	Direct reversible binding to catalytic site only
Monitoring	APTT, ACT	APTT (may↑INR)	APTT (may↑↑INR)	No coagulation monitoring required
Therapeutic goal	ACT 300–350 seconds	APTT 1.5–2.5 times	APTT 1–5–3 times	N/A
Half-life	25 min	1.3 hr	39–51 min	≈3 hr
Main route of clearance	Renal	Renal	Hepatic	Renal
Dose adjustment for renal↓	Yes	Yes	No	Probable
Dose adjustment for hepatic ↓	No	No	Yes	No
Antibodies	No	Yes	No	No
Dose	For PCI 1 mg/kg bolus then 2.5 mg/kg/h×4 hr, may continue at 0.2 mg/kg/hr for 20 hr For HIT 0.2 mg/kg/hr	0.4 mg/kg bolus then 0.1 mg/kg/hr	2 μg/kg/min	Undecided, will be based on outcomes of clinical trials

ACT, activated clotting time; AF, atrial fibrillation; APTT, activated partial thromboplastin time; DVT, deep venous thrombosis; HIT heparin-induced thrombocytopenia; INR, international normalized ratio; LMWH, low-molecular-weight heparin; N/A, not applicable; PCI, percutaneous coronary intervention; PE-Rx, pulmonary embolus treatment; UA, urinalysis. For HIT, avoid LMWH because of high degree of cross-reactivity.

inhibitors of thrombin and are effective against both circulating thrombin and clot-bound thrombin [57,58]. In addition, they have several other advantages over heparin including no binding to plasma proteins and lack of neutralization by platelet factor 4. This latter property helps to maintain their pharmacologic activity when in close proximity to thrombi that are rich in platelets. Because of their fibrin specificity they may be associated with a lower risk of bleeding than the indirect thrombin inhibitors, heparin, and LMWHs. They are currently indicated primarily for the management of patients who have developed HIT, especially when undergoing interventional coronary procedures. There are three intravenous agents approved by the Food and Drug Administration (FDA), and they include argatroban (Argatroban), bivalirudin (Angiomax), and lepirudin (Refludan). There is currently one orally active investigational DTI, ximelagatran. Following oral administration it is converted to melagatran, a selective, reversible inhibitor of thrombin [59,60]. The properties of the DTIs are illustrated in Table 75-4. Gender is a predictor of bleeding following invasive cardiac procedures. Based on observations, this risk in women appears to be approximately 2-fold (10.4% vs 4.5%) greater than in men. In one trial, bivalirudin when compared with heparin was associated with a greater reduction in hemorrhagic events in women compared with men [61]. Some of the differences may be due to the age- and weight-dependent differences in the pharmacokinetics of heparin previously discussed. Regardless, the use of DTIs may prove to be more beneficial in women, especially because they may present for intervention older and with smaller body size. There are no published data to suggest that gender is a specific predictor of dose requirement for the DTIs.

B. Dosing

The doses for these agents are illustrated in Table 75-4. The intravenous DTIs are all dosed based on weight, whereas ximelagatran is administered in a fixed dose. Dose ranging studies are currently being performed to determine the optimal dose of ximelagatran. It is close to approval for the prevention of venous thromboembolism in patients undergoing orthopedic surgical procedures. Additional trials are investigating its efficacy for the treatment of venous thromboembolism, atrial fibrillation, and ACSs. If successful, ximelagatran may replace warfarin in some patients because of its more rapid onset of action, lack of drug interactions, and lack of the need for laboratory monitoring.

C. Risks and Adverse Effects

The primary risk from these agents is bleeding. Recent evidence from side by side comparisons with heparin suggest that bivalirudin is safer than heparin [62]. Dosing adjustment is required for several of the DTIs (see Table 75-3).

VIII. Conclusions

Antithrombotic agents are associated with a narrow therapeutic index. Balancing the potential life-saving benefits against the potential life-threatening hemorrhagic complications requires a recognition of the factors responsible for differences in therapeutic response. Gender may be just one of these factors. Fortunately, the clinical response to most antithrombotic agents is evaluated on the basis of a surrogate endpoint, usually a laboratory test, and dosage adjustments usually follow promptly. Further research should include larger numbers of women, and specific attention should be placed on investigating the potential for gender-specific differences in response.

IX. Suggestions for Further Investigations

- Can we apply the results of large-scale clinical trials that consist primarily of men to the treatment of women?
- Because women present more often at an advanced age, is there a mechanism to more equitably compare outcomes?
- Are women more sensitive to the adverse outcomes because of gender or because of other factors such as differences in body weight and size?
- Are women more likely to respond to the therapeutic effect of antithrombotic agents administered in fixed doses (e.g., reteplase or ximelagatran) than men?
- Are women more likely to respond with adverse outcomes with the administration of antithrombotic agents administered in fixed doses?
- Do different therapeutic ranges need to be established on the basis of gender?

Acknowledgement

This work was supported in part by PHRA National Institute on Aging: RO1 AG 15982.

References

1. Maibohm B, Beirle I, Derendorf H. (2002). How important are gender differences in pharmacokinetics? *Clin Pharmacokinet.* 41:320–342.
2. Coller BS. (1998). Monitoring platelet GPIIb/IIIa antagonist therapy. *Circulation.* 97:5–9.
2a. Berkowitz SD, Granger CB, Pieper KS *et al.* (1997). Incidence and predictors of bleeding after contemporary thrombolytic therapy for myocardial infarction. *Circulation.* 95:2508–2516.
3. Hirsh J, Warkentin TE, Shaughnessy SG *et al.* (2001). Heparin and low-molecular-weight heparin. Mechanisms of action, pharmacokinetics, dosing, monitoring, efficacy and safety. *Chest.* 119:64S–94S.
4. Hirsh J, Dalen JE, Anderson DR *et al.* (2001). Oral anticoagulants: Mechanism of action, clinical effectiveness, and optimal therapeutic range. *Chest.* 119:8S–21S.
5. De Denus S, Spinler SA. (2002). Clinical monitoring of direct thrombin inhibitors using the ecarin clotting time. *Pharmacotherapy.* 22:433–435.
6. Antiplatelet Trialists Collaboration. (2002). Collaborative meta-analysis of randomised trials of antiplatelet therapy for prevention of death, myocardial infarction, and stroke in high risk patients. *BMJ.* 324:71–86.
7. Boersma E, Harrington RA, Moliterno DJ *et al.* (2002). Platelet glycoprotein IIb/IIIa inhibitors in acute coronary syndromes: A meta-analysis of all major randomised clinical trials. *Lancet.* 359:189–198.
8. ESPRIT Investigators. (2002). Is glycoprotein IIb/IIIa antagonism as effective in women as in men following percutaneous intervention? Lessons from the ESPRIT trial. *J Am Coll Cardiol.* 40:1085–1091.
9. Cho L, Topol EJ, Balog C *et al.* (2000). Clinical benefit of glycoprotein IIb/IIIa blockade with abciximab is independent of gender: Pooled analysis from RPIC, EPILOG, and EPISTENT trials. Evaluation of 7E3 for the prevention of ischemic complications. Evaluation in percutaneous transluminal coronary angioplasty to improve long-term outcome with abciximab

GP IIb/IIIa blockade. Evaluation of platelet IIb/IIIa inhibitor for stent. *J Am Coll Cardiol.* 36:381–386.
10. The PURSUIT Trial Investigators. (1998). Inhibition of platelet glycoprotein IIb/IIIa with eptifibatide in patients with acute coronary syndromes. Platelet glycoprotein IIb/IIIa in unstable angina: Receptor suppression using integrelin therapy. *N Engl J Med.* 339:436–443.
11. Glaser R, Herrmann HC, Murphy SA *et al.* (2002). Benefit of early invasive management strategy in women with acute coronary syndromes. *JAMA.* 288:3124–3129.
12. CAPRIE Steering Committee. (1996). A randomised, blinded trial of clopidogrel versus aspirin in patients at risk of ischemic events. (CAPRIE). *Lancet.* 348:329–339.
13. The Clopidogrel in Unstable Angina to Prevent Recurrent Events Trial Investigators. (2001). Effects of clopidogrel in addition to aspirin in patients with acute coronary syndromes without ST-segment elevation. *N Engl J Med.* 345:494–502.
14. Patrono C, Coller B, Dalen JE *et al.* (2001). Platelet-active drugs. The relationship among dose, effectiveness, and side effects. *Chest.* 119:39S–63S.
15. Heer T, Schiele R, Schneider S *et al.* (2002). Gender differences in acute myocardial infarction in the era of reperfusion (The MITRA Registry). *Am J Cardiol.* 89:511–516.
16. Lincoff AM, Califf RM, Ellis SG *et al.* (1993). Thrombolytic therapy for women with myocardial infarction: Is there a gender gap? *J Am Coll Cardiol.* 22:1780–1787.
17. Woodfield SL, Lundergan CF, Reiner JS *et al.* (1997). Gender and acute myocardial infarction: Is there a different response to thrombolysis? *J Am Coll Cardiol.* 29:35–42.
18. Malacrida R, Genoni M, Maggioni AP, for the Third International Study of Infarct Survival (ISIS-3) Collaborative Group. (1998). A comparison of the early outcome of acute myocardial infarction in women and men. *N Engl J Med.* 338:8–14.
19. Koh KK, Mincemoyer R, Bui MN *et al.* (1997). Effects of hormone replacement therapy on fibrinolysis in postmenopausal women. *N Engl J Med.* 336:683–690.
20. Patel SR, Parker JA, Grodstein F *et al.* (1998). Similarity in presentation and response to thrombolysis among women and men with pulmonary embolism. *J Thromb Thrombolysis.* 5:95–100.
21. Stone GW, Grines CL, Browne KF *et al.* (1995). Comparison of in-hospital outcome in men versus women treated by either thrombolytic therapy or primary coronary angioplasty for acute myocardial infarction. *Am J Cardiol.* 75:987–992.
22. White HD, Barbash GI, Modan M *et al.* (1993). After correcting for worse baseline characteristics, women treated with thrombolytic therapy for acute myocardial infarction have the same mortality and morbidity as men except for a higher incidence of hemorrhagic stroke. *Circulation.* 88(Pt 1): 2097–2103.
23. Barron HV, Fox NL, Berioli S *et al.* (1999). A comparison of intracranial hemorrhage rates in patients treated with rt-PA and tPA-TNK: Impact of gender, age and low body weight (abstract). *Circulation.* 100:II.
24. Becker RC, Hochman JS, Cannon CP *et al.* (1999). Fatal cardiac rupture among patients treated with thrombolytic agents and adjunctive thrombin antagonists: Observations from the Thrombolysis Inhibition in Myocardial Infarction 9 Study. *J Am Coll Cardiol.* 33:479–487.
25. Maggioni AP, Maseri A, Fresco C *et al.* (1993). On behalf of the GISSI-2 Investigators. Each related increase in mortality among patients with first myocardial infarctions treated with thrombolysis. *N Engl J Med.* 329: 1442–1448.
26. Lewis JL, Burchell HB, Titus JL. (1969). Clinical and pathologic features of post infarction cardiac rupture. *Am J Cardiol.* 23:43–53.
27. Wein TH, Hickenbottom SL, Morgenstern LB *et al.* (2002). Safety of tissue plasminogen activator for acute stroke in menstruating women. *Stroke.* 33:2506–2508.
28. White RH, Zhou H, Woo L, Mungall D. (1997). Effect of weight, sex, age, clinical diagnosis and thromboplastin reagent on steady-stat intravenous heparin requirements. *Arch Intern Med.* 157:2468–2472.
29. Campbell NRC, Hull RD, Brant R *et al.* (1998). Different effects of heparin in males and females. *Clin Invest Med.* 21:71–78.
30. Toss H, Wallentin L, Siegbahn A. (1999). Influences of sex and smoking habits on anticoagulant activity in low-molecular-weight heparin treatment of unstable coronary artery disease. *Am Heart J.* 137:72–78.
31. Menon V, Berkowitz SD, Antman EM *et al.* (2001). New heparin dosing recommendations for patients with acute coronary syndromes. *Am J Med.* 110:641–650.
32. Juergens CP, Semsarian C, Keech AC *et al.* (1997). Hemorrhagic complications of intravenous heparin use. *Am J Cardiol.* 80:150–154.

33. Warkentin TE, Kelton JG. (2001). Temporal aspects of heparin-induced thrombocytopenia. *N Engl J Med.* 344:1286–1292.

34. Warkentin TE, Levine MN, Hirsh J *et al.* (1995). Heparin-induced thrombocytopenia in patients treated with low-molecular-weight heparin or unfractionated heparin. *N Engl J Med.* 332:1330–1335.

35. Turpie AGG, Gallus AS, Hoek JA. (2001). A synthetic pentasaccharide for the prevention of deep-vein thrombosis after total hip replacement. *N Engl J Med.* 344:619–625.

36. Douketis JD, Ginsberg JS, Burrows RF *et al.* (1996). The effects of long-term heparin therapy during pregnancy on bone density. *Thromb Hemost.* 75:254–257.

37. Barbour LA, Kick SD, Steiner JF *et al.* (1994). A prospective study of heparin-induced osteoporosis in pregnancy using bone densitometry. *Am J Obstet Gynecol.* 170:862–869.

38. Ginsberg JS, Greer I, Hirsh J. (2001). Use of antithrombotic agents during pregnancy. *Chest.* 119:122S–131S.

39. Bates SM, Ginsberg JS. (2002). How we manage venous thromboembolism during pregnancy. *Blood.* 100:3470–3478.

40. Chandramouli NB, Rodgers GM. (2001). Management of thrombosis in women with antiphospholipid syndrome. *Clin Obstet Gynecol.* 44:36–47.

40a. Casele HL, Laifer SA, Woelkers DA *et al.* (1999). Changes in the pharmacokinetics of the low-molecular-weight heparin enoxaparin sodium during pregnancy. *Am J Obstet Gynecol.* 181:1113–1117.

41. Ansell J, Hirsh J, Dalen JE *et al.* (2001). Managing oral anticoagulant therapy. *Chest.* 119:22S–38S.

42. Harrison L, Johnston M, Massicotte MP *et al.* (1997). Comparison of 5-mg and 10-mg loading doses in initiation of warfarin therapy. *Ann Intern Med.* 126:133–136.

43. Gage BF, Fihn SD, White RH. (2000). Management and dosing of warfarin therapy. *Am J Med.* 109:481–488.

44. Demirkan K, Stephens MA, Newman KP *et al.* (2000). Response to warfarin and other oral anticoagulants: Effects of disease states. *South Med J.* 93:448–455.

45. Absher RK, Moore ME, Parker MH. (2002). Patient-specific factors predictive of warfarin dosage requirements. *Ann Pharmacother.* 36:1512–1517.

46. Wittkowsky A. (2001). Drug interactions update: Drugs, herbs, and oral anticoagulants. *J Thomb Thrombolysis.* 12:67–71.

47. Shearer MJ. (1995). Vitamin K. *Lancet.* 345:229–234.

48. Redman AR. (2001). Implications of cytochrome P450 2C9 polymorphism on warfarin metabolism and dosing. *Pharmacotherapy.* 21:235–242.

49. Takahashi H, Kashima T, Nomizo Y *et al.* (1998). Metabolism of warfarin enantiomers in Japanese patients with heart disease having different CYP2C9 and CYP 2C19 genotypes. *Clin Pharmacol Ther.* 63:519–528.

50. Leung AYH, Chow HCH, Lie AKW *et al.* (2001). Genetic polymorphism in exon 4 of cytochrome P450 CYP2C9 may be associated with warfarin sensitivity in Chinese patients. *Blood.* 98:2584–2587.

51. VanDerMeer FJM, Rosendaal FR, Vandenbroucke JP *et al.* (1993). Bleeding complications in oral anticoagulant therapy. An analysis of risk factors. *Arch Int Med.* 153:1557–1562.

52. Levine MN, Raskob G, Landefeld S *et al.* (2001). Hemorrhagic complications of anticoagulant therapy. *Chest.* 119:108S–121S.

53. Weibert RT, Le DT, Kayser SR *et al.* (1997). Correction of excessive anticoagulation with low-dose oral vitamin K. *Ann Intern Med.* 125:959–962.

54. Crowther MA, Douketis JD, Steidl L *et al.* (2002). Oral vitamin K lowers the international normalized ratio more rapidly than subcutaneous vitamin K in the treatment of warfarin-associated coagulopathy. *Ann Intern Med.* 137:251–254.

55. Caraballo PJ, Heit JA, Atkinson EJ *et al.* (1999). Long-term use of oral anticoagulants and the risk of fracture. *Arch Intern Med.* 159:1750–1756.

56. Knapen MH, Hellemon-Boode BS, Langenberg-Ledeboer M *et al.* (2000). Effect of oral anticoagulant treatment on markers of calcium and bone metabolism. *Haemostasis.* 30:290–297.

57. Weitz JI, Buller HR. (2002). Direct thrombin inhibitors in acute coronary syndromes. Present and future. *Circulation.* 105:1004–1011.

58. Antman EM. (2001). The search for replacements for unfractionated heparin. *Circulation.* 103:2310–2314.

59. Gustafson D, Nystrom JE, Carlsson *et al.* (2001). The direct thrombin inhibitor melagatran and its oral prodrug H376/95: Intestinal absorption properties, biochemical and pharmacodynamic effects. *Thromb Res.* 101:171–181.

60. Heit JA, Colwell CW, Francis CW *et al.* (2001). Comparison of the oral direct thrombin inhibitor Ximelagatran with enoxaparin as prophylaxis against venous thromboembolism after total knee replacement. A phase 2 dose-finding study. *Arch Intern Med.* 161:2215–2221.

61. Bhatt DL, Cho L, Lincoff AM. (2002). Reduction in percutaneous coronary intervention-related bleeding with bivalirudin is particularly striking in women (abstract). *J Am Coll Cardiol.* 39(Suppl):17A.

62. Kong DF, Topol EJ, Bittl JA *et al.* (1999). Clinical outcomes of bivalirudin for ischemic heart disease. *Circulation.* 100:2049–2053.

76

Pain Medications: Differences Between the Sexes

CHRISTINE MIASKOWSKI, RN, PhD, FAAN AND JON D. LEVINE, MD, PhD
Department of Physiological Nursing, University of California, San Francisco, CA

I. Introduction

The systematic evaluation of sex differences in the prescription, use, and effectiveness of analgesic medications is a relatively new field of inquiry. Much of the research on sex differences has focused on evaluating for differences in pain thresholds and tolerance using experimental paradigms [for reviews see references 1 and 2]. In addition, sex differences in the prevalence of several chronic pain conditions have been reported in the literature [for review see reference 3]. However, it should be noted that although the number of research studies on sex differences in acute and chronic pain is growing, there is a paucity of animal and human research on sex differences in the pharmacologic actions and effects of various analgesic medications [4,5].

Little is known about sex-related differences in the prescription, use, and effectiveness of analgesic medications. The purpose of this chapter is to provide a summary of the research in humans that has evaluated for sex differences in analgesic prescriptions, in the use of analgesic medications, and in the effectiveness of analgesic medications. Although some of the studies on the effectiveness of analgesic medications evaluated for both pharmacokinetic and pharmacodynamic differences in responses, others evaluated only one parameter. This chapter concludes with a discussion of the major directions for future research.

II. Management of Acute and Persistent Pain

Pain is the primary symptom for which men and women seek health care. Several studies and review articles have noted that men and women experience somatic symptoms differently [6–9]. In general, women report more intense, more numerous, and more frequent symptoms than men. These differences have been reported when men and women are evaluated for medical problems or when surveys are done in community settings. This consistent finding regarding sex differences in symptom appraisal appears to hold true for pain as well. Although the exact reasons for these sex differences in the reporting of pain are not known, a number of factors have been suggested and are supported by variable degrees of evidence. These factors include innate differences in somatic and visceral perceptions; differences in symptom labeling, description, and reporting; the socialization process, which leads to sex differences in the readiness to acknowledge and to report discomfort; a sex differential in the incidence of abuse and violence; sex differences in the prevalence of anxiety and depression; and gender bias in research and in clinical practice [6].

III. Sex Differences in Analgesic Prescriptions and Administration

Studies on sex differences in the prescription of analgesic medications by physicians and on the administration of analgesic medications by nurses are limited in number. In a study done over a decade ago, Calderone [10] investigated whether the frequency of administration of pain and sedative medications to patients following coronary artery bypass surgery differed by patient gender. The medical records of 30 male and female patients were reviewed. Patients were matched on age, number of coronary artery bypass grafts, and the location of the graft donor sites. The frequency of administration of pain and sedative medications to these patients for 12 to 72 hours following surgery were evaluated. The results revealed that the male patients received pain medications significantly more frequently than the female patients and that the female patients received sedative medications significantly more frequently than the male patients. Although these results are interesting and indicate the need for additional research in this area, no data were provided on the effectiveness of the analgesic and sedative medications in the male and female patients.

Two studies of patients with persistent pain [11,12] evaluated for gender differences in analgesic prescriptions. In a prospective study of cancer pain in 1308 outpatients with metastatic cancer [11], female oncology patients were found to be at greater risk for inadequate prescription of analgesics and were significantly more likely to experience inadequate pain management than male patients. In a similar study of patients with acquired immunodeficiency syndrome (AIDS) and AIDS-related pain [12], women were found to be at increased risk for inadequate prescription of analgesics and were significantly more likely to experience inadequate pain management than men. Again, these findings suggest the need for systematic investigations regarding the potential gender bias in the prescription and administration of analgesic medications.

IV. Sex Differences in the Use of Analgesic Medications

A. Use of Analgesics for Acute Postoperative Pain

In the area of acute postoperative pain, Miaskowski *et al* [4] provided a review of data from 14 papers that reported on the results of 18 studies that evaluated for sex differences in analgesic use in the postoperative period. The primary aim of these postoperative pain studies was to evaluate the pharmacokinetic and/or pharmacodynamic properties of one or more opioid analgesics that were administered in the immediate postoperative period. All of these studies [13–26] used patient-controlled analgesia (PCA) devices to administer the analgesic medication. Only two of these studies [22,23] stated that one of their specific aims was to evaluate for sex differences in the use of analgesic medications in the postoperative period. It should be noted that most of the postoperative studies [13–21,24–26] did not evaluate analgesic effectiveness directly (e.g., a decrease in pain intensity) but rather used the consumption of analgesic medications as the outcome measure.

In these 18 studies, a total of 2055 patients (1014 males, 1041 females) were evaluated. In most of the studies, the analgesics that were tested were mu-opioid agonists. In approximately 56% (10/18) of these studies, males (n=959) consumed more opioid analgesics in the immediate postoperative period than did females (n=953). In these studies, males used considerably more opioids than females (i.e., on average 2.4 times more opioids, range 1.1 to 5.5 times more). These findings are compatible with the suggestion that a sexual dimorphism exists in the use of opioid analgesics for the management of acute postoperative pain.

B. Use of Analgesics in the General Population

Analgesics are one of the most commonly used drugs in the general population. Several Scandinavian studies of the general population have determined that women use more analgesics than men [27–29]. In a more recent study [30], 19,137 men and women between the ages of 12 and 56 years from the general population in Tromso were asked about their use of analgesic medications in the past 14 days. On average, 28% of the women and 13% of the men had used analgesics. Drug use because of menstrual pain contributed only partly to the sex difference in analgesic use. Large population-based studies are warranted to determine the factors that predict sex differences in analgesic use in the general population.

C. Use of Analgesics for Persistent Pain

Two studies have evaluated for sex differences in the use of opioid analgesics for persistent pain [31,32]. In a study with two groups of patients with persistent pain (i.e., 428 patients with non-cancer pain and 143 patients with cancer-related pain), Turk and colleagues [31] evaluated for sex differences in medications prescribed, treatment history, and coping and adaptation. In the study of patients with non-cancer pain, no significant differences were found between men and women in past treatments, current analgesic use, pain, or disability. However, women were significantly more depressed and were more likely to receive antidepressants than men. No significant differences were found in any of the study variables between the men and women with cancer-related pain.

In a cross-sectional study of data derived from patients with chronic spinal pain who were undergoing evaluation at a multidisciplinary pain treatment center, Fillingim and colleagues [32] evaluated whether pain severity, psychologic status, and physical disability differed as a function of sex and opioid use and whether the clinical correlates of opioid use differed in men and women with chronic back pain. The sample consisted of 240 patients (35% women) with low back, upper back, or neck pain. The results indicated that opioid use was associated with greater self-reported disability and poorer function in both men

and women. However, the association of opioid use with affective distress differed between men and women. The women who were using opioids reported lower affective distress, which was measured using the Multidimensional Pain Inventory [33], whereas the men who were using opioids reported greater affective distress. Opioid use in this population was not associated with pain severity. However, women reported higher pain scores than men. The authors [32] concluded that opioid use and sex were significant predictors of the clinical status of patients with persistent back pain. Additional research is warranted to determine if sex influences the prescription and use of opioid analgesics for the management of persistent pain.

V. Sex Differences in the Effectiveness of Analgesic Medications

A. Nonsteroidal Anti-inflammatory Drugs

Nonsteroidal anti-inflammatory drugs (NSAIDs) are frequently used to manage acute and persistent pain problems. Only one study (34) has evaluated for sex differences in the pharmacokinetics and pharmacodynamics of an NSAID, namely ibuprofen. These investigators induced pain in young, healthy participants using electrical stimulation of the earlobe. This procedure allowed for the measurement of pain detection thresholds and maximal pain tolerance. Only the male participants demonstrated a statistically significant analgesic response to ibuprofen. The sex-related difference in analgesic response could not be attributed to any pharmacokinetic differences (i.e., C_{max}, area under the curve measurement, half-life, clearance, or volume of distribution). Walker and Carmody [34] concluded that the reduced effectiveness of ibuprofen in women compared with men may have clinical significance, particularly as a factor in the reported response variability of NSAIDs [35]. Additional studies are warranted to evaluate for sex differences in analgesic responses to acetaminophen, aspirin, other NSAIDs, and the selective cyclooxygenase 2 (i.e., COX 2) antagonists.

B. Opioid Analgesics

The opioid analgesics available for clinical use can be divided into two major classes based on the predominant opioid receptor subtype at which they are thought to produce analgesic effects, namely, mu or kappa. Most work on sex differences in the effectiveness of opioid analgesics has evaluated kappa-opioid agonists (e.g., pentazocine, nalbuphine, butorphanol).

All of these studies [36–39] were conducted using the same postoperative pain paradigm. All patients underwent standardized surgery by the same surgeon for the removal of third molar teeth. The surgical procedure always included the removal of at least one bony impacted mandibular third molar. This procedure is associated with moderate to severe postoperative pain.

Before surgery, patients received intravenous diazepam and a local anesthetic without vasoconstrictor to obtain a nerve block of short duration. After surgery, each patient was randomly assigned in an open double-blinded fashion, to receive a test drug through an intravenous line. The drug was administered at least 80 minutes after the onset of the local anesthetic and was only given if the patient had a pain rating that was greater than

2.5 cm on a 10-cm visual analogue (VAS) scale. Baseline pain intensity was defined as the VAS pain rating just before the administration of the test drug. The duration of most of the experiments was 5 hours. Following administration of the study drug, pain ratings were taken every 20 minutes for a total of 2.5 hours. The magnitude of the analgesic response for each patient was defined as the difference between the pain rating at each time point following test drug administration and baseline VAS pain rating [4].

The first study [36] evaluated the effects of preoperative administration of baclofen on the analgesia produced by postoperative administration of morphine (predominantly a mu-opioid agonist) or pentazocine (predominantly a kappa-opioid agonist). The results showed that the analgesic efficacy of morphine was enhanced by the preoperative administration of baclofen. No sex differences were found in the analgesic responses to either morphine alone or morphine given in combination with baclofen. In contrast, in the pentazocine experiments, regardless of drug group (i.e., pentazocine alone or pentazocine with baclofen), women reported consistently better analgesic effects. These data suggest that the administration of an analgesic that relieves pain by an action at the kappa-opioid receptor produced better analgesia in women compared with men [36]. This experiment was confirmed with another study that evaluated for sex differences in the analgesic effects of pentazocine administered intravenously [37]. Again, the analgesic efficacy of pentazocine was greater in women than in men.

To determine whether sex differences were associated with kappa-opioid agonists, the analgesic effects of two additional drugs in this class, namely nalbuphine and butorphanol, were compared in men and women who underwent surgery for removal of third molar teeth [38]. Consistent with the findings from our previous studies [36,37], 10 mg of nalbuphine administered intravenously prolonged the duration of analgesia in women

significantly more than it did in men. Similar sex differences were observed with 2 mg of butorphanol [38].

The next study was conducted to determine whether, within a range of doses usually administered in clinical practice, the observed sex differences in analgesia produced by nalbuphine was due to a rightward shift in the dose-response relationship for men compared with women [39]. Specifically, we tested the hypothesis that men, given a sufficiently large dose of nalbuphine, would experience analgesia equivalent to that observed in women. Because there were no previous studies of analgesic efficacy with kappa-opioids, we compared the analgesic effects produced by nalbuphine with those produced by placebo within each sex. In addition, we evaluated for sex differences in placebo responses. Different groups of male and female patients who were experiencing moderate to severe postoperative pain were given either placebo (0.9% saline) or one of three doses of nalbuphine (i.e., 5, 10, or 20 mg).

No sex differences were found in responses to placebo. However, women experienced a significantly greater analgesic response than men for all of the doses of nalbuphine. Unexpectedly, men who received the 5-mg dose of nalbuphine experienced significantly greater pain than those who received placebo. Only the 20-mg dose of nalbuphine in men produced significant analgesia compared with placebo. Although no antianalgesic effect was observed in women, only the 10-mg dose of nalbuphine produced significant analgesia compared with placebo [39]. Taken together, the results of these studies [36–39] support the hypothesis that among patients experiencing postoperative pain, women obtain better analgesia than men from opioid analgesics of the kappa-opioid class.

In a recent study [40], Sarton and colleagues evaluated for sex differences in responses to the analgesic effects of morphine in the setting of experimentally induced pain. Young, healthy men and women received an intravenous injection of morphine

Table 76-1

Research Recommendations to Evaluate for Sex Differences in Analgesic Medications

Analgesic Prescriptions and Administration

- Need to investigate whether a gender bias exists in the prescription of analgesic medications for the management of acute and persistent pain
- Need to investigate whether a gender bias exists in the administration of analgesic medications in acute and chronic care facilities

Analgesic Use

- Need for large population-based studies to evaluate for sex differences in the patterns of analgesic use for the management of acute and persistent pain
- Need to determine the factors that predict analgesic use in men and women

Analgesic Effectiveness

- Need to evaluate for sex differences in the effectiveness of nonopioid, opioids, and co-analgesics for the management of various types of acute and persistent pain
- Need to evaluate for sex differences in the factors (e.g., physiologic, psychologic, sociologic) that predict the effectiveness of nonopioid, opioids, and co-analgesics

Side Effects of Analgesic Medications

- Need to evaluate for sex differences in the side effects of nonopioid, opioids, and co-analgesics in the management of various types of acute and persistent pain
- Need to evaluate for sex differences in the factors (e.g., physiologic, psychologic, sociologic) that predict the side effects of nonopioid, opioids, and co-analgesics

(0.1 mg/kg followed by an infusion of 0.03 mg/kg/hr for 1 hour). Pain threshold and pain tolerance were tested in response to a gradual increase in transcutaneous electrical nerve stimulation. The results indicated sex differences in the analgesic effects of morphine, with greater morphine potency but slower speed of onset and offset in women. Given the paucity of studies on sex differences in the effectiveness of analgesic medications, additional research is warranted to evaluate for sex differences in responses to other opioid analgesics.

VI. Sex Differences in the Side Effects of Analgesic Medications

Two studies were found that evaluated for sex differences in the side effects of analgesic medications [41,42]. The first study evaluated for sex differences in the respiratory effects of morphine [41]. This study was a randomized, double-blind, placebo controlled trial that evaluated steady state ventilatory responses to intravenous morphine (i.e., a bolus dose of $100 \mu g/kg$ followed by a continuous infusion of $30 \mu g/kg/hr$) in a sample of 12 men and 12 women. Sex differences were noted in the respiratory effects of morphine with women having a decreased hypoxic sensitivity to morphine compared with men.

In a second study [42], sex differences in the incidence of nausea and vomiting following the administration of an opioid agonist in the emergency department were evaluated. Significantly more women required the administration of an antiemetic following the administration of an opioid analgesic for pain management in the emergency department. Given the fact, that only two studies could be found that evaluated for gender differences in side effects associated with opioid analgesics, additional research is warranted in this area.

VII. Summary and Conclusions

This review of the research on sex differences in analgesic prescriptions, analgesic use, the effectiveness of analgesic medications, and the side effects associated with analgesic medications clearly indicates the need for additional studies in each of these areas. Table 76-1 provides a list of recommendations for research in each of these areas. Each area warrants substantial focus of attention and careful, deliberate investigations. Only through careful study will it be possible to develop sex specific recommendations on how to improve the management of pain.

VIII. Suggestions for Further Investigations

- Both animal and human studies are needed to determine the mechanisms that underlie sex differences in the effectiveness of analgesic medications.
- Additional work is warranted on the potential for gender bias in the prescription of analgesic medications.

References

1. Riley JL, Robinson ME, Wise EA *et al.* (1998). Sex differences in the perception of noxious experimental stimuli: A meta-analysis. *Pain.* 74:181–187.
2. Berkley KJ. (1997). Sex differences in pain. *Behav Brain Sci.* 20:371–380.
3. Unruh AM. (1996). Gender variations in clinical pain experience. *Pain.* 65:123–167.
4. Miaskowski C, Gear RW, Levine JD. (2000). Sex-related differences in analgesic responses. In *Sex, Gender, and Pain* (Fillingim RB, ed.), pp. 209–230. Seattle: IASP Press.
5. Kest B, Sarton E, Dahan A. (2000). Gender differences in opioid-mediated analgesia: Animal and human studies. *Anesthesiology.* 93:539–547.
6. Barsky AJ, Peekna HM, Borus JF. (2001). Somatic symptom reporting in women and men. *J Gen Intern Med.* 16:266–276.
7. van Wijk CM, Kolk AM. (1997). Sex differences in physical symptoms: The contribution of symptom perception theory. *Soc Sci Med.* 45:231–246.
8. Kroenke K, Price RK. (1993). Symptoms in the community. *Arch Intern Med.* 153:2474–2480.
9. Verbrugge LM, Ascione FJ. (1987). Exploring the iceberg: Common symptoms and how people care for them. *Med Care.* 25:539–569.
10. Calderone KL. (1990). The influence of gender on frequency of pain and sedative medication administered to postoperative patients. *Sex Roles.* 23: 713–725.
11. Cleeland CS, Gonin R, Hatfield AK *et al.* (1994). Pain and its treatment in outpatients with metastatic cancer. *N Engl J Med.* 330:592–596.
12. Breitbart W, Rosenfeld BD, Passik SD *et al.* (1996). The undertreatment of pain in ambulatory AIDS patients. *Pain.* 65:243–249.
13. McQuay HJ, Bullingham RES, Paterson GMC, Moore RA. (1980). Clinical effects of buprenorphine during and after operation. *Br J Anaesth.* 52: 1013–1019.
14. Bullingham RES, McQuay HJ, Dwyer D *et al.* (1981). Sublingual buprenorphine used postoperatively: Clinical observations and preliminary pharmacokinetics analysis. *Br J Clin Pharmacol.* 12:117–122.
15. Watson PJQ, McQuay HJ, Bullingham RES *et al.* (1982). Single-dose comparison of buprenorphine 0.3 and 0.6 mg I.V. given after operation: Clinical effects and plasma concentrations. *Br J Anaesth.* 54:37–43.
16. Bennett R, Batenhorst R, Graves DA *et al.* (1982). Variation in postoperative analgesic requirements in the morbidly obese following gastric bypass surgery. *Pharmacotherapy.* 2:50–53.
17. Tamsen A, Bondesson U, Dahlstrom B, Hartvig P. (1982). Patient controlled analgesic therapy, Part III: Pharmacokinetics and analgesic plasma concentrations of ketobemidone. *Clin Pharmacokinet.* 7:151–165.
18. Tamsen A, Hartvig P, Fagerlund C, Dahlstrom B. (1982). Patient controlled analgesic therapy, Part I: Pharmacokinetics of pethidine in the pre- and postoperative periods. *Clin Pharmacokinet.* 7:149–163.
19. Dahlstrom B, Tamsen A, Paalzow L, Hartvig P. (1982). Patient-controlled analgesic therapy, Part IV: Pharmacokinetics and analgesic plasma concentrations of morphine. *Clin Pharmacokinet.* 7:266–279.
20. Bahar M, Rsen M, Vickers MD. (1985). Self-administered nalbuphine, morphine, and pethidine. *Anesthesia.* 40:529–532.
21. Lehmann KA, Tenbuhs B. (1986). Patient-controlled analgesia with nalbuphine, a new narcotic agonist-antagonist, for the treatment of postoperative pain. *Eur J Clin Pharmacol.* 31:267–276.
22. Gourlay GK, Kowalski SR, Plummer JL *et al.* (1988). Fentanyl blood concentrations–analgesic response relationship in the treatment of postoperative pain. *Anesth Analg.* 67:329–337.
23. Burns JW, Hodsman NBA, McLintock TT *et al.* (1989). The influence of patient characteristics on the requirements for postoperative analgesia: A reassessment using patient-controlled analgesia. *Anesthesia.* 44:2–6.
24. De Kock M, Scholtes JL. (1991). Postoperative PCA in abdominal surgery. Analysis of 200 consecutive patients. *Acta Anaesthesiol Belg.* 42:85–91.
25. Tsui SL, Tong WN, Irwin M *et al.* (1996). The efficacy, applicability, and side effects of postoperative intravenous patient-controlled morphine analgesia: an audit of 1233 Chinese patients. *Anaesth Intens Care.* 24:658–664.
26. Sidebotham D, Dijkhuizen MRJ, Schug SA. (1997). The safety and utilization of patient controlled analgesia. *J Pain Symptom Manage.* 14:202–209.
27. Boethius G. (1977). Recording of drug prescriptions in the county of Jamtland, Sweden. *Acta Med Scand.* 202:241–251.
28. Klaukka T. (1988). Uses of prescription drugs in Finnish primary care. *Scand J Prim Health Care.* 6:43–50.
29. Ahonen R, Enlund H, Klaukka T, Vohlonen I. (1991). Use of analgesics in a rural Finnish population. *J Pharmacoepidemiol.* 2:3–17.
30. Eggen AE. (1993). The Tromso study: Frequency and predicting factors of analgesic drug use in a free-living population (12–56 years). *J Clin Epidemiol.* 46:1297–1304.
31. Turk DC, Okifuji A. (1999). Does sex make a difference in the prescription of treatments and the adaptation to chronic pain by cancer and non-cancer patients? *Pain.* 82:139–148.

32. Fillingim RB, Doleys DM, Edwards RR, Lowery D. (2003). Clinical characteristics of chronic back pain as a function of gender and oral opioid use. *Spine*. 28:143–150.

33. Kerns RD, Turk DC, Rudy TE. (1985). The West Haven-Yale Multidimensional Pain Inventory (WHYMPI). *Pain*. 23:345–356.

34. Walker JS, Carmody JJ. (1998). Experimental pain in healthy human subjects: Gender differences in nociception and in response to ibuprofen. *Anesth Anal*. 86:1257–1262.

35. Walker JS. (1995). NSAIDS: An update on their analgesic effects. *Clin Exp Physiol Pharmacol*. 22:855–860.

36. Gordon NC, Gear RW, Heller PH *et al*. (1995). Enhancement of morphine analgesia by the GABA-B agonist baclofen. *Neuroscience*. 69:345–349.

37. Gear RW, Gordon NC, Heller PH *et al*. (1996). Gender difference in analgesic response to the kappa-opioid pentazocine. *Neurosci Lett*. 205:207–209.

38. Gear RW, Miaskowski C, Gordon NC *et al*. (1996). Kappa-opioid produce significantly greater analgesia in women than in men. *Nat Med*. 2:1248–1250.

39. Gear RW, Miaskowski C, Gordon NC *et al*. (1999). The kappa-opioid nalbuphine produces gender and dose dependent analgesia and antianalgesia in patients with postoperative pain. *Pain*. 83:339–345.

40. Sarton E, Olofsen E, Romberg R *et al*. (2002). Sex differences in morphine analgesia—an experimental study in healthy volunteers. *Anesthesiology*. 93:1245–1254.

41. Dahan A, Sarton E, Teppema L, Olievier C. (1998). Sex-related differences in the influence of morphine on ventilatory control in humans. *Anesthesiology*. 88:903–913.

42. Zun LS, Downey LV, Gossman W *et al*. (2002). Gender differences in narcotic-induced emesis in the ED. *Am J Emerg Med*. 20:151–154.

77

Evaluation of Drugs in Women: Regulatory Perspective

SHIEW-MEI HUANG, PhD*, MARGARET MILLER, PhD**, THERESA TOIGO, RPh, MBA**, MIN C. CHEN, MS, RPh†, CHANDRA SAHAJWALLA, PhD*, LAWRENCE J. LESKO, PhD*, AND ROBERT TEMPLE, MD‡

*Office of Clinical Pharmacology and Biopharmaceutics, Center for Drug Evaluation and Research, Food and Drug Administration, Rockville, MD
** Office of the Commissioner, Food and Drug Administration, Rockville, MD
†Office of Drug Safety, Center for Drug Evaluation and Research, Food and Drug Administration, Rockville, MD
‡Office of Medical Policy, Center for Drug Evaluation and Research, Food and Drug Administration, Rockville, MD

I. Introduction

In the United States, the Food and Drug Administration (FDA) must approve medical products before marketing. For this approval, manufacturers need to submit clinical studies demonstrating that the medical product is safe and efficacious in a population reasonably similar to the population that would be treated after the drug was marketed [1]. Including women in clinical trials and examining clinical trial data for gender differences has, since the mid-1980s, been an integral part of the FDA's consideration of pharmaceutical products [2]. In a recent report, the Institute of Medicine (IOM) [3] supported the importance of studying potential gender differences during drug development. The IOM evaluated sexual differences in non-reproductive biology and concluded that differences in health and illness can be influenced by an individual's genetic and physiologic constitution. The incidence and severity of disease often vary between the sexes, and these differences could influence the safety or efficacy of therapeutic interventions. For example, females may be more likely to recover their language ability following a left hemisphere stroke than their male counterparts [4]. It seems possible that this could affect response to treatment. Females appear to have a greater susceptibility to development of life-threatening ventricular arrhythmia in response to various potassium-channel blocking drugs [5]. In addition to citing many examples of sex difference, the IOM concluded that sex should be considered when designing and analyzing studies in all areas and at all levels of biomedical and health-related research [3].

In its report, the IOM defined a gender difference as a difference between men and women that occurs resulting from cultural or social variations in a particular sex. A sex difference is defined as a difference resulting from the sex chromosome or sex hormones [3]. Because it will often not be clear whether an observed difference in drug safety or efficacy is due to gender or sex, the FDA has used the term gender to describe any difference, cultural/social or genetic/hormonal, between males and females [2].

The clinical investigation of a new pharmaceutical is usually divided into phases. Phase 1 includes the initial studies of the product in humans, generally involving 20 to 80 healthy volunteers or patients, to determine tolerability of various doses of the drug and to measure its absorption, metabolism, excretion, and disposition. The pharmacologic action of the product may also be assessed as an early indication of possible clinical effectiveness. These trials are often, but not always, randomized and placebo-controlled. Phase 2 studies are randomized, controlled clinical trials in several hundred patients (sometimes more) to evaluate the effectiveness of the product, explore dose-response, and determine common side effects, generally in a narrowly defined population. Phase 3 studies include further randomized, controlled clinical studies and other studies in several hundred to several thousand patients to gather additional information about effectiveness and safety, to study a wider range of patients (different stages of disease, on other drugs and with concomitant illnesses), to further assess dose response and, in general, to provide information on how to use the drug that will be incorporated in product labeling [6].

During the last 2 decades, the FDA has encouraged inclusion in clinical trials of a reasonable representation of both genders, of people with ethnic profiles similar to the population that will be using the product, and of people at the extremes of age [1]. Analyses of new drug application (NDA) databases must look for differences among those groups in both favorable and unfavorable responses. Although there has long been a concern that women were excluded from clinical trials, probably based on certain large cardiovascular studies, such as the early Veteran's Administration (VA) hypertension studies and the Physicians Health Study, in fact, women have been included in drug development studies at least since the early 1980's in approximate proportion to the prevalence of disease in them [2].

II. Current Status

A. Participation of Women in Clinical Trials (Safety/Efficacy) of New Medical Products and Gender Differences

Attention to potential gender differences is part of a larger effort by the FDA to ensure that the safety and efficacy of drugs are adequately studied in people who represent the full range of patients who will receive the drugs on marketing. Although the agency has always stated that pharmaceutical products should be tested in the full range of individuals likely to receive the medication once it is on the market, the FDA's 1977 guideline [7] recommending that women of childbearing potential be excluded from the earliest clinical studies allowed critics to suggest that young women might be excluded from drug development studies. That 1977 guideline said that women of childbearing potential could participate in clinical trials only if adequate information on efficacy and relative safety was obtained during early Phase 2 and if the animal fertility and teratology studies were completed. These recommendations were designed to protect the fetus, and there was an exception for potentially life-saving drugs. The document defined a woman "of childbearing potential" very broadly, including all premenopausal women capable of becoming pregnant. It included women on oral, injectable, or mechanical contraception; women who were single; and women whose husbands had been vasectomized [7]. In the 1980s, many women's advocacy groups, particularly the acquired immuno-deficiency syndrome (AIDS) and cancer communities, challenged the FDA's guidance on ethical grounds, claiming that women were being denied access to important therapies. Several groups questioned whether the drug development process, which tended to exclude women of reproductive potential from early clinical trials, produced adequate information about the safety and efficacy of drugs in women [8].

In 1988, the FDA issued a guidance on how to analyze clinical trial data [1] and emphasized the importance of conducting analyses for age, gender, and racial differences. In 1993, the FDA issued a guideline recommending that the effectiveness and adverse effects be analyzed by gender and that the pharmacokinetics (PKs) of a drug be defined in both men and women [2]. At the same time, the FDA revoked the 1977 guideline [7] that had limited participation of women of childbearing potential.

The 1993 "Guideline for the Study and Evaluation of Gender Differences in the Clinical Evaluation of Drugs" reiterated the FDA's expectations regarding including patients of both genders in drug development [2]. An analysis of participation of women in trials showed that the early exclusion of women of childbearing potential did not lead to under-representation of women generally or women younger than 50 in trials, but the agency nonetheless disavowed the 1977 guideline, largely because that guideline removed the ability of women to make decisions that affected their lives. The agency noted that there were ways to reduce fetal exposure through protocol design or contraception and that women, therefore, did not need to be excluded from clinical trials to protect the fetus.

In 1993, the FDA also published a guidance on the agency's use of the refuse-to-file (RTF) option for marketing applications that specifically stated that the agency could exercise its RTF authority if there were inadequate evaluation of safety and/or effectiveness in pertinent subpopulations, including gender, age, and racial groups [9]. Despite repeated encouragement, however, population subgroup analyses were not consistently performed by applicants.

The FDA completed a study [10] to assess the impact of the guideline by reviewing eligibility criteria for gender-based exclusions before and after the 1993 guideline (i.e., 1992 to 1993 [before] and 1994 to 1996 [after]). Eighty-one percent (3526/4352) of new protocols submitted from 1992 to 1996 to four Center for Drug Evaluation and Research (CDER) review divisions were categorized as (1) women (including women with childbearing potential) excluded, (2) women included but women with childbearing potential excluded, and (3) no specific gender-based exclusions. Women or women with childbearing potential were ineligible to participate in 26% (920/3526)

(1992=30%, 1993=26%, 1994=24%, 1995=23%, 1996=21%) of protocols, suggesting a declining rate of exclusion after the guideline. Women or women with childbearing potential were sometimes excluded from all phases of studies, but 40% of the exclusions were from phase 1 studies.

Informal FDA studies from as early as 1983 showed that women have not been excluded from participating in studies to support approval of NDAs. A 1983 study conducted by CDER reviewed a sample of pending NDAs and determined that, when anticancer drugs for exclusively male conditions were excluded, about half (52%) of the overall trial participants were women (Table 77-1, CDER-1). Nonsteroidal anti-inflammatory drugs were studied predominantly in women because arthritis, especially rheumatoid arthritis, is more common in women. Hypnotic and antibiotic drugs were studied in approximately equal proportions in men and women. Cardiac drugs were studied in a two-thirds male population; gender distribution in these NDAs for patients older than age 70 was about equal, but about two thirds of the patients were younger than 60 years, an age group in which angina and heart failure are more prevalent in men than in women.

Similar results were found in a CDER review of 12 NDAs approved in 1988 (see Table 77-1, CDER-2 report). Forty-five percent of the overall trial participants were women. The nonsteroidal anti-inflammatory drug approved was studied predominantly in women, as was nimodipine, for the prevention of vascular spasm after subarachnoid hemorrhage, also a female-predominant condition. The patient populations in the two NDAs to treat cardiac disease were almost two-thirds male. About 70% of the patients in studies for nizatidine and misoprostol were male. These drugs were studied extensively in duodenal ulcer, a predominantly male disease. Three of the drugs (pergolide, an anti-Parkinson's disease drug; astemizole, an antihistamine; and octreotide, a drug for symptoms of carcinoid tumor) were studied in about equal numbers of men and women. For reasons that are not clear, the remaining three drugs, (cefotiam, an intravenous antibiotic, and the topical drugs, naftifine and Photoplex), were studied predominantly in men. Certain tinea infections are more common in men, which could account for the high proportion (72%) of males in studies of naftifine.

In 1992, the General Accounting Office (GAO) analyzed the gender, age, and race distribution of all NDAs approved between January 1988 and June 1991 (see Table 77-1, GAO-1 report). Data were available for 53 of the 63 drugs approved during the 3½ year period. Women generally represented at least 40% of the trial participants for anti-infective, central nervous system, topical, antihistamine, and cancer drugs. Women represented at least 60% of trial participants for anti-inflammatory/analgesic drugs. One notable exception was the application for mefloquine, in which women represented only 11% of the participants. This occurred because the primary studies for mefloquine were conducted in Thai military personnel. Women fairly consistently represented less than 40% of the patients for anti-ulcer drugs (duodenal ulcer is more common in men) but accounted for 55% of the patients in the studies of Dipentum, a drug for ulcerative colitis, a disease more common in women. As in the previously cited FDA reviews, women consistently made up less than 40% of the populations studied for cardiovascular disease.

Table 77-1
Informal FDA Survey of Participation of Women in Clinical Trials

Report [References]	Year Completed	Data Source and Years Covered	Total Number of Applications	Sample for Analysis	% Participation by Women
GAO [49]	2001	NMEs submitted 8/98–12/00	82	36*	52
OWH/CBER[50]	2001	PLAs approved 1995–1999	63	24**	45
OSHI [45]	2001	NMEs approved 1995–1999	185	171†	48
GAO-1 [2]	1992	NDAs approved 1/88–6/91	63	53‡	44
CDER-2 [2]	1989	NDAs approved in 1988	20	12§	45
CDER-1 [2]	1983	Pending NDAs	11	9¶	52

CBER, Center for Biologics Evaluation and Research; CDER, Center for Drug Evaluation and Research; GAO, General Accounting Office; NDAs, new drug applications; NMEs, new molecular entities; OSHI, Office of Special Health Initiatives; OWH, Office of Women's Health; PLAs, product license applications.

*Includes approved and approvable applications that are not solely for pediatric or gender specific indications and for which gender data are available.

**Includes approved therapeutic and vaccine product license applications for which gender data are available. Herceptin, studied exclusively in women with breast cancer, was included in the analysis.

†Includes approved new molecular entities that are not solely for sex specific indications and for which gender data are available.

‡Includes approved applications that are not solely for sex specific indications and for which information was available.

§Includes approved applications that are not orphans or single-dose contrast agents and for which gender data were available.

¶Includes readily available applications that were not solely for a sex-specific indication.

None of the three surveys included antidepressant drugs, a class of drug frequently cited as needing study in women because women are frequently given antidepressants and because of suspected interactions of the drugs with the menstrual cycle. In the 1993 gender guideline [2], the FDA reviewed data on four antidepressants and found that women represented 58 to 65% of patients.

There have been no formal studies to review the methodology used for the by-gender analyses intended to look for differences in safety or effectiveness. An informal study conducted by CDER [11] reviewed 15 of the 25 new molecular entities (NMEs) approved in 1993. Three of the 15 applications had by-gender analysis of efficacy and 10 had by-gender analysis of safety. Three of the 15 applications did not examine gender at all. There was no mention in any application of exploring the relationship of any gender effects to body size and composition, age, or any other confounding factors.

More recent studies confirm that women continue to participate fully in clinical studies supporting NDAs. A 2001 study conducted by the Office of Special Health Issues (OSHI) examined NMEs approved by CDER between 1995 and 1999 (see Table 77-1, OSHI report). Information about clinical trial enrollment data was obtained from FDA medical officers' reviews of 185 NMEs containing descriptions of 2581 clinical trial protocols. Women participated in the clinical trials at nearly the same rate as men when gender-specific products were excluded, and participation differences generally seemed to reflect gender differences in prevalence. Overall, women appeared to have participated in lesser proportions in trials for cardiorenal, oncology, medical imaging, and antiviral drug products generally reflecting the prevalence of the cardiorenal and oncology conditions studied and the greater prevalence of HIV infection in men, and in greater proportions for neuropharmacologic, anesthetic, gastrointestinal and coagulation, anti-infectives, analgesics, and reproductive and urologic drug products. Women represented about half of the participants in three areas: metabolic/endocrine, pulmonary/allergy, and special pathogens/immunology (e.g., quinolone antibiotics, antituberculosis drugs, antirejection drugs).

This study also reviewed the 185 product labels for statements related to gender. Sixty-eight percent (125/185) contained some type of statement related to gender with 69 of those labels (37%) indicating that there were no differences between the genders. Forty-one (22%) indicated that there were gender differences observed. Fifteen (8%) of the labels stated no studies were performed, studies were inadequate, or the product was not indicated in a specific gender. The remaining 60 (32%) had no statements about gender.

A similar study was conducted for biologic products approved by the Center for Biologics Evaluation and Research (CBER) between 1995 and 1999 (see Table 77-1, OWH/CBER report). The Office of Women's Health and CBER reviewed 33 of the 63 approved product license applications (PLAs) containing 218 clinical study summaries. Overall, the representation of females and males in clinical trials appeared to be similar. The average percentage of females and males enrolled into the clinical studies across all PLAs was 45.3% and 54.6%, respectively. When PLAs for which complete gender data were available were analyzed, (n=24) females represented 45% of the participants. This analysis included pediatric vaccines. Some products were predominantly studied in men, such as a recombinant plasminogen activator for management of acute myocardial infarction and a recombinant platelet-derived growth factor (PDGF) for the treatment of lower extremity diabetic ulcers. One product for metastatic breast cancer was studied exclusively in women.

In 2001, the GAO reviewed 36/82 (44%) NMEs submitted to CDER between August 10, 1998 and December 31, 2000 (see Table 77-1, GAO report). All of the applications reviewed included enough women to demonstrate statistically that the drug was effective in women. Overall, women were 52% of the study participants in all the NDAs and were the majority of the participants in more than half of the NDAs reviewed. The GAO report noted that women made up more than one half of all participants in small-scale efficacy and full-scale safety and efficacy trials but only 22% of the participants in the initial small-scale safety studies used to set dosing levels for larger scale trials.

In 1998, the FDA amended its new drug regulations [21 CFR 314.50 (d)(5)(v) and (d)(5)(vi)(a)] to clearly require presentation of effectiveness and safety data for important demographic subgroups, specifically gender, age, and racial subgroups. The FDA also amended its regulations pertaining to investigational drugs [(21 CFR 312.33(a)(2)] to require sponsors to tabulate in their annual reports the numbers of subjects enrolled in clinical studies for drug and biologic products according to age, gender, and race. These new regulations are sometimes referred to as the Demographic Rule [12].

The 2001 GAO report also reviewed Investigational New Drug (IND) annual reports to assess compliance with the IND data presentation requirements in the 1998 Demographic Rule [12]. In a random sample of 100 INDs, the GAO found that 39% did not include the demographic data required by the regulation and that 24% did not tabulate the number of men and women enrolled in clinical drug trials. An FDA study also examined the extent to which IND sponsors complied with the reporting requirements of the 1998 Demographic Rule and found that required information was not submitted for 85% of the IND protocols with data reported [13].

The latest action undertaken by the agency to ensure that new drugs, biologics, and devices are adequately tested in both sexes was the publication of the Clinical Hold Rule [14]. This regulation allows the FDA to stop a clinical trial if the sponsor proposes to exclude patients from participating in the trial for a life-threatening disease solely because of their reproductive potential. The primary intent of this regulation is to ensure that women with life-threatening disease are not automatically denied access to an investigational drug trial because of their childbearing potential [14].

B. Clinical Pharmacology/Biopharmaceutic Studies (Including Drug-Interaction Studies) of New Drugs and Gender Differences

Many publications have suggested that differences in the PKs and pharmacodynamics (PDs) of an orally administered drug may be attributed to gender differences in the absorption, distribution, metabolism, and excretion of the drug and/or receptor sensitivity and that these differences may be affected by individuals' age, body weight (body mass index), menstrual cycle, pregnancy, use of oral contraceptives/hormonal replacement therapy and the other concomitant medications, disease states, and so forth [3,15–22, and references in these publications and discussions in previous chapters].

Gender-related differences in metabolism have been reviewed extensively [15–22]. Cytochrome P450 (CYP) CYP3A enzymes, including CYP3A4 and CYP3A5 (a polymorphically expressed enzyme), are the most abundant CYP enzymes in the liver and the intestinal tract and metabolize approximately half the therapeutic drugs currently on the market. Although data are not entirely consistent, many of the drugs that were primarily metabolized by CYP3A appeared to show a higher clearance in women, whereas those metabolized by other enzymes showed similar or lower clearance in women than men [3,15,23]. When other confounding factors (age, menopause, oral contraceptive use, etc.) are taken into consideration, the differential gender effects on CYP3A enzymes may not always be present.

A review of the clinical pharmacology and biopharmaceutical data in 300 NDAs received at the FDA between 1994 and 2000 was conducted to find any gender-dependent PK or PD information [24,25]. Of the 300 drugs reviewed, 163 had gender-based PK information and 39 had PD information. Of these, 27 drugs were predominantly excreted by the kidneys. The other drugs were metabolized by multiple metabolic enzymes (CYP and transferases), and some were substrates of transporters including P-glycoprotein (P-gp). As shown in Figure 77-1, CYP3A

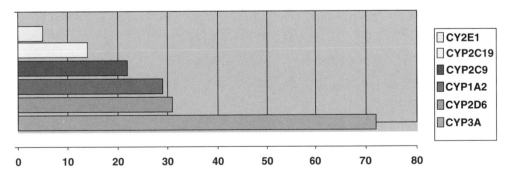

Fig. 77-1 Number of drugs metabolized by cytochrome P450 (CYP) enzyme (data from 163 new drug applications submitted between 1994 and 2000). Note that many drugs are substrates of multiple enzymes, in addition to transferases and transporters.

Table 77-2

Comparative Clearance Data (Body Weight Corrected) in Females (F) and Males (M) of 136 Drugs Metabolized by Various Enzymes and of 27 Drugs Excreted Via the Kidneys

Pathway		Number of Drugs that Showed Clearance Differences of the Following Magnitude				
		>40%	20–40%	<20%	Total	Grand Total
CYP3A	F>M	1	4		5	
	M>F	8	14		22	
	F=M			45	45	72
CYP2C9	F>M	0	2		2	
	M>F	2	5		7	
	F=M			15	15	24
CYP2C19	F>M	0	0		0	
	M>F	1	2		3	
	F=M			11	11	14
CYP2D6	F>M	0	1		1	
	M>F	2	11		13	
	F=M			17	17	31
CYP1A2	F>M	0	2		2	
	M>F	4	6		10	
	F=M			12	12	24
CYP2E1	F>M	0	0		0	
	M>F	0	2		2	
	F=M			3	3	5
Glucuronosyl transferases	F>M	0	2		2	
	M>F	5	16		21	
	F=M			46	46	69
Sulfotransferases	F>M	0	0		0	
	M>F	2	4		6	
	F=M			9	9	15
Renal excretion	F>M	0	0		0	
	M>F	0	5		5	
	F=M			22	22	27

Data from 163 NDAs submitted to Center for Drug Evaluation and Research (CDER) between 1994 and 2000 that contained gender analysis.

CYP, cytochrome P450.

contributed most to the Phase I metabolism of these drugs, followed by CYP2D6, CYP1A2, CYP2C9, CYP2C19, and CYP2E1.

Of the 163 applications in which the effect of gender on PK was evaluated, 51 showed a possible gender effect (i.e., a PK difference between genders of more than 20%; somewhat arbitrarily chosen as describing a difference that was potentially clinically significant). The PK studies were further evaluated to determine the effect of gender on specific drug-metabolizing enzymes. Of the 72 drugs metabolized by CYP3A, 45 drugs showed no gender difference in PK, 5 were cleared more rapidly by women, and 22 were cleared more slowly (Table 77-2). Table 77-2 also lists comparative clearance data in both genders of 136 drugs metabolized by various enzymes and of 27 drugs predominately excreted via the kidneys.

In many cases a 20% difference in clearance will not be clinically important. The survey results showed that (1) the majority (90%) of the PK differences between genders were less than 40%, a difference potentially more important; (2) except for one drug, when PK differences between genders were greater than 40%, females consistently showed higher plasma exposure (i.e., lower clearance); and (3) regardless of the disposition pathways involved, more than 50% of the drugs studied failed to show gender differences (i.e., a difference of <20%). The previously discussed observations are consistent with previous reports [3,15,23] that drugs that are substrates of CYP2C9, CYP2C19, CYP2D6, and CYP1A2 generally showed similar or higher plasma levels in females but contrast with results reported for CYP3A. Many of the earlier reports suggested that for drugs that are substrates for CYP3A, clearance values tended to be higher and plasma levels lower in females. The current survey indicates that, for the majority of drugs metabolized by CYP3A, plasma levels were generally similar or higher in females. The discrepancy could be due to the fact that many of the drugs reviewed in this survey are not predominantly metabolized by CYP3A and have additional pathways. Also some of the CYP3A substrates are substrates of P-gp transporter as well; it has been suggested that males may have higher hepatic expression of P-gp [26] and thus higher clearance of P-gp substrates.

It should be noted that the majority of the previously mentioned 163 gender analyses were based on limited data from a small number (≤12 subjects/group) of young males and young females studied just on one occasion. The studies were probably adequate to detect large gender differences in clearance, but their size makes it difficult to interpret small differences or a finding of no difference. In more recent submissions, additional groups of elderly subjects (>65 years old) have been added to allow the study of PK differences in four distinct groups (young males, elderly males, young females, and elderly females).

Although the FDA has emphasized the importance of examining the effect of (1) menstrual cycle/menopausal status, (2) concomitant estrogen supplementation or systemic contraception on the PK of the drug, and (3) the effect of the drug on oral contraceptives [27], in general the effects of the menstrual cycle, oral contraceptives, and postmenopausal hormonal replacement therapy have not been studied before marketing. Only 2 of the 163 original NDA submissions included the study of effects of menstrual cycle stage on PK.

As indicated earlier, many drugs are substrates of multiple pathways. The effects of a modulator of a particular pathway on the PK of a drug depends on the contribution of the particular pathway to the drug's overall clearance. When a drug is predominantly cleared by a particular pathway, a substantial change in the drug's clearance and its plasma levels would be expected when the drug is co-administered with an inhibitor or inducer of that pathway. A few drugs in recent submissions have been sensitive substrates for CYP3A; these drugs tended to show similar plasma levels in men and women in both young and elderly subjects but greater inhibition in women when a strong CYP3A inhibitor was co-administered. This observation, although limited, is consistent with findings from an earlier study on an interaction between clarithromycin, a CYP3A inhibitor, and midazolam, a CYP3A substrate [28]. That study showed a greater inhibition of midazolam metabolism in women than in men [28]. One possible explanation was higher baseline expression of CYP3A in young women. Although a recent publication failed to show gender differences when tirilazad, a CYP3A substrate, was co-administered with phenobarbital, an inducer of CYP3A [29], a recent submission contained data showing differential extent of induction of the drug with nifedipine in male and female volunteers. The literature has been sparse in addressing gender-related differences in drug interactions. An earlier survey looking at NDAs submitted between 1994 and 1995 showed that females constituted only one third of subjects in drug interaction studies [30]. More data will be needed to fully address possible gender-related differences in drug interactions.

C. Women in Bioequivalence Studies (Studies to Show Equivalent Bioavailability) of Generic Drugs

In the past, bioequivalence (BE) trials have been conducted primarily in males. Bioequivalence studies compare the bioavailability of two drug products, typically an innovator product and a generic product. As a rule, BE is shown when the 90% confidence interval for the ratio of the bioavailability parameters of the two drug products is between 0.8 and 1.25.

A survey of BE studies submitted to CDER between 1977 and 1995 for market access indicated 29 studies included at least six female subjects and at least six male subjects [31]. Of the 29 studies, 26 data sets were available for further analyses to assess gender differences in intrasubject variability and PK differences. The authors concluded that, in general, men and women had similar within-subject variability. Differences in PK parameters (area under the concentration-time curve [AUC], maximum concentration [Cmax]) between men and women should not affect BE studies, which use crossover designs. Thus, although ≥20% differences in such parameters were apparent in one third of the data set, the implication of this is unclear. Moreover, the differences were primarily the result of the greater milligram per kilogram dose in women (when subjects were given the same dose); thus, when body weight was taken into consideration, only 15% showed statistically significant differences. In October 2000, CDER published a guidance document [32] entitled "Bioavailability and Bioequivalence Studies for Orally Administered Drug Products—General Considerations" that recommended that "*in vivo* studies be conducted in individuals representative of the general population, taking into account age, sex, and race factors. If the drug product is intended for use in both sexes, the sponsor should attempt to include similar proportions of males and females in the study." A recent study [33] reviewed demographic data from *in vivo* BE studies in 35 abbreviated new drug applications (ANDAs) submitted to CDER in years 2000 and 2001 (before the publication of the guidance) and 51 studies submitted after the publication of the guidance. The results indicate a small increase (4 to 11%) in the participation of women in BE trials after publication of the guidance. Whether there will be gender-related BE differences remains to be determined and will be elucidated by the growing number of studies conducted in both genders.

D. Gender (or Sex) Differences in Postmarketing Adverse Event Reports

A review of 12 drugs withdrawn from the U.S. market between 1997 and 2001 indicates that serious drug interactions and risk of QT prolongation and torsade de pointes (TdP) were among the critical factors leading to withdrawal of half of them (Table 77-3).

A gender analysis [34–36] of the relevant postmarketing adverse event reports received by the FDA showed that many of these drugs had more reports in females than males (Table 77-4), but in most cases this appeared to reflect more use in women and the cases/use ratios seemed generally similar for most of the adverse event report cases. The exceptions seemed to be mibefradil, a CYP3A and P-gp inhibitor, and astemizole, where TdP and QT prolongation were reported more commonly in women than would have been expected based on their use of these products.

When specific combinations of drugs were reviewed, more rhabdomyolysis cases following use of simvastatin and mibefradil were reported in females (Table 77-5) [34]. Although more TdP cases were reported in females when terfenadine was

Table 77-3
Drugs Withdrawn from the U.S. Market Between 1997 and 2001

Year Withdrawn	Approval	Drug Name*	Use	Risk
1997	1973	Fenfluramine (Pondimin)	Obesity	Heart valve abnormality
1997	1996	Dexfenfluramine (Redux)	Obesity	Heart valve abnormality
1998	1997	Mibefradil (Posicor)	High blood pressure/chronic stable angina	Drug-drug interactions; torsade de pointes
1998	1997	Bromfenac (Duract)	NSAID	Acute liver failure
1998	1985	Terfenadine (Seldane/ Seldane-D)	Antihistamine	Torsade de pointes; drug-drug interactions
1999	1988	Astemizole (Hismanal)	Antihistamine	Torsade de pointes; drug-drug interactions
1999	1997	Grepafloxacin (Raxar)	Antibiotics	Torsade de pointes
2000	2000	Alosetron** (Lotronex)	Irritable bowel syndrome in women	Ischemic colitis; complications of constipation
2000	1993	Cisapride (Propulsid)	Heartburn	Torsade de pointes Drug-drug interactions
2000	1997	Troglitazone (Rezulin)	Diabetes	Acute liver failure
2001	1997	Cerivastatin (Baycol)	Cholesterol lowering	Rhabdomyolysis; Drug-drug interactions
2001	1999	Rapacuronium bromide (Raplon)	Anesthesia	Bronchospasm

*Trade names are in parentheses.
**Reintroduced to the market in 2002 with use restricted to patients severely affected with irritable bowel syndrome.
NSAID, nonsteroidal anti-inflammatory drug.

co-administered with ketoconazole or erythromycin (see Table 77-5), the number of cases was too small to make an adequate gender-based assessment.

The gender difference in drug-induced TdP is the most extensively studied example of a gender-related PD difference in drug toxicity. Torsade de pointes is defined as a polymorphic ventricular tachycardia that occurs following a lengthening of the QT interval [37]. Several studies have identified female gender as a risk factor for drug-induced TdP [5,37–40]. Makkar *et al* [37] found that women made up 70% of all cases of cardiovascular drug-related TdP. Several subsequent studies showed that drug-induced QT prolongation and TdP is more common in women across several diverse classes of drugs including antihistamines, antibiotics, and gastrointestinal prokinetics [5].

E. International Conference on Harmonization

As part of the international effort among Japan, the European Union and the United States, to harmonize technical requirements for registration of pharmaceuticals for human use, in 1996 the FDA published a "Guideline for Industry on the Structure and Content of Clinical Study Reports" (ICH E3) [41]. The guideline is intended to assist sponsors in developing a report that is complete, free from ambiguity, well organized, and easy to review. In addition to presenting detailed information about the study design and conduct, the study report should describe demographic and other potentially predictive characteristics of the study population, and, where the study is large enough to permit this, present data for demographic (e.g., age, sex, race, weight) and other (e.g., renal or hepatic function) subgroups so that possible differences in efficacy or safety can be identified.

Principles outlined in the 1994 "Guideline for Industry Studies in Support of Special Populations: Geriatrics" (ICH E7) [42] are similar to those articulated in the 1989 FDA geriatric guideline [43], the 1993 gender guideline [2], and the 1988 "Guideline for the Format and Content of the Clinical and Statistical Sections of New Drug Applications" [1]. In general, the guidelines do not ask for specific numbers of exposed people in any group. Each, however, maintains that drugs should be studied in all groups for which they will have significant utility and that patients entering clinical trials should be reasonably representative of the population that will later be treated by the drug. The overall databases should be examined for the presence of age- or sex-related differences, (e.g., in adverse event rates, in effectiveness, and in dose-response). If these relatively crude overview analyses show important differences, further evaluation may be needed.

Table 77-4

Comparative Data in Female (F) and Male (M) Patients in Food and Drug Administration (FDA) Postmarketing Adverse Event Reports (AERs) and Drug Use for Drugs Withdrawn from the U.S. Market Between 1997 and 2000

Drug Name	Use*,** %F/%M	Utilization Dates	FDA AERs Cases** %F/%M (Includes All Cases Indicated)		FDA AERs Cases** %F/%M (Only QT Prolongation and Torsade Cases)
Fenfluramine (Pondimin)	83/14	1995–1999	97/3	Valvulopathy cases from fenfluramine-phentermine combination reports received through 8/29/1997	†
Dexfenfluramine (Redux)	77/19	1996–1998	93/7	Valvulopathy cases from FDA-sponsored cardiac ultrasound study in the United States, AERs data not available	†
Mibefradil (Posicor)	47/52	1997–1998	61/22	Torsade de pointes, ventricular arrhythmia, ventricular fibrillation, QT prolongation, cardiac arrest	70/21
Bromfenac (Duract)	56/41	1997–1999	58/42	Fatal liver failure/liver transplant	†
Terfenadine (Seldane/ Seldane-D)	61/33	1994–1999	72/28	All cardiac events for 1995–1999	68/20
Astemizole (Hismanal)	63/32	1994–1999	55/23	All cardiac events	93/7
Grepafloxacin (Raxar)	51/44	1997–1999	54/38	Torsade de pointes, ventricular arrhythmia, ventricular fibrillation, QT prolongation, cardiac arrest	‡
Alosetron (Lotronex)	86/10	2000	99/1	Ischemic colitis/severe constipation	†
Cisapride (Propulsid)	57/40	1994–1999	61/37	Torsade de pointes, ventricular arrhythmia, ventricular fibrillation, QT prolongation, cardiac arrest	66/34
Troglitazone (Rezulin)	53/42	1997–1999	65/35	Acute liver failure	†

Note that, because of the voluntary reporting nature of the FDA's adverse event reporting system, adverse event rates cannot be accurately estimated from these data.

*Use data from IMS Health; National Disease and Therapeutic Index, online data; projected total number of drug appearances during patient visits in office-based practices in the continental United States for drug, stratified by gender.

**Note that, when the sum of %F and %M did not add to 100%, the balance was due to reports with unspecified sex.

†Not reviewed for these drugs.

‡Case number too small for comparison.

F. Valid Analysis

The National Institutes of Health (NIH) Revitalization Act of 1993 directed the NIH to establish guidelines for inclusion of women and minorities in NIH-sponsored clinical research. The National Institutes of Health policies and guidelines related to this law have been updated since the original guideline published in 1994. The National Institutes of Health was directed to ensure that, when women and minorities were included as subjects, trials were designed and carried out in a manner that would provide for "valid analysis" of differences between women and minority groups and other participants in the trial [44]. The National Institutes of Health guidelines (2001) direct investigators to consider appropriate representation of subjects of different genders and race/ethnicity, to provide the opportunity for detecting major qualitative differences, and to identify more subtle differences that may be explored more fully in specifically targeted studies. The guidelines ask that before the design of phase 3 studies, there should be a review of evidence to determine whether clinically important sex and minority based differences are expected. This evidence may include, but is not limited to, data derived from prior animal studies; clinical

Table 77-5

Number of Adverse Drug Reaction (ADR) Reports in Patients Given Mibefradil (a CYP3A and P-gp Inhibitor) or Terfenadine (a CYP3A Substrate) Concomitantly with Other Drugs

Mibefradil Combination	ADR	Females	Males
Cyclosporin	Renal failure	0	1
Lovastatin	Rhabdomyolysis	0	2 (1 unknown)
Simvastatin	Rhabdomyolysis	18 (1 unknown)	8 (1 unknown)
Cerivastatin	Rhabdomyolysis	0	2
Atorvastatin	Rhabdomyolysis	1	0
Cisapride	Torsade	18	6

Terfenadine Combination	ADR	Females	Males
Ketoconazole	Torsade	4	0
Erythromycin	Torsade	3	1

observations; metabolic studies; genetic studies; pharmacology studies; and observational, natural history, epidemiology, and other relevant studies. If men and women are thought likely to respond differently to an intervention, then the phase 3 clinical trial should be designed to answer two separate primary questions, one for men and the other for women, with adequate sample size for each. When prior studies neither support nor negate significant differences of clinical or public health importance, the phase 3 trial should support the sufficient and appropriate accrual of participants by sex and race/ethnicity, so that a valid analysis of the intervention effects can be performed. The NIH defined a valid analysis to mean an unbiased assessment. In defining valid analysis, the NIH policy stated that it should be conducted for both small and large studies and does not need to have a high statistical power for detecting a stated effect. The policy further states that an unbiased process such as randomization should be used to allocate study participants of both sexes/genders to the intervention and control groups, that evaluation of outcomes of study participants should be unbiased, and that unbiased statistical analyses and proper methods of inference should be used to estimate and compare the intervention effects among the sex/gender groups.

G. Labeling Consequences

Many of the gender differences described in labeling are PK differences. A review of the 185 product labels approved between 1995 and 1999 revealed that 125/185 (68%) contained some type of statement related to gender and 41 (22%) indicated that there were actual gender differences [45]. Of the 41 products for which labeling described gender effects, 90% (37/41) were PK differences, 12% (5/41) were safety differences, and 5% (2/41) were efficacy differences. Most of the descriptions of these gender differences appear in the clinical pharmacology or special population sections of the labeling. Table 77-6 lists some examples of the labeling language showing differences in PK parameters. In addition, Table 77-7 lists examples of PD differences between genders and the current labeling language.

In a proposed revision of physician labeling format and content in 2000, significant (or evidence of no) differences between genders would appear in the highlights section, in addition to having this information in the main body of the labeling [46].

III. Recommendations: When to Conduct Gender-Specific Studies

When there are special concerns based on what is known about a particular drug (preclinical data, related drugs), an accelerated gender analysis program may be indicated. For example, when prior information indicates a possible significant gender-specific difference, especially for a drug with a potentially narrow therapeutic ratio, it may be useful to conduct an early PK study to assess the difference in PK between men and women. Based on this data, further clinical trials may be designed that will use different doses for men and women (e.g., clinical trials of dofetilide used a dose adjusted for creatinine clearance [CrCl]). In any case, appropriate analyses of safety and efficacy data by gender and obtaining population PK data should shed light on critical gender differences and the need for dosage or other adjustments.

IV. Conclusion and Future Directions

Although women have been included in drug development in numbers predicted by their disease prevalence whenever this has been examined, the conduct of gender-specific analysis has become standard only in the last decade; these are often referenced in labeling. Pharmacokinetic differences, by far the most common known gender differences, are readily assessed because gender-specific PK data are now regularly obtained. The exclusion of women from early trials in life-threatening conditions because of their childbearing potential was barred by regulation in 1993.

Current practice should ensure the detection of large gender differences in response, but subtle differences may be undetected until they are specifically sought. The profound gender effects of the selective serotonin reuptake inhibitor (SSRI) antidepressants on sexual function in women were significantly underestimated [47,48] for years because usual clinical trials do not assess this function well. The greater susceptibility of women to drugs that cause TdP arrhythmias also took many years to become recognized, as did the potential of CYP3A inducers to render oral

Table 77-6
Labeling Examples of Drugs Showing Gender Differences in PK Parameters

Drug Name (Brand Name)	Labeling Section	Labeling Statement
Atorvastatin (Lipitor)	Clinical pharmacology	Plasma concentrations of atorvastatin in women differ from those in men (approximately 20% higher for C_{max} and 10% lower for AUC); however, there is no clinically significant difference in LDL-C reduction with LIPITOR between men and women.
Dofetilide (Tikosyn)	Clinical pharmacology	Pharmacokinetics in special populations. Women: a population pharmacokinetic analysis showed that women have approximately 12–18% lower dofetilide oral clearances than men (14–22% greater plasma dofetilide levels), after correction for weight and creatinine clearance. In females, as in males, renal function was the single most important factor influencing dofetilide clearance. In normal female volunteers, hormone replacement therapy (a combination of conjugated estrogens and medroxyprogesterone) did not increase dofetilide exposure.
Pioglitazone (Actos)	Clinical pharmacology	The mean C_{max} and AUC values were increased 20 to 60% in females.
Rosiglitazone (Avandia)	Clinical pharmacology	Results of the population pharmacokinetics analysis showed that the mean oral clearance of rosiglitazone in female patients (n = 405) was approximately 6% lower compared with male patients of the same body weight (n = 642).
Temozolomide (Temodar)	Clinical pharmacology	Population PK analysis indicates that women have an approximately 5% lower clearance (adjusted for body surface area) for temozolomide than men.

AUC, area under the concentration-time curve; C_{max}, maximum concentration; LDL-C, LDL-cholesterol; PK, pharmacokinetic.

Table 77-7
Labeling Examples of Drugs Showing Gender Differences in PD Parameters

Drug Name (Brand Name)	Labeling Section	Labeling Statement
Dofetilide (Tikosyn)	Precaution	Use in women. Female patients constituted 32% of the patients in the placebo-controlled trials of Tikosyn. As with other drugs that cause torsade de pointes, Tikosyn was associated with a greater risk of torsade de pointes in female patients than in male patients. During the Tikosyn clinical development program the risk of torsade de pointes in females was approximately 3 times the risk in males. Unlike torsade de pointes, the incidence of other ventricular arrhythmias was similar in female patients receiving Tikosyn and patients receiving placebo. Although no study specifically investigated this risk, in post hoc analyses, no increased mortality was observed in females on Tikosyn compared with females on placebo.
Sertraline (Zoloft)	Clinical trials	Posttraumatic Stress Disorder (PTSD): because PTSD is a more common disorder in women than men, the majority (76%) of patients in these trials were women (152 and 139 women on sertraline and placebo versus 39 and 55 men on sertraline and placebo; Studies 1 and 2 combined). Post hoc exploratory analyses revealed a significant difference between Zoloft and placebo on the CAPS, IES, and CGI in women, regardless of baseline diagnosis of comorbid depression, but essentially no effect in the relatively smaller number of men in these studies. The clinical significance of this apparent gender interaction is unknown at this time
		Depression: analyses for gender effects on outcome did not suggest any differential responsiveness on the basis of sex.
		Obsessive compulsive disorder (OCD): analyses for age and gender effects on outcome did not suggest any differential responsiveness on the basis of age or sex.
		Panic disorder: subgroup analyses did not indicate that there were any differences in treatment outcomes as a function of age, race, or gender.

Continued

Table 77-7

(Continued)

Drug Name (Brand Name)	Labeling Section	Labeling Statement
Pioglitazone (Actos)	Clinical pharmacology	As monotherapy and in combination with sulfonylurea, metformin, or insulin, Actos improved glycemic control in both males and females. In controlled clinical trials, hemoglobin A_{1c} (HbA_{1c}) decreases from baseline were generally greater for females than for males (average mean difference in HbA_{1c} 0.5%). Because therapy should be individualized for each patient to achieve glycemic control, no dose adjustment is recommended based on gender alone.
Rosiglitazone (Avandia)	Clinical pharmacology	As monotherapy and in combination with metformin, Avandia improved glycemic control in both males and females. In metformin combination studies, efficacy was demonstrated with no gender differences in glycemic response.
		In monotherapy studies, a greater therapeutic response was observed in females; however, in more obese patients, gender differences were less evident. For a given body mass index (BMI), females tend to have a greater fat mass than males. Because the molecular target PPAR(gamma) is expressed in adipose tissues, this differentiating characteristic may account, at least in part, for the greater response to Avandia in females. Because therapy should be individualized, no dose adjustments are necessary based on gender alone.
Temozolomide (Temodar)	Clinical pharmacology	Women have higher incidences of grade 4 neutropenia and thrombocytopenia in the first cycle of therapy than men (see adverse reactions).
	Adverse reactions	In clinical trial experience with 110 to 111 women and 169 to 174 men (depending on measurements), there were higher rates of grade 4 neutropenia (ANC < 500 cells/μL) and thrombocytopenia (<20,000 cells/μL) in women than men in the first cycle of therapy (12% vs 5% and 9% vs 3%, respectively).

ANC, absolute neutrophil count; CAPS, clinician-administered PTSD scale part 2; CGI, clinical global impression; IES, impact of event scale.

contraceptives ineffective. It seems certain that further discoveries of gender differences await investigators and that the systematic search for such differences throughout drug development and after marketing will discover them.

V. Suggestions for Further Investigations

- Are there differences of PK between men and women other than those resulting from body weight differences?
- What are the effects of oral contraceptives and hormonal replacement therapy on metabolism of drugs? What drugs affect the efficacy of oral contraceptives?
- In general, are there more adverse event reports in women as compared with men? Is this due to higher percentage of use, higher reporting, or increased sensitivity to certain adverse events in women?
- When should clinical trials be designed to give different doses to men and women (doses adjusted for different gender)?
- When should drugs be labeled differently for women and men?

References

1. Federal Register Notice. (1988). Guideline for the format and content of the clinical and statistical sections of an application. Available July 1988; posted on the Internet in 1997 (http://www.fda.gov/cder/guidance/index.htm) (accessed February 16, 2004).
2. Federal Register Notice. (1993). The study and evaluation of gender differences in the clinical evaluation of drugs. Guideline for the study and evaluation of gender differences in the clinical evaluation of drugs. Federal Register, Notice. 58: 39406–39416; posted on the Internet in 1998 (http://www.fda.gov/cder/guidance/index.htm) (accessed February 16, 2004).
3. Institute of Medicine, Committee on Understanding the Biology of Sex and Gender Differences. (2001). *Exploring the Biological Contributions to Human Health, Does Sex Matter?* (Wizemann TM, Pardue ML, eds.). Washington DC: National Academy Press.
4. Shaywitz BA, Shaywitz, SE, Pugh KR *et al.* (1995). Sex differences in the functional organization of the brain for language. *Nature.* 373:607–609.
5. Ebert SN, Liu XK, Woosley R. (1998). Female gender as a risk factor for drug-induced cardiac arrhythmias: Evaluation of clinical and experimental evidence. *J Womens Health.* 7:547–557.
6. Code of Federal Register (CFR) US Government Printing Office, 312.21.
7. FDA Gender Guideline. (1977). Section on Women of Childbearing Potential. General Consideration for the Clinical Evaluation of Drugs. (HEW publication No. FDA 77–3040).
8. LaRosa JH. (1997). Women's Health Policy and Research. In *Women's Health Across the Lifespan: A Comprehensive Perspective* (Allen KM, Phillips JM eds.), pp. 3–16. Philadelphia: Lippincott.
9. Federal Register Notice. (1993). Guidance on the Agency's use of the refusal-to-file (RTF) option per Code of Federal Register (CFR) 314.101(d)(3), as quoted in the following Federal Register: February 11, 1998 (Volume 63, Number 28), pp. 6854–6862.
10. Toigo T, Struble K, Behrman R *et al.* (1999). Eligibility of Women to Participate in Clinical Trials: The 1993 Gender Guideline, Before And After. Presented at the Annual Drug Information Association Meeting, Baltimore, MD, June 1999.
11. Gender Analysis Workshop. 1995 Transcript pp. 33–43, presentation by Stella Machado, Director Quantitative Methods and Research Staff, CDER.
12. Federal Register Notice. (1998). Final Rule on Investigational New Drug Applications and New Drug Applications.
13. Evelyn B. (2001). Race, Age and Gender: A Review of Demographic Subgroups in Clinical Trials of FDA-Regulated Drugs and Biologics. Presented at the FDA Science Forum, February 2001, Washington DC (http://fda.gov/oc/meeting/2001sciforum.html) (EveLyn B9).
14. Federal Register Notice. (1998). CFR Part 312 [Docket No. 98N–0979] Investigational New Drug Applications; Clinical Holds.

15. Harris RZ, Benet LZ, Schwartz JB. (1995). Gender effects in pharmacokinetics and pharmacodynamics. *Drugs.* 50:222–239.

16. Beierle I, Meibohm B, Derendorf H. (1999). Gender differences in pharmacokinetics and pharmacodynamics. *Int J Clin Pharmacol Ther.* 37:529–547.

17. Meibohm B, Beierle I, Derendorf H. (2002). How important are gender differences in pharmacokinetics? *Clin Pharmacokinet.* 41:329–3342.

18. Gleiter CH, Gundert-Ermy U. (1996). Gender differences in pharmacokinetics. *Eur J Drug Metab Pharmacokinet.* 21(2):123–128.

19. Schwartz JB. (2000). Gender and dietary influences on drug clearance. *J Gend Specif Med.* 3:30–32.

20. Kashuba AD, Nafziger AN. (1998). Physiological changes during the menstrual cycle and their effects on the pharmacokinetics and pharmacodynamics of drugs. *Clin Pharmacokinet.* 34:203–218.

21. Fletcher CV, Acosta EP, Strykowski JM. (1994). Gender differences in human pharmacokinetics and pharmacodynamics. *J Adolesc Health.* 15:619–629.

22. Bonate PL. (1991). Gender-related differences in xenobiotic metabolism. *J Clin Pharmacol.* 31:684–690.

23. Schwartz JB. The influence of sex on pharmacokinetics. *Clin Pharmacokinet.* 42:107–121.

24. Sahajwalla C, Mehta M, Chow W. (2001). OWH report on gender differences in PK and PD of drugs in NDAs submitted to CDER between 1994 and 2000 (manuscript submitted for publication).

25. Miller MA, Hollinger KA. (2002). Gender differences in disease and the safety and efficacy of prescription medicines. Workshop on Biological Variability in Children and Implications for Environmental Risk Assessment: New Perspectives on Ethnicity, Race and Gender, University of Maryland, March 17–19, 2002.

26. Schuetz E, Furyak K, Schuetz J. (1995). Interindividual variation in expression of P-glycoprotein in normal human liver and secondary hepatic neoplasms. *JPET.* 275:1011–1018.

27. Merkatz RB, Temple R, Sobel S et al., Working Group on Women in Clinical Trials. (1993). Women in clinical trials of new drugs—a change in Food and Drug Administration policy. *N Engl J Med.* 329:292–296.

28. Gorski JC, Jones DR, Haehner-Daniels D et al. (1998). The contribution of intestinal and hepatic CYP3A to the interaction between midazolam and clarithromycin. *Clin Pharmacol Ther.* 64:133–143.

29. Fleishaker JC, Pearson LK, Peters GR. (1996). Gender does not affect the degree of induction of tirilazad clearance by phenobarbital. *Eur J Clin Pharmacol.* 50:139–145.

30. Huang S-M, Lesko LJ, Williams RL. (1999). Assessment of the quality and quantity of drug-drug interaction studies in NDA submissions: Study design and data analysis issues. *J Clin Pharmacol.* 39:1006–1014.

31. Chen ML, Lee SC, Ng MJ et al. (2000). Pharmacokinetic analysis of bioequivalence trials: Implications for sex-related issues in clinical pharmacology and biopharmaceutics. *Clin Pharmacol Ther.* 68:510–521.

32. CDER Guidance for Industry. (2003). General BA/BE guidance bioavailability and bioequivalence studies for orally administered drug products—(Issued 3/2003, Posted 3/19/2003); available at http://www.fda.gov/cder/guidance/index.htm (accessed February 16, 2004).

33. Kim CY, Davit BM, Conner DP. (2002). Demographics of subjects in bioequivalence studies of generic drug products. Presented at the American Society of Clinical Pharmacology and Therapeutics, March, 2001, Atlanta, GA, abstract in *Clin Pharmacol Ther.* 71:19.

34. Huang S-M, Booth B, Fadiran E et al. (2000). What have we learned from the recent market withdrawal of terfenadine and mibefradil? Presentation at the 101 Annual Meeting of American Society of Clinical Pharmacology and Therapeutics, March 15–17, 2000, Beverly Hills, CA, abstract in *Clin Pharmacol Ther.* 67:148.

35. Drug Safety. (2001). Most Drugs Withdrawn in Recent Years Had Greater Health Risks for Women. GAO-01–286R. Available at http://www.gao.gov/new.items/d01286r.pdf. January 19, 2001. (Accessed February 16, 2004).

36. Wysowski D, Corken A, Gallo-Torres H et al. (2001). Postmarketing reports of QT prolongation and ventricular arrhythmia in association with cisapride and Food and Drug Administration regulatory actions. *Am J Gastroenterol.* 96:1698–1703.

37. Makkar RR, Fromm BS, Steinman RT et al. (1993). Female gender as a risk factor for torsades de pointes associated with cardiovascular drugs. *JAMA.* 270:2590–2597.

38. Reinoehl J, Frankovich D, Machado C et al. (1996). Probucol-associated tachyarrhythmic events and QT prolongation: Importance of gender. *Am Heart J.* 131:1184–1191.

39. Lehmann MH, Hardy S, Archibald D et al. (1996). Sex difference in risk of torsade de pointes with d,l-sotalol. *Circulation.* 94:2535–2541.

40. Liu XK, Wang W, Ebert SN et al. (1999). Female gender is a risk factor for torsades de pointes in an *in vitro* animal model. *J Cardiovasc Pharmacol.* 34:287–294.

41. ICH E3. (1996). Structure and content of clinical study reports, available at http://www.fda.gov/cder/guidance/index.htm), published July 1996 accessed).

42. ICH E7. (1994). Studies in support of special populations: Geriatrics. Available at http://www.fda.gov/cder/guidance/index.htm, published August 1994 (accessed February 16, 2004).

43. Guidance for Industry. (1989). Guideline for the study of drugs likely be used in the elderly. Available at http://www.fda.gov/cder/guidance/index.htm, issued November 1989, posted on the Internet March 1998 (accessed February 16, 2004).

44. National Institutes of Health (2001). NIH policy and guidelines on the inclusion of women and minorities as subjects in clinical research—amended October 2001. Available at http://grants1.nih.gov/grants/funding/women_min.htm (accessed February 16, 2004).

45. Evelyn B, Toigo T, Banks D. (2001). Women's Participation in Clinical Trials and Gender-Related Labeling: A Review of New Molecular Entities Approved 1995–1999. http://www.fda.gov/cder/reports/womens_health/women_clin_trials.htm.

46. Federal Register Notice. (2000). Labeling guideline (Federal Register 65:247;81082–81131; December 22, 2000).

47. Jacobson F. (1992). Fluoxetine-induced sexual dysfunction and an open trial of yohimbine. *J Clin Psychiatry.* 53:119–122.

48. Clayton AH, Pradko JF, Croft HA et al. (2002). Prevalence of sexual dysfunction among newer antidepressants. *J Clin Psychiatry.* 63:357–366.

49. GAO Report: United States General Accounting Office GAO-01–754. (2001). Report to congressional requesters, women's health—women sufficiently represented in new drug testing but FDA oversight needs improvement. Available at http://www.gao.gov.

50. OWH/CBER: Gruber M. (2001). FDA scholarship in women's health program: Participation of females in clinical trials and gender analysis of data in biological product applications. http://www.fda.gov/cder/clinical/femclin.htm.

78

Gender and Antidepressants

ROBERT R. BIES, PHARMD, PhD, KRISTIN L. BIGOS, BS, AND BRUCE G. POLLOCK, MD, PhD

Departments of Psychiatry, Pharmaceutical Sciences, and Pharmacology, University of Pittsburgh, Pittsburgh, PA

I. Introduction

Antidepressants, like most other medications, are developed without regard for the sex of the patient [1–3]. This is unfortunate, because the dose that is developed for general use typically ignores potential gender differences and may contribute to an increase in inadequate responses or adverse drug reactions in female or male patients [1,4–6]. The prior exclusion of women of child-bearing age from pharmacokinetic studies is especially pertinent for antidepressants because of the marked gender differences in the epidemiology of depression. From puberty until menopause, nearly twice as many women (12%) as men (7%) are affected by a depressive disorder each year [7]. Women also exhibit more atypical symptoms of depression, with greater somatization, increased suicide attempts, and comorbid anxiety, whereas men tend to have more comorbid alcohol or drug abuse and completed suicides [8,9]. Gender-specific differences, which have been found to affect other medications, may also be pertinent to antidepressants. Although the evidence is limited, differences in pharmacokinetics have been shown for several agents (Table 78-1). There is also evidence for gender-related pharmacodynamic differences (Table 78-2). Tables 78-1 and 78-2 were derived from several sources including Medline and PsychInfo searches from 1966 through week 3 (Medline) or week 5 (PsychInfo) of August 2002 under the keywords (and general word searches) sex, gender, pharmacokinetics, and antidepressants in various combinations and a search of the 56th edition of the *Physicians' Desk Reference* [10] for each antidepressant. In general, these tables reflect the paucity of studies evaluating gender-specific differences.

Physiologic differences that may affect pharmacokinetics are discussed in the following section and include average body weight, body water distribution, and the affinity and/or capacity of metabolizing enzymes for the administered drug. Medications could also have effects on the metabolizing pathways for various hormones. The resulting changes in hormone concentrations could contribute to attenuated responses or the occurrence of an adverse event or have a protective effect [6,11–14]. Of particular concern are epidemiologic studies suggesting a possible increase in the risk of breast cancer with use of selective serotonin reuptake inhibitors (SSRIs) [6,14]. An additional underexplored topic is whether exogenous hormone therapy (i.e., oral contraceptives and hormone replacement therapy) may be affected by antidepressants. Conversely, there are very limited data as to whether exogenous hormone therapy alters antidepressant pharmacokinetics or pharmacodynamics. Gender-specific differences that may affect therapy with antidepressants are outlined in detail in the following sections.

II. Nonmetabolic Factors Affecting Drug Disposition

Nonmetabolic factors that affect drug disposition include absorption, distribution (including protein binding), and elimination. Each of these factors is different for men and women. These differences and their potential impact on antidepressant drug disposition are discussed in the following sections.

A. Absorption

Most antidepressants are weak bases; thus, they are most effectively absorbed under less acidic/more basic conditions. Women secrete less gastric acid resulting in a more basic environment that potentially might result in enhanced absorption of antidepressants in the stomach [15]. Colonic transit times are also prolonged in women giving the compounds more time to be absorbed in an environment where the pH favors absorption of weak bases. Women have a slower rate of gastric emptying than men thus increasing antidepressant absorption time [16]. This increase persists even after menopause [17] and is accentuated by exogenous estrogen and progesterone [16,17]. Despite this, enhanced bioavailability in women has not been demonstrated in any bioequivalence trial for antidepressants, although a higher body-weight normalized AUC for bupropion was shown for adolescent women versus men [18].

B. Distribution

The volume of distribution into which an administered drug distributes modulates the amount of drug experienced by the patient. There are substantive differences in body composition between men and women that affect the volume of distribution. Adipose tissue comprises 33% of body weight in young women compared with 18% in young men [19,20]. In elderly women, 48% of body weight is adipose compared with 36% in old men [19,20]. Thus, for lipophilic drugs, there is a much larger volume of distribution possible for those compounds. This can result in a significantly prolonged half-life and a lower observed serum/plasma concentrations of an administered drug. This has been shown for trazodone [21] and bupropion [22] where volume of distribution is increased secondary to increased body fat in women, which is further exaggerated in elderly women.

In addition, Kristensen [23] found that women aged 30 to 39 had significantly lower binding of imipramine than men aged 30 to 39 and women of other age groups. This change was not associated with smoking status or oral contraceptive use. No other data could be found with regard to differential protein binding across sex for any antidepressant.

Table 78-1

Reported Interactions of Gender and Pharmacokinetics for Antidepressants

Antidepressant	Gender Effects
TCAs	Tricyclic antidepressants
Desipramine	Desipramine levels increased 2-fold at midpoint of menstrual cycle [75]. No effect of gender in adolescence on desipramine clearance [97]
Nortriptyline	Women had higher steady state nortriptyline levels, and different nortriptyline to hydroxynortriptyline (OHNT) ratios than men [35] Bayesian optimal sampling modeling did not identify gender as a significant effect in model for PK disposition [98]
Clomipramine	Higher concentrations of desmethylclomipramine (DMC) and lower hydroxylation rates of clomipramine in women vs men. DMC levels are higher and DMC/8-HDMC (hydroxylation ratios) are higher at 8 hours in women than in men [34]
SSRIs	Selective serotonin reuptake inhibitors
Fluvoxamine	Female children had significantly higher AUC_{0-12} and C_{max} than male children 6–11 years old (approximately 3-fold higher AUC and C_{max} in females). Gender difference did not persist in adolescence [10,p. 3257] More pronounced concentration increase in men versus women with dose doubling after 14 weeks of treatment (4.6 fold vs 2.4 fold $p<0.05$) [31]. Plasma drug levels 40–50% lower in men than in women [30]
Sertraline	Lower desmethylsertraline clearance in older men but not in older women [10,p. 2751]. Young women, elderly men, and elderly women had similar terminal elimination half-life (32–37 hours), which were greater than those in young men (22 hours) [28]
Citalopram	Three PK studies (n = 32) showed 1.5 to 2 times higher AUC values for women versus men [10,p. 1365]. Dose-corrected concentrations higher in female adolescents versus males [29]
Others	
Bupropion	AUC, C_{max}, Vd (wt normalized) half-life (terminal) of parent and AUC of metabolite significantly higher in adolescent females compared with males, no difference in CL/F [18]. Half-life longer, Vd larger, and CL slightly lower for elderly women versus young men [22]
Mirtazapine	Longer terminal half-life in women (37 vs 26 hours). No other gender differences reported [10,p. 2483]. One half the plasma concentrations in adult men versus women or elderly men and women [32,33]
Buspirone	No significant gender differences [100,101]
Nefazodone	C_{max}, AUC higher in women seen after first dose, difference does not persist with multiple dosing [10,p. 1104]. Nefazodone and hydroxynefazodone levels 50% higher in elderly women versus elderly men, young men, and young women. All subjects extensive 2D6 metabolizers [27]. Doses may need to be increased in the second and third trimesters [83]
Trazodone	Increased half-life in elderly versus young women (7.6 vs 5.9 hours) secondary to increased V_{area}. No decrease in clearance observed between men and women [21]. Doubling pharmacokinetic levels was observed at midcycle [75]
Venlafaxine	No gender differences reported in PK [10,p.3495;99]

PK, pharmacokinetic.

Table 78-2

Reported Interactions of Gender and Pharmacodynamics for Antidepressants

Antidepressant	Gender Effects
TCAs	Tricyclic antidepressants
Amitriptyline	Response in migraine prophylaxis correlated with female gender [102] In depression, men respond better than women to tricyclic antidepressants [64]
Imipramine	Women have a longer time to response [39] Women more likely to withdraw from therapy on imipramine than on sertraline [39]
Clomipramine	Women show more pronounced antiobsessional effect in response to IV administration [103]

Continued

Table 78-2
(Continued)

Antidepressant	Gender Effects
SSRIs	Selective serotonin reuptake inhibitors
Fluoxetine	Females of reproductive age (<44 yr) more responsive than males [66] Hemispheric asymmetry (EEG, perceptual) and treatment response interacted with gender, being evident among depressed women but not men [104]
Paroxetine	Number of symptoms in discontinuation syndrome in dysthymic patients associated with female gender and age at onset of dysthymia [67]
Sertraline	Women more likely to respond to sertraline than imipramine [39] Gender associated with response for behavioral disturbances in Alzheimer's disease [105]
Citalopram	Response for treatment of alcohol dependence was greater in males (44% decrease) than females (26% decrease) [106]

EEG, electroencephalogram; IV, intravenous.

C. Elimination

The rate of elimination of a drug from the body is often characterized by its half-life. The half-life is a derived parameter that depends on the clearance of the drug from the body and the volume into which the drug distributes [24]; thus, clearance and volume of distribution are the more physiologically relevant parameters. Using volume of distribution and clearance allows one to discern the source of a given effect in examining the differences between sexes. If the half-life increases dramatically, it could be due primarily to an increase in the volume of distribution as shown for bupropion [22] or trazodone [21] and/or a change in the clearance of the drug from the body. Sweet *et al* [22] illustrated how the change in half-life between elderly women and young men could be due to a combination in the change both in the volume of distribution (primary contribution) for bupropion and the change in clearance (minor contribution).

III. Metabolic Differences

Drugs used to treat depression are metabolized by and/or inhibit a wide range of the cytochrome p450 (CYP) enzymes (Table 78-3). Gender differences in CYP isozyme function that affects antidepressant clearance have been reported for CYP3A4 (nefazodone, sertraline, mirtazapine) and CYP1A2 (fluvoxamine). Observation of these differences may be confounded when (1) a drug has a high rate of clearance (e.g., flow limited clearance and/or high intrinsic metabolic capacity), which is the case for most CYP3A4 metabolized antidepressants and/or (2) a drug is a cosubstrate for both CYP3A and the p-glycoprotein multi-drug resistance pump1 (MDR1), which is the case for some CYP3A4 metabolized drugs [25]. High clearance (or flow limited clearance) drugs are dependent on blood flow rate into the eliminating organ (e.g., liver, kidney) and thus indirectly liver size. Because women have a smaller liver and a lower liver blood flow rate compared with men, observed gender differences may not be due to metabolic differences (or differences in enzymatic activity across gender) but rather due to differences in blood flow. Thus, it may be difficult to distinguish the gender effects on liver size and blood flow from actual differences in metabolic activity

across gender. Similarly, the MDR1 pump provides cytosolic access for the compound to metabolizing enzymes. Thus, if one is administered a drug that is a cosubstrate for both the CYP3A4 enzyme and MDR1 pump, an increase in the activity in the MDR1 pump could be mistaken for a decreased CYP3A metabolizing capacity, and conversely a decrease in MDR1 activity could be mistaken for an increased CYP3A metabolizing capacity [25]. The hepatic expression level for p-glycoprotein in women is only 1/3 to 1/2 that of men [25,26], nonetheless differences have been reported for 3A4 metabolized drugs nefazodone [27], sertraline [28], and citalopram [29]. The differences in nefazodone metabolism were evaluated as a comparison of elderly men/women versus younger women. Ronfeld *et al* [28] reported that younger men have a shorter sertraline half-life than women or older men/women, and Reis *et al* [29] showed that citalopram clearance was higher in adolescent males compared with adolescent females, which is consistent with the possibility of the contribution of liver size (i.e., enzymatic capacity) and/or blood flow with changes in disposition. In addition, gender differences in the disposition of the predominately CYP1A2 metabolized drug fluvoxamine (also metabolized by CYP3A4 in a minor pathway) have been demonstrated. Preskorn [30] showed that males had lower plasma levels of fluvoxamine than females. Hartter *et al* [31] demonstrated that the doubling of the fluvoxamine dose while at steady state resulted in a much more dramatic increase in fluvoxamine concentrations in women compared with men. Mirtazapine (metabolized by CYP3A4, 1A2, and 2D6) was reported to have a prolonged half-life in women compared with men [10], and men had half the concentrations of similarly treated women [32,33]. Another study reported higher concentrations of desmethylclomipramine (DMC) and lower hydroxylation rates of clomipramine in women, which resulted in a higher DMC/8-HDMC ratio in women compared with men [34]. Women have also been found to have higher steady state nortriptyline levels and different nortriptyline to hydroxynortriptyline ratios than men [35]. Not only are there effects of gender on the disposition of antidepressants but also antidepressts that inhibit CYP3A enzymes may shift the metabolism of estrogen from CYP3A to CYP1A resulting in the production of less of the highly genotoxic 16-alpha-hydroxyestrone

Table 78-3
Metabolic Pathways for Antidepressant Drugs

Cytochrome P450	Tricyclic and Heterocyclic Antidepressant Substrates	SSRI Substrates	Inhibitors	Inducers
1A2	Amitriptyline Clomipramine Imipramine Mirtazipine**†	Fluvoxamine	Fluvoxamine Citalopram**†	
2B6	Bupropion**			
2C19	Amitriptyline Clomipramine Imipramine Nefazodone	Citalopram**	Fluoxetine Fluvoxamine Paroxetine Citalopram**†	
2C9	Amitriptyline**	Fluoxetine	Fluoxetine Norfluoxetine Fluvoxamine Sertraline Desmethylsertraline Paroxetine	
2D6	Amitriptyline** Clomipramine Desipramine** Imipramine Nortriptyline Venlafaxine** Mirtazapine** Trazodone**	Paroxetine** Fluoxetine** Fluvoxamine	Desipramine**† Clomipramine Bupropion**† Fluoxetine** Norfluoxetine Paroxetine** Sertraline** Citalopram**†	
3A4,5,7	Buspirone Trazodone Nefazodone Amitriptyline**† Venlafaxine**† Mirtazipine**†	Sertraline Citalopram**†	Trazodone Nefazodone** Fluvoxamine** Fluoxetine Norfluoxetine	St. John's wort

*Source: http://medicine.iupui.edu/flockhart/.
**Listed in the *Physicians' Desk Reference* 2002.
†Listed only in *Physicians' Desk Reference* 2002.
SSRI, selective serotonin reuptake inhibitor.

form [11] possibly resulting in a protective effect. Despite these findings, dosing is not typically tailored for women before initiation of therapy.

There are also differences in the phase 2 or conjugating enzymes between men and women. The clearance of oxazepam and temazepam has been reported to be much higher in men than in women [19,36] reflecting a higher rate of glucuronidation or a higher level of activity of the uridyl diphosphate glucuronyl transferase (UDPGT) enzyme system in men. This may result in higher concentrations in women of medications that are metabolized primarily by glucuronidation reactions. However, no differences in conjugating enzyme activity for antidepressants have been demonstrated.

Estrogen is a substrate for both CYP1A2 and CYP3A4 as well as an inhibitor of CYP1A2 [37]; thus, higher levels of both endogenous and potentially exogenously administered estrogens may affect antidepressant metabolism. The concomitant administration of CYP1A2 substrate antidepressants could result in higher plasma levels of either the antidepressant or estrogen and therefore a greater risk of adverse events [38–40].

IV. Effects of Estrogen/Progesterone

A. Exogenous Hormones

The administration of estrogen and progesterone may have specific effects that modulate the response to antidepressants, as shown in Fig. 78-1. In postmenopausal women, estrogen replacement therapy was found to inhibit the clearance of caffeine, a CYP1A2 substrate [37]. Estrogens have some dopamine modulatory [41] and upregulating serotonin and norepinephrine (NE) activity [42–45]. Estrogen's dopamine modulatory effects may be neuroprotective [41], whereas its actions on the serotonin and NE systems may regulate affect.

As reviewed by Joffe and Cohen [46], estrogen may exert its antidepressant effects by modulating the serotonergic system,

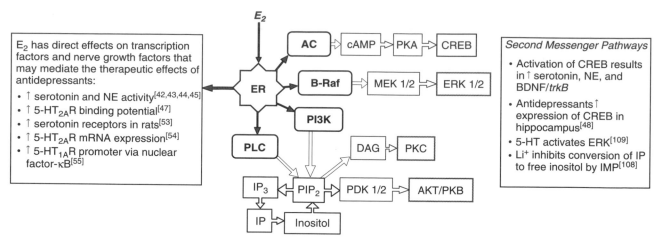

Fig. 78-1 Long-term and rapid actions of estrogen (E_2) in the brain. E_2 acts at the estrogen receptor (ER), which has effects on transcription factors (left) and second messenger pathways (right). Activation of adenylate cyclase (AC) results in the cAMP-dependent activation of protein kinase A (PKA), leading to the phosphorylation and activation of cAMP-responsive element binding protein (CREB). E_2 can also activate the mitogen-activated protein kinase (MAPK) pathway by the activation of the MAPK kinases B-Raf, MEK 1/2, and extracellular regulated kinases 1/2 (ERK 1/2). E_2 can also activate phosphatidylinositol-3 kinase (PI3K) that activates phosphionsitide-dependent kinase (PDK 1/2) and the Akt/protein kinase B (AKT/PKB) pathway through phosphatidylinositol bisphosphate (PIP$_2$). E_2 can also activate phospholipase C (PLC), which cleaves PIP$_2$ to generate inositol 1,4,5-trisphosphate (IP$_3$) and diacylglycerol (DAG), leading to the release of Ca^{+2} and activation of protein kinase C (PKC), respectively. IP$_3$ can also be dephosphorylated to inositol monophosphate (IP) and then dephosphorylated to free inositol by inositol monophosphatase (IMP). (Adapted from Belcher SM, Zsarnovszky A. [2001]. Estrogenic actions in the brain: Estrogen, phytoestrogens, and rapid intracellular signaling mechanisms. *J Pharmacol Exp Ther.* 299:408–414; and Shaldubina A, Agan G, Belmaker RH. [2001]. The mechanism of lithium action: State of the art, ten years later. *Prog NeuroPsychopharmacol Biol. Psychiatry.* 25:855–866.)

and/or by its direct effects on transcription factors and nerve growth factors (NGFs) that may mediate the therapeutic effects of antidepressants. Estrogen and other gonadal hormones may facilitate downregulation of 5-HT$_2$ receptors associated with chronic administration of antidepressants. Exogenous estradiol and progesterone administration in postmenopausal women resulted in a time-delayed upregulation of 5-HT$_{2A}$R binding potential as measured using positron emission tomography (PET) [47]. Duman *et al* [48] proposed a molecular theory of the antidepressant effects of 5-HT and NE systems, by which these systems regulate the cyclic adenosine monophosphate (cAMP)-mediated signal transduction cascade. This cascade activates protein kinases that phosphorylate proteins including cAMP-response element-binding protein (CREB). Long-term use of both SSRIs and selective NE antidepressants has been shown to induce the expression of CREB in the hippocampus [49]. Estradiol can also activate the cAMP cascade, inducing the expression of CREB, and subsequently activating specific target genes including BDNF [50]. BDNF is a NGF involved in neurodevelopment and maintenance of the mature brain, and which itself has antidepressant actions. Long-term administration of antidepressants including SSRIs, monoamine oxidase inhibitors (MAOIs), and atypical and selective NE agents and ECT have been found to increase the expression of BDNF and its receptor (trkB) in the hippocampus [51]. Estradiol administration has also been shown to cause an upregulation of the NGF receptor, trkA [52].

Animal data have also shown that estrogen affects the serotonin system, for example in rats estradiol increased serotonin receptors [53]. Using a genetic animal model for depression, 5-HT$_{2A}$ receptor mRNA expression abnormalities found in rats were reversed in several affected brain areas by 17β-estradiol treatment [54]. Estradiol can upregulate the 5-HT$_{1A}$ receptor promoter via a mechanism involving synergistic activation of nuclear factor-κB and ER$_\alpha$ [55].

A consequence of these changes in neurotransmitter systems is that older postmenopausal women who use estrogens typically report fewer depressive symptoms than nonusers [56]. A meta-analysis of the effect of hormone replacement therapy found that estrogen significantly reduced depressed mood (ES = 0.69) [57]. In a clinical trial of perimenopausal women treated with fluoxetine (20 mg/day), women treated adjunctively with estrogen replacement showed a greater improvement in HAM-D scores (40.1%) than the control group (17.0%) [58].

B. Endogenous Hormones

Changes in serotonin and NE activity in women may modify responses to antidepressants or modes of administration of antidepressants that are effective [42–45]. Most women present with depressive symptoms termed atypical. These atypical reverse neurovegetative symptoms are responsive to different agents than typical symptomatology. Several authors have demonstrated a gender difference in responses to various classes of antidepressants. Estrogens inhibit monoamine oxidase (MAO) activity that may affect the differential responses observed with MAOIs [59–61]. Women tend to demonstrate more atypicality in depression, and patients with significant neurovegetative states tend to respond much more readily to treatment with MAOI versus tricyclic antidepressants (TCAs) [60]. West and Dally [62] suggested that the lower response rates to TCAs compared to MAOI agents observed with depression between men and women might be attributable to the higher rate of atypical reverse neurovegetative symptoms in women. Raskin [63] published a post hoc or second analysis of two large inpatient clinical trials. The first study compared two TCAs (chlorpromazine and imipramine) to placebo. In this study, imipramine was significantly more effective for men than placebo. In women older than 40 years, imipramine response was similar to that seen in men; however, in women younger than 40 years, the imipramine response was no different than placebo. The second study compared phenelzine and diazepam with placebo. They reported a trend toward a better response to phenelzine treatment in young women. Another study of amitriptyline showed that men responded better than women to TCAs [64]. Davidson and Pelton [61] reported on five randomized clinical trials: trial one evaluated phenelzine and imipramine in inpatients; trial two evaluated phenelzine and imipramine in outpatients; trial three evaluated amitriptyline versus bupropion in inpatients; trial four evaluated isocarboxazid at two different dose levels in inpatients; and trial five evaluated isocarboxazid versus placebo in outpatients. These investigators did not find a difference in response across drugs for the entire population studied. However, they did show that depressed women with panic attacks responded better to MAOIs than TCAs, but depressed men with panic attacks responded better to TCAs than to MAOIs. Quitkin et al [59] showed that phenelzine was significantly better than imipramine in the treatment of depression with atypical characteristics. These authors evaluated 400 patients who met the criterion for depression (Diagnostic and Statistical Manual of Mental Disorders, 3rd ed. [DSM-III]) with atypical features who were randomized to imipramine, phenelzine, or placebo. Patients who did not respond to treatment were crossed over to another treatment. Hamilton et al [65] carried out a meta-analysis of 34 trials, where results for men and women were reported separately. The response rate for men to imipramine was 62% versus 51% for women (p < 0.001).

Possible differences in serotonergic activity across gender may also contribute to differential responses to antidepressants. A randomized, parallel group, double-blind comparison trial examining response to imipramine and sertraline in men and women demonstrated that women were much more likely to have a favorable response to sertraline versus imipramine [39]. Conversely, men were more likely to show a favorable response to imipramine versus sertraline [39]. Postmenopausal women showed a similar response rate to both sertraline and imipramine in this study. In other studies, women of reproductive age were more responsive to treatment with fluoxetine than men [66], and the number of symptoms associated with discontinuation of paroxetine was greater in women [67].

V. Menstrual Cycle Effects

A. Nonmetabolic Effects

Cyclic changes in mood as evidenced by premenstrual dysphoric disorder (PMDD) and premenstrual syndrome (PMS) suggest an effect on mood secondary to hormone fluctuation [68]. Menses is accompanied with cognitive effects in 60% of women, lasting 3 to 4 days [69]. As estrogen levels peak, serotonin levels in plasma also peak. This may provide rationale for pulse dosing of antidepressants [44,70–73] or may actually exacerbate side effects [74] in dysphoric premenstrual syndrome.

B. Metabolic Effects

Kimmel et al [75] showed a doubling in trazodone (3A4) and desipramine (2D6) levels at midcycle. In addition, prolongation of caffeine elimination in the late luteal phase suggests a decreased 1A2 activity during this phase of the menstrual cycle, which could possibly affect fluvoxamine clearance [76,77].

VI. Effects of Pregnancy

A. Nonmetabolic Effects

Although antidepressants are classified as pregnancy category C in the Physicians' Desk Reference [10] (which means some risk to the fetus), there is a high risk of not treating depression in pregnancy or the postpartum period. Failure to treat depression during this period can lead to a high risk of harm either to the infant or the mother [78–80].

During pregnancy, there are increases in total body volume and protein binding and changes in clearance. Antiepileptic drugs (phenytoin, phenobarbitone, carbamazepine) appear to be cleared faster [81] in pregnancy, and appropriate dosing adjustments should be undertaken in these cases. An increased renal clearance of lithium during pregnancy has also been reported, with clearance increasing 30 to 50% [82]. In addition, nortriptyline doses may need to be increased for the second to third trimester [83].

B. Metabolic Effects

During pregnancy, higher estrogen and progesterone levels are experienced and may affect either CYP3A4 (induction by progesterone) and CYP1A2 (inhibition). Lower CYP1A2 activities have been reported during pregnancy, evidenced by the increase in the half-life of caffeine [84]. These changes could affect the clearance of the CYP3A4 metabolized medications sertraline, citalopram, trazodone, fluoxetine and the CYP1A2 metabolized fluvoxamine, amitriptyline, clomipramine, and imipramine.

C. Effects on the Fetus

There are several registries that continue to evaluate the potential impact on the fetus of antidepressant treatment. Pregnancy registries have been used to provide both prospective and retrospective evaluation of teratogenic risk attributable to antidepressant treatment. McElhatton et al [85] evaluated exposure to antidepressants without regard to class, Kulin et al [86] prospectively evaluated pregnancy exposures to fluvoxamine, paroxetine, and sertraline, Pastuszak et al [78] prospectively evaluated TCA and fluoxetine exposure in pregnancy, Chambers et al [87] prospectively evaluated fluoxetine exposure in pregnancy, and Ericsson et al [88] evaluated primarily citalopram exposures. None of these evaluations detected an increased risk of teratogenicity. Ericsson *et al* [88] reported on 986 women who had reported taking antidepressants during pregnancy. There was an excess of high parity births and a reduction in multiple births in the antidepressant exposed group; otherwise there were no differences in parturition compared with women not on antidepressants. There were no other significant effects on pregnancy mediated by antidepressants. Pastuszak *et al* [78] reported that increased risk to the fetus was not associated with fluoxetine exposure in 128 women captured through various registry mechanisms. However, because a small number of pregnancies were evaluated, they may not have been able to detect less frequent effects. The rate of miscarriage in the antidepressant-exposed group was 2-fold higher than those control patients reporting exposure to a nonteratogen. Chambers *et al* [87] reported that there was no increased risk in major fetal anomalies or pregnancy loss with fluoxetine exposure (n = 228). However, these authors discovered an increased risk for perinatal complications with fluoxetine exposure in the third trimester. Kulin *et al* [86] reported on a prospective, case-controlled assessment of exposure during pregnancy to sertraline, fluvoxamine, and paroxetine. There did not appear to be an increase in the teratogenic risk based on the assessment of 267 women exposed to antidepressant. However, the relatively small numbers of exposures assessed may not detect an increased risk of teratogenicity.

Another issue that is related is the potential effect of antidepressant exposure on neural development of the child, which may not manifest itself until much later in life. The impact of TCA (n = 80) and fluoxetine (n = 55) exposure was assessed on neural development in preschool children evaluating IQ and language development between 16 and 86 months of age. No effect on global IQ, language development, or behavioral development was detected [89]. Despite these findings, there is a paucity of data that reflects the risk to neural development in children. Therefore, additional use of birth registries such as Motherisk [90] may help to provide a more definitive evaluation of the risk to the fetus and evaluation of the potential impact or neural development into childhood with antidepressant exposure *in utero*.

VII. Discussion

Tables 78-1 and 78-2 reflect the current evidence for gender-specific effects on antidepressants. Given that women clearly have differences from men in both the presentation of depression (more atypical symptomatology) and physiology that affects the pharmacokinetics of drugs [39,65], it is clear that there is a relative paucity of information on the specific impact on both the disposition pharmacokinetics and pharmacodynamics across drug classes. Twice as many women as men experience depression during their most productive years [7] and the National Institutes of Health (NIH) and FDA have suggested [1,91,92] that more information be made available on gender-related differences. Thus, there is a large research opportunity available to examine these issues. Potential concerns include the antidepressant effect on the metabolism of reproductive hormones that may be associated with an increased risk of breast cancer. There is not sufficient information to indicate definitively what these risks or issues are at the current time [6,14]. The antidepressant

effect of St. John's wort remains controversial [93–95]; nonetheless, it is widely used and has a potent 3A4-inducer effect, which may affect other CYP3A4-metabolized medications. The induction of CYP3A4 may cause oral contraceptive failure secondary to increased estrogen metabolism [96] affecting women in their reproductive years. Thus, the paucity of research on gender-specific differences related to antidepressants is a significant public health deficiency and represents an understudied and necessary research area.

VIII. Suggestions for Further Investigations

- Because it is difficult to obtain intensely sampled pharmacokinetic data from patients in this area and there is a specific need for additional information on gender differences that may only be detectable in a larger sample size than is used in the phase I drug development, where these data are typically collected, population (mixed effects) pharmacokinetic modeling techniques would be very useful to evaluate these issues especially where concentration data are collected under naturalistic conditions when dosing history timing and sample timing are known. This methodology can help to detect differences if they exist from much larger sample sizes.

- Additional information on the teratogenicity and impact on children of antidepressant use during pregnancy is needed and could be collected using birth registries and long-term follow-up as has been done for fluoxetine.

- The shift in estrogen metabolism (either producing a protective or a deleterious effect) must be evaluated in more detail in response to conflicting reports of producing a cancer-protective effect or, in the case of epidemiologic studies, being associated with the development of breast cancer.

References

1. Schmucker DL, Vessell ES. (1993). Underrepresentation of women in clinical drug trials. *Clin Pharmacol Ther*. 54:11–15.
2. Dawkins K, Potter WZ. (1991). Gender differences in pharmacokinetics and pharmacodynamics of psychotropics: Focus on women. *Psychopharmacol Bull*. 27:417–426.
3. Harris RZ, Benet LZ, Schwartz JB. (1995). Gender effects in pharmacokinetics and pharmacodynamics. *Drugs*. 50:222–239.
4. Hamilton J, Parry B. (1983). Sex related differences in clinical drug response: Implications for women's health. *J Am Med Womens Assoc*. 38:126–132.
5. Stewart DE. (1998). Are there special considerations in the prescription of serotonin reuptake inhibitors for women? *Can J Psychiatry*. 43:900–904.
6. Cortecchio M, Kreiger N, Darlington G, Steingart S. (2000). Antidepressant medication use and breast cancer risk. *Am J Epidemiol*. 151:951–957.
7. Regier DA, Narrow WE, Rae DS *et al*. (1993). The de facto US mental and addictive disorders service system. Epidemiologic catchment area prospective 1-year prevalence rates of disorders and services. *Arch Gen Psychiatry*. 50:85–94.
8. Rapaport MH, Thompson PM, Kelsoe JR *et al*. (1995). Gender differences in outpatient research subjects with affective disorders: A comparison of descriptive variables. *J Clin Psychiatry*. 56:67–72.
9. Hirschfeld RMA, Russell JM. (1997). Assessment of treatment of suicidal patients. *N Engl J Med*. 337:910–915.
10. (2002). *Physicians' Desk Reference*. Montvale, NJ: Medical Economics and Thomson Health Care.
11. Thompson DS, Kirshner MA, Klug TL *et al*. (in press). Effect of fluoxetine treatment on the 2:16a-hydroxyestrone ratio in young women. *Ther Drug Monitoring*.

12. Writing Group for the Women's Health Initiative Investigators. (2002). Risks and benefits of estrogen plus progestin in healthy postmenopausal women. Principal results from the women's health initiative randomized controlled trial. *JAMA*. 288:321–333.

13. Hlatky MA, Boothroyd D, Vittinghoff E *et al.* (2002). Heart and Estrogen/Progestin Replacement Study (HERS) Research Group. Quality-of-life and depressive symptoms in postmenopausal women after receiving hormone therapy: Results from the Heart and Estrogen/Progestin Replacement Study (HERS) trial. *JAMA*. 287:591–597.

14. Kelly JP, Rosenberg L, Palmer JR *et al.* (1999). Risk of breast cancer according to use of antidepressants, phenothiazines and antihistamines. *Am J Epidemiol*. 150:861–868.

15. Grossman MI, Kirsner JB, Gillespie IA. (1963). Basal and histalog-stimulated gastric secretion in control subjects and in patients with peptic ulcer or gastric cancer. *Gastroenterology*. 45:14–26.

16. Hutson WR, Roehrkasse RL, Wald A. (1989). Influence of gender and menopause on gastric emptying and motility. *Gastroenterology*. 96:11–17.

17. Wald A, Van Thiel DH, Hoechstetter L *et al.* (1981). Gastrointestinal transit: The effect of the menstrual cycle. *Gastroenterology*. 80:1497–1500.

18. Stewart JJ, Berkel HJ, Parish RC *et al.* (2001). Single-dose pharmacokinetics of bupropion in adolescents: Effects of smoking status and gender. *J Clin Pharmacol*. 41:770–778.

19. Greenblatt DJ, Divoll M, Harmatz JS, Shader RI. (1980). Oxazepam kinetics: Effects of age and sex. *J Pharmacol Exp Ther*. 215:86–91.

20. Greenblatt DJ, Divoll M, Abernethy DR, Shader RI. (1982). Physiologic changes in old age: Relation to altered drug disposition. *J Am Geriatr Soc. Suppl*. 30:S6–S10.

21. Greenblatt DJ, Friedman H, Burstein ES *et al.* (1987) Trazodone kinetics: Effect of age, gender, and obesity. *Clin Pharmacol Ther*. 42:193.

22. Sweet RA, Pollock BG, Kirshner M *et al.* (1995). Pharmacokinetics of single- and multiple-dose bupropion in elderly patients with depression. *J Clin Pharmacol*. 35:876–884.

23. Kristensen CB. (1983). Imipramine serum protein binding in healthy subjects. *Clin Pharmacol Ther*. 34:689–694.

24. Rowland M, Tozer T. (1989). Elimination concepts. In *Clinical Pharmacokinetics: Concepts and Applications*, 2nd Edition (Rowland M, Tozer T, eds.), pp. 170. Malvern, PA: Lea & Febiger.

25. Meibohm B, Beierle I, Deredorf H. (2002). How important are gender differences in pharmacokinetics? *Clin Pharmacokinet*. 41:329–342.

26. Schuetz EG, Furuya KN, Schuetz JD. (1995). Interindividual variation in expression of P-glycoprotein in normal human liver and secondary hepatic neoplasms. *J Pharmacol Exp Ther*. 275:1011–1018.

27. Barbhaiya RH, Buch AB, Green DS. (1996). A study of the effect of age and gender on the pharmacokinetics of nefazodone after single and multiple doses. *J Clin Psychopharmacol*. 16:19–25.

28. Ronfeld RA, Tremaine LM, Wilner KD. (1997). Pharmacokinetics of sertraline and its N-dimethyl metabolite in elderly and young male and female volunteers. *Clin Pharmacokinet*. 32:22–30.

29. Reis M, Olsson G, Carlsson B *et al.* (2002). Serum levels of citalopram and its main metabolites in adolescent patients treated in a naturalistic clinical setting. *J Clin Psychopharmacol*. 22:406–413.

30. Preskorn SH. (1997). Clinically relevant pharmacology of selective serotonin reuptake inhibitors. An overview with emphasis on pharmacokinetics and effects on oxidative drug metabolism. *Clin Pharmacokinet*. 32:1–21.

31. Hartter S, Wetzel H, Hammes E *et al.* (1998). Nonlinear pharmacokinetics of fluvoxamine and gender differences. *Ther Drug Monitoring*. 20:446–469.

32. Timmer CJ, Paanakker JE, Van Hal HJM. (1996). Pharmacokinetics of mirtazapine from orally administered tablets: Influence of gender, age and treatment regimen. *Hum Psychopharmacol*. 11:497–509.

33. Timmer CJ, Sitsen JM, Delbressine LP. (2000). Clinical pharmacokinetics of mirtazapine. *Clin Pharmacokinet*. 38:461–474.

34. Mundo E, Pirola R, Bellodi L *et al.* (2002). Are gender differences in anti-obsessional response related to different clomipramine metabolism? *J Clin Psychopharmacol*. 22:341–342.

35. Dahl ML, Bertilsson L, Nordin C. (1996). Steady-state plasma levels of nortriptyline and its 10-hydroxy metabolite: Relationship to the CYP2D6 genotype. *Psychopharmacology*. 123:315–319.

36. Divoll M, Greenblatt DJ, Harmatz JS, Shader RI. (1981). Effect of age and gender on disposition of temazepam. *J Pharm Sci*. 10:1104–1107.

37. Pollock BG, Wylie M, Stack JA *et al.* (1999). Inhibition of CYP1A2 mediated metabolism by estrogen replacement therapy in post-menopausal women. *J Clin Pharmacol*. 39:936–940.

38. Ford JM, Truman CA, Wilcock GK, Roberts CJ. (1993). Serum concentrations of tacrine hydrochloride predict its adverse effects in Alzheimer's disease. *Clin Pharmacol Ther*. 53:691–695.

39. Kornstein SG, Schatzberg AF, Thase ME *et al.* (2000). Gender differences in treatment response to sertraline versus imipramine in chronic depression. *Am J Psychiatry*. 157:1445–1452.

40. Domecq C, Naranjo C, Ruiz I, Busto U. (1980). Sex-related variations in the frequency and characteristics of adverse drug reactions. *Int J Clin Pharmacol Ther Toxicol*. 18:362–366.

41. Gordon JH, Borison RL, Diamond BI. (1980). Modulation of dopamine receptor sensitivity by estrogen. *Biol Psychiatry*. 15:389–396.

42. Halbreich U, Rojansky N, Palter S *et al.* (1995). Estrogen augments serotonergic activity in postmenopausal women. *Biol Psychiatry*. 37:434–441.

43. Halbreich U. (1997). Role of estrogen in postmenopausal depression. *Neurology*. 48(Suppl 7):S16–S19.

44. Halbreich U, Smoller JW. (1997). Intermittent luteal phase sertraline treatment of dysphoric premenstrual syndrome. *J Clin Psychiatry*. 58:399–402.

45. Halbreich U, Kahn LS. (2001). Role of estrogen in the aetiology and treatment of mood disorders. *CNS Drugs*. 15:797–817.

46. Joffe H, Cohen LS. (1998). Estrogen, serotonin, and mood disturbance: Where is the therapeutic bridge? *Biol Psychiatry*. 44:798–811.

47. Moses EL, Drevets WC, Smith G *et al.* (2000). Effects of estradiol and progesterone administration on human serotonin 2a receptor binding: A PET study. *Biol Psychiatry*. 48:854–860.

48. Duman RS, Heninger GR, Nestler EJ. (1997). Molecular and cellular theory of depression. *Arch Gen Psychiatry*. 54:597–606.

49. Nibuya N, Nestler EJ, Duman RS. (1996). Chronic antidepressant administration increases the expression of cAMP response element binding protein (CREB) in rat hippocampus. *J Neurosci*. 16:2365–2372.

50. Belcher SM, Zsarnovszky A. (2001). Estrogenic actions in the brain: Estrogen, phytoestrogens, and rapid intracellular signaling mechanisms. *J Pharmacol Exp Ther*. 299:408–414.

51. Nibuya M, Morinobu S, Duman RS. (1995). Regulation of BDNF and trkB mRNA in rat brain by chronic electroconvulsive seizure and antidepressant drug treatments. *J Neurosci*. 15:7439–7547.

52. Sohrabji F, Miranda RC, Toran-Allerand CD. (1994). Estrogen differentially regulates estrogen and nerve growth factor receptor mRNAs in adult sensory neurons. *J Neurosci*. 14:459–471.

53. Sumner BEH, Fink G. (1995). Estrogen increases the density of 5-hydroxytryptamine$_{2A}$ receptors in cerebral cortex and nucleus accumbens in the female rat. *J Steroid Biochem Mol Biol*. 54:15–20.

54. Sterlund MK, Overstreet DH, Hurd YL. (1999). The Flinders Sensitive Line rats, a genetic model of depression, show abnormal serotonin receptor mRNA expression in the brain that is reversed by 17β-estradiol. *Mol Brain Res*. 74:158–166.

55. Wissink S, van der Burg B, Katzenellenbogen BS, van der Saag PT. (2001). Synergistic activation of the serotonin-1A receptor by nuclear factor-κB. *Mol Endocrinol*. 15:543–552.

56. Palinkas LA, Barrett-Connor E. (1992). Estrogen use and depressive symptoms in postmenopausal women. *Obstet Gynecol*. 80:30–36.

57. Zweifel JE, O'Brien WH. (1997). A meta-analysis of the effect of hormone replacement therapy upon depressed mood. *Psychoneuroendocrinology*. 22:189–212.

58. Schneider LS, Small GW, Hamilton SH *et al.* (1997). Estrogen replacement and response to fluoxetine in a multicenter geriatric depression trial. Fluoxetine Collaborative Study Group. *Am J Geriatr Psychiatry*. 5:97–106.

59. Quitkin FM, Stewart JW, McGrath PJ *et al.* (1993). Columbia atypical depression: A subgroup of depressives with better response to MAOI than to tricyclic antidepressants or placebo. *Br J Psychiatry Suppl*. 21:30–34.

60. Thase ME, Frank E, Kornstein SG, Yonkers KA. (2000). Gender Differences in Response to Treatments of Depression. In *Gender and Its Effect on Psychopathology* (Frank E, ed.), pp. 103–125. Washington DC: American Psychiatric Press.

61. Davidson J, Pelton S. (1986). Forms of atypical depression and their response to antidepressant drugs. *Psychiatry Res*. 17:87–95.

62. West ED, Dally PJ. (1959). Effect of iproniazid in depressive syndromes. *BMJ*. 1:1491.

63. Raskin A. (1974). Age-sex differences in response to antidepressant drugs. *J Nerv Ment Dis*. 159:120–130.

64. Okiishi CG, Paradiso S, Robinson RG. (2001). Gender differences in depression associated with neurologic illness: Clinical correlates and pharmacologic response. *J Gender Specific Med*. 4:65–72.

65. Hamilton JA, Grant M, Jensvold MF. (1996). Sex and Treatment of Depressions: When Does It Matter? In *Psychopharmacology and Women: Sex, Gender, and Hormones* (Jensvold MF, Halbreich U, eds.), pp. 241–260. Washington DC: Institute for Womens Health.

66. Martenyi F, Dossenbach M, Mraz K, Metcalfe S. (2001). Gender differences in the efficacy of fluoxetine and maprotiline in depressed patients: A double-blind trial of antidepressants with serotonergic or norepinephrinergic reuptake inhibition profile. *Eur Neuropsychopharmacol.* 11:227–232.

67. Bogetto F, Bellino S, Revello RB, Patria L. (2002). Discontinuation syndrome in dysthymic patients treated with selective serotonin reuptake inhibitors: A clinical investigation. *CNS Drugs.* 16:273–283.

68. Thompson DS, Pollock BG. (2001). Psychotropic metabolism: Gender related issues. *Psychiatric Times.* 18:1.

69. Demers LM. (1989). *Premenstrual, Postpartum, and Menopausal Mood Disorders.* Baltimore: Urban and Schwarzenberg.

70. Steiner M, Korzekwa M, Lamont J, Wilkins A. (1997). Intermittent fluoxetine dosing in the treatment of women with premenstrual dysphoria. *Psychopharmacol Bull.* 33:771–774.

71. Sundblad C, Hedberg MA, Ericksson E. (1993). Clomipramine administered during the luteal phase reduces the symptoms of pre-menstrual syndrome: A placebo-controlled trial. *Neuropsychopharmacology.* 9:133–145.

72. Young SA, Hurt PH, Benedek DM, Howard RS. (1998). Treatment of premenstrual dysphoric disorder with sertraline during the luteal phase: A randomized, double-blind, placebo-controlled crossover trial. *J Clin Psychiatry.* 59:76–80.

73. Wikander I, Sundblad C, Andersch B *et al.* (1998). Citalopram in premenstrual dysphoria: Is intermittent treatment during luteal phases more effective than continuous medication throughout the menstrual cycle? *J Clin Psychopharmacol.* 18:390–398.

74. Alpay FB, Turhan NO. (2001). Intermittent versus continuous sertraline therapy in the treatment of premenstrual dysphoric disorders. *Int J Fertil Womens Med.* 46:228–231.

75. Kimmel S, Gonsalves L, Youngs D, Gidwani G. (1992). Fluctuating levels of antidepressants premenstrually. *J Psychosom Obstet Gynaecol.* 13:277–280.

76. Lane JD, Steege JF, Rupp SL, Kuhn CM. (1992). Menstrual cycle effects on caffeine elimination in the human female. *Eur J Clin Pharmacol.* 43:543–546.

77. Kashuba ADM, Nafziger AN. (1998). Physiologic changes during the menstrual cycle and their effects on the pharmacokinetics and pharmacodynamics of drugs. *Clin Pharmacokinet.* 34:203–218.

78. Pastuszak A, Schick-Boschetto B, Zuber C *et al.* (1993). Pregnancy outcome following first-trimester exposure to fluoxetine (Prozac). *JAMA.* 269:2246–2248.

79. Wisner KL, Gelenberg AJ, Leonard H *et al.* (1999). Pharmacologic treatment of depression during pregnancy. *JAMA.* 282:1264–1269.

80. Wisner KL, Zarin D, Holboe ES *et al.* (2000). Risk-benefit decision making for treatment of depression during pregnancy. *Am J Psychiatry.* 157:1933–1940.

81. Bologa M, Tang B, Klein J *et al.* (1991). Pregnancy-induced changes in drug metabolism in epileptic women. *J Pharmacol Exp Ther.* 257:735–740.

82. Schou M, Weinstein MR. (1980). Problems of lithium maintenance treatment during pregnancy, delivery and lactation. *Agressologie.* 21(A):7–9.

83. Wisner KL, Perel J, Wheeler SB. (1993). Tricyclic dose requirements across pregnancy. *Am J Psychiatry.* 150:1541–1542.

84. Aldridge A, Bailey J, Neims AH. (1981). The disposition of caffeine during and after pregnancy. *Semin Perinatol.* 15:310–314.

85. McElhatton PR, Garbis HM, Elefant E *et al.* (1996). The outcome of pregnancy in 689 women exposed to therapeutic doses of antidepressants. A collaborative study of the European Network of Teratology Information Services (ENTIS). *Reprod Toxicol.* 10:285–294.

86. Kulin NA, Pastuszak A, Sage SR *et al.* (1998). Pregnancy outcome following maternal use of the new selective serotonin reuptake inhibitors: A prospective controlled multicenter study. *JAMA.* 279:609–610.

87. Chambers CD, Johnson KA, Dick LM *et al.* (1996). Birth outcomes in pregnant women taking fluoxetine. *N Engl J Med.* 335:1010–1015.

88. Ericsson A, Kallen B, Wiholm B. (1999). Delivery outcome after the use of antidepressants in early pregnancy. *Eur J Clin Pharmacol.* 55:503–508.

89. Nulman I, Rovet J, Stewart DE *et al.* (1997). Neurodevelopment of children exposed *in utero* to antidepressant drugs. *N Engl J Med.* 336:258–262.

90. Loebstein R, Koren G. (1997). Pregnancy outcome and neurodevelopment of children exposed *in utero* to psychoactive drugs: The Motherisk experience. *J Psychiatry Neurosci.* 22:192–196.

91. Merkatz RB, Temple R, Subel S *et al.* (1993). Women in clinical trials of new drugs. A change in Food and Drug Administration policy. The Working Group on Women in Clinical Trials. *N Engl J Med.* 329:292–296.

92. National Institutes of Health. (1992). *Opportunities for Research on Women's Health.* Washington DC: National Institutes of Health, Publication 92–3457A.

93. Lecrubier Y, Clerc G, Didi R, Kieser M. (2002). Efficacy of St. John's wort extract WS 5570 in major depression: A double-blind, placebo-controlled trial. *Am J Psychiatry.* 159:1361–1366.

94. van Gurp G, Meterissian GB, Haiek LN *et al.* (2002). St John's wort or sertraline? Randomized controlled trial in primary care. *Can Fam Physician.* 48:905–912.

95. Hypericum Depression Trial Study Group. (2002). Effect of Hypericum perforatum (St John's wort) in major depressive disorder: A randomized controlled trial. *JAMA.* 287:1807–1814.

96. Armstrong SC, Cozza KL, Cole MA. (2000). Consultation-liaison psychiatry drug-drug interactions update. *Psychosomatics.* 5:310–314.

97. Cohen LG, Biederman J, Wilens T *et al.* (1999). Desipramine clearance in children and adolescents: Absence of effect of development and gender. *J Am Acad Child Adolesc Psychiatry.* 38:79–85.

98. Merle Y, Mentre F. (1999). Optimal sampling times for Bayesian estimation of the pharmacokinetic parameters of nortriptyline during therapeutic drug monitoring. *J Pharmacokinet Biopharm.* 27:85–101.

99. Klamerus KJ, Parker VD, Rudolph RL *et al.* (1996). Effects of age and gender on venlafaxine and O-desmethylvenlafaxine pharmacokinetics. *Pharmacotherapy.* 16:915–923.

100. Mahmood I, Sahajwalla C. (1999). Clinical pharmacokinetics and pharmacodynamics of buspirone, an anxiolytic drug. *Clin Pharmacokinet.* 36:277–287.

101. Gammans RE, Westrick ML, Shea JP *et al.* (1989). Pharmacokinetics of buspirone in elderly subjects. *J Clin Pharmacol.* 29:72–78.

102. Ziegler DK, Hurwitz A, Preskorn S *et al.* (1994). Propranolol and amitriptyline in prophylaxis of migraine. Pharmacokinetic and therapeutic effects. *Arch Neurol.* 151:1181–1182.

103. Mundo E, Bareggi SR, Pirola R, Bellodi L. (1999). Effect of acute intravenous clomipramine and antiobsessional response to proserotonergic drugs: Is gender a predictive variable? *Biol Psychiatry.* 45:290–294.

104. Bruder GE, Stewart JW, Tenke CE *et al.* (2001). Electroencephalographic and perceptual asymmetry differences between responders and nonresponders to an SSRI antidepressant. *Biol Psychiatry.* 49:416–425.

105. Lanctot KL, Herrmann N, van Reekum R *et al.* (2002). Gender, aggression and serotonergic function are associated with response to sertraline for behavioral disturbances in Alzheimer's disease. *Int J Geriatr Psychiatry.* 17:531–541.

106. Naranjo CA, Bremner KE, Lanctot KL. (1995). Effects of citalopram and a brief psycho-social intervention on alcohol intake, dependence and problems. *Addiction.* 90:87–99.

107. Belcher SM, Zsarnovszky A. (2001). Estrogenic actions in the brain: Estrogen, phytoestrogens, and rapid intracellular signaling mechanisms. *J Pharmacol Exp Ther.* 299:408–414.

108. Shaldubina A, Agan G, Belmaker RH. (2001) The mechanism of lithium action: State of the art, ten years later. *Prog Neuropsychopharmacol Biol Psychiatry.* 25:855–866.

109. Errico M, Crozier RA, Plummer MR, Cowen DS. (2001). 5-HT$_7$ receptors activate the mitogen activated protein kinase extracellular signal related kinase in cultured rat hippocampal neurons. *Neuroscience.* 102:361–367.

79

Consideration for the Use of Therapeutic Drugs During Pregnancy and the Perinatal Period

MARILYNN C. FREDERIKSEN, MD

Associate Professor, Department of Obstetrics and Gynecology, Northwestern University Medical School, Chicago, IL

Pregnancy is really the ultimate gender difference between males and females. During pregnancy, physiologic changes occur in the woman's body that potentially can alter the way in which drugs are handled. Because of concerns for fetal safety, few pharmacokinetic, pharmacodynamic, or clinical trials are conducted during pregnancy. Currently, most drugs that are marketed in the United States carry the statement in their labeling that

> There are, however, no adequate and well-controlled studies in pregnant women. Because animal reproductive studies are not always predictive of human response, this drug should be used during pregnancy only if clearly needed [1].

Therefore, the decision whether or not to use a drug during pregnancy rests entirely with the practitioner. Assessments of the risks and benefits of a particular agent are usually made on an individual basis in a particular clinical situation. The risk most commonly considered is the fetal risk of teratogenesis or drug-induced malformation. Whether untreated disease in the woman has an effect on either the pregnancy outcome or the offspring is usually not considered. Women are more often than not left untreated in an attempt to avoid a perceived fetal risk related to the use of any pharmacologic agent during pregnancy. Appropriate dosage and frequency of drug administration are also not considered. It is assumed that the usual adult dose is adequate. Few practitioners know whether or not the physiologic changes of pregnancy require drug dosages to be changed.

Maternal physiologic changes occur during gestation to accommodate fetal growth and development. This altered maternal physiology has the potential to affect the pharmacokinetics of drugs. These changes may increase drug distribution volume, decrease drug binding to plasma proteins, alter peak drug concentration and time to peak drug concentration, and cause changes in hepatic and/or renal drug clearance. To extrapolate pharmacokinetic data from drug studies largely conducted in nonpregnant subjects to pregnant women fails to account for the impact of physiologic changes that occur during pregnancy. To disregard these changes in maternal physiology may affect drug efficacy impacting maternal disease and potentially overall pregnancy outcome.

More information is needed today on drugs and drug therapy during pregnancy because the age of reproduction has changed. In the past, pregnancy was mainly undertaken by healthy, younger women. Currently the age of reproduction includes women ranging in age from 10 to approximately 50, and with *in vitro* fertilization and egg donation even older women are undertaking pregnancy. In the United States, the age of a woman's first pregnancy has been steadily rising with an increasing number of first pregnancies occurring after age 30 [2]. The expanded age of reproduction, coupled with pregnancy occurring later in life, effectively increases the number of women who require drug therapy for diseases present before pregnancy and who need to continue therapy during pregnancy. Adequate and well-studied therapies are needed to optimally treat pregnant women with underlying diseases.

I. Physiologic Changes of Pregnancy

Rather than listing the many changes in maternal physiology that are known to occur during pregnancy, this chapter presents the physiologic changes that have the greatest potential to alter the absorption, distribution, and elimination of drugs in the pregnant women and provides examples of studies examining these effects.

A. Cardiovascular Changes

Plasma volume begins to expand by the sixth to eighth week of pregnancy. The increase in plasma volume continues in normal pregnancies until approximately 32 to 34 weeks of pregnancy [3]. This represents an increase in plasma volume of 1200 to 1300 mL for a singleton gestation or approximately 40% higher than the plasma volume of nonpregnant women. For multiple gestations, plasma volume expansion is even greater [4]. There are also significant increases in extracellular fluid space (ECF) and total body water (TBW) that vary somewhat with patient weight [5,6].

The increase in plasma volume is accompanied by a gradual increase in cardiac output. The increase in cardiac output begins in the first trimester of pregnancy. By 8 weeks' gestation, cardiac output can be as much as 50% greater than in the nonpregnant state, and by the third trimester it is at least 30 to 50% above normal [7]. Early in pregnancy, an increase in stroke volume accounts for the increased cardiac output. In later pregnancy, the increase in cardiac output is the result of both elevated maternal heart rate and a continued increase in stroke volume [8].

Regional blood flow changes also occur in pregnant women that can affect drug distribution and elimination. There is an increase in blood flow to the uterus, kidneys, skin, and mammary glands and a compensatory decrease in skeletal muscle blood flow. In a mother at full term, blood flow to the uterus represents about 20 to 25% of cardiac output, and renal blood flow is 20% of cardiac output [9]. There is increased blood flow to the skin to dissipate heat production of the fetus [10]. Blood flow to the mammary glands is increased during pregnancy in preparation for lactation postpartum [11]. Hepatic blood flow has been shown not to change during pregnancy. However, hepatic blood flow, expressed as a percentage of cardiac output, is lower during pregnancy than in the nonpregnant condition because of the increased proportion of blood flow to the uterus and kidneys [12]. With the many increases in blood flow there is a decreased proportion of cardiac output available to skeletal muscle and other vascular beds.

The expansion of plasma volume has the potential to increase the volume of distribution for drugs. The pharmacokinetics of caffeine were studied after oral administration serially during and after pregnancy [13]. In this study, the apparent volume of distribution, or V_d, showed no change when calculated on a liter per kilogram basis to account for the change in weight during and after pregnancy. In a study of a similar drug, theophylline, administered intravenously and examined serially in women during and after pregnancy [14], the steady state distribution volume, or V_{dss}, was increased during the second and third trimesters of pregnancy. However, when distribution volume was normalized for the change in patient weight during pregnancy, no difference was seen. In one study of ampicillin pharmacokinetics during pregnancy, an absolute increase was shown in the volume of distribution of ampicillin, although the study did not include an analysis of the effect of the change in maternal weight on the volume of distribution [15]. A second study of ampicillin pharmacokinetics showed an increase in the V_{dss} on a liters per kilogram basis [16].

This plasma volume expansion has the potential to decrease peak levels of drugs and thereby decrease drug efficacy. In a study of oral ampicillin, the mean peak level was significantly lower during pregnancy as compared with the same women studied after pregnancy [15]. Similarly, in examining enoxaparin pharmacokinetics during pregnancy, a lower mean C_{mas} and lower anti-factor Ten a (Xa) activity was found during pregnancy as compared with studies after pregnancy [17].

The only study examining the pharmacokinetic differences between singleton and twin gestations showed no difference in the V_d of betamethasone, despite higher known plasma volumes for multiple gestations [18].

B. Blood Composition Changes

The concentration of plasma albumin decreases during pregnancy [14,19]. The fall in albumin concentration from 4.2 g/dL in the nonpregnant woman to 3.6 g/dL in the midtrimester of pregnancy has long been attributed to a dilutional effect caused by plasma volume expansion. However, an alternative explanation is that this decrease represents either a reduction in the rate of albumin synthesis or an increase in the rate of albumin clearance. Support for this alternative explanation is found in the fact that the plasma concentrations of total protein [19] and α_1-acid glycoprotein [20], which binds many basic drugs, are relatively unchanged during pregnancy.

The reduction in albumin concentrations potentially can alter the binding of drugs commonly bound to serum albumin. In a study during the second and third trimesters of pregnancy, theophylline protein binding to plasma proteins was reduced to only 11 to 13% of total plasma concentrations, compared with 28% 6-months' postpartum [14]. Although the decrease in the serum concentration of albumin may be thought to account for

these differences, a subsequent study showed that the albumin binding sites for theophylline were actually increased during pregnancy, but the binding affinity constant was significantly lower during pregnancy than in the nonpregnant state [21].

C. Respiratory Changes

Pregnancy is associated with a partially compensated respiratory alkalosis that potentially may affect the protein binding of some drugs. Respiratory changes in pregnancy include a fall in arterial partial pressure of carbon dioxide to 30.9 mm Hg, most likely resulting from a central effect of progesterone [22,23]. In compensation, serum bicarbonate falls and maternal serum pH increases slightly to 7.44 [22]. This change in pH potentially may alter the binding of drugs to plasma proteins.

D. Renal Changes

Accompanied by the increased blood flow to the kidneys is an increase in the glomerular filtration rate (GFR). This increase begins by the sixth week of gestation and gradually continues to rise into the third trimester [24]. This increase in GFR is shown by an increased clearance of inulin and creatinine during pregnancy and by an increased renal clearance of drugs. The tubular reabsorption process, however, does not appear to be changed during pregnancy [25]. For drugs predominantly cleared by the kidney, the increase in GFR will increase drug clearance during pregnancy. Cefuroxime, a cephalosporin predominantly eliminated through the kidneys, was shown to have an elevated clearance in the midtrimester of pregnancy as compared with studies at delivery or postpartum [26]. As a result, plasma cefuroxime concentrations resulting from a 750-mg dose were significantly lower during pregnancy. Tobramycin clearance mirrors the GFR changes in pregnancy with the highest clearance and shortest half-life found in the midtrimester with a fall in clearance in the third trimester and corresponding longer half-life [27].

Even for a drug largely eliminated by hepatic metabolism, the increase in GFR can affect total clearance of drug. For theophylline, a CYP1A2 substrate, the decreased protein binding during pregnancy increases the free fraction of theophylline [14]. The increase in the free fraction of theophylline can then be cleared through the kidney. Renal clearance of theophylline has been shown to parallel the pregnancy associated increase in creatinine clearance and accounts for 30% and 28% of total theophylline elimination in the second and third trimesters, respectively, compared with only 16% 6-months' postpartum [14].

E. Changes in Hepatic Drug Metabolizing

Changes in the activity of hepatic drug metabolizing enzymes also occur during pregnancy and have been shown to affect drug elimination clearance. Although estrogen is the predominant hormone of pregnancy, progesterone, the hormone that sustains the gestation, and other placental hormones can also cause changes in hepatic enzymatic activity. Hepatic N-demethylation activity has been shown to be decreased by progesterone [28]. Using caffeine to examine the changes in hepatic enzymatic activity during pregnancy Bologa *et al* [29], studying both pregnant and nonpregnant epileptic women, found that the activity of CYP1A2, xanthine oxidase, and N-acetyltransferase decreased during pregnancy and that the activity of CYP3A4-mediated 8-hydroxylation was increased during pregnancy. Studying normal healthy women during pregnancy and also using caffeine to examine hepatic enzymatic activity, Tsutsumi et al [30] showed that during pregnancy the activity of XO was unchanged, the activity of CYP1A2 and NAT2 was decreased, and the activity of CYP3A4-mediated 8-hydroxylation was increased. Wadelius et al [31] found that CYP2D6 activity, known to be genetically determined, was actually increased during pregnancy in individuals who were homozygous and heterozygous extensive metabolizers. The activity of this enzyme, however, was decreased in homozygous poor metabolizers.

For hepatically metabolized drugs, pregnancy changes cannot always be predicted. The elimination clearance of caffeine, a CYP1A2 substrate, was shown to decrease by a factor of two by midgestation and by a factor of three in the third trimester compared with the postpartum period [13]. However, the hepatic clearance of theophylline, also a CYP1A2 substrate, was reduced during pregnancy but showed substantially less change because of the pregnancy-associated decrease in theophylline binding to plasma proteins [14]. As a result of the offsetting changes in renal and hepatic clearance, total elimination clearance of theophylline in the third trimester of pregnancy averaged 86% of its value 6-months' postpartum. In this study the reduction in elimination clearance was not statistically significant. However, the combination of a reduced elimination clearance and an increase in theophylline distribution volume significantly prolonged the half-life of theophylline from a mean of 4.4 hours 6-months' postpartum to 6.5 hours in the third trimester of pregnancy.

Methadone, a drug used to treat heroin addiction during pregnancy, is a CYP3A4 substrate. In a study of methadone pharmacokinetics during pregnancy [32], clearance of methadone was shown to be doubled in the midtrimester, falling somewhat in the third trimester. This change was both statistically and clinically significant, resulting in lower methadone plasma levels and symptoms of methadone withdrawal in some women near the end of pregnancy.

The plasma concentrations of most anticonvulsant drugs have been shown to decrease during pregnancy. This is in large part a reflection of the decrease in protein binding that is well documented for phenytoin [33,34], carbamazepine [34], and phenobarbital [35]. However, these drugs are restrictively eliminated, and unbound concentrations of carbamazepine [34,36] remain unchanged during pregnancy reflecting the fact that its intrinsic clearance is unchanged. On the other hand, Tomson et al [34] monitored phenytoin plasma levels serially in 36 women during the first and second trimesters of pregnancy and in the nonpregnant state. Intrinsic clearance was increased in the third trimester of pregnancy, and unbound plasma concentrations were significantly lower than in the nonpregnant state.

Lamotrigine, an anticonvulsant and mood-stabilizing drug, is metabolized through the liver by the phase II biotransformation of glucuronidation. Clearance of lamotrigine has been studied by Tran et al [37] during pregnancy and shown to increase by greater than 50%, necessitating dose adjustment. The clearance of lamotrigine returns rapidly to normal after delivery requiring dose adjustments in the first 2-weeks' postpartum [37,38].

The clearance of citalopram, a selective serotonin reuptake inhibitor (SSRI) metabolized by CYP2C19, 2D6, and 3A4 enzymes, has been studied serially during and after pregnancy and shown to increase in the second and third trimesters of pregnancy. However, dose adjustment was only rarely required [39].

Orally administered nifedipine, another CYP3A4 substrate, has been shown to result in decreased plasma concentrations in women with pregnancy-induced hypertension who were studied during the third trimester of pregnancy but not subsequently studied postpartum [40]. Clearance estimates averaged 2.0 L/hour/kg, compared with a value of 0.49 L/hour/kg reported in a study of nonpregnant subjects. In another study of nifedipine pharmacokinetics in women with pregnancy-induced hypertension, the clearance of nifedipine remained elevated in the immediate postpartum period, averaging 3.3 L/hour/kg in this clinical setting [41].

Betamethasone is metabolized by the liver, and clearance has been shown to be higher in pregnant than in nonpregnant women [42]. In twin gestations, betamethasone has been shown to have a higher clearance and correspondingly shorter half-life than in singleton gestations [18]. This is speculated to be caused by increased metabolism of betamethasone by the two fetoplacental units present in twin pregnancies. The shorter half-life and higher clearance may explain the decreased efficacy of betamethasone in reducing the incidence of respiratory distress syndrome in twins.

F. Gastrointestinal Changes

Because of the action of progesterone on smooth muscle activity, gastric emptying is delayed [43] and gastrointestinal transit time is prolonged [44]. There is also a decrease in gastric acid secretion that results in a correspondingly higher gastric pH [45].

Probably the best study of the effects of gastrointestinal changes occurring during pregnancy is a study of the pharmacokinetics of ampicillin [15], one of the most commonly used drugs in pregnancy. In this study, women were studied while they were pregnant and after pregnancy, serving as their own controls. Ampicillin was given both orally and intravenously, thus examining the bioavailability. Although orally administered ampicillin is only approximately 40% absorbed, no difference in the amount of ampicillin absorption was found. Time to peak drug concentrations (t_{max}) was found to be no different in pregnant and nonpregnant women. Peak drug levels, however, were found to be lower in pregnant women than in nonpregnant women.

First-pass conversion of a prodrug to an active drug has been studied in pregnancy with the drug valacyclovir [46]. Orally administered valacyclovir produced three times higher plasma levels of acyclovir than orally administered acyclovir. However, the plasma levels achieved with valacyclovir were somewhat lower than that reported in normal volunteers.

G. Peripartum Changes

The physiologic changes that begin early in gestation are most pronounced in the third trimester of pregnancy. Further physiologic changes occur during labor and delivery. There is an even further increase in cardiac output [47], while blood flow to muscle mass decreases, and there is a cessation of gastrointestinal activity. The onset of uterine contractions decreases placental blood flow and drug distribution to the fetus. In the postpartum period, maternal pregnancy changes are sustained with an elevated cardiac output, decreased plasma albumin concentration, and increased GFR [48,49]. Hepatic enzymatic activity may rapidly reverse within 24 hours of delivery or may return to normal gradually during the first months after delivery [38,50]. The cardiovascular changes of pregnancy are sustained as long as 12 weeks after delivery [51]. The physiology of the postpartum period appears to have great variability and is largely unstudied.

An intrapartum study of cefuroxime showed a lower clearance than that measured during pregnancy but higher than clearance measured in the remote postpartum period [26]. Morphine clearance has been shown to be markedly increased during labor with a corresponding shortening of its elimination half-life [52]. This shorter half-life affects dosing intervals for pain relief during labor.

Studies in the postpartum period show greater variability in pharmacokinetic parameters than studies in nonpregnant women or normal volunteers do. A study of clindamycin pharmacokinetics demonstrated that there was a 15-fold variation in peak drug concentrations and that t_{max} varied from 1 to 6 hours after oral administration [53]. A study of gentamicin in the postpartum period showed distribution volume estimates that varied from 0.1 to 0.5 L/kg, as compared with distribution volume estimates from studies in nonpregnant subjects that ranged from only 0.2 to 0.3 L/kg [54].

II. Considerations in Studying Drugs During Pregnancy

Studying drugs in pregnancy requires special considerations. Although foregoing all use of pharmacologic agents is held forth as the ideal during pregnancy, studies have shown that most pregnant women use either prescribed or over-the-counter drugs during pregnancy [55,56]. Ethically, drug studies in pregnancy cannot be done in normal pregnant volunteers but only in women who require a drug for a clinical reason. For this reason, study design for these trials must include the ethical argument that the woman would be using the particular agent during pregnancy to treat a medical condition. For Food and Drug Administration (FDA) approval of drugs specific to pregnancy, such as a tocolytic agent, an oxytocic agent, or a drug to treat pregnancy-induced hypertension, studies can only be done during pregnancy. However, drugs commonly used by women of childbearing potential, such as antidepressants, asthma medications, antihypertensive agents, and antihistamines, also can be justifiably studied during pregnancy. Drugs can be studied not only when given for maternal indications (e.g., hypertension or asthma) but when given for fetal indications (e.g., fetal supraventricular tachycardia).

Some subpopulations of pregnant women, however, often have altered physiology that may affect pharmacokinetics. Therefore, to separate the effects of the specific pathophysiology of the subpopulation on the pharmacokinetics of the drug and from those resulting from pregnancy related changes in general, studies in these women should be designed so that maximal

information is obtained. As a preliminary step, population pharmacokinetic techniques can serve as a screening tool to establish the need for further pharmacokinetic studies. For drugs that are chronically administered, these intensive studies should be conducted serially during the second and third trimester of pregnancy and in the postpartum period, so that each woman serves as her own control. Ideally, both an early and a remote postpartum evaluation should be included. For drugs only used during the peripartum period, they need only be studied during that time. Studies should incorporate *in vitro* measurements of drug binding to plasma proteins and use established tracer substances or concurrent noninvasive measures of physiology as reference markers. For bioavailability analysis, the use of the stable isotope method would decrease the number of studies necessary and decrease the biologic variation between studies [57].

III. Suggestions for Further Investigations

- Population PK studies of drugs during pregnancy
- Pharmacokinetics and pharmacodynamics of commonly used drugs during pregnancy and the postpartum period
- Receptor sensitivity tests of commonly used drugs during the perinatal period

References

1. Zinacef (cefuroxime) Labeling. (2003). In *Physicians' Desk Reference*, p. 1696. Montvale, NJ: Thomson PDR.
2. (2000). Births: Preliminary data for 1999. National Vital Statistics Reports, 48(No. 14). Atlanta, GA: Centers for Disease Control and Prevention.
3. Lund CV, Donovan JC. (1967). Blood volume during pregnancy: significance of plasma and red cell volumes. *Am J Obstet Gynecol*. 98:394–403.
4. Hytten F. (1985). Blood volume changes in normal pregnancy. *Clin Haematol*. 14: 601–612.
5. Petersen VP. (1957). Body composition and fluid compartments in normal, obese and underweight human subjects. *Acta Med Scand*. 108:103–111.
6. Plentl AA, Gray MJ. (1959). Total body water, sodium space and total exchangeable sodium in normal and toxemic pregnant women. *Am J Obstet Gynecol*. 78:472–478.
7. Lees MM, Taylor SH, Scott DM, Kerr MR. (1967). A study of cardiac output at rest throughout pregnancy. *J Obstet Gynaecol Br Commonw*. 74:319–328.
8. Robson SC, Hunter S, Boys RJ *et al*. (1989). Serial study of factors influencing changes in cardiac output during human pregnancy. *Am J Physiol*. 256:H1060.
9. Metcalfe J, Romney SL, Ramsey LH, Burwell CS. (1955). Estimation of uterine blood flow in women at term. *J Clin Invest*. 34:1632.
10. Ginsburg J, Duncan SL. (1967). Peripheral blood flow in normal pregnancy. *Cardiovasc Res*. 1:132–137.
11. Thoresen M, Wesch J. (1988). Doppler measurements of changes in human mammary and uterine blood flow during pregnancy and lactation. *Acta Obstet Gynecol Scand*. 67:741–745.
12. Robson SC, Mutch E, Boy RJ, Woodhouse KH. (1990). Apparent liver blood flow during pregnancy: a serial study using indocyanine green clearance. *Br J Obstet Gynaecol*. 97:720–724.
13. Aldridge A, Bailey J, Neims AH. (1981). The disposition of caffeine during and after pregnancy. *Semin Perinatol*. 5:310–314.
14. Frederiksen MC, Ruo TI, Chow MJ, Atkinson AJ Jr. (1986). Theophylline pharmacokinetics in pregnancy. *Clin Pharmacol Ther*. 40:321–328.
15. Philipson A. (1977). Pharmacokinetics of ampicillin during pregnancy. *J Infect Dis*. 136:370–376.
16. Kubacka RT, Johnstone HE, Tan HSI *et al*. (1983). Intravenous ampicillin pharmacokinetics in the third trimester of pregnancy. *Ther Drug Monitoring*. 5:55–60.
17. Casele HL, Laifer SA, Woelders DA, Venkataramanan R. (1999). Changes in the pharmacokinetics of the low-molecular-weight heparin enoxaparin sodium during pregnancy. *Am J Obstet Gynecol*. 181:1113–1117.

18. Ballabh P, Lo ES, Kumari J et al. (2002). Pharmacokinetics of betamethasone in twin and singleton pregnancy. *Clin Pharmacol Ther*. 71:39–45.

19. Mendenhall HW. (1970). Serum protein concentrations in pregnancy: I. Concentrations in maternal serum. *Am J Obstet Gynecol*. 106:388.

20. Wood M, Wood AJJ. (1981). Changes in plasma drug binding and α_1-acid glycoprotein in mother and newborn infant. *Clin Pharmacol Ther*. 29:522–526.

21. Connelly RJ, Ruo TI, Frederiksen MC, Atkinson AJ Jr. (1990). Characterization of theophylline binding to serum proteins in nonpregnant and pregnant women. *Clin Pharmacol Ther*. 47:68–72.

22. Lucius H, Gahlenbeck H, Kleine HO et al. (1970). Respiratory functions, buffer system and electrolyte concentrations of blood during human pregnancy. *Respir Physiol*. 9:311.

23. Lyons HA, Antonio R. (1959). The sensitivity of the respiratory centre in pregnancy and after the administration of progesterone. *Trans Assoc Am Physicians*. 72:173.

24. Davison JM, Hytten FE. (1974). Glomerular filtration during and after pregnancy. *J Obstet Gynaecol Br Commonw*. 81:588–595.

25. Davison JM, Hytten FE. (1975). The effect of pregnancy on the renal handling of glucose. *J Obstet Gynaecol Br Commonw*. 82:374.

26. Philipson A, Stiernstedt G. (1982). Pharmacokinetics of cefuroxime in pregnancy. *Am J Obstet Gynecol*. 142:823–828.

27. Bourget P, Fernandez H, Delouis C, Taburet AM. (1991). Pharmacokinetics of tobramycin in pregnant women, safety and efficacy of a once-daily dose regimen. *J Clin Pharm Ther*. 16:167–176.

28. Gerdin E, Rane A. (1992). N-demethylation of ethylmorphine in pregnant and nonpregnant women and in men: An evaluation of the effects of sex steroids. *Br J Clin Pharmacol*. 34:250–255.

29. Bologa M, Tang B, Klein J et al. (1991). Pregnancy-induced changes in drug metabolism in epileptic women. *J Pharmacol Exp Ther*. 257:735–740.

30. Tsutsumi K, Kotegawa T, Matsuki S et al. (2001). The effect of pregnancy on cytochrome P4501A2, xanthine oxidase, and N-acetyltransferase activities in humans. *Clin Pharmacol Ther*. 70:121–125.

31. Wadelius M, Darj E, Freene G, Rane A. (1997). Induction of CYP2D6 in pregnancy. *Clin Pharmacol Ther*. 62:400–407.

32. Pond SM, Kreek MJ, Tong TG et al. (1985). Altered methadone pharmacokinetics in methadone-maintained pregnancy women. *J Pharmacol Exp Ther*. 233:1–6.

33. Tomson T, Lindbom U, Ekqvist B, Sundqvist A. (1994). Epilepsy in pregnancy: A prospective study of seizure control in relation to free and total plasma concentrations of carbamazepine and phenytoin. *Epilepsia*. 35:122–130.

34. Tomson T, Lindbom U, Ekqvist B, Sundqvist A. (1994). Disposition of carbamazepine and phenytoin in pregnancy. *Epilepsia*. 35:131–135.

35. Chen SS, Perucca E, Lee JN, Richens A. (1982). Serum protein binding and free concentration of phenytoin and phenobarbitone in pregnancy. *Br J Clin Pharmacol*. 13:547–552.

36. Yerby MS, Friel PN, Miller DQ. (1985). Carbamazepine protein binding and disposition in pregnancy. *Ther Drug Monitoring*. 7:269–273.

37. Tran TA, Leppik IE, Blesi K et al. (2002). Lamotrigine clearance during pregnancy. *Neurology*. 59:251–255.

38. Ohman I, Vitois S, Tomson T. (2000). Lamotrigine in pregnancy: Pharmacokinetics during delivery, in the neonate, and during lactation. *Epilepsia*. 41:709–713.

39. Heikkinen T, Ekblad U, Kero P et al. (2002). Citalopram in pregnancy and lactation. *Clin Pharmacol Ther*. 72:184–191.

40. Prevost RR, Aki SA, Whybrew WD, Sibai BM. (1992). Oral nifedipine pharmacokinetics in pregnancy-induced hypertension. *Pharmacotherapy*. 12:174–177.

41. Barton JR, Prevost RR, Wilson DA et al. (1991). Nifedipine pharmacokinetics and pharmacodynamics during the immediate postpartum period in patients with preeclampsia. *Am J Obstet Gynecol*. 165:951–954.

42. Petersen MC, Collier CB, Ashley JJ et al. (1983). Disposition of betamethasone in parturient women after intravenous administration. *Eur J Clin Pharmacol*. 25:803–810.

43. Hunt JN, Murray FA. (1958). Gastric function in pregnancy. *J Obstet Gynaecol Br Emp*. 65:78–83.

44. Parry E, Shields R, Turnbull AC. (1970). Transit time in the small intestine in pregnancy. *J Obstet Gynaecol Br Commonw*. 77:900–901.

45. Gryboski WA, Spiro HM. (1976). The effect of pregnancy on gastric secretion. *N Engl J Med*. 255:1131–1137.

46. Kimberlin DF, Weller S, Whitley RJ et al. (1998). Pharmacokinetics of oral valacyclovir and acyclovir in late pregnancy. *Am J Obstet Gynecol*. 179:846–851.

47. Lees MM, Scott DH, Kerr MG. (1970). Haemodynamic changes associated with labour. *J Obstet Gynaecol Br Commonw*. 77:29–36.

48. Ueland K, Metcalfe J. (1975). Circulatory changes in pregnancy. *Clin Obstet Gynecol*. 18:41.

49. Sims EAH, Krantz KE. (1958). Serial studies of renal function during pregnancy and the puerperium in normal women. *J Clin Invest*. 37:1764.

50. Dam M, Christiansen J, Munck O, Mygind KI. (1979). Antiepileptic drugs: metabolism in pregnancy. *Clin Pharmacokinet*. 4:53–62.

51. Capeless EL, Clapp JF. (1991). When do cardiovascular parameters return to their preconception values? *Am J Obstet Gynecol*. 165:883.

52. Gerdin E, Salmonson T, Lindberg B, Rane A. (1990). Maternal kinetics of morphine during labour. *J Perinat Med*. 18:479–487.

53. Steen B, Rane A. (1982). Clindamycin passage into human milk. *Br J Clin Pharmacol*. 13:661–664.

54. Del Priore G, Jackson-Stone M, Shim EK et al. (1996). A comparison of once-daily and eight hour gentamicin dosing in the treatment of postpartum endometritis. *Obstet Gynecol*. 87:994–1000.

55. Nelson MM, Forfar JO. (1971). Association between drugs administered during pregnancy and congenital abnormalities of the fetus. *BMJ*. 1(5748):523–527.

56. Bonati M, Bortolus R, Marchetti F et al. (1990). Drug use in pregnancy: An overview of epidemiological (drug utilization) studies. *Eur J Clin Pharmacol*. 38:325–328.

57. Strong JM, Dutcher JS, Lee W-K, Atkinson AF Jr. (1975). Absolute bioavailability in man of N-acetylprocainamide determined by a novel stable isotope method. *Clin Pharmacol Ther*. 18:613–622.

80

Weight Reduction Therapies: Anorectants, Thermogenics, and Lipolytics

CHRISTINE A. HALLER, MD

Departments of Medicine and Laboratory Medicine, University of California, San Francisco, CA

I. Introduction

Obesity is an increasingly common condition in the United States, with approximately one in three adults being overweight [1]. Because obesity is linked with a number of health risks including type II diabetes, atherosclerotic cardiovascular disease, hypertension, and certain types of cancer, it is a leading preventable disease, second only to cigarette smoking. Unfortunately, physicians may resist tackling weight loss with their patients, perhaps because of perceived resistance, low success rates, and lack of experience and training in this area. Indeed, motivating patients to change unhealthy dietary and lifestyle patterns can be an enormous hurdle, but, with a rational weight reduction plan and continued encouragement, many men and women can successfully achieve long-term weight loss. There is evidence that even moderate weight loss of 5 to 10% of body weight can significantly reduce obesity-related morbidity and mortality with demonstrated decreases in blood pressure and serum triglycerides and increased levels of high-density lipoprotein (HDL)-cholesterol [2,3].

Easily available nonprescription weight-loss products are an attractive alternative for overweight individuals who struggle to reduce caloric intake and increase physical activity. A 1998 multistate population survey of nearly 15,000 adults found that 7% of respondents used at least one nonprescription weight-loss product in the previous 2 years [4]. Among women, the prevalence of use of weight-loss products in the prior 2 years was 10.9% for nonprescription products and 38.5% for prescription products. Based on body mass index (BMI) calculations [5], approximately one third of study participants were classified as overweight (BMI 25 to 29.9), and 20% were obese (BMI>30).

Studies have demonstrated that pharmacologic treatment of obesity without lifestyle modification typically results in suboptimal weight loss [6]. Because obesity is a multifaceted medical condition, treatment should not be viewed in the narrow context of appetite control. Instead, understanding a patient's external triggers for overeating and his or her history of weight-loss attempts and failures will aid in tailoring an individual weight-loss program with a greater chance of success.

Males and females appear to have different types of obesity and different responses to dieting, as well as discrepant attitudes toward eating and weight reduction. Body fat distribution differs between the genders, with men more likely to exhibit central obesity and women carrying more peripheral body fat, that is on their body frames [7]. Men may substantially reduce central obesity by dietary measures alone, whereas women often require increased exercise along with reduced caloric intake to achieve the same fat loss. In addition, body fat distribution changes in women with reproductive phases and childbearing, and obesity can have adverse consequences on female fertility. Aside from familial patterns of obesity resulting from genetic factors, there is also evidence that mothers' dietary disinhibition, that is habit of overeating, is an independent predictor of daughters' childhood obesity [8].

Psychosocial gender differences regarding eating, dieting, and body image emerge as early as age 9. In general, males show less desire to lose weight than females, with dieting beginning at a higher average BMI in men than women (27.3 vs 24.2, $p < 0.01$) [9]. Males tend to use dieting to achieve specific goals, typically in response to dissatisfaction with their upper body size and shape. In contrast, female children, adolescents, and adults use dieting in an attempt to achieve a cultural norm of thinness that pervades Western societies. Women appear to eat more in times of increased stress and may binge on favorite foods, particularly at night, as an emotional response [10]. Overweight women frequently complain of preoccupation with eating and struggle with discontentment with reduced food intake. Although men may also experience some of the same emotional eating responses, there is a marked gender difference in eating disorders such as bulimia and anorexia nervosa. Only 10% of diagnosed cases of eating disorders in the United States involve males; thus, eating disorders are among the greatest gender discrepancies in medicine and psychiatry [9].

Historically, weight-loss therapies have been problematic, leading to a growing sense of distrust of antiobesity medications. Furthermore, unsafe and unsuccessful fad diets and radical weight-loss schemes have sullied the concept of rational weight reduction techniques. Although there is no magic pill that can melt away fat, there are several pharmacologic options that, when combined with dietary and exercise modifications, can result in successful weight reduction.

Pharmacologic effects of weight-loss drugs are based on three types of mechanisms of action: decreased food intake by suppressing appetite; altered absorption, metabolism, or elimination of food; and increased energy expenditure. Some weight-loss drugs have combined mechanisms of action.

Weight-loss agents may also be considered in the context of federal regulatory categories as being either prescription or over-the-counter (OTC) drugs, or dietary supplements. The requirements for approval, marketing, and postmarketing surveillance of these two categories are vastly different. Table 80-1

Table 80-1
Oral Medications Approved for the Treatment of Obesity

Drug*	Mechanism of Action	Regulation/ DEA Schedule	Recommended Oral Dose/ Duration of Use	Adverse Effects	CI to Use
Diethylpropion (Tenuate)	Increased release of NE and dopamine	Schedule IV	25 mg tid 1 hour before meals, or 75-mg extended-release once in a.m. Few weeks only	Dry mouth, tremor, insomnia, headache, constipation, nervousness, palpitations, hypertension, stroke, arrhythmia	MAOI use within 14 days; severe HTN, symptomatic CV disease, glaucoma, hyperthyroidism
Mazindol (Mazanor, Sanorex)	Inhibits reuptake of NE	Schedule IV	1 mg qd to tid as tolerated before meals, or 2 mg once. Few weeks only	See diethylpropion	See diethylpropion
Orlistat (Xenical)	Inhibits gastric and pancreatic lipases	Prescription drug	120 mg tid with fat-containing meals; and supplemental vitamins >2hr from dosing	Abdominal pain, oily stool, flatus, fecal urgency or incontinence; fat-soluble vitamin loss	Cholestasis, chronic malabsorption, bulimia, anorexia nervosa
Phentermine (Fastin, Phentride, Zantryl, Pro-Fast, Adipex, Ionamin)	Increased release of NE and dopamine	Schedule IV	15–37.5 mg once per day in a.m. Few weeks only	See diethylpropion	See diethylpropion
Sibutramine (Meridia)	Inhibits reuptake of serotonin and NE	Schedule IV	10–15 mg per day in the morning, for no longer than 12 months	Anxiety, dry mouth, insomnia, constipation, headache, hypertension, palpitations, dysmenorrhea	Anorexia nervosa, history of stroke or seizures, uncontrolled HTN, glaucoma, symptomatic CV disease

*Trade names appear in parentheses.
CV, cardiovascular; DEA, United States Drug Enforcement Administration; HTN, hypertension; MAOI, monoamine oxidase inhibitor; NE, norepinephrine; qd, daily; tid, three times daily.

Table 80-2
Dietary Supplements Promoted for Weight Loss

Botanical	Active Constituent	Purported Effects	Scientific Evidence	Adverse Effects	Precautions
Chitosan	Insoluble marine fiber	Binds fat and prevents GI absorption	No supportive evidence	Decreased absorption of fat-soluble vitamins	Shellfish allergy; pregnancy and lactation
Chromium picolinate	Trivalent chromium	Fat loss, lowers serum LDL; improves glucose control; increases lean muscle mass	No evidence that it produces fat loss or increases lean muscle mass	Dermatitis; possibly mutagenic in high doses	Pregnancy and lactation
Citrus aurantium (bitter orange extract)	Synephrine	Increased thermogenesis, increased lipolysis	Insufficient data to substantiate weight-loss claims	Increases blood pressure and arrhythmias in rodents	Hypertension, stroke, cardiac disease, glaucoma
Garcina cambogia	Hydroxycitric acid	Increased fat oxidation; reduced food intake	Studies show not effective in weight reduction	None reported	Only maximum duration of use of 12 weeks has been studied
Guarana	Caffeine	Increased thermogenesis in combination with ephedra	Studies on synthetic caffeine support claims. Inadequate safety studies on guarana	Nausea, vomiting, insomnia, nervousness, palpitations, arrhythmias, diuresis	Peptic ulcer disease; depression, anxiety, arrhythmias, kidney or liver disease

GI, gastrointestinal; LDL, low-density lipoprotein.

summarizes the drugs that are approved by the U.S. Food and Drug Administration (FDA) to treat obesity. Table 80-2 summarizes the dietary supplements and natural products that are currently available as OTC weight-loss remedies. Table 80-3 lists the drugs and herbal supplements that are no longer recommended or have been withdrawn or banned by the FDA for the treatment of obesity because of adverse reactions reported in the United States or internationally.

Table 80-3
Drugs and Supplements That Are Not Endorsed for Treating Obesity or Have Been Withdrawn
or Banned by the FDA Because of Adverse Reactions

Drug*	Mechanism of Action	Adverse Effects	Regulation Status DEA Schedule or Withdrawal Date
Amphetamine	Increased release of NE and dopamine	Dry mouth, tremor, insomnia, headache, sweating, dependence, nervousness, palpitations, hypertension, stroke, arrhythmia, psychosis	Approved with warning label Schedule II
Benzphetamine (Didrex)	Increased release of NE and dopamine	See amphetamine	Schedule III
Dexfenfluramine (Redux)	Promotes central serotonin release, and inhibits its reuptake	Valvular heart disease, primary pulmonary hypertension	Withdrawn Sept. 1997
Dieter's teas contain senna, cascara, aloe, buckthorn	Stimulant laxative herbs that promote colonic evacuation	Diarrhea, vomiting, nausea, abdominal cramps, electrolyte disorders, dependence	FDA required label warning—June 1995
Dinitrophenol	Alters metabolism by uncoupling cellular oxidative phosphorylation	Hyperthermia, cataracts, hepatotoxicity, fatalities	Not approved for treatment of obesity
Ephedra (ma huang)	Increased release of NE and dopamine; increased thermogenesis	See amphetamine	Banned by FDA—April, 2004
Ephedrine/caffeine	Increased release of NE; increased thermogenesis	See amphetamine	Not approved in United States for treatment of obesity
Fenfluramine (Pondimin)	Increased release and decreased reuptake of serotonin	Valvular heart disease, primary pulmonary hypertension	Withdrawn Sept. 1997
Guar Gum (Cal-Ban 3000)	Hygroscopic polysaccharide swells in stomach, producing early satiety	Esophageal and small bowel obstruction, fatalities	Banned by FDA—July 1990
LipoKinetix contains sodium usniate, norephedrine, 3,5-diiodothyronine, yohimbine, caffeine	Unknown	Acute hepatitis	FDA warning—Nov. 2001
Phendimetrazine (Adipost, Bontril, Phendiet-105, Melfiat, Prelu-2)	Increased release of NE and dopamine	See amphetamine	Schedule III
Phenylpropanolamine (Dexatrim, Acutrim)	α-1 Adrenergic agonist	Headache, hypertension, myocardial infarction, intracranial hemorrhage	Withdrawn Nov. 2000

*Trade names appear in parentheses.
DEA, Drug Enforcement Administration; FDA, Food and Drug Administration; NE, norepinephrine.

II. Drugs That Reduce Food Intake and Increase Energy Expenditure

Sympathomimetic drugs that act at noradrenergic and serotoninergic receptors have been demonstrated to be clinically useful in promoting weight loss. A number of monoamines that act at α_1- and β_2-adrenergic receptors are known to reduce food intake [11], and several of these agonists have been approved as pharmaceutical anorexiants. Stimulation of serotonergic receptors in the 5-HT$_1$ and 5-HT-$_2$ family modulates appetite as well. Drugs that stimulate 5-HT release (fenfluramine) or block serotonin reuptake (fluoxetine, fenfluramine) reduce food intake. The pharmacology of the classes of noradrenergic and serotonergic drugs is described in more detail later.

A. Noradrenergic Drugs

Sympathomimetic amines have anorexigenic effects that lead to weight loss, but many have unfavorable side effects that limit their clinical utility. The mechanism of action appears to be a result of central nervous system (CNS) stimulation because of increased release of norepinephrine and dopamine. In addition, amphetamines may reduce taste and olfactory acuity, resulting in reduced appetite, and some derivatives appear to directly suppress the appetite center in the hypothalamus.

Amphetamine was the first stimulant drug in the class of phenyl-ethylamines to be found to have appetite suppressant effects. As early as 1937, amphetamine was promoted as an ideal drug to treat obesity because it decreased appetite while increasing energy and producing a sense of well being [12]. However, the stimulant and euphoriant effects of amphetamine resulted in this drug becoming highly addictive and widely abused, and its therapeutic use as an appetite suppressant fell out of favor.

A number of other amphetamine congeners were explored as suitable alternatives to amphetamine, and several are currently approved for the short-term treatment of obesity. Phenmetrazine was introduced in the 1950s as an anorexiant with less stimulant activity than amphetamine. However, it was subsequently discovered to have significant euphoric effects, and, in large doses, phenmetrazine can produce an amphetamine-like paranoid psychosis. Because of its abuse potential, it is not recommended for the treatment of obesity. Phendimetrazine has been shown in animal studies to have less pronounced central and peripheral nervous system stimulation than phenmetrazine. However, both of these older sympathomimetic appetite suppressants have larger been replaced by phentermine, diethylpropion, and mazindol, which have very little abuse potential. These drugs offer the same anorexigenic properties as amphetamine with a lower therapeutic equivalency than the dose needed to produce stimulant effects, and therefore are less likely to be misused for the purpose of "getting high."

All of the amphetamine congeners produce some degree of central and peripheral nervous system stimulant effects including vasoconstriction, increased cardiac contractility, bronchodilation, mydriasis, urinary bladder sphincter contraction, and increased mental alertness. A number of undesirable effects are associated with use of these drugs as a result of their stimulant actions including dry mouth, palpitations, sweating, headache, hypertension, tremor, irritability, and insomnia. Severe adverse events have included stroke, seizures, cardiac arrhythmias, agitation, and psychosis.

Because tolerance may develop to the anorexigenic effects, these drugs should be used only for a few weeks, as an adjunct to caloric restriction and behavioral modification. Some studies have shown that the rate of weight loss reaches a plateau within a few weeks of initiating treatment and that weight regain is common after stopping therapy [12]. This class of weight-loss drugs has only a temporary weight-loss effect and will not be successful for long-term weight reduction without accompanying changes in diet and exercise patterns.

Phenylpropanolamine (PPA) was a very common ingredient in OTC weight loss and decongestant medications until a case-control study demonstrated a link between PPA and an increased risk of hemorrhagic stroke in women [13]. Phenylpropanolamine is primarily an α_1-adrenergic agonist that results in vasoconstriction and that also appears to act directly on the supraventricular nucleus of the hypothalamus to suppress appetite. A number of serious adverse cardiovascular events including hemorrhagic stroke, myocarditis, and acute myocardial infarction have been reported in association with therapeutic use of PPA [14]. In November of 2000, PPA was voluntarily recalled by drug manufacturers after published results from the Hemorrhagic Stroke Project showed an adjusted odds ratio of 16.58 for the association between use of PPA-containing appetite suppressants and the risk of a hemorrhagic stroke in women [13].

B. Serotonergic Drugs

Several drugs that affect serotonin release and reuptake are currently approved for the treatment of a number of conditions including depression, anxiety, premenstrual dysphoric syndrome, nicotine addiction, and obsessive-compulsive disorder. These drugs all reduce food intake but are not currently approved for the treatment of obesity. Several serotonergic drugs have been used in the past to treat obesity including dexfenfluramine (Redux), fenfluramine (Pondimin), and fenfluramine combined with phentermine (Fen-Phen). Except for phentermine, these drugs have all been withdrawn from the market because of postmarketing reports of serious adverse effects associated with their therapeutic use.

An estimated 3 to 4 million people took the Fen-Phen combination until a case series was published in 1997 that described 24 women with no pre-existing cardiovascular disease who developed atypical cardiac valvulopathy after taking Fen-Phen [15]. Both fenfluramine and dexfenfluramine were promptly withdrawn from the market. The histopathology of the affected heart valves was identical to changes seen with carcinoid syndrome and ergotamine-induced valvulopathy, and the mechanism was postulated to be related to increased levels of circulating serotonin. Primary pulmonary hypertension had previously been reported in patients taking fenfluramine and phentermine alone, as well as in patients taking dexfenfluramine in high doses, and was thought to be a result of the vasoconstrictive actions of serotonin or a result of alterations in pulmonary vascular smooth muscle. Although fenfluramine and phentermine were individually approved as prescription weight-loss drugs, the combination of these drugs was never approved by the FDA for treating obesity. The regulation of phentermine has not changed since the recall of fenfluramine.

The only serotonergic drug currently approved for the treatment of obesity is sibutramine (Meridia). Sibutramine acts by blocking the reuptake of both serotonin and norepinephrine, but it does not promote neuronal release of serotonin. Its clinical effects are a reduction in appetite and increased satiety. This prescription drug is recommended in doses of 10 to 15 mg per day for obese patients with a BMI>30 kg/m^2 without co-morbid conditions, and patients with a BMI>27 kg/m^2 in patients with other disease states such as diabetes, dyslipidemia, or hypertension. Its effectiveness in producing weight loss has been demonstrated in several randomized, double-blind studies [16,17]. In one study of obese patients, long-term sibutramine use (48 weeks) produced equivalent weight loss and comparable safety profiles when given continuously (15 mg/day) or intermittently (12 weeks of sibutramine alternating with 6 weeks of placebo). The rate of weight loss reached a maximum during the first 3 months of continuous therapy and then continued at a slower rate for the remainder of the study. Patients receiving intermittent sibutramine therapy had significantly fewer adverse events compared with patients receiving placebo or continuous therapy [18]. The use of sibutramine for greater than 1 year has not been studied. Whether weight reduction is maintained after cessation of sibutramine is also unknown.

Sibutramine's pharmacologic activity depends on first-pass hepatic metabolism by cytochrome P450 (CYP3A4) into two active metabolites, mono-desmethylsibutramine and di-desmethylsibutramine, with half-lives of 14 and 16 hours, respectively. These metabolites are then inactivated and renally excreted. Medications that inhibit CYP3A4 such as cimetidine, erythromycin, or ketoconazole may decrease clearance of sibutramine. Moderate hepatic or renal impairment does not significantly alter the pharmacokinetics of sibutramine or its active metabolites.

Sibutramine has also been shown in animal and human studies to increase thermogenesis and to enhance satiety. In one randomized, double-blind, placebo-controlled study of 11 healthy nonobese males, a 30-mg dose of sibutramine produced a significant increase in resting energy expenditure in both fasting and nonfasting states [19]. This increased thermogenesis was accompanied by increased plasma epinephrine and glucose and increased heart rate and blood pressure.

The risks versus benefits of sibutramine for the management of obesity remains controversial. Of concern is the aggravation of obesity-related co-morbidities, primarily hypertension, in the setting of modest weight reduction. Since Meridia was approved in 1998, there have been 397 serious adverse reactions reported to the FDA, including 29 deaths, of which 19 were due to cardiovascular causes including 3 women younger than age 30 [20]. Sibutramine was banned in Italy in March of 2002 because of two cardiovascular deaths, and its use as a weight-loss drug is being scrutinized in other European countries as well [21].

Sibutramine should not be taken in combination with monamine oxidase inhibitors, selective serotonin reuptake inhibitors, or any drug that affects serotonin release or reuptake because of the risk of inducing serotonin syndrome, characterized by agitation, hyperthermia, autonomic instability, and myoclonus. Because sibutramine increases thermogenesis and raises heart rate and blood pressure, it should not be used by patients with poorly controlled hypertension, coronary artery disease, glaucoma, or previous stroke. Its use is also contraindicated in patients with anorexia nervosa, severe hepatic or renal dysfunction, or seizure disorder.

III. Drugs that Alter Food Absorption and Elimination

Orlistat (Xenical) was approved by the FDA in 1999 for the treatment of obesity, and it is the only currently approved drug that alters the absorption, distribution, and metabolism of food. Orlistat is a potent inhibitor of gastric and pancreatic lipase, thus reducing lipolysis and increasing fecal fat excretion [22]. Orlistat is not systemically absorbed, but instead it exerts its effects locally in the gastrointestinal tract by covalently binding to the active site of digestive lipases. It, therefore, inhibits hydrolysis of dietary triglycerides and reduces absorption of the products of lipolysis, monoglycerides, and free fatty acids. Many clinical trials have been done with orlistat demonstrating that it reduces gastrointestinal fat absorption by up to 30% [23]. When taken in association with a slightly restricted diet, obese subjects have lost approximately 10% body weight in 1 year [24].

Orlistat is recommended to be taken in doses of 120 mg three times per day in conjunction with a fat-containing meal. If a meal is missed or contains no fat, the dose of orlistat should be skipped. Its actions depend on the dietary intake of lipids, with a maximal effect in persons consuming a high fat diet. Its adverse effects are also correlated with dietary fat consumption and may include abdominal pain, oily stool, fecal incontinence, oily spotting, fecal urgency, flatus, increased defecation, and headache. One placebo-controlled trial in overweight women found that concomitant use of natural fibers (6 g of psyllium mucilloid dissolved in water) reduced the incidence of gastrointestinal side effects of orlistat [25]. In addition, because orlistat reduces absorption of fat-soluble vitamins, a daily multivitamin supplement containing vitamins A, D, K, and beta-carotene should be taken 2 hours before orlistat administration to prevent deficiency.

IV. Dietary Supplements Promoted for Weight Reduction

The use of ephedra and other botanical antiobesity remedies has skyrocketed since the Dietary Supplement Health and Education Act of 1994 (DSHEA) [26] opened the door for widespread marketing and sales of a myriad of "natural" weight-loss products. There is very little federal oversight of these weight-loss dietary supplements because premarket testing for safety and efficacy and postmarketing surveillance of adverse reactions to dietary supplements are not required under the DSHEA. As a result, there is very little published scientific evidence to support the weight-loss claims made by supplement manufacturers.

Most weight-loss supplements are multicomponent products that contain botanicals and trace elements intended to have synergistic effects in promoting weight loss. These products may include components with diuretic actions (sarsaparilla, damiana), stimulant actions (*Ephedra sinica*, guarana, *Citrus aurantium*), and metabolic actions (chromium, *Garcina cambogia*). Potentiation of adverse effects by combining many active ingredients into a single formulation is a pharmacologic concern that cannot be dismissed.

Table 80-2 summarizes the theorized actions and potential risks of some of the most common constituents of weight-loss dietary supplements. Several of these supplements are described in more detail in the following sections.

A. Ephedra/Caffeine

Ephedrine is a bronchodilator that stimulates both α_1- and β-adrenergic receptors and indirectly stimulates release of norepinephrine resulting in increased blood pressure and cardiac output and CNS stimulation. It is rarely used as an OTC bronchodilator because of its adverse effect profile and has largely been replaced by safer drugs. Although never approved in the United States as an anorexigenic drug, it has been studied and shown to be effective in combination with caffeine in decreasing appetite, increasing resting energy expenditure, and promoting weight loss in obese human subjects [27–29]. In one 24-week trial, the combination of 20-mg ephedrine and 200-mg caffeine taken three times per day was more effective that either drug alone in inducing weight reduction and fat loss [30]. This study also showed that undesirable side effects such as tremor, insomnia, and dizziness subside during chronic treatment, whereas the thermogenic actions are preserved. In the United States, drug combinations of caffeine and ephedrine or pseudoephedrine are not allowed under a September 27, 2001 FDA ruling that stated cough and cold combination products containing oral bronchodilators along with other stimulant ingredients are not generally recognized as safe or effective [31].

Botanical products that contain ephedra were formally allowed under the DSHEA but have recently been banned by the FDA. Weight-loss dietary supplements typically contain 12 to 25 mg total ephedrine-group alkaloids derived from extracts of *Ephedra sinica*, the plant source of the Chinese herbal medicine ma huang. Ma huang contains ephedrine and lesser quantities of related alkaloids, including pseudoephedrine, methylephedrine, norephedrine, methylpseudoephedrine, and norpseudoephedrine. Although chemically similar, the various alkaloids have distinctly different pharmacologic profiles including differences in CNS stimulation and cardiovascular effects.

The source of caffeine in weight-loss dietary supplements is typically the seed of the guarana plant, which contains 3 to 5% caffeine and lesser quantities of related methylxanthines, theophylline, theobromine, and numerous other constituents. Only two small studies have been published on the effects of ephedra and herbal caffeine combinations in producing weight loss. The first, an 8-week trial of a dietary supplement containing 72 mg/day ephedrine alkaloids and 240 mg/day caffeine, showed significant weight loss versus placebo, but 23% of the treatment group withdrew from the protocol because of adverse effects, including palpitations, elevated blood pressure, chest pain, and irritability [32]. In a subsequent study by the same research group, herbal versus placebo treatment for 6 months produced significant decreases in body weight, body fat, and low-density lipoprotein (LDL)-cholesterol [33]. In this study, adverse effects did not differ between groups. However, in this study, subjects did not receive the same multicomponent supplement as in the 8-week trial but were given only ma huang and herbal caffeine. It is possible that the multicomponent supplements produce greater adverse effects because of herb-herb interactions or additive pharmacologic actions.

Weight-loss dietary supplements that contain caffeine and ephedra have been associated with nearly 1400 FDA adverse event reports since 1993, including 80 deaths [34]. Adverse events have included psychosis, ischemic and hemorrhagic stroke, seizures, acute myocardial infarction, myocarditis, and sudden death [35–39]. Adverse events related to these dietary supplements sometimes occur in apparently healthy individuals without known risk factors such as cardiovascular disease, hyperthyroidism, seizure, or stroke history [40]. Some of these adverse events have occurred not in obese individuals, but fit athletes, who take ephedra and caffeine-containing products for thermogenesis and performance enhancement.

B. Bitter Orange Extract (Citrus aurantium)

Citrus aurantium is a natural source of synephrine and octopamine, which are structurally similar to norepinephrine and are reported to have α_1-adrenergic agonist actions resulting in vasoconstriction and increased blood pressure [41]. This herbal extract is increasingly being used to replace ephedra in weight-loss dietary supplements. There is only one published human study on the cardiovascular effects of *Citrus aurantium* [42], and no studies have reported on its effects when taken in combination with ephedra alkaloids or caffeine in dietary supplement form. One study showed that high doses of extracts of *Citrus aurantium* can cause ventricular arrhythmias in rats [43]. *Citrus aurantium* has been shown experimentally to inhibit CYP3A4, which suggests the potential for herb-drug interactions [44].

C. Garcinia cambogia

The dried fruit of the Southeast Asian species *Garcinia cambogia* contains 30 to 50% hydroxycitric acid (HCA), which is believed to be the active ingredient of this weight-loss botanical product. Hydroxycitric acid has been demonstrated to have a satiety effect in rats [45], however, studies investigating HCA's effects in promoting weight loss in humans have been disappointing. Although modest weight loss has been observed in some HCA-treated groups [46,47], a larger, more rigorously controlled clinical study of obese subjects found that oral extracts of *Garcinia cambogia* are ineffective for weight loss [48]. In addition, postulated mechanisms for weight-reducing effects of HCA have not been substantiated experimentally. Based on rodent studies, it was hypothesized that HCA increases fat oxidation, depresses *de novo* fatty acid synthesis, and reduces food intake. Results of two human studies on HCA, one in overweight females [47] and one in fasting males [49], have not supported this hypothesis. Adverse reactions have not been reported with oral use of *Garcinia cambogia*.

D. Other Supplements

Other constituents of dietary supplements are promoted to increase loss of body fat while preserving lean muscle mass including chromium picolinate, L-carnitine, dehydroepiandrosterone (DHEA), and pyruvate. Currently, there is insufficient scientific evidence to support use of these substances for weight loss. Chitosan is another weight-loss supplement derived from marine exoskeletons that when ingested is reported to bind with fatty acids and other lipids, preventing lipolysis and absorption. In this way, chitosan would act similarly to orlistat. There is some evidence that dietary chitosan may decrease total serum cholesterol in overweight humans, but it has not been extensively investigated for safety and efficacy [50].

V. The Future of Weight-Loss Medications

Of keen interest is the development of new weight-loss drugs that better target the food intake mechanism and the physiology of body fat storage, mobilization, and metabolism. Also, drugs with greater specificity for β_3-adrenergic receptors as opposed to general sympathetic nervous system activation would optimize lipolysis and limit undesirable stimulant side effects. Several endogenous modulators of food intake and fat utilization are under investigation for development of new antiobesity medications.

A. Leptin

Leptin is a neuropeptide produced by adipose tissue that modulates food intake and energy expenditure via a leptin-signaling pathway in the brain. Deficiencies in leptin production produce extreme obesity, and replacement of this peptide in deficient individuals decreases food intake and results in fat loss [51]. A preliminary randomized, controlled trial in obese and lean humans showed dose-dependent weight loss with sub-cutaneous recombinant leptin but also resulted in injection site reactions at higher doses [52]. Human recombinant leptin (rL) is currently in the late phases of drug development.

B. β_3–Adrenergic Receptor Agonists

Norepinephrine, the neurotransmitter of the sympathetic nervous system, has long been the target of weight-loss drugs with intended actions of promoting thermogenesis, stimulating the CNS, and inhibiting the hypothalamic appetite center. Norepinephrine also may decrease food intake by acting on β_2 and β_3 peripheral adrenoreceptors. β_3 receptors are found primarily in white adipose tissue, liver, and skeletal muscle. β_3 agonists have been observed to increase lipolysis, fat oxidation, energy expenditure, and insulin action. Development of β_3 agonists to treat obesity and diabetes has had disappointing results thus far because of poor bioavailability and limited duration of activity [53]. Recent cloning of the human β_3-adrenergic receptor offers promise for development of novel agonists with greater potency.

VI. Weighing the Risks Versus Benefits of Obesity Medications

The history of weight-reduction drug use had been marred by a number of health catastrophes that have raised to an all-time high the level of skepticism and debate over the safety versus utility of these drugs. In one camp is the opinion that antiobesity drugs do not offer a significant, lasting therapeutic benefit to justify even a very low incidence of adverse events that might be considered acceptable with other medications such as anti-hypertensives, anticonvulsants, or chemotherapeutic agents. On the other hand, uncontrolled weight gain is itself a risk factor for development of a number of diseases, and, therefore, a certain degree of risk would be acceptable if the weight-loss medication had demonstrated efficacy. Unfortunately, many of the adverse events in recent years associated with prescription and nonpre-scription weight-loss medicines have resulted in severe, permanent morbidity and even fatalities. This includes most notably, cardiac valvular disease with Fen-Phen, hemorrhagic stroke with PPA, and pulmonary hypertension with phentermine and dexfenfluramine. In addition, many amphetamine conge-ners have been associated with cardiovascular events including strokes, myocardial infarctions, and cardiac arrhythmias. Confounding the assessment of adverse events reported in asso-ciation with weight-loss drugs is the increased morbidity and mortality associated with obesity-related conditions such as type II diabetes, hypertension, and dyslipidemia.

Most experts agree that pharmacotherapy alone is not an ideal approach for management of obesity and that long-term weight reduction is best achieved with dietary and exercise modifica-tions as the principal treatment and medication as an adjunct [6,10,54]. In the absence of safe and effective prescription weight-loss drugs, obese patients may increasingly turn to inadequately tested alternative medicines or unproven weight-loss quackery. Indeed, recent reports of severe hepatotoxicity associated with a weight-loss supplement called LipoKinetix [55] and the syndrome of Chinese herb nephropathy associated with a Belgian herbal slimming regimen that was inadvertently contaminated with a nephrotoxic herb (Aristolochia fangji) tragi-cally illustrate that natural remedies are not harm-free [56,57].

In summary, weight-loss drugs, like all medications, carry a degree of risk associated with a potential benefit in reducing obesity-related medical complications. However, used inappro-priately in nonobese patients or in the absence of adjunctive weight-reduction therapies such as dietary and lifestyle coun-seling, the risk-benefit profile may become unfavorable shifted.

VII. Suggestions for Further Investigations

- Conduct long-term (>1 year) clinical trials to determine the effectiveness of weight-reduction therapies *after* cessation of medication.
- Characterize the pharmacologic effects of alternative medi-cines and natural products promoted as antiobesity agents.
- Continue to explore novel therapeutics for weight reduction that offer greater selectivity for fat loss and fewer potential adverse effects.

References

1. Kuczmarski RJ, Flegal KM, Campbell SM et al. (1994). Increasing preva-lence of overweight among US adults. The National Health and Nutritional Examination Surveys, 1960 to 1991. JAMA. 272:305–311.
2. Williamson DF, Pamuk E, Thun M et al. (1995). Prospective study of inten-tional weight loss and mortality in never-smoking overweight US white women aged 40–64 years. Am J Epidemiol. 141:1128–1141.
3. Wood PD, Stefanick M, Dreon DM et al. (1988). Changes in plasma lipids and lipoproteins in overweight men during weight loss through dieting as compared with exercise. N Engl J Med. 319:1173–1179.
4. Blanck HM, Khan LK, Serdula MK. (2001). Use of nonprescription weight loss products—Results from a multistate survey. JAMA. 286:930–935.
5. http://www.nhlbisupport.com/bmi/bmicalc.htm (accessed 8/23/02).
6. Wadden TA, Berkowitz RI, Sarwer DB et al. (2001). Benefits of lifestyle modification in the pharmacologic treatment of obesity. Arch Intern Med. 161:218–227.
7. Legato MJ. (1997). Gender-specific aspects of obesity. Int J Fertil. 42: 184–197.
8. Cutting TM, O'Fisher J, Grimm-Thomas K, Birch L. (1999). Like mother, like daughter: Familial patterns of overweight are mediated by mothers' die-tary disinhibition. Am J Clin Nutr. 69:608–613.
9. Andersen AE, Holman JE. (1997). Males with eating disorders: Challenges for treatment and research. Psychopharm Bull. 33:391–397.
10. Meisler JG. (2001). Toward optimal health: The experts discuss weight control drugs. J Womens Health Gender Based Med. 10(2):101–107.
11. Bray GA. (2000). A concise review on the therapeutics of obesity. Nutrition. 16:953–960.
12. Silverstone T. (1986). Clinical use of appetite suppressants. Drug Alcohol Dependence. 17:151–167.
13. Kernan WN, Viscoli CM, Brass LM et al. (2000). Phenylpropanolamine and the risk of hemorrhagic stroke. N Engl J Med. 343:1826–1832.
14. Lake CR, Gallant S, Masson E, Miller P. (1990). Adverse drug effects attributed to phenylpropanolamine: A review of 142 case reports. Am J Med. 89: 195–208.
15. Connolly HM, Crary JL, McGoon MD et al. (1997). Valvular heart disease associated with fenfluramine-phentermine. N Engl J Med. 337:581–588.
16. Lean MEJ. (1997). Sibutramine: A review of clinical efficacy. Int J Obes Relat Metab Disord. 21:30–36.

17. Luque CA, Rey JA. (1999). Sibutramine: A serotonin re-uptake inhibitor for the treatment of obesity. *Ann Pharmacother.* 33:968–978.

18. Wirth A, Krause J. (2001). Long-term weight loss with sibutramine–A randomized controlled trial. *JAMA.* 286:1331–1339.

19. Hansen DL, Toubro S, Stock MJ *et al.* (1998). Thermogenic effects of sibutramine in humans. *Am J Clin Nutr.* 68:1180.

20. http://www.citizen.org/publications/release.cfm?ID = 7160 (accessed 08/23/02).

21. http://www.reutershealth.com/en/index.html (accessed 08/23/02).

22. Carriere F, Renou C, Ransac S *et al.* (2001). Inhibition of gastrointestinal lipolysis by Orlistat during digestion of test meals in healthy volunteers. *Am J Physiol Gastrointest Liver Physiol.* 281:G16–G28.

23. Zhi J, Melia AT, Eggers H *et al.* (1995). Review of limited systemic absorption of Orlistat, a lipase inhibitor, in healthy human volunteers. *J Clin Pharmacol.* 35:1103–1108.

24. Sjostrom L, Rissanen A, Andersen T *et al.* (1998). Randomized placebo-controlled trial of Orlistat for weight loss and prevention of weight regain in obese patients. European Multicentre Orlistat Study Group. *Lancet.* 352:167–172.

25. Cavaliere H, Floriano I, Medeiros-Neto G. (2001). Gastrointestinal side effects of orlistat may be prevented by concomitant prescription of natural fibers (psyllium mucilloid). *Int J Obes Relat Metab Disord.* 25:1095–1099.

26. http://www.health.gov/dietsupp/ch1.htm (accessed 08/23/02).

27. Daly PA, Krieger DR, Dulloo AG *et al.* (1993). Ephedrine, caffeine, and aspirin: Safety and efficacy for treatment of human obesity. *Int J Obes.* 17. S73–S78.

28. Horton TJ, Geissler CA. (1996). Post-prandial thermogenesis with ephedrine, caffeine and aspirin in lean, pre-disposed obese and obese women. *Int J Obes.* 20:91–97.

29. Astrup A, Toubro S, Cannon S *et al.* (1991). Thermogenic synergism between ephedrine and caffeine in healthy volunteers. A double blind placebo controlled study. *Metabolism.* 40:323–329.

30. Astrup A, Breum L, Toubro S *et al.* (1991). The effect and safety of an ephedrine/caffeine compound compared to ephedrine, caffeine and placebo in obese subjects on an energy restricted diet. A double blind trial. *Int J Obes.* 16:269–277.

31. http://www.fda.gov/OHRMS/DOCKETS/98fr/092701a.htm (accessed 08/26/02).

32. Boozer CN, Nasser JA, Heymsfield SB *et al.* (2001). An herbal supplement containing ma huang-guarana for weight loss: A randomized, double-blind trial. *Int J Obes.* 25:316–324.

33. Boozer CN, Daly PA, Homel P *et al.* (2002). Herbal ephedra/caffeine for weight loss. A 6-month randomized safety and efficacy trial. *Int J Obes.* 26:593–604.

34. Centers for Disease Control and Prevention. (1996). Adverse events associated with ephedrine-containing products—Texas, Dec. 1993–Sept. 1995. *JAMA.* 276:1711–1712.

35. Bruno A, Nolte K, Chapin J. (1993). Stroke associated with ephedrine use. *Neurology.* 43:1313–1316.

36. Haller CA, Benowitz NL. (2000). Adverse cardiovascular and central nervous system events associated with dietary supplements containing ephedra alkaloids. *N Engl J Med.* 343:1833–1838.

37. Zaacks SM, Klein L, Tan CD *et al.* (1999). Hypersensitivity myocarditis associated with ephedra use. *J Toxicol Clin Toxicol.* 37:485–489.

38. Doyle H, Kargin M. (1996). Herbal stimulant containing ephedrine has also caused psychosis. *BMJ.* 313:756.

39. Theoharides TC. (1997). Sudden death of a healthy college student related to ephedrine toxicity from a ma-huang containing drink. *J Clin Psychopharmacol.* 17:437–439.

40. Samenuk D, Link MS, Homoud MK *et al.* (2002). Adverse cardiovascular events temporally associated with ma huang, an herbal source of ephedrine. *Mayo Clin Proc.* 77:12–16.

41. Brown CM, McGrath JC, Midgley JM *et al.* (1988). Activities of octopamine and synephrine stereoisomers on α-adrenoceptors. *Br J Pharmacol.* 93:417–429.

42. Penzak SR, Jann MW, Cold JA *et al.* (2001). Seville (sour) orange juice: Synephrine content and cardiovascular effects in normotensive adults. *J Clin Pharmacol.* 41:1059–1063.

43. Calapai G, Firenzuoli F, Saitta A *et al.* (1999). Antiobesity and cardiovascular toxic effects of Citrus aurantium extracts in the rat: A preliminary report. *Fitoterapia.* 70:586–592.

44. Guo LQ, Taniguchi M, Chen QY *et al.* (2001). Inhibitory potential of herbal medicines on human cytochrome P450-mediated oxidation: Properties of umbelliferous or citrus crude drugs and their relative prescriptions. *Jpn J Pharmacol.* 85:399–408.

45. Sullivan AC, Hamilton JG, Miller ON, Wheatley VR. (1972). Inhibition of lipogenesis in rat liver by – hydroxycitrate. *Arch Biochem Biophys.* 150:183–190.

46. Conte AA. (1993). A non-prescription alternative in weight reduction therapy. *Dariutrician.* 23.17–18.

47. Mattes RD, Bormann L. (2000). Effects of – hydroxycitric acid on appetitive variables. *Physiol Behav.* 71:87–94.

48. Heymsfield SB, Allison DB, Vasselli JR, Pietrobelli A. (1998). Garcinia cambogia (hydroxycitric acid) as a potential antiobesity agent. *JAMA.* 280:1596–1600.

49. Kriketos AD, Thompson HR, Greene H, Hill JO. (1999). – Hydroxycitric acid does not affect energy expenditure and substrate oxidation in adult males in a post-absorptive state. *Int J Obes Relat Metabl Disord.* 23:867–873.

50. Mussarelli RA, Jolles P, eds. (1999). *Clinical and Biochemical Evaluation of Chitosan for Hypercholesterolemia and Overweight Control. Chitin and Chitinases.* Switzerland: Birkhauser Verlag Basel.

51. Farooqui IS, Jebb SA, Langmack G *et al.* (1999). Effects of recombinant leptin therapy in a child with congenital leptin deficiency. *N Engl J Med.* 341:879–884.

52. Heymsfield SB, Greenberg AS, Fujioka K *et al.* (1999). Recombinant leptin for weight loss in obese and lean adults. A randomized, controlled, dose-escalation trial. *JAMA.* 282:1568–1575.

53. Weyer C, Gautier JF, Danforth E. (1999). Development of beta 3-adrenoceptor agonists for the treatment of obesity and diabetes—An update. *Diabetes Metab.* 25(1):11–21.

54. Silverstein LJ, Bailey RM, Jeor ST. (1998). The role of weight loss drugs in the treatment of obesity in women. *J Womens Health.* 7:187–188.

55. Favreau JT, Ryu ML, Braunstein G *et al.* (2002). Severe hepatotoxicity associated with the dietary supplement LipoKinetix. *Ann Intern Med.* 136:590–595.

56. Vanherweghem J. (1993). Rapidly progressive interstitial renal fibrosis in young women: Association with slimming regimen containing Chinese herbs. *Lancet.* 341:387–391.

57. Meyer M, Chen T, Bennet W. (2000). Chinese herb nephropathy. *Baylor Univ Med Center Proc.* 13:334–337.

81

Hormone Replacement Therapy: Looking Closely at Low Dose

DONNA SHOUPE, MD

Department of Obstetrics and Gynecology, Keck School of Medicine of the University of Southern California,
Los Angeles, CA

I. Introduction: Current Views of Hormone Replacement Therapy

Although the preponderance of evidence from epidemiologic studies show strong evidence that the use of postmenopausal hormone replacement therapy (HRT) substantially reduces the risk of coronary heart disease in healthy women [1–4], recent randomized prospective trials have brought this view under intense scrutiny [5–8]. There is now increased demand that treatment claims be backed with "gold standard" studies that are randomized, prospective, and blinded to both participants and researchers and that document a statistically significant lower event rate. Biologic, basic science, and observational studies, even though abundant and mutually consistent, are no longer considered relevant by many thought leaders. A potential beneficial role of HRT in preventing dementia, Alzheimer's disease, and cardiovascular disease (CVD) is discarded by many.

Today, there is a great divide among health care providers and scientists in regards to their opinions regarding the indications, benefits, and importance of HRT. A growing number of providers restrict use of HRT to a limited number of years during early menopause solely for the prevention of hot flashes. Continued treatment with vaginal estrogen, presumably for many years, to prevent urogenital atrophy is generally accepted or recommended. In contrast, many providers hold a strong belief that 20 to 40 years of very low estrogen is a serious health threat, resulting in degenerative changes in a host of estrogen-responsive tissues including bone, blood vessels, brain neurons, skin, and vaginal and bladder epithelium. Prospective randomized trials have demonstrated effectiveness of estrogen in preventing hot flushes, bone loss, memory and mood changes, and urogenital atrophy. There is to date a lack of gold standard studies to demonstrate the effectiveness of estrogen as a preventative treatment for CVD, dementia, and Alzheimer's disease. Well-done observational studies have been, until recently, accepted as a way to study the outcomes of lifelong or long-term HRT. The challenge now is to more fully understand the different biologic effects of different types, dosage, and route of administration of each estrogen and each progestin, so that the best combination can be selected for each particular patient type.

II. Types of Hormone Replacement Therapy

Despite the fact that HRT has been associated with a host of beneficial effects, fewer than 20% of postmenopausal women in North America take HRT on a long-term basis [9]. This figure is likely to decline even further in view of the recent high media coverage of the negative outcomes of several recent HRT trials [5,7]. Before publication of these recent studies, one of the major reasons for the poor compliance with HRT was the re-establishment of vaginal bleeding [10] that often accompanied the traditional regimens of continuous combined estrogen with cyclic progestin. The development of a continuous combined replacement therapy was, in great part, an effort to develop regimens that would not stimulate endometrial growth and that would avoid withdrawal bleeding [11]. There are several current continuous combined daily estrogen and progestin options that may or may not eliminate bleeding or have side effects similar to cyclic therapy such as breast tenderness or irritability [12].

Today, there is a new emphasis on finding the most effective low-dose regimens that reduce side effects, in particular bleeding and clotting problems, and yet maintain the beneficial effects on bone and other tissues. Although the perfect HRT has not yet been clearly identified, there are many options of estrogen alone (estrogen replacement therapy [ERT]), continuous combined HRT, and cyclic HRT regimens now available in oral, vaginal, and transdermal preparations. A comprehensive head-to-head comparison of the many regimens now in use proves to be a difficult task. However, it is possible to look at several parameters including bleeding problems, relief of symptoms, side effects, cardiovascular effects, osteoporosis protection, breast cancer, and endometrial cancer risk that are associated with a variety of continuous and cyclic HRT and ERT regimens.

III. Cyclic Versus Continuous Progestins: Bleeding

In many of the high dose cyclic regimens such as conjugated estrogen (CE) 0.625 mg plus monthly 5- or 10-mg cyclic medroxyprogesterone acetate (MPA), up to 80 to 85% of women will experience uterine bleeding and 10% will experience unscheduled bleeding. In continuous regimens, generally the incidence of amenorrhea increases and the incidence of irregular bleeding decreases with longer duration of treatment. In a large, randomized study done with 1724 postmenopausal women at 99 sites during the first year of treatment in users of CE 0.625 mg plus MPA 2.5 or 5.0 mg daily, amenorrhea increased from 52 to 56% in cycle 2 to more than 75 to 87% by cycle 11 [13]. After 8 years of continuous combined estrogen and progestin therapy, another study reports that 35 of 41 postmenopausal women reported prolonged amenorrhea [14]. In a head-to-head comparison study of two current continuous combined preparations, the percentage of postmenopausal women with amenorrhea after 6 months was higher in patients using estradiol 1 mg plus 0.5-mg norethindrone acetate (NA) per day (54.8%

and 56.5%) compared with CE 0.625 plus MPA 2.5 mg per day (17.1% and 34.5%) [15].

The continuous combined regimen containing ethinyl estradiol 5 μg plus NA 1 mg is reported to have close to 80% amenorrhea by the end of 1 year of use. The combination product containing 3-day pulses of norgestimate plus estradiol alternating with progestin-free days [16] reports a 1-year amenorrhea rate at 50%.

A cyclic regimen that is gaining popularity requires only quarterly progestin administration. In a recent report, postmenopausal women taking CE 0.625 mg daily plus monthly MPA were changed to receive MPA for only 14 days every 3 months. This quarterly administration of progestin resulted in longer withdrawal menses 7.7 days (quarterly) versus 5.4 days (monthly) and more women experienced unscheduled bleeding, 15% versus 6.8%, on the quarterly regimen. Despite these problems, women preferred the quarterly regimen by nearly four to one. The quarterly regimen appears to be a good option for women seeking relief from monthly use of progestin and monthly menses [17]. A similar but lower dose cyclic regimen using 0.3 mg CE, 0.25 to 0.5 mg estradiol, or 0.025 mg transdermal estrogen with the cyclic or quarterly administration of a progestin results in less bleeding problems.

A growing number of studies indicate that low-dose or very low-dose estrogen regimens, given with either cyclic or continuous progestin and adequate calcium intake, are effective in preventing bone loss and are associated with less bleeding than standard doses of estrogen. In a recent study, bleeding analysis demonstrated that 88% of women receiving 0.3-mg esterified estrogens or placebo reported either amenorrhea or minimal spotting [18]. This dose is effective for preventing osteoporosis. In a 2-year open-label, randomized study, CE 0.3 mg plus MPA 2.5 mg daily resulted in a 3.2% increase in lumbar bone density and no change in lipids, and the incidence of bleeding was significantly lower compared with a regimen of daily CE 0.625 mg plus MPA 2.5 mg [19]. There is also strong evidence to support use of doses of CE 0.3 mg in women 65 years of age or older [20]. Low-dose transdermal patches releasing 0.025 μg/day estradiol have low rates of bleeding and are approved to prevent bone loss. Even lower dose patches are in development. There is evidence to suggest that addition of low-dose androgens has additive benefit for bones, muscles, and skin and allows for an even further reduction in estrogen dosage.

IV. Cyclic versus Continuous Progestins: Symptoms

In addition to the endometrial protective effects, progestins such as MPA, NA, and micronized progesterone (P) have other beneficial effects that include relief of hot flashes or protection from bone loss. The adverse side effects of the progestins, including mood changes, anxiety, and bloating, vary with the progestin and dosage used. Regimens and combination products now in use are designed to minimize these side effects. In the 36-month Postmenopausal Estrogen/Progestin Interventions (PEPI) trial, there was very little difference between percent adherent to the protocol at the end of the study comparing CE plus either cyclic MPA or cyclic progesterone or continuous combined MPA [21]. Percentage adherent was around 80% in all of these combination regimens compared with 50% in the CE group alone.

V. Cyclic versus Continuous Progestin: Atherosclerosis

Because the major cause of death among women in the United States is CVD, one of the most important parameters on which to judge any replacement regimen is its long-term effect on the risk of atherosclerosis. Unfortunately, there is contradictory evidence, and heath care providers have contradictory opinions regarding the long-term benefits of ERT. Multiple recent prospective trials have failed to demonstrate a beneficial effect of estrogen on reducing cardiovascular events [5,6] or improving angiographic findings [7]. Whether these findings could be explained by the estrogen dose or type and dose of progestin used, by the limited time frame, or because of an older or more diseased study population, is under intense debate. More research is needed to select the HRT products that maximize the known beneficial cardiovascular effects of estrogen while minimizing adverse effects.

In contrast to the negative studies mentioned previously is a 2-year randomized prospective study in early postmenopausal women that demonstrated a protective effect of estradiol 1 mg/day on carotid intima media thickness [22]. In a similar study, postmenopausal women on 0.6- to 2.0-mg estradiol alone or estradiol plus levonorgestrel 0.15 mg for 4.7 years had a significantly lower incidence of carotid plaque (18%) than the untreated group (61%) as measured by Doppler ultrasound and B-mode sonography [23]. Selection of a relatively healthy baseline study population appears to make a big difference in study results.

These studies are consistent with results from multiple observational studies and meta-analyses that report ERT reduces the risk of CVD by 50% [1–4,24,25]. The effect of estrogen plus progestin therapy either by cyclic or continuous regimens on CVD risk is less clear as progestin use was very uncommon during the period when many of the epidemiologic studies addressing this issue were conducted. There are data from the Nurses' Health Study showing that in close to 60,000 postmenopausal nurses followed for 16 years, the age-adjusted relative risk of major coronary disease was 0.45 (confidence interval [CI] 0.34 to 0.60) in users of estrogen alone compared with 0.22 (CI 0.12 to 0.41) in users of estrogen with (mainly cyclic) progestin [2,26]. Interestingly, the age-adjusted relative risk in users of low-dose estrogen of CE 0.3 mg was 0.40 (CI 0.20 to 0.79), which was similar to the age-adjusted relative risk of 0.35 (CI 0.25 to 0.50) in users of standard dose estrogen, conjugated equine estrogen (CEE) 0.625 mg (all comparisons were to no therapy).

The metabolic effect of a progestin in regards to cardiovascular risk factors is generally related to its androgenic potency. The most commonly used progestin, MPA, generally has less androgenic activity than the 19-nortestosterone derivatives like norethindrone and levonorgestrel, but more androgenic activity than progesterone. The addition of MPA in doses currently used is often associated with a variable increase in triglycerides and very-low-density lipoprotein (VLDL), no effect on the estrogen-induced reduction in low-density lipoprotein (LDL)-cholesterol, and an attenuated estrogen-induced increase in high-density lipoprotein (HDL)-cholesterol, principally HDL_2

[27]. Addition of norethindrone or NA tends to lower or block the increase in HDL from oral estrogen but is also associated with a beneficial effect on lowering triglycerides. Treatment with the continuous combination of estradiol 1 mg plus 0.5-mg NA results in an overall decrease in triglycerides, LDL-cholesterol, and total cholesterol. There is also an important 9% reduction in Apo-A, a measurement of LDL particle concentration [28].

Other subfractions of lipoproteins and lipids not commonly measured in many older studies also affect coronary disease risk and are modified by estrogen and progestin therapy. One year of treatment with cyclic CE 0.625 mg per day, 25 days per month, and MPA 10 mg per day for 13 days per month is reported to result in a substantial reduction of plasma levels of lipoprotein (Lp)(a) [29]. Lp(a) is an independent risk factor for myocardial infarction and atherosclerosis [30].

Homocysteine concentration tends to increase in menopausal women compared with premenopausal women and appears to be another independent risk factor for vascular occlusive disease [31]. Multiple studies indicate that HRT reduces homocysteine concentrations in postmenopausal women. Reports using the estrogen plus the progestin, dydrogesterone, indicate similar reductions in homocysteine during cyclic (7 to 11%) compared with continuous combined hormone replacement regimens (13%) [32].

Data from the cynomolgus monkey model suggests that addition of continuous MPA to an estrogen-alone regimen may have a moderately detrimental affect. This monkey model is similar to human beings with respect to pathologic characteristics of the atherosclerotic plaques and the susceptibility to develop main-branch coronary artery atherosclerosis when fed a cholesterol-containing diet. Female monkeys have significantly higher HDL-cholesterol and much less coronary artery atherosclerosis compared with males or ovariectomized female monkeys. While fed an atherogenic diet for 30 months, ovariectomized monkeys were treated with no hormones or several different regimens of 17β-estradiol or CE alone or with cyclically or continuously administered progestins. Those treated with CE or 17β-estradiol alone had a 70% reduction in atherosclerosis extent compared with untreated controls. Treatment with CE plus continuous MPA or MPA alone was not statistically different from controls. Natural progesterone or MPA given parenterally and cyclically did not detract from the beneficial effects of estrogens. Medroxyprogesterone acetate given orally and continuously greatly attenuated the beneficial effects of CE [33,34]. Later studies have shown no negative effect of low dose MPA.

The PEPI study reported only a slight overall negative effect of MPA, given continuously or cyclically; 875 healthy women, aged 45 to 64, were randomly assigned to receive placebo, CE 0.625 mg per day alone, CE plus micronized progesterone 200 mg per day for 12 days per month, CE plus MPA 10 mg per day for 12 days per month, or CE plus daily MPA 2.5 mg. Average increases in HDL-cholesterol were higher in each treatment group compared with placebo but highest in those receiving CE alone or CE plus micronized progesterone [35]. HRT did not affect blood pressure or serum insulin, whereas the age related rise in fibrinogen was attenuated in all active treatment groups. Treatment with CE plus MPA increased 2-hours postchallenged glucose levels [35,36]. This is in contrast to a

double-blind study in which 2-mg estradiol plus 1 mg per day NA, 1-mg estradiol and 0.5-mg NA, and placebo did not change insulin sensitivity in postmenopausal women and other parameters of lipid metabolism were favorable or neutral including no changes in triglycerides, glucose, and C-peptide [37].

The Heart and Estrogen/Progestin Replacement Study (HERS) was the first randomized, placebo-controlled trial to examine the effect of estrogen/progestin in postmenopausal women with known coronary disease. The HERS study group consisted of women with CVD, aged 50 to 79, and studied only one continuous CE and MPA treatment regimen over 4.1 years. The results are difficult to generalize to include women without definite coronary disease or to predict effects of other estrogen/progestin regimens. Although overall coronary heart disease event rates were almost identical between placebo and treatment groups, HDL-cholesterol and triglycerides levels increased significantly and LDL-cholesterol levels decreased among women receiving HRT. The lack of benefit in this trial was primarily due to an excess of thromboembolic events especially during the first year of treatment that overshadowed the protective effect seen in the later years of the study [6].

Complicating the issue are the many other factors influencing atherosclerosis including obesity, exercise, diabetes, smoking, stress, hypertension, and family history or genetic factors. Treatment with statins are very effective in reducing total and LDL-cholesterol, triglycerides levels and are proven effective in decreasing CVD. Treatment with estrogen and progestin plus statins is an excellent option [38,39].

There are a host of known beneficial cardiovascular effects of estrogens. Estrogen replacement therapy increases HDL-cholesterol, lowers LDL, and has beneficial effects on other cardiovascular markers. Direct beneficial effects of estrogen on the arterial wall and on the atherosclerotic process is supported by a large number of studies of blood vessel metabolism [33,34,40,41]. These processes are not necessarily correlated with changes in standard plasma lipoprotein measurements. Demonstration of the beneficial effects of estrogen on vessel walls may be hidden when a study protocol results in a high incidence of clotting problems [42–44]. Beneficial effects appear most convincingly when low dose therapy is started in early menopausal women without significant atherosclerosis.

VI. Cyclic versus Continuous Progestins: Osteoporosis

The first prospective, randomized trial showing a statistically significant reduction in hip fractures was in the Women's Health Initiative (WHI) after treatment for 5.2 years with CE plus MPA compared with placebo. Before the publication of this study, many prospective studies had documented significant increases in hip and spine bone mineral density that often showed a strong relationship between dose and percent increase. Epidemiologic studies report an overall 50% reduced risk of hip fractures in users of HRT or ERT. Generally, the differences between estrogen given with either cyclic and continuous MPA regimens in regards to osteoporosis are not significant. In the PEPI trial [35], CE alone, CE plus cyclic MPA or progesterone, and CEE plus continuous MPA caused an average gain of 2.3% and 5.1% in the hip and spine, respectively. All active regimens were significantly different from placebo where women lost an average of 2.2% of hip bone mineral density (BMD) and 2.8% of spine BMD. Most of the gain (70 to 90%) was gained in the first year of therapy. There was no added benefit of the addition of MPA or progesterone to CEE therapy and no difference between cyclic and continuous regimens.

Progestins that have been demonstrated to have osteoprotection include NA, MPA, and tibolone. Differences between cyclic and continuous regimens are not established. There are higher increases in bone density in the hip and spine noted after treatment with estradiol plus NA compared with the same dose of estradiol alone [45] or bone-sparing effect of treatment with NA alone [46].

VII. Cyclic versus Continuous Progestins: Endometrial Cancer

Postmenopausal estrogen therapy is associated with increasing risk of endometrial cancer, compared with those who are not on HRT. A large body of data suggests that when progestin is added, the risk of developing cancer is reduced to levels similar to or below the risk of those not receiving hormonal therapy [47]. In contrast, however, there is evidence that adding progestin in either a cyclic regimen (10-mg MPA; relative risk [RR] = 2.7) [48,49] or continuous [50] regimen lowers the risk below unopposed estrogen but does not completely eliminate the increased risk of giving estrogen. In the WHI, the incidence of endometrial cancer was not increased in the CE plus MPA group compared with placebo [5].

There is some evidence that continuous combined progestin rather than continuous therapy may offer added protection from endometrial cancer [37]. However, adenocarcinoma of the endometrium is reported in long-term continuous combined regimens [14]. Clearly, it is important to balance the progestin dose with a low estrogen dose.

VIII. Cyclic versus Continuous Progestins: Breast Cancer

Sorting out the effects of cyclic versus continuous therapy on the risk of breast cancer is extremely difficult, especially in view of the varied opinions regarding estrogen alone or estrogen plus any progestin and breast cancer risk. The recent publication of the WHI [5] reported eight extra breast cancers per year per treatment of 10,000 women with CE plus MPA compared with placebo. Although this number was not statistically significant, the trend was of concern to the authors. (When the authors subdivided the patients to reflect the previous HRT treatment, a significant trend was noted.) Three of the five meta-analyses published to date show a duration exposure risk of about 25 to 30% above controls with prolonged use of estrogen in excess of 10 to 15 years [51–53]. That this increase may be detection bias is supported by the data of significantly decreased mortality from breast cancer in those patients who were receiving estrogen therapy before their diagnosis [53,54].

Although the question "Do progestins in general reduce or increase the risk of breast cancer?" is under considerable discussion, a comparison of continuous versus cyclic progestin therapy is less well studied. Few women used progestin before 1986, and progestin use was generally 7 to 14 days per month until the 1990s. Several epidemiologic papers have shown no

change in risk [55,56] with the introduction of progestin to estrogen, a decreased risk [57–59], or an increasing risk [60]. Results from a study from Denmark reported an increasing risk with prolonged duration of estrogen use (RR = 2.32; CI 1.31 to 4.12 after >12 years if used). Cyclic progestin was associated with a nonsignificant increased risk of breast cancer (RR = 1.41; CI 0.93 to 2.13), whereas continuous progestin therapy resulted in a nonsignificant reduction in the RR (RR = 0.63, CI 0.26 to 1.53). Most of the patients in this study were treated with 19-nortestosterone derivatives. Two other studies also report either cyclic regimens with the highest rates of breast cancer or HRT rates that are higher than ERT rates [61,62]. Although no data has linked HRT-associated increases in mammographic breast density to increased risk of breast cancer, awareness of these changes has increased the interest among clinicians. Generally, studies of mammographic densities have reported that from 1 to 19% of women on oral or transdermal estrogen, 10 to 23.5% of women on cyclic HRT, and 19 to 52% of women on continuous HRT have demonstrated increased breast densities after starting therapy [63].

In a study in premenopausal women with benign breast disease, continuous 19-nortestosterone derivatives reduced the risk of developing breast cancer (RR = 0.48; CI 0.26 to 0.93) [64]. In addition, cell culture studies have largely shown that progestins reduce breast cell activity when estrogen is present in the culture medium but may induce some proliferation in estrogen-free media [65]. Use of high-dose MPA after breast cancer may improve long-term survival in women with metastatic breast cancer and improve quality of life [66,67]. In 901 Australian women with breast cancer, 90 (10%) had taken estrogen for relief of symptoms. All were disease-free from the time of diagnosis, 80% had disease in the breast only, and 20% had lymph gland involvement. Most were using continuous combined HRT. No deaths were observed in users, and 7% had recurrence compared with 6% mortality and 17% recurrence of nonusers (RR = 0.4; CI 17 to 0.93). These results suggest that short-term combined continuous use is safe and might be protective [68]. In a case-control study, HRT or ERT therapy also reduced the recurrence rate of breast cancer survivors [69].

Based on these studies, there is evidence that different progestins and different doses have very different effects on the risk of breast cancer and may have very different effects on the development or the rate of growth or spread of breast cancer. Prospective trials are needed to better clarify these findings and determine the risk of adding specific progestins, either cyclic or continuously, to postmenopausal estrogen therapy.

IX. Cyclic versus Continuous Progestins: Oral versus Transdermal

Bleeding patterns with the estradiol plus NA patch are similar to other continuous combined regimens leading to about 60% amenorrhea at 1 year. The standard doses of estrogen-only transdermal patches plus either cyclic progestin or continuous progestin have similar patterns to oral cyclic or continuous therapy [70–72].

Although transdermal estrogen therapy causes less beneficial changes in LDL and HDL-cholesterol, transdermal estradiol has a beneficial effect on decreasing triglycerides, which are often increased following oral therapy. In one study, oral CE 0.625 mg reduced Lp(a) by 20%, whereas transdermal 17β-estradiol 50 μg per day reduced Lp(a) by 12%. Both regimens significantly reduced LDL-cholesterol and total cholesterol. HDL-cholesterol and triglycerides increased only in CEE-treated women [73]. No change in lipids was reported following estrogen only patch plus either cyclic or continuous oral MPA. Irregular spotting and bleeding occurred at similar rates [74].

X. Cyclic versus Continuous Progestins: Other Progestins

The introduction and use of new progestins further complicates a comparison of the difference between cyclic and continuous therapy. The introduction of micronized progesterone (100 mg nightly continuously or 200 mg nightly cyclically) has added another option for HRT. Orally active progestins such as trimegestone [75,76], dydrogesterone [77], and desogestrel [78] are used throughout the world in hormone replacement regimens and may be introduced into the United States. These new progestins have minimal androgenic activity. Regimens using dydrogesterone in either cyclically or continuously (10 mg) are reported safe with bleeding pattern similar to regimens with other progestins [79].

Tibolone, an analogue of norethynodrel, has mild estrogenic, progestogenic, and androgenic effects and has been shown to relieve postmenopausal symptoms, improve mood and libido, and prevent bone loss. Because it does not cause endometrial stimulation, monthly bleeding is avoided. In a head-to-head comparison with cyclical CE plus cyclic regimen, tibolone alone decreased HDL but induced a substantial fall in triglycerides, VLDL, cholesterol, and Lp(a) [80]. Depo-Provera (DMPA) (150 mg intramuscular [IM]) provides substantial endometrial protection; may reduce hot flushes and other menopausal symptoms; and effectively decreases markers of bone resorption, urinary calcium, and hydroxyproline excretion similar to the changes produced by CE [81].

XI. Conclusion

Although unopposed estrogen is the standard of therapy for women following a hysterectomy, women with an intact uterus must generally chose between either continuous or cyclic progestin therapy (Table 81-1) or demonstrate a strong motivation to ensure regular monitoring for endometrial disease. Because the beneficial effects of HRT are predominantly due to the estrogen component, selection of a progestin and a particular dosage regimen can be extremely variable and can primarily focus on minimizing side effects and increasing compliance.

Selection of an estrogen dose must generally take into consideration factors such as symptom relief, bone protection, and other long-term health benefits. Studies indicate, however, that low doses of estrogen can relieve vasomotor symptoms, prevent bone loss [19], and reduce the risk of coronary heart disease. With low dosages of estrogen and progestin, women are less likely to have unacceptable side effects such as bleeding or breast tenderness and thus are less likely to discontinue therapy [82].

Many other factors than those discussed here play a role in developing and selecting the ideal dose for ERT (Table 81-2). Although the introduction of new progestins has complicated

Table 81-1

Partial List of Factors for Comparison of Cyclic versus Continuous Therapy Regimens

Short-term side effects
Incidence and severity of bleeding
Side effects of estrogens
Side effects of progestins
Short-term benefits
Climacteric symptoms
Mood improvements
Potential long-term health benefits
Reduction of atherosclerosis events, CVD
Effect on lipids and lipoproteins, inflammatory markers
Clotting changes
Reduction in hip and spine fractures
Potential long-term health risks
Endometrial cancer
Breast cancer
Clotting parameters

Some of these factors are addressed in this chapter. CVD, cardiovascular disease.

Table 81-2

Beneficial Impact Parameters That Can Be Better Understood with Further Studies Comparing Treatment Outcomes with Different Estrogen and Progestin Combination Products

Now documented by prospective and randomized studies
Urogenital atrophy
Colon cancer
Skin collagen loss
Memory loss
Sleep disturbances
Mood disturbances
Sexual function/libido
Fat distribution/weight gain
Now documented by observational, animal, or basic science research data
Tooth loss
Macular degeneration, blindness
Alzheimer's disease
Parkinson's disease
Cataract formation
Parkinson's disease
Arthritis
Cardiovascular disease

many analysis of continuous versus cyclic therapy, the development and introduction of many new estrogens adds further complication. As further evidence emerges regarding the benefits of different regimens, it may be possible to better identify the strengths and weaknesses of each and better choose the right one for each individual, taking into account her personal risk factors (Table 81-3). Although controversial, some studies suggest

Table 81-3

High-Risk Groups in Whom More Data Are Needed to Determine Which Cyclic or Continuous Hormone Replacement Regimen is Best

Obesity, smokers, diabetes, hypertension
Secondary prevention of CVD
Severe osteopenia or osteoporosis
Alzheimer's disease
High risk for breast cancer
After breast or endometrial cancer
Very old or very young
Clotting disorders

CVD, cardiovascular disease.

that continuous progestin therapy may prove more beneficial in regards to bleeding control, endometrial protection, and breast protection. On the other hand, protection from atherosclerosis may be better using cyclic therapy. Other studies refute both these claims. It is clear that better designed investigations are needed. As doses, types, and routes of administration change for estrogens and progestins, different trends are likely to occur.

For now, the selection of a low dose of estrogen plus progestin that has minimal side effects and addresses a patient's risk factors and symptoms, plus encouragement of a patient to have adequate calcium intake, low carbohydrate and low fat diet, and daily exercise, are recommended.

XII. Suggestions for Further Investigations

- Is there a difference in the effect of estrogen therapy on the progression of atherosclerosis between healthy and diseased vessels?
- What is the lowest dose of estrogen therapy that protects against bone loss and vaginal and bladder atrophy in different individuals based on their body weight, age, and other risk factors?

References

1. Grodstein F, Stampfer M. (1995). The epidemiology of coronary heart disease and estrogen replacement in postmenopausal women. *Prog Cardiovasc Dis.* 38:199–210.
2. Grodstein F, Manson JE, Colditz GA *et al.* (2000). A prospective, observational study of postmenopausal hormone therapy and primary prevention of cardiovascular disease. *Ann Intern Med.* 133:933–941.
3. Grodstein F, Manson JE, Stampfer JM. (2001). Postmenopausal hormone use and secondary prevention of coronary events in the Nurses' Health Study. *Ann Intern Med.* 135:1–8
4. Grady D, Rueben SB, Pettit DB *et al.* (1992). Hormone therapy to prevent disease and prolong life in postmenopausal women. *Ann Intern Med.* 117:1016–1037.
5. The Writing Group for the Women's Health Initiative Investigation. (2002). Risks and benefits of estrogen plus progestin in healthy postmenopausal women. *JAMA.* 288:321–333.
6. Simon JA, Hsia J, Cauley JA *et al.* (2001). Postmenopausal hormone therapy and risk of stroke: The Heart and Estrogen-Progestin Replacement Study (HERS). *Circulation.* 103:638–642.
7. Herrington DM, Reboussin DM, Brosnihan KB *et al.* (2000). Effects of estrogen replacement on the progression of coronary artery atherosclerosis. *N Engl J Med.* 343:522–529.
8. Angerer P, Stork S, Kothny W *et al.* (2001). Effect of oral postmenopausal hormone replacement on progression of atherosclerosis: A randomized, controlled trial. *Arterioscler Tthromb Vasc Biol.* 21:262–268.
9. Brunton SA. (1996). Estrogen replacement therapy (ERT): Results of a patient satisfaction survey on women receiving ERT and implications for treatment. *Todays Ther Trends.* 14:119–130.
10. Bjorn I, Backsrom T. (1999). Drug related negative side effects is a common reason for poor compliance in hormone replacement therapy. *Maturitas.* 32:77–86.
11. Doren M, Reuther G, Minne HW, Schneider HP. (1995). Superior compliance and efficacy of continuous combined oral estrogen-progestogen replacement therapy in postmenopausal women. *Am J Obstet Gynecol.* 173:1446–1451.
12. Udoff L, Langenberg P, Adashi EY. (1995). Combined continuous hormone replacement therapy: A critical review. *Obstet Gynecol.* 86:306–316.
13. Archer DF, Pickar JH, Bottiglioni F. (1994). Bleeding patterns in postmenopausal women taking continuous combined or sequential regimens of conjugated estrogens with medroxyprogesterone acetate. *Obstet Gynecol.* 83:686–692.
14. Leather AT, Studd JW. (1990). Can the withdrawal bleed following oestrogen replacement therapy be avoided? *Br J Obstet Gynaecol.* 97:1071–1074.
15. Johnson JV, Davidson M, Archer D, Bachmann G. (2002). Postmenopausal uterine bleeding profiles with two forms of continuous combined hormone replacement therapy. *Menopause.* 9:16–22.
16. Casper RF, Chapdelaine A. (1993). Estrogen and interrupted progestin: A new concept for menopausal hormone replacement therapy. *Am J Obstet Gynecol.* 168:1188–1196.
17. Ettinger B, Selby J, Citron JT *et al.* (1994). Cyclic hormone replacement therapy using quarterly progestin. *Obstet Gynecol.* 83:693–700.
18. Trabal JF, Lenihan JP Jr, Melchione TE *et al.* (1997). Low-dose unopposed estrogens: Preliminary findings on the frequency and duration of vaginal bleeding in postmenopausal women receiving esterified estrogens over a two-year period. *Menopause.* 3:130–138.
19. Mizunuma H, Okano H, Soda M *et al.* (1997). Prevention of postmenopausal bone loss with minimal uterine bleeding using low dose continuous estrogen/progestin therapy: A 2-year prospective study. *Maturitas.* 27:69–76.
20. Recker RR, Davies KM, Dowd RM, Heaney RP. (1999). The effect of low-dose continuous estrogen and progesterone therapy with calcium and vitamin D on bone in elderly women. A randomized, controlled trial. *Ann Intern Med.* 130:897–904.
21. The Writing Group for the PEPI Trial. (1996). Effects of hormone replacement therapy on endometrial histology in postmenopausal women: The postmenopausal Estrogen/Progestin Interventions (PEPI) trial. *JAMA.* 275:370–375.
22. Hodis HN, Mack WJ, Lobo RA *et al.* (2001). Estrogen in the prevention of atherosclerosis; a randomized double-blind controlled trial. *Ann Intern Med.* 135:939–953.
23. Griewing B, Romer T, Spitzer C *et al.* (1999). Hormone replacement therapy in postmenopausal women: Carotid intima-media thickness and 3-D volumetric plaque quantification. *Maturitas.* 32:33–40.
24. Barrett-Connor E, Grady D. (1998). Hormone replacement therapy, heart disease, and other considerations. *Annu Rev Public Health.* 19:55–72.
25. Stampfer MJ, Colditz GA. (1991). Estrogen replacement therapy and coronary heart disease: A quantitative assessment of the epidemiologic evidence. *Prev Med.* 20:47–63.
26. Grodstein F, Stampfer MJ, Manson JE *et al.* (1996). Postmenopausal estrogen and progestin use and the risk of cardiovascular disease. *N Engl J Med.* 335:453–461.
27. Krauss RM. (1999). Lipids and Lipoproteins and Effects of Hormone Replacement. In *Treatment of the Postmenopausal Woman: Basic and Clinical Aspects,* 2nd Edition (Lobo RA, ed.), pp. 369–376. Philadelphia: Lippincott Williams & Wilkins.
28. Davidson MH, Maki KC, Marx P *et al.* (2000). Effects of continuous estrogen and estrogen-progestin replacement regimens on cardiovascular risk markers in postmenopausal women. *Arch Intern Med.* 160:3315–3325.
29. Soma M, Fumagalli R, Paoletti R *et al.* (1991). Plasma Lp(a) concentration after oestrogen and progestagen in postmenopausal women. *Lancet.* 337:612.
30. Dahlen GH, Guyton JR, Attar M *et al.* (1986). Association of levels of lipoprotein Lp(a), plasma lipids, and other lipoproteins with coronary artery disease documented by angiography. *Circulation.* 74:758–765.
31. Ueland PM, Refsum H, Brattstrom L. (1992). Plasma Homocysteine and Cardiovascular Disease. In *Atherosclerotic Cardiovascular Diseases, Hemostasis and Endothelial Function* (Francis RB, ed.), pp. 183–236. New York: Marcel Dekker.
32. van der Mooren MJ, Mijatovic V, van Baal WM, Stehouwer CD. (1998). Hormone replacement therapy in postmenopausal women with specific risk factors for coronary artery disease. *Maturitas.* 30:27–36.

33. Adams MR, Kaplan JR, Manuck SB *et al.* (1990). Inhibition of coronary artery atherosclerosis by 17β-estradiol in ovariectomized monkeys. Lack of an effect of added progesterone. *Arteriosclerosis.* 10:1051–1057.

34. Adams MR, Register TC, Golden DL *et al.* (1997). Medroxyprogesterone acetate antagonizes inhibitory effects of conjugated equine estrogens on coronary artery atherosclerosis. *Arterioscler Thromb Vasc Biol.* 17:217–221.

35. Writing Group for the PEPI Trial. (1995). Effects of estrogen or estrogen/ progestin regimens on heart disease risk factors in postmenopausal women. *JAMA.* 273:199–208.

36. Espeland MA, Hogan PE, Fineberg SE *et al.* (1998). Effect of postmenopausal hormone therapy on glucose and insulin concentrations. *Diabetes Care.* 21:1589–1595.

37. Kimmerle R, Heinemann L, Heise T *et al.* (1999). Influence of continuous combined estradiol-norethisterone acetate preparations on insulin sensitivity in postmenopausal nondiabetic women. *Menopause.* 6:36–42.

38. Hulley S, Grady D, Bush T *et al.* (1998). Randomized trial of estrogen plus progestin for secondary prevention of coronary heart disease in postmenopausal women. *JAMA.* 280:605–613.

39. Davidson MH, Testolin LM, Maki KC *et al.* (1997). A comparison of estrogen replacement, pravastatin, and combined treatment for the management of hypercholesterolemia in postmenopausal women. *Arch Intern Med.* 157:1186–1192.

40. Wagner JD, Clarkson TM, St. Clair RW *et al.* (1991). Estrogen and progesterone replacement therapy reduces low density lipoprotein accumulation in the coronary arteries of surgically postmenopausal cynomolgus monkeys. *J Clin Invest.* 88:1995–2002.

41. Gruber CJ, Tschugguel W, Schneeberger C, Huber J. (2002). Production and actions of estrogens. *N Engl J Med.* 346:340–352.

42. Viscoli CM, Brass LM, Kernan WN *et al.* (2001). A clinical trial of estrogen-replacement therapy after ischemic stroke. *N Engl J Med.* 345:1243–1249.

43. Castellsague J, Pereq Gutthann S, Garcia Rodriguez LA. (1998). Recent epidemiological studies of the association between hormone replacement therapy and venous thromboembolism: A review. *Drug Safety.* 18:117–123.

44. Grady D, Wenger NK, Herrington D *et al.* (2000). Postmenopausal hormone therapy increases risk for venous thromboembolic disease: The Heart and Estrogen/progestin Replacement Study. *Ann Intern Med.* 132:689–696.

45. Speroff L, Rowan J, Symons J *et al.* (1996). The comparative effect on bone density, endometrium, and lipids on continuous hormones as replacement therapy (CHART study). A randomized controlled trial. *JAMA.* 276:1397–1403.

46. Hornstein MD, Surrey ES, Weisberg GW, Casino LA. (1998). Leuprolide acetate and hormonal add-back therapy in endometriosis: A 12-month study. Lurpon Add-Back study group. *Obstet Gynecol.* 91:16–24.

47. Voigt LF, Weiss NS, Chu J *et al.* (1991). Progestagen supplementation of exogenous oestrogens and risk of endometrial cancer. *Lancet.* 338:274–277.

48. Beresford SA, Weiss NS, Voigt LF, McKnight B. (1997). Risk of endometrial cancer in relation to use of oestrogen combined with cyclic progestagen therapy in postmenopausal women. *Lancet.* 349:458–461.

49. Gruber DM, Wagner G, Kurz C *et al.* (1999). Endometrial cancer after combined hormone replacement therapy. *Maturitas.* 31:237–240.

50. Comerci JT Jr, Fields AL, Runowicz CD, Goldberg GL. (1997). Continuous low-dose combined hormone replacement therapy and the risk of endometrial cancer. *Gynecol Oncol.* 64:425–430.

51. Ettinger B, Friedman GD, Bush T, Quesenberry CP Jr. (1996). Reduced mortality associated with long-term postmenopausal estrogen therapy. *Obstet Gynecol.* 87:6–12.

52. Persson I, Yuen J, Bergkvist L, Schairer C. (1996). Cancer incidence and mortality in women receiving estrogen and estrogen-progestin replacement therapy: Long-term follow-up of a Swedish cohort. *Int J Cancer.* 67:327–332.

53. Schairer C, Adami HO, Hoover R, Persson I. (1997). Cause-specific mortality in women receiving hormone replacement therapy. *Epidemiology.* 8:59–65.

54. Grodstein F, Stampfer JM, Colditz GA *et al.* (1997). Postmenopausal hormone replacement therapy and mortality. *N Engl J Med.* 336:1769–1775.

55. Colditz GA, Hankinson SE, Hunter DJ *et al.* (1995). The use of estrogens and progestins and the risk of breast cancer in postmenopausal women. *N Engl J Med.* 332:1589–1593.

56. Stanford JL, Weiss NS, Voigt LF *et al.* (1995). Combined estrogen and progestin hormone replacement therapy in relation to risk of breast cancer in middle-aged women. *JAMA.* 274:137–142.

57. Ewertz M. (1988). Influence of non-contraceptive exogenous and endogenous sex hormones on breast cancer risk in Denmark. *Int J Cancer.* 42: 832–838.

58. Nachtigall MJ, Smilen SW, Nachtigall RD *et al.* (1992). Incidence of breast cancer in a 22-year study of women receiving estrogen-progestin replacement therapy. *Obstet Gynecol.* 80:827–830.

59. Gambrell RD Jr. (1982). The menopause: Benefits and risks of estrogen-progestogen replacement therapy. *Fertil Steril.* 37:457–474.

60. Bergkvist L, Adami HO, Persson I *et al.* (1989). The risk of breast cancer after estrogen and estrogen-progestin replacement. *N Engl J Med.* 321:293–297.

61. Ross RK, Paganini-Hill A, Wan PC, Pike MC. (2000). Effect of hormone replacement therapy on breast cancer risk: Estrogen versus estrogen plus progestin. *J Natl Cancer Inst.* 92:328–332.

62. Schairer C, Lubin J, Troisi R *et al.* (2000). Menopausal estrogen and estrogen-progestin replacement therapy and breast cancer risk. *JAMA.* 283:485–491.

63. Fiorica JV. (2002). Mammographic breast density and hormone replacement therapy. *Menopausal Med.* 10:2.

64. Plu-Bureau G, Le MG, Sitruk-Ware R *et al.* (1994). Progestogen use and decreased risk of breast cancer in a cohort study of premenopausal women with benign breast disease. *Br J Cancer.* 70:270–277.

65. Clarke CL, Sutherland RL. (1990). Progestin regulation of cellular proliferation. *Endocrin Rev.* 11:266–301.

66. Pannuti F, DiMarco AR, Martoni A *et al.* (1980). Medroxyprogesterone Acetate in Treatment of Metastatic Breast Cancer: Seven Years of Experience. In *Role of Medroxyprogesterone in Endocrine Related Tumors* (Lacobelli S, DiMarco AR, eds.), pp. 73–91. New York: Raven Press.

67. Robustelli della Cuna G, Pavesi L, Preti P, Baroni M. (1988). High doses of medroxyprogesterone acetate in breast cancer, controlled studies. *Adv Clin Oncol.* 1:45–56.

68. Eden JA, Bush T, Nand S, Wren BG. (1995). A case-control study of combined continuous estrogen-progestin replacement therapy among women with a personal history of breast cancer. *Menopause.* 2:67–72.

69. Wren BG, Eden JA. (1996). Do progestogens reduce the risk of breast cancer? A review of the evidence. *Menopause.* 3:4–12.

70. Lubbert H, Nauert C. (1997). Continuous versus cyclical transdermal estrogen replacement therapy in postmenopausal women: Influence on climacteric symptoms, body weight and bleeding pattern. *Maturitas.* 28:117–125.

71. Taskinen MR, Puolakka J, Pyorala T *et al.* (1996). Hormone replacement therapy lowers plasma Lp(a) concentrations: Comparison of cyclic transdermal and continuous estrogen-progestin regimens. *Arterioscler Thromb Vasc Biol.* 16:1215–1221.

72. Soma MR, Osnago-Gadda I, Paoletti R *et al.* (1993). The lowering of lipoprotein (a) induced by estrogen plus progesterone replacement therapy in postmenopausal women. *Arch Intern Med.* 153:1462–1468.

73. Meschia M, Bruschi F, Soma M *et al.* (1998). Effects of oral and transdermal hormone replacement therapy on lipoprotein (A) and lipids: A randomized controlled trial. *Menopause.* 5:157–162.

74. Cano A, Tarin JJ, Duenas JL. (1999). Two-year prospective, randomized trial comparing an innovative twice-a-week progestin regimen with a continuous combined regimen as postmenopausal hormone therapy. *Fertil Steril.* 71:129–136.

75. Ross D, Godfree V, Cooper A *et al.* (1997). Endometrial effects of three doses of trimegestone, a new orally active progestogen, on the postmenopausal endometrium. *Maturitas.* 28:83–88.

76. van Baal WM, Smolders RG, van der Mooren MJ *et al.* (1999). Hormone replacement therapy and plasma homocysteine levels. *Obstet Gynecol.* 94:485–491.

77. van der Mooren MJ, Demacker PN, Thomas CM *et al.* (1993). A 2-year study on the beneficial effects of 17β-oestradiol-dydrogesterone therapy on serum lipoproteins and Lp(a) in postmenopausal women: No additional unfavourable effects of dydrogesterone. *Eur J Obstet Gynecol Reprod Biol.* 52:117–123.

78. Marsh MS, Crook D, Whitcroft SI *et al.* (1994). Effect of continuous combined estrogen and desogestrel hormone replacement therapy on serum lipids and lipoproteins. *Obstet Gynecol.* 83:19–23.

79. Ferenczy A, Gelfand MM. (1997). Endometrial histology and bleeding patterns in post-menopausal women taking sequential, combined estradiol and dydrogesterone. *Maturitas.* 26:219–226.

80. Farish E, Barnes JF, Fletcher CD *et al.* (1999). Effects of tibolone on serum lipoprotein and apolipoprotein levels compared with a cyclical estrogen/ progesterone regimen. *Menopause.* 6:98–104.

81. Lobo RA, McCormick W, Singer F, Roy S. (1984). Depo-medroxyprogesterone acetate compared with conjugated estrogens for the treatment of postmenopausal women. *Obstet Gynecol.* 63:1–5.

82. Ettinger B. (1999). Personal perspective on low-dosage estrogen therapy for postmenopausal women. *Menopause.* 6:273–276.

82

Use of Oral Contraceptives for Contraception

RONALD T. BURKMAN, MD* AND KRISTIN L. DARDANO, MD**

*Chairman, Department of Obstetrics and Gynecology, Baystate Medical Center, Springfield, MA;
Deputy Chairman and Professor, Department of Obstetrics and Gynecology,
Tufts University School of Medicine, Boston, MA

**Senior Staff, Department of Obstetrics and Gynecology, Baystate Medical Center, Springfield, MA; Assistant Professor,
Department of Obstetrics and Gynecology, Tufts University School of Medicine, Boston, MA

I. Overview

The oral contraceptive pill, taken by more than 10 million women in the United States and by more than 90 million worldwide, is one of the most well-studied medications in women and is certainly one of the largest health care interventions for reproductive-aged women. The discovery and evolution of oral contraceptives is a fascinating story of determination and luck [1]. In the early 1900s, Ludwig Haberlandt, a professor of physiology at the University of Innsbruck, Austria, demonstrated that ovarian extracts given orally could prevent fertility in mice. Subsequent chemists including, Russell Marker, eventually prepared several pounds of progesterone in the 1940s and helped to form the pharmaceutical company Syntex. Carl Djerassi, working for the company, discovered that the removal of the 19 carbon from yam-derived progesterone increased the progestational activity of the molecule. This led to the synthesis of norethindrone in 1951 [2,3]. Gregory Pincus, of the Worcester Foundation for Experimental Biology in Massachusetts, shifted his attention from mammalian fertilization to oral contraception for women after a visit from Margaret Sanger, the president of the International Planned Parenthood Federation. Pinkus, working for G.D. Searle Pharmaceutical Company, marketed Enovid (150∝g of mestranol and 9.85 mg norethynodrel) in 1960. The developers had spent significant amounts of time purifying the norethynodrel from its contaminant mestranol. However, the estrogen mestranol was found to aid in cycle control and to act in synergy with the progestin to improve the contraceptive effect. The marketing of the combined estrogen-progesterone oral contraceptive pill was a bold move by G.D. Searle, and other combined formulations manufactured by Syntex and Wyeth pharmaceuticals soon followed.

Despite the introduction of oral contraceptives, unintended or unplanned pregnancies continue to be a major problem in the United States. According to the 1995 National Survey of Family Growth, there were a total of 6.3 million pregnancies in the United States with 49.2% unintended [4]. Among the unintended pregnancies, nearly one half result in a pregnancy termination and more than 10% in spontaneous abortion, a substantial degree of pregnancy wastage [5]. Although this indicates that unintended and unplanned pregnancy carries a significant degree of economic and social consequences, there is also an important public health impact. For example, extrapolating data without any adjustments from the Centers for Disease Control and Prevention estimates of mortality and morbidity associated with pregnancy, each day perhaps one woman dies in the United States because of an unintended pregnancy while about 800 women undergo a caesarean section and 800 women experience a labor-related complication of pregnancy [6]. In addition, about 40% of unintended pregnancies occur among women who do not desire pregnancy but who do not use a method of contraception. About 60% of unintended pregnancies occur among women using some form of birth control with about 1 million of these pregnancies occurring in oral contraceptive users [7]. Such data suggest that many women and couples are inadequately motivated to use contraception, that side effects may be problematic for some, that access may be an issue for others, or that some methods may be difficult for women to use correctly. This latter point is supported by a study of oral contraceptive users in which a personal diary of pill taking was compared with results obtained from an electronic pack [8]. Overall, there was only a 45% agreement between the diary and electronic pack derived data. Although this 3-month study showed that women missed less pills over time, the frequency of missing at least three pills in a given cycle was triple the rate based on electronic pack data compared with self-reported diary data. Such reports suggest that reminder systems that recommend doubling up when one misses pills will fail for some women because they may not even remember they missed a pill. Thus, despite more than 40 years of experience with oral contraceptives, substantial challenges still remain relative to selection of women who can be successful; in addition, these women must be assisted in being successful with the method.

II. Formulations

A. Combination Oral Contraceptives

Combination oral contraceptives contain both an estrogen and progestin in each tablet. In 1960, the Food and Drug Administration approved an oral contraceptive containing 150 µg of the estrogen mestranol and 9.85 mg of the progestin norethynodrel [1,9]. This event had not only medical but also social significance because it provided women with an effective means of controlling their reproductive lives with ultimately an improved potential to achieve gender equality. The oral contraceptive was designed so that the progestin would inhibit ovulation by suppressing the release of luteinizing hormone. Although estrogen can suppress ovulation, it was also shown to be important in stabilizing the endometrium to minimize breakthrough bleeding and spotting. However, with the publication of reports associating oral contraceptives, especially the estrogen content, with venous thromboembolism, the dosages of the steroid components were reduced by the late 1960s. By 1968, most oral contraceptives contained the estrogen ethinyl estradiol at a dose of 50 μg. Currently, most oral contraceptives in use contain between 30 and 35 μg of ethinyl estradiol; a few preparations have 20 μg [10]. Furthermore, there are now several new agents that contain 25 μg of this estrogen. Although dose reduction to 30 to 35 μg of estrogen has resulted in reduced rates of venous thromboembolism, there is no evidence to date that further reductions in the amount of estrogen have any effect on these rates. Reducing the dose to 20 μg in some instances appears to reduce side effects such as nausea, breast tenderness, and fluid retention. However, reducing the estrogen dose to these low levels leads to less endometrial stability resulting in higher rates of breakthrough bleeding and spotting with some of these agents compared with others.

With initial development of oral contraceptives, the progestins were primarily 19-nortestosterone derivatives; most were classified as estranes with chemical structures resembling norethindrone. By the 1970s, newer gonane progestins such as levonorgestrel were introduced that, in general, had higher potency relative to the endometrium compared with estranes. At the same time that the estrogen doses were falling, progestins also underwent reductions to doses ranging between 0.15 to 1 mg. In addition, in the 1980s, a number of new progestins (e.g., desogestrel, gestodene, and norgestimate) were developed in an effort to maintain desired effects on the endometrium but to reduce androgenic effects such as acne, weight gain, and undesired effects on lipids and lipoproteins. Finally, in 2001 another somewhat unique progestin drospirenone received approval for marketing in an oral contraceptive in the United States [11]. This progestin, which is an analogue of spironolactone, has a high binding affinity to the progesterone and mineralocorticosteroid receptors and low binding affinity to the androgen receptors. In theory, oral contraceptives containing this progestin may be associated with less fluid retention and a slight risk of hyperkalemia.

B. Progestin-only Oral Contraceptives

Although combined estrogen-progestin oral contraceptives most effectively interfere with ovulation, the progestin-only minipill offers an estrogen-free alternative. The progestin's contraceptive effect is more dependent on its ability to thin the endometrium, to thicken the cervical mucus and to possibly interfere with tubal transport. Approximately 40% of women ovulate normally, even when the progesterone-only pill is taken correctly. The minipill contains small doses of either norethindrone, levonorgestrel, norgestrel, lynestrenol, or ethynodiol acetate and must be taken at the same time every day, starting on the first day of menses. Failure rates range from 1.1 to 9.6% per 100 women in the first year of use [12]. Unfortunately, although an effective form of oral contraception, there is a high frequency of abnormal uterine bleeding and, therefore, a high discontinuation rate. The pill is well tolerated and contributes

to amenorrhea in lactating women, who desire more protection than lactational amenorrhea can ensure. Changing to a combined estrogen-progestin pill is prudent when menses resume to prevent abnormal bleeding and unintended pregnancy. The progestin-only minipill has not been shown to adversely affect breast-feeding, based on measurements of milk volume and infant growth [13].

III. Efficacy

The efficacy reported for oral contraceptives can be highly variable because many factors can influence reported rates [12,14–16]. In clinical trials, study methodology, subject demographics, various forms of potential bias, and even methods of calculating rates and reporting them can influence results. For example, the commonly used Pearl index (number of pregnancies divided by cumulative months or cycles of exposure with the quotient multiplied by either 1200 if months are used or 1300 if cycles are used) incorporates exposure into the denominator. Thus, studies of longer duration enlarge the denominator and result in lower Pearl indices. Accordingly, this method can be used to compare rates only if studies are of similar duration or if the studies are of short duration (e.g., 1 year). In general, life table analyses give more meaningful results because a separate failure rate is determined for each month of use. Furthermore, this method allows one to compare failure rates far more readily as opposed to the Pearl index [16]. Another important point when one refers to efficacy or failure rates is whether one deems the pregnancy resulting from method or user failure. Method failure measures pregnancy rates when the method has been used correctly, in a consistent manner, and according to the instructions in the package insert. However, compliance data in most studies are derived from self-reporting of patients usually through diaries, an approach that may not be accurate as noted in the introduction section of this chapter. Another issue related to method oral contraceptive failure is the effect of weight. A retrospective cohort study indicated that women in the highest quartile of body weight versus the other three quartiles combined had a relative risk of contraceptive failure of 1.6 [17]. In this study, the cutoff for placing women in this highest quartile was 70.5 kg or about 155 lb. When the relationship between estrogen dose and weight was examined, women using oral contraceptives containing less than 35 μg of ethinyl estradiol and who were in the highest quartile for body weight had the highest relative risk of contraceptive failure. It should be noted that other methods such as Norplant and the transdermal contraceptive patch have also shown higher failure rates for women with the highest body weight [18,19]. In contrast to method failures, user failure rates, also known as typical failure rates, reflect pregnancies that occur when the method is not used correctly. However, even these rates can be highly variable. The typical user failure rate for women older than 30 years who are in higher socioeconomic groups tend to approach that of the method failure rate, whereas women who are teenagers, cohabiting, and unmarried tend to have much higher failure rates, sometimes approaching 30% or higher. With these caveats in mind, most trial data report method pregnancy rates that range between 1 to 3%, whereas recent data on user failures estimate the rate to be 7% [15].

IV. Indications/Noncontraceptive Health Benefits

A. Indications and Proven Noncontraceptive Health Benefits

Oral contraceptives are indicated for the prevention of pregnancy and offer a safe, reliable, effective, and reversible method of contraception. The pill's identification and categorization as a contraceptive leaves many benefits out of its title. Over the last 40 years of use, not only have significant side effects been reduced but many unanticipated benefits have been noted. Health benefits related to preventing pregnancy include reducing the need for abortion and surgical sterilization, reducing the risk of ectopic pregnancy, and decreasing maternal mortality. Approximately half of all unintended pregnancies are aborted, accounting for a rate of 22.9 abortions per 1000 women age 15 to 44 in the United States in 1995 [4]. More widespread oral contraceptive use could significantly decrease the number of abortion procedures performed annually.

Based on a number of epidemiologic studies, oral contraceptives convey about a 90% reduction in risk of ectopic pregnancy [20]. The likely mechanism is through suppression of ovulation, an effect that obviously prevents all types of pregnancy. The rate of ectopic pregnancy has shown a steady rise since 1970 in the United States, such that between one and two ectopic gestations occur for every term delivery in this country. Although mortality associated with ectopic pregnancy is relatively low, morbidity related to medical or surgical treatment and future fertility persist.

Other health benefits include reducing the rates of pelvic inflammatory disease, uterine and ovarian cancer, and anemia. Pelvic inflammatory disease or salpingitis still is a major cause of morbidity for reproductive-aged women. It has been established in a number of epidemiologic studies that use of oral contraceptives will reduce the risk of salpingitis by 50 to 80% compared with women not using contraception or who use a barrier method [20–22]. Interestingly, there is no protective effect against the acquisition of lower genital tract sexually transmitted diseases including *Chlamydia trachomatis* and *Neisseria gonorrhoeae* infections of the uterine cervix. The purported mechanisms by which oral contraceptives exert protection include progestin-induced changes to cervical mucus that make it thick and viscous such that ascent of bacteria is substantially inhibited. Additional theories include reduced menstrual flow such that there is less retrograde menstrual flow to the fallopian tubes and less of an environment that would promote growth of bacterial organisms and possible changes in uterine contractility such that ascent of organisms is less likely.

Endometrial cancer is almost twice as frequent as ovarian cancer with better 5-year survival rates because of earlier appearing symptoms. At least 12 case-control studies and 2 cohort studies have demonstrated that use of oral contraceptives conveys protection against endometrial cancer [23–25]. Overall, the studies suggest up to a 50% reduction in risk, which begins about 1 year following initiation of use. Protection appears to increase with duration of use, and there are data to indicate that the protection persists up to 20 years after oral contraceptive use is discontinued. Protection has been demonstrated for adenocarcinoma, adenosquamous tumors, and adenoacanthomas. However, the strength of the protective effect varies in studies for women with potential risk factors such as obesity and nulliparity. The purported protective mechanism is a reduction in the mitotic activity of endometrial cells by the action of the progestin component. Although ovarian cancer is a relatively uncommon tumor, methods to detect it early are ineffective such that only about one half of women survive for 5 years following diagnosis. At least 22 case-control studies and 3 cohort studies have examined the relationship between oral contraceptive use and ovarian cancer [26–29]. All but two of these studies have shown a protective effect for oral contraceptives. Overall, there appears to be between a 40 to 80% overall decrease in risk among users. The protection begins about 1 year after initiating use and conveys about a 10 to 12% decrease in risk for each year of use. In addition, protection persists for 15 to 20 years after one has discontinued use of oral contraceptives. This protective effect primarily involves epithelial tumors of the ovary. The mechanisms by which oral contraceptives may produce their protective effects include suppression of ovulation thus resulting in a reduced frequency of "injury" to the ovarian capsule and the suppression of gonadotropins. Although the gonadotropin theory is controversial, proponents cite data that high levels of gonadotropins are associated with ovarian cancer in animals and that gonadotropins have been shown to stimulate some human ovarian cancer cell lines.

There are also decreases in menstrual irregularities, benign breast disease, ovarian cysts, and acne and improvements in bone density. There are a number of reports that suggest that most users of combination oral contraceptives have reduced menstrual flow and less dysmenorrhea [30–34]. Menorrhagia is a common complaint among reproductive-aged women. The combination of estrogen and progestin in oral contraceptives essentially stabilizes the endometrium over time. Recent data also indicate that some oral contraceptives can be used to treat menorrhagia and dysfunctional uterine bleeding [35]. Furthermore, because the progestins are 19-nortestosterone derivatives, they are highly potent in respect to their endometrial activity. Thus, for most women, the hormone-free portion of the contraceptive cycle produces orderly, withdrawal bleeding of reduced quantity compared with a normal menstrual cycle. In addition, there is an emerging body of evidence that the continuous use of combination oral contraceptives without a hormone-free interval will result in amenorrhea for many women; a condition that some women prefer [36].

It has been estimated in some studies that up to 75% of young women will experience dysmenorrhea; 15 to 20% of women experience severe pain [33,34]. Oral contraceptives reduce the pain associated with menstruation through two possible mechanisms. First, there are data to suggest that the prostaglandin content of menstrual fluid is reduced, leading to less local endometrial vasoconstriction and ischemia [37]. Second, it has also been shown in oral contraceptive users that there is less uterine contractile activity [38].

Benign breast conditions encompass fibrocystic change, fibroadenoma, galactorrhea, intraductal papilloma, fat necrosis, duct ectasia, lobular hyperplasia, and sclerosing/fibrosing adenosis. The results of several studies reveal a significant decrease in the incidence of benign fibrocystic conditions with oral contraceptive use, with a 30 to 50% decrease overall [39,40]. The occurrence of fibroadenomas, specifically, is decreased among women younger than 45 years. These effects are mainly seen in current and recent long-term users of oral contraceptives. The likely mechanism is through suppression of ovulation and, therefore, inhibition of the breast cell proliferation that normally occurs in the first half of an ovulatory menstrual cycle. Oral contraceptive use has also been demonstrated to decrease the incidence of galactorrhea.

It has been reported that ovarian cysts are the fourth leading cause of hospital admission for gynecologic conditions in the United States [41]. The incidence of ovarian cysts among oral contraceptive users is highly dependent on the steroid dosages in oral contraceptive formulations. Although the data are somewhat inconsistent, there is a clear suggestion that higher dose contraceptives (e.g., 50 µg or greater of ethinyl estradiol) protect against cyst formulation. In contrast, current lower dose formulations appear to have no effect on ovarian cyst formation [42,43]. However, it is important to recognize that many of the recent studies evaluating this issue use ultrasound definitions of cysts as opposed to clinical definitions in which some type of therapy might be indicated. Furthermore, many of these cysts identified in such studies regress over time. Thus, it appears that current low-dose oral contraceptives reduce the frequency of ovulation but may still allow early recruitment of follicles that do not progress to the stage of ovulation. Finally, there are no data to support the use of oral contraceptive in the treatment of existing cysts, although higher dose formulations can be used as a means to prevent cyst formation for women who are plagued by recurrent symptoms resulting from ovarian cyst formation.

At least 25% of reproductive-aged women are affected by acne to a varying degree. Although the condition is not life-threatening, for some women the condition can have significant social and psychologic ramifications. Recently conducted randomized, placebo-controlled clinical trials report that about one half of women demonstrated improvement of their acne while taking a product containing the progestin norgestimate during a 6-month time period [44,45]. Interestingly, about 30% of women receiving a placebo preparation also showed improvement. Overall, the response rate to the oral contraceptive in these studies is similar to that achieved by women using topical agents such as tretinoin or benzoyl peroxide or systemic antibiotics. Although other oral contraceptives may reduce acne, there are insufficient data to indicate their overall effectiveness compared with other measures. There are several purported mechanisms of action by which oral contraceptives reduce acne. Oral contraceptives raise the levels of sex hormone binding globulin that in turn binds testosterone. They also suppress gonadotropins; both of these effects lead to reduced levels of ovarian androgens. In addition, there is some evidence that adrenal output of androgens is also suppressed. Finally, there is some preliminary evidence to suggest that various progestins may also exert effects at the level of the pilosebaceous unit.

One out of every two women will experience an osteoporotic fracture during her lifetime. Bone mineral density in women peaks between the ages of 20 to 25 years, stays constant for about 10 years, and then progressively declines in the later reproductive years [22,46,47]. Accelerated bone loss then occurs in the perimenopausal/menopausal years and during all hypoestrogenic states including premature ovarian failure, gonadal dysgenesis, hypothyroidism, hyperprolactinemia, anorexia nervosa, and exercise-induced amenorrhea. Nineteen studies have revealed a positive effect on bone mineral density and 13 indicated no effect on bone mineral density among oral contraceptive users [46]. No studies have demonstrated a negative effect on bone mineral density. It appears that oral contraceptives are most effective at preventing bone loss during times of low estrogen and have a further protective effect with increased duration of use. Women who have used oral contraceptives for 5 to 10 years or longer are afforded the greatest protection. Most importantly, a population-based case-control study revealed a 25% reduction in hip fracture risk [48]. Estrogens act on bone by increasing calcium absorption, decreasing calcium loss, and directly inhibiting bone reabsorption through inhibition of osteoclasts.

B. Potential Health Benefits: Colorectal Cancer and Rheumatoid Arthritis Protection

Colorectal cancer is the third most common cancer women second only to lung and breast cancer. To date, there have been three studies that suggest up to a 40% reduction in colon and rectal cancer among women who have ever used oral contraceptives [49–51]. However, one other study demonstrated no effect on these cancers with oral contraceptive use [52]. Potential mechanisms of action leading to the protective effect include reduction of bile acid production and concentration and effects on colonic mucosa or flora [53]. A large meta-analysis of nine hospital and population-based studies suggested that oral contraceptives may prevent the progression of rheumatoid arthritis to the more severe varieties [54]. However, this protective effect was noted in the hospital-based studies but not the population-based studies suggesting the possibility of confounding or bias.

V. Contraindications

Table 82-1 lists contraindications to use of an oral contraceptive. Although the table has been divided into absolute and relative contraindications, opinion may vary regarding whether or not a given condition represents an absolute contraindication [9,10]. For example, many practitioners would consider cigarette smoking in women older than 35 years as an absolute contraindication. However, others might, in rare circumstances, consider providing oral contraceptives to someone in this age group who smokes only a few cigarettes a day. Practitioners should be cautioned that use of oral contraception in circumstances when the package insert suggests that use is contraindicated requires careful counseling with the patient regarding her individual risks and benefits and documentation of discussions. In general, most women younger than 35 years have no contraindications to oral contraceptives. Prescribing oral contraceptives to women older than 35 years requires that they either be in good health or that any existing medical condition that *could affect the cardiovascular system be in good control and not be too advanced in severity.*

Table 82-1
Contraindications to Use of Combination Oral Contraceptives

Absolute contraindications

Current or past history of thromboembolism
Cerebral vascular disease
Coronary heart disease
Current or past liver tumor associated with contraceptive
steroid use
Cancer of the breast
Estrogen-dependent tumors
Currently seriously impaired liver function
Undiagnosed uterine bleeding
Suspected pregnancy

Relative contraindications

Severe vascular or migraine headaches especially if neurologic
symptoms are prolonged
Hypertension that is poorly controlled or associated with
vascular disease particularly in women older than 35 years
Diabetes that is poorly controlled or associated with vascular
disease particularly in women older than 35 years
Gallbladder disease
Less than 3 weeks' postpartum
Systemic lupus erythematosus
Lactation
Abdominal or lower extremity surgery contemplated
within 4 to 6 weeks
Presence of lower leg casts or immobilization
Hypertriglyceridemia
History of cholestasis of pregnancy
Older than 35 years with risk factors for cardiovascular disease
(e.g., cigarette smoking) substantially abnormal lipid profile
Use of drugs that may interact with oral contraceptives
(e.g., rifampin)

(Modified from Burkman RT. [1989]. *Handbook of Contraception*,
pp. 23–26. Little, Brown and Company.)

VI. Major Risks

A. Cardiovascular Risk

By the 1970s, it had been established that oral contraceptives
were associated with various types of cardiovascular risks [55,56].
However, with the significant reduction in estrogen and progestin
dosages and the introduction of new formulations, many of the
original estimates require modification.

1. Venous Thromboembolism

Multiple studies by 1980 established that use of combined
oral contraceptives was associated with an increased risk of
venous thromboembolism [55,56]. The reports suggested that
the increase was caused primarily by the estrogen component.
During the 1960s and 1970s, manufacturers began reducing the
dosages of the various active components of oral contraceptives.
This reduction in estrogen dose was associated with a substantial
decrease in risk of venous thromboembolism. Gerstman *et al*

[57] reported a dose-response effect with rates of venous
thromboembolism ranging from 10 events per 10,000 woman-
years for pills with greater than 50 μg estrogen to 4.2 events per
10,000 woman-years for pills with less than 50 μg estrogen.
Manufacturers also introduced new progestins that had different
metabolic profiles to reduce adverse sequelae and side effects.
In late 1995 and early 1996, new data suggested that two of the
newer progestins, gestodene and desogestrel, carried a higher
risk for venous thromboembolism than an older progestin
levonorgestrel [58–61]. Subsequent analyses and reviews have
debated whether these findings are real [62–69]. Table 82-2
provides an estimate of the incidence of venous thromboembolism
for women age 20 to 24 years according to whether women
were using oral contraceptives containing older progestins,
were users of oral contraceptives containing the progestins
gestodene and desogestrel, or were not users of oral contraceptives. As shown, most oral contraceptive use roughly triples
one's risk of venous thromboembolism, whereas gestodene or
desogestrel preparations may increase the risk as much as a
7-fold. Even with the worst case scenario, the attributable risk
(additional cases resulting from the exposure) annually is only
about 18 cases per 100,000 users of gestodene- or desogestrel-
containing oral contraceptives compared with nonusers of oral
contraceptives.

Risk factors for venous thromboembolism include pregnancy,
trauma, immobilization, recent surgery, medical conditions such
as cancer or collagen-vascular disorders, and inherited hemostatic deficiencies. Age has an effect on the risk of venous
thromboembolism. For women aged 40 to 44 years, the risks
listed for venous thromboembolism in Table 82-2 would
approximately double. However, this age-related increase in
risk is independent of oral contraceptive use [70]. Obesity in
a recent World Health Organization analysis was also a risk
factor for venous thromboembolism, although this is not a
consistent finding in all studies [58,70]. There is no evidence
that smoking or the presence of varicose veins among users
of oral contraceptives appreciably affects their relative risk of
venous thromboembolism [71]. Finally, it should be considered

Table 82-2

**Incidence* of Cardiovascular Events Among Low-Dose Oral
Contraceptive** Users by Progestin Type, Ages
20–24 Years Oral Contraceptive Type**

Condition	None	Levonorgestrel/ Norethindrone	Gestodene/ Desogestrel
Venous thromboembolism	3.0	9.6	7.7–21.1
Stroke			
Ischemic	1.0	2.5	2.5
Hemorrhagic	2.0	2.0	2.0
Myocardial infarction	0.2	0.5	0.2

*Incidence per 100,000 annually.
**Less then 50 μg of estrogen with most at 35 μg or less.
(Adapted from International Federation of Fertility Societies. [1999].
Consensus conference on combination oral contraceptives and cardio-
vascular disease. *Fertil Steril*. 71:1S–6S.)

that the mortality resulting from venous thromboembolism among oral contraceptive users is low in reproductive-aged women as shown in Table 82-3. Age affects the risk of death resulting from venous thromboembolism; for women age 35 to 44 years the mortality rates approximately double. For users of gestodene- or desogestrel-containing oral contraceptives, this would equate to an excess of four deaths per 1 million woman-years [65].

The identification of the factor V Leiden mutation in 1993 is another consideration in the relationship between oral contraceptive use and venous thromboembolism [72]. This mutation involves a single amino acid substitution that results in a variant of factor V that is resistant to activated protein C. Clot formation is substantially enhanced and risk of venous thromboembolism also increases because of this mutation. This mutation, which is known as either factor V Leiden or activated protein C resistance, has a prevalence in the general population of about 5% in U.S. Caucasian women, 2.2% in Hispanic Americans, and 1.2% in African Americans, making it the most commonly occurring natural anticoagulant deficiency [73–75]. The risk of venous thromboembolism among oral contraceptive users with factor V Leiden has been estimated recently [76]. Among women with the mutation (at a prevalence of about 5%) who were not using oral contraceptives, there would be 5.7 venous thromboembolism events per 10,000 woman-years. In contrast, among women with the mutation using oral contraceptives, the rate increases to 28.5 events per 10,000 woman-years. The low absolute risk of venous thromboembolism among such women is important to keep in perspective when the issue of screening women before oral contraceptive use is raised [69,75,77]. Recently, Winkler [69] determined that screening 1 million potential users for all known coagulation factor deficiencies or mutations would identify about 50 women at risk but also would result in about 62,000 women having false-positive results.

2. Stroke

Stroke can be separated into two categories—ischemic or thrombotic and hemorrhagic. Earlier literature is difficult to interpret relative to stroke risk because the estrogen dose has been reduced and prescribing practices have changed over time such that women with risk factors are no longer being given oral contraceptives. Recent studies of low-dose oral contraceptives have noted the role of confounders and use more rigorous approaches to both design and analysis such that current risk estimates are probably more accurate [78–89].

a. ISCHEMIC STROKE.   Thrombotic or ischemic stroke risk for current users of low-dose oral contraceptives is relatively low. As shown in Table 82-2, among women age 20 to 24 years, use of oral contraceptives increases overall risk by about two and one-half times compared with nonuse of oral contraceptives [70]. Although mortality is also low, as shown in Table 82-3, for all forms of stroke this risk is strongly affected by risk factors. There is no evidence that type of progestin influences risk or mortality associated with ischemic stroke [70,71]. However, the risk of ischemic stroke is directly proportional to estrogen dose, although this effect is primarily seen in studies completed in developed compared with less-developed countries [70,71, 78,79,87]. Duration of use does not adversely affect a user's risk. Age appears to be a risk factor relatively independent of oral contraceptive use with the relative risk of ischemic stroke doubling as women reach the age of 40 to 44 years [70]. Stroke mortality also increases by about 6-fold once one reaches the age group of 35 to 44 years, although it is unclear whether this increment actually represents an increased likelihood of the presence of an undetected risk factor such as hypertension [71]. Hypertension, cigarette smoking, and migraine headaches interact with oral contraceptive use to increase the risk of ischemic stroke substantially [80,85,88,89]. Of importance is the finding in at least three studies that users of oral contraceptives containing less than 50 μg of estrogen who have regular blood pressure checks do not have a significantly increased risk of ischemic stroke [71,80,82,85].

b. HEMORRHAGIC STROKE.   The risk of hemorrhagic stroke in young women is low, as shown in Table 82-2, and is not increased by use of oral contraceptives in women without risk factors [70,80–82,84,86,87]. The rate of hemorrhagic stroke for nonusers of oral contraceptives rises to 7 per 100,000 annually and to 14 per 100,000 annually among users as women reach the age of 35 to 44 years. There appears to be no relationship among the components of oral contraceptives, dosages, or duration of use and the risk of hemorrhagic stroke. Although hemorrhagic stroke mortality for young women is low (see Table 82-3), mortality can be as high as 25% for women experiencing this condition. In addition to age, the major risk factors for hemorrhagic stroke are cigarette smoking and hypertension. Smoking increases the risk between about 1.5- and 2-fold for non–oral contraceptive users and between 3- and 3.5-fold for oral contraceptive users [80]. In one study, history of hypertension increased the risk by about 5-fold among women in Europe who were not oral contraceptive users compared with non–oral contraceptive using, normotensive women; for hypertensive women in developing countries, the relative risk climbed to 9.4 [80]. For nonhypertensive, current oral contraceptive users, the

Table 82-3
Mortality* from Cardiovascular Events Among Low-Dose Oral Contraceptive** Users by Progestin Type, Ages 15–24 Years Oral Contraceptive Type

Condition	None	Levonorgestrel/ Norethindrone	Gestodene/ Desogestrel
Venous thromboembolism	0.1	0.3	0.2–0.7
Stroke	1.0	1.5	1.5
Myocardial infarction	0.1	0.3	0.1

*Incidence per 100,000 annually.

**Less then 50 μg of estrogen with most at 35 μg or less.

(Adapted from International Federation of Fertility Societies. [1999]. Consensus conference on combination oral contraceptives and cardiovascular disease. *Fertil Steril.* 71:1S–6S.)

risk of hemorrhagic stroke is not elevated, but, with a history of hypertension, the relative risk among users rises to 10.2 in Europe and 14.2 in developing countries [80]. The differential in risk between developed countries and developing countries probably represents differences in access to health services for diagnosis and treatment of hypertension Overall, for women younger than 35 years who do not smoke and who are normotensive, the risk of hemorrhagic stroke is not affected by oral contraceptive use [80].

3. Myocardial Infarction

As shown in Table 82-2, myocardial infarction is a rare condition in the reproductive-aged group. Age influences this risk exponentially with the incidence of myocardial infarction increasing to 30 cases per 100,000 annually among women age 40 to 44 years [70,71]. Other risk factors such as cigarette smoking, hypertension, and diabetes strongly influence the risk of experiencing a myocardial infarction. As shown in Table 82-3, although the mortality resulting from myocardial infarction is low in reproductive-aged women, the case fatality rate is still 30% [71]. The more recent studies of oral contraceptive use and myocardial infarction have shown some increase in risk with oral contraceptive use among women with cardiovascular risk factors [90–95]. Thus, as shown in Table 82-2, although oral contraceptive users overall have some increased risk, it is estimated that 80% of the cases among oral contraceptive users are attributable to cigarette smoking with the remainder occurring in users with other risk factors such as hypertension or diabetes [70]. There is no increased risk of myocardial infarction associated with increasing duration of oral contraceptive use [71,95]. Past use of oral contraceptives does not result in an increased risk of myocardial infarction in later life [91,95–97]. Nonsmoking, nondiabetic oral contraceptive users who have regular blood pressure examinations have no increased risk of myocardial infarction [71]. Although age independently affects risk of myocardial infarction in all women, the relative risk of myocardial infarction for current oral contraceptive users is not increased with aging [71]. Cigarette smoking increases the risk of myocardial infarction in women who do not use oral contraceptives by 3- to 10-fold; a risk that is directly proportional to the number of cigarettes smoked daily [71]. The combination of smoking and oral contraceptive use results in a synergy, which further increases a user's risk of myocardial infarction by about 10-fold. Hypertension increases the relative risk of myocardial infarction in reproductive-aged women by 5- to 10-fold compared with women who have never used oral contraceptives [71]. In addition, the relative risk of myocardial infarction among oral contraceptive users with hypertension is at least three times higher than that of users without hypertension. Use of new low-dose oral contraceptives does not appear to modify the risk of myocardial infarction. One study has even suggested that users of oral contraceptives containing gestodene or desogestrel have a reduced risk of myocardial infarction compared with users of preparations containing the progestin levonorgestrel [60]. This finding has not been confirmed in other studies.

B. Breast Cancer Risk

For several decades, there has been concern regarding the possible association between oral contraceptive use and breast cancer. During this time period, many epidemiologic studies reported conflicting results with the discrepancies probably related to how well biases and confounding were addressed in the individual studies. The ability to control for bias and confounding is particularly important because many of the calculated relative risks are small such that an unrecognized significant bias could essentially weight a study toward a positive association or risk when in fact none existed. It has often been difficult to interpret the results of individual studies in the context of current practice, resulting from changes in dosages and hormones in the formulations against a backdrop of a cancer with a latency period of several years.

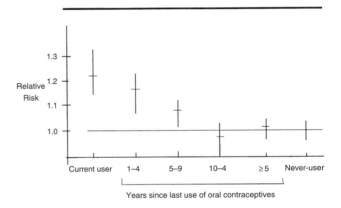

Fig. 82-1   Relative risk of breast cancer with oral contraceptive use. Horizontal bars are point estimates; vertical bars are 95% confidence intervals. Relative risk calculated versus never-use. (Adapted from Collaborative Group on Hormonal Factors in Breast Cancer. [1996]. Breast cancer and hormonal contraceptives: Further results. *Contraception.* 54:1S–106S.)

Table 82-4
Drug Interactions that Alter Oral Contraceptive Concentrations or Effects

Decreased Drug Effect or Concentrations	Increased Drug Effect or Concentrations
Mechanism: increased drug clearance	Mechanism: decreased drug clearance
Anticonvulsants: phenytoin, primidone, and carbamazepine	Antifungals*: ketoconazole, fluconazole, itraconazole, griseofulvin
Antituberculous: Rifampin*	Anticoagulant: warfarin
	Mechanism: inhibited enterohepatic recirculation
	Antibiotics: penicillin, ampicillin, tetracyclines, cephalosporins

*Most potent.
(From Schwartz JB. [1999]. Pharmacy focus. Gender specific therapy: Oral contraceptive therapy in women: drug interactions and unwanted outcomes. *J Gender Specific Med.* 2:26–29.)

In 1996, a collaborative project representing a meta-analysis of the better epidemiologic studies in the literature was published [98]. A total of 54 studies were included in the analysis representing 53,297 women with breast cancer and 100,239 control subjects. Studies had to have had at least 100 women in the study with a diagnosis of breast cancer and the original data had to be available for re-analysis. There were 11 cohort studies, 28 case-control studies with population-based controls, and 15 case-control studies with hospital-based control subjects meeting the criteria. About one third of the cancers were diagnosed in women younger than 45 years and about one half after 1985. Thus, the data probably provide clinicians with the best information that can be applied to their current oral contraceptive users. The relative risk of breast cancer for current users of oral contraceptives compared with never-users was 1.24. This small increase in risk persisted for about 10 years, with disappearance of the risk after that time period. In addition, there was no overall effect of oral contraceptive use by dosage, specific formulation, duration of use, age at first use, age at time of cancer diagnosis, or family history of breast cancer. The comparison of ever-users of oral contraceptives with never-users revealed that the relative risk for tumors that had spread as opposed to localized disease was 0.88. This suggests that although oral contraceptive users face a modest increase in risk of breast cancer, the disease tends to be localized. The pattern of disappearance of risk after 10 years coupled with the tendency toward localized disease suggests that the overall effect may represent detection bias or perhaps a promotional effect. For example, if oral contraceptive users undergo more frequent breast examinations because they are required to see a clinician to get their prescriptions refilled compared with users of other methods, the findings may be due to earlier detection of cancer. A promotional effect would occur if the hormones in oral contraceptives cause growth of cells that have already been transformed into a neoplasm.

More recent information from a case-control study suggests that users of oral contraceptives may, in fact, have no substantial increase in the risk of breast cancer [99,100]. This population-based study from five metropolitan areas across the United States included women between 35 and 64 years of age and involved 4575 breast cancer patients and 4682 control subjects. Because cases had their cancers identified between 1994 and 1998 and controls were interviewed by random-digit dialing proportionally to cases by study site, age, and race, the study provides some estimate of the risk of breast cancer among women using lower dose oral contraceptive formulations. In this study, the relative risk of breast cancer was 1.0 (95% confidence interval [CI] 0.8 to 1.3) among current users of oral contraceptives and 0.9 (95% CI 0.8 to 1.0) for former users. The relative risk did not show any consistent increase by duration of use or with higher estrogen doses. No increase in risk was noted for women with a family history of breast cancer or for women starting oral contraceptive use at an early age. Finally, there were no differences in risk noted between white and black women. Thus, this study indicates no increase in risk of breast cancer associated with oral contraceptive use particularly later in life where the risk is highest.

VII. Side Effects

Combined oral contraceptives offer a low-risk, high-benefit contraceptive option for most reproductive-aged women, including perimenopausal women. The side effects of nausea, breast tenderness, and fluid retention are less common with the lower doses of estrogen. Many gastrointestinal side effects ameliorate over time so patients should be encouraged to try a full 3-month trial of oral contraceptives before discontinuing use. There is no good evidence that oral contraceptives directly cause weight gain; however, estrogens and progestins may act as appetite stimulants or have anabolic steroid effects. There are drug interactions that one should also consider in using oral contraceptives, as shown in Table 82-4. More drugs taken concurrently do not alter the efficacy of oral contraceptives except for certain anticonvulsants and Rifampin. In addition, there is evidence that the herbal remedy St. John's wort may reduce the efficacy of oral contraceptives by increasing the clearance of the progestin component [102].

Even with ideal daily use of oral contraceptives, women with previously normal cycles may have immediate bleeding, midcycle spotting, or absence of menses. Women with a history of irregular menses may have heavy or irregular bleeding initially. More than 50% of women who discontinue oral contraceptives do so within the first 2 months [101]. Patients need to be counseled to expect some change in bleeding and to be reassured that it will likely correct and is not a sign of gynecologic cancer. Patients who have previously and successfully used oral contraceptives are ideal candidates to resume them. Women who have not been compliant in the daily pill taking regimen may not be good candidates, because missing doses of pills increases the unintended pregnancy rate and abnormal bleeding patterns. There are several new options for these women including transdermal contraception, a vaginal ring, and the often forgotten intrauterine contraceptive device.

VIII. Concluding Statements

There is no comparable oral contraceptive for men, because most research on male contraception has involved injectable hormonal approaches. The hypothalamic-pituitary-gonadal axis of the male reproductive tract can be altered to decrease the production of sperm; however, pregnancy rates were still unacceptably high with 9% of subjects' partners conceiving in one study of injectable depomedroxyprogesterone acetate and testosterone enanthanate [103]. Testosterone enanthate can lead to azoospermia when given alone; however, oral preparations are not practical secondary to rapid degradation.

IX. Suggestions for Further Investigations

Oral contraceptives remain a gender-specific, well-studied safe medication that offers reliable contraception and a variety of noncontraceptive benefits. The future of oral contraceptives raises the following questions:

- Will the lower dose formulations (less than 30 µg of estradiol) still offer the same protective benefits against ovarian cancer?
- Can we change patient behavior in terms of being more compliant with oral medications?
- As more information becomes available about risks of postmenopausal hormone replacement therapy, should more

women be encouraged to use oral contraceptives in their forties to help prevent bone loss?

- Does the prevention of ovulation and decrease in androgens related to oral contraceptives affect libido?
- Can an effective, safe, oral preparation be developed for men that leads to reversible azoospermia?

References

1. Speroff L, Darney PD. (1992). *A Clinical Guide for Contraception*, pp. xi, 342. Baltimore: Williams & Wilkins.
2. Goldzieher JW. (1980). Hormonal Contraception–Whence, How and Whither? In *Clinical Uses of Steroids* (Givens J, ed.), p. 375. Chicago: Yearbook Medical Publishers.
3. Medvei VC. (1982). *A History of Endocrinology*, pp. 350. Hingham, MA: MTB Press.
4. Henshaw SK. (1998). Unintended pregnancy in the United States. *Fam Plann Perspect*. 30:24–29, 46.
5. (2002). *Fulfilling the Promise*, p. 50. New York: Alan Guttmacher Institute.
6. Jones WK. (2000). *Safe Motherhood At-A-Glance 2000: Preventing Pregnancy-related Illness*. Atlanta: Centers for Disease Control and Prevention.
7. Piccinino LJ, Mosher WD. (1998). Trends in contraceptive use in the United States: 1982–1995. *Fam Plann Perspect*. 30:4–10, 46.
8. Potter L, Oakley D, de Leon-Wong E, Canamar R. (1996). Measuring compliance among oral contraceptive users. *Fam Plann Perspect*. 28:154–158.
9. Burkman RT. (1989). *Handbook of Contraception and Abortion*, p. 152. Boston: Little, Brown and Company.
10. Hatcher RA, Trussell J, Stewart F et al. (1998). *Contraceptive Technology*, p. 851. New York: Ardent Media.
11. Parsey KS, Pong A. (2000). An open-label, multicenter study to evaluate Yasmin, a low-dose combination oral contraceptive containing drospirenone, a new progestogen. *Contraception*. 61:105–111.
12. Trussell J, Kost K. (1987). Contraceptive failure in the United States: A critical review of the literature. *Stud Fam Plann*. 18:237–283.
13. Tankeyoon M, Dusitsin N, Chalapati S et al. (1984). Effects of hormonal contraceptives on milk volume and infant growth. WHO Special Programme of Research, Development and Research Training in Human Reproduction Task force on oral contraceptives. *Contraception*. 30:505–522.
14. Potter LS. (1996). How effective are contraceptives? The determination and measurement of pregnancy rates. *Obstet Gynecol*. 88:13S–23S.
15. Trussell J, Vaughan B. (1999). Contraceptive failure, method-related discontinuation and resumption of use: Results from the 1995 National Survey of Family Growth. *Fam Plann Perspect*. 31:64–72, 93.
16. Trussell J, Hatcher RA, Cates W et al. (1990). A guide to interpreting contraceptive efficacy studies. *Obstet Gynecol*. 76:558–567.
17. Holt VL, Cushing-Haugen KL, Daling JR. (2002). Body weight and risk of oral contraceptive failure. *Obstet Gynecol*. 99:820–827.
18. Du MK, Chow LP, Zheng HM. (2000). A 10-year follow-up study of contraceptive Norplant implants. *Int J Gynaecol Obstet*. 68:249–256.
19. Audet MC, Moreau M, Koltun WD et al. (2001). Evaluation of contraceptive efficacy and cycle control of a transdermal contraceptive patch vs an oral contraceptive: A randomized controlled trial. *JAMA*. 285:2347–2354.
20. Peterson HB, Lee NC. (1989). The health effects of oral contraceptives: Misperceptions, controversies, and continuing good news. *Clin Obstet Gynecol*. 32:339–355.
21. Mishell DR Jr. (1982). Noncontraceptive health benefits of oral steroidal contraceptives. *Am J Obstet Gynecol*. 142:809–816.
22. Burkman RT Jr. (1994). Noncontraceptive effects of hormonal contraceptives: Bone mass, sexually transmitted disease and pelvic inflammatory disease, cardiovascular disease, menstrual function, and future fertility. *Am J Obstet Gynecol*. 170:1569–1575.
23. Schlesselman JJ. (1997). Risk of endometrial cancer in relation to use of combined oral contraceptives. A practitioner's guide to meta-analysis. *Hum Reprod*. 12:1851–1863.
24. Sherman ME, Sturgeon S, Brinton LA et al. (1997). Risk factors and hormone levels in patients with serous and endometrioid uterine carcinomas. *Mod Pathol*. 10:963–968.
25. Vessey MP, Painter R. (1995). Endometrial and ovarian cancer and oral contraceptives—Findings in a large cohort study. *Br J Cancer*. 71:1340–1342.
26. Hankinson SE, Colditz GA, Hunter DJ et al. (1992). A quantitative assessment of oral contraceptive use and risk of ovarian cancer. *Obstet Gynecol*. 80:708–714.
27. Piver MS, Baker TR, Jishi MF et al. (1993). Familial ovarian cancer. A report of 658 families from the Gilda Radner Familial Ovarian Cancer Registry 1981–1991. *Cancer*. 71:582–588.
28. Risch HA, Marrett LD, Jain M, Howe GR. (1996). Differences in risk factors for epithelial ovarian cancer by histologic type. Results of a case-control study. *Am J Epidemiol*. 144:363–372.
29. Rosenberg L, Palmer JR, Zauber AG et al. (1994). A case-control study of oral contraceptive use and invasive epithelial ovarian cancer. *Am J Epidemiol*. 139:654–661.
30. van Hooff MH, Hirasing RA, Kaptein MB et al. (1998). The use of oral contraceptives by adolescents for contraception, menstrual cycle problems or acne. *Acta Obstet Gynecol Scand*. 77:898–904.
31. Weng LJ, Xu D, Zheng HZ et al. (1991). Clinical experience with triphasic oral contraceptive (Triquilar) in 527 women in China. *Contraception*. 43:263–271.
32. Milman N, Clausen J, Byg KE. (1998). Iron status in 268 Danish women aged 18–30 years: Influence of menstruation, contraceptive method, and iron supplementation. *Ann Hematol*. 77:13–19.
33. Klein JR, Litt IF. (1981). Epidemiology of adolescent dysmenorrhea. *Pediatrics*. 68:661–664.
34. Wilson CA, Keye WR Jr. (1989). A survey of adolescent dysmenorrhea and premenstrual symptom frequency. A model program for prevention, detection, and treatment. *J Adolesc Health Care*. 10:317–322.
35. Davis A, Lippman J, Godwin A et al. (2000). Triphasic norgestimate/ethinyl estradiol oral contraceptive for the treatment of dysfunctional uterine bleeding. *Obstet Gynecol*. 95:S84.
36. Sulak PJ, Caubel P, Lane R. (1999). Efficacy and safety of a constant-estrogen, pulsed-progestin regimen in hormone replacement therapy. *Int J Fertil Womens Med*. 44:286–296.
37. Chan WY, Dawood MY. (1980). Prostaglandin levels in menstrual fluid of nondysmenorrheic and of dysmenorrheic subjects with and without oral contraceptive or ibuprofen therapy. *Adv Prostaglandin Thromboxane Res*. 8:1443–1447.
38. Dawood MY. (1990). Dysmenorrhea. *Clin Obstet Gynecol*. 33:168–178.
39. Brinton LA, Vessey MP, Flavel R, Yeates D. (1981). Risk factors for benign breast disease. *Am J Epidemiol*. 113:203–214.
40. Charreau I, Plu-Bureau G, Bachelot A et al. (1993). Oral contraceptive use and risk of benign breast disease in a French case-control study of young women. *Eur J Cancer Prev*. 2:147–154.
41. Westhoff C, Clark CJ. (1992). Benign ovarian cysts in England and Wales and in the United States. *Br J Obstet Gynaecol*. 99:329–332.
42. Lanes SF, Birmann B, Walker AM, Singer S. (1992). Oral contraceptive type and functional ovarian cysts. *Am J Obstet Gynecol*. 166:956–961.
43. Young RL, Snabes MC, Frank ML, Reilly M. (1992). A randomized, double-blind, placebo-controlled comparison of the impact of low-dose and triphasic oral contraceptives on follicular development. *Am J Obstet Gynecol*. 167:678–682.
44. Redmond GP, Olson WH, Lippman JS et al. (1997). Norgestimate and ethinyl estradiol in the treatment of acne vulgaris: A randomized, placebo-controlled trial. *Obstet Gynecol*. 89:615–622.
45. Lucky AW, Henderson TA, Olson WH et al. (1997). Effectiveness of norgestimate and ethinyl estradiol in treating moderate acne vulgaris. *J Am Acad Dermatol*. 37:746–754.
46. DeCherney A. (1996). Bone-sparing properties of oral contraceptives. *Am J Obstet Gynecol*. 174:15–20.
47. Kuohung W, Borgatta L, Stubblefield P. (2000). Low-dose oral contraceptives and bone mineral density: An evidence-based analysis. *Contraception*. 61:77–82.
48. Michaelsson K, Baron JA, Farahmand BY et al. (1999). Oral-contraceptive use and risk of hip fracture: A case-control study. *Lancet*. 353:1481–1484.
49. Martinez ME, Grodstein F, Giovannucci E et al. (1997). A prospective study of reproductive factors, oral contraceptive use, and risk of colorectal cancer. *Cancer Epidemiol Biomarkers Prev*. 6:1–5.
50. Potter JD, McMichael AJ. (1983). Large bowel cancer in women in relation to reproductive and hormonal factors: A case-control study. *J Natl Cancer Inst*. 71:703–709.
51. Fernandez E, La Vecchia C, Franceschi S et al. (1998). Oral contraceptive use and risk of colorectal cancer. *Epidemiology*. 9:295–300.
52. Troisi R, Schairer C, Chow WH et al. (1997). A prospective study of menopausal hormones and risk of colorectal cancer (United States). *Cancer Causes Control*. 8:130–138.

53. Crandall CJ. (1999). Estrogen replacement therapy and colon cancer: A clinical review. *J Womens Health Gender Based Med.* 8:1155–1166.

54. Spector TD, Hochberg MC. (1990). The protective effect of the oral contraceptive pill on rheumatoid arthritis: An overview of the analytic epidemiological studies using meta-analysis. *J Clin Epidemiol.* 43:1221–1230.

55. Stadel BV. (1981). Oral contraceptives and cardiovascular disease (first of two parts). *N Engl J Med.* 305:612–618.

56. Stadel BV. (1981). Oral contraceptives and cardiovascular disease (second of two parts). *N Engl J Med.* 305:672–677.

57. Gerstman BB, Piper JM, Tomita DK *et al.* (1991). Oral contraceptive estrogen dose and the risk of deep venous thromboembolic disease. *Am J Epidemiol.* 133:32–37.

58. Spitzer WO. (1998). Bias versus causality: Interpreting recent evidence of oral contraceptive studies. *Am J Obstet Gynecol.* 179:S43–S50.

59. Bloemenkamp KW, Rosendaal FR, Helmerhorst FM *et al.* (1995). Enhancement by factor V Leiden mutation of risk of deep-vein thrombosis associated with oral contraceptives containing a third-generation progestagen. *Lancet.* 346:1593–1596.

60. Lewis MA, Heinemann LA, Spitzer WO *et al.* (1997). The use of oral contraceptives and the occurrence of acute myocardial infarction in young women. Results from the Transnational Study on Oral Contraceptives and the Health of Young Women. *Contraception.* 56:129–140.

61. Farmer RD, Lawrenson RA, Thompson CR *et al.* (1997). Population-based study of risk of venous thromboembolism associated with various oral contraceptives. *Lancet.* 349:83–88.

62. Lawrenson R, Farmer R. (2000). Venous thromboembolism and combined oral contraceptives: Does the type of progestogen make a difference? *Contraception.* 62:21S–28S; discussion 37S–38S.

63. Spitzer WO. (2000). Oral contraceptives and cardiovascular outcomes: Cause or bias? *Contraception.* 62:3S–9S; discussion 37S–38S.

64. Vandenbroucke JP, Rosing J, Bloemenkamp KW *et al.* (2001). Oral contraceptives and the risk of venous thrombosis. *N Engl J Med.* 344:1527–1535.

65. Kemmeren JM, Algra A, Grobbee DE. (2001). Third generation oral contraceptives and risk of venous thrombosis: Meta-analysis. *BMJ.* 323:131–134.

66. Farmer RD, Williams TJ, Simpson EL, Nightingale AL. (2000). Effect of 1995 pill scare on rates of venous thromboembolism among women taking combined oral contraceptives: Analysis of general practice research database. *BMJ.* 321:477–479.

67. Jick H, Kaye JA, Vasilakis-Scaramozza C, Jick SS. (2000). Risk of venous thromboembolism among users of third generation oral contraceptives compared with users of oral contraceptives with levonorgestrel before and after 1995: Cohort and case-control analysis. *BMJ.* 321:1190–1195.

68. Skegg DC. (2000). Pitfalls of pharmacoepidemiology. *BMJ.* 321:1171–1172.

69. Winkler UH. (2000). Hemostatic effects of third- and second-generation oral contraceptives: Absence of a causal mechanism for a difference in risk of venous thromboembolism. *Contraception.* 62:11S–20S; discussion 37S–38S.

70. (1999). Consensus conference on combination oral contraceptives and cardiovascular disease. *Fertil Steril.* 71:1S–6S.

71. WHO Scientific Group. (1998). *Cardiovascular Disease and Steroid Hormone Contraception.* Geneva: World Health Organization.

72. Dahlback B, Carlsson M, Svensson PJ. (1993). Familial thrombophilia due to a previously unrecognized mechanism characterized by poor anticoagulant response to activated protein C: Prediction of a cofactor to activated protein C [see comments]. *Proc Natl Acad Sci U S A.* 90:1004–1008.

73. Price DT, Ridker PM. (1997). Factor V Leiden mutation and the risks for thromboembolic disease: A clinical perspective [see comments]. *Ann Intern Med.* 127:895–903.

74. Vandenbroucke JP, van der Meer FJ, Helmerhorst FM, Rosendaal FR. (1996). Factor V Leiden: Should we screen oral contraceptive users and pregnant women? [see comments]. *BMJ.* 313:1127–1130.

75. Winkler UH. (1998). Blood coagulation and oral contraceptives. A critical review. *Contraception.* 57:203–209.

76. Tans G, Curvers J, Middeldorp S *et al.* (2000). A randomized cross-over study on the effects of levonorgestrel- and desogestrel-containing oral contraceptives on the anticoagulant pathways. *Thromb Haemost.* 84:15–21.

77. Schambeck CM, Schwender S, Haubitz I *et al.* (1997). Selective screening for the Factor V Leiden mutation: Is it advisable prior to the prescription of oral contraceptives? *Thromb Haemost.* 78:1480–1483.

78. Heinemann LA, Lewis MA, Thorogood M *et al.* (1997). Case-control study of oral contraceptives and risk of thromboembolic stroke: Results from International Study on Oral Contraceptives and Health of Young Women. *BMJ.* 315:1502–1504.

79. Lidegaard O. (1993). Oral contraception and risk of a cerebral thromboembolic attack: Results of a case-control study. *BMJ.* 306:956–963.

80. (1996). Ischaemic stroke and combined oral contraceptives: Results of an international, multicentre, case-control study. WHO Collaborative Study of Cardiovascular Disease and Steroid Hormone Contraception. *Lancet.* 348:498–505.

81. Hannaford PC, Croft PR, Kay CR. (1994). Oral contraception and stroke. Evidence from the Royal College of General Practitioners' Oral Contraception Study [see comments]. *Stroke.* 25:935–942.

82. Petitti DB, Sidney S, Bernstein A *et al.* (1996). Stroke in users of low-dose oral contraceptives [see comments]. *N Engl J Med.* 335:8–15.

83. Porter JB, Hunter JR, Jick H, Stergachis A. (1985). Oral contraceptives and nonfatal vascular disease. *Obstet Gynecol.* 66:1–4.

84. Schwartz SM, Siscovick DS, Longstreth WT Jr *et al.* (1997). Use of low-dose oral contraceptives and stroke in young women. *Ann Intern Med.* 127:596–603.

85. Schwartz SM, Petitti DB, Siscovick DS *et al.* (1998). Stroke and use of low-dose oral contraceptives in young women: A pooled analysis of two US studies. *Stroke.* 29:2277–2284.

86. Thorogood M, Mann J, Murphy M, Vessey M. (1992). Fatal stroke and use of oral contraceptives: Findings from a case-control study. *Am J Epidemiol.* 136:35–45.

87. Vessey MP, Lawless M, Yeates D. (1984). Oral contraceptives and stroke: Findings in a large prospective study. *BMJ (Clin Res Ed).* 289:530–531.

88. Tzourio C, Tehindrazanarivelo A, Iglesias S *et al.* (1995). Case-control study of migraine and risk of ischaemic stroke in young women. *BMJ.* 310:830–833.

89. Chang CL, Donaghy M, Poulter N. (1999). Migraine and stroke in young women: Case-control study. The World Health Organization Collaborative Study of Cardiovascular Disease and Steroid Hormone Contraception [see comments]. *BMJ.* 318:13–18.

90. Sidney S, Petitti DB, Quesenberry CP Jr *et al.* (1996). Myocardial infarction in users of low-dose oral contraceptives. *Obstet Gynecol.* 88:939–944.

91. Sidney S, Siscovick DS, Petitti DB *et al.* (1998). Myocardial infarction and use of low-dose oral contraceptives: A pooled analysis of 2 US studies. *Circulation.* 98:1058–1063.

92. Lewis MA, Spitzer WO, Heinemann LA et al. (1996). Third generation oral contraceptives and risk of myocardial infarction: An international case-control study. Transnational Research Group on Oral Contraceptives and the Health of Young Women. *BMJ.* 312:88–90.

93. WHO Collaborative Study of Cardiovascular Disease and Steroid Hormone Contraception. (1997). Acute myocardial infarction and combined oral contraceptives: Results of an international multicentre case-control study. *Lancet.* 349:1202–1209.

94. D'Avanzo B, La Vecchia C, Negri E *et al.* (1994). Oral contraceptive use and risk of myocardial infarction: An Italian case-control study. *J Epidemiol Community Health.* 48:324–325.

95. Rosenberg L, Palmer JR, Lesko SM, Shapiro S. (1990). Oral contraceptive use and the risk of myocardial infarction. *Am J Epidemiol.* 131:1009–1016.

96. Stampfer MJ, Willett WC, Colditz GA *et al.* (1988). A prospective study of past use of oral contraceptive agents and risk of cardiovascular diseases. *N Engl J Med.* 319:1313–1317.

97. Croft P, Hannaford PC. (1989). Risk factors for acute myocardial infarction in women: Evidence from the Royal College of General Practitioners' oral contraception study [see comments]. *BMJ.* 298:165–168.

98. Collaborative Group on Hormonal Factors in Breast Cancer. (1996). Breast cancer and hormonal contraceptives: Collaborative reanalysis of individual data on 53,297 women with breast cancer and 100,239 women without breast cancer from 54 epidemiological studies. *Lancet.* 347:1713–1727.

99. Marchbanks PA, McDonald JA, Wilson HG *et al.* (2002). The NICHD Women's Contraceptive and Reproductive Experiences Study: Methods and operational results. *Ann Epidemiol.* 12:213–221.

100. Marchbanks PA, McDonald JA, Wilson HG *et al.* (2002). Oral contraceptives and the risk of breast cancer. *N Engl J Med.* 346:2025–2032.

101. Rosenberg MJ, Waugh MS, Burnhill MS. (1998). Compliance, counseling and satisfaction with oral contraceptives: A prospective evaluation. *Fam Plann Perspect.* 30:89–92, 104.

102. Hall SD, Wang Z, Huang M *et al.* (2003). The interaction between St. John's wort and an oral contraceptive. *Clin Pharmacol Ther.* 74:525–535.

103. Barfield A, Melo J, Coutinho E *et al.* (1979). Pregnancies associated with sperm concentrations below 10 million/ml in clinical studies of a potential male contraceptive method, monthly depot medroxyprogesterone acetate and testosterone esters. *Contraception.* 20:121–127.

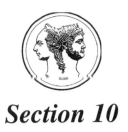

Section 10

INFECTIOUS DISEASE

Scott M. Hammer, MD

Columbia University, Division of Infectious Diseases, New York, NY

Infectious diseases are one of the leading causes of morbidity and mortality worldwide and the leading cause in children and young adults. For the most part, infectious pathogens do not respect gender barriers with relative rather than absolute differences in risks of acquisition, pathogenicity, severity, and response to treatment between men and women. More clear-cut differences can be seen for infectious pathogens for which anatomic or physiologic differences (e.g., pregnancy) play an important role in pathogenic potential.

Given the myriad number of infectious agents, it is not possible nor pertinent to try to provide a detailed discussion of every infecting organism or infectious syndrome. Rather, the purpose of this section is to highlight the major issues in the field across several of the most important microbiologic categories (bacteria, mycobacteria, fungi, viruses, parasites, etc.). Some pathogens and syndromes are dealt with in more depth than others—a reflection of either their relative importance in high-lighting gender–specific issues or the available data in the field.

There are eight chapters in this section, each authored by leaders in their respective fields. The contributions include the following:

- "Bacterial Infections" by S. Tsiouris and F. Lowy leads off this section. In this chapter, urinary tract infections, bacterial vaginosis, listeriosis, and toxic shock syndrome are detailed. These illustrative examples highlight the differential risks between men and women afforded by anatomic consider-ations and pregnancy with respect to bacterial infections.
- "Gender-Specific Issues in Fungal Infections" by N. Kirmani and W. Powderly discusses the most relevant human mycoses. This chapter illustrates the point that for many infectious diseases, small if any differences exist between genders. Where they do exist, anatomic and physiologic differences (e.g., pregnancy again) are the keys to under-standing the spectrum of risk and differential therapeutic considerations.
- "Gender-Specific Issues in HIV Pathogenesis" by R. MClelland and R. Coombs addresses critical aspects of the epidemi-ology, transmission, disease manifestations, treatment, and prevention of human immunodeficiency virus-1 (HIV-1). As a sexually transmitted infection, HIV/AIDS (acquired immune deficiency syndrome) has become the worst infec-tious pandemic the world has experienced. Gender-specific issues are particularly important with respect to susceptibil-ity to infection, viral pathogenesis, prevention approaches, and maternal–fetal transmission. Research in these areas is being pursued intensively on the international level and hopefully will lead to greater control of this devastating infectious disease.
- "Gender-Specific Issues in the Metabolic Complications of HIV Disease and Its Treatment" by M. Gerber and J. Aberg is one of two chapters devoted to this single pathogen. This is appropriate given the global significance of HIV-1. In this context, the potential for metabolic dysfunction induced by the virus or antiretroviral treatment represents a major health consideration. Gender-specific differences in this area are just beginning to be elucidated, but the potential for increased cardiovascular disease risk and osteoporosis have obvious, major medical and public health implications.
- "Gender and Tuberculosis" by C. Zeana and W. El-Sadr is another chapter in this section devoted to a single

pathogen. Again, the shear global burden of this disease, whether viewed as a single infection or as a coinfection with HIV, justifies this focus. This chapter delineates a situation in which epidemiologic data tell us that gender differences exist in the burden of disease but our knowledge of why this difference exists is largely speculative.

- "Gender-Specific Issues in Non-HIV Viral Infections" by M. Sobieszczyk and C. Hay reviews a wide variety of viral pathogens with respect to gender-related issues of risk, pathogenesis, and pregnancy. This chapter highlights the multiplicity and complexity of infectious diseases when viewed in both a general and a gender–specific context.
- "Gender-Specific Issues in Parasitology" by M. Yin and D. Despommier presents a comprehensive view of several pathogens. Despite this breadth, a number of important cross-cutting concepts come to the fore. These include the potential for hormonal differences to influence the cellular immune response to infectious agents, the important role of occupational exposure in differential risks of infection, and (again) the crucial role of pregnancy in gender-specific risk.

- "Sexually Transmitted Infections in Men and Women" by T. Wilkin and M. Chiasson appropriately closes this section. Sexually transmitted infections (STIs) are among the most prevalent infections worldwide, and this chapter focuses on the non–HIV pathogens. It highlights the potential for a wide range of pathogens to be sexually transmitted; acquisition risks that may be based on behavioral differences including economic dependency of women; biologic susceptibility based on anatomic, hormonal, and local immunologic factors; and differences in presentation and outcome (infertility, fetal risk, etc.).

Overall, this section, along with its companion sections in this book, illustrates both the depth of knowledge that exists and the challenges that remain. In this regard, each chapter presents a number of questions that need to be addressed to provide a more complete picture of gender differences in infectious diseases. Answers to these questions inevitably will lead to improved prevention and treatment efforts and a consequent reduction in morbidity and mortality from one of the greatest medical threats faced by the human population.

83

Gender and Bacterial Infections

SIMON J. TSIOURIS, MD* AND FRANKLIN D. LOWY, MD**

*Post-Doctoral Clinical Fellow, Columbia University, College of Physicians and Surgeons, Department of Medicine,
Division of Infectious Diseases, New York, NY
**Professor of Medicine, Columbia University, College of Physicians and Surgeons, Department of Medicine,
Division of Infectious Diseases, New York, NY

I. Introduction

The role of gender in bacterial infections has received limited attention. In this chapter, we highlight certain bacterial infections in which gender plays a role in the epidemiology, pathophysiology, or clinical presentation and management of the disease. The selected topics are chosen to illustrate different issues relating to gender and bacterial infection and are not meant to be a comprehensive list of all bacterial infections with gender-specific issues.

II. Urinary Tract Infection

A urinary tract infection (UTI) is an example of a bacterial infection that affects men and women but whose epidemiology, pathophysiology, and clinical management differ mainly because of anatomic dissimilarities between the sexes. The variation between the male and female genitourinary anatomy explains many of these differences.

A UTI is usually bacterial in origin and can involve the urinary tract anywhere from the distal portion of the urethral meatus to the perinephric fascia and any structure in between including the urethra, the bladder, the ureters as well as the renal pelvis and parenchyma. The topic of urinary tract infections is a large one. This section will focus on the difference that gender makes in the epidemiology and pathophysiology of these infections.

A. Terminology

UTIs can be divided into complicated and uncomplicated UTIs. Uncomplicated UTIs occur most often in persons with normal urinary tracts and are caused by "usual" pathogens, such as *Escherichia coli*, whereas complicated UTIs often are seen in persons with structural or anatomic abnormalities of their urinary tracts and may be the result of antibiotic-resistant bacteria or less common uropathogens such as antimicrobial resistant *Klebsiella spp.* [1]. It is also important to distinguish the anatomic location of the infection. Infections in the lower urinary tract involve the urethra and the urinary bladder. Infections in the upper urinary tract may or may not include the urethra or bladder but do involve the ureters and/or the kidneys.

Another important distinction is the difference between UTI, bacteriuria, and urine culture contamination. In a patient with typical symptoms of a UTI the diagnosis can be confirmed by a clean-catch, midstream, voided urine that grows greater than 10^5 organisms per milliliter [2], especially if pyuria is present. Even 10^4 organisms per milliliter of a uropathogen, such as

E. coli, in a woman with typical symptoms is suggestive of UTI [2]. Bacteriuria, however, implies at least 10^5 organisms per milliliter without symptoms. As discussed later, bacteriuria becomes an important consideration in pregnant women. Finally, urine culture contamination should be suspected in cases where the patient does not have typical UTI symptoms, the growth on urine culture is less than 10^5 organisms per milliliter, or more than one organism is isolated from the sample. Caveats to the previous statements include urine specimens obtained via catheterization, in which case even 10^4 organisms per milliliter should be considered indicative of true bacteriuria or infection, and specimens obtained through suprapubic aspirates, in which case any bacteria recovered are significant [3].

B. Epidemiology

UTIs are much more common in women than men. However, in neonates and infants, the rate of urinary tract infection is as much as 10% higher in males than in females [1,4]. This is the only time period in which incidence of UTI in males exceeds that in females. From adolescence through young adulthood, the incidence and prevalence of UTI is consistently higher in females than in men. In the elderly and institutionalized, the prevalence equalizes between the sexes [5].

A woman's lifetime risk of having a UTI is between 20% and 50% [1]. This risk of UTI increases with age, starting with an incidence of 2–3% at age 15 years and increasing by 1% every decade through age 65 [2].

On a population basis, the most common source of bacteremia in the elderly and the most common infection in nursing home residents (with a prevalence in the range of 20–50% in both men and women) is UTI [4,6,7]. Increased risk of UTI in women has been associated with recent sexual intercourse or use of a spermicide or a diaphragm [8,9].

C. Pathophysiology

Most UTIs in men are complicated. In infants, the higher rate of UTIs found in males is likely the result of a higher incidence of congenital urogenital tract disorders in male than in female infants [10]. Other risk factors leading to higher rates of UTIs in male infants include greater exposure of the male urethra to stool and lack of circumcision, which may lead to colonization of the prepuce with colonic organisms [4]. Once out of infancy, men without anatomic abnormalities have a much smaller chance of developing UTIs than women. Part of this is because the dry epithelium of the glans penis is more difficult for coliform organisms to colonize and the male urethra is considerably longer than the female urethra, making it more difficult for bacteria to reach the bladder [11]. The most common problems leading to complicated UTIs in adult men include benign prostatic hypertrophy and neurogenic bladder, both of which lead to bladder outlet obstruction and urinary retention [4]. Prostatitis, especially chronic prostatitis, can be a particularly challenging problem that complicates UTIs in men. Chronic bacterial prostatitis is the most common cause of recurrent UTI in men and is often difficult to treat [12,13].

The pathophysiology of UTIs in women is different. Most women suffer from uncomplicated UTIs. The process begins when bacteria from the fecal flora migrate and colonize the perineum. From there, they colonize the vaginal introitus and then can ascend the relatively short female urethra to enter the bladder and cause infection [2,14].

The most common causative organism in uncomplicated UTI is *E. coli*. This is a reflection of its predominance as an aerobic Gram-negative rod in the fecal flora [1]. There is evidence that most of the *E. coli* that cause UTIs have two virulence factors, P fimbriae and Type I fimbriae. These pili enhance the ability of *E. coli* to attach to urogenital epithelial structures [15]. Virulence factors like these, along with others, help explain how bacteria can survive to cause infection in the normally unpleasant (from the viewpoint of bacteria) environment of urine with its low pH, changing osmolality, and high organic acid content [14].

D. Bacteriuria in Pregnancy: A Special Case

The prevalence of asymptomatic bacteriuria in pregnancy ranges from 4 to 7% compared to the average prevalence in nonpregnant women from 2 to 4% [16]. Part of the reason for this increase in prevalence results from the condition known as hydroureter which can occur during pregnancy. Hydroureter of pregnancy is likely the result of a combination of factors including mechanical changes such as a shift in position of the bladder from the pelvis to the abdomen which leads to outlet obstruction and hormonal changes which lead to decreased ureteral peristalsis [3].

Of pregnant women 20–40% with asymptomatic bacteriuria will develop symptomatic infections, a higher proportion of which will be upper tract infections such as pyelonephritis [17]. Therefore, treating asymptomatic bacteriuria in pregnancy can reduce the incidence of pyelonephritis during pregnancy. More importantly, these symptomatic infections may lead to increased rates of premature labor and premature delivery [3]. Although there is still debate about whether treating the asymptomatic bacteriuria early in the course of pregnancy actually lowers rates of subsequent preterm delivery and fetal morbidity, most recommendations state that a screening urine culture in the first trimester is appropriate, and treatment of bacteriuria in pregnancy should be part of routine care during pregnancy [3].

E. Clinical Manifestations, Diagnosis, and Treatment

Acute UTI usually presents with dysuria and urinary frequency. Nocturia is often a helpful symptom as well. The urine itself may be cloudy, and, if hematuria is present, the patient may notice red discoloration of their urine. Fever is not a common symptom of lower UTI but sometimes occurs in upper tract infections such as pyelonephritis. Pyelonephritis often is accompanied by costovertebral angle tenderness and flank pain. In cystitis, suprapubic tenderness may be elicited. All of these signs and symptoms may be absent in elderly patients with UTIs, who may only complain of vague gastrointestinal symptoms such as nausea and vomiting [1]. It should be noted, however, that discrimination between upper and lower UTI has limited reliability when based on physical examination alone.

The gold standard for diagnosis of UTI is a combination of typical signs and symptoms along with evidence of pyuria (determined either by microscopic examination of the urine or through the indirect method of leukocyte esterase presence on dipstick) and a voided, clean-catch, midstream urine specimen with greater than 10^5 organisms per milliliter on culture. Many clinicians diagnose and treat UTIs based on symptoms and urine dipstick results alone because of the time and resources needed for urine culture. The importance of a urine culture to help direct appropriate antibiotic therapy should not be overlooked, especially in elderly patients and in patients with complicated or recurrent UTIs [1,2].

Treatment recommendations for UTIs change often as a result of changing antibiotic resistance patterns among bacteria. The physician should be familiar with the resistance patterns of common uropathogens in their areas and choose empiric antibiotics accordingly. Treatment also varies depending on the type of UTI. Uncomplicated UTIs in healthy women are often adequately treated with a 3-day course of trimethoprim-sulfamethoxazole or a 3-day course of a quinolone [1]. Pyelonephritis requires a longer course of antibiotics, on the order of 14 days. Treatment should be guided by culture results, although initial empiric therapy with a quinolone is appropriate. Admission for intravenous antibiotics should also be considered in the very ill or elderly patient with pyelonephritis [1]. Complicated UTIs also deserve a longer course of antibiotics. Any UTI in a man should be treated as a complicated UTI with subsequent urologic follow-up to rule out anatomic abnormalities [4]. Finally, treatment of asymptomatic bacteriuria in pregnancy should involve a 7–10 day course of amoxicillin or nitrofurantoin, assuming the organism grown on culture is sensitive to either amoxicillin or nitrofurantoin, which have both been shown to be effective in treating bacteriuria, followed by a repeat urine culture to prove clearance of bacteriuria [3]. Pregnant women with asymptomatic bacteriuria and organisms resistant to amoxicillin or nitrofurantoin should be treated in consultation with an obstetrician and an infectious diseases specialist to determine which antibiotic the organism is sensitive to (based on results of antibiotic susceptibility testing of the organism) is safest for use in pregnancy.

III. Bacterial Vaginosis

Bacterial vaginosis (BV) is an example of a bacterial infection that is strictly gender specific because of anatomic differences in the reproductive tracts of men and women. BV's clinical limitation to the female sex should not mute its importance as a clinical entity. In fact, the impact that BV can have on outcomes during pregnancy needs to be underscored.

This section will focus on the history, epidemiology, complications, and pathophysiology of the disease. Details regarding diagnosis and treatment have been well described in other sources [18]. BV is now known to be the primary cause of abnormal vaginal discharge the world over [19] and has been associated with numerous conditions affecting the health of women in pregnancy and the health of the fetus, including spontaneous abortion, premature birth, preterm labor, preterm premature rupture of the membranes, postpartum endometritis, and amniotic fluid infection [18,20–23].

A. History

The disease entity we now call bacterial vaginosis was described first in 1894 when it was originally termed "nonspecific" vaginitis because no specific etiologic agent could be identified [18].

BV was first defined as a specific entity separate from other causes of vaginitis by Gardner and Dukes when they described the "clue" cells characteristic of BV [24]. They proposed that a new organism, for which they coined the name *Haemophilus vaginalis,* was solely responsible for the infection. Subsequently, this organism was renamed *Gardnerella vaginalis* in 1980 [25].

Soon after the name change, it became clear that *G. vaginalis* was not the sole pathogen in BV as the importance of anaerobic organisms and other bacteria in the pathophysiology of BV was recognized [26]. Ultimately, the condition was designated as bacterial vaginosis in 1984 [27].

B. Epidemiology

Upwards of 50% of women with BV are asymptomatic. Numerous studies from various nations around the world show that BV can be found in 10–41% of women [18]. Although the rates of BV are highest among women seen and screened at sexually transmitted infections (STIs) clinics [28] and BV most often occurs in sexually active women [29], it is clear that BV is not simply a STI because it has also been detected among virginal women and children [30].

C. Complications

Studies repeatedly show that BV is linked with increased risk of preterm birth, preterm labor, and preterm premature rupture of the membranes [31–33]. Most concerning, the association between BV and preterm birth occurs at low gestational ages [34]. Of great importance for prevention, evidence of BV has been noted to be present weeks to months before preterm birth [35]. In one study, the odds ratio for preterm birth or premature rupture of membranes in pregnant women with BV compared to controls was two by the third trimester [35].

D. Pathophysiology

BV is associated with unique and characteristic changes in the microbiologic milieu of the vagina. The vagina is colonized by acidophilic facultative lactobacilli [36] which are hydrogen peroxide–producing and contribute to the normally low pH of the healthy vagina [37]. In BV, there is a change in the normal flora so that *G. vaginalis* and other species (including *Prevotella spp., Peptostreptococcus spp.,* and others) exist and are found in concentrations 100 to 1000 times greater than concentrations of the same species in the healthy vagina [18]. There are biochemical changes as well, including an elevation in pH of the vaginal fluids and secretions; increases in concentrations of polyamines and organic acids; and increases in concentrations of mucinases, sialidase and immunoglobulin A proteases [10]. These changes are likely important in overcoming the host-defense mechanisms and allowing pathogens to reach the upper reproductive tract and cause the obstetric complications associated with BV [18].

As part of the normal vaginal flora, lactobacilli help maintain a healthy vaginal environment and inhibit the growth of other species of bacteria in part because of their production of hydrogen peroxide, which maintains a low pH in the vaginal secretions [38,39]. What is unclear in the pathogenesis of BV is what change occurs first in the normal vaginal ecosystem. Does a decline in the number of normally present lactobacilli, for reasons yet to be elucidated, lead to an increase in the pH of vaginal secretions (as a result of the lack of lactobacilli-dependent hydrogen peroxide production), thus setting up an environment in which BV-associated bacteria can predominate? Or, conversely, do BV-associated bacteria gain predominance in some other manner and overgrow the lactobacilli, thus leading to an increase in vaginal pH? Some studies suggest that the former may be the case. One study showed that women without hydrogen peroxide–producing lactobacilli as part of their vaginal flora were more likely to develop BV [40].

E. Diagnosis

The mainstay of clinical diagnosis in BV is based on Amsel's criteria (Table 83-1). The presence of at least three of the four criteria is suggestive of a diagnosis of BV. The presence of clue cells on a wet mount examination is the most sensitive and specific indicator of BV of the four criteria that make up Amsel's criteria, with a positive predictive value for BV of 85–90% [41]. Other methods of diagnosis including Papanicolaou smear, Gram stain diagnosis, and culture have had varying sensitivities and specificities but are often too costly and impractical for use in a clinical setting [18].

F. Treatment and Prevention of Complications

Separate studies by McGregor and Morales have shown that treatment of BV in pregnancy with either metronidazole or clindamycin results in a 50% reduction in the risk of preterm

Table 83-1
Amsel's Criteria for the Diagnosis of Bacterial Vaginosis

1. Homogeneous, thin vaginal fluid that adheres to the vaginal walls
2. Vaginal fluid pH >4.5
3. Release of amine odor with alkalinization of vaginal fluid, the "whiff test"
4. Presence of vaginal epithelial cells ("clue" cells) with borders obscured with adherent, small bacteria

Table 83-2

Centers for Disease Control and Prevention Treatment Guidelines for Bacterial Vaginosis in Pregnant Women

Recommended Regimens

Metronidazole 500 mg orally twice a day for 7 days,
OR

Metronidazole gel 0.75%, one full applicator (5 g) intravaginally, once a day for 5 days,
OR

Clindamycin cream 2%, one full applicator (5 g) intravaginally at bedtime for 7 days.

Alternative Regimens

Metronidazole 2 g orally in a single dose,
OR

Clindamycin 300 mg orally twice a day for 7 days,
OR

Clindamycin ovules 100 g intravaginally once at bedtime for 3 days.

birth compared to untreated controls [31,32]. The mainstay of therapy has been metronidazole. It can be given as a one-time oral dose of 2 g with cure rates at 4 weeks of 68–90% [18]. This regimen is the simplest in nonpregnant women with symptomatic BV. See Table 83-2 for the Centers for Disease Control and Prevention (CDC) guidelines for initial and alternative treatment regimens for BV (symptomatic or asymptomatic) in pregnant women.

IV. Listeriosis and Pregnancy

Listeriosis is an example of a bacterial infection that affects the sexes differently because of changes in the hormonal and immune status of women during pregnancy. *Listeria monocytogenes* is a ubiquitous bacterium that can be found in the soil and can contaminate many types of foodstuffs. It is not a common cause of illness in the normal host. In persons with depressed cell-mediated immunity, such as pregnant women, young children, the elderly, persons infected with the human immunodeficiency virus (HIV), and transplant patients receiving immunosuppressive therapy, it can cause life-threatening meningoencephalitis and sepsis and can complicate childbirth [42]. Nonpregnant women and men are, all other things equal, generally equally susceptible to listeriosis. The changes that occur during pregnancy, many of which are still not fully understood, increase the risk of women developing listeriosis.

Despite the gaps in our understanding of the physiologic changes that women undergo during pregnancy and how those changes affect the immune system, the epidemiology of listeriosis during pregnancy has been clearly described and the importance of listeriosis as a clinical entity needs to be recognized by any clinician who cares for women so as to prevent as many cases as possible and be able to treat listeriosis effectively for the benefit of the health of the pregnant woman as well as the fetus.

A. Epidemiology

L. monocytogenes can be cultured from soil and decaying vegetable matter and has been found in the stool of 5% of healthy adults [43]. Other studies have shown that with repeated sampling the recovery rates are much higher, closer to 70% [44]. *L. monocytogenes* has been cultured from multiple food items as well, including but not limited to raw vegetables, raw milk, fish, poultry, and fresh and processed meats at rates from 15 to 70% [43]. Based on these observations, it is believed by some that exposure to *L. monocytogenes* by humans must be a relatively common occurrence [42]. Contaminated food is the usual source of infection in humans. Outbreaks have been linked to contaminated soft cheese, coleslaw, deli meats, hot dogs, pasteurized milk, turkey franks, and alfalfa tablets [42,45]. Two separate surveillance studies on listeriosis conducted by the CDC, one in 1980–1982 and the next in 1986, estimated an annual infection rate of 7.4 cases per million in the United States [46,47]. This translates into about 1850 cases of listeriosis per year, with mortality rates ranging from 20 to 30% [48] for roughly 425 deaths per year. Of these cases, 27% of them occur in pregnant women. The annual rate of infection, or incidence, in pregnant women is estimated at 120 cases per million, a 17-fold increase over that of the general population [49]. An epidemic of listeriosis linked to unpasteurized Mexican style soft cheese that occurred in Los Angeles in 1985 had a total of 142 cases, 65.5% of which were pregnant women [50]. Pregnant women account for 60% of cases in persons 10–40 years of age [42]. Most other cases occur in infants younger than 1 month in age who were infected by vertical transmission; in adults older than 60 years of age; and in persons with depressed immune systems such as persons with hematologic malignancies, AIDS, solid organ transplant recipients, or persons undergoing long-term corticosteroid therapy. The question thus raised is the following: What makes pregnant women more susceptible to infection with *L. monocytogenes*?

B. Pathophysiology

L. monocytogenes is a small, facultative anaerobic, non–spore forming, Gram-positive rod that grows well on routine culture media and forms a small zone of β-hemolysis around its colonies [42,49]. It sometimes can be mistaken for nonpathogenic diptheroids on gram stain but should be easily distinguished because of its unique tumbling motility [49]. *L. monocytogenes* is capable of surviving at much colder temperatures (4–10°C) than most bacteria and can be selectively grown in culture at these low temperatures or by using other selective media [51]. Its ability to survive at these low temperatures plays a role in its ability to multiply within contaminated foods even at refrigerator temperatures.

L. monocytogenes infections occur primarily via the ingestion of contaminated foodstuffs [42]. The inoculum necessary to cause symptomatic illness via the oral route is unknown. The mean incubation period for invasive illness is 23 days (range 11 to 70 days) [42]. *L. monocytogenes* can cross the mucosal barrier of the intestinal wall and enter the epithelial cells of the gastrointestinal tract, likely via active endocytosis. From there, it can reach the bloodstream. Once in the bloodstream,

L. monocytogenes can disseminate widely, particularly to the central nervous system and the placenta [42].

L. monocytogenes has many virulence mechanisms. One of the most important may be its capacity for intracellular survival. *L. monocytogenes* expresses proteins termed internalins, which promote its entry into epithelial cells and hepatocytes [48]. The Listeria is internalized into a phagolysosome. From there, it escapes by utilizing an exotoxin called listeriolysin O to disrupt the phagolysosome's membrane [48]. Once free inside the cytoplasm, *L. monocytogenes* can multiply and become pathogenic. Listeria uses similar mechanisms to survive inside human phagocytic cells, effectively shielding itself from humoral defenses and causing the body to rely on cell-mediated immunity for defense [45]. Listeria protects itself further from detection by the humoral immune system through an ingenious method of cell-to-cell spread via filopod formation, which utilizes the cell's own actin cytoskeleton proteins [48]. To date, no evidence has been brought forth to connect an increased risk of listeriosis with immunoglobulin or complement deficiencies [48]. It therefore follows that persons with impaired cell-mediated immune defenses, such as pregnant women [52,53], may have a higher risk of infection with *L. monocytogenes*. For excellent discussions of the literature pertaining to depression of cell-mediated immunity in pregnancy, please refer to the reviews by Weinberg and Falkoff [52,53].

Another potentially important virulence factor for *L. monocytogenes* is iron [42]. Iron supplementation has been related to increased clinical morbidity from infectious processes, especially malaria [54]. The growth of Listeria is enhanced *in vitro* by the addition of iron [55], and animal studies have shown an increased susceptibility to infection with *L. monocytogenes* in iron-overload states and enhanced lethality in the setting of iron supplementation [56]. What implications this may have in humans is unclear, and further study is needed in this area.

C. Clinical Syndromes

1. Central Nervous System Infection

L. monocytogenes seems to have a particular predilection for the central nervous system, specifically the brainstem and meninges [57]. In 1986, *L. monocytogenes* was the fifth most common cause of bacterial meningitis overall in all age groups [58]; with the advent of vaccination to *Haemophilus influenzae* it is likely to become more common. Of all of the bacterial causes of community-acquired meningitis, *L. monocytogenes* has the highest mortality (~22%), especially in those patients with underlying immunocompromise [42]. It is interesting that meningitis resulting from Listeria in pregnant women is a relatively uncommon finding. The specific characteristics of meningitis/encephalitis caused by *L. monocytogenes* have been well described elsewhere [42,45].

2. Isolated Bacteremia in Pregnant Women and Perinatal Infection

Isolated bacteremia with *L. monocytogenes* can present as a fulminant episode of sepsis or as a flulike illness. The latter syndrome is more commonly encountered in pregnancy and often leads to infection of the placenta and complications that include premature labor and neonatal sepsis [59]. Maternal infection usually occurs in the third trimester but can occur at any time during pregnancy. Vertical transmission can also occur from mother to fetus at the time of delivery [45]. Infection early in gestation has been associated with spontaneous abortion and stillbirth [59] with rates as high as 22% [42]. There is also an increased risk of premature labor. One series described 248 cases of perinatal listeriosis. In that series, 62% of the women had fever as a presenting complaint, premature labor occurred in 50% of the pregnancies, spontaneous abortion occurred in 4%, and intrauterine fetal demise occurred in nearly 11% [49,60]. Maternal listeriosis later in gestation has been associated with two syndromes in the neonate: one is early (<2 days) onset and characterized by septicemia and the other is late (>5 days) onset and characterized by meningitis [49].

3. Other Syndromes and Complications

L. monocytogenes has been associated with other clinical syndromes as well, including endocarditis, localized soft-tissue infections, and febrile gastroenteritis. Complications of infection with *L. monocytogenes* include disseminated intravascular coagulation, acute renal failure, and adult respiratory distress syndrome [42].

D. Diagnosis and Treatment

Diagnosis of infection with *L. monocytogenes* is made by growth of the organism in culture of blood or cerebrospinal fluid. The mainstay of treatment for listeriosis is ampicillin or penicillin in combination with gentamicin. Alternatively, trimethoprim-sulfamethoxazole can be used, especially in those who are penicillin allergic, but with caution in pregnant women, and it may have better activity against the organism [42]. There have been no controlled trials of antibiotics for treatment of listeriosis; other antibiotics, including vancomycin, imipenem, and erythromycin, have shown mixed results [45]. Chloramphenicol, the cephalosporins, tetracycline, and the quinolones should not be used because they have not been shown to be effective.

E. Prevention

Since the outbreak of listeriosis related to the consumption of Mexican-style cheese [50], various government authorities have been trying to reduce the incidence of the disease. In 1986, the CDC in a joint effort with the Food and Drug Administration began to conduct active surveillance of human cases of listeriosis. In 1989, the U.S. Department of Agriculture initiated a zero-tolerance policy aimed at eliminating the sale of contaminated meat and meat products through active surveillance of ready-to-eat processed meats. In a follow-up study conducted in 1993 there was a 44% decrease in the incidence of illness and a 48% decrease in the incidence of death from listeriosis compared to rates in 1989 [61]. The incidence of perinatal listeriosis declined from 17.4 per 100,00 to 8.6 per 100,000, a 51% decrease [61]. New surveillance systems and interventions that are being developed by the CDC, such as the FoodNet and the Enter-net, should ensure that the decreases noted in the 1993 study continue [62,63].

Table 83-3
Recommendations for Preventing Listeriosis

For all persons:

Thoroughly cook raw food from animal sources
Thoroughly wash raw vegetables
Keep uncooked meats separate from other foods
Avoid consuming raw milk or food prepared with raw milk
Wash hands, knives, and cutting boards after handling
raw food

Further recommendations for persons at high risk of
listeriosis: (persons who are immunocompromised secondary
to chemotherapy or human immunodeficiency virus/acquired
immune deficiency syndrome or who are transplant recipients,
elderly persons, and pregnant women)

Avoid soft cheeses
Reheat leftover food or ready-to-eat foods until they are
steaming hot
Reheat cold cuts and deli meats before eating

At the individual level, the CDC published guidelines in 1992 for what persons, especially those at risk for listeriosis, could do to prevent its occurrence [64]. These are summarized in Table 83-3.

V. Toxic Shock Syndrome

Toxic shock syndrome (TSS) is not a bacterial infection; it is a toxin-mediated disease. It does not require clinical infection to be present, but it does depend on the presence of toxin-producing strains of *Staphylococcus aureus*. However, when looking at gender-specific practices and how they affect the expression of disease, TSS can be considered prototypical. TSS is also an example of how good epidemiologic methods can lead to an understanding of the pathophysiology of a disease.

A. History

TSS was first described by Todd *et al* in 1978 [65] as an acute disease that was associated with strains of staphylococci of Phage Group I that produced a unique epidermal toxin. It should be noted that classification of TSS strains of staphylococci by phage group is mostly of historical interest because it is now understood that the ability of a particular strain of staphylococcus to produce toxin is dependent on the presence of a mobile genetic element that contains the genes for toxin production. The syndrome is characterized by fever, hypotension, diffuse or palmar erythema followed by desquamation of the skin of the hands and feet, hyperemia of the mucous membranes, and multiorgan system dysfunction. The first large-scale outbreak of TSS was characterized by a predilection for affecting young women.

B. Epidemiology

In the initial report, seven children were described with the syndrome, all of whom were female. Subsequent surveillance studies proved the strong association of this syndrome with female gender, menstruation, and tampon use. Davis *et al*

[66] described 38 cases in Wisconsin between 1975 and 1980, 37 of whom were women with a mean age of 24.5 years (range 13 to 52). Thirty-five of the cases were matched for age and menstruation with 104 controls. Of the cases, 97% used tampons during the menstrual period that accompanied the onset of TSS. Of controls, 66% used tampons during every menstruation (p < 0.01). Of cases who had vaginal or cervical cultures done, 74% had *S. aureus* isolated as compared with 10% of women visiting family planning clinics [67].

By 1990, 3300 cases of TSS had been reported in the United States. Of these, 95% occurred in women and 90% of those were in menstruating women who used tampons [68]. It was soon discovered that the highest risk for TSS was in those women who were using high-absorbency tampons [69]. Subsequent studies suggested that high oxygen content within the tampon, not just degree of absorbency, played a role in the development of TSS [70]. Since the use of high-absorbency tampons was decreased (high-absorbency tampons were removed from the market in 1980) there has been a concomitant decrease of incidence in TSS in the United States [71]. Figure 83-1, adapted from a *Morbidity and Mortality Weekly Report* review of TSS incidence, depicts the number of reported cases of TSS in the United States from 1979–1990 [72]. It has also become evident that TSS can develop in males and nonmenstruating females and can be associated with focal *Staphylococcus aureus* infection in nongenitourinary sites and with organisms other than *S. aureus* [68].

C. Pathophysiology

TSS, therefore, is a syndrome that predominantly affected young women who used highly absorbent tampons during menstruation. How this set of circumstances predisposed these women to TSS is not exactly clear, but some theories have been proposed. Several pathophysiologic factors may play a role. Among them are microulcerations caused by the superabsorbent tampons in the mucosal epithelium that allowed toxins from the Phage-Type 1 staphylococci to enter the bloodstream [73]. The increased surface area of high-absorbency tampons may also contribute to the promotion of colonization and growth of toxin-producing *S. aureus* and the increased elaboration of toxin. Other mechanisms may involve the ability of *S. aureus* to colonize vaginal mucosae.

Bell proposed the possibility of a pathophysiologic mechanism similar to one already described for *Neisseria gonorrhoeae* [74]. It is known that virulent strains of *N. gonorrhoeae* (specifically those of the transparent phenotype) are more likely to colonize columnar versus squamous cervical epithelium, the former being more prevalent in adolescent women. Furthermore, young women and adolescents have lower progesterone levels during menstruation than older women, as do children in general and all menstruating women during certain portions of their cycle [68]. *N. gonorrhoeae* are known to have greater adherence to vaginal epithelium during phases of the menstrual cycle when estrogen levels are high and progesterone levels are low and have been shown to have decreased virulence in the presence of high levels of progesterone [74]. Bell hypothesized that *S. aureus* may have similar differential affinities for vaginal epithelium leading to the typical association of TSS with menstruation.

Cases of TSS in the United States

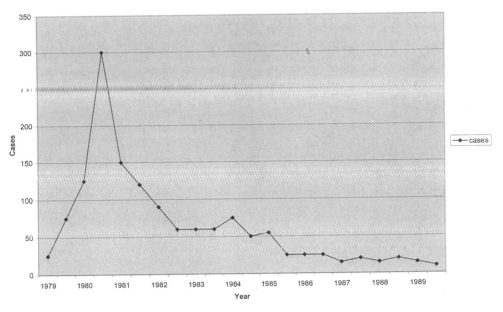

Fig. 83-1 Reported cases of toxic shock syndrome, United States 1979–1990.

Todd has also suggested that children and young persons may be at higher risk for TSS because of a lack of exposure to toxic shock syndrome toxin-1 (TSST-1) and, therefore, a lack of protective antibody or an inability by some persons to form adequate levels of antibodies to TSST-1 [75]. Christensson and Hedström described five cases of recurrent TSS in women who were never able to develop antibody to TSST-1 in acute or convalesscent sera [76].

The syndrome itself, characterized as noted earlier by fever, hypotension, dermal erythema followed by desquamation, and multiorgan failure, is mediated by the toxin, TSST-1, which acts as a super-antigen. TSST-1 binds to the variable region of the beta chain of the T-cell receptor. Through this binding it can activate massive and inappropriate T-cell responses and can directly induce production and release of multiple cytokines including interlekin-1 (IL-1), IL-2, tumor necrosis factor (TNF), and interferon-gamma (IFNγ) [68]. The consequences of this overwhelming and uncontrolled T-cell activation and cytokine release contribute significantly to the clinical characteristics of the syndrome.

D. Treatment and Prevention

Treatment of individuals with TSS consists of providing fluid resuscitation and blood pressure support as well as removing the source of toxin production, in most cases the tampon, and treating any localized *S. aureus* infections with appropriate anti-staphylococcal antibiotics. The rapid association of TSS with high-absorbency tampons and their removal from the market in the late 1970s and 1980s by observant clinicians is an epidemiology and public health success story.

VI. Suggestions for Further Investigations

- Does treating bacteriuria in pregnancy reduce fetal morbidity/mortality?
- Does increase in pH as a result of extrinsic factors contribute to the decline of lactobacilli and the development of BV, or are lactobacilli lost for other reasons and this loss causes an increase in pH, which subsequently contributes to the development of BV?
- Is BV truly a sexually transmitted infection?
- What effect does antibiotic use have on the epidemiology of BV?
- How, on the cellular level, does a fetus/infant, placenta, and/or pregnant woman respond to infection with listeria, and how does this differ from nonimmunocompromised hosts?
- Are there differences by race/ethnicity that make some women more susceptible to TSS?

References

1. Barnett BJ, Stephens DS. (1997). Urinary tract infection: an overview. *Am J Med Sci*. 314(4):245–249.
2. Mulholland SG. (1985). Female urinary tract infection. *Prim Care*. 12(4):661–673.
3. Andriole VT, Patterson TF. (1991). Epidemiology, natural history, and management of urinary tract infections in pregnancy. *Med Clin North Am*. 75(2):359–373.
4. Lipsky BA. (1989). Urinary tract infections in men. Epidemiology, pathophysiology, diagnosis, and treatment. *Ann Intern Med*. 110(2):138–150.
5. Kaye D. (1980). Urinary tract infections in the elderly. *Bull N Y Acad Med*. 56(2):209–220.
6. Ackermann RJ, Monroe PW. (1996), Bacteremic urinary tract infection in older people. *J Am Geriat Soc*. 44(8):927–933.
7. Beck-Sague C, Villarino E, Giuliano D, *et al*. (1994). Infectious diseases and death among nursing home residents: results of surveillance in 13 nursing homes. *Infect Control Hosp Epidemiol*. 15(7):494–496.

8. Hooton TM, Scholes D, Hughes JP, *et al.* (1996). A prospective study of risk factors for symptomatic urinary tract infection in young women. [see comments.] *N Engl J Med.* 335(7):468–474.

9. Foxman B, Frerichs RR. (1985). Epidemiology of urinary tract infection: I. Diaphragm use and sexual intercourse. *Am J Pub Health.* 75(11):1308–1313.

10. Burbige KA, Retik AB, Colodny AH, *et al.* (1984). Urinary tract infection in boys. *J Urol.* 132(3):541–542.

11. Sobel JD. (1997). Pathogenesis of urinary tract infection. Role of host defenses. *Infect Dis Clin North Am.* 11(3):531–549.

12. Meares EM Jr. (1987). Acute and chronic prostatitis: diagnosis and treatment. *Infect Dis Clin North Am.* 1(4):855–873.

13. Sabbaj J, Hoagland VL, Cook T. (1986). Norfloxacin versus co-trimoxazole in the treatment of recurring urinary tract infections in men. *Scand J Infect Dis Suppl.* 48:48–53.

14. Cunha BA. (1981). Urinary tract infections. 1. Pathophysiology and diagnostic approach. *Postgrad Med.* 70(6):141–145.

15. Johnson JR. (1991). Virulence factors in Escherichia coli urinary tract infection. *Clin Microbiol Rev.* 4(1):80–128.

16. Norden CW, Kass EH. (1968). Bacteriuria of pregnancy—a critical appraisal. *Annu Rev Med.* 19:431–470.

17. Kass EH. (1960). Bacteriuria and pyelonephritis in pregnancy. *Arch Intern Med.* 105:194.

18. McGregor JA, French JI. (2000). Bacterial vaginosis in pregnancy. *Obstet Gynecol Surv.* 55(5 Suppl 1):S1–19.

19. Eschenbach DA. (1983). Vaginal infection. *Clin Obstet Gynecol.* 1983. 26(1):186–202.

20. Eschenbach DA, Gravett MG, Chen KC, *et al.* (1984). Bacterial vaginosis during pregnancy. An association with prematurity and postpartum complications. *Scand J Urol Nephrol Suppl.* 86:213–222.

21. Gravett MG, Hummel D, Eschenbach DA, *et al.* (1968). Preterm labor associated with subclinical amniotic fluid infection and with bacterial vaginosis. *Obstet Gynecol.* 67(2):229–37.

22. McGregor JA, *et al.* (1990). Antenatal microbiologic and maternal risk factors associated with prematurity. [see comments.] *Am J Obstet Gynecol.* 163(5 Pt 1):1465–73.

23. Silver HM, Sperling RS, St Clair PJ, *et al.* (1989). Evidence relating bacterial vaginosis to intraamniotic infection. *Am J Obstet Gynecol.* 161(3):808–812.

24. Gardner HL, Dukes CD. (1955). Haemophilus vaginalis vaginitis. *Am J Obstet Gynecol.* 69:962–976.

25. Greenwood. (1980). Transfer of Haemophilus vaginalis Gardner and Dukes to a new genus Gardnerella: G. vaginalis (Gardner and Dukes) comb. *Int J Syst Bacteriol.* 30:170–178.

26. Spiegel CA, Amsel R, Eschenbach D, *et al.* (1980). Anaerobic bacteria in nonspecific vaginitis. *N Engl J Med.* 303(11):601–607.

27. Westrom. (1984). Taxonomy of vaginosis. In: *Bacterial vaginosis.* Mardh PA, ed. Almqvist and Wiksell: Stockholm. 259–260.

28. Embree J, Caliando JJ, McCormack WM. (1984). Nonspecific vaginitis among women attending a sexually transmitted diseases clinic. *Sex Transm Dis.* 11(2):81–84.

29. Barbone F, Austin H, Louv WC, *et al.* (1990). A follow-up study of methods of contraception, sexual activity, and rates of trichomoniasis, candidiasis, and bacterial vaginosis. *Am J Obstet Gynecol.* 163(2):510–514.

30. Bump RC, Buesching WJ 3rd. (1988). Bacterial vaginosis in virginal and sexually active adolescent females: evidence against exclusive sexual transmission. *Am J Obstet Gynecol.* 158(4):935–939.

31. Morales WJ, Schorr S, Albritton J. (1994). Effect of metronidazole in patients with preterm birth in preceding pregnancy and bacterial vaginosis: a placebo-controlled, double-blind study. *Am J Obstet Gynecol.* 171(2):345–347; discussion 348–349.

32. McGregor JA, French JI, Parker R, *et al.* (1995). Prevention of premature birth by screening and treatment for common genital tract infections: results of a prospective controlled evaluation. [see comments.] *Am J Obstet Gynecol.* 173(1):157–167.

33. Hauth JC, Goldenberg RL, Andrews WW, *et al.* (1995). Reduced incidence of preterm delivery with metronidazole and erythromycin in women with bacterial vaginosis. *N Engl J Med.* 333(26):1732–1736.

34. Hillier SL, Martius J, Krohn M, *et al.* (1988). A case-control study of chorioamnionic infection and histologic chorioamnionitis in prematurity. *N Engl J Med.* 319(15):972–978.

35. Gravett MG, Nelson HP, DeRouen T, *et al.* (1986). Independent associations of bacterial vaginosis and Chlamydia trachomatis infection with adverse pregnancy outcome. *JAMA.* 256(14):1899–1903.

36. Mardh PA. (1991). The vaginal ecosystem. *Am J Obstet Gynecol.* 165(4 Pt 2):1163–1168.

37. Giorgi A, Torriani S, Dellaglio F, *et al.* (1987). Identification of vaginal lactobacilli from asymptomatic women. *Microbiologica.* 10(4):377–384.

38. Redondo-Lopez V, Cook RL, Sobel JD. (1990). Emerging role of lactobacilli in the control and maintenance of the vaginal bacterial microflora. *Rev Infect Dis.* 12(5):856–872.

39. Mardh PA, Soltesz LV. (1983). *In vitro* interactions between lactobacilli and other microorganisms occurring in the vaginal flora. *Scand J Infect Dis Suppl.* 40:47–51.

40. Hillier SL, Krohn MA, Rabe LK, *et al.* (1993). The normal vaginal flora, H2O2-producing lactobacilli, and bacterial vaginosis in pregnant women. *Clin Infect Dis.* 16 Suppl 4:S273–281.

41. Thomason JL, Gelbart SM, Anderson RJ, *et al.* (1990). Statistical evaluation of diagnostic criteria for bacterial vaginosis. *Am J Obstet Gynecol.* 162(1):155–160.

42. Lorber B. (1997). Listeriosis. *Clin Infect Dis.* 24(1):1–9; quiz 10–1.

43. Schuchat A, Swaminathan B, Broome CV. (1991). Epidemiology of human listeriosis. [erratum appears in Clin Microbiol Rev. Jul;4(3):396]. *Clin Microbiol Rev.* 4(2):169–183.

44. Kampelmacher EH, Huysinga WT, van Noorle Jansen LM. (1972). The presence of Listeria monocytogenes in feces of pregnant women and neonates. *Zentralbl Bakteriol [Orig A].* 222(2):258–262.

45. Taege AJ. (1999). Listeriosis: recognizing it, treating it, preventing it. *Cleve Clin J Med.* 66(6):375–380.

46. Ciesielski CA, Hightower AW, Parsons SK, *et al.* (1988). Listeriosis in the United States: 1980–1982. *Arch Intern Med.* 148(6):1416–1419.

47. Gellin BG, Broome CV, Bibb WF, *et al.* (1991). The epidemiology of listeriosis in the United States—1986. Listeriosis Study Group. *Am J Epidemiol.* 133(4):392–401.

48. Southwick FS, Purich DL. (1996). Intracellular pathogenesis of listeriosis. *N Engl J Med.* 334(12):770–776.

49. Silver HM. (1998). Listeriosis during pregnancy. *Obstet Gynecol Surv.* 53(12):737–740.

50. Linnan MJ, Mascola L, Lou XD, *et al.* (1988). Epidemic listeriosis associated with Mexican-style cheese. *N Engl J Med.* 319(13):823–828.

51. Hayes PS, Graves LM, Ajello GW, *et al.* (1991). Comparison of cold enrichment and U.S. Department of Agriculture methods for isolating Listeria monocytogenes from naturally contaminated foods. The Listeria Study Group. *Appl Eviron Microbiol.* 57(8):2109–2113.

52. Weinberg ED. (1984). Pregnancy-associated depression of cell-mediated immunity. *Rev Infect Dis.* 6(6):814–831.

53. Falkoff R. (1987). Maternal immunologic changes during pregnancy: a critical appraisal. *Clin Rev Allergy.* 5(4):287–300.

54. Oppenheimer SJ. (2001). Iron and its relation to immunity and infectious disease. *J Nutr* 131(2S-2):616S–633S; discussion 633S–635S.

55. Sword CP. (1966). Mechanisms of pathogenesis in Listeria monocytogenes infection. I. Influence of iron. *J Bacteriol.* 92(3):536–542.

56. Ampel NM, Bejarano GC, Saavedra M Jr. (1992). Deferoxamine increases the susceptibility of beta-thalassemic, iron-overloaded mice to infection with Listeria monocytogenes. *Life Sci.* 50(18):1327–1332.

57. Nieman RE, Lorber B. (1980). Listeriosis in adults: a changing pattern. Report of eight cases and review of the literature, 1968–1978. *Rev Infect Dis.* 2(2):207–227.

58. Wenger JD, Hightower AW, Facklam RR, *et al.* (1990). Bacterial meningitis in the United States, 1986: report of a multistate surveillance study. The Bacterial Meningitis Study Group. *J Infect Dis.* 162(6):1316–1323.

59. Bortolussi R, McGregor DD, Kongshavn PA, *et al.* (1984). Host defense mechanisms to perinatal and neonatal Listeria monocytogenes infection. *Surv Synth Pathol Res.* 3(4):311–332.

60. McLauchlin J. (1990). Human listeriosis in Britain, 1967–85, a summary of 722 cases. 1. Listeriosis during pregnancy and in the newborn. *Epidemiol Infect.* 104(2):181–189.

61. Tappero JW, Schuchat A, Deaver KA, *et al.* (1995). Reduction in the incidence of human listeriosis in the United States. Effectiveness of prevention efforts? The Listeriosis Study Group. *JAMA.* 273(14):1118–1122.

62. Tauxe RV. (1998). New approaches to surveillance and control of emerging foodborne infectious diseases. *Emerg Infect Dis.* 4(3):455–456.

63. Yang S. (1998). FoodNet and Enter-net: emerging surveillance programs for foodborne diseases. *Emerg Infect Dis.* 4(3):457–458.

64. Broome CV. (1993). Listeriosis: Can we prevent it? *ASM News.* 444–446.

65. Todd J, Fishaut M, Kapral F, *et al.* (1978). Toxic-shock syndrome associated with phage-group-I Staphylococci. *Lancet.* 2(8100):1116–1168.

66. Davis JP, Chesney PJ, Wand PJ, *et al.* (1980). Toxic-shock syndrome: epidemiologic features, recurrence, risk factors, and prevention. *N Engl J Med.* 303(25):1429–1435.

67. Shands KN, Schmid GP, Dan BB, *et al.* (1980). Toxic-shock syndrome in menstruating women: association with tampon use and Staphylococcus aureus and clinical features in 52 cases. *N Engl J Med.* 303(25):1436–1442.

68. Chance TD. (1996). Toxic shock syndrome: role of the environment, the host and the microorganism. *Br J Biomed Sci.* 53(4):284–289.

69. Berkley SF, Hightower AW, Broome CV, *et al.* (1987). The relationship of tampon characteristics to menstrual toxic shock syndrome. *JAMA.* 258(7):917–920.

70. Lanes SF, Rothman KJ. (1990). Tampon absorbency, composition and oxygen content and risk of toxic shock syndrome. *J Clin Epidemiol.* 43(12):1379–1385.

71. Anon. (1990). Reduced incidence of menstrual toxic shock syndrome. *MMWR Morb Mortal Wkly Rep.* 39:421–423.

72. Anon. (1990). Reduced incidence of menstrual toxic-shock syndrome—United States, 1980–1990. *MMWR Morb Mortal Wkly Rep.* 39(25):421–423.

73. Friedrich EG Jr, Siegesmund KA. (1980). Tampon-associated vaginal ulcerations. *Obstet Gynecol.* 55(2):149–156.

74. Bell TA. (1982). Gonorrhea in female adolescents: potential analogies to toxic shock syndrome. *Ann Intern Med.* 96(6 Pt 2):924–925.

75. Todd JK. (1988). Toxic shock syndrome. *Clin Microbiol Rev.* 1(4):432–446.

76. Christensson B, Hedstrom SA. (1985). Serological response to toxic shock syndrome toxin in Staphylococcus aureus infected patients and healthy controls. *Acta Pathol Microbiol Immunol Scand [B].* 93(2):87–90.

84

Gender-Specific Issues in Fungal Infections

NIGAR KIRMANI, MD AND WILLIAM G. POWDERLY, MD

Division of Infectious Diseases, Department of Medicine, Washington University School of Medicine, St. Louis, MO

I. Introduction

Fungi are eukaryotic organisms that inhabit water, soil, or decaying organic matter. There are more than 50,000 species, of which less than 300 cause human disease. Systemic infection occurs only with a handful; the rest cause cutaneous and subcutaneous disease. Fungi grow as yeast (unicellular) or filamentous (mold) forms. The fungal filamentous colony (mycelium) is made up of branching, threadlike filaments (hyphae). Hyphae are either septate or without cross walls, features that are useful in diagnosis. Yeasts are unicellular with a rigid cell wall that divides by budding, although some species divide by binary fission. Many pathogenic fungi are dimorphic (e.g., *Coccidioides immitis*, *Blastomyces dermatitidis*, *Histoplasma capsulatum*), which means they can grow either as yeasts or molds, depending on conditions such as pH, carbon dioxide or glucose concentration, and temperature. The transition frequently occurs when a free-living organism becomes a parasite (e.g., the mold form is found in the environment and the yeast form develops at human body temperature).

This chapter will describe the common systemic mycoses, both opportunistic and endemic. Most fungal infections do not differ in their epidemiology, pathogenesis, or clinical manifestations between men and women. However, there are some relevant gender-specific issues, such as genital tract infection, the effect of pregnancy on some fungal infections, and the use of antifungal agents in special situations, that will be highlighted.

II. Opportunistic Fungi

Opportunistic fungi are less pathogenic fungi that cause disease when host resistance is diminished. They may be part of the endogenous flora or inhaled from the environment.

Patients at high risk for opportunistic fungal infections include those with organ or bone marrow transplants, malignancies, human immunodeficiency virus (HIV) infection, burns, trauma, or long-term use of intravenous catheters and broad-spectrum antibiotics. The most important host defect that affects response to these fungi is neutropenia; cure is extremely difficult without functioning white cells. Some features of the major opportunistic fungi are summarized in Table 84-1.

A. Cryptococcosis

Cryptococcus neoformans is an encapsulated yeast found on rotted fruits and vegetables and in the excreta of birds, particularly pigeons. Infection is acquired by inhalation; symptomatic infection is rare except in individuals with impaired immunity. Prior to the AIDS epidemic, the overall incidence was 0.8 cases per million persons per year [1]. Early in the epidemic about 5% of patients infected with HIV in the Western World developed disseminated cryptococcosis; the disease is more prevalent in sub-Saharan Africa and Southern Asia. Most cases of infection are seen at very low CD4 lymphocyte counts (<50 cells/mm^3). Recent data suggest cryptococcosis is less common, occurring in 2–3% of patients [2]. Improved antiretroviral therapy has led to a decline in the incidence and has led to more frequent use of azole antifungals.

The response to the initial pulmonary infection is granulomatous inflammation, followed by clearance of infection and latency in immunocompetent hosts. Most primary infections are asymptomatic. In immunocompromised hosts, acute infection with or without disseminated cryptococcosis develops. There is a special tropism for the central nervous system (CNS); the reasons for this are unclear.

Table 84-1
Common Opportunistic Fungi

Disease	Fungus	Predisposing Factors	Route of Entry	Organ Involvement	Diagnosis
Cryptococcosis	*Cryptococcus neoformans*	Immunosuppression, HIV	Inhalation	Lung, central nervous system, blood, skin, bone	Antigen in cerebrospinal fluid and serum, culture
Candidiasis	*Candida albicans*, Non-albicans species	Immunosuppression, broad-spectrum antibiotics, foreign bodies	Endogenous in gastrointestinal tract	Mucosal (oral, vaginal), blood, liver, spleen, kidney, other organs	Culture
Aspergillosis	*Aspergillus fumigatus*	Immunosuppression, neutropenia	Inhalation	Lungs, central nervous system, sinuses, invasion of other organs	Culture, biopsy
Zygomycosis	Mucor	Diabetes, burns, immunosuppression	Inhalation, cutaneous exposure	Blood vessels, noses, sinuses, eye, central nervous system, lungs	Culture, biopsy

The most common presentation is subacute meningitis or meningoencephalitis. Fever, malaise, headache, lethargy, altered mental status, and memory loss are common symptoms; neck stiffness and photophobia are seen in only one-third of patients [3]. Pulmonary involvement occurs in about 50% of patients [4]. Disseminated cryptococcosis with skin, prostate, or eye involvement is more frequent in patients with HIV [5]. Infection of any organ can occur, including bone and joint involvement and peritonitis [6].

Analysis of the cerebrospinal fluid (CSF) shows a few lymphocytes, slightly low glucose, and elevated protein. The CSF opening pressure is elevated, is of prognostic significance, and should always be measured. India ink examination of CSF outlines the polysaccharide capsule and is positive in 80% of patients with AIDS and 50% of non-AIDS patients with meningitis [7]. The organism can be isolated on most routine fungal media. Detection of cryptococcal polysaccharide antigen by latex agglutination in the serum is highly sensitive and specific (>90%) and has been used as a screening test in febrile HIV-positive patients. A positive antigen titer warrants antifungal therapy [8]. The chest x-ray may show pulmonary infiltrates, nodules, or lymphadenopathy.

Untreated, cryptococcal meningitis is fatal. The best outcome in patients with HIV is with amphotericin B (0.7 mg/kg) for 2 weeks, followed by fluconazole 400 mg orally for 8 weeks [9]. This regimen reduces mortality to <10%, with sterilization of cultures in 70% of patients. The addition of 5-flucytosine (5-FC) 100 mg/kg/day to amphotericin may decrease risk of relapse. Initial therapy with fluconazole is associated with a 50% response rate. Sterilization of CSF takes longer with azole therapy [10]. Lipid preparations of amphotericin do not show superior efficacy but are associated with less toxicity [11]. Reduction of intracranial pressure by repeated lumbar puncture, lumbar drain, or shunt should be considered if the opening CSF pressure is >25 cm of water [12].

Relapse rates in AIDS patients with cryptococcal meningitis are 50–60% when antifungal therapy is discontinued. Lifelong suppressive therapy with fluconazole 200 mg daily should be initiated after completion of initial therapy, although it is possible to discontinue antifungal therapy in patients whose immune function is restored with antiretroviral therapy [13]. There are no guidelines for suppressive therapy in patients without HIV infection, although fluconazole 200 mg daily is usually given for 6–12 months to cover the 10–15% possibility of relapse within the first year.

B. Candidiasis

Candida species are normal flora of the human gastrointestinal (GI) tract and are isolated from the oral cavity of up to 50% of healthy individuals. The majority (70–80%) are *Candida albicans*, followed by *C. glabrata* and *C. tropicalis* [14]. Colonization of the GI tract increases in patients taking a broad spectrum of antibiotics, corticosteroids, and other immunosuppressive therapy, and in those with diabetes and HIV infection. In addition, local trauma (dentures, mucositis, radiation), neutropenia, debilitation, and extremes of age and malignancy (acute leukemia, bone marrow transplantation) predispose patients to increased frequency and severity of Candida infections [15]. Mucosal and skin infections can occur in normal hosts (vaginitis, diaper rash), whereas oropharyngeal candidiasis and invasive infection are seen in patients with impaired immunity.

1. Oropharyngeal Candidiasis

Colonization with Candida leads to symptomatic infection in patients predisposed by debility or depressed immunity. Clinical manifestations range from none to oral discomfort, burning tongue, or dysphagia, especially in patients with HIV. The classic presentation is of creamy white plaques on an erythematous base that can be wiped off with a tongue blade. Denture stomatitis can occur in up to 60% of patients with dentures and presents with erythema and edema of the palate at the point of contact [16]. Other oral manifestations where Candida may be a colonizer or invader are angular cheilitis and chronic oral leukoplakia [17]. Microscopic examination with 10% potassium hydroxide establishes the diagnosis; cultures are not essential.

The presence of dysphagia, odynophagia, or retrosternal pain should raise suspicion for esophageal involvement. The combination of oral candidiasis and these symptoms is a specific and sensitive predictor of esophageal involvement in patients with AIDS [18]. Esophageal candidiasis occurs more frequently in women infected with HIV. White plaques, hyperemia and friability of the mucosa, and ulceration are seen on endoscopy, which is the diagnostic method of choice because it can differentiate between the various causes of esophagitis [19]. Patients with HIV can be treated empirically, and endoscopy should be reserved for those who fail to respond [20].

The azole antifungals are the treatment of choice for oropharyngeal candidiasis, and 80% of patients with uncomplicated disease respond to treatment. Clotrimazole troches can be used for mild disease; moderate or severe disease requires systemic therapy [21]. Fluconazole (50–100 mg) and itraconazole suspension (100–200 mg) are equivalent in acute treatment, whereas ketoconazole therapy is rarely used because of hepatotoxicity. Oral or intravenous fluconazole or itraconazole is used for esophagitis [22]. Intravenous amphotericin B can be used in patients with severe disease or those refractory to treatment with the azoles. The new echinocandin caspofungin may be an alternative option. In some patients with advanced HIV infection and frequent recurrences of oropharyngeal candidiasis secondary prophylaxis may be warranted. Daily, thrice weekly, or weekly fluconazole are effective in decreasing recurrences in these patients [23]. This has led to emergence of resistance in *Candida albicans* and also to the emergence of non-albicans Candida species (*C. glabrata, C. dublinensis, C parapsilosis, C. krusei*) that are inherently less susceptible to the azoles [24]. Management of these patients is more difficult and involves introduction of more effective antiretroviral therapy. Higher doses of fluconazole (up to 800 mg), itraconazole suspension, and oral suspensions of amphotericin B have had moderate success [25]. Intravenous amphotericin B or caspofungin are alternative options.

2. Vulvovaginal Candidiasis

Candida species are part of the lower genital tract flora of 10–20% of asymptomatic, healthy women. It is estimated that

75% of women of childbearing age will develop an episode of vulvovaginal candidiasis (VVC), and 50% of those will have a recurrence [26]. Candida is the second most common cause of vulvovaginitis, after bacterial vaginosis. Virulence factors that enhance colonization of the vagina and facilitate tissue invasion are listed in Table 84-2.

The incidence of VVC increases with pregnancy, contraceptive use, diabetes, use of broad-spectrum antibiotics, and HIV infection (CD4 counts <200 cells/mm^3). Estrogen therapy and pregnancy enhance germination (yeast to mycelial transformation) and adherence of Candida to vaginal epithelial cells. Lactobacilli in normal vaginal flora resist colonization and prevent germination of Candida; suppression by broad-spectrum antibiotics increases both colonization and symptomatic vaginitis [30]. Uncontrolled diabetes also precipitates VVC. Other factors that may predispose to VVC are wearing tightly fitted clothing, eating diets high in sugar, using intrauterine devices, and having reduced cell-mediated immunity [31]. Table 84-3 lists some of the predisposing factors for VVC. More than 90% of VVC is caused by *Candida albicans*, even in patients with recurrent VVC. Except in patients with advanced HIV infection, the majority of patients with recurrent VVC have azole-susceptible strains of *Candida albicans*. Non-albicans species produce similar clinical manifestations; however, they are more resistant to treatment.

The most frequent symptom is vulvar and/or vaginal pruritus. Vulvar pain, dyspareunia, and dysuria are slightly less common. A thick, curdlike vaginal discharge, erythema and edema of the labia and vulva, and white plaques adherent to the vaginal

Table 84-2
Virulence Factors in Vulvovaginal Candidiasis

- *Candida albicans* adheres to vaginal cells in higher number than *C. tropicalis* and *C. krusei* [27].
- Nongerminating mutants of *C. albicans* are incapable of inducing experimental vulvovaginal candidiasis [28].
- A proteinase enzyme with the ability to cause disease is present in higher amounts in symptomatic women than in asymptomatic women [29].
- Erythrocyte-binding surface receptors facilitate binding of iron and enhance virulence.

Table 84-3
Predisposing Factors for Vulvovaginal Candidiasis

Definite	Probable
• Age—rare before menarche	• Sexual activity—increased incidence of vulvovaginal candidiasis
• Pregnancy—third trimester	
• Contraceptives—increased vaginal colonization	• Tight, poorly ventilated clothing
• Diabetes mellitus	
• Broad-spectrum antibiotics—eliminate protective flora	

mucosa are generally seen. In some patients, there is minimal discharge but severe pruritus and erythema. A transient rash, erythema, and pruritus of the penis can be seen in 20% of male partners of women with recurrent VVC [32].

Clinical signs and symptoms are not specific enough to make an etiologic diagnosis of vaginitis. A wet-mount examination of vaginal secretions should be performed to look for presence of yeast, "clue" cells, or motile trichomonads. However, approximately 50% of women who are culture positive will be negative on microscopy [33]. The addition of 10% potassium hydroxide increases sensitivity of microscopy to 60–70%. The Pap smear is not reliable for diagnosis (only 25% of cases are positive). Vaginal culture should be performed when microscopy is negative and clinical suspicion is high. Measuring the vaginal pH helps distinguish Candida vaginitis (pH less than 4.5) from bacterial vaginosis and trichomonas vaginitis, in which the pH is >4.5.

Topical antifungal agents are the mainstay of treatment. Topical azoles achieve an 85–90% cure rate (symptomatic and mycologic cure), which is better than the 75–80% cure with topical nystatin preparations [34]. Except for some burning with initial application, there are no side effects of topical treatment. Shorter courses of topical therapy (3-day or even single-dose regimens) are effective in mild to moderate disease. Oral azoles (itraconazole 200 mg bid×1 day or fluconazole 150 mg×1 dose) are effective but not superior to topical therapy, although many women prefer oral therapy. Adverse effects and drug interactions are a concern with systemic therapy. Complicated VVC (severe infection in abnormal host, non-albicans Candida species) requires longer duration of therapy (at least 7 days) [35]. Most topical agents are effective in pregnancy, although response is slower and recurrences are more frequent [36]. Prolonged duration (1–2 weeks) of therapy is often required. Oral azoles are **contraindicated** in pregnancy.

Recurrent VVC (four or more attacks per year) is an extremely troublesome problem in some women. Persistence of a few organisms after treatment is common, with relapses occurring as a result of breakdown of local protective immunity in the vagina [37]. A predisposing factor is rarely identified. Antifungal resistance is rarely a cause of recurrent VVC. Chronic suppressive therapy with fluconazole 100 mg orally or clotrimazole 500 mg suppositories is effective, but symptoms return in 50% of women when treatment is discontinued [35]. For refractory or azole-resistant infection, topical boric acid (600 mg intravaginally daily for 2 weeks) has been used successfully in some cases [38].

3. Invasive Candidiasis

The incidence of nosocomial fungal infection has risen in the past two decades. Candida is now the fourth leading cause of bloodstream infections, accounting for 8% of such infections [39]. The proportion of infections resulting from non-albicans Candida has also increased dramatically, accounting for 48% of all episodes of candidemia. The increased frequency of candidemia can be attributed to increasing immunosuppression, prolonged hospital stay, broad-spectrum antibiotic therapy, and invasive procedures and devices. Patients at high risk for developing invasive candidiasis are neonates, patients who have undergone burns and bone marrow transplantation or abdominal surgery, those receiving parenteral nutrition, cancer patients with neutropenia, and transplant recipients [40]. Non-albicans species, including *C. krusei* and *C. parapsilosis*, have emerged in patients receiving fluconazole prophylaxis. Candidemia caused by *C. parapsilosis* is generally catheter-related or associated with intravenous drug abuse [41].

Candidemia may result in seeding of the eye, bone, kidney, meninges, heart valves, or joints. Candida peritonitis occurs in association with peritoneal dialysis catheters or bowel perforation. Endophthalmitis from retinal seeding can lead to blindness; a careful ophthalmologic examination is mandatory in patients with candidemia [42]. Candida endocarditis is characterized by large vegetations and a high risk of embolization, necessitating surgery in addition to antifungal therapy. Hepatosplenic candidiasis with multiple abscesses is seen in immunocompromised patients recovering from neutropenia, and it may be difficult to treat. Fluconazole or the lipid-based preparations of amphotericin B are used for treatment.

Mortality rates from candidemia range from 50–80%, and attributable mortality is as high as 38% [43]. Treatment is recommended for **all cases of candidemia**. Removal of infected devices is necessary but usually is insufficient to clear fungemia. Fungemia with *C. albicans* in non-neutropenic patients can be treated with amphotericin B (0.5–0.6 mg/kg/day) or fluconazole (400 mg/day) [44]. For non-albicans species, higher fluconazole doses (800 mg/day) or amphotericin B (0.7–1.0 mg/kg/day) is used. Prior to identification of species, amphotericin B should be started empirically in all patients in whom yeast is isolated from blood cultures. Isolation of *C. lusitaniae* warrants a switch to fluconazole because this organism demonstrates innate resistance to amphotericin B. Flucytosine has been added to amphotericin B in patients with endophthalmitis, CNS infection, or persistent fungemia. Lipid-based preparations of amphotericin are less nephrotoxic but do not demonstrate superior efficacy. Caspofungin has excellent activity against Candida species and has been shown to be as effective as amphotericin for invasive candidiasis [45].

C. Aspergillosis

Aspergillus species are among the most common molds in the environment, found in decomposing vegetable matter and potted plants, including marijuana. There are more than 180 species, of which only a few cause human disease. The infective form is the conidia, which are aerosolized and inhaled. In tissues, filamentous forms invade blood vessels and cause local tissue destruction and hematogenous spread. *Aspergillus fumigatus* is the most frequent pathogen and causes 90% of invasive infections. It has small conidia (2–3 µm), which are more likely to bypass entrapment by local respiratory defenses [46]. Conidia are ingested and killed by pulmonary macrophages. Hyphae are damaged and sometimes killed extracellularly by neutrophils. Both these killing functions are impaired by corticosteroids. In immunosuppressed patients, vascular invasion with necrosis and hemorrhage is seen in tissues, along with abundant hyphal elements. *Aspergillus flavus* has been implicated in sinusitis, *A. niger* has been implicated in otomycosis, and *A. nidulans* causes infection in patients with chronic granulomatous disease [47].

A wide variety of clinical disease is seen, ranging from allergic to invasive aspergillosis [48]. Hypersensitivity to aspergillus antigens manifesting as worsening asthma, pulmonary infiltrates, eosinophilia, and precipitating immunoglobulin G (IgG) and IgE antibodies is the hallmark of allergic bronchopulmonary aspergillosis. Corticosteroids are required to control the inflammatory response. A randomized trial in 2000 demonstrated improvement in pulmonary function with the addition of itraconazole, 200–400 mg/day given over 16–32 weeks [49].

Aspergilloma, or fungus ball, can develop in any preexisting cavity and consists of a mass of hyphae protected within fibrin and cellular debris. Cough, hemoptysis, wheezing, and weight loss can occur. Up to 10% of aspergillomas may resolve spontaneously. Surgical resection, embolization in nonoperable patients, and intracavitary amphotericin are therapeutic options; however, aspergillomas are often difficult to treat [50]. Fungus balls can also appear in normal lungs; these represent a progressive infection—semi-invasive or chronic necrotizing aspergillosis. Patients at risk have diabetes and chronic obstructive pulmonary disease. Unlike aspergilloma, this condition requires antifungal therapy, generally with itraconazole [51]. Otomycosis with *A. niger* is seen in patients with chronic otitis externa. Topical amphotericin B (3%), flucytosine (10%), clotrimazole, or econazole is used for treatment.

Sinusitis with aspergillus can be allergic or invasive. In immunocompetent hosts, an allergic inflammatory response leads to edema and obstruction without fungal invasion of bone. Drainage, nasal corticosteroids, and saline douches are the treatment [52]. Invasive sinusitis occurs in immunocompromised hosts, especially those with neutropenia and bone marrow transplantation. Fever, cough, epistaxis, or headache may be presenting symptoms. Hyphae can invade mucosa and bone, leading to infarction and spread to the orbit or brain. Computed tomography (CT) scans or magnetic resonance imaging (MRI), along with biopsy and culture, are essential to identify the causative organisms. Surgical debridement and resection of necrotic tissue, along with systemic antifungal therapy with amphotericin B and withdrawal of immunosuppression, are essentials of treatment. Despite aggressive measures, mortality remains high, ranging from 20–100%, depending on the underlying disease [53].

Tracheobronchitis resulting from aspergillus occurs more frequently in patients with HIV and lung transplant recipients. Manifestations range from obstructive bronchial involvement with large mucoid aspergillus-containing casts to ulcerative or pseudomembranous tracheobronchitis. Cough, fever, hemoptysis, and wheezing or stridor can occur. Bronchoscopy with bronchial biopsy, microscopy, and culture is essential for diagnosis. Systemic antifungal therapy with amphotericin B is necessary [54].

Invasive aspergillosis has increased in the past three decades as the number of patients undergoing organ or bone marrow transplantation, intensified chemotherapy regimens, and HIV infection has increased. Neutropenia and graft vs host disease are risk factors [55]. Most patients (80–90%) have pulmonary disease. Presenting features are respiratory symptoms (cough, chest pain, hemoptysis, pleural rub) in 50% of cases, fever in 32%, and neurologic symptoms (seizures, hemiparesis, stupor) in 27% [56]. About 20% of patients may be asymptomatic in the first several days of infection. Consolidation with cavitation; nodular lesions; wedge-shaped, pleural based lesions; and diffuse infiltrates may be seen on radiographs and CT scans. Nodules surrounded by low attenuation (the "halo" sign) or cavitation ("air-crescent" sign) are distinctive for invasive fungal disease and represent lung tissue full of hyphae beyond the area of infarction. A CT scan or MRI of the brain should be performed to rule out cerebral aspergillosis. Diagnosis requires demonstration of septate hyphae in lung tissue along with positive respiratory culture for aspergillus or a positive culture from a sterile site. A positive respiratory tract culture in a high-risk patient is predictive of disease [57]. Studies of circulating markers of infection (ELISA [enzyme-linked immunosorbent assay], PCR [polymerase chain reaction]) are under way and look promising [58]. Above all, the diagnosis rests on a very high index of suspicion and prompt work-up of patients at high risk for invasive aspergillosis.

Therapy requires the initiation of systemic antifungal agents and withdrawal of immunosuppression. High-dose amphotericin B (1.0–1.5 mg/kg/day) has been the mainstay of treatment. The lipid-based formulations of amphotericin B are useful in patients at risk for nephrotoxicity. Itraconazole is acceptable alternative therapy but requires careful attention to problems with absorption and potential drug interactions. It can be used to switch to oral therapy after an initial course of amphotericin B. There are two new and exciting developments in treatment of aspergillus infection. Caspofungin, a new echinocandin, has been approved as a salvage agent for failure of therapy or drug toxicities. Voriconazole, a new triazole, has been approved for use as a first-line agent, based on a randomized trial showing superior efficacy compared to amphotericin B [59]. The possibility of using combination therapy (e.g., amphotericin B and echinocandins or echinocandins plus voriconazole) has generated much interest and should become clearer in the future. The most important factor influencing response to treatment, however, is recovery of host immunity.

D. Mucormycosis (Zygomycosis)

Zygomycetes include two different orders, the Mucorales and Entomophthorales, which cause distinct diseases. Mucorales are ubiquitous fungi that grow on decaying matter. However, human disease is rare in immunocompetent hosts. Risk factors for developing mucormycosis include diabetes, ketoacidosis, corticosteroid therapy, neutropenia, organ transplantation, malnourishment, deferoxamine therapy, intravenous drug use, and traumatic inoculation [60]. Infection is generally acquired by inhalation of spores, although direct inoculation into abraded skin can result in primary cutaneous mucormycosis. Spores germinate into hyphae, which cause local invasion and grow through blood vessel walls, leading to thrombosis and tissue necrosis. Neutrophils are important in host defense, along with macrophages that ingest spores and inhibit their germination. Acidosis can affect phagocytic and chemotactic functions of neutrophils. The importance of iron, which is used by the fungus to enhance its growth, is emphasized by the development of rapidly fatal cases of mucormycosis in patients receiving deferoxamine therapy [61].

The anatomic site involved determines the clinical manifestations of mucormycosis. The most common site is rhinocerebral (50%), followed by pulmonary (10%), cutaneous (10%), and gastrointestinal (2%). Rhinocerebral mucormycosis is seen most frequently in patients with diabetic ketoacidosis, immunosuppression, neutropenia, and organ transplantation. Facial pain, headache, fever, malaise, nasal congestion, and bloody rhinorrhea may be presenting symptoms. Invasion of the orbit leads to periorbital swelling and numbness, blurred vision, chemosis, diplopia, proptosis, and loss of vision from the thrombosis of the retinal artery. Extension into the brain can occur via the optic nerve or cavernous sinus, with ophthalmoplegia and ptosis, and is a poor prognostic sign. A CT scan or MRI can best define the extent of infection and may show fluid in the sinuses, abnormalities of soft tissues, and destruction of bone [62].

Pulmonary mucormycosis is seen in patients with neutropenia, bone marrow transplantation, and prolonged corticosteroid therapy. Fever, dyspnea, and cough are presenting symptoms, followed by hemoptysis. Consolidation with cavitation, nodular infiltrates, or pulmonary infarction can occur, with invasion into pericardium, chest wall. or mediastinal blood vessels [63].

Cutaneous mucormycosis occurs secondary to direct inoculation (an outbreak caused by contaminated elastic bandages occurred in the 1970s) or by dissemination from a site of primary infection. Contamination of devitalized tissues or burns has been described [64]. Gastrointestinal mucormycosis involving the stomach, ileum, or colon has been described in patients with extreme malnutrition [65]. It is often fatal, but fortunately it is rare. CNS disease occurs by extension from the sinuses or after open head trauma. Disseminated mucormycosis is associated with a very high mortality and is seen in severely immunocompromised patients [66].

A high index of suspicion in a host at risk for mucormycosis is essential for early diagnosis. A black eschar or black nasal discharge, altered mental status, diplopia, or vision loss in a susceptible host should prompt aggressive diagnostic evaluation with radiography and biopsy of any suspicious lesion. Demonstration of the organism in tissue, along with culture from specimens, is required. Fungi appear as broad (10–20 μm diameter), nonseptate hyphae that branch at right angles. Distinguishing characteristics from aspergillus and Candida are listed in Table 84-4.

Successful therapy requires the early initiation of antifungal agents, surgical debridement, and reversal of the underlying disease. This includes rapid correction of hyperglycemia and acidosis and discontinuation of corticosteroids and other immunosuppressives, at least temporarily. Amphotericin B is the standard treatment; higher than usual doses are needed because the fungus is relatively resistant. A dose of 1–1.5 mg/kg/day is used with a

Table 84-4
Characteristics of Mucor, Aspergillus, and Candida in Tissue

Features	Mucormycosis	Aspergillus	Candida
Fungal elements	Hyphae	Hyphae	Pseudohyphae
Width	Broad (15–20 μm)	Narrow (4–5 μm)	Narrow (2–3 μm)
Septations	Aseptate	Septate	Septate
Branching	90° angle	45° angle	

(Modified from Gonzalez CE, Rinaldi MG, Sugar AM. [2002]. Zygomycosis. *Infect Dis Clin N Am.* 16:895–914.)

total dose of 2 g or higher. Lipid formulations of amphotericin B have been used successfully and are associated with less nephrotoxicity; doses up to 10 mg/kg/day have been used [67]. The addition of flucytosine or rifampin to amphotericin B is not recommended. None of the available azoles have activity against mucormycosis, although the investigational azole, posaconazole, shows promise in early studies.

Aggressive surgical debridement of necrotic tissue is essential. Survival of patients with medical therapy alone is much worse than patients treated with the combined medical and surgical approach [68]. Early diagnosis and treatment has decreased the overall mortality of 50%; recently, survival rates up to 85% have been reported [69].

III. Endemic Mycoses

Endemic mycoses can be acquired by immunocompetent hosts during travel to, or residence in, distinct geographic locations where these fungi are distributed. Histoplasmosis, coccidioidomycosis, and blastomycosis are fungi endemic to various locations in the United States.

A. Histoplasmosis

Histoplasma capsulatum is the most common endemic mycosis in the United States, found in the Midwest and Southeast, especially along the Mississippi and Ohio River valleys. It has emerged as an opportunistic pathogen among patients with HIV living in these areas. Mycelial forms are found in the soil and are particularly associated with bird roosts, chicken coops, and bats. Construction, excavation, and spelunking have been associated with exposure and infection [70]. The disease is more common in men. Histoplasma is a dimorphic fungus (i.e., it grows as mycelia at ambient temperature and as yeast at 37°C); the transition is a critical step in infectivity of the fungus [71]. In tissue, yeast cells are found within macrophages, where they are protected from the host immune response. Caseating or noncaseating granulomas develop, in which calcium is deposited. Yeast cells may remain viable within calcified lesions for years and can reactivate when immunity wanes [72].

More than 90% of primary infections are asymptomatic. Symptomatic infection follows inhalation of a heavy inoculum, resulting in three different forms of illness—acute, chronic, and disseminated. Acute pulmonary histoplasmosis presents as a flulike illness with cough, pleuritic chest pain, fever, and fatigue, occurring 1–3 weeks after exposure. Arthralgias, erythema nodosum, and pericarditis can occur. Diffuse reticulonodular infiltrates and mediastinal lymphadenopathy are seen on radiographs. Most individuals recover without treatment [73]. Some patients develop an exuberant granulomatous or fibrotic response to histoplasma antigens, leading to mediastinal fibrosis with obstruction. Chronic (or cavitary) pulmonary histoplasmosis usually develops in patients with underlying lung disease. Cavitary upper lobe lesions are found in 90% of cases. Symptoms include fever, productive cough, hemoptysis, dyspnea, and weight loss [74].

Progressive disseminated histoplasmosis (PDH) is unusual, except in immunocompromised hosts or at the extremes of age. Acute PDH is seen in infants and patients with HIV or hematologic malignancies. Fever, cough, dyspnea, and malaise are presenting symptoms. Hepatosplenomegaly, lymphadenopathy, oropharyngeal and skin ulcers, gastrointestinal ulcers, and meningitis can occur. The CD4 count is less than 200 cells/mm^3 in patients with HIV. The mortality is 100% if untreated [75]. Subacute and chronic PDH present with weight loss, fatigue, oropharyngeal ulcers, and hepatosplenomegaly and are distinguished from acute PDH by the chronicity of the symptoms. Adrenal involvement, chronic meningitis, cerebral mass, endocarditis, or GI involvement may also be seen [76].

Definitive diagnosis of histoplasmosis requires culturing the fungus from clinical specimens. *Histoplasma capsulatum* requires several weeks to grow, although nucleic acid probes shorten the time to species identification. Cultures are positive in 85% of patients with disseminated infections. Bone marrow (75%); blood (50–70%); alveolar lavage (70%); or biopsy of lung, mouth, skin, or GI lesions (25%) are the most useful sites [77]. Histopathologic examination with silver stains is a useful adjunct. Peripheral blood smears may show intracellular yeasts in 30–45% of patients with acute PDH. Detection of polysaccharide antigen in the urine or serum can establish the diagnosis rapidly. Urine antigen can be detected in 90% of patients with PDH, 40% with cavitary disease, and 20% with acute pulmonary histoplasmosis [78]. It is also useful in monitoring response to therapy because an increasing antigen level predicts relapse. Serologic assays, such as immunodiffusion (ID) and complement fixation (CF), are also useful. The CF test is more sensitive but less specific than ID. It is positive 2–6 weeks after infection; a single titer ≥1:32, or a fourfold increase in titer is highly suggestive of active infection. Two major precipitin bands can be detected by ID. The H band is specific for acute disease, but it is positive in only 10% of cases. The M band can be detected in 80% of individuals after exposure to the fungus but can persist for many months after initial infection. Serologic assays are negative in 50% of immunosuppressed patients, especially those with HIV [79].

Antifungal therapy consists of amphotericin B or the azoles itraconazole or ketoconazole. Itraconazole is preferred because of fewer problems with side effects and drug interactions. Fluconazole is only moderately effective and more likely to be associated with relapse, and it should be avoided in immunosuppressed patients.

Acute pulmonary histoplasmosis is self-limited and does not require antifungal therapy. If the illness is prolonged for 3–4 weeks, or there are diffuse pulmonary infiltrates with hypoxia, itraconazole 200 mg once daily should be given for 6–12 weeks. Hospitalized patients may be treated initially with amphotericin B for 7–14 days prior to switching to itraconazole. Pericarditis is treated with antiinflammatory therapy. Granulomatous mediastinitis with severe obstructive complications should be treated with amphotericin B (0.7–1.0 mg/kg/day) followed by a switch to itraconazole for 6–12 months. Fibrosing mediastinitis is difficult to treat; a trial of itraconazole for 3 months is reasonable [80].

Chronic pulmonary histoplasmosis is a progressive illness and should be treated with itraconazole 200 mg once or twice daily for 12–24 months. Amphotericin B (0.7 mg/kg/day) should be used for severely ill hospitalized patients or for those who fail or are intolerant to itraconazole. Fluconazole is less effective than either itraconazole or amphotericin; if intolerance necessitates its use, the dose given should be 400–800 mg/day [81].

Patients with acute PDH should be treated with amphotericin B 0.7–1.0 mg/kg/day emergently. Once the patient responds, itraconazole 200 mg once or twice daily can be given for 6–18 months to patients who do not have HIV infection. If amphotericin B is used for the entire course, a total dose of 35 mg/kg should be given over 2–4 months. For patients with less severe disease, itraconazole for 6–18 months can be given [82].

Treatment of acute PDH in patients with HIV is given in two phases—induction and maintenance. Amphotericin B is the treatment of choice for hospitalized patients and those with meningeal involvements and is given for 12 weeks. For patients with mild to moderate symptoms, itraconazole 200 mg three times daily for 3 days is followed by 200 mg twice daily for 12 weeks. All patients should be placed on maintenance therapy for life to prevent relapse of infection. Itraconazole 200 mg once or twice daily is the suppressive therapy of choice [83].

Patients with CNS histoplasmosis should be treated with amphotericin B. Unfortunately, the mortality is 20–40% even with treatment and 50% of patients relapse within 2 years. Amphotericin B (0.7–1.0 mg/kg/day) to complete a 35 mg/kg total dose over 3–4 months should be given, followed by fluconazole 800 mg daily for 12 months. Itraconazole does not enter the CSF fluid in high concentrations, although the role of CSF drug concentrations in the outcome of fungal meningitis is unclear [84].

B. Coccidioidomycosis

Coccidioides immitis is a dimorphic fungus that is endemic to the soil of the southwestern United States, Mexico, and parts of Central and South America. An increase in migration and travel to endemic areas has led to increased numbers of cases in the past few decades, with 100,000 infections estimated annually [85]. Infection is acquired by inhalation of arthroconidia, although rare cases of cutaneous inoculation have been reported. Windstorms, dust clouds and excavation, and other outdoor activities have been associated with accompanying infection. In the lungs, arthroconidia transform into spherules, which may be large (up to 75 μm diameter) and are associated with acute inflammation with neutrophils and eosinophils, followed by granulomatous lesions with lymphocytes and multinucleated giant cells. Control of infection depends on T lymphocytes; patients who are T-cell deficient develop severe infection [86].

Most infections (50–60%) are asymptomatic or mild. Approximately 40% of patients develop fever, cough, chest pain, fatigue, shortness of breath, weight loss, headache, and migratory arthralgias 1–3 weeks after exposure. A papular rash can occur; other skin manifestations include erythema nodosum and erythema multiforme, which are more frequent in females. Pulmonary infiltrates, hilar adenopathy, and pleural effusions may be seen on radiographs [87]. A high inoculum exposure may lead to diffuse pulmonary infiltrates and a fulminant, septic picture—this presentation is seen in patients with HIV with CD4 counts of less than 100 cells/mm^3 [88]. Most infections

resolve over several weeks to months without complications. About 4% result in pulmonary nodules. Thin wall cavities may develop, which usually close within 2 years. Severe pulmonary disease with chronic fibrocavitary pneumonia can develop in patients with diabetes, in patients who smoke cigarettes, and in patients with preexisting pulmonary fibrosis [89].

Disseminated disease is rare, occurring in 0.5% of all infections. Patients at high risk for dissemination include patients with HIV, organ transplant recipients, patients receiving corticosteroid therapy, and patients of African American and Filipino ancestry. Men are more likely to develop disseminated infection; pregnant women, especially during the third trimester, and women in the immediate postpartum period are also at risk for disseminated infection [90]. The skin is the most common site of dissemination; other sites include bone and joint involvement and CNS involvement, especially with meningitis. Hydrocephalus is a common complication of meningitis; it is fatal within 2 years if untreated [91].

Definitive diagnosis requires isolation of *C. immitis* from clinical specimens, which usually require 5–7 days incubation. Cultures are highly infectious and should not be opened except in an appropriate chamber. Spherules may be seen by calcofluor, hematoxylin eosin, or silver stains. Serologic assays are commonly used for diagnosing primary coccidioidomycosis. The immunodiffusion tube precipitin uses heated coccidioidin antigen and detects IgM antibodies; up to 90% of patients have antibodies within the first 3 weeks of infection. The CF test detects IgG antibodies, which develop 4–12 weeks after infection and can persist for prolonged periods. CF antibodies can be detected in other body fluids, and are especially useful in diagnosing coccidioidal meningitis. A titer ≥1:16 has been associated with disseminated disease, and increasing CF titers are found with worsening disease. Skin testing is a useful epidemiologic tool, but the antigen is no longer available [92].

A thorough assessment of patient risk factors and extent of disease is necessary to assess need for treatment. Antifungal agents include amphotericin B (0.5–0.7 mg/kg/day), ketoconazole (400 mg/day), fluconazole (400–800 mg/day), and itraconazole (200 mg bid). In general, amphotericin B is used initially in patients with progressive infection.

Most patients with primary respiratory infection do not require antifungal therapy but should be followed closely. However, this is controversial, and some authorities advocate treatment of all symptomatic patients. All patients at increased risk for dissemination should be treated, initially with amphotericin B if they have severe disease, followed by fluconazole or itraconazole for 3–6 months. During pregnancy, amphotericin B is indicated because the azoles are teratogenic. Factors indicating severity include night sweats of longer than 3 weeks duration, weight loss of more than 10%, extensive infiltrates, CF titer more than 1:16, inability to work, or symptoms persisting for longer than 2 months [93].

Patients with diffuse pneumonia (bilateral reticulonodular or miliary infiltrates) should be treated with amphotericin B followed by oral azoles for 1 year. Patients with immunodeficiency need to continue taking azole prophylaxis. Solitary pulmonary nodules can be followed, whereas enlarging pulmonary cavities should be resected. Chronic fibrocavitary pneumonia is treated with oral azoles for 1 year [94].

Disseminated coccidioidomycosis is treated with oral azoles or with amphotericin B if lesions are worsening. Surgical debridement is an important adjunctive measure. Coccidioidal meningitis is treated with fluconazole 400–800 mg. Some authorities add intrathecal amphotericin B initially because response may be more prompt. Azole therapy should be continued indefinitely. Intrathecal amphotericin (0.01–1.5 mg) is also indicated for patients who fail to respond to fluconazole or itraconazole. A shunt is frequently needed for decompression of hydrocephalus [95].

C. Blastomycosis

Blastomyces dermatitidis is a dimorphic fungus that is endemic to areas bordering the Mississippi and Ohio Rivers, the Great Lakes, and the St. Lawrence River. The organism is difficult to isolate unless specific environmental conditions (moist soil, decaying vegetation) are present. Sporadic cases in rural areas have occurred in men with outdoor occupations; outbreaks associated with recreational activities, crop harvesting, and construction projects have been described with no sex predilection. The organism is acquired by inhalation; rare cases of primary cutaneous blastomycosis have occurred after dog bites or accidental inoculation [96]. In the lung, conversion to the yeast form occurs at 37°C. The host inflammatory response consists of neutrophil and noncaseating granulomas; intraepidermal microabscesses and pseudoepitheliomatous hyperplasia is characteristic of skin lesions. Hematogenous dissemination leads to extrapulmonary blastomycosis in two-thirds of patients.

Acute pulmonary infection is asymptomatic in 50% of individuals. The incubation period is 30–45 days; fever, fatigue, night sweats, myalgias, arthralgias, and cough are presenting symptoms. Lobar consolidation or diffuse infiltrates are seen on radiographs. Hilar adenopathy and pleural effusions are uncommon. Some cases may be self-limited, although how frequently this occurs is unclear [97].

The majority of patients present with chronic pneumonia. Symptoms include low-grade fever, productive cough, hemoptysis, weight loss, and pleuritic chest pain. Lobar consolidation (sometimes with cavitation), nodules or mass lesions, pleural effusions, and miliary infiltrates can be seen. The disease is indolent and progressive.

Skin lesions are the most common manifestation of extrapulmonary blastomycosis (40–80%) and are either verrucous or ulcerative. The former are crusted, heaped-up lesions often mistaken for squamous cell carcinoma. Ulcerative lesions are raised with friable granulomatous tissue [98]. Skeletal lesions involving the long bones, vertebrate, and ribs occur in 7–40% of patients [99]. Genitourinary tract involvement (prostatitis and epididymitis) is seen in 10–30% of patients. CNS disease manifesting as abscess or meningitis occurs in less than 5% of patients. However, 40% of patients with HIV with blastomycosis have CNS disease [100]. Blastomycosis during pregnancy is infrequent, but it is associated with disseminated disease. Perinatal and transplacental infection has been described [101].

Definitive diagnosis of blastomycosis requires isolation of the organism from clinical specimens. Isolation on Sabouraud agar can take up to 4 weeks. Direct examination of sputum with addition of 10% KOH may show large (8–20 μm) yeast with refractile cell walls and broad-based buds. Bronchoscopy with bronchial washings can be positive in more than 90% of patients. The methenamine silver stain and periodic acid Schiff (PAS) stain are best for histopathologic tissue examination because the yeast forms are difficult to see with hematoxylin and eosin stains [102].

Serologic diagnosis for blastomycosis is unsatisfactory. The complement fixation test is neither sensitive nor specific. The immunodiffusion test is better for disseminated (88%) than localized (33%) diseases but does not become positive for more than 50 days after onset of symptoms [103]. An enzyme immunoassay and radioimmunoassay detecting a 120-kD cell wall protein are more sensitive but are not widely available [104]. There is no available skin test for blastomycosis.

Most cases of blastomycosis are treated with antifungal therapy because the disease is often progressive and mortality is as high as 90% if untreated. The exception is a few cases of acute pulmonary blastomycosis that may be self-limited, although identification of these patients is difficult. If therapy is withheld, patients should be followed closely for many years for evidence of progressive disease. All patients with life-threatening disease (such as acute respiratory distress syndrome) should be treated with amphotericin B 0.7–1.0 mg/kg/day (total dose 1.5–2.5 g). Patients may be switched to itraconazole 200–400 mg/day for at least 6 months. Alternatives include ketoconazole 400–800 mg/day. However, itraconazole is superior to the other azoles. Patients with mild to moderate pulmonary disease can be treated with itraconazole 200–400 mg/day for 6 months [105].

All patients with disseminated disease should be treated. For those with CNS infection, amphotericin B (0.7–1.0 mg/kg/day, total dose 2 g or more) should be used because CSF penetration of itraconazole is poor. Lipid formulations of amphotericin B have been used successfully in disseminated disease. Fluconazole at high doses (800 mg/day) may be an alternative in patients intolerant of amphotericin B because of its excellent CSF penetration [106]. Amphotericin B (total dose 1.5–2.5 g) followed by itraconazole is used for patients with life-threatening disseminated disease without CNS involvement; mild to moderate disease can be treated with itraconazole for 6 months. Patients with osteomyelitis should be treated with an azole for at least 1 year because they are more likely to relapse [107].

Blastomycosis in patients with HIV is associated with mortality rates of 30–40% and should be treated with amphotericin B (total dose 1.5–2.5 g). Patients who do not have CNS disease could be switched to itraconazole. Relapse is common in immunosuppressed patients, requiring chronic suppressive therapy with itraconazole [108]. All pregnant women with blastomycosis should be treated with amphotericin B promptly. The azoles should be avoided because of embryotoxicity.

IV. Antifungal Agents

The mainstay of treatment of systemic mycosis has been amphotericin B, an effective but toxic agent. The introduction of the azoles provided safer oral agents for the treatment of many fungal infections, including superficial mycosis. In the past few years, a new class of agents, the echinocandins, and newer azoles with a broader spectrum of activity have expanded therapeutic options for fungal infections. This section will briefly describe currently available antifungal agents and discuss their use in special situations (e.g., pregnancy).

Antifungal agents can act on the cell membrane (polyenes, azoles, allylamines), cell wall (echinocandins), nuclear division (griseofulvin), or nucleic acid synthesis (5-FC).

A. Polyenes

The polyene macrolide antibiotics bind to ergosterol in the fungal cell membrane, causing increased permeability and the formation of pores in the membrane. Leakage of potassium ions and other molecules lead to irreversible fungal cell damage. Included in this class are amphotericin B and nystatin.

1. Amphotericin B

Amphotericin B was long considered the "gold standard" for the treatment of systemic mycosis. It is poorly absorbed from the GI tract and does not penetrate the CSF, requiring intrathecal administration if used for fungal meningitis. The use of amphotericin is associated with considerable toxicity. Immediate hypersensitivity reactions (fever, chills, tachypnea, hypotension) can occur soon after the first infusion of amphotericin and have led to the use of a test dose. These are not allergic reactions and can be ameliorated with premedication with acetaminophen or hydrocortisone. Nephrotoxicity is dose-dependent and frequent. An increase in the serum creatinine to 2–3 mg/dl is frequent and should not lead to discontinuation of therapy. Nausea, hypokalemia, hypomagnesemia, and anemia are other side effects. Amphotericin B is effective in infections caused by mucor, aspergillus, coccidioides, cryptococcus, histoplasma, and candida, including non-albicans species. One exception is *Candida lusitaniae*, which is intrinsically resistant. The dose of amphotericin B is generally between 0.5–1.0 mg/kg/day but varies with the fungus treated. Patients with mucormycosis or invasive aspergillosis require 1.0–1.5 mg/kg, whereas 0.3 mg/kg may be sufficient for esophageal candidiasis [109].

There are three lipid complexed preparations of amphotericin—amphotericin B colloidal dispersion (ABCD), amphotericin B lipid complex (ABLC), and liposomal amphotericin B (AmBisome). These agents are less nephrotoxic but do not demonstrate superior clinical efficacy. They are extremely expensive and are generally reserved for patients intolerant of amphotericin B or for those with renal dysfunction [110].

2. Nystatin

The clinical use of nystatin is limited to topical applications to the skin and mucous membranes, localized candidiasis, and oral administration to suppress Candida in the gut in patients with impaired immunity.

B. Azoles

Azoles inhibit fungal lipid synthesis by binding to 14 demethylase (a cytochrome P450 enzyme), leading to accumulation of C-14 methylsterols and reduced concentrations of ergosterol. Important drug interactions can result from inhibition of cytochrome P450, including decreased synthesis of testosterone and cortisol. The triazoles (fluconazole, itraconazole) have greater selectivity against fungi, and less endocrine disturbances than imidazoles (ketoconazole), and are widely used.

1. Ketoconazole

Ketoconazole is used in the treatment of superficial cutaneous infections (ringworm, tinea versicolor) and chronic mucocutaneous candidiasis, although its use is limited by side effects. These include gynecomastia, nausea, hepatotoxicity, and drug interactions (cyclosporine, warfarin, dilantin, oral hypoglycemics, and many others) [111].

2. Fluconazole

Fluconazole is readily absorbed from the GI tract and penetrates the CSF. It is used in oropharyngeal and vaginal candidiasis and to treat candidemia in immunocompetent patients who are not severely ill. It is very useful in induction and maintenance therapy of cryptococcal meningitis in patients with HIV. It is also useful for coccidioidal meningitis and disseminated coccidioidomycosis, although higher doses (800 mg) are required. It is not effective against aspergillus, mucor, or Pseudallescheria. Adverse effects include vomiting, diarrhea, rash, and alopecia. Drug interactions are common and should be carefully monitored, especially in transplant recipients receiving fluconazole prophylaxis [112].

3. Itraconazole

Absorption of itraconazole is erratic and dependent on food and gastric acid. The cyclodextrin suspension is better absorbed and used preferentially. An intravenous form is now available. It has limited CSF penetration. It is used in the treatment of blastomycosis, histoplasmosis, coccidioidomycosis, sporotrichosis, onychomycosis, and aspergillosis. Adverse effects include nausea, abdominal discomfort, headache, and elevated liver enzymes. Significant drug interactions can occur. An assay for monitoring serum itraconazole levels is available [113].

4. Voriconazole

Voriconazole is a newly licensed, broad-spectrum triazole with a spectrum of action similar to itraconazole. It is well absorbed orally and metabolized in the liver by cytochrome P450 enzymes. It showed superior efficacy when compared to amphotericin B for invasive aspergillosis in a recent randomized trial [114]. It is also approved for refractory infection with Scedosporium and fusarium species. Visual disturbances are a frequent side effect but are transient. Other adverse effects include hallucinations, increased liver enzymes, and photosensitivity. Concurrent use of voriconazole with sirolimus, quinidine, rifampin, rifabutin, carbamazepine, and long-acting barbiturates should be avoided [115].

C. Flucytosine

Flucytosine interferes with DNA synthesis by inhibiting thymidylate synthetase. It is well absorbed orally and penetrates the CSF. Its usefulness is limited by the rapid development of resistance; for this reason, it is generally used in combination with amphotericin B for the treatment of cryptococcal meningitis and (possibly) systemic candidiasis. Adverse effects include bone marrow suppression, GI upsets, and hepatotoxicity [116].

D. Echinocandins

Echinocandins are a new class of antifungal agents that block the synthesis of beta (1,3)-glucan, a polysaccharide component of the cell wall of many fungi. Caspofungin is the first licensed agent in this class, and others are under investigation. It is active against aspergillus and Candida species and is used in patients refractory or intolerant of amphotericin B. Adverse effects include fever, rash, nausea, and vomiting. It is embryotoxic in animals. An initial dose of 70 mg is followed by daily doses of 50 mg administered intravenously [117].

E. Drugs Used for Superficial Mycoses

Topical azoles are useful in treating ringworm of the body, foot, hand, and perineum as well as tinea versicolor.

1. Topical Azoles for Vaginitis

Topical azoles are highly effective in the treatment of VVC. A wide variety of preparations are available over the counter. Both cream and tablets are effective; however, they should be inserted deep in the vagina. Manual insertion, rather than an applicator, is preferred in pregnancy. Persistence of azoles in vaginal secretions has allowed for shorter (3-day or single-dose) regimens. Table 84-5 lists some of the available vaginal preparations.

F. Allylamines

Allylamines prevent ergosterol synthesis by inhibiting squalene epoxidase, resulting in squalene accumulation and membrane disruption. Terbinafine is the first orally active allylamine. It is well absorbed and concentrated in the dermis, epidermis, and adipose tissue. It is used orally in the treatment of onychomycosis; the cream is effective for ringworm. Adverse effects include nausea, abdominal pain, and elevated liver enzymes. It is extremely expensive.

G. Griseofulvin

Griseofulvin was the first orally active antifungal agent isolated. It interferes with nucleic acid synthesis. It inhibits dermatophytes but has no effect on Candida or systemic mycoses. It is used in ringworm and onychomycosis, although relapse is frequent. A hypersensitivity reaction with fever, rash, and serum sickness can occur, along with headaches and gastrointestinal upsets.

V. Use of Antifungal Agents in Pregnancy

The safest approach is to avoid exposure to drugs during pregnancy; however, this is not always possible. Fungal infection

Table 84-5
Topical Agents for Vulvovaginal Candidiasis

Drugs (Trade Name)	Formulation	Dose
Butoconazole (Femstat, Gynazole)	2% cream	5 g × 3 days
Clotrimazole (Mycelex, Lotrimin)	1% cream	5 g × 7–14 days
	100 mg vag. tabs	1 tab × 7 days or 2 tabs × 3 days
Clotrimazole	500 mg vag. tabs	1 tab single dose
Econazole (Spectrazole)	150 mg vag. tabs	1 tab × 3 days
Fenticonazole (Lomexin)	2% cream	5 g × 7 days
Miconazole (Monistat, Micatin)	2% cream	5 g × 7 days
	100 mg vag. supp.	1 supp. × 7 days
	200 mg vag. supp.	1 supp. × 3 days
	1200 mg vag. supp.	1 supp. single dose
Terconazole (Terazole)	0.4% cream	5 g × 7 days
	0.8% cream	5 g × 3 days
	80 mg vag. supp.	1 supp. × 3 days
Tioconazole (Vagistat)	2% cream	5 g × 3 days
	6.5% cream	5 g single dose
Nystatin	1,000,000 units vag. tabs	1 tab × 14 days

requiring treatment occurs in women regardless of pregnancy, and there are clearly infections that are more frequent or more severe in pregnancy. VVC is more frequent, refractory to therapy, and likely to relapse in pregnant women. Pregnant women are also more likely to develop disseminated disease when they become infected with coccidioidomycosis or blastomycosis. Antifungal treatment in pregnancy requires careful attention to risks and benefits of therapy and knowledge of the effect on mother and fetus [118].

A. Topical Therapy in Pregnancy

The imidazoles are not absorbed systemically and are considered safe for use in pregnancy when used topically in the treatment of ringworm, tinea versicolor, and cutaneous candidal infections. The polyenes (nystatin) are also not absorbed, but they are not as effective. Terbinafine cream is effective but has higher systemic absorption after local application. None of these preparations have been associated with fetal or maternal problems.

For VVC, the imidazoles and nystatin can be used. The experience with nystatin in pregnancy is more extensive, and no increase in fetal malformations or deaths has been reported. The imidazoles are more efficacious and have lower relapse rates [119]. No adverse effects have been associated with the use of miconazole, clotrimazole, butoconazole, or terconazole during pregnancy, including first-trimester exposures, and they are recommended for use [120].

B. Systemic Therapy in Pregnancy

The use of systemic antifungal agents in pregnancy has been limited to life-threatening infection. Amphotericin B is the most widely used antifungal agent in pregnancy. It crosses the placenta and enters the fetal circulation [121]. No major fetal adverse effects have been described, although isolated case reports describe azotemia, anemia, rash, respiratory failure, and a single case of congenital malformation [122]. Far more common are maternal side effects, including nephrotoxicity, nausea and vomiting, and infusion-related fever and chills. There is less experience with the lipid-based preparations of amphotericin B, although animal studies have not shown any detrimental effect on the fetus.

The use of azoles in pregnancy is contraindicated. Systemic ketoconazole is teratogenic and embryotoxic and should be avoided in pregnancy. The use of high-dose fluconazole (400 mg) for coccidioidomycosis has been associated with congenital malformations and is assigned to risk category C in pregnancy [123]. However, 150 mg or less of fluconazole has not been associated with miscarriage or congenital malformations [124]. Itraconazole is embryotoxic and teratogenic in animals and is assigned to risk category C.

Flucytosine is metabolized to 5-fluorouracil, crosses the placenta, and is teratogenic in rats. It should probably be avoided in pregnancy. Griseofulvin is also teratogenic and crosses the placenta and should be avoided as well. There are little data on the use of terbinafine in pregnancy.

VI. Suggestions for Further Investigations

- Why do some women develop recurrent VVC? Is it possible to predict who is at risk for developing recurrent VVC?
- Why do pregnant women develop disseminated coccidioidomycosis? Is there an immunologic defect specific for this fungus?

References

1. Friedman GD. (1983). The rarity of cryptococcosis in Northern California: the 10-year experience of a large defined population. *Am J Epidemiol.* 177:230–234.
2. Sorvillo F, Beall G, Turner PA, *et al.* (1997). Incidence and factors associated with extrapulmonary cryptococcosis among persons with HIV infection in Los Angeles County. *AIDS.* 11:673–679.
3. Powderly WG. (1993). Cryptococcal meningitis and AIDS. *Clin Infect Dis.* 17:837–842.
4. Driver JA, Saunders CA, Heinze-Lacey B, *et al.* (1995). Cryptococcal pneumonia in AIDS: is cryptococcal meningitis preceded by clinically recognizable pneumonia? *J Acquir Immune Defic Syndr Hum Retrovirol.* 9:168–171.
5. Pema K, Diaz J, Guerra LG, *et al.* (1994). Disseminated cutaneous cryptococcosis: comparison of clinical manifestations in the pre-AIDS and AIDS eras. *Arch Intern Med.* 154:1032–1034.
6. Behrman RE, Masci JR, Nicholas P. (1990). Cryptococcal skeletal infections: case report and review. *Rev Infect Dis.* 12:181–190.
7. Perfect JR, Casadevall A. (2002). Cryptococcosis. *Infect Dis Clin N Am.* 16:837–874.
8. Feldmeser M, Harris C, Reichberg S, *et al.* (1996). Serum cryptococcal antigen in patients with AIDS. *Clin Infect Dis.* 23:827–830.
9. Van der Horst CM, Saag NS, Cloud GA, *et al.* (1997). Treatment of AIDS-associated acute cryptococcal meningitis: a four-arm, two step clinical trial. *N Engl J Med.* 337:15–21.
10. Robinson PA, Bauer M, Leal MA, *et al.* (1999). Early mycological treatment failure in AIDS-associated cryptococcal meningitis. *Clin Infect Dis.* 28:89–92.
11. Sharkey PK, Graybill JR, Johnson ES, *et al.* (1996). Amphotericin B lipid complex compared with amphotericin B in the treatment of cryptococcal meningitis in patients with AIDS. *Clin Infect Dis.* 22:315–321.
12. Bach MC, Tally PW, Godofsky EW. (1997). Use of cerebrospinal fluid shunts in patients having acquired immunodeficiency syndrome with cryptococcal meningitis and uncontrollable intracranial hypertension. *Neurosurgery.* 41:1280–1282.
13. Powderly WG, Saag MS, Cloud GA, *et al.* (1992). A controlled trial of fluconazole or amphotericin B to prevent relapse of cryptococcal meningitis in patients with the acquired immunodeficiency syndrome. *N Engl J Med.* 326:793–798.
14. Cohen R, Roth FJ, Delgado F, *et al.* (1969). Fungal flora of the normal human small and large intestine. *N Engl J Med.* 280:638–641.
15. Vasquez JA, Sobel JD. (2002). Mucosal candidiasis. *Infect Dis Clin N Am.* 16:793–820.
16. Lockhart SR, Joly S, Vargas K, *et al.* (1999). Natural defenses against *Candida* colonization breakdown in the oral cavities of the elderly. *J Dent Res.* 78:857–868.
17. Russotto SB. (1980). The role of *Candida albicans* in the pathogenesis of angular cheilosis. *J Prosthet Dent.* 44:243–246.
18. Darouiche RO. (1998). Oropharyngeal and esophageal candidiasis in immunocompromised patients: treatment issues. *Clin Infect Dis.* 26:259–274.
19. Wheeler RR, Peacock Jr JE, Cruz JM. (1987). Esophagitis in the immunocompromised host: role of esophagoscopy in diagnosis. *Rev Infect Dis.* 9:88–96.
20. Rabeneck L, Laine L. (1994). Esophageal candidiasis in patients infected with the human immunodeficiency virus. A decision analysis to assess cost-effectiveness of alternative management strategies. *Arch Intern Med.* 154:2705–2710.
21. Pons VG, Greenspan D, Koletar S, *et al.* (1993). Comparative study of fluconazole and clotrimazole troches for the treatment of oral thrush in AIDS. *J Acquir Immune Defic Syndr.* 6:1311–1316.
22. De Wot S, Goossens H, Clumeck N. (1993). Single-dose versus 7 days of fluconazole treatment for oral candidiasis in human immunodeficiency virus-infected patients: a prospective, randomized pilot study. *J Infect Dis.* 168:1332–1333.
23. Powderly WG, Finkelstein D, Feinberg J, *et al.* (1995). A randomized trial comparing fluconazole with clotrimazole troches for the prevention of fungal infections in patients with advanced human immunodeficiency virus infection. *N Engl J Med.* 443:700–705.
24. Fichtenbaum CJ, Powderly WG. (1998). Azole-resistant candidiasis. *Clin Infect Dis.* 26:556–565.
25. Philips P, Zemcov J, Mahmood W, *et al.* (1996). Itraconazole cyclodextrin solution for fluconazole-refractory oropharyngeal candidiasis in AIDS: correlation of clinical response with *in vitro* susceptibility. *AIDS.* 10:1369–1376.
26. Geiger AM, Foxman B. Risk factors in vulvovaginal candidiasis: A case-control study among college students. *Epidemiology.* (1996). 7:182.
27. Sobel JD, Myers P, Levison ME, *et al.* (1981). *Candida albicans* adherence to vaginal epithelial cells. *J Infect Dis.* 143:76.
28. Sobel JD, Muller G, Buckley H. (1984). Critical role of germination in the pathogenesis of experimental candidal vaginitis. *Infect Immun.* 44:576.
29. DeBernardis F, Agatens L, Ross IK, *et al.* (1990). Evidence for a role for secreted aspartate proteinase of *Candida albicans* in vulvovaginal candidiasis. *J Infect Dis.* 161:1276.
30. Sobel JD, Chaim W. (1996). Vaginal microbiology of women with acute recurrent vulvovaginal candidiasis. *J Clin Microbiol.* 34:2497–2499.
31. Elgebe IA, Elgebe I. (1983). Quantitative relationships of *Candida albicans* infections and dressing patterns in Nigerian women. *Am J Public Health.* 73:450–452.
32. Sobel JD, Faro S, Force RW, *et al.* (1998). Vulvovaginal candidiasis: epidemiologic, diagnostic and therapeutic considerations. *Am J Obstet Gynecol.* 178:203–211.
33. Bertholf ME, Stafford MJ. (1983). Colonization of *Candida albicans* in vagina, rectum, and mouth. *J Family Pract.* 16:919.
34. Reef S, Levine W, McNeil M, *et al.* (1995). Treatment options for vulvovaginal candidiasis: Background paper for development of 1993 STD treatment recommendations. *Clin Infect Dis.* 20:80.
35. Sobel JD. (2001). Candida vaginitis. In: *Infectious Diseases in Women.* Faro S, Soper D, eds. 39–54.

36. McNellis D, McLeod M, Lawson J, *et al.* (1977). Treatment of vulvovaginal candidiasis in pregnancy: A comparative study. *Obstet Gynecol.* 50:674.

37. Fidel PL Jr, Sobel JD. (1996). Immunopathogenesis of recurrent vulvovaginal candidiasis. *Clin Microbiol Rev.* 9:335.

38. Jovanovic R, Congema E, Ngujen HT. (1991). Antifungal agents versus boric acid for treating chronic mycotic vulvovaginitis. *J Reprod Med.* 36:593.

39. Beck-Sagué CM, Jarvis WM. (1993). The National Nosocomial Infections Surveillance System: secular trends in the epidemiology of nosocomial fungal infections in the United States, 1980–1990. *J Infect Dis.* 167:1247–1251.

40. Wey SB, Mori M, Pfaller MA, *et al.* (1989). Risk factors for hospital acquired candidemia: a matched case-control study. *Arch Intern Med.* 149:2349–2353.

41. Abi-Said D, Anaissie E, Uzun O, *et al.* (1997). The epidemiology of hematogenous candidiasis caused by different *Candida* species. *Clin Infect Dis.* 24:1122–1128.

42. Bouza E, Cobo-Soriano R, Rodriguez-Creixems M, *et al.* (2000). A prospective search for ocular lesions in hospitalized patients with significant bacteremia. *Clin Infect Dis.* 30:306–312.

43. Jarvis WR. (1995). Epidemiology of nosocomial fungal infections, with emphasis on Candida species. *Clin Infect Dis.* 20:1526–1530.

44. Rex JH, Walsh TJ, Sobel JD, *et al.* (2000). Practice guidelines for the treatment of candidiasis. Infectious Diseases Society of America. *Clin Infect Dis.* 30:662–678.

45. Mora-Duarte J, Betts R, Rotstein C, *et al.* (2002). Comparison of caspofungin and amphotericin B for invasive candidiasis. *N Engl J Med.* 347:2020–2029.

46. Tronchin G, Bouchara JP, Ferron M, *et al.* (1995). Cell surface properties of *Aspergillus fumigatus* conidia; correlation between adherence, agglutination, and rearrangements of the cell wall. *Can J Microbiol.* 41:714–721.

47. Marr KA, Carter RA, Crippa F, *et al.* (2002). Epidemiology and outcome of mould infections in hematopoietic stem cell transplant recipients. *Clin Infect Dis.* 34:909–917.

48. Marr KA, Patterson T, Denning D. (2002). Aspergillosis. Pathogenesis, clinical manifestations, and therapy. *Infect Dis Clin N Am.* 16:875–894.

49. Stevens DA, Schwartz HJ, Lee JY, *et al.* (2000). A randomized trial of itraconazole in allergic bronchopulmonary aspergillosis. *N Engl J Med.* 342:756–762.

50. Kawamura S, Maesaki S, Tomono K, *et al.* (2000). Clinical evaluation of 61 patients with pulmonary aspergilloma. *Intern Med.* 39:209–212.

51. Denning DW. (2001). Chronic forms of pulmonary aspergillosis. *Clin Microbiol Infect.* 7(suppl 2):25–31.

52. Washburn RG. (1998). Fungal sinusitis. *Curr Clin Top Infect Dis.* 18:60–74.

53. Talbot GH, Huang A, Provencher M. (1991). Invasive *Aspergillus* rhinosinusitis in patients with acute leukemia. *Rev Infect Dis.* 13:219–232.

54. Kemper CA, Hostetler JS, Follansbee SE, *et al.* (1993). Ulcerative and plaque-like tracheobronchitis due to infection with *Aspergillus* in patients with AIDS. *Clin Infect Dis.* 17:344–352.

55. Wald A, Leisenring W, van Burik J, *et al.* (1997). Epidemiology of *Aspergillus* infections in a large cohort of patients undergoing bone marrow transplantation. *J Infect Dis.* 175:1459–1466.

56. Jantunen E, Ruutu P, Niskanen L, *et al.* (1997). Incidence and risk factors for invasive fungal infections in allogeneic BMT recipients. *Bone Marrow Transplant.* 19:801–808.

57. Horvath JA, Dummer S. (1996). The use of respiratory-tract cultures in the diagnosis of invasive pulmonary aspergillosis. *Am J Med.* 100:171–178.

58. Kawamura S, Maesaki S, Noda T, *et al.* (1999). Comparison between PCR and detection of antigen in sera for diagnosis of pulmonary aspergillosis. *J Clin Microbiol.* 37:218–220.

59. Hebrecht R, Denning DW, Patterson TF, *et al.* (2002). Voriconazole versus amphotericin B for primary therapy of invasive aspergillosis. *N Engl J Med.* 347:408–415.

60. Kontoyianis DP, Wessel VC, Bodey GP, *et al.* (2000). Zygomycosis in the 1990s in a tertiary-care cancer center. *Clin Infect Dis.* 30:851–856.

61. Boelaert JR, de Locht M, Van Cutsem J, *et al.* (1993). Mucormycosis during deferoxamine therapy is a siderophore mediated infection: *in vitro* and *in vivo* animal studies. *J Clin Invest.* 91:1979–1986.

62. Gonzalez CE, Rinaldi MG, Sugar AM. (2002). Zygomycosis. *Infect Dis Clin N Am.* 16:895–914.

63. McAdams HP, Rosado de Christenson M, Strollo DC, *et al.* (1997). Pulmonary mucormycosis: Radiologic findings in 32 cases. *Am J Radiol.* 168:1541–1548.

64. Leong KW, Crowley B, White B, *et al.* (1997). Cutaneous mucormycosis due to *Absidia corymbifera* occurring after bone marrow transplantation. *Bone Marrow Transplant.* (19:513–515.

65. Singh N, Gayowsky T, Singh J, *et al.* (1995). Invasive gastrointestinal zygomycosis in a liver transplant recipient: case report and review of zygomycosis in solid-organ transplant recipients. *Clin Infect Dis.* 20:617–620.

66. Kontoyianis DP, Vartivarian S, Anaissie EJ, *et al.* (1994). Infections due to *Cunninghamella bertholetiae* in patients with cancer: report of three cases and review. *Clin Infect Dis.* 18:925–928.

67. Gonzalez CE, Couriel DR, Walsh TJ. (1997). Disseminated zygomycosis in a neutropenic patient: successful treatment with amphotericin B lipid complex and granulocyte colony-stimulating factor. *Clin Infect Dis.* 24:192–196.

68. Tedder M, Spratt JA, Anstadt MP, *et al.* (1994). Pulmonary mucormycosis: results of medical and surgical therapy. *Ann Thorac Surg.* 57:1044–1050.

69. Parfrey NA. (1986). Improved diagnosis and prognosis of mucormycosis: A clinicopathologic study of 33 cases. *Medicine (Baltimore).* 65:113–123.

70. Cano MVC, Hajjeh RA. (2001). The epidemiology of histoplasmosis: a review. *Semin Respir Infect.* 16:109–118.

71. Medoff G, Kobayashi GS, Painter A, *et al.* (1987). Morphogenesis and pathogenicity of *Histoplasma capsulatum*. *Infect Immun.* 55.1355–1358.

72. Baughman RP, Kim CK, Vinegar A, *et al.* (1986). The pathogenesis of experimental pulmonary histoplasmosis. Correlative studies of histopathology, bronchoalveolar lavage, and respiratory function. *Am Rev Respir Dis.* 134:771–776.

73. Wheat J. Histoplasmosis. (1997). Experience during outbreaks in Indianapolis and review of the literature. *Medicine (Baltimore).* 76:339–353.

74. Wheat LJ, Wass J, Norton J, *et al.* (1984). Cavitary histoplasmosis occurring during two large urban outbreaks: Analysis of clinical, epidemiologic, roentgenographic, and, laboratory features. *Medicine (Baltimore).* 63:201–209.

75. Sarosi GA, Johnson PC. (1992). Disseminated histoplasmosis in patients infected with human immunodeficiency virus. *Clin Infect Dis.* 14(suppl):S60–S67.

76. Goodwin RA Jr, Shapiro JL, Thurman GH, *et al.* (1980). Disseminated histoplasmosis: Clinical and pathologic correlations. *Medicine (Baltimore).* 59:1–31.

77. Wheat LJ, Connolly-Stringfield PA, Baker RL, *et al.* (1990). Disseminated histoplasmosis in the acquired immune deficiency syndrome: clinical findings, diagnosis and treatment, and review of the literature. *Medicine (Baltimore).* 69:361–374.

78. Wheat LJ, Kobler RB, Tewari RP. (1986). Diagnosis of disseminated histoplasmosis by detection of *Histoplasma capsulatum* antigen in serum and urine specimens. *N Engl J Med.* 314:83–88.

79. Wheat LJ. (2001). Laboratory diagnosis of histoplasmosis: update 2000. *Semin Respir Infect.* 16:131–140.

80. Wheat J, Sarosi G, McKinsey D, *et al.* (2000). Practice guidelines for the management of patients with histoplasmosis. *Clin Infect Dis.* 30:688–695.

81. McKinsey DS, Kauffman CA, Pappas PG, *et al.* (1996). Fluconazole therapy for histoplasmosis. *Clin Infect Dis.* 23:996–1001.

82. Dismukes WE, Bradsher RW Jr, Cloud GC, *et al.* (1992). Itraconazole therapy for blastomycosis and histoplasmosis. NIAID Mycoses Study Group. *Am J Med.* 93:489–497.

83. Wheat J, Hafner R, Wulfson M, *et al.* (1993). Prevention of relapse of histoplasmosis with itraconazole in patients with the acquired immunodeficiency syndrome. NIAID Clinical Trials & Mycoses Study Group Collaborators. *Ann Intern Med.* 118:610–616.

84. Wheat LJ, Batteiger BE, Sathapatayavongs B. (1990). *Histoplasma capsulatum* infections of the central nervous system: a clinical review. *Medicine (Baltimore).* 69:244–260.

85. Kirkland TN, Fierer J. (1996). Coccidioidomycosis: A reemerging infectious disease. *Emerg Infect Dis.* 2:192–199.

86. Ampel NM, Dols CL, Galgiani JN. (1993). Coccidioidomycosis during human immunodeficiency virus infection. Results of a prospective study in coccidioidal endemic area. *Am J Med.* 94:235–240.

87. Standaert SM, Schaffner W, Galgiani JN, *et al.* (1995). Coccidioidomycosis among visitors to a *Coccidioides immitis*-endemic area: An outbreak in a military reserve unit. *J Infect Dis.* 171:1672–1675.

88. Arsura EL, Bellinghausen PL, Kilgore WB, *et al.* (1998). Septic shock in coccidioidomycosis. *Crit Care Med.* 26:62–65.

89. Sarosi GA, Parker JD, Doto IL, *et al.* (1970). Chronic pulmonary coccidioidomycosis. *N Engl J Med.* 283:325–329.

90. Walker MP, Brody CZ, Resnik R. (1992). Reactivation of coccidioidomycosis in pregnancy. *Obstet Gynecol.* 79:815–817.

91. Vincent T, Galgiani JN, Huppert M, *et al.* (1993). The natural history of coccidioidal meningitis: VA-Armed Forces Cooperative Studies. 1955–1958. *Clin Infect Dis.* 16:247–254.

92. Wieden MA, Galgiani JN, Pappagianis D. (1983). Comparison of immunodiffusion techniques with standard complement fixation assay for quantitation of coccidioidal antibodies. *J Clin Microbiol.* 18:529–534.

93. Galgiani JN, Ampel NM, Catanzaro A, *et al.* (2000). Practice guidelines for the treatment of coccidioidomycosis. *Clin Infect Dis.* 30:658–661.

94. Stevens DA. (1994). Itraconazole and fluconazole for treatment of coccidioidomycosis. *Clin Infect Dis.* 18:470.

95. Galgiani JN, Cloud GA, Catanzaro A, *et al.* (1998). Fluconazole (FLU) versus itraconazole (ITRA) for coccidioidomycosis: randomized, multicenter, double-blinded trial in nonmeningeal progressive infections [abstract 100]. *Clin Infect Dis.* 27:939.

96. Klein BS, Vergeront JM, Davis JP. (1986). Epidemiologic aspects of blastomycosis, the enigmatic systemic mycosis. *Semin Respir Infect.* 1:29–39.

97. Chapman SW, Lin AC, Hendricks DA, *et al.* (1997). Endemic blastomycosis in Mississippi: Epidemiological and clinical studies. *Semin Respir Infect.* 12:219–228.

98. Mercurio MG, Elewski BE. (1992). Cutaneous blastomycosis. *Cutis.* 50:422–424.

99. MacDonald PB, Black GB, MacKenzie R. (1990). Orthopaedic manifestations of blastomycosis. *J Bone Joint Surg (Am).* 72:860–864.

100. Pappas PG, Pottage JC, Powderly WG, *et al.* (1992). Blastomycosis in patients with acquired immunodeficiency syndrome. *Ann Intern Med.* 116:847–853.

101. MacDonald D, Alguire PC. (1990). Adult respiratory distress syndrome due to blastomycosis during pregnancy. *Chest.* 98:1527–1528.

102. Lemos LB, Baliga M, Taylor BD, *et al.* (1995). Bronchoalveolar lavage for diagnosis of fungal disease: Five years experience in a southern United States rural area with many blastomycosis cases. *Acta Cytol.* 39:1101–1111.

103. Klein BS, Kuritsky WAC, Kaufman L, *et al.* (1986). Comparison of enzyme immunoassay, immunodiffusion and complement fixation in detecting antibody in human serum to the A antigen in *B. dermatitidis. Am Rev Respir Dis.* 133:144–148.

104. Soufleris AJ, Klein BS, Courtney BT, *et al.* (1994). Utility of anti-WI-1 serological testing in the diagnosis of blastomycosis in Wisconsin residents. *Clin Infect Dis.* 19:87–92.

105. Chapman SW, Bradsher RW, Campbell GD, *et al.* (2000). Practice guidelines for the management of patients with blastomycosis. *Clin Infect Dis.* 30:679–683.

106. Pappas PG, Bradsher RW, Kaufman CA, *et al.* (1997). Treatment of blastomycosis with higher dose fluconazole. *Clin Infect Dis.* 25:200–205.

107. Bradsher RW. (1996). Histoplasmosis and blastomycosis. *Clin Infect Dis.* 22:5102–5111.

108. Pappas PG, Threikeld MG, Bedsole GD, *et al.* (1993). Blastomycosis in immunocompromised patients. *Medicine (Baltimore).* 72:311–325.

109. White MH, Anaissie EJ, Kusne S, *et al.* (1997). Amphotericin B colloidal dispersion vs amphotericin B as therapy for invasive aspergillosis. *Clin Infect Dis.* 24:635–642.

110. Wong-Beringer A, Jacobs RA, Gugliemo JB. (1998). Lipid formulations of amphotericin B: Clinical efficacy and toxicities. *Clin Infect Dis.* 27:603–618.

111. Sugar AM, Alsip SG, Galgiani JN, *et al.* (1987). Pharmacology and toxicity of high-dose ketoconazole. *Antimicrob Agents Chemother.* 31:1874–1878.

112. Zervos M, Meunier F. (1993). Fluconazole (Diflucan): A review. *Int J Antimicrob Agents.* 3:147–170.

113. Stevens DA. (1999). Itraconazole in cyclodextrin solution. *Pharmacotherapy.* 19:603–611.

114. Walsh TJ, Pappas P, Winston DJ, *et al.* (2002). Voriconazole compared with liposomal amphotericin B for empirical antifungal therapy in patients with neutropenia and fever. *N Engl J Med.* 346:225–234.

115. Denning DW, Riband P, Milpied N, *et al.* (2002). Efficacy and safety of voriconazole in the treatment of acute invasive aspergillosis. *Clin Infect Dis.* 34:563–571.

116. Polak A, Scholer HJ, Wall M. (1982). Combination therapy of experimental candidiasis and aspergillosis in mice. *Chemotherapy.* 28:461.

117. Kurtz MB, Rex JH. (2001). Glucan synthase inhibitors as antifungal agents. *Adv Protein Chem.* 56:463–475.

118. King CT, Rogers D, Cleary JD, *et al.* (1998). Antifungal therapy during pregnancy. *Clin Infect Dis.* 27:1151–1160.

119. Eliot BW, Howat RC, Mack AE. (1979). A comparison between the effects of nystatin, clotrimazole and miconazole on vaginal candidiasis. *Br J Obstet Gynaecol.* 86:572–577.

120. Centers for Disease Control and Prevention. (1998). 1998 Guidelines for treatment of sexually transmitted diseases. *MMWR Morb Mortal Wkly Rep.* 47:78.

121. Gallis HA, Drew RH, Pickard WW. (1990). Amphotericin B: 30 years of clinical experience. *Rev Infect Dis.* 12:308–329.

122. Dean JD, Wolf JE, Ranzini AC, *et al.* (1994). Use of amphotericin B during pregnancy: case report and review. *Clin Infect Dis.* 18:364–368.

123. Pursley TJ, Blomquist IK, Abraham J, Andersen HF, Bartley JA. Fluconazole-induced congenital anomalies in three infants. *Clin Infect Dis.* (1996). 22:336–340.

124. Mastroiacovo P, Mazzone T, Botto LD, *et al.* (1996). Prospective assessment of pregnancy outcomes after first-trimester exposure to fluconazole. *Am J Obstet Gynecol.* 175:1645–1650.

85

Sex and Gender-Specific Issues in HIV Pathogenesis

R. SCOTT MCCLELLAND, MD, MPH* AND ROBERT W. COOMBS, MD, PhD, FRCPC**

*Department of Medicine, University of Washington, Seattle, WA
**Departments of Medicine and Laboratory Medicine, University of Washington, Seattle, WA

I. Epidemiology

A. Background

In 1981 the recognition of unusual clusters of *Pneumocystis* pneumonia (PCP) caused by a fungal pathogen *Pneumocystis carinii* (now referred to as *P. jiroveci* [1]) and Kaposi's sarcoma (later found to be caused by a viral pathogen HHV-8) among men who have sex with men (MSM) heralded the beginning of the acquired immune deficiency syndrome (AIDS) epidemic [2,3]. Within the same year, the first cases of a similar syndrome were identified in women [4]. A striking feature shared by the patients with these unusual illnesses was a severe defect in cell-mediated immunity, which predisposed them to infection with intracellular pathogens and certain malignancies. The retrovirus responsible for AIDS was identified 2 years later [5,6], and was initially called human T-cell leukemia virus type III (HTLV-III) because of similarity to other known retroviruses. This virus was subsequently renamed the human immunodeficiency virus type 1 (HIV-1).

The early HIV-1 epidemic was most evident among MSM. Additional groups at risk for infection, including injection drug users (IDU), recipients of blood products, and heterosexual contacts of individuals with other risk factors, were soon identified. Initial prevention efforts in response to the spread of HIV-1 were directed toward MSM, IDU, and blood product safety. The greatest prevention success has been in the area of blood safety; screening has virtually eliminated blood products as a means of transmission in developed countries.

The past decade has witnessed increasing numbers of HIV-1 infections acquired through heterosexual contact. By 1992 the annual percent increase in AIDS cases attributed to heterosexual contact was higher than for any other risk category [7]. Among women, heterosexual contact with men who have other risk factors for HIV-1 has become the most common route for HIV-1 acquisition [8]. Women who are younger, economically disadvantaged, minorities, and from the southern United States are at especially high risk for infection with HIV-1 [9,10]. As with other sexually transmitted infections (STIs), in discordant couples the risk to an uninfected female partner is greater than the risk to an uninfected male [11,12]. Social and behavioral factors also place women at increased risk. Women often have an earlier sexual debut, have sex with older male partners, are the victims of sexual coercion, and may not be able to negotiate condom use [13].

B. HIV-1 Prevalence and Trends in the United States

In 2001 there were estimated to be more than 460,000 people living with HIV-1 in the United States, and 99% of these infections were in adults [14]. The proportion of cases in women has increased from 11% to 25% in the past decade, and minority women are disproportionately affected [15] (Fig. 85-1). By the end of the 1990s, new infection rates for African American, Hispanic, and white women were 51.2, 16.3, and 2.5 per 100,000. respectively. Increasing rates of HIV-1 infection among young minority women are of particular concern. Whereas HIV-1 seroprevalence declined for virtually all population groups studied in the United States between 1993 and 1997, the HIV-1 seroprevalence among female Job Corps applicants actually increased from 0.29% to 0.52%. This represents an increase in HIV-1 seroprevalence in a population of socially and economically disadvantaged women between the ages of 16 and 21 years old. The figures are particularly sobering because they are the results of routine screening, rather than testing initiated by recognized risk factors for HIV-1 infection. The HIV-1 seroprevalence figures continue to reflect the widening ethnic divide in the prevalence of HIV-1 in the United States. Whereas the observed overall 1988–1994 seroprevalence in white women aged 18–59 years was 1:1,667, the seroprevalence in African American women was 1:182. African American men are at even higher risk with a seroprevalence of 1:56, which contrasts with that for white men of 1:286. However, the estimated seroprevalence rates for African American women and men are considerably higher at 1:135 and 1:37, respectively [16].

Heterosexual contact is now the dominant mode of transmission among women diagnosed with AIDS, representing 39% of cases diagnosed between July 2000 and June 2001 [14]. IDU accounted for 23% of cases in women, whereas only about 1% of women had acquired infection as a result of hemophilia, coagulation disorders, or receipt of infected blood products or tissue. Among the remaining 37% of women, the risk factor for HIV-1 was not reported or not identified, or in rare instances infections occurred through exposures such as health care, laboratory, or household exposure. The large percentage of women without an identified risk factor for HIV-1 suggests that many women may be unaware of their partners risk for HIV-1.

The geographic distribution of HIV-1 cases in the United States differs according to the predominant modes of transmission, reflecting three distinct epidemics [9]. Heterosexually acquired HIV-1 is most prevalent in the Northeast and the South. The overall prevalence of HIV-1 among heterosexual patients in STI clinics is 2.3%; the rate in women is less than 2%, whereas the rate in men is less than 3%. The geographic distribution of heterosexually acquired HIV-1 reflects the risk associated with heterosexual contact with individuals with other risk factors, particularly IDUs. Among IDUs, the rates are highest in cities in the Northeast and South. The overall rate of HIV-1 infection

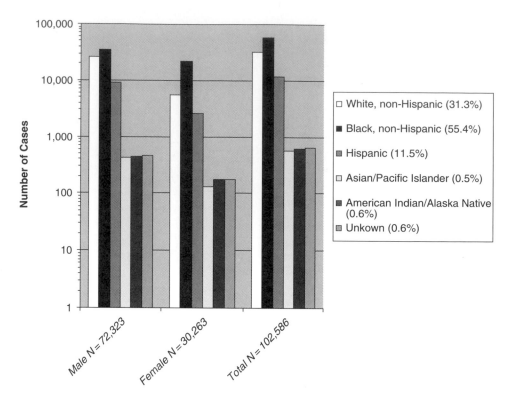

Fig. 85-1 Estimated number and percentage of persons with a new diagnosis of HIV infection, by sex and race/ethnicity from 29 states with HIV reporting between 1999 and 2002. (Adapted from Centers for Disease Control and Prevention. [2003]. MMWR. 52[47]:1145–1148).

among people entering drug treatment centers is 18%, and it is slightly lower among female than among male IDUs. Finally, among MSM high rates of infection are found in metropolitan areas throughout the country. At surveillance STI clinics, the overall rate for MSM is 26%.

C. Summary

Two decades after the initial recognition of AIDS in the United States, three distinct epidemics have emerged. The most important modes of HIV-1 transmission among women are heterosexual contact and IDU. Women who are socially or economically disadvantaged are particularly at risk, highlighting an urgent need for a renewed focus on both HIV-1 prevention and treatment for women.

II. Pathogenesis

A. Virology

HIV is a retrovirus belonging to the lentivirus family [17]. Retroviruses are unique in their ability to use reverse transcriptase, an enzyme that produces a DNA provirus from viral RNA. The available evidence supports the evolution of HIV-1 from an ancestral primate virus [18,19].

Infection with HIV-1 is a dynamic process, even during the period of clinical latency. The entire viral life cycle can be completed in 2 days, and it is estimated that untreated individuals

may produce more than 10^{10} viral particles per day [20,21]. Because reverse transcriptase is relatively error-prone, there is a rapid development of a diverse population of viral variants called quasispecies [22]. The genetic diversity of the virus has important implications for viral escape from the immune response as well as development of resistance to antiretroviral medications.

In addition to the development of quasispecies within infected individuals, there are broader genetic variations in HIV-1 that are observed in different regions. Three main groups of HIV-1 have been recognized: M (major), O (outlier), and N (new). Within group M, nine subtypes, A through K, and at least four major recombinants have been distinguished. Subtype B is the most common in the United States and Europe [23]. There may be differences between the subtypes in relation to infectivity and pathogenicity, but the overall data are too limited to support any strong influence of subtype on either disease progression or transmission [24].

B. Natural History of HIV-1 Infection

Initial infection with HIV-1 is followed by a high level of viral replication and an acute decline in the CD4 lymphocyte count [25]. A potentially important difference between women and men is evident at this early stage of infection among HIV-1 infected individuals in Kenya. Men have a homogeneous viral population early in infection, whereas many women have a heterogeneous viral population. This may be the result of infection with multiple subtypes during a single exposure [26]. The long-term effect of this difference is not yet known and needs to be confirmed in other populations.

Acute HIV-1 infection is accompanied by a mononucleosis-like syndrome, the acute retroviral syndrome, in 40–90% of cases [27–31]. Symptoms of the acute retroviral syndrome are shown in (Table 85-1). These symptoms generally last for less than 14 days [32]. At this time, there is no evidence to support major sex differences in the clinical presentation of acute infection [33]. Clinical improvement is accompanied by a decrease in the viral load and an increase in CD4 lymphocyte count [25]. This partial immunologic control of the infection is probably related to CD8 positive HIV-1 specific cytotoxic T lymphocytes (CTLs) [34–36]. Humoral immunity, with development of neutralizing anti-HIV-1 antibodies, may also be important [37]. However, the immune response is not capable of eradicating HIV-1, and the infection enters a chronic stage.

In untreated individuals infected with HIV-1, the virus and the immune system reach an equilibrium that can be evaluated in terms of the viral set point [38–42]. During this time, ongoing HIV-1 replication leads to a gradual reduction in the CD4 lymphocyte count, which may result either from a cytopathic effect of the virus on infected cells or to virus-specific killing of infected cells by CTLs [25]. In chronic HIV-1 infection, the plasma viral load is the strongest predictor of disease progression, and the accuracy of prediction is further improved by including the CD4 cell count [40] (Table 85-2).

Women tend to have plasma viral loads that are less than half that of men, even after adjustment for CD4 lymphocyte count [43,44]. The difference is particularly evident earlier in disease,

when the CD4 cell count is greater than 200 cells/mcL. These findings suggest that it may be necessary to revise the thresholds for initiating antiretroviral therapy downward in women [45]. The most recent recommendations for initiation of antiretroviral therapy in adults appropriately place increased emphasis on the

Table 85-1

Features of the Acute Retroviral Syndrome

Symptom, Sign, or Laboratory Abnormality	Frequency (%)
Fever	>80–90
Fatigue	>70–90
Rash	>40–80
Headache	32–70
Lymphadenopathy	40–70
Pharyngitis	50–70
Myalgia or arthralgia	50–70
Nausea, vomiting, or diarrhea	30–60
Night sweats	50
Aseptic meningitis	24
Oral ulcers	10–20
Genital ulcers	5–15
Thrombocytopenia	45
Leukopenia	40
Elevated hepatic enzyme levels	21

(Adapted from Kahn JO, Walker BD. [1998]. Acute human immunodeficiency virus type 1 infection. *N Engl J Med*. 339:33–39.)

Table 85-2

Three-, Six-, and Nine-Year Probability of AIDS-Free Survival in Untreated Patients Based on Viral Load and CD4 Cell Count

CD4 cell count	Plasma HIV-1 RNA	3 years (%)	6 years (%)	9 years (%)
0–200 cells/μL	10,001–30,000 copies/mL	50	25	10
	>30,000 copies/mL	14	1	0
201–350 cells/μL	501–3,000 copies/mL	93	74	59
	3,001–10,000 copies/mL	91	52	27
	10,001–30,000 copies/mL	62	26	11
	>30,000 copies/mL	34	9	6
351–500 cells/μL	501–3,000 copies/mL	96	74	40
	3,001–10,000 copies/mL	90	57	29
	10,001–30,000 copies/mL	83	40	16
	>30,000 copies/mL	50	20	5
>500 cells/μL	<500 copies/mL	94	82	70
	501–3,000 copies/mL	96	81	56
	3,001–10,000 copies/mL	92	70	42
	10,001–30,000 copies/mL	84	50	25
	>30,000 copies/mL	66	28	14

Groups that were too small to provide estimates of AIDS-free survival were omitted.
(Adapted from Mellors JW *et al*. [1996]. Prognosis in HIV-1 infection predicted by the quantity of virus in plasma. *Science*. 272:1167–1170.) Women with the same viral load as men have a 1.6-fold higher risk of developing AIDS (95% confidence interval: 1.10–2.32); or conversely, women with one-half the viral load of men have a similar risk of progression to AIDS [43].

CD4 lymphocyte count in guiding early treatment decisions [46]. These recommendations may be more helpful for clinical decision-making in women than previous versions, which placed more emphasis on plasma viral load.

The median duration of clinical latency in patients infected with HIV-1 is about 10 years [47]. Of patients, 5–10% are long-term nonprogressors, who remain asymptomatic without major declines in CD4 cell count for 15 years or more. However, it is now evident that these patients do show gradually progressive immunosuppression but over longer periods. Conversely, about 10% of individuals have a rapid progression, developing AIDS within 5 years or less of infection.

As the CD4 lymphocyte count declines, there is a progressive decrease in cell-mediated immunity that leads to increased risk of infection and malignancy. Early symptoms, prior to the onset of more severe immunosuppression, include recurrent vaginal candidiasis and persistent generalized lymphadenopathy [48]. As immune dysfunction worsens, the disease enters a late stage marked by an increase in the plasma viral load and more rapid depletion of CD4 lymphocytes [49]. In the United States, the diagnosis of AIDS is based on clinical criteria and/or a CD4 lymphocyte count less than 200 cells/mcL. Without treatment, patients eventually die from complications of opportunistic infections or malignancies. Survival in women with HIV-1 is the same as in men when adjusted for differences in the utilization of health care services [50]. The more rapid progression of disease in women that has been described in some studies is likely related to differences in access to health care.

C. Menstrual Cycle and Genital Shedding of HIV-1

The hormonal changes of the menstrual cycle could influence the levels of HIV-1 replication [51]. In fact, the effect of the menstrual cycle on HIV-1 RNA levels in the blood and genital tract are likely different. Although some studies show an effect of the menstrual cycle on plasma levels of HIV-1, others clearly do not [52,53]. In contrast, the genital tract shedding of HIV-1 is influenced by the menstrual cycle with higher virus levels in the endocervical canal prior to menses followed by a nadir in the follicular phase [53]. The effect of the menstrual cycle on genital HIV-1 shedding may be directed through local cytokine production or other hormone-related changes in cellular composition and endocervical canal fluid characteristics [54]. As a consequence of local genital factors that include sex hormones, cytokines, and microbial flora, the viral populations may differ genetically between the genital tract and blood [55,56]. Thus, the maintenance of a normal vaginal flora may be an important factor in controlling HIV-1 acquisition or transmission [51].

D. Response to Antiretroviral Therapy

Antiretroviral therapy (ART), using combinations of three or more antiretroviral drugs, changes the natural history of HIV-1 infection by suppressing viral replication and allowing some degree of immune reconstitution [57]. The introduction of combination ART in the United States and in Europe has led to substantial decreases in AIDS-related death [58]. The CD4 lymphocyte count appears to be the most important determinant of prognosis in patients receiving ART [59]. The factors associated with clinical progression after starting ART include a CD4 cell count <200/mcL, viral RNA >100,000 copies/mL of plasma, age >50 years, injection drug use, and a diagnosis of AIDS [59]. However, after starting ART, the CD4 and viral RNA response at 6 months but not the baseline values are strongly predictive of disease progression [60]. Although women may achieve virologic suppression at a faster rate than men and possibly have a more durable response, there is no evidence that these sex differences in treatment response translate into differences in clinical progression [59–61]. To date there is no evidence that genetic differences between the sexes influences the effects of the MDR1 3435C/T polymorphism or the CCR5 delta 32 mutation on treatment response or disease progression [62,63].

E. Summary

The etiology of the subtle virologic differences between men and women is not understood. However, the preponderance of evidence to date indicates that these virologic differences are not clinically important and neither influences the current recommendations to initiate antiretroviral therapy at a CD4 cell count of between 200 and 350 cells/mcL nor affects the clinical response once therapy is started. The influence of sex hormones and the reproductive health of women and girls on HIV replication, genital tract infection, and both vertical and horizontal transmission are important areas of ongoing research.

III. Prevention

Historically, the main modes of transmission of HIV-1 to women include heterosexual contact, injection drug use, and exposure to blood products. Screening of blood products has virtually eliminated this mode of transmission in developed countries. The following section will focus on prevention of transmission through sexual contact and injection drug use. Three general approaches to transmission including avoidance of exposure, reduction of transmission risk with exposure, and treatment to abort early infection are considered (Table 85-3).

A. The ABCs of Sexual Transmission Risk Reduction

Heterosexual transmission is now the most common source of infection for women diagnosed with AIDS [8]. The risk of acquiring HIV-1 from a single episode of penile–vaginal intercourse is about 1/1000 and is somewhat higher for male-to-female transmission [64,65]. The risk of male-to-female transmission may be increased in the presence of female-recipient factors including younger age and the presence of cervical ectopy and STI [66–68]. However, the presence of normal vaginal flora with a predominance of hydrogen peroxide–producing Lactobacillus species may be protective [69]. The risk of male-to-female sexual transmission is also influenced by male-partner factors including plasma HIV-1 viral load, CD4 lymphocyte count, use of antiretroviral therapy, circumcision status, and STI [70–72].

Table 85-3
Interventions to Reduce the Risk of HIV-1 Transmission

	Sexual Transmission	Injection Drug Use/Percutaneous Transmission
Avoid exposure	Abstinence • Delay sexual debut	Abstinence • Drug treatment • Methadone programs
Reduce risk of exposure	Monogamy Nonpenetrative sex Barrier contraception • Male latex condom • Female polyurethane condom* • Diaphragm* • Cervical cap* Microbicide* Vaccine*	Clean needles and injecting equipment • Needle exchange • Safe injecting practice
Treatment to abort early infection	Postsexual exposure prophylaxis* • Combination of antiretroviral medications	Post–needle-injury prophylaxis** • Combination of antiretroviral medications

*Currently under investigation.
**Available data on post–needle-injury prophylaxis is from exposure in health care workers.

The ABCs of sexual transmission risk reduction refers to a pneumonic for the main methods of decreasing sexual transmission:

A—abstinence
B—be faithful (mutual fidelity)
C—condoms
S—STI treatment and prevention

In the future, microbicides that inactivate or kill the virus may provide an important, female-controlled means of reducing the risk of sexual transmission [73]. Each of these approaches is considered in detail in the following section.

1. Behavioral Interventions

The risk of sexual transmission of HIV-1 can be eliminated through abstinence. This option may be particularly effective in adolescents and young women. Substantial decreases in HIV-1 prevalence have been achieved with 1- to 2-year delays in the onset of sexual intercourse in high HIV-1 prevalence areas [74]. The practice of nonpenetrative sex may reduce the risk of sexual transmission. There are also behavioral components to the utilization of other preventive measures, such as negotiation with partners about condom use. Finally, mutual fidelity within concordant seronegative couples is an option that minimizes risk.

2. Barrier Contraceptives

Correct use of latex condoms is the most effective means of HIV-1 prevention after abstinence and mutual fidelity [75]. A 100% condom use campaign among sex workers was an important part of an effective HIV-1 reduction program in Thailand [76]. In addition to proven efficacy, advantages of the male condom include low cost and wide availability. However, potential disadvantages of condoms must be considered in light of the specific circumstances of individual women. First, this method

of HIV-1 prevention is not female controlled and it may be difficult for some women to negotiate condom use with their partners. Second, some potential condom users may be concerned about decreases in sensation or adverse consequences in relation to desire and mood. Third, women involved in sex work may be concerned over loss of clients or may receive increased pay for sex without a condom. Finally, latex condoms should not be used with oil-based lubricants, which may increase the risk of condom breakage.

The female condom is a relatively new form of barrier contraception, consisting of a polyurethane sheath with outer and inner rings to assist with fitting and insertion. To date, there are inadequate data on the efficacy of the female condom for HIV-1 prevention. However, because the female condom prevents exposure to semen in a fashion similar to the male condom, it seems plausible that it may be effective in preventing HIV-1 transmission when used correctly. A major advantage of this method is that it is female initiated. In addition, the female condom can be inserted up to several hours before intercourse and may be used with any oil- or water-based lubricant. The disadvantages of the female condom include greater cost, less availability, and similar concerns to the male condom in terms of sensation and mood.

3. Treatment and Prevention of Sexually Transmitted Infections

There is epidemiologic evidence that STIs, particularly genital ulcer disease, frequently precede HIV-1 seroconversion [77]. Although there is likely to be some association because of higher risk individuals being infected with both HIV-1 and another STI, the available evidence suggests an independent effect of STIs on HIV-1 risk [67]. A community-based program for treatment of STIs in Tanzania reduced the incidence of HIV-1 infection by 42% [78]. STIs may increase HIV-1 susceptibility through direct effects on HIV-1 replication, disruption of normal epithelial barriers, and recruitment of HIV-1 susceptible inflammatory cells to the genital mucosa.

Recent data implicate herpes simplex virus type 2 (HSV-2) as an important risk factor for HIV-1 transmission [79]. Women and men who are seropositive for HSV-2 have a much higher risk of also being HIV-1 seropositive [80,81]. Studies are under way to determine whether treatment to reduce the frequency of recurrences of HSV-2 can reduce the risk of acquiring HIV-1.

4. Microbicides

The use of microbicides that inactivate or kill HIV-1 could provide an important female-controlled method of HIV-1 prevention [73]. In contrast to barrier contraceptives, women could potentially use a microbicide without requiring the cooperation of their sexual partner.

Early microbicide research focused on the spermicidal agent nonoxynol-9, with disappointing results [82,83]. Increased transmission of HIV-1 was seen among women using nonoxynol-9, possibly as a result of mucosal irritation or ulceration related to use of the product [84]. However, there are many other potential microbicides. Presently, 56 new products are in various stages of clinical testing [75]. These agents have multiple potential mechanisms of action including creating a physical barrier, inhibiting viral fusion and entry into cells, and providing direct virucidal effects.

B. Postsexual Exposure Prophylaxis

The effectiveness of postsexual exposure prophylaxis for HIV-1 is not known. Despite this, care providers may face questions about postsexual prophylaxis, particularly in the setting of sexual assault [85]. Decisions about the use of antiretroviral medications in this setting must be made on a case-by-case basis. Factors to be considered include the risk of HIV-1 infection in the source, the risk of transmission if the assailant is positive, and the efficacy and safety of postexposure prophylaxis regimens.

The Centers for Disease Control and Prevention (CDC) recommend prophylaxis with zidovudine and lamivudine in cases of sexual assault [86]. The addition of Indinavir, a protease inhibitor, is recommended if the source is infected with HIV-1 resistant to reverse transcriptase inhibitors. Based on experience with occupational exposure, postexposure prophylaxis is most likely to be effective if it can be initiated within 2 hours of exposure, but it may be considered up to 72 hours after exposure. Treatment should be continued for 1 month.

C. Women Who Have Sex with Women

Among women with HIV-1 who report a history of sex with women, the vast majority have additional risk factors including sex with high-risk men, injection drug use, or receipt of blood products [87]. The CDC has reported no confirmed cases of female-to-female sexual transmission. Although transmission by this route would seem to be uncommon, exposure of mucous membranes to infected fluids could allow transmission. Thus, safe sexual practices that minimize the risk of exposure to

potentially infected fluids should be encouraged for women who have sex with women.

D. Reducing the Transmission Risk Associated with Injection Drug Use

The risk of a single exposure to an infected needle has been estimated from data on occupational exposure as close to 3/1000 and increases with large-bore needle stick, visible blood on the needle, deep needle stick, not wearing gloves, and high viral load in the HIV-1 infected index patient [88]. The risk of exposure related to injection drug use is likely to be at least as high as from occupational exposure because the infected needle is frequently inserted directly into a vein. It is also important to keep in mind that IDUs can be exposed to HIV-1 through sharing other injecting equipment including syringes, cookers, and cottons.

Several interventions have demonstrated efficacy in reducing the risk of HIV-1 infection among IDUs [75]. Access to drug treatment programs can reduce drug abuse and HIV-1 transmission, and such programs should remain a high priority for public funding even in difficult economic times. Access to needle-exchange services decreases the rate of HIV-1 infection in IDUs and does not increase the rate of drug use [75]. However, care providers for women should be aware that women are less likely than men to use these services. The harm reduction philosophy holds that IDUs should be instructed in safe injecting practices and counseled to avoid sharing needles or other equipment.

E. The Search for an HIV-1 Vaccine

Novel approaches to vaccine development have generated new hope for the development of an HIV-1 vaccine [75,89]. However, despite some progress, there is little hope that a vaccine will be available for wide-scale use before the end of 2010 [89]. Furthermore, it is possible that initial vaccines against HIV-1 may have only 30–50% efficacy.

Several factors have made the development of a vaccination against HIV-1 a particularly difficult task. Because the virus attacks the immune system, the use of a live attenuated vaccine is potentially unsafe. In addition, it is not known what constitutes a protective immune response against HIV-1, which makes the study of candidate vaccines difficult. Third, there are multiple subtypes of virus, referred to as clades, which differ in their geographic distribution. Locally appropriate vaccines may need to be developed for different parts of the world. Vaccine development must be accompanied by plans for vaccination programs that will make the vaccines available to all who need them.

F. Summary

With the expanding epidemic of HIV-1 among young minority women in the United States, there is an urgent need to provide women with information about the risk of HIV-1 infection and with the information and resources that will allow them to protect themselves. Women's health providers can play an essential role in HIV-1 prevention. They can assist women with recognizing their risk for HIV-1 infection and can offer HIV-1 counseling and testing where appropriate. Providers can also teach women about how HIV-1 is transmitted and provide multiple options for HIV-1 prevention.

From a public health perspective, the increase in HIV-1 infection rates among young minority women should be viewed as a very concerning sign of a worsening epidemic in the United States. Prevention options that are currently available have proven efficacy when implemented as part of an integrated approach to HIV-1. Prevention efforts must be broad based and sustained to succeed [75]. In addition, effective prevention should focus on the populations at greatest risk, including economically and socially disadvantaged, marginalized, or stigmatized groups, and should include interventions for youth. Prevention programs should enlist the help of people living with HIV-1. Political will, leadership, and adequate sustained funding will be essential to reverse the recent and concerning trends in HIV-1 infection among women.

IV. Suggestions for Further Investigations

Biological sex differences relevant to HIV infection are generally under appreciated. However, sex and gender influences the HIV/AIDS pandemic at nearly all levels, including vulnerability to infection, prevention behaviors, disease manifestation and progression, access to treatment, pharmacology of antiretroviral drugs, antiretroviral treatment, and vaccine responses [90]. Major areas with research gaps related to sex and gender have been identified and include [90,91]:

- Normative data for different populations and physiological sites
- Mechanisms of viral transmission that focus on the interaction between the genital tract and immune system
- The effect of sex hormones on transmission, immunology, and vaccine responses throughout the life cycle of men and women

Every effort must be made to encourage interdisciplinary collaborations that recognize the importance of sex-specific studies in HIV virology, immunology, and vaccine development.

References

1. Stringer JR, Beard CB, Miller RF, *et al.* (2002). A new name (*Pneumocystis jiroveci*) for Pneumocystis from humans. *Emerg Infect Dis.* 8:891–896.
2. CDC. Pneumocystis pneumonia—Los Angeles. (1981). *MMWR Morb Mortal Wkly Rep.* 30:250–252.
3. CDC. (1981). Kaposi's sarcoma and pneumocystis pneumonia among homosexual men—New York City and California. *MMWR Morb Mortal Wkly Rep.* 30.
4. CDC. (1981). Follow-up on Kaposi's sarcoma and Pneumocystis pneumonia. *MMWR Morb Mortal Wkly Rep.* 30:409–410.
5. Ho DD, Schooley RT, Rota TR, *et al.* (1984). HTLV-III in the semen and blood of a healthy homosexual man. *Science.* 226:451–453.
6. Zagury D, Bernard J, Leibowitch J, *et al.* (1984). HTLV-III in cells cultured from semen of two patients with AIDS. *Science.* 226:449–451.
7. CDC. (1993). Update: Acquired immunodeficiency syndrome—United States, 1992. *MMWR Morb Mortal Wkly Rep.* 42:547–551, 557.
8. CDC. (1996). *HIV/AIDS Surveillance Report.* Vol 8. Atlanta: U.S. Department of Health and Human Services, Public Health Service, Centers for Disease Control and Prevention.
9. CDC. (2001). *HIV prevalence trends in selected populations in the United States: Results from national serosurveillance, 1993–1997.* Atlanta: Centers for Disease Control and Prevention. 1–51.
10. Neal JJ, Fleming PL, Green TA, *et al.* (1997). Trends in heterosexually acquired AIDS in the United States, 1988 through 1995. *J Acquir Immune Defic Syndr. Hum Retrovirol.* 14:465–474.
11. Carpenter LM, Kamali A, Ruberantwari A, *et al.* (1999). Rates of HIV-1 transmission within marriage in rural Uganda in relation to the HIV sero-status of the partners. *AIDS.* 13:1083–1089.
12. European Study Group. (1992). European Study Group on Heterosexual Transmission of HIV. Comparison of female to male and male to female transmission of HIV in 563 stable couples. *BMJ.* 304:809–813.
13. Lindegren ML, Hanson C, Miller K, *et al.* (1994). Epidemiology of human immunodeficiency virus infection in adolescents, United States. *Pediatr Infect Dis J.* 13:525–535.
14. CDC. (2001). HIV/AIDS Surveillance Report, Vol 13. Atlanta: Department of Health and Human Services, Public Health Service, Centers for Disease Control and Prevention.
15. Karon JM, Fleming PL, Steketee RW, *et al.* (2001). HIV in the United States at the turn of the century: an epidemic in transition. *Am J Public Health.* 91:1060–1068.
16. Smith DK, Gwinn M, Selik RM, *et al.* (2000). HIV/AIDS among African Americans: progress or progression? *AIDS.* 14:1237–1248.
17. Chiu IM, Yaniv A, Dahlberg JE, *et al.* (1985). Nucleotide sequence evidence for relationship of AIDS retrovirus to lentiviruses. *Nature.* 317:366–368.
18. Letvin NL. (1992). Nonhuman primate models for HIV vaccine development. *Immunodefic Rev.* 3:247–260.
19. Gao F, Yue L, White AT, *et al.* (1992). Human infection by genetically diverse SIVSM-related HIV-2 in west Africa. *Nature.* 358:495–499.
20. Ho DD, Neumann AU, Perelson AS, *et al.* (1995). Rapid turnover of plasma virions and CD4 lymphocytes in HIV-1 infection. *Nature.* 373:123–126.
21. Wei X, Ghosh SK, Taylor ME, *et al.* (1995). Viral dynamics in human immunodeficiency virus type 1 infection. *Nature.* 373:117–122.
22. Wong-Staal F, Shaw GM, Hahn BH, *et al.* (1985). Genomic diversity of human T-lymphotropic virus type III (HTLV-III). *Science.* 229:759–762.
23. Brodine SK, Mascola JR, Weiss PJ, *et al.* (1995). Detection of diverse HIV-1 genetic subtypes in the USA. *Lancet.* 346:1198–1199.
24. Alaeus A. (2000). Significance of HIV-1 genetic subtypes. *Scand J Infect Dis.* 32:455–463.
25. Fauci AS, Pantaleo G, Stanley S, *et al.* (1996).Immunopathogenic mechanisms of HIV infection. *Ann Intern Med.* 124:654–663.
26. Long EM, Martin HL Jr, Kreiss JK, *et al.* (2000). Gender differences in HIV-1 diversity at time of infection. *Nat Med.* 6:71–75.
27. Cooper DA, Gold J, Maclean P, *et al.* (1985). Acute AIDS retrovirus infection. Definition of a clinical illness associated with seroconversion. *Lancet.* 1:537–540.
28. Tindall B, Barker S, Donovan B, *et al.* (1988). Characterization of the acute clinical illness associated with human immunodeficiency virus infection. *Arch Intern Med.* 148:945–949.
29. Fox R, Eldred LJ, Fuchs EJ, *et al.* (1987). Clinical manifestations of acute infection with human immunodeficiency virus in a cohort of gay men. *AIDS.* 1:35–38.
30. Schacker T, Collier AC, Hughes J, *et al.* (1996). Clinical and epidemiologic features of primary HIV infection. *Ann Intern Med.* 125:257–264.
31. Kahn JO, Walker BD. (1998). Acute human immunodeficiency virus type 1 infection. *N Engl J Med.* 339:33–39.
32. Quinn TC. (1997). Acute primary HIV infection. *JAMA.* 278:58–62.
33. Vanhems P, Routy JP, Hirschel B, *et al.* (2002). Clinical features of acute retroviral syndrome differ by route of infection but not by gender and age. *J Acquir Immune Defic Syndr.* 31:318–321.
34. Borrow P, Lewicki H, Hahn BH, *et al.* (1994). Virus-specific CD8 + cytotoxic T-lymphocyte activity associated with control of viremia in primary human immunodeficiency virus type 1 infection. *J Virol.* 68:6103–6110.
35. Koup RA, Safrit JT, Cao Y, *et al.* (1994). Temporal association of cellular immune responses with the initial control of viremia in primary human immunodeficiency virus type 1 syndrome. *J Virol.* 68:4650–4655.
36. Musey L, Hughes J, Schacker T, *et al.* (1997). Cytotoxic-T-cell responses, viral load, and disease progression in early human immunodeficiency virus type 1 infection. *N Engl J Med.* 337:1267–1274.
37. Lathey JL, Pratt RD, Spector SA. (1997). Appearance of autologous neutralizing antibody correlates with reduction in virus load and phenotype switch during primary infection with human immunodeficiency virus type 1. *J Infect Dis.* 175:231–232.
38. Henrard DR, Phillips JF, Muenz LR, *et al.* (1995). Natural history of HIV-1 cell-free viremia. *JAMA.* 274:554–558.

39. Schacker T, Zeh J, Hu HL, *et al*. (1998). Frequency of symptomatic and asymptomatic herpes simplex virus type 2 reactivations among human immunodeficiency virus-infected men. *J Infect Dis*. 178:1616–1622.

40. Mellors JW, Rinaldo CR Jr, Gupta P, *et al*. (1996). Prognosis in HIV-1 infection predicted by the quantity of virus in plasma. *Science*. 272:1167–1170.

41. O'Brien TR, Blattner WA, Waters D, *et al*. (1996). Serum HIV-1 RNA levels and time to development of AIDS in the Multicenter Hemophilia Cohort Study. *JAMA*. 276:105–110.

42. Lyles RH, Munoz A, Yamashita TE, *et al*. (2000). Natural history of human immunodeficiency virus type 1 viremia after seroconversion and proximal to AIDS in a large cohort of homosexual men. Multicenter AIDS Cohort Study. *J Infect Dis*. 181:872–880.

43. Farzadegan H, Hoover DR, Astemborski J, *et al*. (1998). Sex differences in HIV-1 viral load and progression to AIDS. *Lancet*. 352:1510–1514.

44. Sterling TR, Vlahov D, Astemborski J, *et al*. (2001). Initial plasma HIV-1 RNA levels and progression to AIDS in women and men. *N Engl J Med*. 344:720–725.

45. Napravnik S, Poole C, Thomas JC, *et al*. (2002). Gender difference in HIV RNA levels: a meta-analysis of published studies. *J Acquir Immune Defic Syndr*. 31:11–19.

46. Yeni PG, Hammer SM, Carpenter CC, *et al*. (2002). Antiretroviral treatment for adult HIV infection in 2002: updated recommendations of the International AIDS Society-USA Panel. *JAMA*. 288:222–235.

47. Collaborative Group on AIDS. (2000). Collaborative Group of AIDS Incubation and Survival. Time from HIV-1 seroconversion to AIDS and death before widespread use of highly-active antiretroviral therapy: a collaborative re-analysis. *Lancet*. 355:1131–1137.

48. Hanson DL, Chu SY, Farizo KM, *et al*. (1995). Distribution of CD4+ T lymphocytes at diagnosis of acquired immunodeficiency syndrome-defining and other human immunodeficiency virus-related illnesses. The Adult and Adolescent Spectrum of HIV Disease Project Group. *Arch Intern Med*. 155:1537–1542.

49. Fauci AS. (1988). The human immunodeficiency virus: infectivity and mechanisms of pathogenesis. *Science*. 239:617–622.

50. Chaisson RE, Keruly JC, Moore RD. (1995). Race, sex, drug use, and progression of human immunodeficiency virus disease. *N Engl J Med*. 333:751–756.

51. Coombs RW, Reichelderfer PS, Landay AL. (2003). Recent observations on HIV type-1 infection in the genital tract of men and women. *AIDS*. 17:455–480.

52. Greenblatt RM, Ameli N, Grant RM, *et al*. (2000). Impact of the ovulatory cycle on virologic and immunologic markers in HIV-infected women. *J Infect Dis*. 181:82–90.

53. Reichelderfer PS, Coombs RW, Wright DJ, *et al*. (2000). Effect of menstrual cycle on HIV-1 levels in the peripheral blood and genital tract. WHS 001 Study Team. *AIDS*. 14:2101–2107.

54. Al-Harthi L, Kovacs A, Coombs RW, *et al*. (2001). A menstrual cycle pattern for cytokine levels exists in HIV-positive women: implication for HIV vaginal and plasma shedding. *AIDS*. 15:1535–1543.

55. Zhu T, Wang N, Carr A, *et al*. (1996). Genetic characterization of human immunodeficiency virus type 1 in blood and genital secretions: evidence for viral compartmentalization and selection during sexual transmission. *J Virol*. 70:3098–3107.

56. Ellerbrock TV, Lennox JL, Clancy KA, *et al*. (2001). Cellular replication of human immunodeficiency virus type 1 occurs in vaginal secretions. *J Infect Dis*. 184:28–36.

57. O'Brien WA, Hartigan PM, Martin D, *et al*. (1996). Changes in plasma HIV-1 RNA and CD4+ lymphocyte counts and the risk of progression to AIDS. Veterans Affairs Cooperative Study Group on AIDS. *N Engl J Med*. 334:426–431.

58. Palella FJ Jr, Delaney KM, Moorman AC, *et al*. (1998). Declining morbidity and mortality among patients with advanced human immunodeficiency virus infection. HIV Outpatient Study Investigators. *N Engl J Med*. 338:853–860.

59. Egger M, May M, Chene G, *et al*. (2002). Prognosis of HIV-1-infected patients starting highly active antiretroviral therapy: a collaborative analysis of prospective studies. *Lancet*. 360:119–129.

60. Egger M, Chene G, Sterne JA, *et al*. (2003). Prognostic importance of initial response in HIV-1 infected patients starting potent antiretroviral therapy: analysis of prospective studies. *Lancet*. 362:679–686.

61. Moore AL, Mocroft A, Madge S, *et al*. (2001). Gender differences in virologic response to treatment in an HIV-positive population: a cohort study. *J Acquir Immune Defic Syndr*. 26:159–163.

62. Fellay J, Marzolini C, Meaden ER, *et al*. (2002). Response to antiretroviral treatment in HIV-1-infected individuals with allelic variants of the multidrug resistance transporter 1: a pharmacogenetics study. *Lancet*. 359:30–36.

63. Valdez H, Purvis SF, Lederman MM, *et al*. (1999). Association of the CCR5delta32 mutation with improved response to antiretroviral therapy. *JAMA*. 282:734.

64. Lurie P, Miller S, Hecht F, *et al*. (1998). Postexposure prophylaxis after non-occupational HIV exposure: clinical, ethical, and policy considerations. *JAMA*. 280:1769–1773.

65. Mastro TD, de Vincenzi I. (1996). Probabilities of sexual HIV-1 transmission. *AIDS*. 10 Suppl A:S75–82.

66. Quinn TC. (1996). Global burden of the HIV pandemic. *Lancet*. 348:99–106.

67. Martin HL Jr, Nyange PM, Richarson BA, *et al*. (1998). Hormonal contraception, sexually transmitted diseases, and risk of heterosexual transmission of human immunodeficiency virus type 1. *J Infect Dis*. 178:1053–1059.

68. Moss GB, Clemetson D, D'Costa L, *et al*. (1991). Association of cervical ectopy with heterosexual transmission of human immunodeficiency virus: results of a study of couples in Nairobi, Kenya. *J Infect Dis*. 164: 588–591.

69. Martin HL, Richardson BA, Nyange PM, *et al*. (1999). Vaginal lactobacilli, microbial flora, and risk of human immunodeficiency virus type 1 and sexually transmitted disease acquisition. *J Infect Dis*. 180:1863–1868.

70. Quinn TC, Wawer MJ, Sewankambo N, *et al*. (2000). Viral load and heterosexual transmission of human immunodeficiency virus type 1. Rakai Project Study Group. *N Engl J Med*. 342:921–929.

71. Kapiga SH, Lyamuya EF, Lwihula GK, *et al*. (1998). The incidence of HIV infection among women using family planning methods in Dar es Salaam, Tanzania. *AIDS*. 12:75–84.

72. Musicco M, Lazzarin A, Nicolosi A, *et al*. (1994). Antiretroviral treatment of men infected with human immunodeficiency virus type 1 reduces the incidence of heterosexual transmission. Italian Study Group on HIV Heterosexual Transmission. *Arch Intern Med*. 154:1971–1976.

73. van de Wijgert J, Coggins C. (2002). Microbicides to prevent heterosexual transmission of HIV: ten years down the road. *Beta*. 15:23–28.

74. Buve A, Carael M, Hayes RJ, *et al*. (2001). Multicentre study on factors determining differences in rate of spread of HIV in sub-Saharan Africa: methods and prevalence of HIV infection. *AIDS*. 15 Suppl 4:S5–14.

75. UNAIDS. (2002). Report on the global HIV/AIDS epidemic. *UNAIDS*. 1–226.

76. UNAIDS. (2001). *AIDS Epidemic Update*. 1–36.

77. Wasserheit JN. (1992). Epidemiological synergy. Interrelationships between human immunodeficiency virus infection and other sexually transmitted diseases. *Sex Transm Dis*. 19:61–77.

78. Grosskurth H, Mosha F, Todd J, *et al*. (1995). Impact of improved treatment of sexually transmitted diseases on HIV infection in rural Tanzania: randomised controlled trial. *Lancet*. 346:530–536.

79. Wald A, Link K. (2002). Risk of human immunodeficiency virus infection in herpes simplex virus type 2-seropositive persons: a meta-analysis. *J Infect Dis*. 185:45–52.

80. Auvert B, Ballard R, Campbell C, *et al*. (2001). HIV infection among youth in a South African mining town is associated with herpes simplex virus-2 seropositivity and sexual behaviour. *AIDS*. 15:885–898.

81. Weiss HA, Buve A, Robinson NJ, *et al*. (2001). The epidemiology of HSV-2 infection and its association with HIV infection in four urban African populations. *AIDS*. 15 Suppl 4:S97–108.

82. Kreiss J, Ngugi E, Holmes K, *et al*. (1992). Efficacy of nonoxynol 9 contraceptive sponge use in preventing heterosexual acquisition of HIV in Nairobi prostitutes. *JAMA*. 268:477–482.

83. Roddy RE, Zekeng L, Ryan KA, *et al*. (1998). A controlled trial of nonoxynol 9 film to reduce male-to-female transmission of sexually transmitted diseases. *N Engl J Med*. 339:504–510.

84. Stafford MK, Ward H, Flanagan A, *et al*. (1998). Safety study of nonoxynol-9 as a vaginal microbicide: evidence of adverse effects. *J Acquir Immune Defic Syndr. Hum Retrovirol*. 17:327–331.

85. Fong C. (2001). Post-exposure prophylaxis for HIV infection after sexual assault: when is it indicated? *Emerg Med J*. 18:242–245.

86. Bamberger JD, Waldo CR, Gerberding JL, *et al*. (1999). Postexposure prophylaxis for human immunodeficiency virus (HIV) infection following sexual assault. *Am J Med*. 106:323–326.

87. CDC. HIV/AIDS and U.S. (1999). Women who have sex with women. At: http://www.cdc.gov/hiv/pubs/facts/wsw.htm.

88. CDC. (1995). Case-control study of HIV seroconversion in health-care workers after percutaneous exposure to HIV-infected blood—France, United Kingdom, and United States, January 1988–August 1994. *MMWR Morb Mortal Wkly Rep*. 44:929–933.

89. Ho DD, Huang Y. (2002). The HIV-1 vaccine race. *Cell*.110:135–138.

90. Forum for Collaborative HIV Research. (2002). Sex and gender issues in HIV disease. At: http://www.hivforum.org.

91. National Institutes of Health Fiscal Year 2003 Plan for HIV-Related Research. (2003). At: http://www.nih.gov/od/oar.

86

Gender-Specific Issues in the Metabolic Complications of HIV Disease and Its Treatment

MARISA TUNGSIRIPAT-GERBER, MD* AND JUDITH A. ABERG, MD**

*Washington University School of Medicine, St. Louis, MO
**Associate Professor of Medicine, Principal Investigator AIDS Clinical Trials Unit, New York, NY

I. Introduction

Women continue to be the fastest-growing segment of adults with acquired immune deficiency syndrome (AIDS) in the United States. In 2000, 25% of new AIDS cases were in women [1]. Studies done in the mid-1980s suggested that the prognosis for women was significantly less than for men. These studies, however, really were a marker for poor access to care and late diagnosis. Although a few studies have demonstrated that the plasma human immunodeficiency virus (HIV) viral load is less in women than in age-matched men, there are no data to demonstrate a gender difference in prognosis or progression of HIV [2,3]. Nevertheless, gender-specific issues affect HIV disease and its treatment. Perhaps not the least significant of the gender issues are the nonmedical issues. Many biologic and social theories exist for possible causes that make women more vulnerable to HIV infection than men. Fear, isolation, and lack of information remain key factors contributing to the increase in heterosexual acquisition of HIV, especially among women with color. Socioeconomic constraints may place women at harm as they exchange sex for material goods for themselves and their children. Despite these aspects, relatively less is known about HIV and its impact on women because women tend to be less likely to participate in research. For example, in 1997, only 12% of the National Institute of Allergy and Infectious Disease's AIDS Clinical Trials Group (ACTG) trial subjects in non–pregnancy-related trials were women [4].

The intent of this chapter is to focus on the medical aspects in which gender affects the metabolic complications of HIV disease. The gender-specific issues regarding HIV pathogenesis will be excluded because they will be addressed in a separate chapter. There are numerous case reports and descriptions of the complications of HIV and its treatment, but much remains unknown and even less is known about the gender differences. This chapter summarizes some of the current descriptions and controversies regarding the metabolic complications of HIV and HIV therapy. Specific metabolic syndromes reviewed in this chapter are lipodystrophy, glucose intolerance, hyperlipidemia, lactate acidosis, and bone demineralization.

II. Lipodystrophy

The term lipodystrophy often is used to describe any alteration in the distribution of adipose tissue in individuals with HIV. For our discussion,/ we will use that definition. Some experts use the term more broadly to encompass all of the potentially associated metabolic abnormalities and not just fat redistribution.

It remains unclear whether there is one syndrome with phenotypic variations or multiple unrelated subsyndromes. The prevalence of fat redistribution has been reported in 2–84% of individuals with HIV [5]. The lack of a standard definition likely accounts for much of the wide variation in prevalence. Both central obesity and peripheral fat wasting are observed in the setting of normal adrenal function [6]. Lipohypertrophy refers to central obesity, visceral fat accumulation, dorsocervical fat accumulation or "buffalo hump," breast enlargement, and benign lipomatosis [7]. Lipoatrophy refers to peripheral fat wasting, which is characterized as loss of buttock fat, loss of subcutaneous fat in the extremities with venous prominence, and facial thinning.

In addition to initial reports describing these observations in male patients, these findings have also been specifically described in women [8]. Changes in body habitus have been reported in a study of 21 women undergoing highly active antiretroviral therapy (HAART) [9]. Carpenter et al published a study of 21 women with self-reported changes in body habitus and a control group who were followed for 3.5 years. The women were evaluated by physical examination, anthropometric measurements, serum lipid assays, and endocrine assays over 3.5 years to address the issue of the timing of the morphologic changes in women undergoing HAART. Although morphologic changes were described over the first year the affected individuals were evaluated, in 10 of the 14 patients who were available for follow-up, changes in body habitus were stable over the subsequent 2.5 years [10]. Galli et al have reported evidence for correlation between gender and the morphologic alterations of fat redistribution. In a study of 2258 patients by a multivariate analysis including duration of antiretroviral therapy, age, viral load, and use of combination antiretroviral therapy, female gender was the strongest independent risk factor associated with an increased risk of development of a morphologic abnormality [11]. At least one morphologic abnormality was seen in 33.2% of the patients in this study. The morphologic abnormalities of abdominal fat accumulation, buffalo hump, and fat loss in legs, glutei, arms, and neck all showed a strong statistical correlation with female gender. In this study there was no significant gender difference in lipoatrophy, but there was a significant increase in women with fat accumulation and having both fat accumulation and lipoatrophy as defined by patient self-report and confirmed by physician physical examination.

Because the syndrome of lipodystrophy was identified at approximately the same time as the widespread use of protease inhibitors (PIs), the pathogenesis of lipodystrophy was initially attributed to PIs. Lipodystrophy has been described as an association with all PIs [12,13]. However, the first case of a patient developing a buffalo hump was reported prior to the introduction of HAART [6,14]. Subsequently, the syndrome of lipodystrophy also has been described in patients naïve to PIs [8]. Furthermore, lipodystrophy also has been directly associated with nucleoside analogue reverse transcriptase inhibitors (NRTIs) [15–17].

HIV itself in the absence of HAART has also been associated with lipoatrophy. This hypothesis is supported by the HIV Outpatient Study (HOPS) data. Lichtenstein *et al* prospectively evaluated a cohort of 337 individuals with HIV for the development of lipoatrophy over 21 months. Forty-four patients (13.1%) developed lipoatrophy by diagnosis, based on a standardized interview and physician assessment. Patients with a CD4+ T-cell count consistently less than 200 cells/mm^3 were reported to have a relatively high rate of lipoatrophy (30.8%). They also found no association between lipoatrophy and antiretroviral medication [18].

Studies have also been severely limited by the lack of diagnostic criteria of lipodystrophy. Many of the studies depend on either patient self-report, physician subjective assessment, or a combination of patient/physician report. Although dual-energy x-ray absorptiometry (DEXA), computerized tomography (CT), and magnetic resonance imaging have been evaluated, no objective variable is consistently reliable for the diagnosis of lipodystrophy. In central obesity, a waist-to-hip ratio greater than 0.85 in women is associated with increased adverse outcomes, including cardiovascular disease [19]. An abdominal circumference of greater than 102 cm in men and 88 cm in women is advocated by some in the National Cholesterol Education Program (NCEP) treatment guidelines as a better tool because waist-to-hip ratios can be increased by a decreased hip circumference [19]. The ratio of greater that 0.4 of intraabdominal to total abdominal adipose tissue area has been to proposed identify lipodystrophy by CT [20]; however, variability in technique makes it difficult to use. DEXA cannot discriminate between intraabdominal and subcutaneous adiposity. There are no widely accepted diagnostic definitions for dorsocervical fat pads and benign symmetric lipomatosis.

There are no known therapies. Current strategies include stopping the offending agent or switching antiretroviral therapy, but this remains problematic because the exact offending agents(s) is or are not known. Multiple studies of antiretroviral "switching" to evaluate lipodystrophy have demonstrated favorable virologic and immunologic outcomes; however, these studies are limited by subjective endpoints of self-report or physician assessment for measuring the effects on lipodystrophy [21]. To date, only one study has clearly demonstrated an improvement in lipodystrophy. Carr *et al* evaluated 111 individuals with HIV and lipoatrophy who were undergoing antiretroviral therapy regimens including zidovudine or stavudine. The subjects were randomly assigned to switch from the zidovudine or stavudine to abacavir while continuing all other antiretroviral therapy without change. They found a significant increase in limb fat in the abacavir group in comparison to the placebo group by DEXA measurement of limb fat mass [22]. In addition, dietary modifications, exercise, insulin-sensitizing agents, anabolic steroids, and cosmetic surgery have all been tried as therapeutic interventions [13].

III. Glucose Intolerance

Glucose intolerance has been associated with HIV and/or its therapy. The following definitions according to the American Diabetes Association for a non-HIV population are also used in the HIV-positive population [23]. Insulin resistance is defined as a condition in which higher than normal concentrations of insulin are needed to exert its normal physiologic effects. The term impaired glucose tolerance is defined as an elevated blood sugar of 140–199 mg/dL measured 2 hours after a 75-g oral glucose load, as given in a glucose tolerance test. Impaired fasting glucose refers to a fasting blood sugar level in the 110–125 mg/dL range. Diabetes mellitus is a fasting blood sugar greater than or equal to 126 or a 2-hour glucose level greater than or equal to 200 in a glucose tolerance test.

From an epidemiologic standpoint, individuals with HIV may be at a higher risk for diabetes than HIV-negative counterparts. Currier *et al* studied incidence rates of diabetes mellitus in men and women older than age 18 with and without HIV. They reported that individuals with HIV were 3.32 times more likely to have diabetes [24]. Hadigan *et al* also described that patients with lipodystrophy were more likely to have impaired glucose tolerance and diabetes than controls. This study evaluated the metabolic and clinical features of 71 individuals with HIV compared with 213 healthy control subjects who were matched for age and body mass index. The measured parameters in this study were fasting glucose, insulin, lipid levels, oral glucose tolerance tests, and anthropometric measurements [25].

All PIs may be associated with hyperglycemia, hyperlipidemia, or both. In fact, up to 40% of patients taking PI-containing regimens will have impaired glucose tolerance [26]. Two published studies described 6–7% of subjects given PIs developed symptomatic diabetes mellitus and 16% developed impaired glucose tolerance [27,28].

Much remains unknown regarding the pathogenesis of glucose intolerance as it relates to HIV and its therapy. The proposed pathogenesis is by the direct effect of PIs on the impairment of glucose tolerance. Possible indirect mechanisms may be related to fat redistribution. One hypothesis of the mechanism of indinavir-induced insulin resistance is inhibition of cellular glucose uptake by interfering with the cellular glucose transporter Glut-4 and/or inhibition of peroxisome proliferator activated receptor-gamma (PPAR-gamma) expression [29,30]. However, the PIs amprenavir and atazanavir do not appear to directly induce insulin resistance [31,32]. "Non-HIV" risk factors may also play a role in the development of diabetes in patients with HIV. Yoon *et al* found in a case-control study that traditional diabetes mellitus risk factors of body mass index, family history, and alanine aminotransferase levels were associated with diabetes by multivariate analysis. Hepatitis C virus coinfection and prior or current PI usage was found to be more common in cases than controls [33].

According to the International AIDS Society-USA (IAS-USA) guidelines, screening fasting glucose levels are recommended prior to initiation of HAART, including PIs, every 3–6 months after initiating therapy and annually thereafter [26]. Falutz *et al* report that the oral glucose tolerance test (OGTT) may be the most reliable screening test [34]. The routine use of the OGTT for screening, however, may be limited by practical implications in a clinical setting.

Although IAS-USA guidelines for the metabolic complications of HIV exist, the text of the guidelines themselves point out that the recommendations are based on expert opinion and extrapolation from data from the HIV-negative population. Diet, exercise, and insulin-sensitizing medications such as metformin or thiazolidinedione are recommended therapeutic options. Sulfonureas are potential therapeutic options; however, in the IAS-USA guidelines, they are noted as being potentially not as useful because the mechanism of glucose intolerance in HIV is thought to be insulin resistance. Additional options include avoiding or substituting alternatives to PI, especially in patients with preexisting abnormalities of blood glucose or risk factors for diabetes mellitus [26,35–37].

Many unanswered questions exist. Insulin resistance in HIV-negative individuals is associated with increased cardiovascular complications. It is not clear whether in individuals who are HIV-positive if a drug-induced or lipodystrophy-associated insulin resistance would have the same effect. It is not known if the individuals with insulin resistance will ultimately develop frank diabetes mellitus. Furthermore, the role of treatment of individuals with elevated insulin levels in the presence of normal fasting blood sugar is not clarified because the clinical significance of this is not known.

IV. Dyslipidemia

The development of dyslipidemia has been associated with HIV disease and its therapy. The question regarding whether individuals with HIV are at risk of developing coronary heart disease (CHD) and subsequent myocardial infarction (MI) remains unanswered. The data available on the development of CHD are limited by its retrospective nature, short duration of follow-up, potential confounding factors, and biased ascertainment. We will review select publications to demonstrate the current knowledge of this field as well as to emphasize the need for prospective longitudinal observational cohort studies addressing these issues.

There have been a few retrospective cohort studies to evaluate the risk of CHD and whether it can be attributed to HIV or its treatments. A study by Klein et al reviewed a Kaiser Permanente dataset for CHD-related ICD-9 primary discharge diagnosis codes among 4159 patients with HIV compared with 39,877 patients not known to be infected with HIV. CHD rates were higher in men with HIV versus the control group. The difference in rates was 6.5 events/1000 person years in men with HIV vs 3.8 events/1000 person years in controls [38]. Mary-Krause et al reported a dose-related higher MI incidence rate in their study cohort who had been exposed to PIs. Fifty-four patients were diagnosed with MI of 19,795 men exposed to PIs in the French Hospital Database. Of these patients, the highest MI incidence rates were noted among the cohort patients who were exposed to PIs for at least 18 months [39]. In contrast, Bozzette et al found no association between antiretroviral therapy and cardiovascular or cerebrovascular morbidity and mortality in their analysis of the Veterans Administration (VA) cohort. They analyzed the data of 36,766 individuals with HIV from the Immunology Case Registry of the VA AIDS Service; other VA databases; and the national death index for hospital admissions, cardiovascular and cerebrovascular events, and all-cause mortality. They noted that although the use of antiretroviral therapy increased over time, the rates of cardiovascular and cerebrovascular events and overall mortality declined [40].

The increased risk for progression of ischemic cardiovascular disease has been described prospectively. Wall et al followed 111 individuals with HIV and 25 controls for measurement of cardiovascular risk by ATP3 Framingham score. The median risk for progression of CHD in 10 years was 4% in the HIV-infected cohort and 1% in the HIV-negative cohort [41]. Specifically in females, Pernerstorfer-Schoen et al have described that although the female gender typically has a lower low-density lipoprotein:high-density lipoprotein (LDL:HDL) ratio than males and similar baseline levels of triglycerides (TG) to males, in AIDS the initiation of combined antiretroviral therapy increased the LDL:HDL: ratio, serum triglycerides, and serum insulin levels specifically in the female subjects with HIV [42]. On the contrary, the ES40002 study presented by Kumar demonstrated that the men were much more likely to have increased LDL and TG levels. Kumar et al reported significant increases in LDL and total cholesterol of subjects taking PI-containing regimens compared with subjects on all-nucleoside-containing regimens [43].

All PIs have been implicated to increase total cholesterol, LDL, and TG levels, but there appears to be significant differences among them with atazanavir showing little effect, indinavir increasing LDL and insulin, and ritonavir increasing TG. There have also been studies suggesting that the NRTIs and non-nucleoside analogue reverse transcriptase inhibitors (NNRTIs) may also play a role. Association of PIs with lipid alterations have been described at the 9th Conference on Retroviruses and Opportunistic Infections. Van Leth et al reported that patients undergoing NRTI- and NNRTI-containing regimens were less likely to have dyslipidemia and had a 2.09-fold chance of having an elevated HDL-c when compared to patients undergoing PI-containing regimens [44]. However, in the ES40002 study, the switch from zidovudine to stavudine resulted in increased LDL and TG levels [43].

These studies do not address if the increase in lipid translates into increased cardiovascular risk. Holmberg et al, Mary-Krause et al, and Wall et al have all described increased MI incidence rates in association with patients taking PIs [39,41,45]. However, Mauss et al propose that a large subgroup of patients with hypercholesterolemia undergoing antiretroviral therapy may have a lower cardiovascular risk than previously expected. The analysis of very-low-density lipoprotein (VLDL) composition in this subgroup of patients revealed a large TG-rich VLDL particle that resembled particles found in familial hypertriglyceridemia, which is associated with low coronary, risk rather than particles found in familial combined hyperlipidemia, which is associated with high risk for coronary artery disease [46].

One proposed etiology of lipid alterations in HIV is related to circulating cell adhesion molecules (CAMS). Increased CAMS have been associated with coronary disease and cerebrovascular disease in the general population. Increased concentrations of CAMS have been described in women with HIV by Bausserman *et al* [47]. Another proposed etiology for the alteration in lipid status with HIV is genetic susceptibility. Individuals with apolipoprotein E-2 genotype have higher triglyceride levels and may subsequently be predisposed to dramatic changes in cholesterol and TG levels with exposure to antiretroviral therapy [26].

Elevated C-reactive protein (CRP) levels are markers of inflammation that have been associated with an increase in CHD risk in the general population. Furthermore, data in a recently published study by Ridker *et al* of apparently healthy women suggest that CRP is a stronger predictor of cardiovascular events than the LDL cholesterol [48]. In the HIV population, Henry *et al* reported observations of elevated CRP levels in a cohort of virologically suppressed HIV-infected individuals when compared with expected values from the general population [49]. In this study, CRP levels were also associated with increased age, higher fibrinogen levels, lower HDL levels, higher TG levels, higher insulin levels, and higher Framingham CHD scores.

The recommended evaluation for dyslipidemia is a fasting lipid profile prior to initiation of antiretroviral therapy and a fasting lipid profile 3 months after initiation of therapy. The fasting lipid profile is recommended to be repeated yearly if the 3-month value is within normal limits. There are no guidelines for therapy specifically for the individual with HIV. Beyond NCEP guidelines for the general population are proposed interventions of switching antiretroviral therapy and lipid-lowering therapy.

Treatment of lipid-lowering agents according to NCEP guidelines is complicated by interactions with antiretroviral medication. The concern is that many "statins" as well as PIs and NNRTIs are metabolized by the cytochrome P450 CYP34A isoenzymes, which could result in excessively high levels of statins, placing patients at risk for developing rhabdomyolysis. Pravastatin starting at 20 mg/day is a preferred choice because it does not have significant cytochrome P450 interactions [50]. Atorvastatin starting at 10 mg/day is the recommended agent by the ACTG expert committee for concurrent use with PI and NNRTI [51]. Concurrent use is felt to be acceptable with indinavir, saquinavir, ritonavir, and amprenavir. Fichtenbaum *et al* described that in the presence of ritonavir/saquinavir, atorvastatin acid levels increased by 347% and total active atorvastatin levels increased by 79%, simvastatin acid levels increased by 3059%, and pravastatin levels decreased by 47% [53].

Fibrates have been described to be safe for use in patients with PI-associated hypertriglyceridemia. [54]. The ACTG 5087 trial evaluated the efficacy and safety of fenofibrate compared with pravastatin in a prospective trial of 174 subjects. The subjects were initially randomized to either agent alone then treated with both agents after 12 weeks if the subject had not achieved NCEP goals. The study found that although monotherapy with pravastatin or fenofibrate alone was safe, it was not likely to be effective in achieving NCEP goals. The data for dual therapy at 28 weeks, however, showed significant additional lipid-lowering activity, especially in subjects who were initially randomized to fenofibrate [55]. Bile sequestrants are not recommended because of the potential for interference with drug absorption of antiretroviral medication. Niacin is not recommended because of its potential for worsening insulin resistance pending results of pilot safety and tolerability trials.

Studies "switching" a PI for abacavir, efavirenz, and nevirapine have shown mixed results [21]. The largest switch study with metabolic data to date was presented by Fisac *et al*. The study described 92 patients who switched from a PI regimen to three different randomized PI-sparing regimens. The 12-month data showed an improvement in lipid profile in all three arms [56]. A promising option is Atazanavit, a PI that has been shown to have a superior lipid profile to current PIs [57,58].

V. Lactic Acidosis

Hyperlactatemia and lactate acidosis have been associated with HIV disease and its therapy. Hyperlactatemia is defined as higher than 2 mmol/mL with or without acidosis. This is often accompanied by microvesicular steatosis of the liver as demonstrated by CT or biopsy [59]. Nucleoside metabolic dysfunction syndrome is defined as lactic acidosis, peripheral wasting, lipoatrophy, abdominal distension, weight loss, fatigue, nausea, and abdominal pain. Abnormal liver function tests are common. The spectrum of disease can range from asymptomatic hyperlactatemia to life-threatening lactic acidosis.

The incidence of hyperlactatemia has been reported at 1.3 per 1000 patient years [60]. Although lactic acidosis and hyperlactatemia can occur with all NRTIs, stavudine, didanosine (DDI), and zalcitabine (ddC) are the most common offenders.

Female gender specifically has been found to have a predisposition for life-threatening lactate acidosis in case reports [61]. Fatal lactic acidosis and steatosis have been specifically described in pregnant women receiving d4T and DDI [62].

Other predisposing factors to hyperlactatemia and lactate acidosis include age, obesity, and ethanol intake. Age is thought to result in cumulative oxidative damage to mitochondria and therefore predisposes patients to mitochondrial dysfunction. Obesity has been shown to lead to uncoupling of oxidative phosphorylation from the respiratory chain and reduce the efficiency of adenosine triphosphate (ATP) synthesis by the electron transport chain. Ethanol has been shown to induce ultrastructural changes in hepatic mitochondria and to induce fatty liver. This may be synergistic with NRTIs.

The proposed pathogenesis of NRTI-associated hyperlactatemia is via mitochondrial dysfunction. Although the therapeutic target of NRTIs is HIV reverse transcriptase, they also inhibit mitochondrial DNA (mtDNA) polymerase gamma. This inhibition of mtDNA polymerase gamma can lead to impairment of the ability of the mitochondria to provide ATP to the cell by inhibiting the electron transport and oxidative phosphorylation pathways. Tissues that transport and phosphorylate NRTIs or rely heavily on mitochondrial oxidative phosphorylation will accumulate the largest number of mtDNA polymerase gamma impairments and therefore would be predisposed to the most toxicity. In settings of impaired oxygen delivery and impaired mitochondrial function, ATP production switches to anaerobic glycolysis. This is less efficient and can sustain metabolism for only a short period. Lactate eventually forms, accumulates, and diffuses out to the systemic circulation. Lactate acidosis occurs as the utilization of ATP produced by this pathway liberates hydrogen ions, leading to a drop in pH.

The diagnosis of nucleoside metabolic dysfunction syndrome is made by an elevated lactate level in the setting of an appropriate clinical syndrome. The primary therapeutic intervention is cessation of nucleoside analogue. The lactate acidemia typically resolves over 3–6 months. No specific treatment guidelines are available because there are not enough available data. Suggestions from anecdotal reports advocate thiamine; riboflavin [63]; L-carnitine [64]; coenzyme-Q; and vitamins C, E, and A.

VI. Bone Demineralization

Osteoporosis disproportionately affects women in the general population. Osteoporosis occurs in approximately 25% of women and 13% of men older than age 50 years in the United States [65]. Female gender is a major risk factor for osteoporosis [65]. Bone disorders including avascular necrosis have been described in association with HIV and its treatment [66].

Bone demineralization is further classified as osteopenia and osteoporosis. A Working Group of the World Health Organization (WHO) gives the following definitions for bone demineralization by T-score measurements from DEXA scan [67]. DEXA results are typically expressed in T-scores and Z-scores. The T-score is the score given to a bone mineral density (BMD) measurement when compared with the BMD values from sex-matched reference population of approximately 30 years of age. The Z-score is a similar score, but the measurements are compared with a sex- and age-matched reference population. The T-score is the score that is routinely used to diagnose osteoporosis.

Osteopenia is defined as a T-score as measured by between 1 standard deviation and 2.5 standard deviations below the mean peak value in young adults. Osteoporosis is a T-score lower than 2.5 standard deviations below the mean peak value in young adults. A limitation of the DEXA scan is a variability of 3–6% in the reproducibility of DEXA results because of differences in technique, machine reading, and technologist. Established osteoporosis is osteoporosis in the presence of fragility fractures.

Changes in bone mineralization have been reported to be more prevalent in individuals with HIV than in individuals without HIV. Romeyn et al were among the first to describe this alteration of bone demineralization in 1999. A study of 20 men who were HIV-positive described nine men (46%) with evidence of osteopenia and eight men (40%) with evidence of osteoporosis [68]. Tebas et al described in a study of 64 male and female patients that subjects on regimens including PIs had a higher incidence of osteopenia and osteoporosis by WHO definitions [69]. Mondy et al presented a longitudinal cohort study with 128 patients with HIV that found that 47% of the subjects had osteopenia or osteoporosis. There was no reported association of antiretroviral class, however [70].

In addition to the described association of bone loss and PIs, greater-than-expected bone demineralization has also been described in studies presented at the 8th CROI of individuals with HIV naïve to therapy [71,72]. Thus, it is less clear if the primary mechanism of bone demineralization is the result of HIV or its treatment.

In addition to the described association of osteoporosis with HIV, a number of traditional "non-HIV" risk factors for osteoporosis have been described. The National Osteoporosis Foundation lists the following factors to identify women as individuals at risk for fracture: low body weight (<58 kg), current smoker, first-degree relative with low-trauma fracture, and personal history of low-trauma factor [73]. Other known risk factors include female gender, increasing age, race/ethnicity, alcohol usage, caffeine intake, lack of weight-bearing exercise, low estrogen in women, low testosterone levels in men, and medication use [65]. Aniston et al described that PI use is independently associated with decreased bone mineral density in females with HIV [74]. However, it is important to note that perimenopausal women who were HIV-seronegative had higher rates of osteoporosis compared with women who were HIV-positive.

The mechanism of bone loss in osteoporosis relates to the coupling process of bone remodeling. Bone is remodeled continuously during adulthood through the resorption of old bone by osteoclasts and the subsequent formation of new bone by osteoblasts. In osteoporosis, a reduction of skeletal mass is caused by an imbalance between bone resorption and bone formation. Starting around the fourth or fifth decade of life, both men and women lose bone at a rate of 0.3–0.5% per year [75].

Although many theories exist, the pathogenesis of how HIV or PI therapy specifically affects bone demineralization is not known. Hypogonadism, deficiencies of growth hormone levels, deficiencies of insulin-like growth factor (IGF)-1, and high cytokine levels have been postulated to be the cause of HIV-associated osteoporosis because these alterations have been shown in individuals positive for HIV [65].

Currently recommendations for therapy of osteoporosis specifically in individuals with HIV have not yet been defined. As in HIV-negative individuals, elimination of modifiable risk factors of smoking, physical inactivity, and malnutrition have been advocated. Calcium (1000 mg/day) and vitamin D (400–1000 IU/day) should be part of the treatment regimen. As in HIV-negative populations, bisphosphonates, hormone replacement therapy, and calcitonin have been used to treat osteoporosis. Specifically in individuals with HIV, switching antiretroviral therapy has been suggested. Because it remains unclear which agent(s) is/are responsible, no recommendations regarding altering HIV therapy solely to affect bone demineralization can be made.

VII. Suggestions for Further Investigations

- Do HIV-associated metabolic complications translate into increased risk of development of cardiovascular or cerebrovascular disease?
- Case reports of life-threatening hyperlactatemia have been described in females more than males. Why?
- What is the etiology of HIV-associated fat redistribution?
- How is HIV-associated osteopenia and osteoporosis in females affected by menopause?

References

1. Summary of notifiable diseases—United States, 2000. (2002). *MMWR Morb Mortal Wkly Rep.* 49:i–xxii, 1–100.
2. Sterling TR, Vlahov D, Astemborski J, *et al.* (2001). Initial plasma HIV-1 RNA levels and progression to AIDS in women and men. *N Engl J Med.* 344:720–725.
3. Moore RD, Cheever L, Keruly JC, *et al.* (1999). Lack of sex difference in CD4 to HIV-1 RNA viral load ratio. *Lancet.* 353:463–464.

4. Newman M, Wofsy CB. (1999). Women and HIV Disease. In: Sande MA, Volberding P, eds. *The Medial Management of AIDS*. Philadelphia: WB Saunders Company, 537–554.

5. Safrin S, Grunfeld C. (1999). Fat distribution and metabolic changes in patients with HIV infection. *AIDS*. 13:2493–2505.

6. Lo JC, Mulligan K, Tai VW, *et al*. (1998). "Buffalo hump" in men with HIV-1 infection. *Lancet*. 351:867–870.

7. Dank JP, Colven R. (2000). Protease inhibitor-associated angiolipomatosis. *J Am Acad Dermatol*. 42:129–131.

8. Gervasoni C, Ridolfo AL, Trifiro G, *et al*. (1999). Redistribution of body fat in HIV-infected women undergoing combined antiretroviral therapy. *AIDS*. 13:465–471.

9. Dong KL, Bausserman LL, Flynn MM, *et al*. (1999). Changes in body habitus and serum lipid abnormalities in HIV-positive women on highly active antiretroviral therapy (HAART). *J Acquir Immune Defic Syndr*. 21:107–113.

10. Mahajan AP, Tashima KT, Bausserman LL, *et al*. (2001). Plateau in body habitus changes and serum lipid abnormalities in HIV-positive women on highly active antiretroviral therapy: a 3.5-year study. *J Acquir Immune Defic Syndr*. 28:332–335.

11. Galli M, Veglia F, Angarano G. (2001). Correlation between gender and morphologic alterations in treated HIV patients, The 1st IAS Conference of Pathogenesis and Treatment, Buenos Aires, Argentina, Abstract 505, July 8–11.

12. Roth VR, Kravcik S, Angel JB. (1998). Development of cervical fat pads following therapy with human immunodeficiency virus type 1 protease inhibitors. *Clin Infect Dis*. 27:65–67.

13. Wanke CA, Falutz JM, Shevitz A, *et al*. (2002). Clinical evaluation and management of metabolic and morphologic abnormalities associated with human immunodeficiency virus. *Clin Infect Dis*. 34:248–259.

14. Schambelan M. (1998). Buffalo Hump in HIV-infected Patients on Antiretroviral Therapy, 5th Conference on Retroviruses and Opportunistic Infections. Chicago: Abstract 409.

15. Saint-Marc T, Partisani M, Poizot-Martin I, *et al*. (2000). Fat distribution evaluated by computed tomography and metabolic abnormalities in patients undergoing antiretroviral therapy: preliminary results of the LIPOCO study. *AIDS*. 14:37–49.

16. Saint-Marc T, Partisani M, Poizot-Martin I, *et al*. (1999). A syndrome of peripheral fat wasting (lipodystrophy) in patients receiving long-term nucleoside analogue therapy. *AIDS*. 13:1659–1667.

17. Mallal SA, John M, Moore CB, *et al*. (2000). Contribution of nucleoside analogue reverse transcriptase inhibitors to subcutaneous fat wasting in patients with HIV infection. *AIDS*. 14:1309–1316.

18. Lichtenstein K, Delaney K, Ward D. (2002). Incidence, Prevalence, and Pathogenic Correlates of Insulin Resistance and Lipodystrophy Syndrome, 9th Conference on Retroviruses and Opportunistic Infections. Seattle: Abstract 684a–T.

19. Expert Panel on Detection, Evaluation, and Treatment of High Blood Cholesterol in Adults. (2001). Executive Summary of The Third Report of The National Cholesterol Education Program (NCEP) Expert Panel on Detection, Evaluation, and Treatment of High Blood Cholesterol in Adults (Adult Treatment Panel III). *JAMA*. 285:2486–2497.

20. Miller KD, Jones E, Yanovski JA, *et al*. (1998). Visceral abdominal-fat accumulation associated with use of indinavir. *Lancet*. 351:871–875.

21. Drechsler H, Powderly WG. (2002). Switching Effective Antiretroviral Therapy: A Review. *Clin Infect Dis*. 35:1219–1230.

22. Carr A, Workman C, Smith DE, *et al*. (2002). Abacavir substitution for nucleoside analogs in patients with HIV lipoatrophy: a randomized trial. *JAMA*. 288:207–215.

23. Standards of medical care for patients with diabetes mellitus. *Diabetes Care*. (2000). 23 Suppl 1:S32–42.

24. Currier JS, Boyd F, Kawabata H. (2002). Diabetes Mellitus in HIV-infected individuals, 9th Conference on Retroviruses and Opportunistic Infections. Seattle: Abstract 677–T.

25. Hadigan C, Meigs JB, Corcoran C, *et al*. (2001). Metabolic abnormalities and cardiovascular disease risk factors in adults with human immunodeficiency virus infection and lipodystrophy. *Clin Infect Dis*. 32:130–139.

26. Schambelan M, Benson CA, Carr A, *et al*. (2002). Management of metabolic complications associated with antiretroviral therapy for HIV-1 infection: recommendations of an International AIDS Society-USA panel. *J Acquir Immune Defic Syndr*. 31:257–275.

27. Carr A, Samaras K, Thorisdottir A, *et al*. (1999). Diagnosis, prediction, and natural course of HIV-1 protease-inhibitor-associated lipodystrophy, hyperlipidaemia, and diabetes mellitus: a cohort study. *Lancet*. 353:2093–2099.

28. Dever LL, Oruwari PA, Figueroa WE, *et al*. (2000). Hyperglycemia associated with protease inhibitors in an urban HIV-infected minority patient population. *Ann Pharmacother*. 34:580–584.

29. Noor MA, Lo JC, Mulligan K, *et al*. (2001). Metabolic effects of indinavir in healthy HIV-seronegative men. *AIDS*. 15:F11–18.

30. Caron M, Auclair M, Vigouroux C, *et al*. (2001). The HIV protease inhibitor indinavir impairs sterol regulatory element-binding protein-1 intranuclear localization, inhibits preadipocyte differentiation, and induces insulin resistance. *Diabetes*. 50:1378–1388.

31. Dube MP, Qian D, Edmondson-Melancon H, *et al*. (2002). Prospective, intensive study of metabolic changes associated with 48 weeks of amprenavir-based antiretroviral therapy. *Clin Infect Dis*. 35:475–481.

32. Sension M. (2002). Absence of Insulin Resistance Through Week 24 With Atazanvir Once Daily and Efavirenz Once Daily, Each With Twice-Daily Fixed-Dose ZDV + 3TC, 4th International Workshop on Adverse Drug Reactions and Lipodystrophy in HIV. San Diego: Poster.

33. Yoon C, Gulick R, Hoover D. (2002). Incidence, Prevalence, and Pathogenic Correlates of Insulin Resistance and Lipodystrophy Syndrome, 9th Conference on Retroviruses and Opportunistic Infections. Seattle: Abstract 678–T.

34. Falutz JM, Gardiner R. (2002). Incidence, Prevalence, and Pathogenic Correlates of Insulin Resistance and Lipodystrophy Syndrome, 9th Conference on Retroviruses and Opportunistic Infections. Seattle: Abstract 676–T.

35. Walli RK, Michl GM, Bogner JR, *et al*. (2001). Improvement of HAART-associated insulin resistance and dyslipidemia after replacement of protease inhibitors with abacavir. *Eur J Med Res*. 6:413–421.

36. Martinez E, Garcia-Viejo MA, Blanco JL, *et al*. (2000). Impact of switching from human immunodeficiency virus type 1 protease inhibitors to efavirenz in successfully treated adults with lipodystrophy. *Clin Infect Dis*. 31:1266–1273.

37. Martinez E, Conget I, Lozano L, *et al*. (1999). Reversion of metabolic abnormalities after switching from HIV-1 protease inhibitors to nevirapine. *AIDS*. 13:805–810.

38. Klein D, Hurley LB, Quesenberry CP, *et al*. (2002). Do protease inhibitors increase the risk for coronary heart disease in patients with HIV-1 infection? *J Acquir Immune Defic Syndr*. 30:471–477.

39. Mary-Krause M, Cotte L, Simon A, *et al*. (2003). Increased risk of myocardial infarction with duration of protease inhibitor therapy in HIV-infected men. *AIDS*. 17:2479–2486.

40. Bozzette SA, Ake C, Tam HK, *et al*. (2003). Cardiovascular and cerebrovascular events in patients treated for human immunodeficiency virus infection. *NEJM*. 348:702–710.

41. David MH, Hormung R, Fichtenbaum CJ. (2002). Ischemic cardiovascular disease in persons with human immunodeficiency virus infection. *Clin Infect Dis*. 34:98–102.

42. Pernerstorfer-Schoen H, Jilma B, Perschler A, *et al*. (2001). Sex differences in HAART-associated dyslipidaemia. *AIDS*. 15:725–734.

43. Kumar P, Rodriguez-French A, Thompson M. (2002). Prospective Study of Hyperlipidemia in ART-Naive Subjects Taking Combivir/Abacavir (COM/ ABC), COM/Nelfinavir(NFV), or Stavudine(d4T)/ Lamivudine(3TC)/NFV (ESS40002), 9th Conference on Retroviruses and Opportunistic Infections. Seattle: Abstract 33.

44. van Leth F, Friis-Moeller N, Weber R. (2002). Distinguishable Lipid Profiles between PI and NNRTI Therapy May Carry Different Risk of Cardiovascular Disease, 9th Conference on Retroviruses and Opportunistic Infections. Seattle: Abstract 34.

45. Holmberg SD, Moorman AC, Williamson JM, *et al*. (2002). Protease inhibitors and cardiovascular outcomes in patients with HIV-1. *Lancet*. 360:1747–1748.

46. Mauss S, Stechel J, Willers R, *et al*. (2003). Differentiating hyperlipidaemia associated with antiretroviral therapy. *AIDS*. 17:189–194.

47. Bausserman LL, Tashima KT, Dispigno M. (2002). Circulating Cell Adhesion Molecules are Elevated in HIV+ Women, 9th Conference on Retroviruses and Opportunistic Infections. Seattle: Abstract 693–T.

48. Ridker PM, Rifai N, Rose L, *et al*. (2002). Comparison of C-Reactive Protein and Low-Density Lipoprotein Cholesterol Levels in the Prediction of First Cardiovascular Events. *N Engl J Med*. 347:1557–1565.

49. Henry K, Zackin R, Dube M. (2002). ACTG 5056: C-Reactive Protein (CRP) Levels and Cardiovascular Risk Status for a Cohort of HIV-1-Infected Persons Durably Suppressed on an Indinavir(IDV)-Containing Regimen, 9th Conference on Retroviruses and Opportunistic Infections. Seattle: Abstract 694–T.

50. Neuvonen PJ, Kantola T, Kivisto KT. (1998). Simvastatin but not pravastatin is very susceptible to interaction with the CYP3A4 inhibitor itraconazole. *Clin Pharmacol Ther*. 63:332–341.

51. Dube MP, Stein JH, Aberg JA, *et al.* (2003). Guidelines for the evaluation and management of dyslipidemia in human immunodeficiency virus (HIV)-infected adults receiving antiretroviral therapy; recommendations of the HIV Medical Association of the Infectious Disease Society of America and the Adult AIDS Clinical Trials Group. *Clin Infect Dis.* 37:613–627.

53. Fichtenbaum CJ, Gerber JG, Rosenkranz SL, *et al.* Pharmacokinetic interactions between protease inhibitors and statins in HIV seronegative volunteers: ACTG Study A5047. *AIDS.* (2002). 16:569–577.

54. Miller J, Brown D, Amin J, *et al.* (2002). A randomized, double-blind study of gemfibrozil for the treatment of protease inhibitor-associated hypertriglyceridaemia. *AIDS.* 16:2195–2200.

55. Aberg JA, Zackin R, Evans S. (2002). A Prospective, Multicenter, Randomized Trial Comparing the Efficacy and Safety of Fenofibrate versus Pravastatin in HIV-infected Subjects with Lipid Abnormalities: ACTG 5087, 40th Annual Meeting of IDSA. Chicago: Abstract 26.

56. Pisac C, Fumero E, Crespo M. (2002). Metabolic and body composition changes in patients switching from protease inhibitor-containing regimen to Abacavir (ABC), Efavirenz (EFV) or Nevirapine (NVP). Twelve-month results of a randomized study (LIPNEFA), XIV International Aids Conference. Barcelona, Spain: Abstract ThPe7354.

57. Sanne I, Piliero P, Squires, *et al.* (2003). Results of a phase 2 clinical trial at 48 weeks (AI424-007): a dose-ranging, safety, and efficacy comparative trial of atazanavir at three doses in combination with didanosine and stavudine in antiretroviral-naïve subjects. *J Acquir Immune Defic Syndr.* 32:18–29.

59. Miller KD, Cameron M, Wood LV, *et al.* (2000). Lactic acidosis and hepatic steatosis associated with use of stavudine: report of four cases. *Ann Intern Med.* 133:192–196.

60. Fortgang IS, Belitsos PC, Chaisson RE, *et al.* (1995). Hepatomegaly and steatosis in HIV-infected patients receiving nucleoside analog antiretroviral therapy. *Am J Gastroenterol.* 90:1433–1436.

61. Boxwell DE, Styrt BA. (1999). Lactic acidosis (LA) in patients receiving nucleoside reverse transcriptase inhibitors (NRTIs). 39th Interscience Conference on Antimicrobial Agents and Chemotherapy. San Francisco: Abstract 1284.

62. Marcus K, Truffa D, Boxwell DE. (2002). Recently Identified Adverse Events Secondary to NRTI Therapy in HIV-Infected Individuals: Cases from the FDA's Adverse Event Reporting System (AERS), 9th Conference on Retroviruses and Opportunistic Infections. Seattle: Abstract LB14.

63. Fouty B, Frerman F, Reves R. (1998). Riboflavin to treat nucleoside analogue-induced lactic acidosis. *Lancet.* 352:291–292.

64. Carr A, Cooper DA. (2000). Adverse effects of antiretroviral therapy. *Lancet.* 356:1423–1430.

65. Chaonie M. (2001). Osteoporosis and HIV disease. *Beta.* 14:26–34.

66. Miller KD, Masur H, Jones EC, *et al.* (2002). High prevalence of osteonecrosis of the femoral head in HIV-infected adults. *Ann Intern Med.* 137:17–25.

67. Kanis JA, Melton LJ 3rd, Christiansen C, *et al.* (1994). The diagnosis of osteoporosis. *J Bone Miner Res.* 9:1137–1141.

68. Romeyn M, Ireland J. (2001). Bone loss in HIV—not a protease inhibitor effect, 4th International Conference on Nutrition and HIV Infection., Cannes, France, Poster 50.

69. Tebas P, Powderly WG, Claxton S. (2000). Accelerated Bone Mineral Loss in HIV-Infected Patients Receiving Potent Antiretroviral Therapy, 7th Conference on Retroviruses and Opportunistic Infections. San Francisco: Abstract 207.

70. Mondy K, Yarasheski K, Powderly W, *et al.* (2003). Longitudinal evolution of bone mineral density and bone markers in human immunodeficiency virus-infected individuals. *Clin Infect Dis.* 36:482–490.

71. Lawal A, Engelson E, Wang J, *et al.* (2001). Equivalent Osteopenia in HIV-infected individuals studied before and during the era of highly active antiretroviral therapy. *AIDS.* 15:278–280.

72. Knobel H, Guelar A, Carmona A, *et al.* (2001). Osteopenia in HIV-infected patients: is it the disease or is it the treatment? *AIDS.* 15:807–808.

73. Eastell R. (1998). Treatment of postmenopausal osteoporosis. *N Engl J Med.* 338:736–746.

74. Arnsten J, Freeman R, Santoro N. (2002). Bone Mineral Density and Protease Inhibitor Use in Older HIV-Infected Women, 9th Conference on Retroviruses and Opportunistic Infections. Seattle: Abstract 717–T.

75. Manolagas SC, Jilka RL. (1995). Bone marrow, cytokines, and bone remodeling. Emerging insights into the pathophysiology of osteoporosis. *N Engl J Med.* 332:305–311.

87

The Effect of Gender on the Epidemiology, Clinical Presentation, and Management of Tuberculosis

COSMINA ZEANA, MD* AND WAFAA EL-SADR, MD, MPH**

*Assistant Attending, Division of Infectious Diseases, Harlem Hospital Center, Clinical Instructor Medicine,
Columbia University College of Physicians and Surgeons, New York, NY
**Director of Infectious Diseases Division, Harlem Hospital Center; Professor of Clinical Medicine and Epidemiology,
Columbia University College of Physicians and Surgeons, New York, NY

I. Introduction

The magnitude of the global tuberculosis (TB) epidemic is enormous. TB is the most frequent cause of death worldwide as the result of a single infectious agent, and in 1993 the World Health Organization (WHO) declared TB a global public health emergency [1]. About one-third of the world's population is infected with *Mycobacterium tuberculosis (M. tuberculosis)* and an estimated 8 million new cases and 2 million deaths occur yearly from the disease [1]. However, the prevalence of infection is not the same for males and females. It is estimated that around 1300 million males and 900 million females are infected with *M. tuberculosis* [1]. Each year more men than women are diagnosed with and reported to have TB. There is an ongoing debate regarding the reasons for this gender difference. Possible explanations include biologic factors, differential exposure patterns to TB cases for men and women, gender differences in access to health care services, and underdiagnosis or underreporting by health services of TB in women. This chapter explores the impact of gender on different aspects of TB including prevalence of infection and active disease; clinical presentation; diagnosis, treatment, and response to treatment; access to health care; and attitudes toward the disease.

A. Pathogenesis

TB is caused by bacteria belonging to the *M. tuberculosis* complex. The disease usually affects the lungs, although in as many as one-third of cases, other organs are involved (extrapulmonary TB) [2].

M. tuberculosis is most commonly transmitted from a patient with infectious pulmonary TB to other persons by droplet nuclei, which are aerosolized by coughing, sneezing, or speaking. Other routes of transmission of *M. tuberculosis*, such as through skin or the placenta, are uncommon and of no epidemiologic significance. The probability of contact with a source case of TB, the intimacy and duration of that contact, the degree of infectiousness of the case, and the environment of the contact are all important determinants of transmission. Several studies of close contacts have clearly demonstrated that patients with TB whose sputum contains acid-fast bacilli (AFB) visible by microscopy play the greatest role in the spread of the infection. These patients have cavitary pulmonary disease or TB of the respiratory tract and produce sputa containing as many as 10^5

organisms/ml. Transmission can less commonly occur from patients with negative smears.

Only a small fraction of those who are infected with *M. tuberculosis* develop the disease. An infected individual has a 10% lifetime risk of developing TB. This risk increases to 10% per year if the person is coinfected with human immunodeficiency virus (HIV) [2]. Unlike the risk of acquiring infection with *M. tuberculosis*, the risk of developing TB after being infected depends largely on endogenous factors, such as the individual's innate susceptibility to disease and the level of function of cell-mediated immunity.

B. Clinical Manifestations

Symptoms and signs of TB are often nonspecific and insidious, consisting mainly of fever, night sweats, weight loss, anorexia, and weakness. However, in the majority of cases of pulmonary TB, cough with or without hemoptysis eventually develops. Physical findings are not specific, in general underestimating the extent of the illness, and may be absent despite of extensive disease.

Diagnosis of active pulmonary disease is based on the clinical picture, abnormalities on chest radiography, the presence of AFB on microscopic examination of the sputa, and sputum cultures. Extrapulmonary TB is often difficult to diagnose and requires isolation of the organism from the site involved.

Before effective drugs were available, 50% of patients with active pulmonary TB died within 2 years and only 25% were cured [3]. With the advent of chemotherapy, successful treatment became a realistic goal for all patients. Five drugs are considered the first-line agents for the treatment of TB: isoniazid, rifampin, pyrazinamide, ethambutol, and streptomycin. Most patients with TB are treated with short-course regimens, which are divided into an initial or bactericidal phase (first 2 months) and a continuation or sterilizing phase. The treatment regimen of choice for virtually all forms of TB in both adults and children consists of a 2-month initial phase of isoniazid, rifampin, ethambutol, and pyrazinamide followed by a 4-month continuation phase with isoniazid and rifampin. Treatment can be given daily throughout the course, although intermittent regimens (either three times weekly throughout the course or a daily initial phase followed by twice- or thrice-weekly treatment during the continuation phase) produce similar results [2]. In practice, treatment failure occurs because of drug resistance or an inappropriate regimen but most importantly because of nonadherence with treatment. Nonadherence may occur as health returns and motivation for continued intake of medications declines. Non-adherence is recognized worldwide as the most important impediment to TB cure, with resultant TB relapse and development of resistance. Therefore, WHO recommends direct observed treatment (DOT) for all cases of active TB. Supervision of medication ingestion increases the proportion of patients completing treatment and greatly lessens the chance of relapse and acquired drug resistance. The number of countries implementing DOTs (at least in part) is 127 (out of 211) [1].

II. Gender-Specific Issues

A. Epidemiology

In most of the world, more men than women are diagnosed with TB and die from it. The male-to-female notification ratio of TB cases ranges from 1.5 to 2.1 [1]. TB is nevertheless a leading infectious cause of death among women. In 1998 more than 3 million women contracted the disease, accounting for about 17 million disability adjusted life years (DALY) [4]. TB is the greatest single infectious cause of death in women worldwide, with about three-fourths of a million deaths in 1998 [5]. Overall more women die from TB than from all causes of maternal death [4]. Because TB affects women mainly in their economically and reproductive active years, the impact of the disease is also strongly felt by their children and families.

The reason for the global gender difference in the prevalence of TB is still unknown. There are two main hypotheses to explain this discrepancy [6]. First, the observed differences could be real and gender related. Thus, biologic factors could account for the gender difference in infection with M. tuberculosis and/or progression to active disease. Sociocultural factors could influence opportunities for exposure to M. tuberculosis as well as conditions that foster progression to disease and reactivation. Alternatively, it has been hypothesized that underdiagnosis and underreporting of TB in women, especially those in low-income countries, are responsible for the previously mentioned gender difference in TB prevalence. Various factors, including self-image, status in family and society, access to resources, and manifestation and expression of stigma associated with TB, may influence care-seeking behavior in women. Subsequent sections in this chapter elaborate further on these possible causes.

1. Prevalence of Latent Tuberculosis Infection

The prevalence of M. tuberculosis infection (number of cases of M. tuberculosis infection per population at risk) is assessed with the tuberculin skin test (TST), utilizing purified protein derivative (PPD). Technical problems with TST testing, including standardization of tuberculin, technique of administration, and reading of the test result, have been described [7]. Furthermore, interpretation of TST results must also consider the effect of nonspecific cross-reactions with environmental mycobacteria and Mycobacterium bovis, transient or waning tuberculin sensitivity, as well as the effect of prior vaccination with bacillus Calmette-Guerin (BCG) and the immune status of the individual [8,9]. Despite these caveats, a number of tuberculin surveys worldwide yield a remarkably consistent picture of gender and age differences in the prevalence of M. tuberculosis infection and annual risk of infection.

Examination of data from tuberculin surveys undertaken in 15 countries around the world by the International Tuberculosis Campaign from 1948 to 1951, prior to widespread BCG vaccination, showed that the prevalence of M. tuberculosis infection was nearly equal in males and females at younger ages [10]. Between the ages of 10 and 16 years, prevalence of M. tuberculosis infection among males began to exceed that among females. From age 15 years onward, the prevalence of infection is almost universally higher among males than females [11–15]. Prevalence surveys carried out by WHO in Africa during the same era found similar age- and gender-related patterns in infection prevalence [16].

More comprehensive investigations performed between 1961 and 1968 in the Bangalore district of India found the same prevalence of infection among females and males until the age of 14 years, after which the prevalence among males was 20–71% higher than among females [17]. This pattern was also found in a study carried out in Chingleput, India [18].

The Korean prevalence surveys revealed similar results. Six surveys since 1965 have consistently shown than among persons aged 0–9 years who are not BCG vaccinated, the prevalence of TST positivity was similar in both sexes, whereas males older than age 15 years had a 3–30% higher prevalence than females [19–24]. In addition to prevalence data, studies have assessed gender difference in annual risk of infection. In a study of Dutch schoolchildren, Sutherland et al reported little or no difference in the annual risk of infection between boys and girls aged 6 to 12 years [25]. However, among children between the ages of 12 and 18 years, there was an excess annual risk of infection of 10.2 among males.

There are two main hypotheses to explain the observed age-dependent difference in prevalence of M. tuberculosis infection and annual risk of infection between males and females [26]. First, it has been suggested that males in general have higher risk of acquiring M. tuberculosis infection because of a wider social network that would lead to a greater exposure to the organism. This difference in social mixing patterns is considered to be of importance after puberty, following the differentiation of gender roles [27]. An alternative explanation is that TST may have different sensitivity in men and women, caused by differences in the gender-specific immune response to M. tuberculosis infection. A lesser delayed type hypersensitivity response to infection in women could account for the lower prevalence of tuberculin test positivity in women compared with men [28]. This hypothesis is supported by a study from Japan examining tuberculin sensitivity in an elderly population, with no prior BCG vaccination, with or without human T-cell lymphotropic virus type 1 (HTLV-1) [29]. It was found that women who were HTLV-1 negative were more likely to have a negative PPD reaction compared to men who were HTLV-1 negative. Another study of schoolchildren in Kuwait found that boys had a delayed-type hypersensitivity reaction to more mycobacterial antigens than girls; they also had larger scars after BCG revaccination [30]. In addition, Kurasawa showed that fewer male patients with TB disease had a negative tuberculin reaction compared to women [31]. The results of these studies indicate that TST testing may be less sensitive in women. More research is needed to verify these findings.

2. Incidence of Tuberculosis

WHO requests all countries to provide an annual report on the number of new TB cases registered. Incidence of TB disease is defined as the number of new cases of TB per population at risk. Worldwide, more male than female TB cases are notified to WHO. This has been described in both industrialized and developing countries [1]. In 2001, women represented 35% of the new smear-positive reported cases. The percentage of males among new notifications in 2001 for each region was as follows: Africa, 60%; Americas, 62%; Eastern Mediterranean, 65%; Europe, 71%; South East Asia, 61%; and Western Pacific, 64% [11]. It is not known whether this is a true difference in the incidence of TB, the result of underdiagnosis and underreporting of female cases, or a combination of these factors.

Age- and gender-specific prevalence rates (number of cases of TB per population at risk per unit time) of smear-positive TB were compared in a retrospective study with age- and gender-specific notification rates from 14 countries in 1996 [32]. The female-to-male ratios of notification was less than 1 in all countries except Samoa and decreased with increasing age in all countries except Syria. The female-to-male crude prevalence ratios by WHO region were approximately 0.3 in South-East Asia, approximately 0.5 in the Western Pacific region, and approximately 1 in sub-Saharan Africa. The authors concluded that the overall gender differences in TB notification rates were largely the result of gender differences in TB prevalence. Still, because of methodologic weaknesses it is not possible to obtain conclusive evidence from this study. The African prevalence studies used in the analysis were carried out many years before the notification rates. Moreover, the cases notified were reported primarily from the public sector, with cases treated within the private sector not accurately reflected in the reported notification rates. Of concern is also the validity of estimating prevalence based on smear sputum positivity, which assumes similar sensitivity of sputum testing in men and women, and a similar duration of sputum positivity among men and women. These issues will be discussed later in this chapter.

A retrospective epidemiologic analysis of sex-specific TB incidence rates in San Francisco from 1991 to 1996 suggested that the observed differences in TB rates between sexes are the result of a difference in transmission dynamics rather than diagnosis or reporting biases [33]. The male-to-female ratio in this study was 2.1 (similar to the global distribution ratio) and remained unchanged after stratification for HIV status. Further analyses revealed differences in sex-specific rates after the age of 14 years, and the highest male-to-female ratios were noted in U.S.-born, white, and black patients with TB. DNA fingerprinting was performed on organisms from 85% of the culture-positive cases. The incidence of clustered cases was higher among men compared to women, indicating recent, ongoing transmission to be more likely among men. The authors concluded that ongoing transmission of TB among U.S.-born men is one of the factors that explain the difference in gender-specific rates of disease in San Francisco.

The lower notification rates reported among women living in low-income countries compared to women from industrialized countries raised the possibility that women are being underreported in these areas [7]. This hypothesis is supported by a study from Nepal comparing passive and active case findings of TB. Women represented 28% of the 159 cases who presented to a clinic (passive case finding), whereas with active case finding, 46% of 111 cases identified were among women [34]. A similar gender differential in the outcome of active and passive case findings has been described in studies of malaria and leishmaniasis [35,36]. Reasons for undernotification of women include inadequate care-seeking as a result of time and financial constraints, status in family and society, self-image, and stigma associated with TB. These differences are attributed to larger societal gender inequities such as women's insufficient access to income, legal rights, social status, and education. Traditional and religious customs underlie many of these inequities. TB is a symptom of global poverty, and 70% of the world's poor are female.

B. Progression from Infection to Disease

Comparison of infection rates with disease rates among women in their reproductive years suggests that women may have a higher rate of progression to disease, whereas men have higher rates of progression at older ages [27,37]. In a prospective study performed in Bangalore, India, all subjects were initially screened for *M. tuberculosis* infection and disease and then followed with active screening for TB on three subsequent occasions [17]. Over the 8 years of the study, 134 subjects with a positive TST test developed TB. Females had a 130% higher risk than men of progression from infection to disease between the ages of 10 and 44 years. At older ages, men's rates of progression were 2.5-fold greater than among women of the same age. A higher rate of progression in reproductive-age women was also reported in two other studies [38,39]. The 3017 participants assigned to placebo in a trial of isoniazid prophylaxis among Alaskan Inuits were found to have similar rates of development of TB disease among boys and girls up to the age of 10 years [38]. After this age up to 39 years, women had rates 25% higher than men. The rates equalized for both genders in the older age groups. Finally, in a study from Puerto Rico, passive follow-up over an average of 18.7 years of 82,269 unvaccinated, TST-positive persons yielded 1400 cases of TB [39]. Overall, the rate of progression to disease was 17% higher in females, and the male rate was higher only in the 1- to 6-year old age group.

A similar age and gender pattern in progression from infection to disease was noted in four studies carried out in high-income countries. A study from Denmark found that women aged 25 to 34 years progressed to TB at a rate 71% higher than men of the same age. Between 35 to 44 years the rate was 22% higher in women. However, this was reversed after the age of 45 years to 67% higher rates in men than women [40].

Passive follow-up of TST-positive persons in Ontario, Canada, showed that women had up to 30% higher rates of disease progression than men, whereas men older than age 40 years had rates of progression more than twice as high as women [41].

In a prospective study from Norway, rates of disease progression were the same for men and women between 15 and 19 years old, but they were 25–30% higher in women 20 to 29 years old. After the age of 30 years, rates were 30% higher in men [42].

Finally, a study performed in the United States between 1950 and 1970 yielded a different age and gender pattern in African American women compared to white women [43]. African

American women aged 20 to 39 years had rates of progression to disease 25–30% higher than men, whereas men older than age 40 years had progression rates 17–25% higher. In contrast, in the white subjects, men's rates of progression following infection were higher than women's at all ages.

Holmes *et al.* explored possible explanations for the higher rate of progression from *M. tuberculosis* infection to disease in young women observed in these studies [6]. In early literature, it was commonly believed that the stresses of pregnancy lead to a decreased immunity and hence higher vulnerability for progression to TB. Extensive reviews of older studies indicate that there is probably little or no relationship between pregnancy and progression to disease [44,45]. A more recent case-control study comparing history of pregnancy or childbirth over the previous 6-months between patients with and without TB found no difference in prior pregnancy, supporting the lack of association between TB and pregnancy [46].

Another possible explanation of higher disease progression in these young women is the apparent lower prevalence of *M. tuberculosis* infection in women than men during and after adolescence resulting in more recent acquisition of *M. tuberculosis* infection prior to development of disease [6]. It has been documented that the risk of progression to disease is higher in the first and second year after *M. tuberculosis* infection [47]. Lastly, higher rates of disease progression in this group of women could be the result of higher utilization of health services by women in their reproductive years [6].

In the case of older men, it has been postulated that risk factors for TB such as alcohol abuse and smoking may be more common compared with women and contribute to the higher progression rates reported by these studies.

C. Diagnosis

1. Recognition of Symptoms

The severity and types of symptoms associated with an illness have an effect on health-seeking practices. Illness typically proceeds along a course from a person experiencing symptoms to the decision to seek help and subsequently to take treatment either for relief or cure. The global strategy for TB control recommended by WHO is based on passive case-detection (i.e., ascertainment dependent on patient's presentation to the health care system). Therefore, the patient's perceived symptoms are a crucial parameter that influences case detection. Gender differentials in the experience and expression of illnesses may play an important role in access to care and diagnosis of active TB cases.

Unlike affluent societies, women in resource-constrained countries were less likely than men to report sick and must negotiate more obstacles before accessing health care services [48,49]. A sociologic study undertaken in India in the 1960s found that women with radiologic abnormalities consistent with TB were less likely to report respiratory symptoms than men [50]. In another study from Vietnam investigating symptoms among 757 men and 270 women with smear-positive pulmonary TB, fewer women than men reported each of the following symptoms: cough, sputum production, and hemoptysis. At follow-up 1 month later, more women than men reported resolution of cough and sputum production [51].

Another possible explanation for the gender differences in disease incidence may be gender bias in sputum examination. A study carried out by the National Tuberculosis Program in Malawi in 1995–1996 evaluated gender differences in relation to sputum submission in patients with suspected TB [52]. During a 12-month period, 26,624 new patients with suspected TB submitted sputum samples, 3,282 of which were smear-positive. The proportion of males who submitted sputum was 52% compared with 48% among females. Among males, 53% were smear-positive compared with 47% among females. These later differences were statistically significant. One possible explanation for the observed discrepancies is that men are better able to produce good quality sputum as a result of higher rates of coexisting lung pathology and smoking history. Rates of sputum submission per 100,000 adults were also significantly higher for males than females except in the 15- to 24-year-old age group, where more women were asked to submit sputum compared to men.

Other investigators have suggested that the sensitivity of the sputum examination may differ by gender. A study investigating sputum microscopy in patients with chest symptoms in Africa showed that the probability of finding AFB on the sputum smear was less among women suspected to have TB compared with men. This difference was more pronounced with increasing age [53]. The authors suggested that women may have a higher prevalence of nonspecific respiratory symptoms than men. An alternative explanation is that men are able to produce better-quality sputum compared with women.

These findings are consistent with an earlier survey in India that showed the prevalence of sputum positivity to be higher in male patients presenting with symptoms suggestive of TB compared with women [54]. Other possible reasons for lower sputum positivity in women remain to be investigated.

2. Delay in Diagnosis

A study conducted in 23 randomly selected districts in four provinces of Vietnam in 1996 compared health-seeking behavior between men and women and measured delays in TB diagnosis [55]. Total delay was defined as the time from the first symptoms to TB diagnosis; patient-related delay was defined as the time from onset of first disease symptoms until first visit to a doctor or a hospital; and doctor-related delay was defined as the time from the first visit to a medical doctor or a hospital to TB diagnosis. In addition, delay to first health care provider (from onset of symptoms to first visit to any health care provider) and provider-related delay (from first visit to any health care provider to TB diagnosis) were also investigated. In this study the mean total time to diagnosis of TB was significantly longer for women (13.3 weeks) than men (11.4 weeks). This delay may have significant consequences to the patient and may result in further transmission of *M. tuberculosis* to others. Physician-related delay and health care provider's delay in making the diagnosis were also significantly longer for women than for men. To receive a correct diagnosis of TB, women had to visit more providers than men (average 1.7 versus 1.5). In this study patient's delay did not differ by gender. Similar results were found in studies from Africa [56].

A reason for the underdiagnosis of TB in women in high-income countries, where access is more readily available, may be provider bias (i.e., health care providers are less likely to consider the diagnosis in women). A retrospective study of patients discharged from the hospital with a diagnosis of *Pneumocystis carinii* pneumonia between 1987 and 1990 found that the physicians' suspicion of TB among female patients decreased from 76 to 71% over the 4-year period [57]. After controlling for confounding variables by multiple logistic regression, the odds that TB would be suspected by the provider early (in the first two hospital days) increased 1.8-fold among men but not in women. In contrast to the previous results, studies from Japan and Malaysia reported that delay in obtaining care by patients with TB tended to be longer in men than in women [58,59], whereas in Australia there were no gender differences [60].

3. Health Care–Seeking Behavior

Health seeking and treatment behavior of men and women suffering from TB is largely determined by how patients and those around them perceive the symptoms, regard the diagnosis, accept the treatment, and adhere to it. Gender may influence each of these and may affect diagnosis of the disease and its outcome. Among affluent societies, in general, women have higher levels of utilization of health services [48].

An extensive analysis of typical health-seeking behavior in men and women, performed in Vietnam in 1996, explored the main contributing factors to delays in health seeking [61]. In summary, three major contributing factors were identified. First, stigma associated with the disease and resultant denial and concealment played an important role in the health-seeking pattern of women. Stigma may not only affect individual behavior—the whole family may suffer from social stigma and its negative consequences. Stigma may lead to delays for both sexes in seeking care but more so for women. Second, participants expressed concern regarding cost of diagnosis and treatment, which led to delay or total avoidance of health care facilities. Third, health facilities did not respond to patients' expectations in terms of resources and human competence at public health facilities. Women were believed to be more sensitive to deficiencies in conditions of facilities and attitudes of staff and often chose private health facilities and self-medication, all factors further delaying the diagnosis of TB.

A population-based survey in the Ha Tay province, Vietnam, showed that among individuals with long-term cough, women are more likely to choose less-qualified health care as their first choice [62]. More than 70% of the men and women did not seek hospital care for their cough, showing a general tendency to choose other providers at the expense of better-equipped hospital facilities. However, although both men and women were disadvantaged, women had a longer delay to reach the hospital than men, suggesting that women are at greater risk of not receiving effective health care. Typically, men were reported to neglect their symptoms until seeking hospital care directly, whereas women were more likely to report visiting private practitioners or self-medicating before seeking public health services or hospital care. Similar findings were reported from a study of patients with TB in Pakistan [63]. Women faced more challenges in receiving adequate TB treatment than men for various reasons including restrictions on the movement

of women in Pakistan and a general unwillingness to pay for treatment for women.

The choice of health care provider is also influenced by gender. A cross-sectional analysis of newly diagnosed TB cases in a rural area of Nepal showed that women were more likely to visit and to believe in traditional healers, which might lead to longer delays in TB diagnosis [64]. In the latter study, 35% of the women visited traditional healers before diagnosis, compared to 18% of the men, and women were more likely to receive more complicated charms from traditional healers. Women were found to have a significantly longer delay before diagnosis of TB (median 2.3 months for men and 3.3 months for women). Women were rarely diagnosed within 1 month if they visited a traditional healer first, and an extensive delay of more than 7 months was related to an initial visit to a traditional healer. From patient interviews, women indicated that they were heavily loaded with various jobs, household chores, and the care of young children in their home. These burdens might deprive them of the time and opportunity to visit distant government medical facilities. Several other studies performed in urban and rural areas in South Asia showed women's preference for private practitioners including paramedics as well as traditional healers [65–68].

Thus, it appears that gender-related barriers to TB care may vary greatly based on the setting. Understanding the variety and details of these barriers is a crucial factor for the development of effective TB control programs based on gender-sensitive strategies that take into account the observed sex differences in health-seeking behavior.

D. Treatment

1. Outcomes of Tuberculosis

Gender differences have also been described in the prognosis and outcome of active TB cases. The National Tuberculosis Institute study in Bangalore, India, examined gender differentials in the case-fatality rates for TB (death from TB per population with TB per unit time) [69]. Females aged 5 to 24 years had a case-fatality rate 27–41% greater than males of the same age group, whereas case-fatality rates were similar at age 25 years and older.

In a study investigating vital records between 1957 and 1976 in Nagpur, India, females between 15 and 34 years of age had TB-attributed mortality rates (deaths from TB per population per unit time) that were 10–36% higher than men of the same age [70]. Subsequently, after 35 years of age, men's mortality rates were several times higher. Similar results were obtained from a survey in China that found that women from birth through the age of 29 years had higher TB-related mortality than men of the same age [71]. Men older than 25 years had higher mortality rates than women. This pattern of mortality in low-income settings is similar to that observed in industrialized countries such as Iceland [72], Denmark [40], and the United States [73].

One proposed explanation for the observed higher mortality from TB among young to early-middle-aged women compared to men is the higher rate of progression from infection to disease among women of this age group.

The differential in outcome of treated TB cases (i.e., case-fatality rate) cannot be explained by gender differences in the pharmacokinetic of antituberculous medications. Studies have shown that the concentrations of orally administered isoniazid, ethambutol, ethionamide, and pyrazinamide in plasma as well as intrapulmonary tissues were not affected by gender [74–77].

Other reasons for the excess case fatality may be the result of health care–seeking behavior or provider practices, as elucidated in Sections 2.3 and 2.6.

2. Adherence to Treatment

Compliance or adherence to treatment is an important issue in TB control, not only for the successful cure of the individual patient but also from a public-health perspective. Defaulting from treatment can result in delay in sputum conversion to smear-negativity, higher relapse rates, and the emergence of resistance to antituberculous medications. Adherence, or compliance, is a complex concept that should be seen as a chain of responsibilities involving the patient, the treating doctors, and public health officers.

The reasons for inability to adhere to treatment have been reported to be different for men and women. A study performed in Bombay, India, showed that men dropped out because of pressures to return to wage work or as a result of alcohol and drug addiction, whereas women dropped out because of the pressures of housework and the strain of keeping their condition secret [78]. Other studies confirmed these results and showed that men had higher default rates than women and that the rates of default are higher in the older (older than age 45 years) age group [79–84]. Defaulting in the first month of treatment had been found to be a reliable predictor of default or dropout [85].

A qualitative study performed in Tamatave, Madagascar, explored factors determining compliance to TB treatment [86]. Default appeared to be significantly linked to male sex, transportation time, patient information, and the quality of communication between patients and health workers. Similar results were obtained from studies carried out in South Africa, Hong Kong, and Vietnam [87–89].

The apparent better adherence to TB treatment in women compared to men could reflect selection bias. The barriers to diagnosis in women described earlier may exclude women who are most likely to default, and those who make it to diagnosis and treatment are the ones most likely to have the necessary support and access to resources to complete treatment [28].

E. Knowledge and Attitudes Toward Tuberculosis

Important factors contributing to patients' adherence to TB treatment are their beliefs, knowledge, and attitudes toward the disease. Numerous studies showed that patients had misconceptions and limited knowledge about the disease and its treatment, leading to poor compliance to treatment [90–95].

A study performed in San Francisco in 1993 analyzed attitudes regarding TB and TB control among homeless adults [96]. Of 292 persons interviewed, more than 60% had misconceptions about transmission, in particular confusion with transmission of HIV. Higher TB knowledge score and male sex were associated

with a favorable attitude toward directly observed therapy. In this study women were less in agreement with stringent TB control measures to ensure adherence with treatment among patients with active disease. Further work needs to be done to understand whether this represents a true sex difference in attitudes toward TB control measures.

F. Socioeconomic Impact of Tuberculosis

Qualitative studies on gender differentials in TB carried out in Vietnam also explored the social consequences of TB [97]. The economic burden for the family was believed to be heaviest when the husband had the disease because men are often the major generators of family income. The social consequences reflected the general power structure of the society. Men were in general well-treated and supported, whereas women were often left without support and even rejected by the family. TB was also found to be a reason for divorce.

Another study, performed in India, quantified the socioeconomic impact of TB on patients and their families from the costs incurred by patients in rural and urban areas. In this analysis, the total direct cost incurred by women was higher than that for men [98]. Indirect cost could not be computed for unemployed women because the household activities performed by women cannot be measured in traditional financial terms. TB in women affects child survival and family welfare. Care of children was found to be most affected in both rural and urban settings; 58% of female patients expressed the inability to feed their children or take care of their daily activities and education. Of the children 11% had discontinued school as a result of the burden caused by the parent's illness and 8% took up employment to support the family.

III. Conclusion

This chapter reviews gender differences in various aspects of TB such as prevalence of infection and active disease; clinical presentation; diagnosis, treatment, and response to treatment; barriers to care; and attitudes toward the disease. The analysis of gender differences in TB hopefully will lead to increased awareness of discrepancies in health care and encourage the organization of gender-sensitive TB control programs. Little is known about how the currently recommended models for the control and treatment of TB affect women and men differently. Understanding gender-related differences is essential in the design of a gender-sensitive protocol for a successful global TB control program. Increased awareness of gender inequalities in health care should lead to research efforts to understand inequities in health and health care utilization.

IV. Suggestions for Further Investigations

- What genetic/biologic factors could explain the differences between men and women in the acquisition of TB, progression of infection to disease, and response to treatment?
- Is diagnosis of infection with the use of the TST less sensitive in women compared with men, and, if so, what better tests to diagnose TB infection can we use?

- Are reasons for compliance with TB treatment different between men and women?
- What are ways of addressing gender differentials in access to health and TB care?

References

1. World Health Organization. (2001). Global Tuberculosis Control. *WHO Report* Geneva: WHO. 1–181.

2. Raviglione MC, O'Brien RJ. (1998). Tuberculosis. In: *Harrison's principles of internal medicine*. New York: McGraw-Hill. 1004–1014.

3. Styblo K. (1980). Recent advances in epidemiological research in tuberculosis. *Adv Tuberc Res.* 20:1–63.

4. Uplekar M, Rangan S, Ogden J. (1999). *Gender and Tuberculosis Control: Towards a Strategy for Research and Action*. Geneva: WHO. 1–33.

5. Howson CP, Harrison PF, Hotra D, Law M. (1996). *In Her Lifetime: Female Morbidity and Mortality in Sub-Saharan Africa*. National Academy Press, Washington, DC.

6. Holmes CB, Hausler H, Nunn P. (1998). A review of sex differences in the epidemiology of tuberculosis. *Int J Tuberc Lung Dis.* 2(2):96–104.

7. Murray CJL, Styblo K, Rouillon A. (1990). Tuberculosis in developing countries: burden, intervention and cost. *Bull Int Union Tuberc Lund Dis.* 65(1):6–26.

8. Nyboe J. (1957). Interpretation of tuberculosis infection age curves. *Bull World Health Organ.* 17:319–339.

9. Rieder HL. (1995). Methodological issues in the estimation of the tuberculosis problem from tuberculin surveys. *Tuberc Lund Dis.* 2:114–121.

10. Sutherland I. (1976). Recent studies in the epidemiology of tuberculosis, based on the risk of being infected with tubercle bacilli. *Adv Tuberc Res.* 19:1–63.

11. Dolin P. (1998). Tuberculosis epidemiology from a gender perspective. In: Diwan V, Thorson A, Winkhurst A, eds. *Gender and tuberculosis*. Nordic School of Public Health, Goteborg. 29–40.

12. World Health Organization. (1961). Tuberculosis survey in Tunisia. WHO, Alexandria.

13. World Health Organization. (1956). Tuberculosis survey in the Somalilands. WHO, Copenhagen.

14. World Health Organization. (1958). A tuberculin survey in Tangayika. WHO, Copenhagen.

15. World Health Organization. (1963). A tuberculosis prevalence survey in Saigon, Vietnam. WHO, Manila.

16. Roelsgaard E, Iversen E, Blocher C. (1964). Tuberculosis in tropical Africa: an epidemiological study. *Bull World Health Organ.* 30:459–518.

17. Gothi GD, Nair SS, Olakowski T, *et al.* (1974). Tuberculosis in a rural population of South India: a five year epidemiological study. *Bull World Health Organ.* 51:473–488.

18. Baily GVJ, Narain R, Mayurnath S, *et al.* (1980). Trial of BCG vaccines in South India for tuberculosis prevention: tuberculosis prevention trial. *Ind J Med Res.* 72(suppl):1–74.

19. Ministry of Health and Social Affairs and the Korean National Tuberculosis Association. Report on the first tuberculosis prevalence survey in Korea. (1965).

20. Ministry of Health and Social Affairs and the Korean National Tuberculosis Association. Report on the second tuberculosis prevalence survey in Korea. (1970).

21. Ministry of Health and Social Affairs and the Korean National Tuberculosis Association. Report on the third tuberculosis prevalence survey in Korea. (1975).

22. Ministry of Health and Social Affairs and the Korean National Tuberculosis Association. Report on the forth tuberculosis prevalence survey in Korea. (1980).

23. Ministry of Health and Social Affairs and the Korean National Tuberculosis Association. Report on the fifth tuberculosis prevalence survey in Korea. (1985).

24. Ministry of Health and Social Affairs and the Korean National Tuberculosis Association. Report on the sixth tuberculosis prevalence survey in Korea. (1990).

25. Sutherland I, Bleiker MA, Meijer J, *et al.* (1983). The risk of tuberculous infection in the Netherlands from 1967 to 1979. *Tubercle.* 64:241–253.

26. Thorson A, Diwan VK. (2001). Gender inequalities in tuberculosis: aspects of infection, notification rates, and compliance. *Curr Opin Pulm Med.* 7:165–169.

27. Hundelson P. (1996). Gender differential in tuberculosis: the role of socio-economic and cultural factors. *Tuberc Lund Dis.* 77:391–400.

28. Fine PEM. (1993). Immunities in and to tuberculosis: implications for pathogenesis and vaccination. In: Porter JDH, McAdam KPWJ, eds. *Tuberculosis back to future*. Chichester: Wiley and Sons. 53–78.

29. Hisada M, Stuver SO, Okayama A, *et al.* (1999). Gender differences in skin reactivity to purified protein derivatives among carriers of HTLV-1 in Japan. *JAIDS.* 22:302–307.

30. Shaaben MA, Abdul AM, Cross ER, *et al.* (1990). Revaccination with BCG: its effect on skin tests in Kuwaiti senior school children. *Eur Resp J.* 3:187–91.

31. Kurasawa T. (1990). Tuberculin skin tests of patients with active pulmonary tuberculosis and non-tuberculosis pulmonary disease. *Kekkaku.* 65:47–52.

32. Borgdorff MW, Nagelkerke NJ, Dy C, *et al.* (2000). Gender and tuberculosis: a comparison of prevalence surveys with notification data to explore sex differences in case detection. *Int J Tuberc Lung Dis.* 4(2):123–132.

33. Martinez AN, Rhee JT, Small PM, *et al.* (2000). Sex differences in the epidemiology of tuberculosis in San Francisco. *Int J Tuberc Lung Dis.* 4(1):26–31.

34. Cassels A, Heineman E, LeClerq S. (1982). Tuberculosis case-finding in eastern Nepal. *Tubercle.* 63:173–185.

35. Ettling MB, Thimasarn K, Krachaiklin S, *et al.* (1989). Evaluation of malaria clinics in Maesot, Thailand: Use of serology to assess coverage. Transactions of the Royal Society of Tropical medicine and Hygiene. 83:325–331.

36. WHO. (1996). Gender and leishmaniasis in Columbia, a re-definition of existing concepts? Geneva: WHO, Gender and Tropical Diseases Resource Paper. 2:1.

37. Murray CJL. (1991). Social, economic and operational research on tuberculosis: recent studies and some priority questions. *Bull Int Union Tuberc Lung Dis.* 66(4):149–156.

38. Comstock GW, Ferebee SH, Hammes LM. (1967). A controlled trial of community-wide isoniazid prophylaxis in Alaska. *Am Rev Respir Dis.* 95:935–943.

39. Comstock GW, Livesay VT, Woolpert SF. (1974). The prognosis of a positive tuberculin reaction in childhood and adolescence. *Am J Epidemiol.* 99:131–138.

40. Groth-Petersen E, Knudsen J, Wilbek E. (1959). Epidemiological basis of tuberculosis eradication in an advanced country. *Bull World Health Organ.* 21:5–49.

41. Grybowski S, Allen EA. (1964). Challenge of tuberculosis in decline: a study based on the epidemiology of tuberculosis in Ontario, Canada. *Am Rev Resp Dis.* 90:707–720.

42. Gedde-Dahl T. (1952). Tuberculosis infection in the light of tuberculin matriculation. *Am J Hyg.* 56:139–214.

43. Comstock GW, Edwards PQ. (1975). The competing risks of tuberculosis and hepatitis for adult tuberculin reactors. *Am Rev Respir Dis.* 111:573–577.

44. Snider D. (1984). Pregnancy and tuberculosis. *Chest.* 86:10S–13S.

45. Hamedah MA, Glassroth J. (1992). Tuberculosis and pregnancy. *Chest.* 101:1114–1120.

46. Espinal M, Reingold AL, Lavandera M. (1996). Effect of pregnancy on the risk of developing active tuberculosis. *J Infect Dis.* 173:488–491.

47. Styblo K. (1991). Epidemiology of tuberculosis. Selected papers. *The Netherlands: KNCV.* 24:1–136.

48. Nathanson CA. (1997). Sex, illness and medical care: A review of data-theory and method. *Soc Sci Med.* 11(3):50–65.

49. Rangan S, Uplekar M. (1998). Gender perspectives of access to health and tuberculosis care. In: Diwan VK, Thorson A, Winkist A, eds. *Gender and Tuberculosis*. The Nordic School of Public Health, Goteborg. 3:107–125.

50. Banerji D, Anderson S. (1963). A sociological awareness of symptoms among persons with pulmonary tuberculosis. *Bull World Health Organ.* 29:665–683.

51. Long NH, Diwan VK, Winkvist A. (2000). Differences in symptoms suggesting pulmonary tuberculosis among men and women. In: Long NH, ed. *Gender specific epidemiology of tuberculosis in Vietnam* [Ph.D. thesis]. Stockholm: Karolinska Institute. IV:1–10.

52. Boeree MJ, Harries AD, Godschalk P, *et al.* (2000). Gender differences in relation to sputum submission and smear-positive pulmonary tuberculosis in Malawi. *Int J Tuberc Lung Dis.* 4(9):882–884.

53. Rieder HL, Arnadottir T, Tardencilla Gutierrez AA, *et al.* (1997). Evaluation of a standardized recording tool for sputum smear microscopy for acid-fast bacilli under routine conditions in low income countries. *Int J Tuberc Lung Dis.* 1(4):339–345.

54. Nayar S, Narang P, Tyagi NK. Field trial of short term intermittent chemotherapy against tuberculosis. Department of Community Medicine and Department of Microbiology, MG Institute of Medical Sciences, Sevagram, Wardha (unpublished).

55. Long NH, Johansson E, Lonnroth K, *et al.* (1999). Longer delays in tuberculosis diagnosis among women in Vietnam. *Int J Tuberc Lung Dis.* 3(5):388–393.

56. Needham DM, Foster SD, Tomlinson G, *et al.* (2001). Socio-economic, gender and health services factors affecting diagnostic delay for tuberculosis patients in urban Zambia. *Trop Med Int Health.* 6(4):256.

57. Cegielski JP, Goetz MB, Jacobson JM, *et al.* (1997). Gender differences in early suspicion of tuberculosis in hospitalized, high-risk patients during 4 epidemic years, 1987 to 1990. *Infect Control Hosp Epidemiol.* 18:237–243.

58. Niijima T, Yamagishi F, Suzuki K. (1990). Patient's delay in the primary treatment cases of pulmonary tuberculosis detected by subjective symptoms. *Kekkaku.* 65:609–613.

59. Hooi LN. Case-finding for pulmonary tuberculosis in Penang. *Med J Malaysia.* 1994;49:223–230.

60. Pirkis JE, Speed BR, Young AP, *et al.* (1996). Time to initiation of anti-tuberculosis treatment. *Tuberc Lund Dis.* 77:401–406.

61. Johansson E, Long NH, Diwan VK, *et al.* (2000). Gender and tuberculosis control. Perspectives on health seeking behavior among men and women in Vietnam. *Health Policy.* 52133–52151.

62. Thorson A, Hoa NP, Long NH. (2001). Health-seeking behaviour of individuals with a cough of more than 3 weeks. *Lancet.* 9244:1823–1824.

63. Khan A, Walley J, Newell J. (2000). Tuberculosis in Pakistan: socio-cultural constraints and opportunities in treatment. *Soc Sci Med.* 50:247–254.

64. Yamasaki-Nakagawa M, Ozasa K, Yamada N, *et al.* (2001). Gender differences in delays to diagnosis and health care seeking behaviour in a rural area of Nepal. *Int J Tuberc Lung Dis.* 5(1):24–31.

65. Duggal R, Amin S. (1989). Cost of health care: a household survey in an Indian district. The Foundation for Research in Community Health, Bombay.

66. Vora A. (1994). Women's health, population and development: concerns and perspectives. Anubhav. 3:22–23.

67. Health Development Manpower Research Project. (1977). Rural health needs: Report of a study in the primary care unit (district) of Tanahu, Nepal. Tribhuvan University, Kathmandu.

68. Mathias AR. (1991). An exploratory study of the utilization by women of two health posts in Latlitpur district, Nepal. Ph.D. thesis, Nuffield Institute for Health, International Division, University of Leeds.

69. Olakowski T. (1973). A tuberculosis longitudinal survey, National Tuberculosis Institute, Bangalore WHO Project: India 0103. World Health Organization Regional Office for South East Asia.

70. Rao GR. (1982). Tuberculosis mortality in an urban complex in central India: a study of long-term trends. *Tubercle.* 63:187–193.

71. Ministry of Public Health of the People's Republic of China. (1985). National random survey for the epidemiology of tuberculosis in 1984–85.

72. Sigurdsson S. (1950). Tuberculosis in Iceland: epidemiological studies. Public Health Technical Monograph No. 2, Federal Security Agency, United States Government Printing Office. 1–53.

73. Centers for Disease Control and Prevention. (1993). Tuberculosis statistics in the United States, 1992. Atlanta, Georgia: CDC, Division of Tuberculosis Elimination.

74. Conte JE Jr, Golden JA, McQuitty M, *et al.* (2002). Effects of gender, AIDS, and acetylator status on intrapulmonary concentrations of isoniazid. *Antimicrob Agents Chemother.* 46(8):2358–2364.

75. Conte JE Jr, Golden JA, Kipps J, *et al.* (2001). Effects of AIDS and gender on steady-state plasma and intrapulmonary ethambutol concentrations. *Antimicrob Agents Chemother.* 45(10):2891–2896.

76. Conte JE Jr, Golden JA, McQuitty M, *et al.* (2000). Effects of AIDS and gender on steady-state plasma and intrapulmonary ethionamide concentrations. *Antimicrob Agents Chemother.* 44(5):1337–1341.

77. Conte JE Jr, Golden JA, Duncan S, *et al.* (1999). Intrapulmonary concentrations of pyrazinamide. *Antimicrob Agents Chemother.* 43(6):1329–1333.

78. Nair D, George A, Chacko KT. (1997). Tuberculosis in Bombay: new insights from poor urban patients. *Health Policy Plan.* 12(1):77–85.

79. Gothi GD, Savic D, Baily GVJ, *et al.* (1971). Collection and consumption of self administered anti-tuberculous drugs under programme conditions. *Ind J Tub.* 18:107–113.

80. Singh G, Banerji SC, Mathur SK. (1976). A study of defaulters in anti-tuberculosis therapy. *Ind J Tub.* 42:98–102.

81. Sharma SK, Patodi RK, Sharma PK, *et al.* (1979). A study in default in drug intake by patients of pulmonary tuberculosis in Indore, MP. *Ind J Prev Soc Med.* 10:123–128.

82. Padmanabhan VK, Sivaramakrishnan PR, Umashankar V. (1990). A study of lost cases put on short course chemotherapy under programme conditions. *Lung Ind.* 8:156–159.

83. Geethakrishnan K. (1990). Case holding and treatment failures under a TB clinic operating in rural setting. *Ind J Tub.* 37:145–148.

84. Suhadev M, Ganapathy S, Sivasubramaniam S, *et al.* (1995). A retrospective study of "noncompliant" patients in controlled trials of short course chemotherapy. *Ind J Tub.* 42:221–225.

85. Jagota P, Sreenivas TR, Parimala N. (1996). Improving treatment compliance by observing differences in treatment irregularity. *Ind J Tub.* 43:75–80.

86. Comolet TM, Rakotomalala R, Rajaonarioa H. (1998). Factors determining compliance with tuberculosis treatment in an urban environment, Tamatave, Madagascar. *Int J Tuberc Lung Dis.* 2(11):891–897.

87. Connolly C, Davies GR, Wilkinson D. (1999). Who fails to complete tuberculosis treatment? Temporal trends and risk factors for treatment interruption in a community-based directly observed therapy programme in a rural district of South Africa. *Int J Tuberc Lung Dis.* 3(12):1081–1087.

88. Chan-Yeung M, Noerjojo K, Chan SL, *et al.* (2002). Sex differences in tuberculosis in Hong Kong. *Int J Tuberc Lung Dis.* 6(1):11–18.

89. Johansson E, Long NH, Diwan VK, *et al.* (1999). Attitudes to compliance with tuberculosis treatment among women and men in Vietnam. *Int J Tuberc Lung Dis.* 3(10):862–868.

90. Liam CK, Lim KH, Wong CM, *et al.* (1999). Attitudes and knowledge of newly diagnosed tuberculosis patients regarding the disease, and factors affecting treatment compliance. *Int J Tuberc Lung Dis.* 3(4):300–309.

91. Liefooghe R, Michiels N, Habib S, *et al.* (1995). Perception and social consequences of tuberculosis: a focus group study of tuberculosis patients in Sialkot, Pakistan. *Soc Sci Med.* 41:1685–1692.

92. Liefooghe R, Baliddawa JB, Kipruto EM, *et al.* (1997). From their own perspective. A Kenyan community's perception of tuberculosis. *Trop Med Int Health.* 2:809–821.

93. Kim SC, Jin BW, Shimao T, *et al.* (1985). Study on knowledge of tuberculosis and attitudes towards the disease. *Bull Int Union Tuberc.* 60(3–4):131–132.

94. Menzies R, Rocher I, Vissandjee B. (1993). Factors associated with compliance in treatment of tuberculosis. *Tuberc Lund Dis.* 74:32–37.

95. Long NH, Johansson E, Vinod KD, *et al.* (1999). Different tuberculosis in men and women: beliefs from Focus groups in Vietnam. *Soc Sci Med.* 49(6):815–822.

96. Peterson Tulsky J, Castle White M, *et al.* (1999). Street talk: knowledge and attitudes about tuberculosis and tuberculosis control among homeless adults. *Int J Tuberc Lung Dis.* 3(6):528–533.

97. Long NH. (2000). Gender specific epidemiology of tuberculosis in Vietnam [Ph.D. thesis]. Stockholm: Karolinska Institute.

98. Rajeswari R, Balasubramanian R, Muniyandi M, *et al.* (1999). Socio-economic impact of tuberculosis on patients and family in India. *Int J Tuberc Lung Dis.* 3(0):869–877.

88

Gender-Specific Issues in Non-HIV Viral Infections

MAGDALENA E. SOBIESZCZYK, MD AND CHRISTINE M. HAY, MD

Division of Infectious Diseases, University of Rochester Medical Center, Rochester, NY

Gender-specific effects of viral infections may be the result of differences in pathophysiology, differences in exposure or risk factors, and effects specific to pregnancy. Although these differences have been noted for many years, for most infections the exact mechanisms behind gender-specific differences have yet to be elucidated. This chapter will examine the following:

1. Gender-specific manifestations of viral infections resulting from differences in pathophysiology
2. Gender-specific manifestations of viral infections resulting from differences in exposures or risk factors
3. Manifestations specific to pregnancy

I. Human Lymphotropic Viruses: HTLV-1 and HTLV-2

The first human retrovirus, human T-cell lymphotropic virus type 1 (HTLV-1) was discovered in 1979, derived from the lymphocytes of a patient originally thought to have an aggressive form of cutaneous T-cell lymphoma. Two years later, HTLV-2 was isolated from the cells of a patient with atypical hairy cell leukemia. Morphologically, HTLV-1 and HTLV-2 are type C viruses, which make up a group of retroviruses known as the primate T-cell leukemia/lymphoma virus. Both are single-stranded RNA viruses with a genome that undergoes reverse transcription into a DNA provirus that integrates into a host T-cell genome. This integration process allows the retrovirus to cause lifelong infection, evade immune clearance, and produce diseases of long latency.

There is 65% overall nucleotide homology between HTLV-1 and HTLV-2. Based on sequencing data, HTLV-1 is composed of three types: Cosmopolitan, Melanesian, and Zairian, which are present in widely scattered populations in the world. Two best-studied areas are the islands of southwestern Japan and the Caribbean basin. HTLV-1 infection has also been reported in central and West Africa, Melanesia, and parts of South America and the Middle East. HTLV-2, however, consists of type A, B, and C and is reported mainly in intravenous drug users and their sexual contacts. Endemic areas include the United States, Europe, South America, and Southeast Asia. HTLV seroprevalence can range from 5–30%, depending on the population in question, but clinical disease develops in only about 3–5% of carriers of HTLV-1 over their lifetime.

There is a wide range of clinical conditions linked to HTLV-1. The best-described associations include adult T-cell leukemia/lymphoma (ATL), a proliferative disorder of T-cells characterized by lymphadenopathy, hypercalcemia, lytic bone lesions, skin involvement, and hepatomegaly. HTLV-1 has also been linked to the HTLV-associated myelopathy or tropical spastic paraparesis (HAM/TSP), a chronic neurologic syndrome associated with demyelination of the long motor neurons of the spinal cord.

Other HTLV-1 associated clinical syndromes include infective dermatitis, polymyositis, uveitis and arthritis, Sjörgen syndrome, and infiltrative pneumonitis. HTLV-2 does not have any clearly documented disease associations other than a link to HAM/TSP. It has been associated with atypical hairy cell leukemia and mycosis fungoides, yet there is no clear evidence confirming an etiologic role of HTLV-2 in these disorders. Routes of transmission of HTLV-1 and HTLV-2 are similar and include sexual intercourse, administration of blood products, and mother-to-child transfer.

Laboratory diagnosis of infection rests on an enzyme-linked immunosorbent assay (ELISA) screen; there is, however, cross reactivity between HTLV-1 and HTLV-2 in the assay, and the virus subtype is distinguished by Western blot. Polymerase chain reaction (PCR) assay to quantify the level of virus is used in research settings.

A. Manifestations Specific to Pregnancy

In endemic areas, seropositive persons are clustered around families, reflecting predominance of mother-to-child and male-to-female transmission. Breast-feeding is the predominant route of vertical transmission and occurs through ingestion of infected milkborne lymphocytes. According to epidemiologic studies from Japan, 15–20% of children of seropositive mothers acquire HTLV-1 through breast-feeding [1], whereas only 1–2% of bottle-fed infants of mothers positive for HTLV-1 become infected. Transmission appears to increase with the number of months that the infant has nursed. Recent data from Japan suggest that babies who were short-term breast-feeders (for 6 months or less) showed a statistically significant lower seroconversion rate than long-term breast-feeders: 3.9% vs 20.3% [2,3].

There may be other factors implicated in the mother-to-child transmission. Two separate studies from Japan and France identified maternal anti-HTLV-1 antibody titer and maternal HTLV-1 proviral load as additional risk factors; higher levels of both were associated with increased risk of HTLV-1 seropositivity in children [4,5].

The antibody titers correlate with the proviral burden. This may explain the paradoxic finding of high antibody titers among women who transmit HTLV-1 to their infants through prolonged breast-feeding; transplacental maternal antibodies appear to protect the infant from infection in the first months of life, but subsequently the infants become infected via maternal virus transmitted in breast milk.

Intrauterine transmission occurs rarely; the placenta can be infected by HTLV-1, but the infection does not reach the fetus.

The placenta has been known to be a barrier against intrauterine transmission, perhaps by mechanism of apoptosis; it has been reported that the incidence of apoptosis-positive cells in placentas from pregnant women who were HTLV-1 seropositive was higher than that from women who were HTLV-1 seronegative [6]. HTLV-2 is also found in breast milk, and although there are no good studies of mother-to-child transmission, the finding that seropositive children had seropositive mothers supports this route of infection.

B. Gender-Specific Manifestations Resulting from Differences in Exposure or Risk Factors

HTLV-1 seroprevalence is characterized by an age-dependent increase that is similar in diverse geographic areas. Among children, the prevalence rate of both sexes is low, about 1%, and the male-to-female ratio is 1. Starting with adolescence, however, the prevalence increases and infection rates between males and females diverge, with female rates exceeding male rates. This trend continues into adulthood, and whereas male rates plateau by the age of 40 years, female rates continue to increase and peak at about age 60 years [7]. The reason for this divergence is ascribed to the fact that although sexual transmission is bidirectional, male-to-female transmission occurs 10 times much more efficiently. For example, some studies report that after 10 years of sexual contact with an infected partner, a woman has a 61% likelihood of being infected, as opposed to only 0.4% for a man [8]. In a Japanese cohort study of 100 discordant couples practicing unprotected sexual intercourse, there were seven seroconversions during 5 years of observation. Uninfected females were 3.9 times more likely to become infected than uninfected males [9].

Similar differences in prevalence were noted among pregnant women. A study of young pregnant women (<30 years old) in French Guiana demonstrated that factors such as high gravidity, a high parity, and a negative Rhesus factor were independently linked to an increased risk of HTLV-1 seropositivity [10]. It has been postulated that the increase in HTLV-1 prevalence rates in the younger than 30 age group could be the result of high levels of sexual transmission in this population. In Jamaica or French West Indies, for example, women who were HTLV-1 seropositive were slightly more likely to have had more than three lifetime sex partners, earlier age at first sexual intercourse, and a history of sexually transmitted diseases [10–12]. In many studies an increased risk of seropositivity has been seen with increasing age but also with prior miscarriages, caesarian sections, and high gravidity. These factors are known to be associated with a low socioeconomic level, and they could reflect sexual activity and a high number of lifetime sexual partners [10]. Sexual transmission of HTLV-2 has been difficult to study.

C. Gender-Specific Manifestations

HTLV-1–associated myelopathy, or tropical spastic paresis, affects mainly adults, with a female-to-male predominance of 3:1. It has been shown that HAM/TSP incidence increases with age and is higher in women between 40 and 59 years of age compared with men in the same age group. With HTLV-1 infection, the lifetime risk of developing HAM/TSP was estimated to be 1.9% overall and is slightly higher in women (1.8%) than in men (1.3%) [13]. Thus, the higher prevalence of HTLV-1 in women living in endemic areas does not fully explain the preponderance of female HAM/TSP, suggesting that other cofactors may be present. It has been postulated that the overrepresentation of females and the increase in incidence with age are indicative of the predominance of infections acquired through sexual transmission [13,14].

HTLV-1 infection is also considered a risk factor for ATL. A male predominance in ATL has been shown to exist in Japan, perhaps because of an earlier average age of infection among males. The overall ATL mortality was shown to be higher for males than females. Reasons for this difference have not been elucidated [15].

II. Polyomavirus

Human polyomaviruses, JC and BK, named after patients from whom the initial virus isolates were obtained, were first isolated in 1971. Polyomaviruses are members of the Papovaviridae family, which are unenveloped icosahedral nucleocapsids with a double-stranded DNA genome.

They are worldwide in distribution, and approximately 60–80% of adults in United States and Europe have antibodies to JC or BK virus. The infection is acquired in childhood, persists in the kidneys, and is asymptomatic in the majority of patients. The seroprevalence of both viruses increases sharply during childhood. The route of transmission is not known, and the only detailed information about transmission comes from studies of nonprimate agents. The BK and JC viruses have been detected in human and mice tonsillar tissue as well as murine intestinal endothelial cells, suggesting oral or respiratory mode of transmission. Clinically, primary infection in childhood is largely asymptomatic and only rarely associated with upper-respiratory or urinary tract disease. Following primary infection the viruses remain latent in the kidney. Both BK and JC viruses can be detected in mononuclear cells in peripheral blood, bone marrow, and the central nervous system (CNS).

Reactivation of infection occurs most commonly with immunosuppression, and viral shedding increases with age and levels of immunosuppression. The BK virus has been linked to ureteral stenosis and hemorrhagic cystitis in renal or bone marrow transplant recipients; however, the majority of renal transplant recipients with JC or BK virus viruria have no symptoms. JC virus has been shown to have tropism for oligodendrocytes and to cause progressive multifocal leukoencephalopathy in older patients with underlying hematologic malignancies and in patients with HIV.

BK and JC viruses are slow growing in tissue culture, which hampers isolation of the virus from clinical specimen. Cytologic examination of urinary epithelial cells, looking for intranuclear inclusions, can be used to detect BK and JC virus viruria. PCR, however, is the most sensitive method of detecting BK or JC virus in the cerebrospinal fluid (CSF) and in the urine.

A. Manifestations Specific to Pregnancy

Asymptomatic viruria with JC and BK virus occurs primarily in immunosuppressed patients and pregnant women; in humans with intact immune function it is a rare occurrence. The high seroprevalence of JC and BK virus antibodies in the absence of seroconversion in pregnancy suggests that viral excretion represents reactivation of previously acquired infection [15a]. About 5% of pregnant women demonstrate a fourfold rise in antibody titers to BK virus, and about 9–15% have a similar increase in JC virus antibody titers. Virus shedding occurs primarily during the third trimester of pregnancy and usually ceases in the immediate postpartum period [16,17]. Both JC and BK virus shedding may occur, although JC virus viruria is more common [17].

Pregnant women tend to have more severe manifestations of infections in which cell-mediated immunity is important. Compared to pregnant controls, women with reactivation of the virus tended to have a monocytosis earlier in pregnancy, a lower neutrophil count, and a significant lymphopenia [7,16]. The only detailed data concerning polyomavirus transmission comes from nonprimate studies: perinatal transmission of virus can occur in mice if the mother develops a primary infection during pregnancy. At present there is no definitive evidence that perinatal transmission of polyomavirus occurs in the setting of maternal viruria. In one study immunoglobulin M (IgM) to BK virus was detected in three of six infants whose mothers had serologic evidence of BK virus infection during pregnancy [7]. However, more recent serologic studies have failed to demonstrate evidence of congenital infection by BK virus [18].

III. Parvovirus B19

Human parvovirus B19, a small, nonenveloped, single-stranded DNA virus, was first discovered in 1974 during evaluation of tests for hepatitis B surface antigen. This virus can be propagated only in human or primate erythroid cells. It is cytotoxic and in normal hosts has been shown to lead to an acute but self-limited cessation of red blood cell production. In immunocompetent children B19 is the cause of erythema infectiosum; in adults it may lead to acute symmetric polyarthropathy. In patients with underlying hemolytic disorders, infections lead to transient aplastic crises. In the immunocompromised host B19 viremia manifests as pure red-cell aplasia and chronic anemia, whereas in the fetus the virus can lead to death in utero, hydrops fetalis, or congenital anemia. Parvovirus B19 infection is prevalent throughout the world, and by the age of 15 years old the prevalence of antibody is quoted to be more than 50% [7].

Outbreaks of infections occur most commonly during late winter and spring, and the infection is probably spread by a respiratory route; the virus can also be found in serum and has been transmitted by blood and blood products. Laboratory diagnosis of parvovirus B19 infection is best accomplished with a PCR assay; antibody assays (IgM) can aid in diagnosing acute infection but are not reliable for diagnosing chronic infection in immunocompromised patients.

A. Manifestations Specific to Pregnancy

Infection during the second trimester when the red blood cell turnover is high and immune response is deficient can lead to fetal death in utero, hydrops fetalis, congenital anemia, and myocarditis. By the third trimester, a more effective fetal immune response to the virus accounts for the decrease in fetal loss.

There is no convincing evidence for congenital abnormalities after maternal B19 infections, only case reports of congenital ocular and neurologic abnormalities. Pregnant women are commonly exposed to B19 through other children; about 30% of maternal infections are vertically transmitted to the fetus, and fetal death occurs in 2–10% of maternal infections [19,20].

The risk of fetal death with maternal exposure is between 2 and 10% [7]. Thus, the Centers for Disease Control and Prevention recommend that pregnant health care workers should not care for patients with transient aplastic crises or with chronic B19 infection [21].

B. Gender-Specific Manifestations

Parvovirus B19 infection is common in childhood. It can also occur in adult life; in women of childbearing age in the United States an annual seroconversion rate of 1.5% has been documented [7]. Clinical manifestation of the disease range from asymptomatic or subclinical infections to a biphasic illness with symptoms during the viremic and immune complex–mediated stages of the disease. A large proportion of adults, especially women, experience arthralgia or frank arthritis with painful joints, swelling, and stiffness [7].

IV. Measles

Measles, caused by the rubeola virus, is a highly contagious infection usually seen in children. The measles virus virions are pleomorphic spheres with an inner nucleocapsid that is a coiled helix of protein and RNA.

Measles occurs throughout the world and prior to the introduction of vaccine, the infection was endemic in developed and developing countries. At that time, measles epidemics occurred every 2 years and typically lasted 3 to 4 months, peaking in late spring. Since the vaccine was licensed in 1963, the incidence of measles in the United States has decreased by almost 99%. It is an airborne virus spread by droplets of infected respiratory-tract secretions. Patients are most infectious during the late prodromal phase when cough and coryza are at their peak.

The illness is characterized by a prodromal phase of malaise, cough, coryza, fever, and anorexia. Toward the end of the prodrome, Koplik's spots appear on the buccal mucosa, preceding the onset of maculopapular rash. The entire illness lasts 7–10 days and the rash resolves.

Morbidity and mortality are highest in infants, the elderly, and patients of low socioeconomic status. Natural measles induces lifelong immunity, and reexposure is almost always asymptomatic [7]. In developed countries complications occur in only about 10% of cases; the most common ones include otitis media, pneumonia, acute disseminated encephalomyelitis, subacute sclerosing panencephalitis and inclusion-body encephalitis. Myocarditis, pericarditis, conjunctivitis, and keratitis can also occur.

Diagnosis is clinical; infection can also be documented by a fourfold increase in measles antibody titer in acute and convalescent serum. Treatment is supportive, and great emphasis is placed on preventive measures such as passive immunization of exposed persons within 6 days of exposure and active immunization between the ages of 12 to 15 months and the second dose on school entry. Contraindications to measles vaccination include pregnancy.

A. Manifestations Specific to Pregnancy

In most countries, maternal antibodies confer protection against measles during the first 6 months of life and the disease may be modified by waning levels of antibody that persist for an additional 6–9 months [7]. Because vaccinated mothers have lower levels of antibody to the measles virus than do mothers who have had natural measles, these infants will become susceptible to measles at an earlier age.

Postnatally acquired neonatal measles is rare. The high prevalence of passively acquired maternal antibodies results in protection of most newborns. In the absence of maternal antibodies, measles in the neonate is often a severe disease with the majority of deaths associated with pneumonia.

Measles, unlike rubella (German measles), does not cause congenital abnormalities in the fetus. There have been, however, reports of spontaneous abortion and premature delivery [7]. Passive immunization with immunoglobulin is recommended at birth for infants born to women with active disease.

Maternal antibody levels have obvious implications for infants' immunity and timing of vaccinations. Measles antibody titers are lower in women vaccinated as children than in women who have had natural measles, and the children of vaccinated women lose transplacentally acquired measles antibodies before 1 year of age. Therefore vaccination can be routinely given as early as 12 months of age because most women of childbearing age were vaccinated as children.

The morbidity and mortality of measles are higher in pregnant women mostly because of an increased risk of measles virus pneumonia during the third trimester and puerperium [22].

Interstitial pneumonitis resulting from viral replication and inflammation in the lower-respiratory tract is more severe in pregnancy [23]. For example, during a resurgence of measles in 1989–1991, a number of pregnant women developed measles. Out of 50% of those who required hospitalization, 54% had respiratory complications (primary measles pneumonia) requiring admission to an intensive care unit. There was one death in this group [22]. Likewise, during a 1951 epidemic in Greenland, pregnant women had 4.8% mortality compared to 1.0% mortality in nonpregnant women. Death was associated with left-ventricular failure and pulmonary edema [7].

V. Mumps

Mumps virus is a member of the Paramyxoviridae family, and its virion is an irregularly shaped spherical particle with a single-stranded RNA genome. Mumps is a disease of school-aged children and has a worldwide distribution. It is commonly acquired at school and spread to susceptible family members. Infection is rare in infants younger than 1 year old, presumably as a result of passively acquired maternal antibodies. The virus is transmitted via direct contact, droplet nuclei, or fomites and enters through the nose or mouth; the peak period of contagion is at the onset of parotitis. The virus replicates in the epithelial cells of the upper-respiratory tract and is spread to regional lymph nodes; primary viremia follows during which the virus is seeded to parotid glands, the CNS, pancreatic tissue, and seminiferous tubules. The clinical syndrome develops after an incubation period of 16–18 days; symptoms may be nonspecific at first, soon followed by tenderness and enlargement of the parotid gland. CNS involvement is the most common extrasalivary manifestation of mumps, but clinical meningitis or encephalitis occurs in only 0.1–10% cases [8]. Complications of infection include epididymoorchitis, oophoritis, pancreatitis, migratory polyarthritis, and (rarely) myocarditis or hearing loss.

Diagnosis is made on the basis of a history of exposure followed by parotid swelling and parotitis. Laboratory confirmation may be obtained by documenting an increase in IgM antibodies. The virus can also be isolated from the saliva, the CSF, or urine of infected patients. Mumps can be efficiently prevented by use of the Jerryl Lynn strain of live mumps vaccine. It is administered as part of the measles–mumps–rubella vaccine and is given in two doses. It is contraindicated in pregnant women or in significantly immunocompromised patients.

A. Gender-Specific Manifestations

Symptomatic gonadal involvement occurs in 25–38% of postpubertal men and is rarely documented in women. Some reports note that up to 5% of postpubertal women develop oophoritis [7]. Ovarian involvement may be underdiagnosed because unless a careful pelvic examination is documented, abdominal and pelvic pain may be attributed to pancreatic infection. Symptoms include fever, nausea, vomiting, and abdominal pain. Impaired fertility and premature menopause, albeit rare, have been reported [7]. About 15% of females infected with the virus complain of breast swelling and tenderness, and the incidence of mastitis doubles among postpubertal women [7].

Mumps was the most common cause of encephalitis in the United States until 1975. Although men and women have the same frequency of development of parotitis, CNS involvement (encephalitis or meningitis) has a clear male predominance (threefold).

B. Manifestations Specific to Pregnancy

Maternal infection during the first trimester can lead to bloodborne infection of the placenta and ultimately to fetal wastage. A proliferative necrotizing villitis with decidual cells containing intracytoplasmic inclusions has been described in the products of spontaneous and induced abortions [24].

Siegel and Fuerst have documented that second- and third-trimester mumps infections were not associated with increased fetal mortality [25]. Although there is no clear connection between mumps infection during pregnancy and congenital defects, there may be a possible association between mumps during the first trimester and low birth weight.

Mumps virus is excreted in breast milk, but few cases of prenatal mumps have been described [8]. However, transplacental transfer of maternal neutralizing antibodies has been clearly demonstrated and accounts for the rarity of mumps in young infants as well as lack of response to immunization in this age group. Antibody titers in maternal and cord serum are identical [26].

VI. Alphaviruses

The alphaviruses are RNA viruses in the Togaviridae family that are mostly mosquitoborne and cause a wide range of diseases in humans and animals. The main target organs are muscle, brain, reticuloendothelial system, and the joints. Serologically these viruses can be divided into six antigenic complexes: Eastern Equine Encephalitis (EEE), Venezuelan Equine Encephalitis (VEE), Sindbis (western equine encephalitis, or WEE, virus is the most notable one), Semliki Forest (Chikungunya and Ross River virus are notable human pathogens), Barmah Forest, Middleburg, and Ndumu antigenic complex. Clinically, these viruses can be divided into those that are associated with fever, rash, and polyarthritis (Chikungunya virus, Ross River virus, and O'nyong-nyong virus are the most important ones) or those that are associated with encephalitis. Alphaviruses are limited in their geographic spread by the range of their respective arthropod vectors. EEE virus infection, for example, occurs along the eastern and Gulf coasts of the United States; some cases have been documented in South America and Canada. WEE viruses are distributed primarily in states west of Mississippi and in corresponding Canadian provinces, whereas VEE infection has been documented primarily in South and Central America, reaching Texas. Infections secondary to encephalitis-causing alphaviruses are manifested by headaches, high fever, nausea, and vomiting; respiratory symptoms may occur as well.

There is no specific treatment for any of the alphavirus infections. Prevention depends primarily on control of vector mosquito populations.

A. Manifestations Specific to Pregnancy

Alphaviruses can be transmitted transplacentally in mice as well as humans. In mice, the virus infects the placenta, where it persists and spreads to the fetus despite the development of maternal antibody. The timing of maternal infection has implications for the fetus. In humans no fetal abnormalities were observed in infants infected with Ross River virus at 11–19 weeks of gestation; however, earlier infection has lead to fetal death [27].

Infections with the VEE virus have been associated with increases in spontaneous abortion [28] associated with cerebral necrosis and calcifications similar to those seen in toxoplasmosis. Infections acquired early in pregnancy have been associated with fetal hydrencephaly, porencephaly, and cerebral dysgenesis. Similarly, transplacental transmission has been documented for WEE, resulting in perinatal infection within the first week of life.

B. Gender-Specific Manifestations

WEE in older children and adults shows a male preponderance: male patients are two to three times more likely to develop disease than are female patients [29]. In contrast, there are some data that among alphaviruses associated primarily with polyarthritis and rash, the Ross River virus may show a female preponderance of polyarthritis [30,31].

VII. Viral Respiratory Infections: Coronavirus, Parainfluenza, Respiratory Syncytial Virus, Adenovirus, and Rhinovirus

A. Gender-Specific Manifestations

Gender does appear to influence the severity of respiratory syncytial virus (RSV) infection. There are epidemiologic data from Chapel Hill, North Carolina, to suggest that boys younger than 6 years of age had a higher rate of RSV lower-tract disease: 2.4 per 100 compared with 1.5 per 100 for girls. The greater severity of infection in male children is suggested by the preponderance of boys admitted to the hospital with lower respiratory–tract disease [8].

Similar data were derived from the Cleveland Family Study, an investigation conducted from 1948 to 1957 that followed almost 100 families to identify common respiratory illness. The investigators found that the highest number of illnesses occurred in young children, and they were the most likely introducers of infections. Mothers were the next most likely common introducers. More recent studies conducted in Michigan focused again on the family and demonstrated that illnesses were more frequent in boys than in girls up to 3 years of age. After the age of 3 years old, the incidence became more frequent in females. Females between ages 20–29 years had a greater increase in frequency in total respiratory illnesses compared to males.

Another relevant observation emerging from theses studies was that women who did not work outside the home had higher rates of respiratory illness than women who worked out of the home. Overall, women working out of the home still had a higher frequency of illness than males [32–34].

VIII. Varicella-Zoster Virus

Varicella-zoster virus (VZV) is the virus that causes chickenpox (varicella) and shingles (zoster). VZV is a member of the Herpesviridae family and the alpha subfamily, which also includes herpes simplex virus types 1 and 2 and herpes B virus. Like all herpesviruses, it induces lifelong latency in the host. Initial infection with VZV leads to the clinical syndrome of chickenpox in most susceptible hosts, although infection can be subclinical, especially in young children. Primary VZV infection in adults tends to be a more severe illness than in children, and in individuals with impaired cell-mediated immunity fatal outcomes can be seen. After primary infection, latent VZV can be demonstrated in the dorsal root ganglia. Prior to an outbreak of shingles, VZV reactivates in the dorsal root ganglion and travels down the sensory nerves to the skin, where it causes the characteristic painful rash of shingles. Whereas chickenpox is primarily a disease of children, shingles is primarily a disease of adults. Decreased cell-mediated immunity puts individuals at increased risk of zoster, and outbreaks may be more severe and last longer than in nonimmunocompromised individuals. VZV infections occur worldwide and affect both sexes equally. Morbidity and mortality of primary VZV infection is more severe in adults than in children. Pneumonitis, the most frequent complication of varicella infection, is 25 times more common in adults than in children and accounts for most of the fatalities ascribed to VZV infection.

A. Manifestations Specific to Pregnancy

1. Maternal Effects

Primary varicella infection during pregnancy is associated with more severe disease than in other immunocompetent adults. In particular, the third trimester of pregnancy is associated with an increased risk of varicella pneumonitis and increased mortality. Before specific antiviral therapy was available for VZV, the mortality rate of varicella pneumonia was 11.4–15% in nonpregnant adults but increased to 36–41% in pregnant women [35]. Better supportive care and specific antiviral therapy have decreased this mortality to 13–14% [36], and more recent reports show further reductions [37]. Maternal smoking, 100 or more skin lesions, and the third trimester of pregnancy are associated with a higher risk of varicella pneumonia [38]. Because of these findings, varicella–zoster immune globulin (VZIG) is recommended as prophylaxis for pregnant women who are VZV seronegative who have had significant exposure to chickenpox. VZIG provides passive immunization against VZV and is effective in preventing or ameliorating disease in children. It is effective if given within 72 hours of exposure and may be effective if given up to 96 hours after exposure, but once disease is established, its efficacy is questionable. A new formulation of VZIG appears to result in higher maternal antibody levels and is comparable in efficacy and safety to standard VZIG. Acyclovir may also be used to protect against VZV infection and to treat established infection. Data on outcomes from 1129 prospectively followed acyclovir-exposed pregnancies (712 involving first-trimester exposure) were reported to a voluntary registry from June 1984 through December 1997. The data fail to show an increase in the number of birth defects identified among the fetuses exposed to acyclovir when compared with those expected in the general population. In addition, no pattern of defects was seen, suggesting that maternal acyclovir use in pregnancy is safe [39]. Varicella vaccine was licensed in 1995 to prevent chickenpox. Because it is a live-virus vaccine, its use is contraindicated in pregnancy. The Vaccine Adverse Event Reporting System (VAERS) had received 87 reports of inadvertent vaccination of pregnant women as of July 25, 1998. None of these exposures resulted in characteristic features of congenital varicella syndrome in the exposed fetuses [40]. It is interesting that 19 pregnant women received varicella vaccine by mistake (instead of VZIG) after chickenpox exposure, suggesting that health care workers need to be educated to eliminate confusion between these agents.

2. Fetal Effects

Maternal chickenpox in pregnancy can lead to fetal varicella in up to 10% of infections occurring before 24 weeks of pregnancy [41]. These infections are usually benign and self-limiting, but in up to 2% of cases occurring between 13 and 20 weeks of gestation, a characteristic constellation of findings known as the congenital varicella syndrome (CVS) may occur [42]. This syndrome is often severe and is characterized by skin lesions, limb hypoplasia, microcephaly, prematurity, chorioretinitis, mental retardation, and early death. Despite advances in the field, the syndrome remains difficult to predict. Negative PCR results for VZV in amniotic fluid is associated with a favorable outcome; however, a positive test correlates poorly with the development of CVS and it is not clear that the benefit of the test outweighs the risk of amniocentesis [41]. It is recommended that pregnant women who develop chickenpox during pregnancy be counseled about the risk of CVS.

Maternal chickenpox in the perinatal period can result in neonatal varicella infection, which is often severe and can result in mortality rates up to 30%. The risk is greatest to infants born 7 days or less after the appearance of maternal varicella because they receive a large transplacental viral inoculum without passive transfer of maternal antibody. Babies exposed to maternal varicella in the first 28 days of life also have increased risk of severe infections. VZIG is therefore recommended for all infants exposed to maternal varicella from 7 days prior to delivery up to 28 days after birth. Infants of mothers with zoster during the perinatal period are protected by maternal antibody and are not at increased risk of serious infection. Similarly, infants born to seropositive mothers who are exposed to chickenpox in their siblings are not at increased risk of serious infection.

IX. Cytomegalovirus

Cytomegalovirus (CMV) is a beta subgroup herpesvirus that is found all over the world and has infected almost all people by late adulthood. Although usually asymptomatic, primary CMV infection can be characterized by a mononucleosis-like syndrome of fever, lymphadenopathy, and lymphocytosis, especially in young adults. Like all herpesviruses, CMV establishes latent infection with polymorphonuclear cells, T cells, vascular tissue, renal cells, and salivary glands, all potentially harboring the virus. Reactivation, except in the case of immunocompromised individuals, is usually asymptomatic, and although reinfections can occur, they too are usually asymptomatic. Complications in the immunocompetent host are rare but can include pneumonia, hepatitis, Guillain-Barré syndrome, meningoencephalitis, myocarditis, thrombocytopenia, and rash. Patients with the acquired immunodeficiency syndrome (AIDS) and bone marrow and solid organ transplants are at highest risk of complications from CMV infection. In patients with AIDS, CMV infection of the retina, CNS, and gastrointestinal tract are of particular importance. CMV has multiple different potential routes of infection. It is shed asymptomatically in saliva, urine, semen, and cervicovaginal secretions. Transmission can occur during intrauterine life, during the perinatal period, through breast milk, through close personal contact, through sexual intercourse, through blood transfusions, and through organ donation.

A. Manifestations Specific to Pregnancy

1. Maternal Effects

Symptomatic primary CMV infection is seen more commonly in pregnant women than in all other groups except for solid organ recipients [43]. In a study of a cohort of pregnant women with primary CMV infection, 59.8% had at least one clinical or laboratory manifestation and 31.4% had a flulike illness or persistent fever [44], suggesting that it may be possible to diagnose infection in these patients. Fever, lymphadenopathy, splenomegaly, hepatitis, and atypical lymphocytosis are the most common features of primary CMV infection in pregnant women.

2. Fetal Effects

CMV is the most common intrauterine infection affecting babies in this country. Congenital infection is most common in infants born to women with primary CMV infection during pregnancy. Preexisting maternal immunity results in a 69% reduction in the risk of congenital CMV infection [43]. Congenital infection occurs in approximately 30–40% of infants born to mothers with primary infection, and of these, about 10% will have clinical disease at birth [45]. Clinical disease includes varying degrees of cytomegalic inclusion disease, which may include jaundice; hepatosplenomegaly; petechial rash; multiple organ involvement; and CNS findings of microcephaly, chorioretinitis, and cerebral calcifications. Mortality with CNS involvement is high. Of the 90% of affected infants who are asymptomatic at birth, 5–17% will develop long-term sequelae including subtle effects on hearing and intelligence. Congenital infections resulting from recurrent maternal infection are much less severe as are postnatally acquired infections.

X. Epstein-Barr Virus

Epstein-Barr virus (EBV) is a member of the gamma herpesvirus family and is the etiologic agent of classic infectious mononucleosis. EBV infects B lymphocytes, which are also the site of latent virus infection [46]. EBV is found all over the world. Infection rates are highest in young children in developing countries; in the developed world approximately 50% of the population remains susceptible into the second decade of life [47]. Infection is spread through close personal contact, often with an asymptomatic shedder. In children younger than age 5 years, primary infection is usually asymptomatic but can present with upper-respiratory symptoms, pharyngitis, adenopathy, diarrhea, and abdominal complaints. In older children and adults, EBV primary infection often leads to classic infectious mononucleosis, which is characterized by malaise, headache, fever, pharyngitis, and cervical lymphadenopathy. Severe fatigue, nausea, vomiting, facial edema, and rashes can occur in more severe forms of the illness. Up to 90% of infected individuals will have mild hepatitis [48], and up to 50% will have splenomegaly. Serious complications found equally in either gender include airway obstruction from massive lymphoid hyperplasia, Guillain-Barré syndrome, facial nerve palsy, meningoencephalitis, aseptic meningitis, hemolytic anemia, pneumonia, myocarditis, pancreatitis, and glomerulonephritis.

A. Gender-Specific Manifestations

Splenic rupture is a rare but potentially fatal complication of EBV infection that occurs almost exclusively in young males [49]. The X-linked lymphoproliferative syndrome occurs in previously healthy males with a defect in the gene that encodes for signal transduction in T lymphocytes [50]. These individuals appear to have a selective immunodeficiency to EBV and when exposed, develop fulminant EBV infection. Bone marrow transplant, chemotherapy, and cord stem cell transplants are currently used to treat the disorder.

XI. Human Herpes Virus 8

This DNA gamma herpesvirus similar to Ebstein-Barr virus has been implicated in several important human neoplasms. The site of viral replication has not been completely elucidated, but viral DNA has been detected in saliva, semen, and peripheral blood mononuclear cells. Antibodies to this virus are found in diverse populations all over the world. Recently it has been isolated in tissues from all four forms of Kaposi's sarcoma (KS): classic, iatrogenic, endemic African, and HIV-associated. KS is characterized by bluish-red, well demarcated, painless nodules in the skin, lungs, viscera and the biliary system [8,51]. Classically it occurs in elderly people, particularly men, of Mediterranean, Middle Eastern, or Eastern European descent. It has been recognized as an AIDS-associated malignancy particularly common among homosexual men infected with HIV-1. Other less common diseases it is associated with include primary effusion lymphoma arising exclusively in patients with AIDS or Castleman's disease seen both in HIV-positive and HIV-negative patients.

A. Gender-Specific Manifestations

The epidemiology of KS reveals a male predominance of this disease; as mentioned earlier the classic, typically benign form of this disease is found predominantly in males. Incidence rates reported in Denmark, Sweden, and Wales are considerably lower in women than in males [52]. In the United States, a gender ratio of 4 was documented between 1970 and 1979. Similarly, HIV-seropositive homosexual and bisexual men are approximately 10 times more likely than the general healthy population to develop KS [51,53]. This suggests that gender may be a risk factor for development of KS.

Worldwide, occasional cases of classic KS have been reported in children, and among those cases data suggest male predominance. For example, a study of Tanzanian children before and during the AIDS epidemic reports 126 cases of KS. Of those children with pediatric KS, 126 (84%) were male and 24 (16%) were female. The gender ratio was 5.1:1 and 5.4:1 during the endemic and epidemic periods, respectively, and the highest occurrence of PKS was observed in the 0- to 5-years-of age group [54].

XII. Human Herpesvirus 6

Human herpesvirus (HHV) 6 and HHV 7 are two lymphotropic viruses representative of the Roseolovirus genus within the Betaherpesviririnae subfamily. HHV 6 infects nearly all humans by the age of 2 years. It is found in circulating lymphocytes during primary infection, in monocyte-macrophages during the convalescent phase, or in healthy individuals. This virus has the capacity to persist in the human host; evades immune surveillance and can be transmitted very efficiently. Clinically it causes sixth disease, or roseola infantum, characterized by fever followed by a diffuse exanthems. HHV 6 has neurotropic and neuroinvasive properties. The virus has been found in the CSF of many children with aseptic meningoencephalitis (either as a sequela of sixth disease or independently) and in infants with febrile seizures [8].

A. Manifestations Specific to Pregnancy

Given the very high seroprevalence of HHV 6 in the first 2 years of life, both horizontal (via saliva) and vertical transmission have been implicated as the two possible mechanisms. Intrauterine transmission has been documented and the virus has been isolated in cord blood specimen. Interestingly enough, however, despite the high seroprevalence of infection among the general adult population, the rate of fetal HHV 6 or HHV 7 infection during pregnancy is less than 1% of all births [55,56]. Intrauterine transmission has been documented by HHV 6 DNA detection in cord blood specimens of apparently healthy newborns and in fetuses following spontaneous abortions; however, no clear causation has been established. Because the viral genome has been documented in cervical swabs of about 20% of pregnant women, the possibility of intrapartum transmission has also been suggested [57].

Vertical transmission of HHV 6 may be symptomatic at birth; there are a few case reports in literature of early neonatal afebrile seizures resulting from a congenital HHV 6 variant B infection with subsequent neurologic impairments [58].

XIII. Influenza Virus

Influenza viruses belong to the family Orthomyxoviridae and are classified into three distinct groups—influenza A virus, B virus, and C virus—based on antigenic differences. The virus causes an acute, usually self-limited, febrile illness that occurs in outbreaks during winter months. Most common symptoms of fever, myalgias, and cough are often difficult to distinguish from symptoms caused by RSV, adenovirus, or other respiratory viruses [8]. Influenza attack rates are higher in children than adults, and pulmonary complications are more frequent in the elderly than in any other age group. CNS complications, specifically Reye's syndrome, have been described following influenza in children.

A. Manifestations Specific to Pregnancy

Historical data from 1918 and 1957 pandemics have shown that severe influenza infections, with concurrent pulmonary symptoms, have resulted in a marked mortality in pregnant women and were associated with abortions, premature deliveries, and intrauterine growth delays. These data have not been confirmed in larger, case-controlled studies. There are some recent data as to whether maternal influenza infection in the second and third trimester of pregnancy can result in transplacental transmission or an increase in complications of pregnancy. One study in particular reported that although intercurrent influenza infection was found in about 115 of pregnancies, none of the cord sera from maternal cases were positive for virus-specific IgM antibodies; likewise IgG antibodies did not persist in any of the infants past 6 months after birth. Most importantly, there were no significant differences in pregnancy outcomes between cases and controls [59].

In psychiatric literature there is considerable discussion as to whether prenatal exposure to influenza is a risk factor for adult schizophrenia. In most epidemiologic studies, fluctuations in the incidence of influenza have been compared with the birth dates of patients with schizophrenia, based on the assumption that the risk of the mother being infected with the virus was associated with occurrence of an influenza epidemic during the pregnancy [60]. To date there is only one retrospective study that has attempted to answer this question. The study looked at more than 900 patients with schizophrenia born in France between 1949 and 1981, using nonschizophrenic siblings as controls, and documented that significantly more patients with schizophrenia than controls had been exposed to the virus during the fifth month of pregnancy [60]. Currently inactivated influenza vaccine is recommended for routine use in women who will be in the second or third trimesters of pregnancy. The basis for this recommendation is the high risk of exposure and disease resulting from influenza viruses in pregnant women as well as the impact of influenza virus infection on the fetus and infant derived mostly from historical data [61].

XIV. Rubella Virus

Rubella virus belongs to the Togaviridae family with its RNA genome, and it is closely related to alphaviruses. No vector is required for its transmission. Rubella is only moderately contagious, in contrast to measles, and the virus is spread in droplet forms. Infants with congenital rubella shed large quantities of the virus for many months. Persons who have been vaccinated do not transmit the virus to others.

Rubella virus causes an acute exanthemous infection in children and adults; symptoms include rash, fever, and lymphadenopathy and can cause birth defects following fetal infections.

A. Manifestations Specific to Pregnancy

Vaccines that are contraindicated because of the theoretic risk of fetal transmission include measles, mumps, and rubella [62], although the observed risk of congenital rubella after immunization has so far not been found. The theoretic risk of congenital complications after immunization is 2%, contrasted with a 30% or greater risk after maternal rubella infection in the first trimester [63]. However, because the rubella virus can cross the placenta, it is advised that women vaccinated against rubella avoid becoming pregnant for at least 3 months after the administration of vaccine [8,62]. The minimal risk to the fetus does not mandate automatic termination of a pregnancy following vaccination.

1. Fetal Effects

Congenital rubella can be quite devastating to the fetus, leading to death, low birth weight, deafness, congenital heart disease, and mental retardation. The specific effects on the fetus depend on the time of infection. The most vulnerable time period is during the first 2 months of gestation, when the fetus has a 65–90% chance of being affected (spontaneous abortion or congenital defects) [64]. During the third month of fetal life the chance of developing a single congenital defect decreases to about 30–35%. It is generally held that, for maternal illness occurring after the 20th week of gestation, the fetal damage is reduced to deafness occurring at 1–2% [65].

Whether reinfection with rubella that occurs during pregnancy can result in transmission has been debated for a long time.

Many of the case reports documenting high rates of fetal defects actually refer to primary maternal infections; in subclinical cases of reinfection the rate of fetal complications may be nonexistent [66].

B. Gender-Specific Manifestations

Complications of rubella are quite rare and include arthritis of the small joints of upper extremities and knees and seem to affect predominantly women. Rubella vaccination itself has also been found to be associated with joint complications, particularly in women. In 2001 an analysis of the Vaccine Adverse Events Reporting System database concluded that such an association was indeed observed following immunizations from 1991 to 1998 [67].

XV. Lymphocytic Choriomeningitis Virus

The lymphocytic choriomeningitis virus belongs to the arenaviruses family; its reservoir is the *Mus domesticus* and *Mus musculus,* the house mouse. LCMV infection in humans occurs only in Europe and the Americas with cases occurring most commonly in the autumn, during times of lower humidity. Infections among humans are associated with substandard, mouse-infested, inner-city dwellings and the cleaning of rodent-infested barns. Most infections occur among young adults. The mode of transmission is not clear, but it most likely involves aerosolized virions, direct contact with rodents, and rodent bites [68].

The initial signs and symptoms of LCMV infection include fever and headaches that come on insidiously, resolve for 2–4 days, only to return with increased intensity. During the second febrile episode patients may exhibit signs of meningitis with a predominantly lymphocytic CSF profile; encephalomyelitis may ensue with psychosis, paraplegia, and abnormalities in cranial and autonomic nervous system function. Other complications include orchitis, myocarditis, and arthritis. Diagnosis can be made with IgM ELISA of serum and CSF. Treatment of arenavirus infection is mostly supportive but may include administration of Ribavirin in very severe infections. Prevention of spread by household rodent control is crucial in limiting transmission of the disease.

A. Considerations Specific to Pregnancy

It has been shown that arenaviruses readily invade the fetus and can lead to fetal infection. The initial case report of intrapartum infection in the 1950s involved an infant who was born in England 12 days after maternal illness developed, became febrile and lethargic, and died at 12 days of age [69].

Additional studies from Germany, Lithuania, and France have documented the association of intrauterine LCMV infection with the occurrence of spontaneous abortion as well as with congenital hydrocephalus, microcephalus, and chorioretinitis in live-born infants [68].

These sequelae of fetal infection have only been recognized within the last decade in the United States. Since then there have been little more than 50 documented cases of congenital LCMV infection worldwide. Rodent exposure was noted in 18

out of 38 mothers of infected infants. The transplacental infection of the fetus presumably occurred during symptomatic maternal viremic illness, primarily during the first and second trimesters, and was documented in 21 out of 33. Mice infected in utero asymptomatically shed LCMV in their feces, urine, saliva, breast milk, and semen and transmit the infection to humans (and hamsters) by direct contact or inhalation. Therefore, pregnant women should be advised to avoid contact with these rodents and their secretions, as they are similarly counseled to avoid contact with cat litter to prevent congenital toxoplasmosis [68,70,71].

XVI. Suggestions for Further Investigations

- What is the biologic basis for gender-based differences in the response to viral infection?
- What can be done to protect pregnant women from serious viral infections?
- What is the future of herpesvirus vaccines, especially against those herpesviruses most likely to result in fetal damage? Can reactivation of latent infections be prevented?

References

1. Kajiyama W, Kashiwagi S, Ikematsu H, *et al.* (1986). Intrafamilial transmission of adult T cell leukemia virus. *J Infect Dis.* 154(5):851–857.
2. Oki T, Yoshinaga M, Otsuka H, *et al.* (1992). A sero-epidemiological study on mother-to-child transmission of HTLV-I in southern Kyushu, Japan. *Asia Oceania J Obstet Gynaecol.* 18(4):371–377.
3. Takezaki T, Tajima K, Ito M, *et al.* (1997). Short-term breast-feeding may reduce the risk of vertical transmission of HTLV-I. The Tsushima ATL Study Group. *Leukemia.* 11(Suppl 3):60–62.
4. Manns A, Miley WJ, Wilks RJ, *et al.* (1999). Quantitative proviral DNA and antibody levels in the natural history of HTLV-I infection. *J Infect Dis.* 180(5):1487–1493.
5. Ureta-Vidal A, Angelin-Duclos C, Tortevoye P, *et al.* (1999). Mother-to-child transmission of human T-cell-leukemia/lymphoma virus type I: implication of high antiviral antibody titer and high proviral load in carrier mothers. *Int J Cancer.* 82(6):832–836.
6. Fujino T, Nagata Y. (2000). HTLV-I transmission from mother to child. *J Reprod Immunol.* 47(2):197–206.
7. Richman D, Whitely R, Hayden F, eds. (2002). *Clinical Virology.* Washington, DC: ASM Press.
8. Mandell G, Bennett J, Dolin R, eds. (2000). *Principles and Practice of Infectious Disease,* Vol. 2. Philadelphia: Churchill Livingstone: 1865.
9. Stuver SO, Tachibana N, Okayama A, *et al.* (1993). Heterosexual transmission of human T cell leukemia/lymphoma virus type I among married couples in southwestern Japan: an initial report from the Miyazaki Cohort Study. *J Infect Dis.* 167(1):57–65.
10. Tuppin P, Lepere JF, Carles G, *et al.* (1995). Risk factors for maternal HTLV-I infection in French Guiana: high HTLV-I prevalence in the Noir Marron population. *J Acquir Immune Defic Syndr Hum Retrovirol.* 8(4):420–425.
11. Dowe G, Smilkle MF, Thesiger C, *et al.* (2001). Bloodborne sexually transmitted infections in patients presenting for substance abuse treatment in Jamaica. *Sex Transm Dis.* 28(5):266–269.
12. Rouet F, Herrmann-Storck C, Courouble G, *et al.* (2002). A case-control study of risk factors associated with human T-cell lymphotrophic virus type-I seropositivity in blood donors from Guadeloupe, French West Indies. *Vox Sang.* 82(2):61–66.
13. Maloney EM, Cleghorn FR, Morgan OS, *et al.* (1998). Incidence of HTLV-I-associated myelopathy/tropical spastic paraparesis (HAM/TSP) in Jamaica and Trinidad. *J Acquir Immune Defic Syndr Hum Retrovirol.* 17(2):167–170.
14. Zaninovic V. (1986). Spastic paraparesis: a possible sexually transmitted viral myeloneuropathy. *Lancet.* 2(8508):697–698.
15. Hisada M, Okayama A, Spiegelman D, *et al.* (2001). Sex-specific mortality from adult T-cell leukemia among carriers of human T-lymphotropic virus type I. *Int J Cancer.* 91(4):497–499.

16. Coleman DV, Gardner SD, Mulholland C, et al. (1983). Human polyomavirus in pregnancy. A model for the study of defence mechanisms to virus reactivation. Clin Exp Immunol. 53(2):289–296.

17. Coleman DV, Wolfendale MR, Daniel RA, et al. (1980). A prospective study of human polyomavirus infection in pregnancy. J Infect Dis. 142(1):1–8.

18. Gibson PE, Field AM, Gardner SD, et al. (1981). Occurrence of IgM antibodies against BK and JC polyomaviruses during pregnancy. J Clin Pathol. 34(6):674–679.

19. Nomura T, Kusuhara K, Hara T. (2002). Human fetal infection with parvovirus B19: maternal infection time in gestation, viral persistence and fetal prognosis. Pediatr Infect Dis J. 21(12):1133–1136.

20. Valeur-Jensen AK, Pedersen CB, Westergaard T, et al. (1999). Risk factors for parvovirus B19 infection in pregnancy. JAMA. 281(12):1099–1105.

21. Hogue CJ, Strauss LT, Buehler JW, et al. (1989). Overview of the National Infant Mortality Surveillance (NIMS) project. MMWR CDC Surveill Summ. 38(3):1 16.

22. Atmar RL, Englund JA, Hammill H. (1992). Complications of measles during pregnancy. Clin Infect Dis. 14(1):217–226.

23. Ali ME, Albar HM. (1997). Measles in pregnancy: maternal morbidity and perinatal outcome. Int J Gynaecol Obstet. 59(2):109–113.

24. Garcia AG, Pereira JM, Vidigal N, et al. (1980). Intrauterine infection with mumps virus. Obstet Gynecol. 56(6):756–759.

25. Siegel M, Fuerst HT. (1966). Low birth weight and maternal virus diseases. A prospective study of rubella, measles, mumps, chickenpox, and hepatitis. JAMA. 197(9):680–684.

26. Hodes D, Brunell PA. (1970). Mumps antibody: placental transfer and disappearance during the first year of life. Pediatrics. 45(1):99–101.

27. Aaskov JG, Nair K, Lawrence GW, et al. (1981). Evidence for transplacental transmission of Ross River virus in humans. Med J Aust. 2(1):20–21.

28. Rivas F, Diaz LA, Cardenas VM, et al. (1997). Epidemic Venezuelan equine encephalitis in La Guajira, Colombia, 1995. J Infect Dis. 175(4): 828–832.

29. Bianchi TI, Aviles G, Monath TP, et al. (1993).Western equine encephalomyelitis: virulence markers and their epidemiologic significance. Am J Trop Med Hyg. 49(3):322–328.

30. Hazelton RA, Hughes C, Aaskov JG. (1985). The inflammatory response in the synovium of a patient with Ross River arbovirus infection. Aust N Z J Med. 15(3):336–339.

31. Hawkes RA, Boughton CR, Naim HM, et al. (1985). A major outbreak of epidemic polyarthritis in New South Wales during the summer of 1983/1984. Med J Aust. 143(8):330–333.

32. Monto AS, Ullman BM. (1974). Acute respiratory illness in an American community. The Tecumseh study. JAMA. 227(2):164–169.

33. Monto AS, Sullivan KM. (1993). Acute respiratory illness in the community. Frequency of illness and the agents involved. Epidemiol Infect. 110(1):145–160.

34. Monto AS. (2002). Epidemiology of viral respiratory infections. Am J Med. 112 Suppl 6A:4S–12S.

35. Harris RE, Rhoades ER. (1965). Varicella pneumonia complicating pregnancy. Report of a case and review of literature. Obstet Gynecol. 25:734–740.

36. Smego RA Jr, Asperilla MO. (1991). Use of acyclovir for varicella pneumonia during pregnancy. Obstet Gynecol. 78(6):1112–1116.

37. Harger JH, Ernest JM, Thurnau GR, et al. (2002). Frequency of congenital varicella syndrome in a prospective cohort of 347 pregnant women. Obstet Gynecol. 100(2):260–265.

38. Harger JH, Ernest JM, Thurnau GR, et al. (2002). Risk factors and outcome of varicella-zoster virus pneumonia in pregnant women. J Infect Dis. 185(4):422–427.

39. White AD, Andrews EB. (1999). The Pregnancy Registry program at Glaxo Wellcome Company. J Allergy Clin Immunol. 103:S362–S363.

40. Wise RP, Salive ME, Braun MM, et al. (2000). Postlicensure safety surveillance for varicella vaccine. JAMA. 284(10):1271–1279.

41. Mouly F, Mirlesse V, Meritet JF, et al. (1997). Prenatal diagnosis of fetal varicella-zoster virus infection with polymerase chain reaction of amniotic fluid in 107 cases. Am J Obstet Gynecol. 177(4):894–898.

42. Enders G, Miller E, Cradock-Watson J, et al. (1994). Consequences of varicella and herpes zoster in pregnancy: prospective study of 1739 cases. Lancet. 343(8912):1548–1551.

43. Fowler KB, Stagno S, Pass RF, et al. (1992). The outcome of congenital cytomegalovirus infection in relation to maternal antibody status. N Engl J Med. 326(10):663–667.

44. Nigro G, Anceschi MM, Cosmi EV. (2003). Clinical manifestations and abnormal laboratory findings in pregnant women with primary cytomegalovirus infection. BJOG. 110(6):572–577.

45. Raynor BD. (1993). Cytomegalovirus infection in pregnancy. Semin Perinatol. 17(6):394–402.

46. Higuchi M, Izumi KM, Kieff E. (2001). Epstein-Barr virus latent-infection membrane proteins are palmitoylated and raft-associated: protein 1 binds to the cytoskeleton through TNF receptor cytoplasmic factors. Proc Natl Acad Sci U S A. 98(8):4675–4680.

47. Niederman JC, McCollum RW, Henle G, et al. (1968). Infectious mononucleosis. Clinical manifestations in relation to EB virus antibodies. JAMA. 203(3):205–209.

48. Chetham MM, Roberts KB. (1991). Infectious mononucleosis in adolescents. Pediatr Ann. 20(4):206–213.

49. Aldrete JS. (1992). Spontaneous rupture of the spleen in patients with infectious mononucleosis. Mayo Clin Proc. 67(9):910–912.

50. Coffey AJ, Brooksbank RA, Brandau O, et al. (1998). Host response to EBV infection in X-linked lymphoproliferative disease results from mutations in an SH2-domain encoding gene. Nat Genet. 20(2):129–135.

51. Iscovich J, Boffetta P, Franceschi S, et al. (2000). Classic kaposi sarcoma: epidemiology and risk factors. Cancer. 88(3):500 517.

52. Hjalgrim H, Melbye M, Lecker S, et al. (1996). Epidemiology of classic Kaposi's sarcoma in Denmark between 1970 and 1992. Cancer. 77(7):1373–1378.

53. Friedman-Kien AE, Saltzman BR, Cao YZ, et al. (1990). Kaposi's sarcoma in HIV-negative homosexual men. Lancet. 335(8682):168–169.

54. Amir H, Kaaya EE, Manji KP, et al. (2001). Kaposi's sarcoma before and during a human immunodeficiency virus epidemic in Tanzanian children. Pediatr Infect Dis J. 20(5):518–521.

55. Boutolleau D, Fernandez C, Andre E, et al. (2003). Human herpesvirus (HHV)-6 and HHV-7: two closely related viruses with different infection profiles in stem cell transplantation recipients. J Infect Dis. 187(2):179–186.

56. Adams O, Krempe C, Kogler G, et al. (1998). Congenital infections with human herpesvirus 6. J Infect Dis. 178(2):544–546.

57. Ando Y, Kakimoto K, Ekuni Y, et al. (1992). HHV-6 infection during pregnancy and spontaneous abortion. Lancet. 340(8830):1289.

58. Lanari M, Papa I, Venturi V, et al. (2003). Congenital infection with human herpesvirus 6 variant B associated with neonatal seizures and poor neurological outcome. J Med Virol. 70(4):628 632.

59. Irving WL, James DK, Stephenson T, et al. (2000). Influenza virus infection in the second and third trimesters of pregnancy: a clinical and seroepidemiological study. BJOG. 107(10):1282–1289.

60. Limosin F, Rouillon F, Payan C, et al. (2003). Prenatal exposure to influenza as a risk factor for adult schizophrenia. Acta Psychiatr Scand. 107(5):331-335.

61. Englund JA. (2003). Maternal immunization with inactivated influenza vaccine: rationale and experience. Vaccine. 21(24):3460–3464.

62. Sur DK, Wallis DH, O'Connell TX. (2003). Vaccinations in pregnancy. Am Fam Physician. 68(2):299–304.

63. Anon. (1987). Rubella vaccination during pregnancy—United States, 1971-1986. MMWR Morb Mortal Wkly Rep. 36(28):457–461.

64. Tang JW, Aarons E, Hesketh LM, et al. (2003). Prenatal diagnosis of congenital rubella infection in the second trimester of pregnancy. Prenat Diagn. 23(7):509–512.

65. Best J, Bantawala J. (2000). Rubella. In Arie J. Zuckerman AJ, Banatvala JE, Pattison JR, eds. Principles and Practice of Clinical Virology, 4th ed. Chichester: John Wiley. 387–418.

66. Boue A, Nicolas A, Montagnon B. (1971). Reinfection with rubella in pregnant women. Lancet. 1(7712):1251–1253.

67. Geier DA, Geier MR. (2001). Rubella vaccine and arthritic adverse reactions: an analysis of the Vaccine Adverse Events Reporting System (VAERS) database from 1991 through 1998. Clin Exp Rheumatol. 19(6):724–726.

68. Barton LL, Mets MB. (2001). Congenital lymphocytic choriomeningitis virus infection: decade of rediscovery. Clin Infect Dis. 33(3):370–374.

69. Komrower GM, Williams BL, Stones PB. (1955). Lymphocytic choriomeningitis in the newborn; probable transplacental infection. Lancet. 268(6866):697–698.

70. Wright R, Johnson D, Neumann M, et al. (1997). Congenital lymphocytic choriomeningitis virus syndrome: a disease that mimics congenital toxoplasmosis or Cytomegalovirus infection. Pediatrics. 100(1):E9.

71. Barton LL, Mets MB, Beauchamp CL. (2002). Lymphocytic choriomeningitis virus: emerging fetal teratogen. Am J Obstet Gynecol. 187(6):1715–1716.

89

Gender-Specific Issues in Parasitology

MICHAEL YIN, MD* AND DICKSON D. DESPOMMIER, PhD**

*Division of Infectious Diseases, Columbia University, New York, NY
**Mailman School of Public Health, Columbia University, New York, NY

I. Introduction

Gender-specific differences in parasitic diseases are related to risk of infection within social roles and gender-based occupations, differences in biologic susceptibility and clinical manifestation, and affect on female reproductive health and neonatal transmission. This chapter reviews the current knowledge of the association between gender and the epidemiology and clinical manifestations of a few parasitic infections that have particular significance for women. Three specific topics will be discussed in greater detail because of their clinical importance: female genital schistosomiasis (FGS), malaria in pregnancy, and toxoplasmosis in pregnancy.

II. Medical Ecology

Environment plays an enormous role in the transmission of infectious diseases. This is particularly true for parasitic diseases involving eukaryotic organisms that have complex life cycles involving other organisms [1]. The physical setting in which each is acquired is defined by the science of medical ecology (www.medicalecology.org). Many parasitic infections require intermediate hosts, vectors (e.g., mosquitoes), and reservoirs, all of which are essential to help to maintain their presence in the peridomestic environment. Human behavior plays an equally large role in the acquisition of tropical infectious diseases. Gender-specific issues arise when that behavior differs from male to female. Agriculture is an important human activity that illustrates these differences.

Infection by Schistosomes often occurs during the practice of traditional rice farming because the infectious *cercariae* swim on the surface of freshwater. Ordinarily, men carry out the heavy work of plowing with oxen while women do most of the planting, weeding, and harvesting. Women tend to spend longer periods of time in the rice paddies and often have higher rates and levels of Schistosome infection. Similarly, women are more often engaged in the harvesting of cyprinoid fishes (i.e., grass carp) from freshwater ponds, which is an activity associated with higher rates of Schistosome infection. From Thailand there is anecdotal evidence that acquisition of *Fasciolopsis buski* (a large intestinal fluke) infection is higher in women because women facilitate the preparation of water chestnuts by peeling back the tough, outer husk with their teeth. Inadvertently, they ingest the metacercariae of *F. buski* that encyst on the husks and acquire the infection.

III. Gender Differences in Biologic Susceptibility

It is widely recognized that significant differences in rate of acquisition and burden of parasitic infection (protozoa and helminths) exist between male and female animals during experimental infections using a wide range of host species. These differences are presumably related to differences in sex-specific hormones and hormone levels. Translating these findings to humans, however, has not been straightforward. The inability to perform experiments limits the data to epidemiologic findings. Hence, although it is strongly suspected that similar differences occur between men and women for the same kinds of infectious agents, proof of concept is often lacking.

Much of the research has been focused on characterizing the immune response according to the Th1/Th2 (T helper) paradigm. T helper cells that secrete interleukin-2 (IL-2), interferon gamma (IFN-γ), and lymphotoxin-alpha (LT-α) are classified as Th1 cells, and T helper cells that secrete IL-4, IL-5, IL-6, and IL-13 are classified as Th2 cells [4]. Generally, a Th1 response promotes cell-mediated immunity and is protective during chronic infections with intracellular bacterial and protozoan pathogens. A Th2 response promotes isotype switching to immunoglobulin G_1 (IgG$_1$) and IgE and is protective against extracellular pathogens such as nematodes and cestodes [5,6]. In mouse models, there is a Th2 bias during pregnancy with fetoplacental tissue spontaneously producing IL-4, IL-5, and IL-10 [7,8]. Evidence suggests that progesterone promotes Th2 cell expansion and production of IL-4 by established Th1 cell clones [9]. In pregnant mice, high progesterone levels have also been associated with suppression of natural killer (NK) cell activity and inhibition of tumor necrosis factor-alpha (TNF-α) production [10–12]. Similarly, high estrogen levels in pregnant mice have been associated with down-regulation of TNF-α and INF-γ and reduction of NK cell activity [8,13–16]. The difficulty in generalizing the associations between sex hormones and immunity found in animal models of pregnancy to women is not only in the translation of animal findings to humans, but also that estrogen and progesterone levels are vastly different at various stages of a woman's life (childhood, the follicular and luteal phases of the menstrual cycle, pregnancy, and menopause). Associations observed during pregnancy, when progesterone and estradiol levels are at peak levels, cannot be extrapolated to predict immunologic response during other physiologic conditions.

Studies on Leishmania parasites, which live intracellularly and have been instrumental in understanding the Th1/Th2 paradigm, provide an example of the difficulty with interpreting results from animal studies. Leishmaniasis describes a group of diseases that display a range of clinical manifestations depending on the species of parasite and the host's immune response [17]. Epidemiologic studies of *Leishmania spp.* among children, where gender roles may contribute less to differential transmission than among adults, suggest that boys are more likely than girls to develop visceral leishmaniasis [18] and cutaneous leishmaniasis [19]. Many experimental animal studies have also suggested that gender differences and sex hormones may be important determinants of the host response and clinical outcome [8,20]; however, results are difficult to generalize because they differ according to the species of parasite and clinical outcome. For example, male B10/129 and DBA/2 mice are more resistant than females to cutaneous infection with *Leishmania major* [21,22]; whereas, male DBA/2 were more susceptible to *L. mexicana* infection [21]. Male BALB/2 and DBA/2 mice are more susceptible to systemic infection with *L. major* [17], whereas pregnant C57BL/6 mice exhibit a Th2 cytokine bias and are more susceptible to cutaneous *L. major* infection [23].

Experimental animal models of infections with helminths also reveal interesting sex differences that are difficult to translate to humans. For example, female mice acquire *Trichinella spiralis* differently than male mice. Males become infected in a more uniform manner with respect to the number of worms that establish in the gut tract [24]. Females behave more erratically with respect to worm burden. Some female mice acquire large numbers of worms, whereas others receiving the same dose acquire far fewer worms. These results could be fully explained in terms of female-specific hormone levels. Other parasitic helminths (*Trichuris spp. Nippostrongylus brasiliensis*) give the same results in experimental infections.

IV. Medically Important Parasitic Diseases and Gender-Related Issues

Table 89-1 summarizes gender-specific differences in several medically important parasitic diseases. Behavioral or biologic differences resulting in differential transmission or clinical manifestation are presented in the first column. Reproductive

Table 89-1

Parasite	Differences in Transmission or Clinical Manifestation	Reproductive Morbidity
Nematodes		
Enterobius vermicularis (pinworms)		Female genital tract migration does not increase sterility; case report of human embryo invasion [25]
Trichuris trichiura (whipworm)		Anemia during pregnancy [26]
Ascaris lumbricoides		Anemia during pregnancy; congenital infections rare [27]
Necator americanus, Ancylostoma duodenale (hookworm)		Anemia during pregnancy [26]
Strongyloides stercoralis		Reduced gastrointestinal motility during pregnancy may predispose women to hyperinfection syndromes [28]
Trichinella spiralis		During acute infection, *T. spiralis* can be found in the placenta and breast milk [29]
Wuchereria bancrofti		Rare congenital infection [30,31]
Cestodes		
Echinococcus granulosus		Rare presentation of pelvic hydatid cysts obstructing pregnancy [32,33]
Trematodes		
Schistosoma haematobium and S. japonicum	Female genital schistosomiasis causing abdominal pain, dysmenorrhea, and infertility [34]	Placental infection is frequent but does not cause intrauterine growth restriction or prematurity [35]
Giardia lamblia		Severe maternal infection can rarely compromise fetal growth [36]
Entameba histolytica		Amebiasis during pregnancy may be more severe [37]
Toxoplasma gondii		Congenital toxoplasmosis incidence: 1/1000–1/10,000 live births in the United States [38,39]

Continued

Table 89-1

(Continued)

Parasite	Differences in Transmission or Clinical Manifestation	Reproductive Morbidity
Malaria	Prevalence usually lower in women because of occupational roles [3]	Anemia and low birth-weight babies [3]
Trypanosoma cruzi (Chagas disease)	Prevalence of myocardial manifestations lower in women, etiology unclear [2]	Congenital infection in 1–4% with chronic infection [2], can occur with both acute and chronic infection
Trypanosoma brucei rhodesiense, *T. brucei gambiense* (African sleeping sickness)		Intrauterine infections are rare, can cause prematurity and spontaneous abortion [40]
Leishmania spp. (cutaneous, mucocutaneous, visceral leishmaniasis)	Prevalence of cutaneous leishmaniasis may be higher in boys than girls [19]	Congenital infections rare [41]
Trichomonas vaginalis	Self-limited infection more common in men possibly secondary to micturition or the trichomonacidal action of prostatic secretions [42,43]	Infertility and increase in preterm labor associated with *T. vaginalis* infection in observational studies [44], but treatment of *T. vaginalis* does not decrease rate of preterm labor [45]

morbidity, including infertility, maternal nutrition and its impact on fetal health, and neonatal transmission is addressed in the second column.

V. Special Topics

A. *Female Genital Schistosomiasis*

FGS is characterized by the presence of schistosomal eggs and worms in the genital organs. Clinical manifestations range from vaginal bleeding and pelvic pain to infertility, ectopic pregnancies, and vesicovaginal fistulas depending on the localization of the eggs and the host immunologic response. Despite significant progress in the field of schistosomiasis, the natural history, pathophysiology, and immunology of genital schistosomiasis is imperfectly understood [46].

1. Epidemiology

Schistosomiasis is a series of related diseases caused by four trematode species: *Schistosoma haematobium*, *S. mansoni*, *S. japonicum*, and *S. mekongi*. The species differ in the areas of endemicity, host selection, and migratory patterns of schistosomula and oviposition, resulting in different patterns of acute and chronic disease. *S. haematobium* is prevalent in most parts of Africa and in parts of the Middle East [1]. The adult worm has a predilection for migrating to the venous plexus that drains the bladder; therefore, deposition of its eggs causes pathology predominantly in genitourinary organs. *S. mansoni* is prevalent throughout sub-Saharan Africa, Egypt and Sudan, parts of the Middle East, northeastern parts of South America, and the Caribbean [1]. *S. japonicum* is prevalent in China, Malaysia, Philippines, Japan, and Indonesia, and *S. mekongi* is found in the Mekong river in southeast Asia [1]. The adult worms of *S. mansoni* and *S. japonicum* migrate to the mesenteric veins;

therefore, their eggs are deposited predominantly in the intestines and liver, resulting in intestinal and hepatic fibrosis [1].

It is still unclear to what extent *S. japonicum* and *S. mansoni* cause genital lesions. Genital lesions caused by *S. japonicum* seem to be rare, although ovarian involvement may be more common [46]. *S. mansoni* eggs have been discovered in the vagina, cervix, and uterus but only rarely in the vulva, fallopian tubes, or ovaries [46]. The reason for this dichotomy is unclear.

The frequency of FGS is inferred from postmortem studies and a few population-based studies. From postmortem studies, the prevalence of genital lesions associated with schistosomiasis ranges from 2–83% for the upper reproductive tract and 33–75% for the lower reproductive tract, depending on the area of endemicity studied and the methodology of sample processing [46]. From more recent population-based studies, the point-prevalence of FGS of the cervix/vagina ranges between 33% and 75%. In an endemic district in Tanzania, 239/657 (36%) of participating women had evidence of urinary schistosomiasis, and 134/359 (37%) of women consenting to gynecologic examination had biopsy evidence of genital schistosomiasis [47]. Of note, only 56% of the women with biopsy-proven FGS had detectable schistosome eggs in their urine. Women with higher concentrations of eggs in their urine were more likely to have evidence of FGS [47].

2. Pathogenesis

Infection in the human host is initiated when the cercariae penetrates unbroken skin through hair follicles. After penetration, cercariae shed their tails and transform into schistosomulae and migrate to the capillaries of the lung; they remain there and acquire the ability to incorporate host serum proteins onto their tegumental surface, allowing them to evade immunological detection by host cells [1]. After several days, the schistosomulae migrate from lungs through the bloodstream into the liver where they mature into adult worms. They find and mate with worms of the opposite sex, remaining in copula for their lifespan, migrate into the mesenteric circulation, and begin producing eggs.

The adult *S. haematobium* travels against the venous blood flow to reach the first portosystemic anastomoses, the anorectal plexus. From there, the worms migrate to the perivesical plexus and plexus uterovaginalis either by traversing the rectovaginal septum or through abundant vascular links [34]. Changes in pelvic vasculature that occur during puberty and pregnancy increase the likelihood that adult worms will migrate to the genital organs and deposit eggs [1,48]. In tissue, the eggs induce the formation of a perioval granuloma, a delayed-type hypersensitivity reaction, which eventually leads to destruction of soft tissue, fibrosis, and the formation of scars [34].

3. Clinical Presentation

The clinical manifestation of genital schistosomiasis varies according to the affected organs. Involvement of the fallopian tubes and/or ovaries may cause infertility by inducing a sterile salpingitis followed by local fibrosis and tubal occlusions or by causing hilar obstruction and adhesions resulting in anovulation [34,49]. Schistosomal involvement of the uterus has been associated with uterine fibroids and premature deliveries [50]. Cervical lesions can be polymorphous, ranging from ulcerative lesions to nodular or cauliflower-like growth, and can be misdiagnosed as malignancies. In one cross-sectional study, cervical lesions were visible on colposcopy in 75% of subjects with biopsy-proven genital schistosomiasis. Vaginal lesions are similarly polymorphous and may result in debilitating rectovaginal and vesiculovaginal fistulae. Menstrual disturbances, abdominal pain, and abdominal masses have been associated with ovarian and uterine involvement, and dysmenorrhea, leukorrhea, dyspareunia, and postcoital bleeding have been associated with cervical and vaginal involvement; however, none of these self-reported symptoms are specific enough to aid in diagnosis [34].

4. Diagnosis

Diagnosis of genital schistosomiasis is usually made through the incidental finding of schistosome eggs during routine biopsies taken during gynecological examination [34]. The value of most diagnostic procedures is unknown, and resources for diagnosis are often unavailable in endemic areas.

The gold standard for diagnosis of lower reproductive tract schistosomiasis is the quantitative compressed biopsy technique (QCBT), in which a forceps biopsy is taken from a suspicious lesion and examined for schistosome eggs [51]. In an individual with high clinical likelihood for FGS but a macroscopically normal cervix and vagina, several biopsies can be taken and examined by QCBT with reasonable yield [34,51]. Examination of routinely obtained cervical specimens has inadequate sensitivity, and examination of urine cannot substitute for a gynecological examination because FGS frequently occurs in women with no urinary egg secretion. Noninvasive assays such as vaginal fluid antigen assays are under investigation.

Schistosomiasis of the upper reproductive tract can be made through histologic examination of material taken during laparoscopy. Transabdominal ultrasound has been used to identify echogenic foci or masses and enlargement of the reproductive organs associated with schistosomiasis [52]; however, the diagnostic specificity of these findings and its utility in monitoring treatment are still unclear [34].

5. Treatment and Prevention

Praziquantel is the drug of choice for most species of schistosomes but is only active against adult worms and schistosomulae and not eggs. Treatment, however, accelerates the resolution of egg-induced pathology by eliminating further deposition of eggs and possibly by modulating host immune response [53]. In patients with hepatosplenic schistosomiasis, markers of liver fibrosis decreased within 2–6 months after repeated treatment with praziquantel [54].

There are case reports documenting regression or disappearance of genital lesions after treatment, although no controlled studies exist. A single dose of praziquantel (40 mg/kg) in a small clinical study done in Malawi resulted in resolution of symptoms in most patients after 9 weeks and regression of genital lesions after more time [55]. Because complete resolution of all egg-induced pathology requires elimination of all worms, Poggensee recommends repeated administration of praziquantel, four to five doses of 40 mg/kg each spaced 48 hours, for moderately to heavily infected women [34].

Prevention of schistosomiasis at the personal level requires that individuals never come into contact with infested fresh water, which is practical advice only for temporary visitors to endemic areas. Control at the community level has been directed at eradication of snail vectors with biologic agents, public health education, sanitation, and chemotherapy [1]. Although praziquantel is not considered teratogenic or mutagenic, it is not recommended in pregnancy or in lactating women; therefore, certain women would not be included in control programs [34].

The need for a vaccine against schistosomes is urgent, and development is under way. In a recent human trial of Sh28GST (derived from *S. haematobium* and African species), women receiving the vaccine candidate had a different pattern of responses than men. In women, IgA dominated the antibody response, whereas TGF-β was the most abundant interleukin generated [56]. The authors speculated that differences are related to either hormone production (estradiol) or pattern of chronic infection. In field studies by the same group, it was shown that women with low (i.e., chronic) levels of infection had elevated levels of IgA directed mainly against epitopes of the naturally occurring Sh28GST protein within the adult worm [57]. These results, taken together, suggest that women may regulate *S. haematobium* infection better than similarly aged men under the same environmental conditions.

B. Malaria in Pregnancy

With more than one-half of the world's population living in endemic areas, the World Health Organization (WHO) report in 1998 estimated 500 million new cases of malarial infection and 1.5 to 2.7 million deaths from malaria each year. Man is commonly infected by four species of the parasite: *Plasmodium falciparum*, *P. vivax*, *P. ovale*, and *P. malariae*. Greater than 90% of malaria deaths occur in sub-Saharan Africa, affecting mostly children younger than the age of 5 years, although significant morbidity also occurs among pregnant women, especially in primigravidae.

1. Epidemiology

Both the prevalence and density of malarial parasitemia are increased in pregnant women compared to age-matched, nonpregnant women residing in the same area [29,58]. In young Nigerian women, Gilles *et al* found that parasitemia was 4–12 times more common during pregnancy than pre-pregnancy or post-pregnancy, and mean parasite densities were 1775 mm^3 in pregnant women compared to 140 mm^3 in nonpregnant women [59]. The prevalence of infection and density of parasitemia is also greater in the primigravidae than multigravidae. According to Brabin and Rogerson, a weighted relative risk for the increased malaria prevalence in African primigravidae across 21 studies is 1.90 (95% confidence interval 1.82–1.98) [60]. Placental parasitemia is also more prevalent in primigravidae than multigravidae [58,61].

Malaria in pregnancy has been associated with an increased risk of severe anemia, increased maternal mortality, low birth-weight infants, and infant death. In an analysis of the burden of *P. falciparum*-associated anemia in pregnant women in sub-Saharan Africa, Guyatt and Snow reported a median prevalence of 8.2% for severe anemia in all-parity pregnant women. Studies suggest that 7.3–26% of these cases are attributable to infection with malaria [62]. Primigravidae living in endemic areas are at even higher risk of anemia than multigravidae [60]. Intervention studies of malaria chemoprophylaxis have demonstrated a significant increase of mean hemoglobin values with different regimens [63,64]. Maternal morbidity from malaria is low in closely monitored communities in holoendemic regions [60]. Mortality may be increased in hypoendemic and/or unstable regions. In an urban setting in Mozambique where the women may have had low levels of prenatal immunity to malaria, the overall maternal mortality was 320 per 100,000 live births, of which 37 (15.5%) were attributed to malaria [65].

Infection with either *P. falciparum* or *P. vivax* during pregnancy is associated with an increased risk of having a low birth-weight infant [60]. Brabin estimates the increased low birth-weight prevalence attributable to *P. falciparum* malaria to be 10% in low endemic areas to more than 50% in holoendemic areas [60,66]. It is unclear whether low birth weight is primarily a result of intrauterine growth restriction or preterm delivery. Low birth weight is also more common when there is evidence of placental infection. Infant mortality, especially neonatal mortality, is associated with low birth weights. In rural Malawi where malaria is holoendemic, McDermott estimated that low birth weight contributed to 80% of neonatal deaths, 45.7% of perinatal deaths, and 37.8% of infant mortality [67].

Congenital malaria occurs less frequently than postnatal infection in endemic areas. The incidence has been estimated to be 1–4% of pregnancies and is higher when the mother is symptomatic from malaria during the pregnancy. The placenta serves as an adequate barrier against the parasite despite frequent placental involvement, and maternal IgG antibody most likely has a role in preventing the establishment of infection in parasites that reach the fetal circulation [29]. When it does occur, the clinical onset of disease in a congenitally infected infant can be delayed for weeks to months [29,68].

2. Pathophysiology

When the infected female anopheles mosquito bites, she injects salivary fluids that contain sporozoites into the wound. The sporozoites are cleared from the circulation within a half an hour and reach the parenchymal cells of the liver. Inside the hepatocyte, the parasite undergoes asexual division and produces a large number of progeny called merozoites. When merozoites are released into the bloodstream, they invade erythrocytes and form ringlike early trophozoites that enlarge and begin asexual division to form a schizont composed of merozoites. The erythrocytic cycle is complete when the cell ruptures and merozoites are released into the bloodstream to invade other erythrocytes. Usually this cycle is synchronous and periodic, resulting in periodic fevers in the host. *P. falciparum*, *P vivax*, and *P. ovale* complete the cycle from merozoite infection to erythrocyte rupture within 48 hours, and *P. malariae* completes the cycle within 72 hours. Falciparum malaria is the primary form of malaria in sub-Saharan Africa and has a more fulminant course because it can invade all erythrocyte stages and can reach very high levels of parasitemia. *P. falciparum* is also able to sequester in large numbers in the placenta. *P. vivax* exclusively invades reticulocytes and does not accumulate in the placenta, resulting in a less severe clinical course. Unlike *P. falciparum*, *P. vivax* forms hypnozoites in the liver that can cause relapses ranging from weeks to months after the initial infection [1].

Pregnancy modulates the immune system, but studies have not clearly provided evidence that a pregnancy-related immunologic defect causes increased susceptibility to malaria [69]. A comprehensive review of the immunity to malaria during pregnancy was published in 2001 [69]. A series of experiments by Fried and Duffy offer a plausible explanation of how multigravidas are protected against the more serious effects of falciparum infection. They have shown that a distinct subpopulation of *P. falciparum* can bind selectively to chondroitin sulphate A (CSA), which is expressed on placental villi [70]. Multigravidae posses an antibody that can inhibit this binding, whereas primigravidae and men do not [71]. Therefore, the development of antibodies to this phenotype may inhibit the binding of placental parasites to CSA and protect against sequestration of malaria parasites in subsequent pregnancies [69].

The mechanisms by which malaria affect fetal development are not clearly defined and could relate to multiple factors. In falciparum infection, it has been postulated that heavy infiltration of parasites in the placenta results in diminished transport of oxygen, nutrients, and maternal antibody to the fetus,. It also has been suggested that local release of cytokines causes alterations of fetal metabolism [29,60,72]. *P. vivax* does not sequester in placenta but has been associated with low birth weight; therefore, systemic effects from cytokine release or maternal anemia appear to be contributory.

3. Clinical Presentation

The presentation of malaria depends on the stage of pregnancy, previous history of malaria exposure, and general maternal health and nutrition. In women living in holoendemic areas with high levels of immunity, most malarial infections are asymptomatic. In nonimmune women, or semi-immune women such as those in areas of unstable endemism or returning to holoendemic areas after prolonged absence, disease can be symptomatic and severe [73]. Severe hemolytic anemia, acute pulmonary edema, premature labor, and hypoglycemia as a result of malaria infection and/or treatment have all been reported with increased frequency in pregnant women with malaria [60,74].

4. Treatment and Prevention

Treatment of malaria in pregnant women is especially challenging given the limited data on fetal toxicity, maternal tolerability, and efficacy, especially on placental parasite clearance. Several antimalarials can be used safely in pregnant patients: chloroquine, quinine, sulfadoxine–pyrimethamine, mefloquine, chlorproguanil and dapsone (Lapdap), artesunate, and artemether. The following antimalarial medications should not be used in pregnancy: halofantrine, atovaquone–proguanil, tetracyclines, primaquine, and the combination mefloquine–sulfadoxine–pyrimethamine (MSP) [75]. Decisions about treatment are based on the known resistance profiles, treatment of complicated versus uncomplicated infection, and availability. A thorough review of antimalarial drug profiles and treatment guidelines was published in 2001 [75].

Chemoprophylaxis is recommended in nonimmune or semi-immune pregnant women visiting an endemic area. Recommendations will depend on the sensitivity of malaria in the region of travel. Chloroquine and proguanil are known to be safe at any stage of pregnancy. Most other antimalarial agents have restrictions for use during the first trimester as a result of preclinical toxicologic studies in laboratory animals that demonstrated teratogenic effects [76]. The safety of mefloquine, chloroquine–proguanil, or sulfadoxine–pyrimethamine has been inferred from a 1998 study that examined the fetal outcomes of 236 pregnant women who had been accidentally administered these agents as chemoprophylaxis during the first trimester [77].

Numerous trials of chemoprophylaxis during pregnancy have been performed in holoendemic areas in an attempt to affect various maternal and fetal outcomes, but doubt remains over its impact and cost-effectiveness [76]. A Cochrane review of 15 randomized studies concluded that chemoprophylaxis with various regimens during pregnancy was associated with fewer episodes of fever and higher birth weights in infants [78]. Most studies did not have the power to assess other outcomes such as maternal anemia, neonatal deaths, and preterm births. Currently, WHO recommends intermittent antimalarial chemoprophylaxis with sulfadoxine–pyrimethamine to pregnant women in areas with high risk of P. falciparum infection during pregnancy and where P. falciparum is susceptible to sulfadoxine–pyrimethamine [79]. These recommendations are based on the success of a studies conducted in Malawi [80], as well as in Kenya, an area of less intense transmission [81].

C. Toxoplasmosis in Pregnancy

Toxoplasma gondii infection acquired during pregnancy places the fetus at risk for an infection that can cause devastating damage to its CNS, which is often clinically undetectable at birth. Maternal infection is also predominantly asymptomatic. Toxoplasmosis is one of the most challenging infections to manage in pregnancy because controversies still remain in areas of prevention, diagnosis, and treatment.

1. Epidemiology

The serologic prevalence of T. gondii infection varies widely between geographic locales and cultures. In the United States, 23% of adolescents and adults have serologic evidence of infection with T. gondii [82]. Prevalence of antibodies in pregnant women or women of childbearing age also vary considerably, ranging from 3% to 30% in series from cities within the United States [83]. The incidence of acute T. gondii infection acquired during pregnancy is 1.6–2.3% in France, where serologic screening of pregnant women is compulsory [84]. Prenatal screening is not mandatory in the United States, but the incidence of maternal infection acquired during pregnancy has been estimated at 0.2–1%, and the incidence of congenital infection has been estimated to range from 1/1000 to 1/8000 live births [38]. One study of neonatal screening in New England reported an incidence for congenital toxoplasmosis of 1/10,000 live births [39]. Calculating the burden of disease, there are approximately 500–1400 congenital infections among the 4.2 million annual live births in the United States [83].

2. Pathogenesis

Toxoplasma is an obligate intracellular protozoan that exists in three forms: the oocyst that contains two sporozoites and is the product of sexual cycles in cats; the tachyzoite that is the asexual invasive form; and the tissue cyst that contains bradyzoites [38]. Most commonly, humans are infected by either ingestion of sporulated oocysts that are shed from the intestines of infected cats or by ingestion of tissue cysts found in undercooked meats. After disruption of the cyst wall in the intestinal tract, bradyzoites are released and differentiate into tachyzoites. Tachyzoites can invade virtually any cell type causing cell death and tissue destruction and disseminate through invasion of adjacent cells and via the bloodstream [38]. Cysts are formed as early as the first week of infection and can persist throughout the life of the mammalian host [38]. The most common sites of latent infection appear to be the brain, skeletal, and heart muscles.

Congenital transmission occurs in the setting of maternal parasitemia and results from the invasion of the placenta by tachyzoites and entrance into the fetal circulation. Fetal transmission depends on the burden of maternal parasitemia, the maturity of the placenta, the competency of the maternal immune response, and whether the mother was treated during acute infection. Therefore, the incidence of congenital infection is greater if the mother is acutely infected during the second or third trimester, correlating with the development of a mature placenta and less time for the development of an immune response [83]. Using PCR testing of amniotic fluid to diagnose congenital toxoplasmosis, Hohlfeld found that the incidence was less than 2% when maternal infection occurred during the first 10 weeks of gestation and rose sharply from weeks 15 to 34 to 67% when maternal infection occurred during weeks 31–34 [85]. Reported incidences vary between studies as a result of different screening criteria and treatment of maternal infection. However, the clinical outcome of the neonate is better when maternal infection occurs during the second or third trimesters. Acute maternal infection during weeks 10–24 of gestation, therefore, was associated with the highest risk of developing severe congenital toxoplasmosis, whereas infection occurring 6 months prior to conception to 10 weeks after conception and greater than 24 weeks after conception was associated with lower risk [83].

3. Clinical Presentation

In an immunocompetent host, infection with *T. gondii* acquired before pregnancy does not confer increased risk of fetal transmission; however, in immunocompromised pregnant women there is a risk of reactivation and congenital transmission. There are insufficient data to quantify the risk of congenital transmission by women with the human immunodeficiency virus (HIV) who have chronic toxoplasma infection, and available studies report conflicting results [38].

Clinical manifestations of acute infection in immunocompetent individuals may be undetected. The most commonly recognized manifestation is a localized, nontender, self-limited lymphadenopathy that is not associated with fever and resolves within 6 months [38]. Ocular toxoplasmosis (chorioretinitis) in an adult is usually the result of congenital infection that presents clinically in the second or third decade rather than a manifestation of acute infection. In rare cases, acute infection can present as myocarditis, pericarditis, hepatitis polymyositis, pneumonitis, or encephalitis with a fulminant course.

The clinical spectrum of congenital toxoplasmosis ranges from normal appearance at birth to chorioretinitis, epilepsy, psychomotor or motor retardation, hydrocephalus, and intracranial calcifications [86]. Left untreated, as many as 85% of infants with subclinical infection at birth will develop signs and symptoms over subsequent years, presenting at a mean age of 3.7 years, and most commonly with chorioretinitis [87].

4. Diagnosis

In the United States, where routine screening is not implemented, maternal infection is most often diagnosed as a result of routine serologic testing by the physician, testing done as a result of patient concern, or when there is clinical signs suggestive of acute toxoplasmosis [38]. The goal of maternal testing is to determine the acuity of the infection because the risk of congenital toxoplasmosis is negligible if maternal infection occurred before pregnancy.

After acute infection, IgM and IgG generally increase within 1–2 weeks. IgM increases rapidly and decreases at variable rates to disappear after a few months, although in some cases will persist for longer than a year [38]. IgG usually peaks at 1–2 months and gradually declines with persistent low titers for life [88]. The strength with which IgG binds to *T. gondii* shifts from low to high avidity at about 5 months after infection. IgG avidity tests have been used to determine the chronicity of infection and are widely used in Europe. Similarly, the differential agglutination test (AC/HS) can make inferences about the chronicity of infection based on the observation that

different tachyzoite antigen preparations vary in their ability to recognize antibodies in sera from patients with recent or chronic infection [38]. Assays for IgA and IgE may sometimes be helpful in narrowing the time of infection when used in conjunction with IgM and IgG results [88].

In most cases, the diagnosis of acute toxoplasmosis requires demonstration of an increase in titers in serial specimens (taken at least 3 weeks apart and run in parallel) [38]. In specific situations, a combination of tests such as the Toxoplasma Serological Profile (Sabin-Feldman dye test, double sandwich IgM ELISA, IgA ELISA, IgE ELISA, and AC/HS test) offered at the Toxoplasma Serology Laboratory of the Palo Alto Medical Foundation Research Institute (TSL-PAMFRI) can be used to establish the chronicity of infection [89]. A negative IgM taken within the first 24 weeks of gestation essentially rules out an acute infection. A negative IgM and a positive IgG in the first two trimesters suggests past infection but in the third trimester could be consistent with an acute infection acquired early in pregnancy with a rapid IgM decline, and further serologic testing (e.g., IgA, IgE, AC/HS avidity) may be helpful [89]. A positive IgM test requires further testing with confirmatory serologic testing at a reference laboratory because nonreference laboratories can have false positivity rates of up to 60%.

If a diagnosis of acute infection is established or highly suspected, prenatal diagnosis of congenital toxoplasmosis based on ultrasonography, and PCR on amniotic fluid is advised. The sensitivity of PCR on amniotic fluid varies with gestational age at the time of amniocentesis, and the reliability before 18 weeks is unknown. Romand reports an overall sensitivity of 64%, specificity of 100%, positive predictive value of 100%, and negative predictive value of 87.8% for the diagnosis of congenital toxoplasmosis [90].

Diagnosis in the newborn should be obtained from peripheral blood because the umbilical cord could be contaminated with maternal blood. Maternal IgG that is transferred to the infant should disappear within 6–12 months of life; therefore, a negative IgG test at 1 year essentially rules out congenital toxoplasmosis [89].

5. Treatment

Treatment of acute acquired infection in immunocompetent adults is rarely necessary unless severe disease develops. Treatment in the pregnant woman, therefore, is primarily to prevent transmission to the fetus and to limit the severity of congenital disease if transmission has occurred. Treatment of the fetus is recommended when infection is established or highly probable.

There are no randomized trials on the efficacy of treatment administered during pregnancy to prevent transmission of maternal infection to the fetus. Older observational studies have indicated that treatment may reduce the frequency of maternal transmission by as much as 60% [91]. In 1999 Foulon published results from a multicenter European cohort study of 144 women who had toxoplasma seroconversion during pregnancy and were offered treatment with spiramycin or a combination of pyrimethamine and sulfadiazine [92]. The infants were followed for 1 year after birth for clinical and serologic sequelae. Of the women, 64/144 (44%) gave birth to congenitally infected infants: transmission occurred in 72% of the mother–infant pairs that did not receive antibiotic therapy, and transmission occurred in 39% of the mother–infant pairs who received therapy. After adjusting for the gestational age of maternal infection, neither the administration of antibiotics or time lapse between infection and start of antibiotics were predictive of maternal transmission. However, antibiotics were associated with decreased incidence of severe infant sequelae. Although inconclusive, most experts agree that the data support treatment of acute maternal infection to prevent transmission and limit the sequelae of congenital infection. Spiramycin is recommended for prevention of fetal transmission, and the combination of pyrimethamine and sulfadiazine is recommended for treatment once fetal infection is established [38].

6. Prevention

Epidemiologic studies have identified a long list of possible risk factors for *T. gondii* infection: owning cats, cleaning cat litter, eating raw or undercooked meat, gardening, eating raw vegetables prepared outside the home, having poor hand hygiene, and travel outside of Europe or United States [93–96]. Studies suggest that cat ownership may be less important as a risk factor than ingestion of undercooked meats and unwashed vegetables in pregnant women [95]. House cats that are not fed raw meat are at low risk of *T. gondii* infection, and once infected, they only shed oocysts in their stool for several weeks.

Primary prevention of toxoplasmosis in pregnant women involves the application of specific hygienic measures concerning proper preparation of raw meats, fruits, and vegetables; using gloves when gardening; avoiding direct contact with cat litter; keeping the cat indoors; and feeding it only commercial or well-cooked table food. One Belgian study suggests that educational efforts alone could significantly decrease seroconversion rates in pregnant women [97]. In the mid-1970s, screening programs were implemented in France and Austria to institute preventive measures for seronegative women and to ensure early diagnosis and treatment of infection acquired during pregnancy. In both countries, a decline in the incidence of congenital infections has been observed; however, without an unscreened comparison group it is difficult to determine the proportion of decline attributable to the screening programs [82].

Although findings of European studies suggest that *T. gondii* screening programs can prevent cases of congenital toxoplasmosis, the American College of Obstetricians and Gynecologists (ACOG) does not recommend routine screening. Opponents of routine screening caution that routine testing of a low-risk population will result in more false positive tests, which may lead to hazardous testing (amniocentesis) and inappropriate treatment. They also argue that there is inadequate evidence on efficacy of treatment for prevention of transmission [98].

VI. Suggestions for Further Investigations

- How important are occupational differences in the gender-specific acquisition of parasitic infections?
- What overall effects do intestinal helminth infections have on fetal development? Does female genital schistosomiasis increase risk of HIV transmission? Would diagnosis and treatment of female genital schistosomiasis in endemic areas decrease HIV transmission?
- What diagnostic modalities for female genital schistosomiasis are available for resource-poor areas where schistosomiasis is endemic?

References

1. Despommier DD. Parasitic diseases, 4th ed. (2000). New York: Apple Trees Productions. xii:345.
2. Dias JC. (1996). Tropical diseases and the gender approach. *Bull Pan Am Health Organ.* 30(3):242–260.
3. Reuben R. (1993). Women and malaria—special risks and appropriate control strategy. *Soc Sci Med.* 37(4):473–480.
4. Johnson RM, Brown EJ. (2000) Cell-mediated immunity in host defense against infectious diseases. In: Mandell GL, Bennett JE, Dolin R, eds. *Principles and Practice of Infectious Diseases.* Philadelphia: Churchill Livingstone. 112–146.
5. Bancroft AJ, Else KJ, Sypek JP, *et al.* (1997). Interleukin-12 promotes a chronic intestinal nematode infection. *Eur J Immunol.* 27(4):866–870.
6. Rotman HL, Schnyder-Candrian S, Scott P, *et al.* (1997). IL-12 eliminates the Th-2 dependent protective immune response of mice to larval Strongyloides stercoralis. *Parasite Immunol.* 19(1):29–39.
7. Lin H, Mosmann TR, Guilbert L, *et al.* (1993). Synthesis of T helper 2-type cytokines at the maternal-fetal interface. *J Immunol.* 151(9):4562–4573.
8. Roberts CW, Walker W, Alexander J. (2001). Sex-associated hormones and immunity to protozoan parasites. *Clin Microbiol Rev.* 14(3):476–488.
9. Piccinni MP, Giudizi MG, Biagiotti R, *et al.* (1995). Progesterone favors the development of human T helper cells producing Th2-type cytokines and promotes both IL-4 production and membrane CD30 expression in established Th1 cell clones. *J Immunol.* 155(1):128–133.
10. Baley JE, Schacter BZ. (1985). Mechanisms of diminished natural killer cell activity in pregnant women and neonates. *J Immunol.* 134(5):3042–3048.
11. Furukawa K, Itoh K, Okamura K, *et al.* (1984). Changes in NK cell activity during the estrous cycle and pregnancy in mice. *J Reprod Immunol.* 6(6):353–363.
12. Miller L, Hunt JS. (1998). Regulation of TNF-alpha production in activated mouse macrophages by progesterone. *J Immunol.* 160(10):5098–5104.
13. Deshpande R, Khalili H, Pergolizzi RG, *et al.* (1997). Estradiol down-regulates LPS-induced cytokine production and NFkB activation in murine macrophages. *Am J Reprod Immunol.* 38(1):46–54.
14. Seaman WE, Blackman MA, Gindhart TD, *et al.* (1978). beta-Estradiol reduces natural killer cells in mice. *J Immunol.* 121(6):2193–2198.
15. Seaman WE, Gindhart TD. (1979). Effect of estrogen on natural killer cells. *Arth Rheum.* 22(11):1234–1240.
16. Fox HS, Bond BL, Parslow TG. (1991). Estrogen regulates the IFN-gamma promoter. *J Immunol.* 146(12):4362–4367.
17. Mock BA, Nacy CA. (1988). Hormonal modulation of sex differences in resistance to Leishmania major systemic infections. *Infect Immun.* 56(12):3316–3319.
18. Shiddo SA, Aden Mohamed A, Akuffo HO, *et al.* (1995). Visceral leishmaniasis in Somalia: prevalence of markers of infection and disease manifestations in a village in an endemic area. *Trans R Soc Trop Med Hyg.* 89(4):361–365.
19. Jones TC, Johnson WD Jr, Barretto AC, *et al.* (1987). Epidemiology of American cutaneous leishmaniasis due to Leishmania braziliensis braziliensis. *J Infect Dis.* 156(1):73–83.
20. Travi BL, Osorio Y, Melby PC, *et al.* (2002). Gender is a major determinant of the clinical evolution and immune response in hamsters infected with Leishmania spp. *Infect Immun.* 70(5):2288–2296.
21. Alexander J. (1988). Sex differences and cross-immunity in DBA/2 mice infected with L. mexicana and L. major. *Parasitol.* 96(Pt 2):297–302.
22. Giannini MS. (1986). Sex-influenced response in the pathogenesis of cutaneous leishmaniasis in mice. *Parasite Immunol.* 8(1):31–37.
23. Krishnan L, Guilbert LJ, Wegmann TG, *et al.* (1996). T helper 1 response against Leishmania major in pregnant C57BL/6 mice increases implantation failure and fetal resorptions. Correlation with increased IFN-gamma and TNF and reduced IL-10 production by placental cells. *J Immunol.* 156(2):653–662.
24. Gould SE. (1970). *Trichinosis in Man and Animal.* Springfield: Charles C. Thomas.

25. Mendoza E, *et al.* (1987). Invasion of human embryo by Enterobius vermicularis. *Arch Pathol Lab Med.* 111(8):761–762.

26. Nurdia DS, Sumarni S, Suyoko, *et al.* (2001). Impact of intestinal helminth infection on anemia and iron status during pregnancy: a community based study in Indonesia. *Southeast Asian J Trop Med Public Health.* 32(1):14–22.

27. Chu WG, Chen PM, Huang CC, *et al.* (1972). Neonatal ascariasis. *J Pediatr.* 81(4):783–785.

28. Lee RV. (1988). Parasites and pregnancy: the problems of malaria and toxoplasmosis. *Clin Perinatol.* 15(2):351–363.

29. Maldonado YA. (2001). Protozoan and helminth infections (including Pneumocystis carinii). In: Remington JS, Klein JO, eds. *Infectious Diseases of the Fetus and Newborn Infant.* Philadelphia: W. B. Saunders. 867–912.

30. Bloomfield RD, Suarez JR, Malangit AC. (1978). Transplacental transfer of Bancroftian filariasis. *J Natl Med Assoc.* 70(8):597–598.

31. Pires ML, Ferreira RS, Araujo S, *et al.* (1991). [Transplacental passage of Wuchereria bancrofti microfilariae in newborns of microfilaremic mothers]. *Rev Inst Med Trop Sao Paulo.* 33(2):91–95.

32. Jasper P, Peedicayil A, Nair S, *et al.* (1989). Hydatid cyst obstructing labour: a case report. *J Trop Med Hyg.* 92(6):393–395.

33. Rahman MS, Rahman J, Lysikiewicz A. (1982). Obstetric and gynaecological presentations of hydatid disease. *Br J Obstet Gynecol.* 89(8):665–670.

34. Poggensee G, Feldmeier H. (2001). Female genital schistosomiasis: facts and hypotheses. *Acta Trop.* 79(3):193–210.

35. Renaud R, Brettes P, Carrie J, *et al.* (1971). [Bilharziasis of the internal female genital organs]. Rev Fr Gynecol Obstet. 66(1):1–18.

36. Roberts NS, Copel JA, Bhutani V, *et al.* (1985). Intestinal parasites and other infections during pregnancy in Southeast Asian refugees. *J Reprod Med.* 30(10):720–725.

37. Abioye AA. (1973). Fatal amoebic colitis in pregnancy and puerperium: a new clinico-pathological entity. *J Trop Med Hyg.* 76(4):97–100.

38. Liesenfeld O, Remington JS. (2001). Toxoplasmosis. In: Martens MG, Faro S, Soper D, eds. *Infectious Diseases in Women.* Philadelphia: W. B. Saunders.

39. Guerina NG, Hsu HW, Meissner HC, *et al.* (1994). Neonatal serologic screening and early treatment for congenital Toxoplasma gondii infection. The New England Regional Toxoplasma Working Group. [see comments.]. *N Engl J Med.* 330(26):1858–1863.

40. Ikede BO, Elhassan E, Akpavie SO. (1988). Reproductive disorders in African trypanosomiasis: a review. *Acta Trop.* 45(1):5–10.

41. Eltoum IA, Zijlstra EE, Ali MS, *et al.* (1992). Congenital kala-azar and leishmaniasis in the placenta. *Am J Trop Med Hyg.* 46(1):57–62.

42. Krieger J. (1995). Trichomoniasis in men: old issues and new data. *Sex Transm Dis.* 22:83–96.

43. Rein M. (2000). Trichomonas vaginalis. In: Mandell GL, Bennett JE, Dolin R, eds. *Principles and Practices of Infectious Diseases.* Philadelphia: Churchill Livingstone. 2894–2897.

44. El-Shazly AM, El-Naggar HM, Soliman M, *et al.* (2001). A study on Trichomoniasis vaginalis and female infertility. *J Egypt Soc Parasitol.* 31(2):545–553.

45. Klebanoff MA, Carey JC, Hauth JC, *et al.* (2001). Failure of metronidazole to prevent preterm delivery among pregnant women with asymptomatic Trichomonas vaginalis infection. *N Engl J Med.* 345(7):487–493.

46. Feldmeier H, Poggensee G, Krantz I, *et al.* (1995). Female genital schistosomiasis. New challenges from a gender perspective. *Trop Geogr Med.* 47(2 Suppl):S2–15.

47. Poggensee G, Krantz I, Kiwelu I, *et al.* (2000). Screening of Tanzanian women of childbearing age for urinary schistosomiasis: validity of urine reagent strip readings and self-reported symptoms. *Bull World Health Organ.* 78(4):542–548.

48. Moore GR, Smith CV. (1989). Schistosomiasis associated with rupture of the appendix in pregnancy. *Obstet Gynecol.* 74(3 Pt 2):446–448.

49. Berry A. (1966). A cytopathological and histopathological study of bilharziasis of the female genital tract. *J Pathol Bacteriol.* 91(2):325–338.

50. Leutscher P, Ravaoalimalala VE, Raharisolo C, *et al.* (1998). Clinical findings in female genital schistosomiasis in Madagascar. *Trop Med Int Health.* 3(4):327–332.

51. Helling-Giese G, Sjaastad A, Poggensee G, *et al.* (1996). Female genital schistosomiasis due to Schistosoma haematobium. Clinical and parasitological findings in women in rural Malawi. *Acta Trop.* 62(4):239–255.

52. Richter J, Poggensee G, Helling-Giese G, *et al.* (1995). Transabdominal ultrasound for the diagnosis of Schistosoma haematobium infection of the upper female genital tract: a preliminary report. *Trans R Soc Trop Med Hyg.* 89(5):500–501.

53. Brindley PJ, Sher A. (1987). The chemotherapeutic effect of praziquantel against Schistosoma mansoni is dependent on host antibody response. *J Immunol.* 139(1):215–220.

54. Zwingenberger K, Harms G, Poggensee U, *et al.* (1990). Re-infection in human schistosomiasis mansoni: a prospective field study 18 months after praziquantel therapy. *Ann Trop Med Parasitol.* 84(5):457–465.

55. Richter J, Poggensee G, Kjetland EF, *et al.* (1996). Reversibility of lower reproductive tract abnormalities in women with Schistosoma haematobium infection after treatment with praziquantel—an interim report. *Acta Trop.* 62(4):289–301.

56. Remoue F, Rogerie F, Gallissot MC, *et al.* (2000). Sex-dependent neutralizing humoral response to Schistosoma mansoni 28GST antigen in infected human populations. *J Infect Dis.* 181(5):1855–1859.

57. Remoue F, To Van D, Schacht AM, *et al.* (2001). Gender-dependent specific immune response during chronic human Schistosomiasis haematobia. *Clin Exp Immunol.* 124(1):62–68.

58. McGregor IA. (1984). Epidemiology, malaria and pregnancy. *Am J Trop Med Hyg.* 1984. 33(4):517–525.

59. Gilles HM, Lawson JB, Sibelas M, *et al.* (1969). Malaria, anaemia and pregnancy. *Ann Trop Med Parasitol.* 63(2):245–263.

60. Brabin B, Rogerson S. (2001). The epidemiology and outcome of maternal malaria. In: Duffy PE, Fried M, eds. *Malaria in Pregnancy.* London: Taylor and Francis. 27–52.

61. McGregor IA, Wilson ME, Billewicz WZ. (1983). Malaria infection of the placenta in The Gambia, West Africa; its incidence and relationship to stillbirth, birthweight and placental weight. *Trans R Soc Trop Med Hyg.* 77(2):232–244.

62. Guyatt HL, Snow RW. (2001). The epidemiology and burden of Plasmodium falciparum-related anemia among pregnant women in sub-Saharan Africa. *Am J Trop Med Hyg.* 64(1–2 Suppl):36–44.

63. Greenwood BM, Greenwood AM, Snow RW, *et al.* (1989). The effects of malaria chemoprophylaxis given by traditional birth attendants on the course and outcome of pregnancy. *Trans R Soc Trop Med Hyg.* 83(5):589–594.

64. Nosten F, ter Kuile F, Maelankiri L, *et al.* (1994). Mefloquine prophylaxis prevents malaria during pregnancy: a double-blind, placebo-controlled study. [see comments.]. *J Infect Dis.* 169(3):595–603.

65. Granja AC, Machungo F, Gomes A, *et al.* (1998). Malaria-related maternal mortality in urban Mozambique. *Ann Trop Med Parasitol.* 92(3):257–263.

66. Brabin B. (1991). An assessment of low birthweight risk in primiparae as an indicator of malaria control in pregnancy. *Int J Epidemiol.* 20(1): 276–283.

67. McDermott JM, Slutsker L, Steketee RW, *et al.* (1996). Prospective assessment of mortality among a cohort of pregnant women in rural Malawi. *Am J Trop Med Hyg.* 55(1 Suppl):66–70.

68. Hindi RD, Azimi PH. (1980). Congenital malaria due to Plasmodium falciparum. *Pediatrics.* 66(6):977–979.

69. Duffy PE. (2001). Immunity to malaria during pregnancy: different host, different parasite. In: Duffy PE, Fried M, eds. *Malaria in Pregnancy.* London: Taylor and Francis. 71–126.

70. Fried M, Duffy PE. (1996). Adherence of Plasmodium falciparum to chondroitin sulfate A in the human placenta. [see comments.]. *Science.* 272(5267):1502–1504.

71. Fried M, Duffy PE. (1998). Maternal malaria and parasite adhesion. *J Molec Med.* 76(3–4):162–171.

72. Bray RS, Anderson MJ. (1979). Falciparum malaria and pregnancy. *Trans R Soc Trop Med Hyg.* 73(4):427–431.

73. Silver HM. (1997). Malarial infection during pregnancy. *Infect Dis Clin North Am.* 11(1):99–107.

74. Nathwani D, Currie PF, Douglas JG, *et al.* (1992). Plasmodium falciparum malaria in pregnancy: a review. *Br J Obstet Gynecol.* 99(2):118–121.

75. Nosten F, McGready R. (2001). The treatment of malaria in pregnancy. In: Duffy PE, Fried M, eds. *Malaria in Pregnancy.* London: Taylor and Francis. 223–240.

76. Mutabingwa TK, Leopoldo V, Nosten F. Chemoprophylaxis and other protective measures: preventing pregnancy malaria. In: Duffy PE, Fried M, eds. *Malaria in Pregnancy.* London: Taylor and Francis. 189–222.

77. Phillips-Howard PA, Steffen R, Kerr L, *et al.* (1998). Safety of mefloquine and other antimalarial agents in the first trimester of pregnancy. *J Travel Med.* 5(3):121–126.

78. Garner P, Gulmezoglu AM. (2002). Prevention versus treatment for malaria in pregnant women. *Cochrane Database Syst Rev.* (2).

79. Anon. (2000). WHO Expert Committee on Malaria. *World Health Organization Technical Report Series*. 892:i–v.

80. Schultz LJ, Steketee RW, Macheso A, *et al.* (1994). The efficacy of antimalarial regimens containing sulfadoxine-pyrimethamine and/or chloroquine in preventing peripheral and placental Plasmodium falciparum infection among pregnant women in Malawi. *Am J Trop Med Hyg*. 51(5):515–522.

81. Shulman CE, Dorman EK, Cutts F, *et al.* (1999). Intermittent sulphadoxine-pyrimethamine to prevent severe anaemia secondary to malaria in pregnancy: a randomised placebo-controlled trial. *Lancet*. 353(9153):632–636.

82. Jones JL, Lopez A, Wilson M, *et al.* (2001). Congenital toxoplasmosis: a review. *Obstet Gynecol Surv*. 56(5):296–305.

83. Remington JS, *et al.* (2001). Toxoplasmosis. In: Remington JS, Klein JO, eds. *Infectious Diseases of the Fetus and Newborn Infant*, pp. 205–346. Philadelphia: W.B. Saunders.

84. Ioannel D, Niel G, Costagliola D, *et al.* (1988). Epidemiology of toxoplasmosis among pregnant women in the Paris area. *Int J Epidemiol*. 17(3):595–602.

85. Hohlfeld P, Daffos F, Costa JM, *et al.* (1994). Prenatal diagnosis of congenital toxoplasmosis with a polymerase-chain-reaction test on amniotic fluid. *N Engl J Med*. 331(11):695–699.

86. Montoya JG, Remington JS. (2000). Toxoplasma gondii. In: Mandell GL, Bennett JE, Dolin R, eds. *Principles and Practice of Infectious Diseases*. Philadelphia: Churchill Livingstone. 2858–2888.

87. Wilson CB, Remington JS, Stagno S, *et al.* (1980). Development of adverse sequelae in children born with subclinical congenital Toxoplasma infection. *Pediatrics*. 66(5):767–774.

88. Wong SY, Remington JS. (1994). Toxoplasmosis in pregnancy. [see comments.]. *Clin Infect Dis*. 18(6):853–861; quiz 862.

89. Montoya JG. (2002). Laboratory diagnosis of Toxoplasma gondii infection and toxoplasmosis. *J Infect Dis*. 185 Suppl 1:S73–82.

90. Romand S, Wallon M, Franck J, *et al.* (2001). Prenatal diagnosis using polymerase chain reaction on amniotic fluid for congenital toxoplasmosis. *Obstet Gynecol*. 97(2):296–300.

91. Desmonts G, Couvreur J. (1999). Congenital toxoplasmosis: a prospective study of the offspring of 542 women who acquired toxoplasmosis during pregnancy: pathophysiology of congenital disease. In: Thalhammer O, Baumgarten K, Pollak A, eds. *Perinatal Medicine*, Vienna: Georg Thieme. 51–60.

92. Foulon W, Villena I, Stray-Pedersen B, *et al.* (1999). Treatment of toxoplasmosis during pregnancy: a multicenter study of impact on fetal transmission and children's sequelae at age 1 year. *Am J Obstet Gynecol*. 180(2 Pt 1): 410–415.

93. Baril L, Ancelle T, Goulet V, *et al.* (1999). Risk factors for Toxoplasma infection in pregnancy: a case-control study in France. *Scand J Infect Dis*. 31(3):305–309.

94. Kapperud G, Jenum PA, Stray-Pedersen B, *et al.* (1996). Risk factors for Toxoplasma gondii infection in pregnancy. Results of a prospective case-control study in Norway. *Am J Epidemiol*. 144(4):405–412.

95. Cook AJ, Gilbert RE, Buffolano W, *et al.* (2000). Sources of toxoplasma infection in pregnant women: European multicentre case-control study. European Research Network on Congenital Toxoplasmosis. [see comments.]. *BMJ*. 321(7254):142–147.

96. Weigel RM, Dubey JP, Dyer D, *et al.* (1999). Risk factors for infection with Toxoplasma gondii for residents and workers on swine farms in Illinois. *Am J Trop Med Hyg*. 60(5):793–798.

97. Foulon W, Naessens A, Lauwers S, *et al.* (1988). Impact of primary prevention on the incidence of toxoplasmosis during pregnancy. *Obstet Gynecol*. 72(3 Pt 1):363–366.

98. Bader TJ, Macones GA, Asch DA. (1997). Prenatal screening for toxoplasmosis. *Obstet Gynecol*. 90(3):457–464.

90

Sexually Transmitted Infections in Men and Women

TIMOTHY WILKIN, MD, MPH* AND MARY ANN CHIASSON, DrPH**

*Instructor of Medicine, Division of International Medicine and Infectious Diseases,
Weill Medical College of Cornell University, New York, NY
**Vice-President for Research and Evaluation, Medical and Health Research Association of NYC, Inc.;
Associate Professor of Clinical Epidemiology (in Medicine), Mailman School of Public Health,
Columbia University, New York, NY

I. Introduction

This chapter will discuss the current state of knowledge of the association of biologic sex with the manifestations, complications, and epidemiology of sexually transmitted infections (STIs), biologic and behavioral factors for both men and women that modify susceptibility, and considerations for STI prevention and control. Current recommendations for treatment of common STIs including considerations for pregnancy are listed in Table 90-1 [1]. Although the response to these treatments is similar in men and women, the complications for certain STIs are very gender specific, with women confronting the possibilities of infertility, ectopic pregnancy, cancer, and neonatal transmission of pathogens. As a result, the Centers for Disease Control and Prevention (CDC) recommend that sexually active women, especially young women, be screened annually for STIs including cervical cytology; men are tested for STIs only when they have symptomatic infection.

II. Gender Differences in Biologic Susceptibility

In addition to the anatomic differences between men and women, there are many more subtle biologic differences that influence the relative risk of STI acquisition and transmission. In men biologic risk factors associated with STIs remain relatively constant throughout life, although behavioral factors (e.g., condom use) may change dramatically. Male circumcision status is one of the most important characteristics associated with variable risk of STI and the only factor discussed in detail in this section. The bulk of the discussion focuses on changes that occur in the female genital tract from birth through menopause.

A. Circumcision

Male circumcision has been identified as an important factor in the acquisition of certain STIs, especially the human immunodeficiency virus (HIV). Both cross-sectional and prospective studies have found an association between being uncircumcised and acquisition of HIV [2–7]. This effect is independent of the increased risk of genital ulcer disease in uncircumcised men that is also associated with HIV acquisition [3,4,8]. Circumcision of adult males is being studied in randomized trials as a strategy to prevent sexual transmission of HIV in Africa.

Uncircumcised males are at higher risk for penile infection with high-risk (or oncogenic) types of human papillomavirus (HPV) [9,10] and penile cancer, a rare sequela of that infection [11]. This may put their female partners at risk for infection with high-risk HPV, cervical squamous intraepithelial lesions (SIL, a precursor to invasive disease) and cervical carcinoma. Among women who report sexual intercourse with only one sexual partner, having an uncircumcised male partner is associated with a higher risk of cervical SIL [12]. In a study pooling five international case-control studies, monogamous women having a male sexual partner with a previous history of multiple sexual partners had increased odds of cervical cancer if that partner was uncircumcised compared to having a partner who was circumcised [9]. A conflicting result has been found for low-risk types of HPV with circumcision being associated with an increased prevalence of genital warts, a manifestation of that infection [13]. In a study comparing risk factors for infection with high-risk and low-risk types of HPV, there was a trend for an association between high-risk HPV and being uncircumcised but not for low-risk HPV for unclear reasons [10]. Data are conflicting on an association between genital herpes and being uncircumcised, with some studies finding an association [14,15] and others not finding an association [16]. Studies have consistently found an association between being uncircumcised and increased risk of infection with both syphilis and *Neisseria gonorrhoeae* but not *Chlamydia trachomatis* [13,14,17–19]. Lack of circumcision was associated with a poorer response to treatment for chancroid [20].

The mechanism by which circumcision alters the risk of STIs is not completely understood. In the case of HIV, the foreskin contains large numbers of dendritic cells, which are a target cell for HIV [21]. When compared to an uncircumcised penis, the glans of a circumcised penis has a thicker cornified epithelium that is more resistant to ulcerations from either infection or trauma during sexual intercourse that can serve as a portal for other infectious agents [4]. The inner surface of the foreskin is nonkeratinized and may be vulnerable to viral infections; and the foreskin may act as a reservoir for sexually transmitted infectious pathogens that could lead to urethritis [22]. Finally, being uncircumcised is associated with a nonspecific balanitis, increasing the susceptibility to STIs [13].

B. Puberty

Unlike in men, in women the biologic susceptibility to STIs varies throughout a woman's reproductive life cycle. Changes

Table 90-1
Treatment Guidelines for Curable Sexually Transmitted Infections

Infection	Primary Regimens	Alternative Regimens	Regimens to be Used During Pregnancy
Chancroid	Azithromycin 1 g orally in a single dose OR Ceftriaxone 250 mg intramuscularly in a single dose OR Ciprofloxacin 500 mg orally twice daily for 3 days OR Erythromycin base 500 mg orally three times daily for 7 days	—	Ceftriaxone 250 mg intramuscularly in a single dose
Gonococcal infection (urethritis, cervicitis, pharyngitis, *proctitis)	Cefixime 400 mg orally in a single dose** OR Ceftriaxone 125 mg intramuscularly in a single dose OR Ciprofloxacin 500 orally in a single dose† OR Ofloxacin 400 mg orally in a single dose† OR Levofloxacin 250 mg orally in a single dose†	Spectinomycin 2 g intramuscularly in a single dose	Cefixime 400 mg orally in a single dose Ceftriaxone 125 mg intramuscularly in a single dose Spectinomycin 2 g intramuscularly in a single dose (alternative, if unable to take cephalosporin)
Chlamydia trachomatis infection (cervicitis, urethritis, pharyngitis, and proctitis)	Azithromycin 1 g orally in a single dose OR Doxycycline 100 mg orally twice daily for 7 days‡	Erythromycin base 500 mg orally four times daily for 7 days OR Erythromycin ethylsuccinate 800 mg orally four times a day for 7 days OR Ofloxacin 300 mg orally twice a day for 7 days OR Levofloxacin 500 mg orally once daily for 7 days	Erythromycin base 500 mg orally four times daily for 7 days OR Amoxicillin 500 mg orally three times daily for 7 days OR Azithromycin 1 g orally in a single dose (alternative)
Syphilis (primary, secondary, and early latent)	Benzathine penicillin G 2.4 million units intramuscularly in a single dose	Efficacy of alternative regimens not established§	Benzathine penicillin G 2.4 million units intramuscularly in a single dose
Syphilis (tertiary, late latent)	Benzathine penicillin G 2.4 million units intramuscularly once weekly for 3 doses	Efficacy of alternative regimens not established§	Benzathine penicillin G 2.4 million units intramuscularly once weekly for 3 doses
Neurosyphilis	Aqueous crystalline penicillin G 3–4 million units intravenous every 4 hours for 10–14 days	Procaine penicillin 2.4 million units intramuscularly once daily with probenecid 500 mg orally four times daily, both for 10–14 days	Aqueous crystalline penicillin G 3–4 million units intravenous every 4 hours for 10–14 days
Trichomonas (vaginitis or urethritis)	Metronidazole 2 g orally in a single dose	Metronidazole 500 mg twice daily for 7 days	Metronidazole 2 g orally in a single dose¶

*Gonococcal pharyngitis is more difficult to eradicate than cervical, urethral, or rectal infections. Either ceftriaxone or ciprofloxacin should be used.

**Cefixime production has been halted in the United States as of 2002. No other satisfactory oral cephalosporins are available.

†Fluoroquinolones such as ciprofloxacin, levofloxacin, or ofloxacin should not be used in areas with high rates of quinolone-resistant gonococcus such as Asia, Hawaii, or California.

‡Observed single-dose therapy is preferable to assure adherence.

§Other antibiotics with activity against *T. pallidum* include azithromycin, doxycycline, and ceftriaxone. The dose and length of therapy is not well established.

¶*T. vaginalis* has been associated with preterm labor, but treatment of asymptomatic infection in pregnant women actually resulted in a higher incidence of preterm labor [131].

(From Anonymous. [2002]. Sexually transmitted diseases treatment guidelines 2002. Centers for Disease Control and Prevention. *MMWR Recomm Rep.* 51[No. RR-6].)

in the anatomy, physiology, and cellular morphology of the genital tract beginning with puberty, continuing through the normal monthly hormonal fluctuations of the menstrual cycle, during pregnancy, and following menopause modulate susceptibility to various pathogens.

1. Vagina

The changes in cell type that occur in the female genital tract during development influence the likelihood of infection with specific pathogens. Some pathogens, including C. trachomatis and N. gonorrhoeae, infect or attach to columnar or cuboidal epithelial cells [23], whereas others (HPV, genital herpes, and Trichomonas vaginalis) are associated with stratified squamous epithelium [24]. T. pallidum attaches to multiple cell types including both squamous and columnar epithelia. At birth, the neonatal vagina is lined with the stratified squamous epithelium of adulthood as a result of intrauterine exposure to maternal estrogen; the neonatal vagina is resistant to perinatally transmitted C. trachomatis and N. gonorrhoeae [25]. During the first month of life, the squamous epithelium lining the neonate's vagina is replaced by columnar epithelium, which is susceptible to C. trachomatis and N. gonorrhoeae [25]. Colonization of the neonatal vagina with T. vaginalis can spontaneously resolve as the epithelial lining of the vagina is replaced with columnar cells [26].

The ecosystem of the vagina is complex and dynamic. At puberty the vaginal pH is lowered from 6.5 to 7.5 to the more acidic pH of 4.0–4.5 normally found in women from menarche to menopause. Numerous organisms, both facultative and anaerobic, have been recovered from normal vaginal fluid of asymptomatic women without vaginitis [28]. However, Lactobacillus species are the most common bacteria found, and hydrogen peroxide–generating lactobacilli contribute to the control of vaginal flora [29]. Peroxide itself may also provide protection from STIs [30]. Lactobacillus species appear to inhibit microorganisms, such as T. vaginalis and selected anaerobic bacteria associated with bacterial vaginosis, and to inhibit genital infections including those associated with C. trachomatis [31–33]. Vaginal fluids produced during sexual excitement, cervical mucus, and semen are all of normal or basic pH and may temporarily neutralize vaginal fluid, increasing the risk of infection. Lactobacillus species are required to maintain the normal vaginal ecosystem including flora and the acidic pH.

2. Cervix

The gradual changes in cellular composition and morphology of the cervix that occur during development account, in part, for the increased susceptibility to STIs observed in adolescents. The extension of the friable columnar epithelium of the endocervix out over the visible exocervix, referred to as ectopy or ectropion, is a hallmark of the immature cervix of adolescence. Throughout adolescence, the columnar epithelium of the lower genital tract is gradually replaced by thicker stratified squamous epithelium through squamous metaplasia with the squamocolumnar junction gradually advancing to and then into the endocervical os. In adult women, the external surface of the portio vaginalis of the cervix is covered by stratified squamous epithelium identical to that of the vagina. Although cervical ectopy is a normal feature of the immature cervix of adolescence, it can also be induced by exogenous factors including oral contraceptives [34,35] and cervicitis resulting from infection with C. trachomatis, cytomegalovirus, T. vaginalis, N. gonorrhoeae, and herpes simplex virus (HSV).

In addition to the critical role it plays in conception, cervical mucus may both directly and indirectly protect the genital tract from infection. The estrogen-related changes of the cervix that occur during adolescence also result in changes in the composition and quantity of mucus secreted from the specialized epithelium of the endocervical canal. Mucus secretion is greatly increased in puberty but is thinner than the viscous fluid found in the endocervical canal of adult women. The thinner mucus of adolescence may allow organisms to penetrate more easily and attach to mucosal sites or may permit entry to the upper genital tract. Mucus may also provide an appropriate support medium for other nonspecific microbial defenses including lysozyme, lactoferrin, zinc, fibronectin, and complement [36].

C. Menstrual Cycle

The steroid hormones—estradiol, estrone, estrone-sulfate, and progesterone—show wide fluctuations across the menstrual cycle. For example, mean plasma levels of estradiol vary from a low of 44 pg/ml (range 20–120) at menses to a high of 250 pg/ml (range 150–600) just before ovulation [37]. Normal physiologic variation in the vagina in response to fluctuating hormone levels during the menstrual cycle has been described in several studies. Eschenbach et al. [38] and Patton et al [39] examined genital tissue, vaginal fluid, and vaginal microbial flora in asymptomatic women not using vaginal or systemic contraception at three stages of the menstrual cycle: menstrual phase (days 1–5), preovulatory phase (days 7–12), and postovulatory phase (days 19–24). The volume of vaginal discharge increased and the amount of cervical mucus decreased over the menstrual cycle. The rate of heavy growth of Lactobacillus increased over the menstrual cycle, whereas the concentration of non-Lactobacillus species tended to be higher at menses, providing evidence that the vaginal flora becomes less stable at this time. The heavy growth of non-Lactobacillus species during menses could be the result of the presence of an additional substrate in menstrual blood. Other investigators [40] have found that a greater number of sexual partners and more frequent vaginal intercourse are also associated with changes in vaginal flora. The vaginal pH is somewhat higher during menses (pH = 4.6) but otherwise remains stable over the cycle at 4.4 [38].

Vaginal biopsies from participants in the study described above [38] showed a small statistically, but probably not clinically, significant reduction in the number of vaginal epithelial cells over the menstrual cycle. Immune cell populations in the vaginal tissues including Langerhans cells, macrophages, CD4+ or CD8+ lymphocytes and neutrophils remained stable throughout the three phases of menstrual cycle examined. B lymphocytes were not observed in the vaginal tissues [39].

The proliferative phase of the cycle (within 14 days of the beginning of the last menstrual period, between menses and ovulation) appears to be an independent risk factor for onset of salpingitis and endometritis, and, in about half the women with disseminated gonococcal infection, onset of symptoms occurs within 7 days of menses [23]. In a study of women hospitalized with acute salpingitis between 1981 and 1984, the majority of women with chlamydial and/or gonococcal infection had onset of symptoms within 7 days of onset of menses [41]. A more recent study of risk factors for endometritis among women with cervical N. gonorrhoeae or C. trachomatis or bacterial vaginosis reported similar findings. Women who were in the proliferative phase of their menstrual cycle had a significantly increased likelihood of endometritis [42]. Subclinical pelvic inflammatory disease (PID) [43] and acute PID are also associated with the proliferative phase of the menstrual cycle [44].

Several explanations for the association between the proliferative phase and endometritis and other upper genital tract infections most commonly caused by C. trachomatis and N. gonorrhoeae have been proposed. The most straightforward of these is the failure of the endocervical barrier because of loss of cervical mucus during menses [41,42]. Another possible explanation for increased upper genital tract and disseminated gonococcal infection relates to the absolute requirement that gonococci have iron for growth. Dissemination of gonococcal infection may be the result of provision of iron during menses in the form of hemin and transferrin, which permits rapid growth of the organism [36]. Extracellular iron is unlikely to be an important factor in the growth of C. trachomatis, however, because, unlike N. gonorrhoeae, it is an intracellular parasite. Hormonal changes that occur during the menstrual cycle may play a role instead in chlamydial infections. Animal data support this explanation because estradiol treatment of guinea pigs results in a chlamydial infection of increased intensity and duration [41,45] and the majority of in vitro studies suggest that infection of mammalian cells by pathogenic chlamydiae is promoted by estrogens, which are at the highest levels of the menstrual cycle just before menstruation [46,47]. The relationship between menstrual cycle phase and upper genital tract infection may be further confounded by vaginal douching, which is also a risk factor for infection [48], because women may be more likely to douche following menses.

D. Exogenous Hormones

The effects of oral contraceptives and depot medroxyprogesterone acetate (DMPA) on cervical and vaginal mucosa and vaginal flora have been well described, but findings on the relationship of their use to the incidence of upper genital tract infections are contradictory. The difficulty in establishing consistent associations between contraceptive use and infection is in part because both the infection (outcome) and contraceptive use (risk factor) are so closely related to sexual behavior (potential confounder). This makes it a challenge to determine whether the association is simply the result of more high-risk sexual behavior in women using nonbarrier contraceptives. It is also very problematic that few studies take into account the probability of a woman's exposure to potential pathogens by measuring STI prevalence in male partners.

The use of oral contraceptives causes an increase in cervical ectopy [34,35] and small changes in vaginal flora but has minimal effect on vaginal epithelium and vaginal and cervical discharge [49]. Oral contraceptives are associated with an increased incidence of C. trachomatis [50]; however, in one study they were found to protect against PID in women infected with C. trachomatis but not with N. gonorrhoeae [51]. In contrast, women using DMPA experience hypoestrogenism, which causes a decrease in peroxide-producing Lactobacilli colonization and a slight thinning of the vaginal epithelium [52]. These women also have an increased incidence of chlamydial infection as well as an increased incidence of trichomoniasis and PID [50]. A 2001 study of the risk of upper genital tract disease and PID reported no association between contraceptive method (oral contraceptives or DMPA) and decreased likelihood of upper genital tract disease [53]. In a single prospective study, the use of hormonal contraceptives (oral contraceptives or DMPA) was not found to increase the cervical shedding of HSV in already infected women [54].

Contradictory results also have been reported from numerous studies examining the association between hormonal contraceptive use and HPV infection [55], even when potential confounding by sexual behavior is statistically controlled for in the analysis. In contrast, data supporting a moderate positive association between cervical cancer and long-term oral contraceptive use in women with HPV are more consistent [56,57], although this association is not found in all studies [58]. Much less is known about the effect of hormone replacement therapy. In one study, exogenous estrogen use was positively associated with cervical adenocarcinoma but not squamous cell carcinomas in women with HPV [59].

E. Pregnancy

Dramatic hormonal and anatomic changes occur during pregnancy that have important effects on STI acquisition, pathogenesis, and disease manifestations. During pregnancy the placenta produces huge amounts of estrogen and progesterone. In addition, the anatomy of the genital tract undergoes dramatic changes related to the growing fetus and the surge in estrogen and progesterone. Vaginal walls become thickened and engorged with blood, and the glycogen content of the vagina increases with a concomitant decrease in vaginal pH. The columnar epithelial cells of the endocervix extend to ectocervix (cervical ectopy), and this tissue is friable and bleeds easily, thereby increasing susceptibility to infection [60]. The attachment of the chorion to the endometrial decidua with obliteration of the uterine cavity after the 12th week of pregnancy may obstruct the route for ascending intraluminal spread of gonococci [61]. After the 16th week of pregnancy, the fetal membranes rest over the internal cervical opening, and infection of the membranes (chorioamnionitis), caused by a variety of organisms, is more common [62].

High levels of estrogens such as those that occur during pregnancy may depress cell-mediated immunity, impair the activity of natural killer cells, and suppress some aspects of neutrophil function [46]. The depressed cellular immune response of pregnancy may protect the fetus from rejection but may also promote maternal susceptibility to infectious agents including C. trachomatis [63]. HPV persists during pregnancy and declines in the postpartum period [64]. It is conventional wisdom that HPV-associated genital lesions can progress during pregnancy, presumably because of accelerated HPV replication.

Genital warts can increase in size to such an extent that they mechanically obstruct labor [65], but the natural history of cervical intraepithelial neoplasia during pregnancy is unclear [66].

In pregnant women, cervical mucus thickens and forms a semi-solid plug that occludes the endocervical canal. Not only does the cervical mucus plug serve as a mechanical barrier to the uterine cavity, but it also exhibits antimicrobial activity against anaerobic microbes. Secretory leukoprotease inhibitor, lysozyme, lactoferrin, and neutrophil defensins are all present in concentrations sufficient for antimicrobial activity [67,68].

F. Menopause

There are few studies on the prevalence of risk factors for STIs other than HIV in menopausal and postmenopausal women [69,70]. The very low levels of estrogen following menopause can result in atrophic vaginitis, which may increase susceptibility to STIs and increase vaginal transmission of HIV [71].

III. Bacterial Infections

A. Neisseria gonorrhoeae

Approximately 360,000 cases of *N. gonorrhoeae* were reported to the CDC in 2001 [72]. *N. gonorrhoeae* causes a mucopurulent urethritis in men and a mucopurulent cervicitis in women [73]. Most men with gonococcal urethritis develop symptomatic infection within 5 days of exposure, whereas less than half of women develop symptomatic cervicitis. Other possible sites of infection include the pharynx and rectum. Complications of *N. gonorrhoeae* can include disseminated infection characterized by acute monoarticular arthritis, tenosynovitis, and rash; PID in women; and epididymitis in men.

More cases of *N. gonorrhoeae* have been reported in men than women, probably as a result of their higher rate of symptoms prompting medical care and an increased rate of *N. gonorrhoeae* among men who have sex with men; this difference is decreasing with increased screening of asymptomatic women [73]. A probability sample of adults aged 18–35 years in the Baltimore area suggested that the number of asymptomatic untreated adults with *N. gonorrhoeae*, *C. trachomatis*, or both approached or exceeded the number actually diagnosed [74]. African American women in this study had a higher prevalence of both infections compared to African American men, but there was not a gender difference for other races. In a study from Seattle, young urban African American women had the highest incidence of *N. gonorrhoeae* [75].

Although the CDC recommends annual screening for curable STIs for all sexually active women, especially young women (under age 25), men do not routinely undergo screening for STIs. A study that empirically derived the reproductive rate for men (an estimate of the spread of the infection) with *N. gonorrhoeae* suggested that asymptomatic men spread *N. gonorrhoeae* to more women than did symptomatic men and they may be responsible for the continued persistence of this infection in a given population [76]. The advent of urine-based tests for *N. gonorrhoeae* and *C. trachomatis* has altered the setting of screening for these conditions by eliminating the need for a pelvic examination for women and a urethral swab for men.

Examples of new approaches are screening through the mail [77], through community-based organizations [78], and in other nonclinical settings such as prisons and entertainment venues [79–81].

Men and women have differing complications from *N. gonorrhoeae*, with disseminated gonococcal infection being more common in women than men [82]. One likely explanation for this difference is that women are more likely to have undiagnosed asymptomatic infection, allowing a longer opportunity for dissemination of the infection prior to treatment. Cervical infection with *N. gonorrhoeae* in pregnant women has been associated with premature rupture of membranes and spontaneous abortion [73]. The most important complication for neonates is gonococcal conjunctivitis, which has been dramatically reduced in industrialized countries by screening pregnant women for *N. gonorrhoeae* and by prophylactic administration of 1% silver nitrate eye drops to all newborns. All pregnant women should be screened for cervical *N. gonorrhoeae* at the first prenatal visit and again in the third trimester for those women at higher risk, including those living in areas with a higher incidence of this infection (see Table 90-2).

B. Chlamydia Trachomatis

More than 750,000 cases of *C. trachomatis* were reported to the CDC in 2001 [72]. Similar to *N. gonorrhoeae*, *C. trachomatis* also causes a mucopurulent urethritis in men and cervicitis in women and can also infect rectal and pharyngeal tissues [83]. Urogenital chlamydial infections are less likely to be symptomatic in both men and women than those caused by *N. gonorrhoeae*. Complications of *C. trachomatis* include PID in women and epididymitis in men, both of which occur more frequently with *C. trachomatis* than with *N. gonorrhoeae*. *C. trachomatis* also causes a reactive arthritis and is associated with Reiter's syndrome (conjunctivitis, arthritis, and urethritis).

Table 90-2
STI Screening in Pregnancy

Initial Evaluation
HIV serology, *Neisseria gonorrhoeae* and *Chlamydia trachomatis* testing, syphilis serology, hepatitis B surface antigen, cervical cytology
Hepatitis C serology for higher risk women
Subsequent Evaluations
Repeat syphilis serology at 28 weeks in areas of higher prevalence and in higher risk women
Repeat human immunodeficiency virus serology, *N. gonorrhoeae*, and *C. trachomatis* testing and hepatitis B surface antigen at 36 weeks in higher risk women
Controversial
Repeat pap smear later in pregnancy, herpes simplex virus type-specific serologies

(From Anonymous. [2002]. Sexually transmitted diseases treatment guidelines 2002. Centers for Disease Control and Prevention. *MMWR Recomm Rep.* 51[No. RR-6].)

The epidemiology of *C. trachomatis* in men is less well characterized than that of women, but more information has been forthcoming with the use of urine-based amplification tests. Several studies found no difference in the prevalence of *C. trachomatis* by gender including young intravenous drug users (5.2%) [84] and street youth in Montreal (6.6%) [85]. Young African American women in Baltimore were found to have a higher prevalence of *C. trachomatis* than young African American men, but this gender difference was not seen for other groups [74]. Young women aged 16–24 years entering a national job training program had a 12% prevalence of *C. trachomatis*, which was associated with age, with younger women having the highest prevalence [86]. Young male army recruits had a prevalence of 5.3% that did not vary according to age [87].

Women had higher inclusion-forming units observed in quantitative chlamydial cultures (a measure of infectiousness) [88]. The reason for the gender difference in infectivity is not known, but possible explanations include an artifact of the sampling technique, differential sex hormones, or the flushing effect of urine in men. However using urine-based amplification techniques, it appears that male-to-female transmission is similar to female-to-male transmission [89]. As discussed previously, men do not enter care with the same frequency as women and are less likely to be screened for *N. gonorrhoeae* or *C. trachomatis*. Most sexually active young men are practicing unprotected intercourse, but few view themselves at risk [90]. Most young men with *C. trachomatis* are asymptomatic and should be a focus for interventions to reduce the incidence of this infection.

Reactive arthritis from infection with *C. trachomatis* is more common in men than women despite a similar occurrence of reactive arthritis from enteric infections and is probably caused by disseminated infection in the joints [91]. Men, especially those with reactive arthritis, were found to have a humoral response to fewer *C. trachomatis* antigens than women. Pregnant women with chlamydial cervicitis can transmit the infection to their infants during birth [1]. Neonatal infection can present as ophthalmia neonatorum, which is not prevented by the 1% silver nitrate drops used to avert gonococcal conjunctivitis, and as pneumonia around 1–3 months of life. Similar to *N. gonorrhoeae*, all pregnant women should be screened for *C. trachomatis* cervicitis at the first prenatal visit and again in the third trimester for women at higher risk (see Table 90-2).

C. Syphilis

Syphilis is a systemic infection with the bacterium *Treponema pallidum* [92]. The manifestations in the untreated individual are classified as follows:

- Primary syphilis—a painless ulcer (or chancre) at the site of inoculation
- Secondary syphilis—disseminated infection including rash, mucocutaneous lesions, and lymphadenopathy
- Tertiary syphilis—dementia; gummatous lesions; cardiac, auditory, and ophthalmic abnormalities
- Latent syphilis—serologic evidence without clinical manifestations (early latent being syphilis acquired within the past year and late latent being syphilis acquired greater than 1 year prior)

Approximately 6100 cases of primary or secondary syphilis, 8700 cases of early latent syphilis, and 17,000 cases of late latent or tertiary syphilis were reported to the CDC in 2001 [72]. Women are less likely than men to present during primary syphilis probably because women are less likely than men to notice the painless ulcer associated with primary syphilis that would prompt an individual to seek medical attention [93].

According to the CDC, the rates of primary or secondary syphilis have been higher in men than women with a peak male-to-female ratio of 3.5:1 in 1980 [94]. Since that time, the ratio has decreased because of a declining syphilis epidemic in men who have sex with men (which has began reversing [95]) and an increasing syphilis epidemic among women in the rural South. However, a national seroepidemiologic study conducted as part of the National Health and Nutrition Examination Survey did not show a gender difference in the prevalence of syphilis [96]. Both African American women in the rural South involved in the trade of sex for drugs [97] and female intravenous drug users [98] have a higher prevalence of syphilis than their male counterparts.

In both a study of untreated patients with clinical syphilis from Norway and a collection of autopsy studies, late complications such as cardiovascular syphilis or neurosyphilis were twice as common in men as women [99,100]. Women having any stage of syphilis can transmit the infection to their offspring with the risk being highest in primary and secondary syphilis [92]. Congenital syphilis can manifest as late abortion, stillbirth, or neonatal disease and rarely occurs before 4 months *in utero*. The most common abnormalities associated with neonatal disease are bone lesions, liver disease, and rash. The CDC recommends that all pregnant women receive testing for syphilis at their first prenatal visit. For those women at increased risk of syphilis or who live in areas of high syphilis endemicity, syphilis testing should be repeated at 28 weeks of pregnancy and again at delivery [1]. Early diagnosis and treatment of syphilis in the mother should prevent neonatal infection. Current CDC guidelines appear efficacious in preventing neonatal syphilis; an open-label, noncomparative study found that 334 of 340 (98.3%) infants born to women treated accordingly for syphilis prior to delivery had no evidence of neonatal syphilis [101].

D. Chancroid

Chancroid is an ulcerative STI caused by the organism *Haemophilus ducreyi* [102]. The lesions begin as tender papules, which then erode to become painful, nonindurated ulcers. One-half of lesions are associated with unilateral, tender lymphadenopathy that can progress to draining sinuses if left untreated. The diagnosis of chancroid can be difficult, and isolation of the organism requires a special culture medium. A presumptive diagnosis is often made on clinical appearance and negative tests for HSV and syphilis [1].

Chancroid occurs as outbreaks in the United States but is endemic in many parts of the world, and it is associated with a higher risk of HIV [1]. Notably, there were only 38 cases of chancroid reported to the CDC in 2001, down from a high of 5000 in 1988 [72]. The epidemiology of chancroid has a striking gender difference, with 90% of reported cases occurring in men [102]. Women may have an inapparent carrier state or overlooked lesions. Commercial sex workers are an important feature of *H. ducreyi* epidemiology and may infect many male partners [103]. Women are less likely than men to progress from the papule stage to pustules when experimentally inoculated with *H. ducreyi*, and this lower likelihood of progressive infection may also explain the differential epidemiology [103].

IV. Viral Infections

A. *Human Papillomavirus*

HPV causes a variety of lesions of the skin and mucous membranes including common warts of the skin, plantar warts, genital warts (or condyloma acuminatum), squamous intraepithelial lesions, and invasive anogenital carcinoma including cervical, vaginal, vulvar, perineal, penile, and anal cancers [104]. There are more than 100 types of HPV, approximately 30 of which infect the anogenital area and are spread principally through sexual contact. Anogenital types of HPV are divided into high risk (those types that have been associated with anogenital malignancies) and low risk (those types associated with condyloma only). Most HPV infections are subclinical and can be either transient or persistent.

The majority of epidemiologic studies of HPV are among women. Major risk factors for HPV among women are earlier age at onset of sexual activity, higher lifetime number of sexual partners, younger age, and presence of other STIs such as HIV or HSV [105]. Similar risk factors have been found for penile HPV in men [10]. In a population-based study of antibodies to HPV-16, women had a higher prevalence compared to men (18% vs 8%) and the risk factors for HPV-16 antibodies were similar for both men and women [106]. Cervical carcinoma is the most important sequela of genital high-risk HPV infection in women. In the United States and other developed countries, the rate of this disease has fallen dramatically since the advent of routine Papanicolaou screening for SILs of the cervix, but cervical carcinoma remains the most common malignancy for women in many developing countries [107,108]. Annually, 3.5 million women are diagnosed with cytologic abnormalities requiring follow-up in the United States [109]. Although HPV is the most important cofactor in developing cervical SIL and cervical cancer, direct testing for HPV has only recently been included in the routine algorithm for managing cervical cytologic abnormalities [110]. Women with high-risk HPV are also at risk for vaginal and vulvar cancer, especially those who have HIV [111].

Overall, women are at higher risk for cancers of the anus than are men, but men with a history of receptive anal intercourse are at the highest risk [112]. Researchers have proposed screening for premalignant lesions of the anus, similar to cervical cancer screening for women, in certain groups including men who have sex with men, all individuals with HIV, and women who are HIV-negative with other genital HPV-associated lesions [113]. The benefit of this screening is limited by the unclear efficacy of treating anal SILs to prevent invasive carcinoma.

Pregnant women having genital condyloma are at risk of transmitting HPV to their newborns [1]. Most infections of the newborn are subclinical, but a small percentage can lead to recurrent respiratory papillomatosis, of which there are an estimated 800–1500 cases annually. This disease is characterized by recurring exophytic lesions throughout the respiratory tract and is extremely debilitating and difficult to treat. It is associated mostly with HPV types 6 and 11, which are low-risk types causing condyloma. Most infections of neonates take place at the time of delivery. However, routine caesarian section is not recommended for women with genital condyloma because of the low incidence of recurrent respiratory papillomatosis.

B. *Herpes Simplex Virus*

There are two types of herpes simplex viruses—HSV-1- and HSV-2 [1]. Both types of HSV establish lifelong infection characterized by latency in the dorsal root ganglion and ability for recurrent clinical disease. HSV-1 infection typically presents as vesicles or ulcers in the orolabial area, whereas HSV-2 infects the genital area; however, crossover infection is not unusual. HSV-1 infection is extremely common, with approximately 62% of adults in the United States having HSV-1–specific immunoglobulin G (IgG) compared to 22% of adults having HSV-2–specific IgG [114,115]. For both types of HSV, the clinical course is extremely variable, and most individuals with serologic evidence of HSV-2 infection do not recall a history of compatible clinical disease [115].

Animal models of HSV have suggested some interesting sex-specific differences in HSV infection. In the mouse corneal inoculation model of HSV, investigators found that male wild-type mice had a higher mortality than female wild-type mice [116]. Female interferon-gamma knockout and interferon-gamma receptor knockout mice had the same mortality as the female wild type mice, whereas the same experiments in male mice revealed significantly higher mortality for both types of interferon-gamma knockout mice. The same investigators found that although there was no difference in reactivation for male and female wild-type mice (hyperthermic stress model), both types of male interferon-gamma knockout mice had a much higher rate of reactivation compared to male wild-type mice. Female interferon-gamma knockout mice had a similar rate of reactivation to female wild-type mice. This led investigators to conclude that some immunomodulatory effects of interferon-gamma may be sex-specific. A study of male and female mice inoculated with HSV in the pinna found no difference in primary infection or reactivation of HSV [117].

Epidemiologic studies of HSV-1 and HSV-2 have been greatly improved by the use of more reliable type-specific IgG assays. Gender has not been associated with HSV-1 seropositivity [115,118], but women consistently have been found to have a higher rate of HSV-2 seropositivity than men [114,115,119,120]. This association remained significant after controlling for age, number of sexual partners, and other factors relating to HSV-2 seropositivity. The reasons for the differential rates of HSV-2 are unclear, but they may result from the higher rate of male-to-female transmission compared to female-to-male transmission and a higher frequency of recurrent genital HSV lesions in men increasing the likelihood of transmission [121–123]. In a prospective study for a failed HSV vaccine, women were more likely than men to have symptomatic primary HSV-2 infection (44% vs 32%) [122]. Two studies of a different HSV vaccine found that the vaccine was effective in preventing symptomatic infection in women seronegative for both HSV-1 and HSV-2 but not in seronegative men [124]. Although this may have been secondary to a small number of new HSV infections in men limiting statistical power, an alternate theory is that women were more likely to have a type-1 T helper (Th1) response to the vaccine than men, which is important for control of HSV infection. The association of gender with the frequency of reactivation is unclear, with recurrent HSV-2 genital lesions lasting longer in men in one study [125] but not in another [126].

One of the major complications associated with HSV infection is neonatal infection transmitted at the time of delivery. Neonatal herpes can manifest as mucocutaneous lesions, disseminated infection, and central nervous system infection. The mortality for neonatal central nervous system infection in the absence of therapy is 65%. The risk of neonatal infection ranges from 44% for infants born vaginally to women experiencing a primary HSV infection to less than 1% for women with a history of recurrent herpes with no active lesions [127]. Performing a caesarian section on mothers having asymptomatic shedding of HSV (a positive HSV culture without genital lesions) at the time of delivery was associated with a reduction of neonatal herpes. No cases of neonatal herpes developed in this study in infants born to mothers having visible genital herpetic lesions probably because all such women had a caesarian section. Other options for preventing neonatal herpes include serologic testing of pregnant women and their sexual partners to identify women at risk for primary infection of either HSV-1 or HSV-2 and treatment with acyclovir to prevent recurrences and asymptomatic viral shedding at term. Currently, there is no firm recommendation on the use of acyclovir during pregnancy. Acyclovir reduces HSV recurrences at delivery for women with a history of HSV prior to pregnancy [128] and reduces both HSV recurrences and caesarian sections for women acquiring HSV during pregnancy [129].

V. Other Organisms and Syndromes

A. Trichomonas Vaginalis

T. vaginalis is a protozoan that causes vaginitis with discharge, vulvovaginal soreness, and dysuria in women, but it does not cause endocervical disease [130]. The prevalence of T. vaginalis in women varies widely from 5% to 10% in the general population to 50% in STI clinics. Infection in men manifests most commonly as urethritis, with prostatitis and penile ulceration occurring less often. Many clinicians will test for T. vaginalis or treat empirically in those men with urethritis who fail to respond to treatment for N. gonorrhoeae and C. trachomatis. It is found in 5–15% of men with nongonococcal urethritis and is isolated in 14–60% of male partners of infected females and 67–100% of female partners of infected males. T. vaginalis has been associated with preterm labor, but treatment of asymptomatic infection in pregnant women actually resulted in a higher incidence of preterm labor [131].

B. Pelvic Inflammatory Disease

PID is a syndrome characterized by infection of the upper female genital tract (uterus, fallopian tubes, ovaries, and peritoneum) that spreads from an initial infection in the cervix and vagina [132]. More than 1 million women are treated annually in the United States for symptomatic PID. It is firmly associated with two STIs: N. gonorrhoeae and C. trachomatis. PID as a consequence of infection with C. trachomatis is thought to be less symptomatic than PID related to N. gonorrhoeae. Other organisms associated with PID include Mycoplasma hominis, M. genitalium, and Ureaplasma urealyticum [133]. PID dramatically increases a woman's risk for tubal infertility, ectopic pregnancy, and chronic pelvic pain [132].

C. Epididymitis

Epididymitis is an inflammation of the epididymis caused by infection or trauma that presents as painful, unilateral swelling of the testicle [1]. There are more than 500,000 cases annually in the United States, and the infectious etiologies typically vary according to age [134]. Sexually active men younger than age 35 years tend to have epididymitis as a consequence of urethral infection with C. trachomatis or N. gonorrhoeae, but many of these men may not have concurrent signs or symptoms of urethritis. Men older than 35 years, men practicing insertive anal intercourse, and men having structural abnormalities of the urinary tract may have epididymitis as a result of coliform bacteria, such as Escherichia coli, or Pseudomonas aeruginosa. Bilateral epididymitis is associated with male infertility.

VI. STI Behavioral Risks, Prevention, and Control

A. Behavioral Risks

Behavioral risks for STI acquisition in adolescents and adults include early age at initiation of sexual intercourse, multiple sexual partners, frequency of intercourse, high-risk sexual partners and practices, and irregular condom use [135,136]. A history of childhood sexual abuse and adult intimate partner violence are also associated with an increased incidence and prevalence of STIs in women [137]. In a large case-control study, abused women were found to experience an increase in gynecologic (e.g., STIs, vaginal bleeding, vaginal infections, etc.) and other problems, suggesting the importance of routine universal screening and sensitive in-depth assessment of women frequently presenting with these problems [138,139].

The rates of many STIs are highest among adolescents for both behavioral and biologic reasons. Less is known about the STI risks of older adults because those older than age 60 years are often excluded from sexual behavior surveys despite the fact that 17% of the female and 14% of the male population of the United States is in this age group, according to the U.S. Bureau of the Census (www.census.gov/population/socdemo/age/pp1–147tab01.txt). A 1992 national survey of sexual behavior with a sample limited to 18 to 59 year olds found that 66% of men and 49% of women ages 50–59 report having sex at least a few times a month, suggesting that it is important to examine sexual behavior in those age 60 years and older [140]. Additionally, a study examining the reasons that people older than age 50 presented to genitourinary medicine clinics found striking differences in sexual risk between women and men. Men were likely to present for a sexual health screen, often with minimal or no symptoms, following an extramarital or casual liaison, whereas women more commonly had symptoms causing diffi-culties with sexual intercourse with their regular partner [141].

B. Primary Prevention

For those who have sex outside a mutually monogamous relationship, correct, consistent use of male latex, polyurethane, or other synthetic condoms is a crucial component of STI prevention [1], yet researchers are just beginning to explore how the attitudes and characteristics of U.S. men influence their willingness to protect themselves and their partners from STIs and unwanted pregnancies [142]. Used consistently and correctly, male latex condoms have been shown to prevent transmission of HIV and other STIs transmitted by fluids from urogenital mucosal surfaces including *N. gonorrhoeae*, *C. trachomatis*, and *T. vaginalis*. Because condoms do not cover all areas of exposed skin, they are not likely to be as effective in preventing STIs transmitted by skin-to-skin contact (HSV, HPV, syphilis, and chancroid) [1]. Other primary pre-vention strategies for STIs include abstinence, mutual monogamy, full compliance with STI treatment protocols, and reduction in number of sex partners. Screening those at high risk for bacterial (curable) STIs and treatment of those infected and their sex partners has always played an important role in the public health response to control of STIs.

Recent evidence indicates that vaginal spermicides containing nonoxynol-9 (N-9) are not effective in reducing the incidence of HIV infection, cervical *N. gonorrhoeae*, or *C. trachomatis*, and N-9 has been associated with the development of genital ulcers or lesions, which may actually facilitate HIV transmission [143]. Although the need for safe and effective vaginal micro-bicides is great, N-9–containing products are no longer likely contenders. Two randomized-controlled trials, however, have demonstrated success in reducing episodes of unprotected vaginal intercourse and STI transmission through targeted behavioral interventions [144,145].

C. Sexually Transmitted Infection Control

Because most STI care in the United States takes place in the private sector rather than in publicly funded STI clinics operated by state and local health departments [146,147], medical care providers have a broader role in the control of STIs than just the diagnosis and treatment of symptomatic disease. A recent multisite survey of providers found that sexual histories were obtained from every patient regardless of reason for visit in only 57% of sites [148]. Thus, development and implementation of provider interventions that foster standardized sexual history elicitation in primary care settings are important first steps in controlling STIs. A national survey of more than 4000 physicians in five medical specialties (obstetrics/gynecology, internal medicine, general or family practice, emergency medicine, or pediatrics) found that fewer than 20% screened all male patients and less than one-third screened all female patients (pregnant and non-pregnant) for four STIs (syphilis, *N. gonorrhoeae*, *C. trachomatis*, and HIV). Ob-gyns were the exception, with 80% or more screening all pregnant women [47]. However, even this level of screening is below standard practice guidelines that all pregnant women should be screened [1]. On the positive side, nearly

80% of physicians advised patients not to have sex during treat-ment, to use a condom, and to tell partners to seek care for diag-nosis and treatment. In general, less than one-half the physicians reported patients with STIs to the state or local health department as required in all states for syphilis, *N. gonorrhoeae*, and *C. trachomatis* and in most for HIV. The national STI surveillance system relies on case reports to health departments from physi-cians and laboratories. Complete and accurate surveillance data are essential in monitoring the incidence of STIs and are used to target limited resources in the most cost effective manner.

VII. Suggestions for Further Investigations

- Should there be universal STI screening for men? Universal screening programs for STIs have been recommended for women only. Few data are available on the benefits of screening men for STIs as well. Research is needed on the societal impact of universal screening in an effort to dramatically reduce or eliminate curable bacterial STIs.
- Will there be an HPV vaccine for men? There are promising results from studies of a vaccine for HPV type 16 [149]. This study was done only in young women because they have the highest incidence of new infections with high-risk types of HPV. However, future research should include the efficacy of vaccination in men because they are generally the source of infection for women.
- What is the role of hormonal contraception in STIs? Despite the use of hormonal contraceptives for several decades, their effect on STI acquisition is still uncertain. Fortunately, large cohort studies are under way that should address this issue.
- What is the sexual behavior and what are STI risks in those older than age 60 years? There is a paucity of data available in this area, including the effect of hormone replacement on women's susceptibility to STIs. As the median age of the population continues to rise, this issue will become more significant.
- What is the role of STI in male infertility? Given the high frequency of epididymitis, STIs may be an important cause of male infertility that has not been studied adequately to date.
- What is the role of biologic sex in animal models of STI? Given the interesting gender differences seen in animal models of HSV, continued research in this area is warranted.

References

1. Anonymous. (2002). Sexually transmitted diseases treatment guidelines 2002. Centers for Disease Control and Prevention. *MMWR Recomm Rep.* 51(No. RR-6).
2. Auvert B, Buve A, Lagarde E, *et al.* (2001). Male circumcision and HIV infection in four cities in sub-Saharan Africa. *AIDS.* Suppl 4:S31–40.
3. Cameron DW, Simonsen JN, D'Costa LJ, *et al.* (1989). Female to male trans-mission of human immunodeficiency virus type 1: risk factors for seroconversion in men. *Lancet.* 2:403–407.
4. Lavreys L, Rakwar JP, Thompson ML, *et al.* (1999) Effect of circumcision on incidence of human immunodeficiency virus type 1 and other sexually transmitted diseases: a prospective cohort study of trucking company employees in Kenya. *J Infect Dis.* 180:330–336.
5. Seed J, Allen S, Mertens T, *et al.* (1995). Male circumcision, sexually trans-mitted disease, and risk of HIV. *J Acquir Immune Defic Syndr Hum Retrovirol.* 8:83–90.
6. Simonsen JN, Cameron DW, Gakinya MN, *et al.* (1988). Human immunodefi-ciency virus infection among men with sexually transmitted diseases. Experience from a center in Africa. *N Engl J Med.* 319:274–278.

7. Telzak EE, Chiasson MA, Bevier PJ, *et al.* (1993). HIV-1 seroconversion in patients with and without genital ulcer disease. A prospective study. *Ann Intern Med.* 119:1181–1186.

8. Jessamine PG, Plummer FA, Ndinya-Achola JO, *et al.* (1990). Human immunodeficiency virus, genital ulcers and the male foreskin: synergism in HIV-1 transmission. *Scand J Infect Dis.* Suppl. 69:181–186.

9. Castellsague X, Bosch FX, Munoz N, *et al.* (2002). Male circumcision, penile human papillomavirus infection, and cervical cancer in female partners. *N Engl J Med.* 346:1105–1112.

10. Svare EI, Kjaer SK, Worm AM, *et al.* (2002). Risk factors for genital HPV DNA in men resemble those found in women: a study of male attendees at a Danish STD clinic. *Sex Transm Infect.* 78:215–218.

11. Maden C, Sherman KJ, Beckmann AM, *et al.* (1993). History of circumcision, medical conditions, and sexual activity and risk of penile cancer. *J Natl Cancer Inst.* 85:19–24.

12. Agarwal SS, Sehgal A, Sardana S, *et al.* (1993). Role of male behavior in cervical carcinogenesis among women with one lifetime sexual partner. *Cancer.* 72:1666–1669.

13. Cook LS, Koutsky LA, Holmes KK. (1994). Circumcision and sexually transmitted diseases. *Am J Public Health.* 84:197–201.

14. Parker SW, Stewart AJ, Wren MN, *et al.* (1983). Circumcision and sexually transmissible disease. *Med J Aust.* 2:288–290.

15. Taylor PK, Rodin P. (1975). Herpes genitalis and circumcision. *Br J Vener Dis.* 51:274–277.

16. Bassett I, Donovan B, Bodsworth NJ, *et al.* (1994). Herpes simplex virus type 2 infection of heterosexual men attending a sexual health centre. *Med J Aust.* 160:697–700.

17. Diseker RA 3rd, Peterman TA, Kamb ML, *et al.* (2000). Circumcision and STD in the United States: cross sectional and cohort analyses. *Sex Transm Infect.* 76:474–479.

18. Moses S, Bailey RC, Ronald AR. (1998). Male circumcision: assessment of health benefits and risks. *Sex Transm Infect.* 74:368–373.

19. Todd J, Munguti K, Grosskurth H, *et al.* (2001). Risk factors for active syphilis and TPHA seroconversion in a rural African population. *Sex Transm Infect.* 77:37–45.

20. Tyndall MW, Agoki E, Plummer FA, *et al.* (1994). Single dose azithromycin for the treatment of chancroid: a randomized comparison with erythromycin. *Sex Transm Dis.* 21:231–234.

21. Hussain LA, Lehner T. (1995). Comparative investigation of Langerhans' cells and potential receptors for HIV in oral, genitourinary and rectal epithelia. *Immunology.* 85:475–484.

22. Aral SO, Holmes KK. (1999). Social and behavioral determinants of the epidemiology of STDs: Industrialized and developing countries. In: Holmes KK, Sparling PE, Mardh PA, eds. *Sexually Transmitted Diseases.* New York: McGraw Hill Health Professions Division. 39–76.

23. Hook EW, Handsfield HH. (1999). Gonococcal infections in the adult. In: Holmes KK, Sparling PE, Mardh PA, eds. *Sexually Transmitted Diseases.* New York: McGraw Hill Health Professions Division. 451–466.

24. Aral SU, Holmes KK. (1999). Social and behavioral determinants of the epidemiology of STDs: Industrialized and developing countries. In: Holmes KK, Sparling PE, Mardh PA, eds. *Sexually Transmitted Diseases.* New York: McGraw Hill Health Professions Division. 39–76.

25. Hammerschlag MR, Alpert S, Rosner I, *et al.* (1978). Microbiology of the vagina in children: normal and potentially pathogenic organisms. *Pediatrics.* 62:57–62.

26. Krieger JN, Alderete JF. (1999). *Trichomonas Vaginalis* and Trichomoniasis. In: Holmes KK, Sparling PE, Mardh PA, eds. *Sexually Transmitted Diseases.* New York: McGraw Hill Health Professions Division. 587–604.

27. Laufer MR. (1998). The Physiology of Puberty. In: Emans SJ, Laufer MC, Goldstein D, eds. *Pediatric and Adolescent Gynecology.* Philadelphia: Lippincott Williams and Wilkins. 109–140.

28. Eschenbach DA. (1983). Vaginal infection. *Clin Obstet Gynecol.* 26:186–202.

29. Klebanoff SJ, Hillier SL, Eschenbach DA, *et al.* (1991). Control of the microbial flora of the vagina by H2O2-generating lactobacilli. *J Infect Dis.* 164:94–100.

30. Hillier SL, Krohn MA, Klebanoff SJ, *et al.* (1992). The relationship of hydrogen peroxide-producing lactobacilli to bacterial vaginosis and genital microflora in pregnant women. *Obstet Gynecol.* 79:369–373.

31. Saigh JH, Sanders CC, Sanders WE Jr. (1978). Inhibition of Neisseria gonorrhea by aerobic and facultatively anaerobic components of the endocervical flora: evidence for a protective effect against infection. *Infect Immun.* 19:704–710.

32. Martius J, Krohn MA, Hillier SL, *et al.* (1988). Relationships of vaginal Lactobacillus species, cervical Chlamydia trachomatis, and bacterial vaginosis to preterm birth. *Obstet Gynecol.* 71:89–95.

33. Hawes SE, Hillier SL, Benedetti J, *et al.* (1996). Hydrogen peroxide-producing lactobacilli and acquisition of vaginal infections. *J Infect Dis.* 174:1058–1063.

34. Harrison HR, Costin M, Meder JB, *et al.* (1985). Cervical Chlamydia trachomatis infection in university women: relationship to history, contraception, ectopy, and cervicitis. *Am J Obstet Gynecol.* 153:244–251.

35. Critchlow CW, Wolner-Hanssen P, Eschenbach DA, *et al.* (1995). Determinants of cervical ectopia and of cervicitis: age, oral contraception, specific cervical infection, smoking, and douching. *Am J Obstet Gynecol.* 173:534–543.

36. Cohen MS, Anderson DJ. (1999). Genitourinary mucosal defenses. In: Holmes KK, Sparling PE, Mardh PA, eds. *Sexually Transmitted Diseases.* New York: McGraw Hill Health Professions Division. 173–190.

37. Stenchever MA, Droegemueller W, Herbst AL, *et al.*, eds. (2001). Reproductive endocrinology. In: *Comprehensive Gynecology.* St. Louis: Mosby. 71–124.

38. Eschenbach DA, Thwin SS, Patton DL, *et al.* (2000a) Influence of the normal menstrual cycle on vaginal tissue, discharge, and microflora. *Clin Infect Dis.* 30:901–907.

39. Patton DL, Thwin SS, Meier A, *et al.* (2000). Epithelial cell layer thickness and immune cell populations in the normal human vagina at different stages of the menstrual cycle. *Am J Obstet Gynecol.* 183:967–973.

40. Schwebke JR, Weiss H. (2001). Influence of the normal menstrual cycle on vaginal microflora. *Clin Infect Dis.* 32:325.

41. Sweet RL, Blankfort-Doyle M, Robbie MO, *et al.* (1986). The occurrence of chlamydial and gonococcal salpingitis during the menstrual cycle. *JAMA.* 255:2062–2064.

42. Korn AP, Hessol NA, Padian NS, *et al.* (1998). Risk factors for plasma cell endometritis among women with cervical Neisseria gonorrhoeae, cervical Chlamydia trachomatis, or bacterial vaginosis. *Am J Obstet Gynecol.* 178:987–990.

43. Wiesenfeld HC, Hillier SL, Krohn MA, *et al.* (2002). Lower genital tract infection and endometritis: insight into subclinical pelvic inflammatory disease. *Obstet Gynecol.* 100:456–463.

44. Hillier SL, Kiviat NB, Hawes SE, *et al.* (1996). Role of bacterial vaginosis-associated microorganisms in endometritis. *Am J Obstet Gynecol.* 175:435–441.

45. Rank RG, White HJ, Hough AJ Jr, *et al.* (1982). Effect of estradiol on chlamydial genital infection of female guinea pigs. *Infect Immun.* 38:699–705.

46. Styrt B, Sugarman B. (1991). Estrogens and infection. *Rev Infect Dis.* 13:1139–1150.

47. Sonnex C. (1998). Influence of ovarian hormones on urogenital infection. *Sex Transm Infect.* 74:11–19.

48. Wolner-Hanssen P, Eschenbach DA, Paavonen J, *et al.* (1990a). Association between vaginal douching and acute pelvic inflammatory disease. *JAMA.* 263:1936–1941.

49. Eschenbach DA, Patton DL, Meier A, *et al.* (2000b). Effects of oral contraceptive pill use on vaginal flora and vaginal epithelium. *Contraception.* 62:107–112.

50. Baeten JM, Nyange PM, Richardson BA, *et al.* (2001). Hormonal contraception and risk of sexually transmitted disease acquisition: results from a prospective study. *Am J Obstet Gynecol.* 185:380–385.

51. Wolner-Hanssen P, Eschenbach DA, Paavonen J, *et al.* (1990b). Decreased risk of symptomatic chlamydial pelvic inflammatory disease associated with oral contraceptive use. *JAMA.* 263:54–59.

52. Miller L, Patton DL, Meier A, *et al.* (2000). Depomedroxyprogesterone-induced hypoestrogenism and changes in vaginal flora and epithelium. *Obstet Gynecol.* 96:431–439.

53. Ness RB, Soper DE, Holley RL, *et al.* (2001). Hormonal and barrier contraception and risk of upper genital tract disease in the PID Evaluation and Clinical Health (PEACH) study. *Am J Obstet Gynecol.* 185:121–127.

54. McClelland RS, Wang CC, Richardson BA, *et al.* (2002). A prospective study of hormonal contraceptive use and cervical shedding of herpes simplex virus in human immunodeficiency virus type 1-seropositive women. *J Infect Dis.* 185:1822–1825.

55. Koutsky LA, Kiviat NB. (1999). Genital human papillomavirus. In: Holmes KK, Sparling PE, Mardh PA, eds. *Sexually Transmitted Diseases.* New York: McGraw Hill Health Professions Division. 347–359.

56. Moreno V, Bosch FX, Munoz N, *et al.* (2002). Effect of oral contraceptives on risk of cervical cancer in women with human papillomavirus infection: the IARC multicentric case-control study. *Lancet.* 359:1085–1092.

57. Berrington A, Jha P, Peto J, *et al.* (2002). Oral contraceptives and cervical cancer. *Lancet.* 360:410.

58. Lacey JV Jr, Brinton LA, Abbas FM, *et al.* (1999). Oral contraceptives as risk factors for cervical adenocarcinomas and squamous cell carcinomas. *Cancer Epidemiol Biomarkers Prev.* 8:1079–1085.

59. Lacey JV Jr, Brinton LA, Barnes WA, *et al.* (2000). Use of hormone replacement therapy and adenocarcinomas and squamous cell carcinomas of the uterine cervix. *Gynecol Oncol.* 77:149–154.

60. Singer A. (1975). The uterine cervix from adolescence to the menopause. *Br J Obstet Gynaecol.* 82:81–99.

61. Watts DH, Brunham RC. (1999). Sexually transmitted diseases, including HIV infection in pregnancy. In: Holmes KK, Sparling PE, Mardh PA, eds. *Sexually Transmitted Diseases.* New York: McGraw Hill Health Professions Division. 1089–1132.

62. Bolan G, Ehrhardt AA, Wasserheit JN. (1999). Gender perspectives and STDs. In: Holmes KK, Sparling PE, Mardh PA, eds. *Sexually Transmitted Diseases.* New York: McGraw Hill Health Professions Division. 117–127.

63. Brunham RC, Martin DH, Hubbard TW, *et al.* (1983). Depression of the lymphocyte transformation response to microbial antigens and to phytohemagglutinin during pregnancy. *J Clin Invest.* 72:1629–1638.

64. Fife KH, Katz BP, Brizendine EJ, *et al.* (1999). Cervical human papillomavirus deoxyribonucleic acid persists throughout pregnancy and decreases in the postpartum period. *Am J Obstet Gynecol.* 180:1110–1114.

65. Cunningham FG, Gant NF, Leveno KJ, *et al.*, eds. (2001a). Sexually transmitted diseases. In: *Williams Obstetrics.* New York: McGraw Hill Medical Publishing Division. 1485–1513.

66. Cunningham FG, Gant NF, Leveno KJ, *et al.*, eds. (2001b). Neoplastic diseases. In: *Williams Obstetrics.* New York: McGraw Hill Medical Publishing Division. 1439–1459.

67. Hein M, Helmig RB, Schonheyder HC, *et al.* (2001). An *in vitro* study of antibacterial properties of the cervical mucus plug in pregnancy. *Am J Obstet Gynecol.* 185:586–592.

68. Hein M, Valore EV, Helmig RB, *et al.* (2002). Antimicrobial factors in the cervical mucus plug. *Am J Obstet Gynecol.* 187:137–144.

69. Nagashima T. (1987). A high prevalence of chlamydial cervicitis in postmenopausal women. *Am J Obstet Gynecol.* 156:31–32.

70. Golmeier D, Ridgway GL, Oriel JD. (1981). Chlamydial vulvovaginitis in a postmenopausal woman. *Lancet.* 2:476–477.

71. Peterman TA, Stoneburner RL, Allen JR, *et al.* (1988). Risk of human immunodeficiency virus transmission from heterosexual adults with transfusion-associated infections. *JAMA.* 259:55–58.

72. Anonymous. (2002). Centers for Disease Control and Prevention. Sexually Transmitted Disease Surveillance, 2001. Atlanta, GA: U.S. Department of Health and Human Services. September 2002.

73. Sparling PF, Handsfield HH. (2000). *Neisseria gonorrhoeae.* In: Mandell GL, Bennett JE, Dolin R, eds. *Principles and Practice of Infectious Diseases.* Philadelphia: Churchill Livingstone. 2242–2258

74. Turner CF, Rogers SM, Miller HG, *et al.* (2002). Untreated gonococcal and chlamydial infection in a probability sample of adults. *JAMA.* 287:726–733.

75. Rice RJ, Roberts PL, Handsfield HH, *et al.* (1991). Sociodemographic distribution of gonorrhea incidence: implications for prevention and behavioral research. *Am J Public Health.* 81:1252–1258.

76. Potterat JJ, Dukes RL, Rothenberg RB. (1987). Disease transmission by heterosexual men with gonorrhea: an empiric estimate. *Sex Transm Dis.* 14:107–110.

77. Bloomfield PJ, Kent C, Campbell D, *et al.* (2002). Community-based chlamydia and gonorrhea screening through the United States mail, San Francisco. *Sex Transm Dis.* 29:294–297.

78. Jones CA, Knaup RC, Hayes M, *et al.* (2000). Urine screening for gonococcal and chlamydial infections at community-based organizations in a high-morbidity area. *Sex Transm Dis.* 27:146–151.

79. Debattista J, Clementson C, Mason D, *et al.* (2002). Screening for Neisseria gonorrhoeae and Chlamydia trachomatis at entertainment venues among men who have sex with men. *Sex Transm Dis.* 29:216–221.

80. Pack RP, Diclemente RJ, Hook EW 3rd, *et al.* (2000). High prevalence of asymptomatic STDs in incarcerated minority male youth: a case for screening. *Sex Transm Dis.* 27:175–177.

81. Mertz KJ, Schwebke JR, Gaydos CA, *et al.* (2002). Screening women in jails for chlamydial and gonococcal infection using urine tests: feasibility, acceptability, prevalence, and treatment rates. *Sex Transm Dis.* 29:271–276.

82. Holmes KK, Counts GW, Beaty HN. (1971). Disseminated gonococcal infection. *Ann Intern Med.* 74:979–993.

83. Jones RP, Batteiger BE. (2000). *Chlamydia trachomatis* (Trachoma, Perinatal Infections, Lymphogranuloma Venereum, and Other Genital Infections). In: Mandell GL, Bennett JE, Dolin R, eds. *Principles and Practice of Infectious Diseases.* Philadelphia: Churchill Livingstone. 1989–2004.

84. Latka M, Ahern J, Garfein RS, *et al.* (2001). Prevalence, incidence, and correlates of chlamydia and gonorrhea among young adult injection drug users. *J Subst Abuse.* 13:73–88.

85. Haley N, Roy E, Leclerc P, *et al.* (2002). Risk behaviours and prevalence of Chlamydia trachomatis and Neisseria gonorrhoeae genital infections among Montreal street youth. *Int J STD AIDS.* 13:238–245.

86. Mertz KJ, Ransom RL, St. Louis ME, *et al.* (2001). Prevalence of genital chlamydial infection in young women entering a national job training program, 1990–1997. (2001). *Am J Public Health.* 91:1287–1290.

87. Cecil JA, Howell MR, Tawes JJ, *et al.* (2001). Features of *Chlamydia trachomatis* and *Neisseria gonorrhoeae* infection in male Army recruits. *J Infect Dis.* 184:1216–1219.

88. Eckert LO, Suchland RJ, Hawes SE, *et al.* (2000). Quantitative *Chlamydia trachomatis* cultures: correlation of chlamydial inclusion-forming units with serovar, age, sex, and race. *J Infect Dis.* 182:540–544.

89. Quinn TC, Gaydos C, Shepherd M, *et al.* (1996). Epidemiologic and microbiologic correlates of Chlamydia trachomatis infection in sexual partnerships. *JAMA.* 276:1737–1742.

90. Ku L, St. Louis M, Farshy C, *et al.* (2002). Risk behaviors, medical care, and chlamydial infection among young men in the United States. *Am J Public Health.* 92:1140–1143.

91. Bas S, Scieux C, Vischer TL. (2001). Male sex predominance in *Chlamydia trachomatis* sexually acquired reactive arthritis: are women more protected by anti-chlamydia antibodies? *Ann Rheum Dis.* 60:605–611.

92. Tramont EC. (2000). *Treponema pallidum* (Syphilis). In: Mandell GL, Bennett JE, Dolin R, eds. *Principles and Practice of Infectious Diseases.* Philadelphia: Churchill Livingstone. 2474–2490.

93. Rompalo AM, Joesoef MR, O'Donnell JA, *et al.* (2001). Clinical manifestations of early syphilis by HIV status and gender: results of the syphilis and HIV study. *Sex Transm Dis.* 28:158–165.

94. Nakashima AK, Rolfs RT, Flock ML, *et al.* (1996). Epidemiology of syphilis in the United States, 1941–1993. *Sex Transm Dis.* 23:16–23.

95. Anonymous. (2002). Primary and secondary syphilis—United States, 2000–2001. *MMWR Morb Mortal Wkly Rep.* 51:971–973.

96. Hahn RA, Magder LS, Aral SO, *et al.* (1989). Race and the prevalence of syphilis seroreactivity in the United States population: a national seroepidemiologic study. *Am J Public Health.* 79:467–70.

97. Thomas JC, Kulik AL, Schoenbach VJ. (1995). Syphilis in the South: rural rates surpass urban rates in North Carolina. *Am J Public Health.* 85:1119–1122.

98. Muga R, Roca J, Tor J, *et al.* (1997). Syphilis in injecting drug users: clues for high-risk sexual behaviour in female IDUs. *Int J STD AIDS.* 8:225–228.

99. Clark EG, Danbolt N. (1964). The Oslo study of the natural course of untreated syphilis. *Med Clin North Am.* 48:613–621.

100. Rosahn PD. (1947). Autopsy study in syphilis. *J Vener Dis.* 649(suppl 21).

101. Alexander JM, Sheffield JS, Sanchez PJ, *et al.* (1999). Efficacy of treatment for syphilis in pregnancy. *Obstet Gynecol.* 93:5–8.

102. Hand WL. (2000). *Haemophilus* Species (including Chancroid). In: Mandell GL, Bennett JE, Dolin R, eds. *Principles and Practice of Infectious Diseases.* Philadelphia: Churchill Livingstone. 2378–2382.

103. Bong CT, Harezlak J, Katz BP, *et al.* (2002). Men are more susceptible than women to pustule formation in the experimental model of *Haemophilus ducreyi* infection. *Sex Transm Dis.* 29:114–118.

104. Bonnez W, Reichman RC. (2000). Papillomaviruses. In: Mandell GL, Bennett JE, Dolin R, eds. *Principles and Practice of Infectious Diseases.* Philadelphia: Churchill Livingstone. 1630–1644.

105. Koutsky L. (1997). Epidemiology of genital human papillomavirus infection. *Am J Med.* 102:3–8.

106. Stone KM, Karem KL, Sternberg MR, *et al.* (2002). Seroprevalence of human papillomavirus type 16 infection in the United States. *J Infect Dis.* 186:1396–1402.

107. Anonymous. (1996). National Institutes of Health: Cervical Cancer. *NIH Consensus Statement.* 14:1–38.

108. Parkin DM, Bray FI, Devesa SS. (2001). Cancer burden in the year 2000. The global picture. *Eur J Cancer.* 37(Suppl 8):S4–66.

109. Jones BA, Davey DD. (2000). Quality management in gynecologic cytology using interlaboratory comparison. *Arch Pathol Lab Med.* 124:672–681.

110. Wright TC Jr, Cox JT, Massad LS, *et al.* (2002). 2001 Consensus Guidelines for the management of women with cervical cytological abnormalities. *JAMA.* 287:2120–2129.

111. Conley LJ, Ellerbrock TV, Bush TJ, et al. (2002). HIV-1 infection and risk of vulvovaginal and perianal condylomata acuminata and intraepithelial neoplasia: a prospective cohort study. Lancet. 359:108–113.

112. Daling JR, Weiss NS, Hislop TG, et al. (1987). Sexual practices, sexually transmitted diseases, and the incidence of anal cancer. N Engl J Med. 317:973–977.

113. Palefsky JM. (2000). Anal squamous intraepithelial lesions in human immunodeficiency virus-positive men and women. Semin Oncol. 27.471–479.

114. Fleming DT, McQuillan GM, Johnson RE, et al. (1997). Herpes simplex virus type 2 in the United States, 1976 to 1994. N Engl J Med. 337:1105–1111.

115. Siegel D, Golden E, Washington AE, et al. (1992). Prevalence and correlates of herpes simplex infections. The population-based AIDS in Multiethnic Neighborhoods Study. JAMA. 268:1702–1708.

116. Han X, Lundberg P, Tanamachi B, et al. (2001). Gender influences herpes simplex virus type 1 infection in normal and gamma interferon mutant mice. J Virol. 75:3048–3052.

117. Blondeau JM, Embil JA, McFarlane ES. (1989). Herpes simplex virus infections in male and female mice following pinna inoculation: responses to primary infection and artificially induced recurrent disease. J Med Virol. 29:320–326.

118. Stock C, Guillen-Grima F, de Mendoza JH, et al. (2001). Risk factors of herpes simplex type 1 (HSV-1) infection and lifestyle factors associated with HSV-1 manifestations. Eur J Epidemiol. 17:885–890.

119. Varela JA, Garcia-Corbeira P, Aguanell MV, et al. (2001). Herpes simplex virus type 2 seroepidemiology in Spain: prevalence and seroconversion rate among sexually transmitted disease clinic attendees. Sex Transm Dis. 28:47–50.

120. Wald A, Koutsky L, Ashley RL, et al. (1997). Genital herpes in a primary care clinic. Demographic and sexual correlates of herpes simplex type 2 infections. Sex Transm Dis. 24:149–155.

121. Benedetti J, Corey L, Ashley R. (1994). Recurrence rates in genital herpes after symptomatic first-episode infection. Ann Intern Med. 121:847–854.

122. Langenberg AG, Corey L, Ashley RL, et al. (1999). A prospective study of new infections with herpes simplex virus type 1 and type 2. Chiron HSV Vaccine Study Group. N Engl J Med. 341:1432–1438.

123. Mertz GJ, Benedetti J, Ashley R, et al. (1992). Risk factors for the sexual transmission of genital herpes. Ann Intern Med. 116:197–202.

124. Stanberry LR, Spruance SL, Cunningham AL, et al. (2002). Glycoprotein D-adjuvant vaccine to prevent genital herpes. N Engl J Med. 347:1652–1661.

125. Wald A, Zeh J, Selke S, et al. (2000). Reactivation of genital herpes simplex virus type 2 infection in asymptomatic seropositive persons. N Engl J Med. 342:844–850.

126. Sacks SL, Tyrrell LD, Lawee D, et al. (1991). Randomized, double-blind, placebo-controlled, clinic-initiated, Canadian multicenter trial of topical edoxudine 3.0% cream in the treatment of recurrent genital herpes. Canadian Cooperative Study Group. J Infect Dis. 164:665–672.

127. Brown ZA, Wald A, Morrow RA, et al. (2003). Effect of serologic status and cesarean delivery on transmission rates of herpes simplex virus from mother to infant. JAMA. 289:203–209.

128. Brocklehurst P, Kinghorn G, Carney O, et al. (1998). A randomised placebo controlled trial of suppressive acyclovir in late pregnancy in women with recurrent genital herpes infection. Br J Obstet Gynaecol. 105:275–280.

129. Scott LL, Hollier LM, McIntire D, et al. (2002). Acyclovir suppression to prevent recurrent genital herpes at delivery. Infect Dis Obstet Gynecol. 10:71–77.

130. Krieger JN, Alderete JF. (1999). Trichomonas vaginalis and trichomoniasis. In: Holmes KK, Sparling PE, Mardh PA, eds. Sexually Transmitted Diseases. New York: McGraw Hill Health Professions Division. 587–604.

131. Klebanoff MA, Carey JC, Hauth JC, et al. (2001). Failure of metronidazole to prevent preterm delivery among pregnant women with asymptomatic Trichomonas vaginalis infection. N Engl J Med. 345:487–493.

132. Weström L, Eschenbach D, (1999). Pelvic Inflammatory Disease. In Holmes KK, Sparling PE, Mardh PA, eds. Sexually Transmitted Diseases. New York: McGraw Hill Health Professions Division. 783–809.

133. Taylor-Robinson D, Horner PJ. (2001). The role of Mycoplasma genitalium in non-gonococcal urethritis. Sex Transm Infect. 77:229–231.

134. Berger RE. (1999). Acute epididymitis. In: Holmes KK, Sparling PE, Mardh PA, eds. Sexually Transmitted Diseases. New York: McGraw Hill Health Professions Division. 847–858.

135. Aral SO. (1994). Sexual behavior in sexually transmitted disease research. An overview. Sex Transm Dis. 21:S59–64.

136. Lewis LM, Melton RS, Succop PA, et al. (2000). Factors influencing condom use and STD acquisition among African American college women. J Am Coll Health. 49:19–23.

137. Plichta SB, Abraham C. (1996). Violence and gynecologic health in women <50 years old. Am J Obstet Gynecol. 174:903–907.

138. Campbell J, Jones AS, Dienemann J, et al. (2002). Intimate partner violence and physical health consequences. Arch Intern Med. 162:1157–1163.

139. Family Violence Prevention Fund (1999). Preventing domestic violence: Clinical guidelines on routine screening. San Francisco: Family Violence Prevention Fund.

140. Michael RT, Gagnon JH, Laumann EO, et al. (1994). Sex in America: A Definitive Survey. Boston: Little, Brown and Company. 116.

141. Tobin JM, Harindra V. (2001). Attendance by older patients at a genitourinary medicine clinic. Sex Transm Infect. 77:289–291.

142. Forste R, Morgan J. (1998). How relationships of U.S. men affect contraceptive use and efforts to prevent sexually transmitted diseases. Fam Plann Perspect. 30:56–62.

143. Richardson BA. (2002). Nonoxynol-9 as a vaginal microbicide for prevention of sexually transmitted infections: it's time to move on. JAMA. 287:1171–1172.

144. Shain RN, Piper JM, Newton ER, et al. (1999). A randomized, controlled trial of a behavioral intervention to prevent sexually transmitted disease among minority women. N Engl J Med. 340:93–100.

145. Kamb ML, Fishbein M, Douglas JM Jr, et al. (1998). Efficacy of risk-reduction counseling to prevent human immunodeficiency virus and sexually transmitted diseases: a randomized controlled trial. Project RESPECT Study Group. JAMA. 280:1161–1167.

146. Brackbill RM, Sternberg MR, Fishbein M. (1999). Where do people go for treatment of sexually transmitted diseases? Fam Plann Perspect. 31:10–15.

147. St. Lawrence JS, Montano DE, Kasprzyk D, et al. (2002). STD screening, testing, case reporting, and clinical and partner notification practices: a national survey of US physicians. Am J Public Health. 92:1784–1788.

148. Bull SS, Rietmeijer C, Fortenberry JD, et al. (1999). Practice patterns for elicitation of sexual history, education, and counseling among providers of STD services: results from the gonorrhea community action project (GCAP). Sex Transm Dis. 26:584–589.

149. Koutsky LA, Ault KA, Wheeler CM, et al. (2002). A controlled trial of a human papillomavirus type 16 vaccine. N Engl J Med. 347:1645–1651.

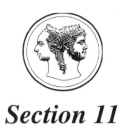

Section 11

BONE

John Bilezikian, MD

Professor of Medicine and of Pharmacology and Chief, Division of Endocrinology,
College of Physicians and Surgeons, Columbia University, New York, NY

As is the case so many times in the study of disease and disease processes, the sex that suffers the most gets the most attention. In metabolic bone diseases, it is the female sex that has been the focus of investigative and clinical efforts. Without doubt, osteoporosis, the most important of the metabolic bone diseases, afflicts women to a much greater extent than men. In fact, until about 10 or 20 years ago, convention could have said, without too much qualification, that men do not "get" osteoporosis. Not surprisingly, therefore, research funds have been directed toward women in the quest for greater understanding of this disease. In addition, pharmaceutical companies have invested most of their efforts to develop drugs for osteoporosis that will have primary indications for women. If one casually peruses the literature, for example, less than 5% of original research on osteoporosis is devoted to men. More than 30,000 women have been enrolled in clinical trials, a figure that far outdistances the 1000 men or so who have been part of osteoporosis trials.

The point is, however, that osteoporosis occurs in men and women. It does not occur with the same frequency as it does in women but certainly more often than commonly believed. In the United States, the female-to-male ratio is about 4:1. So men "get it," as do women and the male figures do add up. The estimates of 12 to 15 million Americans with osteoporosis includes 2 to 3 million men. These relative frequencies make a key basic point. We need to understand more about how the disease presents among women versus men and to gain insights into the basic differences that account for these different numbers.

Men achieve greater bone mass than women, so it is said. However, if one examines that statement carefully, it is total bone mass not bone density that gives men this edge. During growth and development, true bone density, as expressed in grams/cm³ (a volumetric quantity) is not very much different between the sexes and does not change appreciably in the long bones during puberty. It is areal density, as expressed in grams/cm², that changes in puberty with males achieving substantially more areal density than females. This is an important difference among males and females because areal density defines a biomechanical property. When areal density is greater, even though volumetric density is the same, the bone will have greater strength. Thus, the male bone is a stronger bone at peak bone mass.

It has been assumed that this difference in areal density is an androgen effect. Androgens stimulate periosteal bone growth to a greater extent than do estrogens. With aging, in fact, periosteal bone growth compensates for cortical thinning better in the male than in the female, again a function of androgens. Thus, the thinning bones of males are actually stronger than the thinning bones of females. Of course, the menopause marks another fundamental difference between women and men. With the exception of a disease, men do not experience a period of acute and then chronic androgen deficiency, although androgen levels do fall with age in men. Women undergo the menopause, an event that sets into motion a cascade of biochemical and cellular processes that lead to a period of accelerated bone loss. This period of accelerated bone loss further separates the sexes insofar as aging and skeletal strength is concerned.

However, it is too simplistic to argue that women and men have different skeletons because one is endowed with androgens and the other is endowed, until the middle years, with estrogens. Androgens are found in women; estrogens are present in men.

Insights into how important estrogens are to the acquisition and maintenance of peak bone mass in the male come from seminal studies of estrogen-deficient men who were born that way. These gene-knockout experiments of nature, both with regard to the estrogen alpha receptor gene and the aromatase gene, have provided information about the importance of estrogens to male skeletal health that we never knew before. We now know that the estrogen-deficient male does not achieve peak bone mass, does not close his epiphyses (he grows continually, achieving great height), does not experience a pubertal growth spurt, and in fact has markedly reduced bone density. Further observations have established that estrogens in the male are also important for the maintenance of bone mass. The natural loss of bone mass with aging in the male is more a function of declining estrogen levels than it is of declining androgen levels. The cellular bases for these differences, that is how the sex steroids differentially affect bone cells, is a focus of intense study.

Even the fundamental concept of defining osteoporosis by dual-energy x-ray absorptiometry (DXA) is not clear among men and women. The highly touted and generally accepted definition of osteoporosis, provided by the World Health Organization (WHO), was meant to apply specifically to Caucasian women. It is not clear, therefore, that the operational definition of osteoporosis in Caucasian women (T-score ≤ 2.5) is the right definition for men or for any other group. It is also not clear what normative database should be used. The epidemiology of osteoporotic fractures provides some evidence for using a gender-based T-score (men are compared with men at peak bone mass) and a gender-independent T-score (men are compared with women at peak bone mass). We need more information about this point to adjust our clinical antennae as we begin to see more and more men with T-scores in the osteoporotic range.

In an interesting twist, men who present with osteoporosis, especially in their middle years, are assumed to have a secondary cause for osteoporosis. This is ironic. Although men are generally ignored, when they develop osteoporosis, a concerted effort is advised to understand its cause. We conduct a vigorous search for a cause of osteoporosis in men. However, women who present with osteoporosis in their middle years are assumed to have the disease without regard to cause. In women, it is generally assumed to be due to aging and/or the menopause. This is an absurdly odd situation. A potential underlying cause of osteoporosis should be sought just as vigorously in women as in men. Regrettably, we have almost no knowledge about how secondary causes of osteoporosis may affect the sexes differently. Glucocorticoid-induced osteoporosis, the most important secondary cause of osteoporosis, has been assumed to affect women and men similarly. However, we do not know this. The list goes on: bone loss syndromes associated with thyroid hormone excess, primary hyperparathyroidism, Cushing's disease, and acromegaly are all assumed to be similar among the sexes. However, in none of these disorders do we have information to bring to bear on this subject.

Clinical trials of osteoporotic drugs have not addressed hypotheses with regard to possible differences among the sexes. Head-to-head comparisons of drugs for osteoporosis among men and women have not been a focus of anyone's attention. We do not know of dosage differences, pharmacokinetic differences, or target organ differences among the therapeutics that are used for the treatment of osteoporosis in women and men.

It is with this background that the following chapters might shed some insight into differences among the sexes in metabolic bone disorders. The chapters provide insight but also point out numerous areas in which our knowledge is sadly lacking. Hopefully, in the next decade, this imbalance will be rectified by focusing more attention on similarities and differences among the sexes with regard to basic bone biology, aging, the sex steroids, diseases of the aging skeleton, and therapeutics.

91

Corticosteroid-Induced Osteoporosis: A Comprehensive Review

ALEXANDRA PAPAIOANNOU, MD, FRCP(C)*, ANN CRANNEY, MD, FRCP(C)**,
AND JONATHAN D. ADACHI, MD, FRCP(C)†

*Associate Professor, Department of Medicine, McMaster University, Hamilton, Ontario, Canada
**Associate Professor, Department of Medicine, University of Ottawa, Ottawa, Ontario, Canada
†Professor, Department of Medicine, McMaster University, Hamilton, Ontario, Canada

I. Introduction

Since Harvey Cushing first noted the coexistence of excess cortisol and loss of skeletal mass more than 50 years ago [1], it has been accepted that supraphysiologic doses of corticosteroids cause clinically significant bone loss. Corticosteroid-induced bone loss has become a serious concern because of widespread use for the treatment of disease. High-dose oral corticosteroids are used to treat people with a variety of medical conditions including rheumatic diseases such as rheumatoid arthritis, polymyalgia rheumatica, systemic lupus erythematosus and vasculitis; inflammatory lung diseases such as asthma; gastrointestinal diseases including inflammatory bowel disease and chronic liver disease; skin diseases, in particular pemphigus; and more recently in those who have undergone transplantation. Reductions in bone mass have even been reported in men on higher doses of glucocorticoid replacement therapy for Addison's disease [2]. Clinically significant bone loss occurs in most men and women exposed to corticosteroids. Fractures at the spine and hip have been reported with corticosteroid use [3]. Between 30 and 50% of patients taking long-term corticosteroids will experience fractures [4].

Today, fractures resulting from corticosteroid-induced osteoporosis may be prevented. A number of well–designed, randomized, double-blind, placebo-controlled trials have been conducted that demonstrate preservation and in some instances actual increases in bone mass with treatment. Some have even demonstrated reductions in fracture risk in both men and women. As a result it is extremely important for clinicians to appreciate the very high risk for vertebral fracture in particular, in postmenopausal women and in older men on corticosteroids.

II. Epidemiology

Bone loss occurs rapidly within the first 6 to 12 months of beginning corticosteroid therapy; thereafter, the rate of loss slows to two to three times that of normal [5–7]. This is seen in both sexes. Initially trabecular rather than cortical bone is affected more severely by corticosteroids [3,8]. Interestingly, cortical bone loss as reflected by changes in femoral neck bone density is particularly evident during the second year of corticosteroid therapy [9,10], and in epidemiologic studies far greater losses are seen at the hip than the spine [11]. There also appears to be a close relationship between the rate of bone loss and the dose of corticosteroid [7]. Significant trabecular bone loss occurs with prednisone doses greater than 7.5 mg/day in most patients [7,12] but may also be seen in those on low-dose therapy [13]

and in those on high-dose, inhaled corticosteroids [14,15]. Some recovery of bone may be seen in the spine once doses of prednisone fall below 7.5 mg/day [7]. In one study, rates of bone loss increased with doses of prednisone between 5 and 10 mg daily and with inhaled steroids [5]. A similar study examining vertebral fracture rates compared systemic corticosteroid therapy with inhaled therapy and control subjects and showed that the greatest deleterious effects occurred with systemic followed by inhaled corticosteroids [16]. Thus, although lower doses of corticosteroids may be safer than higher doses [17] and inhaled corticosteroids are less likely to cause bone loss than oral corticosteroids, there may be no truly safe dose [5,18].

Corticosteroids alter the usual risk factors for osteoporosis. Young people taking corticosteroids lose bone as rapidly as older people. This is particularly evident when one compares the bone mineral density (BMD) results in the placebo groups between premenopausal and postmenopausal women in many of the clinical trials [19,20]. Postmenopausal women taking corticosteroids, however, have a greater fracture risk, presumably because they are susceptible to age- and menopause-related bone loss and have other risk factors, placing them at higher risk for fracturing. Bone loss may occur even in those that are on stable doses of estrogen [10]. Men are equally susceptible to bone loss caused by corticosteroids [12,16,19–21], and in one study the rate of loss was greater in men than in women [5]. In rheumatoid arthritis, it is likely that the inflammatory disease activity and immobilization contribute to bone loss [17], and high doses of corticosteroids may well exacerbate this bone loss [22]. Controversy exists about the effects of repeated use of intermittent high-dose corticosteroids, intra-articular corticosteroids, and inhaled corticosteroids on bone metabolism. Most of the concern is raised from deleterious effects noted from bone marker data. However, more recent bone density and epidemiologic data have raised concerns for both men and women. Intermittent high-dose or pulse therapy does alter bone markers. A recent study suggests that intermittent oral pulse therapy in men leads to similar vertebral fracture risk as is seen with inhaled corticosteroids [16]. Both groups show greater risk than control subjects but were not as likely to fracture as those on continuous therapy [16]. In part this may reflect the short nature of the studies and a reduced total cumulative dose. With intra-articular injections, osteocalcin levels decline and then fully recover over the course of 15 to 30 days. Bone density data is sparse; however, it does suggest that even with chronic, continuous inhaled use of corticosteroids, bone loss occurs and is particularly evident in postmenopausal women at the hip and spine [23]. Losses were intermediate between those on oral corticosteroids and never users' of corticosteroids [23]. As a result most would agree that both inhaled and intermittent corticosteroids are safer than continuous oral use, and studies examining vertebral fracture risk confirm these concerns [16]. Fracture data from epidemiologic studies do raise concern [18]. These concerns may be specific to individual products [24].

Fracture rates increase with duration of corticosteroid use [25]. Anywhere from 30 to 50% of chronic corticosteroid users will sustain a fracture [4].

In summary, significant trabecular bone loss occurs in both men and women at corticosteroid doses equivalent to 7.5 mg or greater of prednisone. Trabecular bone loss occurs early in the course of treatment and appears to be dose related. Cortical loss is particularly evident during the second year of therapy and may be related to total cumulative dose and duration. Furthermore, corticosteroids modify risk factors for osteoporosis and may even alter the normally protective effects of postmenopausal women on stable hormone replacement therapy (HRT).

III. Patterns of Corticosteroid Use

Corticosteroids are used across by men and women with an assorted array of diseases. Most trials have had a preponderance of patients with rheumatic diseases, in particular rheumatoid arthritis and polymyalgia rheumatica [19,20,26]. As a result the preponderance of study subjects were women. Those with rheumatoid arthritis treated with corticosteroids are at high risk for fracture; the disease itself and menopausal status are independent risk factor for fractures. Corticosteroids are used in rheumatoid arthritis as intermittent oral or intravenous pulses, as intra-articular injections, or as long-term low dose treatment. Many feel that it is the total cumulative dose of corticosteroids that is most important in increasing the risk for fracture. With polymyalgia rheumatica, corticosteroids are used on average for 18 months. Significant bone loss is seen with corticosteroids within the first 6 months of treatment initiation. Therefore, the duration of use in polymyalgia rheumatica is abundant time for significant bone loss to occur.

In patients with inflammatory bowel disease the use of corticosteroids is probably the most important risk factor for the development of osteoporosis. In one trial that measured the BMD of 84 consecutive patients with inflammatory bowel disease [27], corticosteroid users were at significantly greater risk of osteopenia with 58% having osteopenia versus 28% in nonusers. The rate of bone loss in inflammatory bowel disease has been studied in several longitudinal studies [28–31]. The early annual rate of bone loss appears to be more important in the spine and varies from 3 to 6%. Postmenopausal women suffer from the greatest rates of bone loss [31]. Bone loss is most closely related to corticosteroid use [30,32,33]. In a study of patients with Crohn's disease and ulcerative colitis, there was a greater prevalence of osteopenia among patients with Crohn's disease [33]; however, using stepwise discriminant analysis, corticosteroid use was found to be the most important factor predicting diminished BMD rather than disease type.

In asthma, corticosteroids are used as intermittent oral and intravenous pulses, topically as inhaled steroids or as chronic intermediate- to low-dose therapy. Oral corticosteroids lead to

bone loss [23] and fractures [3]; however, recent studies suggest that inhaled corticosteroids also lead to bone loss at a rate that is intermediate to those that have never been on corticosteroids and oral users [23]. In a study of men 50 years of age and older, oral corticosteroids lead to the greatest fracture risk followed by those on inhaled corticosteroids followed by those who did not take any corticosteroids [16]. Intermittent use of oral corticosteroids lead to similar fracture risk compared with those who had been on inhaled therapy [16]. Fractures, although they may in part be attributable to corticosteroid use, may also be attributed to the underlying disease [18].

Prolonged, high doses of corticosteroids are used in the treatment of dermatologic patients with pemphigus and dermatomyositis, resulting in increased rates of bone loss. These patients are often on high prolonged doses of corticosteroids and as a result are at greatly increased fracture risk.

IV. Pathophysiology of Corticosteroid-induced Osteoporosis

Although our understanding of osteoporosis has increased, the pathophysiology of corticosteroid-induced osteoporosis is not well understood. Data elicited from clinical trials regarding the mechanisms of corticosteroid-induced osteoporosis are very difficult to interpret because most have examined corticosteroid-induced osteoporosis in patients with a wide variety of complicated systemic disorders of varying severity that in themselves may cause bone disease. In addition, the risk of developing osteoporosis appears to be variable from disease to disease and depends on a number of factors including the dose of a corticosteroid prescribed and the duration of exposure, sex of the patient, and the menopausal status.

The cause of corticosteroid-induced osteoporosis is multifactorial and occurs in addition to normal age- and menopause-associated bone loss. Two abnormalities in bone metabolism are said to occur; the first is a reduction in bone formation and the second is an increase in bone resorption. That they both play a role is not in doubt. Controversy exists as to the relative contribution of each to the development of osteoporosis.

Reduced bone formation has been attributed to the direct inhibitory effects of corticosteroids on osteoblasts. Even moderate doses of corticosteroids inhibit the osteoblast synthesis of bone collagen and the conversion of precursor cells into functioning osteoblasts [34–36]. Furthermore, corticosteroids substantially reduce protein synthesis affecting osteoid formation [37]. A decrease in osteoid seams, a low mineral apposition rate, and reduced mean wall thickness are seen on bone biopsy [35]. The reduction in mean wall thickness is thought to be due to a shortened osteoblast lifespan [35]. Reductions in the bone turnover marker osteocalcin are consistent with a decrease in bone formation; however, it should be recognized that decreases in osteocalcin may overestimate the effects of corticosteroids on collagen synthesis [38–41]. Corticosteroids may further affect osteoblasts by modulating their responses to parathyroid hormone (PTH), prostaglandins, cytokines, growth factors, and 1,25-dihydroxyvitamin D. Compared with normal aging, bone loss in corticosteroid-induced osteoporosis is greater [35,42]. Recent work by Manolagas' group has demonstrated an increase in osteoblast apoptosis [43]. Their group is the first to clearly

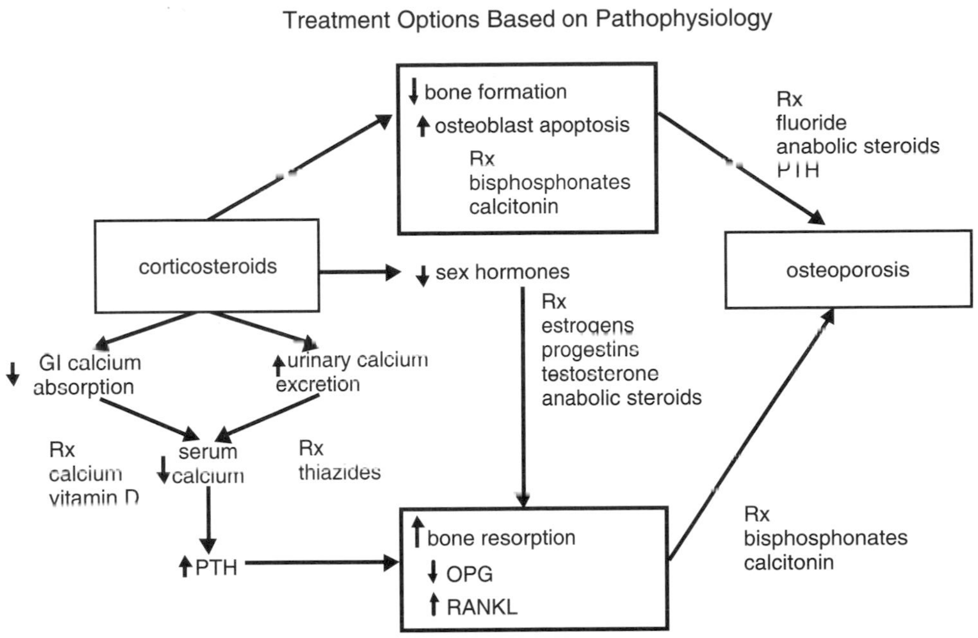

Treatment Options Based on Pathophysiology

Fig. 91-1 Treatment options based on the pathophysiology of corticosteroid-induced osteoporosis.

demonstrate osteoblast cell death resulting from corticosteroids and to provide strong evidence that the loss of osteoblast function plays a major role in corticosteroid-induced bone loss [43]. In addition, their group showed diminished bone formation and turnover, as determined by histomorphometric analysis of tetracycline-labeled vertebrae, and impaired osteoblastogenesis and osteoclastogenesis, as determined by *ex vivo* bone marrow cell cultures [43]. There was a 3-fold increase in osteoblast apoptosis in vertebrae, and apoptosis was shown in 28% of the osteocytes in metaphyseal cortical bone. Decreased production of osteoclasts explains the reduction in bone turnover, whereas decreased production and apoptosis of osteoblasts would account for the decline in bone formation and trabecular width. Furthermore, accumulation of apoptotic osteocytes may contribute to osteonecrosis.

The effects of corticosteroids on bone resorption have been controversial. It has been postulated that bone resorption is PTH mediated [44–47] and may occur as a result of secondary hyperparathyroidism that is a consequence of decreased intestinal calcium absorption [48–51] and increased urinary excretion of calcium [52,53]. It has been shown that the osteoclastic response to corticosteroids is abolished after parathyroidectomy, suggesting that increased bone resorption is, in part, controlled by PTH [44]. Others have suggested that an increase in bone resorption may result from secondary hyperparathyroidism and that this occurs as a consequence of decreased intestinal calcium absorption [48–51,54] and increased urinary excretion of calcium [52,53]. Most studies, however, have not found any increases in PTH levels and its role has been challenged. It has been argued that elevated PTH levels were seen in assays that measured hormone fragments [45–47,52,55], whereas no change was seen with assays that measured intact PTH [39] or midregion fragments [41,56–58].

The effect of corticosteroids on net intestinal calcium absorption is also controversial. Radioisotope studies have indicated that calcium absorption may decrease [59,60], increase [61], or remain unchanged [62] in response to corticosteroids. These contradictory results may be explained by the fact that corticosteroids act differently on individual intestinal segments. It has been reported that, although duodenal calcium absorption is depressed [63–66], corticosteroids may stimulate calcium absorption in the colon [67,68]. In addition, corticosteroids may alter calcium absorption in a dose-dependent manner [69]. Thus, conflicting results may be caused by differences in dosages. In the patient with inflammatory bowel disease this is further complicated by the segment of bowel that is affected by disease.

In addition to decreased calcium absorption, corticosteroids may increase urinary calcium excretion. Hypercalciuria is most likely due to increased skeletal calcium mobilization and decreased renal tubular reabsorption and results from a PTH-independent mechanism [41] or indirectly by increased filtered calcium load due to an increased calcium load due to increased bone resorption [70].

Corticosteroids may alter vitamin D metabolism, although the evidence in support of this is not convincing and is complicated by the fact that in elderly populations vitamin D levels may be low whether they are on corticosteroids or not. Normal 25-hydroxyvitamin D concentrations have been found in those on corticosteroids compared with matched controls. Prednisone depresses calcium absorption from the gastrointestinal tract without depressing serum 25-hydroxyvitamin D levels [71,72]. Corticosteroids may reduce serum levels of 1,25-dihydroxyvitamin D [73]; however, they do not alter the conversion of 25-hydroxyvitamin D to 1,25-dihydroxyvitamin D [51,63]. Seeman *et al* [48] confirmed the absence of significant abnormalities in vitamin D metabolism. Godschalk *et al* [74] found that corticosteroids reduced the number of vitamin D receptors, suggesting that this might be the mechanism by which these drugs antagonize vitamin D action, although this has yet to be confirmed. Ho *et al* [75] studied the effects of the vitamin D receptor genes in patients treated with a cumulative dose of 1.8 g per year or a minimum dose of 5 mg of prednisolone or equivalent per day. They did not find any significant differences in BMD between the genotypes even after adjustments for numerous potential confounding variables. They suggested that the vitamin D receptor genotype may not be a means of identifying patients at greater risk of corticosteroid-induced bone loss.

Corticosteroids alter gonadal function by inhibiting pituitary gonadotrophin secretion and, combined with their direct effect on the ovaries and testes, may lead to a reduction in the production of estrogen and testosterone. They blunt the secretion of luteinizing hormone in response to luteinizing hormone releasing hormone in both men and women [76,77] and inhibit follicle stimulating hormone–induced estrogen production in women and decrease testosterone production in men [78–80]. Levels of androstenedione and estrone are further suppressed as a result of the reduced adrenal production of androstenedione, caused by the suppression of ACTH and the resultant adrenal atrophy [81]. In fact, estrogen deficiency and corticosteroids may have an additive effect in increasing the rate of bone loss [82].

Corticosteroids may have a more direct effect on osteoclasts through their effect on osteoprotegerin (OPG) and the receptor activator of nuclear factor-κ ligand (RANKL). Data are consistent with the hypothesis that corticosteroids promote osteoclastogenesis by inhibiting OPG and concurrently stimulating RANKL production by osteoblastic lineage cells, thereby enhancing bone resorption [70,83,84]. Serum OPG is suppressed by corticosteroids [70,83,84]. In one study, markers of bone metabolism, including serum OPG, osteocalcin, bone-specific alkaline phosphatase activity, PTH, tartrate-resistant acid phosphatase, and BMD, were measured before and during the treatment period in a study if those initiating corticosteroids [70].

Corticosteroids significantly reduced BMD of the lumbar spine in the 6-month treatment period with serum OPG significantly decreased by within 2 weeks and serum tartrate-resistant acid phosphatase markedly increased. On the other hand, there were no remarkable changes in serum PTH. Serum osteocalcin and bone-specific alkaline phosphatase were transiently reduced during the treatment period. In this study only serum OPG was positively and independently correlated with percentage BMD of age-matched reference [70]. These findings imply that glucocorticoid-induced bone loss develops rapidly via enhanced bone resorption and suppressed bone formation. Moreover, the increased bone resorption caused by corticosteroids may be, at least in part, mediated by inhibition of OPG not by incremental increases in PTH

Evidence suggests that when bone loss occurs, trabecular rather than cortical bone is affected earlier and more severely by corticosteroids [3,8]. It is not surprising then that fractures affecting the ribs, vertebrae, and pelvis occur early after corticosteroids are initiated [85]. Cortical bone loss as reflected by femoral neck does occur and is most noticeable after the first year of treatment [9–11].

V. Risk Factors

Risk factors that should be examined in patients receiving corticosteroids include family history, hormonal status, fracture history, age, other medications that may interfere with normal bone metabolism, and lifestyle habits [76,86–91]. A family history should be completed to determine the existence of bone disease in the patient's ancestry and should include history of osteoporosis, early menopause, longevity, and fractures. Those with a low BMD and a prevalent fracture are at greatest risk to have yet another fracture. The longer the duration and the greater the dose of corticosteroids, the greater the rate of bone loss. All medications that interfere with normal bone metabolism should be noted and avoided if possible. Lifestyle risk factors, such as diet, alcohol use, physical activity, and smoking, should be identified and treated appropriately. Other potential causes of bone loss such as hyperparathyroidism, hyperthyroidism, osteomalacia, and multiple myeloma should be ruled out.

VI. Risk Assessment

A. Biochemical Assessment

A number of biochemical parameters are altered in corticosteroid-induced osteoporosis. However, they have not been shown to have an impact on clinical management of patients with this condition. Bone-specific alkaline phosphatase and osteocalcin levels are low in most patients on corticosteroids. Doses of prednisone as low as 2.5 mg will suppress osteocalcin levels [92] as will inhaled and intra-articular corticosteroids. Measurements of urinary calcium concentrations are useful in assessing calcium balance, susceptibility to secondary hyperparathyroidism, and potential treatment options for corticosteroid-treated patients [53,74,92]. With corticosteroid use, urine calcium excretion is initially high, then falls over time. Urinary hydroxyproline, pyridinoline, deoxypyridinoline, and carboxy- and aminotelopeptide excretions are indicators of bone resorption and along with urinary calcium may help predict those who will develop corticosteroid-induced osteoporosis [93].

B. Radiologic Assessment

Distinctive features of corticosteroid-induced osteoporosis can be seen on x-ray films [85]. In corticosteroid-induced osteoporosis, vertical and horizontal trabeculae are equally thin, producing a uniformly translucent appearance of the vertebrae, whereas in postmenopausal osteoporosis, horizontal trabeculae are lost out of proportion to vertical trabeculae, leading to a "corduroy stripe" appearance [4]. Abundant pseudocallus formation at the site of stress fractures is a hallmark of corticosteroid-induced osteoporosis [4] and is most frequently seen at the end plates of collapsed vertebrae or around stress fractures in the ribs or pelvis. The basis for this is a reduction in osteoblastic activity and increased production of cartilaginous callus that becomes highly mineralized in an amorphous fashion. Radiologic assessment is important at the time of corticosteroid initiation. The presence of a vertebral compression fracture identifies those who are greatest risk for fracture [94–96] and makes treatment to prevent subsequent fractures mandatory. In men this may be particularly important because their bone mass may be falsely elevated because of degenerative changes and x-ray changes may be the only evidence that they are at higher fracture risk.

C. Bone Density Assessment

Trabecular bone loss occurs early in the course of corticosteroid therapy, although both trabecular and cortical loss occur over time. Early changes in BMD can be detected in the lumbar spine and femoral neck using DXA or quantitative computed tomography [97] The rate of bone loss is greatest during the first year of therapy [4,7]. Bone loss is identifiable by 6 months with DXA, and, on average, 5% of bone mass is lost within the first year of therapy. During the second year of treatment, bone loss continues to occur but at a slower rate and indeed recovery may be seen and seems to be related to the dose of corticosteroid [7].

Bone mineral density measurements have been used to assess the risk of fractures in corticosteroid-treated patients. Although these measurements are accurate and precise, they may underestimate the fracture risk in patients receiving corticosteroids. With the use of corticosteroids, bone strength may not be related to bone mass as directly as it is in primary osteoporosis. For instance, in postmenopausal women, a decrease in BMD of one standard deviation is associated with a 2-fold increase in fracture risk [98]. The incremental increase in fracture risk may be greater in postmenopausal women who are treated with corticosteroids [99] simply because they may have a number of other independent risk factors that contribute to fracture risk. In men, degenerative changes and areal bone density rather than volumetric measurements may suggest that their bone density is greater than it really is; thus, x-rays should be obtained, particularly in men.

VII. Clinical Manifestations

Bone loss occurs rapidly within the first 6 to 12 months of beginning corticosteroid therapy; thereafter the rate of loss slows to two to three times that of normal [5–7]. Initially trabecular rather than cortical bone is affected more severely by corticosteroids [3,8]. Interestingly, cortical bone loss as reflected by changes in femoral neck bone density, is particularly evident during the second year of corticosteroid therapy [9,10], and may be of particular concern with longer term corticosteroid use. There also appears to be a close relationship between the rate of bone loss and the dose of corticosteroid [7]. Significant trabecular bone loss occurs with prednisone doses greater than 7.5 mg/day in most patients [7,12]. Some recovery of bone may be seen in the spine once doses of prednisone fall below 7.5 mg/day [7]. In one study, rates of bone loss increased with doses of prednisone between 5 and 10 mg daily and with inhaled steroids [5]. In yet another study, inhaled corticosteroids also lead to bone loss intermediate to those who were on oral corticosteroids and those who had never been on them [23]. Thus, although lower doses and inhaled corticosteroids may be safer than higher doses [17], there is still no truly safe dose [5].

Corticosteroids alter the usual risk factors for osteoporosis. Young people taking corticosteroids lose bone more rapidly than older people and premenopausal women in their forties [12]. After menopause, fracture risk is greater for women taking corticosteroids, presumably because they are susceptible to age- and menopause-related bone loss. Bone loss may occur even in those that are on stable doses of estrogen [10]. Men are equally susceptible to bone loss caused by corticosteroids [12]. In rheumatoid arthritis, it is likely that the inflammatory disease activity, loss of muscle mass, and immobilization contribute to bone loss [17], and high doses of corticosteroids may well exacerbate this bone loss [22].

In summary, significant trabecular bone loss occurs in most patients at corticosteroid doses equivalent to 7.5 mg or greater of prednisone. Bone loss occurs early in the course of treatment and appears to be dose related. Cortical loss is evident during the second year of therapy and is likely to get progressively greater with increasing time on corticosteroids. Furthermore, corticosteroids modify risk factors for osteoporosis and may even alter the normally protective effects of those on stable HRT. Fractures occur in up to 50% of those on long-term corticosteroids. Spine, rib, and pelvic fractures occur earlier in the course of corticosteroid with other nonvertebral fractures occurring with more prolonged use.

VIII. Therapeutic Options

Therapeutically, complete discontinuation of corticosteroids would reduce the risk of bone loss and subsequent fractures, but in practice the termination of corticosteroid therapy is often clinically difficult or impossible. Patients who have discontinued corticosteroid therapy exhibit a rebound increase in osteoblastic function and new bone formation [7,34,100,101]. Unfortunately, even with this increase in bone formation, BMD seldom returns to the level seen before corticosteroids were instituted. If corticosteroid therapy must be continued, the lowest possible dose should be used. Alternate-day corticosteroid therapy may be less toxic than daily administration; nonetheless, bone loss still has been detected in individuals receiving alternate-day treatment [102].

In those in whom ongoing corticosteroid therapy is necessary, therapy to prevent fractures need to be considered. Unfortunately few receive any preventive treatment. In men, it is seldom recognized that corticosteroid use may place them at increased risk for fracture. Indeed the use of any therapy to prevent the devastating effects of corticosteroids was abysmal with only 8 to 14% receiving some form of therapy [103,104]. These studies do not even address whether the treatment given was the most effective available. The need for a well thought out systematic approach to preventive therapy is essential if we are to decrease the number of fractures occurring in those on corticosteroids.

A. General

For the most part, studies in corticosteroid-induced osteoporosis have been conducted in postmenopausal women, with some studies men mostly as a subset in larger clinical trials. The efficacy of therapy in preventing corticosteroid-induced osteoporosis should be interpreted in light of when drug therapy was initiated in the course of corticosteroid use. Primary prevention studies refer to trials in which treatment occurs at the same time or shortly after corticosteroid use is initiated. Treatment studies are those in which patients begin following chronic corticosteroid use. As a result, prevention studies examine the efficacy of drug therapy in patients before rapid corticosteroid-induced bone loss, whereas treatment studies determine the efficacy in patients in whom bone loss has already occurred. The main goal in the prevention and treatment of corticosteroid-induced bone loss is to stabilize bone mass, in some instances to increase bone mass, and ultimately to reduce fracture risk. Efforts to prevent fractures should be made in light of the risk for fracturing. For many, the addition of a corticosteroid may be the straw that breaks the camel's back because they often have other independent risks for fracture. At greatest risk are postmenopausal women [105]. Of the recent bisphosphonate clinical trials, incident fractures occurred most frequently in postmenopausal women and least frequently in premenopausal women with men being at intermediate risk [10,19–21,106,107]. Their risk factors may include their postmenopausal status, age, increased susceptibility to falling as a result of decreases in muscle mass, reductions in balance and eyesight, and in some their underlying disease. With the addition of corticosteroids and the resultant loss of bone that accompanies treatment initiation, their risk for fracture is extremely high and it could be argued that treatment should be instituted regardless of bone density.

B. Bisphosphonates

Substantial data exist supporting the use of bisphosphonates in corticosteroid-induced osteoporosis. Indeed, in a recent meta-analysis that examined calcitonin, vitamin D, fluoride, and bisphosphonates in corticosteroid-treated patients, bisphosphonate therapy was found to have a larger bone density treatment effect at the lumbar spine as compared with either fluoride, calcitonin, or vitamin D [108]. The efficacy of bisphosphonates was enhanced further when used in combination with vitamin D. Vitamin D and calcitonin were more effective than no therapy/calcium and were of similar efficacy, but both were significantly less effective than the bisphosphonates.

Many randomized controlled clinical trials [10,19–21,26, 106,107,109–120], including both prevention and treatment, of bisphosphonates have been evaluated in corticosteroid-treated patients. In general, patients suffered from a variety of underlying diseases that required corticosteroid therapy. For the most part, patients were given calcium and/or vitamin D supplements throughout the study.

Of the prevention studies [19–21,26,109–111,113,115,119], etidronate, alendronate, risedronate, clodronate, and intravenous pamidronate have been conducted. Therapy resulted in significant differences between treatment and placebo in lumbar spine BMD in favor of bisphosphonate treatment. In addition bisphosphonate-treated patients were found to have small increases in femoral neck BMD, whereas decreases were observed in placebo-treated patients [10,19–21,109,111,113,119]. This held true for premenopausal and postmenopausal women and men when they were included in the studies.

Of the treatment studies [10,20,106,116,117], etidronate, alendronate, and risedronate have been examined. In the studies, lumbar spine BMD increased from baseline in the bisphosphonate groups, whereas it decreased or remained stable, depending on the use of vitamin D and calcium supplementation, in the placebo

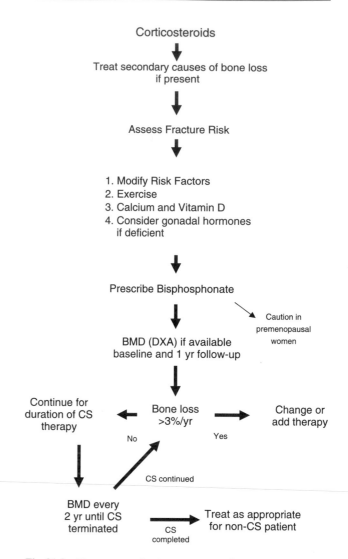

Fig. 91-2   Management of patients commenced on corticosteroids.

groups following therapy. These differences were statistically significant. Of the studies reporting data on the femoral neck [10,20,106,116,117], the largest studies found significant differences between the treatment groups, in favor of bisphosphonate therapy [10,20,106]. Furthermore, results from the alendronate trials demonstrated significant differences between groups in BMD of the trochanter in favor of alendronate-treated patients after 1 [20] and 2 [10] years of treatment. Once again these findings were applicable to men and women.

Ideally, bisphosphonates should protect patients from skeletal fractures. Studies have been conducted that identified incident fractures [10,19–21,106,107,109,116,118]. A number of fracture trials found a reduced vertebral fracture incidence with bisphosphonate therapy. Among the postmenopausal women in the cyclical etidronate study of Adachi et al, etidronate-treated postmenopausal women experienced an 85% reduction in the proportion of patients with vertebral fractures compared with the placebo group [19,121]. In part this was due to differences in baseline BMD [121]. In the study by Saag et al [20], new vertebral fractures were uncommon. Most new fractures occurred among postmenopausal women. Overall, there was a trend to fewer vertebral fractures in the pooled alendronate-treated group [20]. In the 2-year follow-up of these patients there were fewer patients with new vertebral fractures in the alendronate group versus the placebo group [10]. When the risedronate prevention and treatment studies were pooled, a significant reduction in vertebral fracture was seen with the data from both sexes [120]. In addition in a separate publication, vertebral fracture reduction was seen in men [107]. Bisphosphonate treatment consistently improves axial BMD in corticosteroid-treated patients, with a smaller detectable benefit to the appendicular skeleton. The patient populations studied to date have, of practical necessity, been heterogeneous as to morbidity, corticosteroid dose and duration, and initial skeletal status. This does, however, make these studies generalizeable to the patient population seen in practice. Treatment of established corticosteroid-induced bone loss results in restoration of lumbar spine BMD at least as effectively, if not more so, than the use of bisphosphonates for primary prevention.

Saag *et al* [20] also reported that in postmenopausal women on stable estrogen therapy, treatment with alendronate resulted in a significant increase in lumbar spine BMD when compared with placebo. In the second year there was a decline in bone mass in the group treated with estrogen and placebo, whereas the estrogen- and alendronate-treated groups had an increase in lumbar spine BMD [10]. These data suggest that bone loss occurs during the second year on prednisone therapy even when patients are on estrogen therapy. This was most noticeable in the spine. This loss of bone, however, may be prevented by alendronate suggesting that even in the estrogen-treated patient a bisphosphonate, in this case alendronate, should be considered.

Cyclical etidronate, alendronate, and risedronate therapies reduce incident vertebral fractures in patients treated with corticosteroids, generally speaking, within the first year of treatment. This is most evident in postmenopausal women, who are at greatest risk for fracture, but is also evident in men. In the future, the results of comparison trials may help determine the role of specific bisphosphonates in the treatment and prevention of corticosteroid-induced osteoporosis.

In summary, the bisphosphonates have been shown to stabilize bone mass and in some instances to actually increase bone density in the spine and hip in those commencing and on long-term therapy. They have been shown to be effective in those on high and low doses of corticosteroids, in men, and in both premenopausal and postmenopausal women. They are the only agents that have been shown to significantly reduce vertebral fractures and to reduce them in men and women.

C. Hormone Replacement Therapy

Two intervention studies have been performed evaluating HRT in the treatment of corticosteroid-induced osteoporosis [122,123]. Of these, one study was a retrospective cohort study [122]. In these studies, the patients were postmenopausal women suffering from either rheumatoid arthritis or asthma. The average age of the patients ranged from 56 to 68 years. No primary prevention studies have been completed. The results of the studies indicated that mean BMD of the lumbar spine increased in the hormone replacement treatment groups, whereas it decreased in the placebo

groups. The differences between treatment groups were significant. One study described data for femoral neck BMD [123]. An insignificant difference was found between treatment groups.

Contrary findings were observed in a 2-year study of alendronate in patients on corticosteroids [10]. A small number of women who were on stable estrogen and placebo therapy continued to lose bone mass in the lumbar spine over the course of 2 years. In contrast those who were on stable estrogen and alendronate had an increase in BMD. In addition to their beneficial effects on bone, HRT has been shown to reduce low-density lipoprotein (LDL) cholesterol and is one of the few therapies that increases high-density lipoprotein (HDL) cholesterol. This is of benefit in the corticosteroid-treated patient who is at increased risk of cardiovascular disease. Theoretically the use of hormone replacement may prevent the development of corticosteroid-induced cardiovascular disease. Other beneficial effects including their benefits in the treatment of menopausal and urogenital symptoms need to be discussed, as well as potential problems such as the development of deep venous thrombosis, pulmonary emboli, bleeding, and breast cancer.

In summary, HRT exhibited a positive effect on lumbar spine BMD in the only randomized controlled trial of treatment in corticosteroid-induced osteoporosis. Data on the effects of hormone therapy in the hip are at best equivocal. At present we do not have any firm data on the effects of HRT on those commencing corticosteroids. Beneficial effect on lipids may prevent the late-stage cardiovascular disease seen in those on long-term corticosteroids. Unfortunately even with the potential additional benefits, long-term compliance may still be a major difficulty given the complex decision-making process both patients and physicians go through when discussing HRT. Although selective estrogen receptor modulator therapy such as raloxifene has been shown to be effective in the treatment of postmenopausal osteoporosis [124], further research is needed to elucidate their role in the management of corticosteroid-induced osteoporosis.

D. Calcitonin

There have been randomized, placebo-controlled, trials that have assessed the efficacy of calcitonin in corticosteroid-induced osteoporosis [104,125–130]. For the most part these trials have been conducted in postmenopausal women. Calcitonin was administered intranasally or subcutaneously. The prevention trials [104,125,126] demonstrated that lumbar spine BMD decreased from baseline in both treatment groups but to a lesser extent in the calcitonin-treated when compared with the placebo groups. Bone mineral density data on femoral neck, trochanter, Ward's triangle, distal radius, and whole body have also been reported. No significant differences were found between treatment groups at these sites following therapy.

Three of the four treatment studies measured lumbar spine BMD [127,128,130]. Lumbar spine BMD increased from baseline in the active treatment groups, whereas it decreased in the placebo groups. Two studies demonstrated significant differences between treatment groups [127,128]. Data on distal radius [129] and femoral neck [130] BMD have been reported. A significant difference between the increase in BMD in the calcitonin group and the decrease in the placebo group at both sites has been shown.

One of the potential additional benefits of calcitonin beyond improving bone mass is that it may relieve pain associated with vertebral fracture. Ringe and Welzel [129] found that the amount of pain experienced by those treated with calcitonin was significantly less than the placebo group, and the difference persisted for the duration of the study.

In summary, studies of calcitonin efficacy in corticosteroid-induced osteoporosis suggest that calcitonin produces a beneficial effect on bone density. This appears to be true in both the prevention and treatment of corticosteroid-induced osteoporosis. The most consistent positive changes are seen in the spine. Studies with greater patient populations will be necessary to prove a reduction in fracture risk.

E. Fluoride

Four intervention studies assessing fluoride therapy in the treatment of corticosteroid-induced osteoporosis have been done [131–134]. The studies use either sodium fluoride or monofluorophosphate with similar results with either preparation. One trial compared the advantage of adding sodium fluoride with cyclical etidronate therapy [131]. Patients had various underlying conditions that required corticosteroid therapy. No primary prevention studies have been completed.

On average, vertebral BMD substantially increased in fluoride-treated patients after 18 to 24 months of therapy, whereas it remained stable or slightly increased from baseline in the placebo-treated patients. Differences between treatment groups were significant after therapy. Femoral neck BMD decreased from baseline in both treatment and placebo groups [131, 132,134].

In summary, fluoride seems to increase BMD at the spine without protecting the hip from the effects of corticosteroids. There may be an added benefit for the spine in using fluoride in combination with an antiresorptive agent, but no benefit has been seen in the appendicular skeleton. Fluoride therapy has not been shown to prevent fractures in corticosteroid-induced osteoporosis. Indeed, further investigation is required because studies in primary osteoporosis in postmenopausal women have not conclusively demonstrated fracture benefit. In high doses fluoride may result in an increase in nonvertebral fractures.

F. Anabolic Therapy

Three randomized controlled studies have used anabolic therapy in the treatment of corticosteroid-induced osteoporosis [135–137]. One study each examined human PTH, testosterone, and nandrolone decanoate. The testosterone trial examined men, whereas the other two enrolled postmenopausal women. No primary prevention studies have been completed. The results of the studies indicated that BMD of the lumbar spine [135,136] and forearm [137] increased in the treatment groups, whereas it decreased in the placebo groups following therapy. The differences between groups were significant. Human PTH was found to have no effect on femoral neck, trochanter, total hip, and distal radius BMD [135]. Furthermore, testosterone therapy was found to have no effect on whole body BMD following therapy [136].

In conclusion, anabolic therapy may have some benefit in the treatment of corticosteroid-induced bone loss. The prevention of corticosteroid-induced osteoporosis with these agents still must be determined.

G. Calcium and Vitamin D and Its Analogues

Seven controlled studies have been identified that examine the effects of vitamin D or its analogues in corticosteroid-treated patients [7,125,138–142]. In these studies, patients in the active treatment groups received calcium supplements ranging from 450 to 1000 mg/day. Calcium supplements were administered to patients in the placebo groups in four studies [125,139, 141,142]. In the other trials, no medication was given.

Of the seven studies, three were prevention [7,125,139] with one study evaluating calcitriol [125], another alfacalcidol [139], and the third vitamin D [7]. The results of the three trials indicated that lumbar spine BMD decreased from baseline in both treatment groups but to a lesser extent in the active treatment groups as compared with the placebo groups. In the vitamin D trial, the differences between groups were not significant following therapy, whereas in the active vitamin D metabolites alfacalcidol and calcitriol trial significant differences between treatment and control groups were noted. The calcitriol study also assessed data on the femoral neck and distal radius. At these skeletal sites, no significant differences were found between the treatment groups and placebo.

Four treatment studies have been done [138,140–142]. Of these, three examined vitamin D and one calcitriol. They showed that lumbar spine BMD increased from baseline in the active treatment groups in all three studies, whereas it decreased in the placebo group in one trial following therapy. One study demonstrated a significant difference in lumbar spine BMD between the treatment groups [140]. This study also demonstrated significant differences between treatment groups in trochanter BMD, in favor of vitamin D therapy. One treatment and both prevention studies evaluated fracture rates [7,125,142]. In these studies, all patients had spinal x-rays performed. No significant differences in fracture rates were found between groups following therapy.

Although most studies investigating vitamin D treatment did not report side effects associated with therapy, the few studies that did report side effects frequently reported hypercalciuria. Because side effects may occur, urinary calcium levels should be checked before instituting therapy and they should be monitored every 3 months while taking vitamin D. Serum calcium should also be monitored regularly, and if hypercalcemia develops the calcium and vitamin D dose should be reduced appropriately.

In an earlier meta-analysis, vitamin D plus calcium was found to be superior to no therapy or calcium alone in the management of corticosteroid-induced osteoporosis. Vitamin D was less effective than some other osteoporosis therapies. It was concluded however that treatment with vitamin D plus calcium, as a minimum, should be recommended to patients receiving long-term corticosteroids [143].

In conclusion, although it is likely that vitamin D and its analogues have some benefit in the prevention of corticosteroid-induced osteoporosis, it is quite clear that these agents cannot completely prevent corticosteroid-induced bone loss. Nonetheless, vitamin D therapy has been shown to maintain spine and hip

BMD in patients who are taking chronic corticosteroids and is an important adjunctive therapy. It is also important to remember that a large number of those on corticosteroids are elderly and in many instances housebound. In this population, vitamin D deficiency is common, and the use of vitamin D and calcium is essential.

H. Thiazide Diuretics

Thiazides or other calcium-retaining diuretics have not been subjected to prospective, randomized, controlled trials using BMD or fracture rates as a primary outcome measure in corticosteroid-induced osteoporosis. The major effect of thiazide diuretic administration is to reduce calcium excretion via increased tubular calcium reabsorption in the distal tubule. In a study of corticosteroid-treated patients, 50 mg of hydrochlorothiazide given twice daily also increased intestinal calcium absorption [65]. Nonetheless, thiazide diuretics are not without risk. They may aggravate hypokalemia in corticosteroid-treated patients [144], and there is a risk of hypercalcemia developing in those patients treated with a combination of vitamin D and thiazides. Despite their apparent widespread use, there is a lack of clinical data with appropriate long-term outcome measures supporting the use of thiazide diuretics in corticosteroid-induced osteoporosis.

I. Summary of Therapeutic Options

Based on currently available data, bisphosphonates appear to be the drugs of choice for the prevention and/or treatment of corticosteroid-induced osteoporosis. In fact, the data for the bisphosphonates are more compelling than for any other agent. The efficacy of bisphosphonates is enhanced further with concomitant use of vitamin D. Although HRT is extensively used in the treatment of primary osteoporosis, data for its effectiveness when used alone in corticosteroid-induced osteoporosis are limited. Indeed the data regarding its benefit in preventing bone loss in those commencing corticosteroids are still lacking. Of concern for the busy clinician is the lack of compliance with the use of hormone replacement. On the other hand HRT may be of benefit in reducing the risk of coronary artery disease and because of its efficacy in those on chronic low-dose corticosteroid therapy, it should be considered in all postmenopausal women. If bisphosphonate therapy is contraindicated, calcitonin may be an effective alternative, particularly in those with acute back pain secondary to vertebral fractures. For patients who have been treated but continue to lose bone, fluoride and anabolic therapy should be considered. Although vitamin D and its analogues appear to have weak positive effects on bone in those receiving corticosteroids, they may not be potent enough to be used alone. As such, these agents should be administered in combination with other medications. Presently, little evidence is available to support the use of thiazide diuretic. In the future, the results of long-term clinical and comparison trials may provide us with more definitive treatment strategies.

IX. Patient Management

Practically speaking all patients either commencing or on chronic corticosteroids need to receive counseling about the risks to their bone health. Because it is well accepted that bone loss is most rapid in the first 6 to 12 months of corticosteroid therapy, it is important that preventive measures be initiated concurrently with corticosteroids. In this manner, bone mass may well be maintained through what normally is a phase of rapid bone loss. The preservation of bone mass is crucial because the loss that occurs in the first 6 to 12 months is rarely fully regained, even after the discontinuation of corticosteroid therapy [13].

The clinical approach to the patient on corticosteroids should begin with an assessment of the individual's risk factors. Risk factors that should be considered include BMD at the lumbar spine and femoral neck, family history, hormonal status, fracture history, age, and other medications that may interfere with normal bone metabolism. In addition, lifestyle risk factor assessment should include diet, alcohol, physical activity, and smoking habits. Assessing risk factors allows the clinician to develop some perspective of the individual's unique susceptibility to bone loss and fracture during and after corticosteroid use. Appropriate procedures should be taken to modify lifestyle risk factors including diet, alcohol use, physical activity, and smoking. If possible, BMD measurements (at all sites if feasible) and a lateral thoracic and lumbar spinal x-ray film should be completed. Bone density measurement should be performed not just as a diagnostic tool (because the evidence that a T-score value for BMD can be used to determine the relative risk of fracture in corticosteroid-treated patients is limited) but also as a tool for the clinical assessment of intervention efficacy. A lateral spine x-ray film should be obtained as an instrument for the evaluation of fracture status.

The presence of secondary causes of osteopenia or osteoporosis should also be determined and treated (e.g., multiple myeloma, hypercalciuria, hyperparathyroidism, etc.). To aid with the diagnosis of secondary causes of osteopenia or osteoporosis, standard laboratory investigations should include a complete blood count, serum measures of creatinine, alkaline phosphatase, calcium, and phosphorus. In patients older than 65 years, measures of serum protein electrophoresis and lipids and a urinary calcium-to-creatinine ratio may also be justified. Laboratory measures may be later used to assess treatment efficacy or to identify complications of therapy, such as hypercalcemia.

The risk of osteoporosis increases as the corticosteroid dose increases, but the exact relationship between the dose, duration, and fracture risk in individuals cannot accurately be determined. Pragmatically, patients receiving daily doses of corticosteroids greater than 7.5 mg/day of prednisone or its equivalent for 3 months or longer should be treated. As a general rule, all patients receiving any dose of corticosteroids for prolonged periods of time should have their BMD monitored because significant bone loss has been found in patients receiving corticosteroids at doses lower than 7.5 mg/day [13,140]. Although it is difficult to determine the relationship of corticosteroid dose and duration to the development of osteoporosis, it is felt that the risk of corticosteroid-induced osteoporosis increases as the cumulative corticosteroid dose increases [145,146]. Given that short courses of steroid therapy (<3 months) can cause significant bone loss [125,147,148], preventive measures should be taken.

In general, patients only need to continue calcium and vitamin D supplements for the duration of short-term corticosteroid therapy. However, treatment beyond calcium and vitamin D supplements is needed if corticosteroid therapy goes beyond 3 months, if it is anticipated that the duration of corticosteroid therapy will be longer than 3 months, or in the treatment of chronic corticosteroid use. In patients beginning therapy for corticosteroids, calcium intake should be approximately 1500 mg/day, as a total of both dietary and supplemental sources. To ensure proper calcium absorption, vitamin D should also be concurrently prescribed at a dose of 400 to 500 IU/day in younger individuals (<65 years) and 800 to 1000 IU/day in older patients (>65 years). The activated forms of vitamin D, including 1-alphahydroxyvitamin D and 1,25 dihydroxyvitamin D have been shown to be more effective than plain vitamin D in the prevention of bone loss. If these therapies are used, monitoring of serum and urine calcium should be undertaken to avoid clinically significant hypercalcemia and hypercalciuria.

Corticosteroids have muscle wasting effects that decrease muscular strength [149–153]; thus, patients should be advised on exercises to maintain or increase their muscle mass and strength. This is especially important in the elderly, in whom the risk of falling is greatly increased by weakened musculature [154,155]. A number of investigations have shown that exercise assists in counteracting the muscle wasting effects of corticosteroids [156–158]. Physical therapy should include postural training and back extension exercises to strengthen the low back musculature and thus potentially reduce the risk of fracture. Back flexion exercises should be avoided in high-risk patients with low bone mass, because they may produce vertebral compression fractures. For those with low bone mass, exercise training should be supervised by a qualified physical therapist familiar with exercise regimens for individuals at high risk of fracture.

For courses of corticosteroid therapy greater than 3 months, a bisphosphonate should be prescribed. If there is evidence of hypogonadism, sex hormone levels should be measured in both men and women. If an individual is deficient, attempts should be made to correct the imbalance because this deficiency will negatively affect bone mass. With oligomenorrheic or amenorrheic premenopausal women, the cause of the menstrual dysfunction should be determined. For women with low estrogen levels, birth control pills with adequate levels of estrogen (at least 50 μg estradiol) or HRT should be prescribed. For hypogonadal men, testosterone replacement should be considered. In the case of postmenopausal women, HRT may also be administered based on an individual's desire or contraindications. Whether the addition of hormone replacement adds to the bone mass achieved with those already on a bisphosphonate therapy is unknown. Nonetheless, the fact that it may offer further benefit and the other potential benefits of ovarian hormone therapy make it a valuable mainstay to therapy. Premenopausal women who do not plan to conceive may also be prescribed bisphosphonates. For premenopausal women with future plans for childbirth, other agents such as calcitonin should be considered first. It is important that patients are aware that there are theoretical risks to the developing fetus with bisphosphonate therapy, even years following its termination. This is due to the drug's extremely long half-life in bone tissue.

After 1 year of therapy, a follow-up bone density assessment should be performed. Because of a very conservative estimate of the precision error seen in most clinical DXA units of 1.5% at the lumbar spine, if bone loss has occurred at a rate greater than 3% per year at any site measured, the intervention should be changed or another added. If bone loss has been less than 3% per year, treatment should continue for the duration of corticosteroid therapy plus 3 years afterward in those with low bone mass. Bone mineral density should then be reassessed every 2 years until corticosteroid therapy is terminated. If at any time, bone loss is greater than 3%, therapy should be adjusted accordingly. Once corticosteroid therapy is discontinued, the patient should be assessed and managed in the manner appropriate for a patient not using corticosteroids.

X. Conclusion

Fractures and bone loss are common in both men and women on corticosteroids. With more elderly patients being treated with corticosteroids for a variety of illnesses, the prevalence of corticosteroid-induced osteoporosis, fractures, and associated morbidity and mortality can only increase unless aggressive intervention is undertaken. This starts with patient and physician awareness and education about the risks and benefits of corticosteroid therapy and the need to prevent the devastating fractures caused by corticosteroids. Ideally, discontinuation of corticosteroid therapy should be undertaken where possible. If corticosteroids must be used, then one would hope to be able to prevent fractures by using agents that achieve rapid response and that stabilize (or build) bone mass. Patients at particular risk for osteoporotic fractures include postmenopausal women, elderly men and women, those with a history of previous fracture or a family history of hip fracture, and those with a low bone density at disease onset. In these individuals, one may be able to reduce the risk of fractures by using the lowest effective corticosteroid dose and by using preventive agents such as the bisphosphonates at the time corticosteroids are instituted. In those requiring treatment, the bisphosphonates remain the treatment of choice. Hormone replacement therapy for postmenopausal women and calcitonin are alternatives to bisphosphonate-intolerant persons. Vitamin D is a valuable adjunct to the bisphosphonates. Adequate intake of calcium and an exercise program might also be beneficial but need to be used in conjunction with other therapy.

References

1. Cushing H. (1932). The basophil adenomas of the pituitary body and their clinical manifestations. *Bull Johns Hopkins Hosp.* 20:137–195.
2. Zelissen PM, Croughs RJ, van Rijk PP, Raymakers JA. (1994). Effect of glucocorticoid replacement therapy on bone mineral density in patients with Addison disease. *Ann Intern Med.* 120:207–210.
3. Adinoff AD, Hollister JR. (1983). Steroid-induced fractures and bone loss in patients with asthma. *N Engl J Med.* 309:265–268.
4. Lukert BP, Raisz LG. (1990). Glucocorticoid-induced osteoporosis: Pathogenesis and management. *Ann Intern Med.* 112:352–364.
5. Saito JK, Davis JW, Wasnich RD, Ross PD. (1995). Users of low-dose glucocorticoids have increased bone loss rates: A longitudinal study. *Calcif Tissue Int.* 57:115–119.
6. Gennari C. (1985). Glucocorticoids and Bone. In *Bone and Mineral*, 3rd Edition (Peck WA, ed.), pp. 213–232. Amsterdam: Elsevier Publishers B.V.

7. Adachi JD, Bensen WG, Bianchi F *et al.* (1996). Vitamin D and calcium in the prevention of corticosteroid induced osteoporosis: A 3 year followup. *J Rheumatol.* 23:995–1000.

8. Hahn TJ, Boisseau VC, Avioli LV. (1974). Effect of chronic corticosteroid administration on diaphyseal and metaphyseal bone mass. *J Clin Endocrinol Metab.* 39:274–282.

9. Brown JP, Olszynski WP, Hodsman A *et al.* (2001). Positive effect of etidronate therapy is maintained after drug is terminated in patients using corticosteroids. *J Clin Densitom.* 4:363–371.

10. Adachi JD, Saag KG, Delmas PD *et al.* (2001). Two-year effects of alendronate on bone mineral density and vertebral fracture in patients receiving glucocorticoids: A randomized, double-blind, placebo-controlled extension trial. Arthritis Rheum. 44:202–211.

11. van Staa TP, Leufkens HG, Abenhaim L *et al.* (2000). Use of oral corticosteroids and risk of fractures. *J Bone Miner Res.* 15:993–1000.

12. Ruegsegger P, Medici TC, Anliker M. (1983). Corticosteroid-induced bone loss. A longitudinal study of alternate day therapy in patients with bronchial asthma using quantitative computed tomography. *Eur J Clin Pharmacol.* 25:615–620.

13. Laan RF, van Riel PL, Van De Putte LB *et al.* (1993). Low-dose prednisone induces rapid reversible axial bone loss in patients with rheumatoid arthritis. A randomized, controlled study. *Ann Intern Med.* 119:963–968.

14. Wong CA, Walsh LJ, Smith CJ *et al.* (2000). Inhaled corticosteroid use and bone-mineral density in patients with asthma. *Lancet.* 355:1399–1403.

15. (2000). Effect of inhaled triamcinolone on the decline in pulmonary function in chronic obstructive pulmonary disease. *N Engl J Med.* 343:1902–1909.

16. McEvoy CE, Ensrud KE, Bender E *et al.* (1998). Association between corticosteroid use and vertebral fractures in older men with chronic obstructive pulmonary disease. *Am J Respir Crit Care Med.* 157:704–709.

17. Sambrook PN, Eisman JA, Champion GD *et al.* Determinants of axial bone loss in rheumatoid arthritis. *Arthritis Rheum.* 30:721–728.

18. van Staa TP, Leufkens HG, Cooper C. (2001). Use of inhaled corticosteroids and risk of fractures. *J Bone Miner Res.* 16:581–588.

19. Adachi JD, Bensen WG, Brown J *et al.* (1997). Intermittent etidronate therapy to prevent corticosteroid-induced osteoporosis. *N Engl J Med.* 337:382–387.

20. Saag KG, Emkey R, Schnitzer TJ *et al.* (1998). Alendronate for the prevention and treatment of glucocorticoid-induced osteoporosis. Glucocorticoid-Induced Osteoporosis Intervention Study Group. *N Engl J Med.* 339:292–299.

21. Cohen S, Levy RM, Keller M *et al.* (1999). Risedronate therapy prevents corticosteroid-induced bone loss: A twelve-month, multicenter, randomized, double-blind, placebo-controlled, parallel-group study. *Arthritis Rheum.* 42:2309–2318.

22. Dykman TR, Gluck OS, Murphy WA *et al.* (1985). Evaluation of factors associated with glucocorticoid-induced osteopenia in patients with rheumatic diseases. *Arthritis Rheum.* 28:361–368.

23. Marystone JF, Barrett-Connor EL, Morton DJ. (1995). Inhaled and oral corticosteroids: Their effects on bone mineral density in older adults. *Am J Public Health.* 85:1693–1695.

24. Pauwels RA, Yernault JC, Demedts MG, Geusens P. (1998). Safety and efficacy of fluticasone and beclomethasone in moderate to severe asthma. Belgian Multicenter Study Group. *Am J Respir Crit Care Med.* 157:827–832.

25. Michel BA, Bloch DA, Fries JF. (1991). Predictors of fractures in early rheumatoid arthritis. *J Rheumatol.* 18:804–808.

26. Jenkins EA, Walker-Bone KE, Wood A *et al.* (1999). The prevention of corticosteroid-induced bone loss with intermittent cyclical etidronate. *Scand J Rheumatol.* 28:152–156.

27. Abitbol V, Roux C, Chaussade S, Guillemant S *et al.* (1995). Metabolic bone assessment in patients with inflammatory bowel disease. *Gastroenterology.* 108:417–422.

28. Motley RJ, Crawley EO, Evans C *et al.* (1988). Increased rate of spinal trabecular bone loss in patients with inflammatory bowel disease. *Gut.* 29:1332–1336.

29. Roux C, Abitbol V, Chaussade S *et al.* (1995). Bone loss in patients with inflammatory bowel disease: A prospective study. *Osteoporos Int.* 5:156–160.

30. Motley RJ, Clements D, Evans WD *et al.* (1993). A four-year longitudinal study of bone loss in patients with inflammatory bowel disease. *Bone Miner.* 23:95–104.

31. Clements D, Motley RJ, Evans WD *et al.* (1992). Longitudinal study of cortical bone loss in patients with inflammatory bowel disease. *Scand J Gastroenterol.* 27:1055–1060.

32. Silvennoinen JA, Karttunen TJ, Niemela SE *et al.* (1995). A controlled study of bone mineral density in patients with inflammatory bowel disease. *Gut.* 37:71–76.

33. Bernstein CN, Seeger LL, Sayre JW *et al.* (1995). Decreased bone density in inflammatory bowel disease is related to corticosteroid use and not disease diagnosis. *J Bone Miner Res.* 10:250–256.

34. Bressot C, Meunier PJ, Chapuy MC *et al.* (1979). Histomorphometric profile, pathophysiology and reversibility of corticosteroid induced osteoporosis. *Met Bone Dis Rel Res.* 1:303–311.

35. Dempster DW, Arlot MA, Meunier PJ. (1983). Mean wall thickness and formation periods of trabecular bone packets in corticosteroid-induced osteoporosis. *Calcif Tissue Int.* 35:410–417.

36. Ishida Y, Heersche JN. (1998). Glucocorticoid-induced osteoporosis: Both *in vivo* and *in vitro* concentrations of glucocorticoids higher than physiological levels attenuate osteoblast differentiation. *J Bone Miner Res.* 13:1822–1826.

37. Peck WA, Brandt J, Miller I. (1967). Hydrocortisone-induced inhibition of protein synthesis and uridine incorporation in isolated bone cells *in vitro.* *Proc Natl Acad Sci U S A.* 57:1599–1606.

38. Caporali R, Gentile S, Caprotti M, Montecucco C. (1991). Serum osteocalcin (bone Gla-protein) and steroid osteoporosis in rheumatoid arthritis. *J Rheumatol.* 18:140–149.

39. Prummel MF, Wiersinga WM, Lips P *et al.* (1991). The course of biochemical parameters of bone turnover during treatment with corticosteroids. *J Clin Endocrinol Metab.* 72:382–386.

40. Kotowicz MA, Hall S, Hunder GG *et al.* (1990). Relationship of glucocorticoid dosage to serum bone Gla-protein concentration in patients with rheumatologic disorders. *Arthritis Rheum.* 33:1487–1492.

41. Nielsen HK, Thomsen K, Eriksen EF *et al.* (1988). The effects of high-dose glucocorticoid administration on serum bone gamma carboxyglutamic acid-containing protein, serum alkaline phosphatase and vitamin D metabolites in normal subjects. *Bone Miner.* 4:105–113.

42. Stellon AJ, Webb A, Compston JE. (1988). Bone histomorphometry and structure in corticosteroid treated chronic active hepatitis. *Gut.* 29:378–384.

43. Weinstein RS, Jilka RL, Parfitt AM, Manolagas SC. (1998). Inhibition of osteoblastogenesis and promotion of apoptosis of osteoblasts and osteocytes by glucocorticoids. Potential mechanisms of their deleterious effects on bone. *J Clin Invest.* 102:274–282.

44. Jee WS, Park HZ, Roberts WE, Kenner GH. (1970). Corticosteroid and bone. *Am J Anat.* 129:477–479.

45. Fucik RF, Kukreja SC, Hargis GK *et al.* (1975). Effect of glucocorticoids on function of the parathyroid glands in man. *J Clin Endocrinol Metab.* 40:152–155.

46. Lukert BP, Adams JS. (1976). Calcium and phosphorus homeostasis in man. Effect of corticosteroids. *Arch Intern Med.* 136:1249–1253.

47. Hahn TJ, Hahn BH. (1976). Osteopenia in patients with rheumatic diseases: Principles of diagnosis and therapy. *Semin Arthritis Rheum.* 6:165–188.

48. Seeman E, Kumar R, Hunder GG *et al.* (1980). Production, degradation, and circulating levels of 1,25-dihydroxyvitamin D in health and in chronic glucocorticoid excess. *J Clin Invest.* 66:664–669.

49. Hahn TJ, Halstead LR, Baran DT. (1981). Effects off short term glucocorticoid administration on intestinal calcium absorption and circulating vitamin D metabolite concentrations in man. *J Clin Endocrinol Metab.* 52:111–115.

50. Klein RG, Arnaud SB, Gallagher JC *et al.* (1977). Intestinal calcium absorption in exogenous hypercortisonism. Role of 25-hydroxyvitamin D and corticosteroid dose. *J Clin Invest.* 60:253–259.

51. Kimberg DV, Baerg RD, Gershon E, Graudusius RT. (1971). Effect of cortisone treatment on the active transport of calcium by the small intestine. *J Clin Invest.* 50:1309–1321.

52. Suzuki Y, Ichikawa Y, Saito E, Homma M. (1983). Importance of increased urinary calcium excretion in the development of secondary hyperparathyroidism of patients under glucocorticoid therapy. *Metabolism.* 32:151–156.

53. Need AG. (1987). Corticosteroids and osteoporosis. *Aust N Z J Med.* 17:267–272.

54. Favus MJ, Walling MW, Kimberg DV. (1973). Effects of 1,25-dihydroxycholecalciferol on intestinal calcium transport in cortisone-treated rats. *J Clin Invest.* 52:1680–1685.

55. Eastell R, Reid DM, Compston J *et al.* (1998). A UK Consensus Group on management of glucocorticoid-induced osteoporosis: An update. *J Intern Med.* 244:271–292.

56. Pearce G, Tabensky DA, Delmas PD *et al.* (1998). Corticosteroid-induced bone loss in men. *J Clin Endocrinol Metab.* 83:801–806.

57. Jennings BH, Andersson KE, Johansson SA. (1991). The assessment of the systemic effects of inhaled glucocorticosteroids. The effects of inhaled budesonide vs oral prednisolone on calcium metabolism. *Eur J Clin Pharmacol.* 41:11–16.

58. Bikle DD, Halloran B, Fong L *et al.* (1993). Elevated 1,25-dihydroxyvitamin D levels in patients with chronic obstructive pulmonary disease treated with prednisone. *J Clin Endocrinol Metab.* 76:456–461.

59. Williams GA, Bowser EN, Henderson WJ, Uzgiries V. (1960). Calcium absorption in the rat in relation to excessive vitamin D and cortisone. *Proc Soc Exp Bio Med.* 5:354–358.

60. Hahn TJ, Halstead LR, Strates B *et al.* (1980). Comparison of subacute effects of oxazacort and prednisone on mineral metabolism in man. *Calcif Tissue Int.* 31:109–115.

61. Lekkerker JF, Van Woudenberg F, Doorenbos HD. (1972). Influence of low dose of sterol therapy on calcium absorption. *Acta Endocrinol (Copenh).* 69:488–496.

62. Sjoberg HE. (1970). Retention of orally administered 47-calcium in man under normal and diseased conditions studied with a whole-body counter technique. *Acta Med Scand Suppl.* 509:1–28.

63. Favus MJ, Kimberg DV, Millar GN, Gershon E. (1973). Effects of cortisone administration on the metabolism and localization of 25-hydroxycholecalciferol in the rat. *J Clin Invest.* 52:1328–1335.

64. Lindgren U, Lindholm S, Sarby B. (1978). Short-term effects of 1-alpha-hydroxy-vitamin D3 in patients on corticosteroid treatment and in patients with senile osteoporosis. *Acta Med Scand.* 204:89–92.

65. Adams JS, Wahl TO, Lukert BP. (1981). Effects of hydrochlorothiazide and dietary sodium restriction on calcium metabolism in corticosteroid treated patients. *Metabolism.* 30:217–221.

66. Findling JW, Adams ND, Lemann J Jr *et al.* (1982). Vitamin D metabolites and parathyroid hormone in Cushing's syndrome: Relationship to calcium and phosphorus homeostasis. *J Clin Endocrinol Metab.* 54:1039–1044.

67. Lee DB. (1983). Unanticipated stimulatory action of glucocorticoids on epithelial calcium absorption. Effect of dexamethasone on rat distal colon. *J Clin Invest.* 71:322–328.

68. Binder HJ. (1978). Effect of dexamethasone on electrolyte transport in the large intestine of the rat. *Gastroenterology.* 75:212–217.

69. Ferretti JL, Bazan JL, Alloatti D, Puche RC. (1978). The intestinal handling of calcium by the rat *in vivo*, as affected by cortisol. Effect of dietary calcium supplements. *Calcif Tissue Res.* 25:1–6.

70. Sasaki N, Kusano E, Ando Y *et al.* (2002). Changes in osteoprotegerin and markers of bone metabolism during glucocorticoid treatment in patients with chronic glomerulonephritis. *Bone.* 30:853–858.

71. Hahn TJ, Halstead LR, Teitelbaum SL, Hahn BH. (1979). Altered mineral metabolism in glucocorticoid-induced osteopenia. Effect of 25-hydroxyvitamin D administration. *J Clin Invest.* 64:655–665.

72. Hahn TJ, Halstead LR, Haddad JG Jr. (1977). Serum 25-hydroxyvitamin D concentrations in patients receiving chronic corticosteroid therapy. *J Lab Clin Med.* 90:399–404.

73. Chesney RW, Mazess RB, Hamstra AJ *et al.* (1978). Reduction of serum-1, 25-dihydroxyvitamin-D3 in children receiving glucocorticoids. *Lancet.* 2:1123–1125.

74. Godschalk M, Levy JR, Downs RW Jr. (1992). Glucocorticoids decrease vitamin D receptor number and gene expression in human osteosarcoma cells. *J Bone Miner Res.* 7:21–27.

75. Ho YV, Briganti EM, Duan Y *et al.* (1999). Polymorphism of the vitamin D receptor gene and corticosteroid-related osteoporosis. *Osteoporos Int.* 9: 134–138.

76. Sakakura M, Takebe K, Nakagawa S. (1975). Inhibition of luteinizing hormone secretion induced by synthetic LRH by long-term treatment with glucocorticoids in human subjects. *J Clin Endocrinol Metab.* 40:774–779.

77. Luton JP, Thieblot P, Valcke JC *et al.* (1977). Reversible gonadotropin deficiency in male Cushing's disease. *J Clin Endocrinol Metab.* 45:488–495.

78. Hsueh AJ, Erickson GF. (1978). Glucocorticoid inhibition of FSH-induced estrogen production in cultured rat granulosa cells. *Steroids.* 32:639–648.

79. Doerr P, Pirke KM. (1976). Cortisol-induced suppression of plasma testosterone in normal adult males. *J Clin Endocrinol Metab.* 43:622–629.

80. Schaison G, Durand F, Nakagawa S. (1987). Effect of glucocorticoids on plasma testosterone in men. *Acta Endocrinol (Copenh).* 89:126–131.

81. Crilly RG, Cawood M, Marchall DH, Nordin BE. (1978). Hormonal status in normal, osteoporotic and corticosteroid-treated postmenopausal women. *J R Soc Med.* 71:733–736.

82. Goulding A, Gold E. (1988). Effects of chronic prednisolone treatment on bone resorption and bone composition in intact and ovariectomized rats and in ovariectomized rats receiving beta-estradiol. *Endocrinology.* 122:482–487.

83. Vidal NO, Brandstrom H, Jonsson KB, Ohlsson C. (1998). Osteoprotegerin mRNA is expressed in primary human osteoblast-like cells: Down-regulation by glucocorticoids. *J Endocrinol.* 159:191–195.

84. Hofbauer LC, Gori F, Riggs BL *et al.* (1999). Stimulation of osteoprotegerin ligand and inhibition of osteoprotegerin production by glucocorticoids in human osteoblastic lineage cells: Potential paracrine mechanisms of glucocorticoid-induced osteoporosis. *Endocrinology.* 140:4382–4389.

85. Maldague B, Malghem J, de Deuxchaisnes C. (1984). Radiologic aspects of glucocorticoid-induced bone disease. *Adv Exp Med Biol.* 171:155–190.

86. Arden NK, Baker J, Hogg C *et al.* (1996). The heritability of bone mineral density, ultrasound of the calcaneus and hip axis length: A study of post-menopausal twins. *J Bone Miner Res.* 11:530–534.

87. Morrison D, Capewell S, Reynolds SP *et al.* (1994). Testosterone levels during systemic and inhaled corticosteroid therapy. *Respir Med.* 88:659–663.

88. Ross PD, Davis JW, Epstein RS, Wasnich RD. (1991). Pre-existing fractures and bone mass predict vertebral fracture incidence in women. *Ann Intern Med.* 114:919–923.

89. Kimble RB. (1997). Alcohol, cytokines, and estrogen in the control of bone remodeling. *Alcohol Clin Exp Res.* 21:385–391.

90. Ernst E. (1998). Exercise for female osteoporosis. A systematic review of randomised clinical trials. *Sports Med.* 25:359–368.

91. Egger P, Duggleby S, Hobbs R *et al.* (1996). Cigarette smoking and bone mineral density in the elderly. *J Epidemiol Community Health.* 50:47–50.

92. Nielsen HK, Charles P, Mosekilde L. (1988). The effect of single oral doses of prednisone on the circadian rhythm of serum osteocalcin in normal subjects. *J Clin Endocrinol Metab.* 67:1025–1030.

93. Garnero P, Shih WJ, Gineyts E *et al.* (1994). Comparison of new biochemical markers of bone turnover in late postmenopausal osteoporotic women in response to alendronate treatment. *J Clin Endocrinol Metab.* 79:1693–1700.

94. Ettinger B, Black DM, Mitlak BH *et al.* (1999). Reduction of vertebral fracture risk in postmenopausal women with osteoporosis treated with raloxifene: Results from a 3-year randomized clinical trial. Multiple Outcomes of Raloxifene Evaluation (MORE) Investigators. *JAMA.* 282: 637–645.

95. Black DM, Arden NK, Palermo L *et al.* (1999). Prevalent vertebral deformities predict hip fractures and new vertebral deformities but not wrist fractures. Study of Osteoporotic Fractures Research Group. *J Bone Miner Res.* 14:821–828.

96. Ross PD, Genant HK, Davis JW *et al.* (1993). Predicting vertebral fracture incidence from prevalent fractures and bone density among non-black, osteoporotic women. *Osteoporos Int.* 3:120–126.

97. Seeman E, Wahner HW, Offord KP *et al.* (1982). Differential effects of endocrine dysfunction on the axial and the appendicular skeleton. *J Clin Invest.* 69:1302–1309.

98. Marshall D, Johnell O, Wedel H. (1996). Meta-analysis of how well measures of bone mineral density predict occurrence of osteoporotic fractures. *BMJ.* 312:1254–1259.

99. Luengo M, Picado C, Del Rio L *et al.* (1991). Vertebral fractures in steroid dependent asthma and involutional osteoporosis: A comparative study. *Thorax.* 46:803–806.

100. Hough S, Teitelbaum SL, Bergfeld MA, Avioli LV. (1981). Isolated skeletal involvement in Cushing's syndrome: Response to therapy. *J Clin Endocrinol Metab.* 52:1033–1038.

101. Riggs BL, Jowsey J, Kelly PJ. (1966). Quantitative microradiographic study of bone remodeling in Cushing's syndrome. *Metabolism.* 15:773–780.

102. Gluck OS, Murphy WA, Hahn TJ, Hahn B. (1981). Bone loss in adults receiving alternate day glucocorticoid therapy. A comparison with daily therapy. *Arthritis Rheum.* 24:892–898.

103. Walsh LJ, Wong CA, Pringle M, Tattersfield AE. (1996). Use of oral corticosteroids in the community and the prevention of secondary osteoporosis: A cross sectional study. *BMJ.* 313:344–346.

104. Peat ID, Healy S, Reid DM, Ralston SH. (1995). Steroid induced osteoporosis: An opportunity for prevention? *Ann Rheum Dis.* 54:66–68.

105. Sambrook PN. (2000). Corticosteroid osteoporosis: Practical implications of recent trials. *J Bone Miner Res.* 15:1645–1649.

106. Reid DM, Hughes RA, Laan RF et al. (2000). Efficacy and safety of daily risedronate in the treatment of corticosteroid-induced osteoporosis in men and women: A randomized trial. European Corticosteroid-Induced Osteoporosis Treatment Study. *J Bone Miner Res.* 15:1006–1013.

107. Reid DM, Adami S, Devogelaer JP, Chines AA. (2001). Risedronate increases bone density and reduces vertebral fracture risk within one year in men on corticosteroid therapy. *Calcif Tissue Int.* 69:242–247.

108. Amin S, LaValley MP, Simms RW, Felson DT. (2002). The comparative efficacy of drug therapies used for the management of corticosteroid-induced osteoporosis: A meta-regression. *J Bone Miner Res.* 17:1512–1526.

109. Roux C, Oriente P, Laan R et al. (1998). Randomized trial of effect of cyclical etidronate in the prevention of corticosteroid-induced bone loss. Ciblos Study Group. *J Clin Endocrinol Metab.* 83:1128–1133.

110. Mulder H, Struys A. (1994). Intermittent cyclical etidronate in the prevention of corticosteroid-induced bone loss. *Br J Rheumatol.* 33:348–350.

111. Wolfhagen FH, van Buuren HR, den Ouden JW et al. (1997). Cyclical etidronate in the prevention of bone loss in corticosteroid-treated primary biliary cirrhosis. A prospective, controlled pilot study. *J Hepatol.* 26:325–330.

112. Skingle SJ, Crisp AJ. (1994). Increased bone density in patients on steroids with etidronate. *Lancet.* 344:543–544.

113. Boutsen Y, Jamart J, Esselinckx W, Devogelaer JP. (2001). Primary prevention of glucocorticoid-induced osteoporosis with intravenous pamidronate and calcium: A prospective controlled 1-year study comparing a single infusion, an infusion given once every 3 months, and calcium alone. *J Bone Miner Res.* 16:104–112.

114. Gonnelli S, Rottoli P, Cepollaro C et al. (1997). Prevention of corticosteroid-induced osteoporosis with alendronate in sarcoid patients. *Calcif Tissue Int.* 61:382–385.

115. Nordborg E, Schaufelberger C, Andersson R et al. (1997). The ineffectiveness of cyclical oral clodronate on bone mineral density in glucocorticoid-treated patients with giant-cell arteritis. *J Intern Med.* 242:367–371.

116. Pitt P, Li F, Todd P et al. (1998). A double blind placebo controlled study to determine the effects of intermittent cyclical etidronate on bone mineral density in patients on long-term oral corticosteroid treatment. *Thorax.* 53:351–356.

117. Geusens P, Dequeker J, Vanhoof J et al. (1998). Cyclical etidronate increases bone density in the spine and hip of postmenopausal women receiving long term corticosteroid treatment. A double blind, randomised placebo controlled study. *Ann Rheum Dis.* 57:724–727.

118. Worth H, Stammen D, Keck E. (1994). Therapy of steroid-induced bone loss in adult asthmatics with calcium, vitamin D, and a diphosphonate. *Am J Respir Crit Care Med.* 150:394–397.

119. Reid IR, King AR, Alexander CJ, Ibbertson HK. (1988). Prevention of steroid-induced osteoporosis with (3-amino-1-hydroxypropylidene)-1, 1-bisphosphonate (APD). *Lancet.* 1(8578):143–146.

120. Wallach S, Cohen S, Reid DM et al. (2000). Effects of risedronate treatment on bone density and vertebral fracture in patients on corticosteroid therapy. *Calcif Tissue Int.* 67:277–285.

121. Adachi JD, Pack S, Chines AA. (1997). Intermittent etidronate and corticosteroid-induced osteoporosis (abstract). *N Engl J Med.* 337:1921.

122. Lukert BP, Johnson BE, Robinson RG. (1992). Estrogen and progesterone replacement therapy reduces glucocorticoid-induced bone loss. *J Bone Miner Res.* 7:1063–1069.

123. Hall GM, Daniels M, Doyle DV, Spector TD. (1994). Effect of hormone replacement therapy on bone mass in rheumatoid arthritis patients treated with and without steroids. *Arthritis Rheum.* 37:1499–505.

124. Delmas PD, Bjarnason NH, Mitlak BH et al. (1997). Effects of raloxifene on bone mineral density, serum cholesterol concentrations, and uterine endometrium in postmenopausal women. *N Engl J Med.* 337:1641–1647.

125. Sambrook P, Birmingham J, Kelly P et al. (1993). Prevention of corticosteroid bone loss. *Osteoporos Int.* 3(Suppl 1):141–143.

126. Adachi JD, Bensen WG, Bell MJ et al. (1997). Salmon calcitonin nasal spray in the prevention of corticosteroid-induced osteoporosis. *Br J Rheumatol.* 36:255–259.

127. Luengo M, Picado C, Del Rio L et al. (1990). Treatment of steroid-induced osteopenia with calcitonin in corticosteroid-dependent asthma. A one-year follow-up study. *Am Rev Respir Dis.* 142:104–107.

128. Luengo M, Pons F, Martinez de Osaba MJ, Picado C. (1994). Prevention of further bone mass loss by nasal calcitonin in patients on long term glucocorticoid therapy for asthma: A two year follow up study. *Thorax.* 49:1099–1102.

129. Ringe JD, Welzel D. (1987). Salmon calcitonin in the therapy of corticoid-induced osteoporosis. *Eur J Clin Pharmacol.* 33:35–39.

130. Kotaniemi A, Piirainen H, Paimela L et al. (1996). Is continuous intranasal salmon calcitonin effective in treating axial bone loss in patients with active rheumatoid arthritis receiving low dose glucocorticoid therapy? *J Rheumatol.* 23:1875–1879.

131. Lems WF, Jacobs JW, Bijlsma JW et al. (1997). Is addition of sodium fluoride to cyclical etidronate beneficial in the treatment of corticosteroid induced osteoporosis? *Ann Rheum Dis.* 56:357–363.

132. Lems WF, Jacobs WG, Bijlsma JW et al. (1997). Effect of sodium fluoride on the prevention of corticosteroid-induced osteoporosis. *Osteoporos Int.* 7:575–782.

133. Guaydier-Souquieres G, Kotzki PO, Sabatier JP et al. (1996). In corticosteroid-treated respiratory diseases, monofluorophosphate increases lumbar bone density: A double-masked randomized study. *Osteoporos Int.* 6:171–177.

134. Rizzoli R, Chevalley T, Slosman DO, Bonjour JP. (1995). Sodium mono-fluorophosphate increases vertebral bone mineral density in patients with corticosteroid-induced osteoporosis. *Osteoporos Int.* 5:39–46.

135. Lane NE, Sanchez S, Modin GW et al. (1998). Parathyroid hormone treatment can reverse corticosteroid-induced osteoporosis. Results of a randomized controlled clinical trial. *J Clin Invest.* 102:1627–1633.

136. Reid IR, Wattie DJ, Evans MC, Stapleton JP. (1996). Testosterone therapy in glucocorticoid-treated men. *Arch Intern Med.* 156:1173–1177.

137. Adami S, Fossaluzza V, Rossini M et al. (1991). The prevention of corticosteroid-induced osteoporosis with nandrolone decanoate. *Bone Miner.* 15:73–81.

138. Bernstein CN, Seeger LL, Anton PA et al. (1996). A randomized, placebo-controlled trial of calcium supplementation for decreased bone density in corticosteroid-using patients with inflammatory bowel disease: A pilot study. *Aliment Pharmacol Ther.* 10:777–786.

139. Reginster JY, Kuntz D, Verdickt W et al. (1999). Prophylactic use of alfacalcidol in corticosteroid-induced osteoporosis. *Osteoporos Int.* 9:75–81.

140. Buckley LM, Leib ES, Cartularo KS et al. (1996). Calcium and vitamin D3 supplementation prevents bone loss in the spine secondary to low-dose corticosteroids in patients with rheumatoid arthritis. A randomized, double-blind, placebo-controlled trial. *Ann Intern Med.* 125:961–968.

141. Bijlsma JW, Raymakers JA, Mosch C et al. (1988). Effect of oral calcium and vitamin D on glucocorticoid-induced osteopenia. *Clin Exp Rheumatol.* 6:113–119.

142. Dykman TR, Haralson KM, Gluck OS et al. (1984). Effect of oral 1,25-dihydroxyvitamin D and calcium on glucocorticoid-induced osteopenia in patients with rheumatic diseases. *Arthritis Rheum.* 27:1336–1343.

143. Amin S, LaValley MP, Simms RW, Felson DT. (1999). The role of vitamin D in corticosteroid-induced osteoporosis: A meta-analytic approach. *Arthritis Rheum.* 42:1740–1751.

144. Alon U, Costanzo LS, Chan JC. (1984). Additive hypocalciuric effects of amiloride and hydrochlorothiazide in patients treated with calcitriol. *Miner Electrolyte Metab.* 10:379–386.

145. Aman S, Hakala M, Silvennoinen J et al. (1998). Low incidence of osteoporosis in a two year follow-up of early community based patients with rheumatoid arthritis. *Scand J Rheumatol.* 27:188–193.

146. Kroger H, Honkanen R, Saarikoski S, Alhava E. (1994). Decreased axial bone mineral density in perimenopausal women with rheumatoid arthritis—a population based study. *Ann Rheum Dis.* 53:18–23.

147. Sambrook P, Birmingham J, Kempler S et al. (1990). Corticosteroid effects on proximal femur bone loss. *J Bone Miner Res.* 5:1211–1216.

148. Locascio V, Bonucci E, Imbimbo B et al. (1990). Bone loss in response to long-term glucocorticoid therapy. *Bone Miner.* 8:39–51.

149. Mckay LI, DuBois DC, Sun YN et al. (1997). Corticosteroid effects in skeletal muscle: Gene induction/receptor autoregulation. *Muscle Nerve.* 20:1318–1320.

150. Van Balkom RH, Zhan WZ, Prakash YS et al. (1997). Corticosteroid effects on isotonic contractile properties of rat diaphragm muscle. *J Appl Physiol.* 83:1062–1067.

151. Gibson JN, Poyser NL, Morrison WL et al. (1991). Muscle protein synthesis in patients with rheumatoid arthritis: Effect of chronic corticosteroid therapy on prostaglandin F2 alpha availability. *Eur J Clin Invest.* 21:406–412.

152. Danneskiold-Samsoe B, Grimby G. (1986). Isokinetic and isometric muscle strength in patients with rheumatoid arthritis. The relationship to clinical parameters and the influence of corticosteroid. *Clin Rheumatol.* 5:459–567.

153. Danneskiold-Samsoe B, Grimby G. (1986). Muscle morphology and enzymes in proximal and distal muscle groups of lower limb from patients with corticosteroid treated rheumatoid arthritis: The relationship to maximal isokinetic muscle strength. *Clin Sci (Lond).* 71:685–691.

154. Shaw JM, Snow CM. (1998). Weighted vest exercise improves indices of fall risk in older women. *J Gerontol A Biol Sci Med Sci.* 53:M53–M58.

155. Nelson ME, Fiatarone MA, Morganti CM *et al.* (1994). Effects of high-intensity strength training on multiple risk factors for osteoporotic fractures. A randomized controlled trial. *JAMA*. 272:1909–1914.

156. Hickson RC, Davis JR. (1981). Partial prevention of glucocorticoid-induced muscle atrophy by endurance training. *Am J Physiol*. 241: E226–E232.

157. Hickson RC, Kurowski TT, Andrews GH *et al.* (1986). Glucocorticoid cytosol binding in exercise-induced sparing of muscle atrophy. J Appl Physiol. 60:1413–1419.

158. Czerwinski SM, Kurowski TG, O'Neill TM, Hickson RC. (1987). Initiating regular exercise protects against muscle atrophy from glucocorticoids. *J Appl Physiol*. 63:1504–1510.

92

Anabolic Therapy of Osteoporosis in Women and in Men

MISHAELA R. RUBIN, MD* AND JOHN P. BILEZIKIAN, MD**

*Department of Medicine, College of Physicians and Surgeons, Columbia University, New York, NY
**Professor of Medicine and of Pharmacology and Chief, Division of Endocrinology,
College of Physicians and Surgeons, Columbia University, New York, NY

I. Introduction

Osteoporosis is the most prevalent metabolic bone disease in the world [1]. The prevalence of the disease is much greater in women, although it is becoming increasingly well-recognized in men [2]. Based on recent data from the National Osteoporosis Foundation, about 28 to 32 million women and 10 to 12 million men in the United States have either osteopenia (low bone mass) or osteoporosis [3]. The basic pathogenesis of osteoporosis in women and men is fundamentally similar. Bone is lost because of an imbalance, in both sexes, between bone resorption and formation. The remodeling process by which skeletal strength is maintained leads to bone loss because with aging less new bone is formed when old bone is resorbed. The net effect is bone loss.

However, despite common themes in underlying pathogenesis, osteoporosis clearly differs in men and women with regard to some pathophysiologic elements. In women, the imbalance between bone resorption and formation accelerates dramatically at menopause. Estrogen loss precipitates an increase in bone remodeling. Because bone remodeling in the adult skeleton leads to net loss of bone (more bone is resorbed than formed for each bone remodeling unit), when bone turnover is accelerated, as is the case at the time of menopause, bone loss is accelerated [4]. Men have no equivalent, well-defined midlife event that leads to acute loss of sex steroids, although it is now clear that estrogen deficiency in the male, a more gradual process, is also profoundly detrimental to his skeletal health [5]. For this and a variety of other reasons, women fracture more often than men [6]. The purpose of this chapter is 2-fold: first, we review discrepancies between the two sexes in relation to osteoporosis, and, second, we compare the mechanisms of the two available categories of osteoporosis therapy, antiresorptive and anabolic agents.

II. Skeletal Differences Between Women and Men

The first manifestations of male and female skeletal dimorphism are detected at puberty. As boys and girls enter puberty, they both experience an increase in bone size resulting from an enlargement of the outer diameter of bone and a concomitant widening of the medullary diameter. The result is an increase in areal bone density (g/cm^2) but not a major increase in volumetric density (g/cm^3) of the long bones. Nevertheless, the enlarged cross-sectional diameter gives bone, for the same volumetric density, greater strength [7,8]. The increase in bone size is believed to be primarily an effect of androgens. The mechanical

effect places cortical mass further from the neutral axis of long bone, thus conferring greater resistance to bending. Although these changes in geometry occur in both sexes, they occur to a substantially greater extent in the growing male skeleton than in the growing female skeleton. This is due in part to the fact that as the female skeleton grows, thickening of the inner bone shaft adjacent to the marrow, or endocortical apposition, predominates. This is stimulated primarily by estrogen, which simultaneously acts to inhibit periosteal apposition. A more complete discussion of the ways in which the sex steroids affect geometrical, densitometric, and structural parameters of bone are found in Chapter 94.

In both genders, thinning of the bone cortex occurs over time. Bone resorption occurs in men and women on the endocortical and trabecular surfaces of the mineralized skeleton, producing bone loss and cortical and trabecular thinning [9]. The amount of bone lost on the inner surfaces of bone with aging is equivalent in men and women [10]. To offset bone loss on the inner endocortical surface of bone, compensatory new bone formation occurs on the outer periosteal surface [11]. The male skeleton is more adept than the female skeleton at this compensatory process, leading to male bones that actually enlarge with aging [12]. Despite the age-related thinning of cortices, for the same degree of volumetric bone loss, the aging male bone maintains its strength better because of this geometric adjustment [8]. When bone density is measured by dual–energy x-ray absorptiometry (DXA) (a two-dimensional test), age-related bone loss appears to be slower in the male than in the female because the loss in true bone density (g/cm^3) is compensated more effectively by an increase in areal density (g/cm^2). Although bone mass measurements with technologies like DXA have been criticized because they do not measure true bone density, they do nevertheless provide information that takes into account changes in bone size, an important determinant of bone strength. A densitometer that measures volumetric density directly such as quantitative computed tomography (QCT) is not influenced by changes in bone size.

III. The Importance of Bone Mineral Density and Other Bone Qualities

Osteoporosis is defined in densitometric terms because reduced bone mass is the most important predictor of fracture risk [13]. In this critical respect, therefore, bone mineral density (BMD) reflects bone quality. As BMD decreases, fracture risk

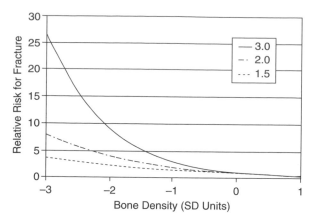

Fig. 92-1 Exponential relationship between bone density and fracture risk. Curves are shown for odds ratios 1.5, 2.0, and 3.0 per standard deviation (SD) change in bone density. (From Faulkner KG. [2000]. Bone matters: Are density increases necessary to reduce fracture risk? *J Bone Miner Res.* 15:183–187, with permission.)

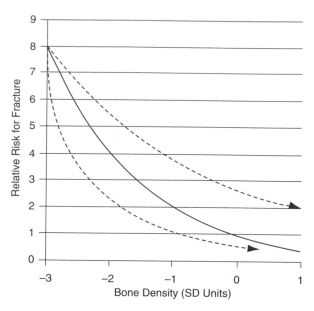

Fig. 92-2 Hysteresis effect for bone density (shown in standard deviation units) and fracture risk. The fracture risk curve based on observational data is shown as the solid line, indicating the increase in risk for a given decrease in bone density. The dashed lines represent potential variations in the bone density/fracture risk relationship as bone density increases (and fracture risk decreases) resulting from therapeutic intervention. Note that the density/fracture risk curve is not necessarily bidirectional. (From Faulkner KG. [2000]. Bone matters: Are density increases necessary to reduce fracture risk? *J Bone Miner Res.* 15:183–187, with permission.)

increases [14,15] (Fig. 92-1). The correlation between bone density and bone strength, in subjects who have not been treated for osteoporosis, is linear and powerful [16].

However, bone density is only one of several measures of bone strength. Factors other than BMD contribute to aggregate fracture risk. In some situations, high BMD is not necessarily beneficial as shown well by the experience with fluoride in the treatment of osteoporosis. Moreover, in patients with identical bone densities, fracture risk can be variable depending on age [17], gender [18], and race [19]. Although BMD alone does not predict fracture risk completely, improvements in BMD, in response to therapy do not completely account for the reduction in fracture risk [14] (Fig. 92-2). Small increases in BMD with antiresorptive agents can lead to impressive decreases in fracture rate. [21,22] Clearly, there are other factors that contribute to increased and decreased fracture risk. Other determinants of bone quality, including microarchitecture, turnover, microfractures, and mineralization, have thus emerged as important contributors to fracture risk and therapeutic benefit.

IV. Antiresorptives

Until now, the mainstay of therapy for osteoporosis in women, and more recently in men, has been antiresorptive in mechanism. Drugs such as estrogen, raloxifene, alendronate, risedronate, and calcitonin all inhibit osteoclast-mediated bone loss and, thus, reduce bone turnover [23–26]. By reducing bone turnover, these antiresorptive drugs allow bone formation to proceed more completely while bone resorption is inhibited. The remodeling space containing unmineralized bone is replaced in part by more mineralized bone. The measured parameter is an increase in bone density, but there is no net increase in bone formed. The increase in bone density is variable depending on the site and the drug, but typically ranges between 4 to 8% over 3 years [20,29]. Both sexes respond to these antiresorptives with a reduction in fracture risk [18,30].

Antiresorptive drugs reduce the occurrence of fracture to a greater extent than would be predicted by the magnitude of

the increase in BMD alone [21,22]. As much as 30 to 50% of the decrease in fracture risk with antiresorptives cannot be accounted for by changes in BMD [31,32]. This disproportionate reduction in fracture risk with only a modest increase in bone mass could be explained by considering the power function of the relationship between bone mass and fracture risk [33]. For example, data with raloxifene predict a 10% reduction in fracture risk for an average 2.5% gain in BMD, but instead a 50% decrease in fracture risk is observed [34]. Moreover, if all the antiresorptive agents are considered over the wide spectrum of their effects on bone density, they all seem to reduce vertebral fracture incidence to a similar degree [21,22,31,32,34,35]. Finally, the majority of the effect of bisphosphonates on fracture reduction is achieved during the early phase of treatment [35,36], well before changes in BMD have reached their maximum [37]. To account further for these observations, it is possible that the relationship between fracture incidence and an increase in BMD is not the same as the relationship between fracture incidence and a decrease in BMD. Such concerns between two variables when considered in the "forwards and backwards" directions have been considered by Faulkner [14].

A. Bone Turnover and Antiresorptives

In normal bone remodeling, osteoclast precursors are initially activated, leading to bone cavities and removal of old bone. Osteoblasts then proceed to lay down unmineralized osteoid, which eventually becomes fully mineralized bone. In a high turnover state, such as estrogen deficiency, many active remodeling sites are underfilled throughout the skeleton. High bone turnover increases the number of resorption cavities, which act as stress-risers, along the length of trabeculae [38]. These sites of active bone turnover can be points of weakness when the vertical strut is exposed to force. It is a weak link in a chain. As a function of how many weak links are present, the likelihood of fracture is increased. Bone turnover has been shown to correlate with fractures directly and independently of BMD [39,40]. Increased turnover, together with decreased BMD, better predict fracture than does either factor alone. It is thus logical to expect that when bone turnover is reduced by antiresorptive agents, the number and depth of resorption sites and thus stress-risers will decrease [41]. There will be fewer sites at which forces can lead to breakage; the bone will be stronger. For the bisphosphonates, reduced bone turnover occurs, in part, through induction of osteoclast apoptosis [42]. Hochberg et al [43] have shown that the antifracture efficacy of antiresorptive drugs can be explained best by considering both increases in bone density and reductions in bone turnover.

B. Microarchitecture and Antiresorptives

Microarchitectural changes also contribute to fracture risk [44]. Increased osteoclast activity that is associated with high bone turnover states in postmenopausal women leads to perforation of cancellous plates, loss of trabeculae, and trabecular discontinuity [45]. Because much of the strength of cancellous bone is derived from its microarchitectural organization, the loss of trabecular connectivity predisposes to vertebral fracture. Preserving the trabecular network (i.e., preventing a loss in number of trabeculae) is even more important for bone strength than maintaining trabecular thickness [46]. When the trabecular network becomes discontinuous because of perforations, more likely to occur in the context of excessive remodeling, bone strength is affected without any necessary change in bone density. With aging, preferential loss of horizontal trabeculae in vertebrae occurs [47]. Bracing of structural elements is analogous to the function of architectural "flying buttresses"; a slender column will buckle depending on the length of the column. With additional horizontal trabecular elements, the effective length of the column is decreased and the effective strength is increased. The horizontal trabeculae thus act as cross-ties. Their loss leaves the vertical trabeculae, which are subject to compressive force, vulnerable to buckling and failure [48]. The lack of cross-ties dramatically reduces the strength of the remaining trabeculae, because the strength of the trabeculae is inversely proportional to the square of its effective length [49]. A doubling of effective length weakens the trabeculae by a factor of four. Evidence has recently been provided that argues for microarchitectural effects following the use of bisphosphonates. Recent work in minipigs [48] and in human subjects with the bisphosphonate risedronate show that cross-ties are preserved and plate-like structures of trabeculae are maintained. There is no evidence at this time, however, that the bisphosphonates actually improve microarchitectural qualities of bone. Nevertheless, the fact that they preserve these elements is an important observation.

C. Changes in Mineralization and Antiresorptives

Mineralization is mainly a passive process that follows the deposition of the organic matrix. It is enhanced when bone remodeling is retarded. There are two phases to mineralization. Initially, soon after osteoid is formed, mineralization follows rapidly. The second phase is a slower one, progressing until mineralization is complete. With inhibition of bone turnover, antiresorptive drugs provide more opportunity for secondary mineralization [50–52]. Changes in mineral content, as measured by ash fraction, have a profound effect on increasing bone strength [53]. Using newer methods such a quantitative back scattered electron imaging (qBEI), Roschger et al [54] showed that the bisphosphonate alendronate increases mineralization of bone. With conventional technology such as DXA, this property of the bisphosphonates is measured as part of the increase in BMD.

D. Osteocytes and Antiresorptives

The health of the osteocyte probably plays an important role in fracture prevention. The osteocyte acts as a mechanosensor and regulates the bone remodeling process [55]. Antiresorptive drugs prevent osteocyte apoptosis [56], providing another mechanism through which bone strength is enhanced.

V. Anabolics

Anabolic agents represent an important new advance in the therapy of osteoporosis for both men and women. The concept of an anabolic agent is based on a therapeutic mechanism entirely distinct from inhibition of bone resorption. Anabolic agents directly stimulate bone formation, at least in the early phases of their action, and improve the microarchitecture of bone. Bone is literally reconstructed, an effect not observed with the antiresorptives. Hence, anabolic agents have the potential to increase bone mass to a greater extent than antiresorptives. The potential of anabolic agents to improve the microarchitectural qualities of bone suggests that they might reduce fracture risk to a greater extent than the antiresorptives. The most promising anabolic agent to date is parathyroid hormone (PTH).

A. Basic Principle Accounting for Parathyroid Hormone as an Anabolic Therapy for Osteoporosis

Continuous secretion of PTH elicits a catabolic response in the skeleton, particularly at cortical sites. The demonstration of preferential cortical bone loss in primary hyperparathyroidism illustrates well this general catabolic action of PTH at a site enriched in cortical bone, such as the distal one third of the radius. [57,58]. On the other hand, when PTH is administered in low dose and intermittently, its anabolic properties predominate. This effect is observed most dramatically in the cancellous skeleton. In contrast to bisphosphonates, where gains in BMD can be attributed to a reduction in the remodeling space and increased mineralization of bone [51], new bone is likely to be formed with PTH. Microarchitectural qualities, such as enhanced connectivity, can be shown directly and are illustrated subsequently.

B. Cellular and Regulatory Mechanisms of Teriparatide Action

Possible cellular mechanisms for the anabolic effects of PTH include stimulation of growth factors, especially insulin-like growth factor-1 (IGF-1) [59–66], and unique subsets of bone-forming genes [67], including gene expression of osteocalcin and tartrate-resistant acid phosphatase (TRAP) [68]. In addition, intermittent PTH appears to prevent osteoblast and osteocyte apoptosis [69] and to prevent an increase in receptor activator of nuclear factor-κ ligand (RANKL), an osteoclast-enhancing cytokine [70,71]. An extensive animal literature supports increases in cancellous bone with PTH administration [61–66,69,72,73]. Recent animal data also suggest that cortical bone might be similarly enhanced [74–76]. Basic fibroblast growth factor (FGF-2) has also been found to be a critical mediator of the anabolic effect of PTH on bone in mice [77]. Most recently, it was shown that the L-type calcium channel mediates mechanically induced bone adaptation to PTH *in vivo* [78]. Lane *et al* [79] have found that administration of PTH in glucocorticoid-induced osteoporosis (GIO) might increase osteoclast activity by stimulating osteoblast production of RANKL, the osteoclast-enhancing cytokine [79].

C. Therapy of Osteoporosis with Teriparatide

Most of the data with PTH as an anabolic agent in human subjects comes from use of the fragment PTH (1–34), a molecule that is foreshortened from the full-length, intact 1–84 hormone but which appears to contain all the known anabolic properties of PTH. This fragment is known generically as teriparatide. Teriparatide refers either to synthetic human PTH (1–34) or recombinant human PTH (1–34). In this discussion, PTH is referred to as teriparatide because the data reviewed are either based on the synthetic or the recombinant molecule.

In November, 2002, rhPTH (1–34) was approved by the Food and Drug Administration (FDA) for the treatment of osteoporosis in postmenopausal women and in men with osteoporosis at high risk for fracture. Although information is available at two low doses of teriparatide, only the 20 μg dose is approved for use. Reviewed here are data for both the specific agent that was approved and for synthetic hPTH (1–34).

D. Teriparatide as Monotherapy in Postmenopausal Osteoporosis

As a single therapy, PTH has been studied in postmenopausal osteoporotic women. One randomized, placebo-controlled trial demonstrated a nearly 7% increase (p < 0.001) in spine BMD with virtually no change in femoral BMD and a slight decrease in total body BMD [81,82]. The seminal clinical trial of Neer *et al* tested daily administration of 20 or 40 μg of subcutaneous teriparatide in 1637 women with postmenopausal osteoporosis (i.e., low BMD and fractures) in a randomized, placebo-controlled design [92]. Median follow-up was 21 months. For the two doses of PTH, spine BMD increased 10 to 14%. Femoral BMD also increased significantly by approximately 3%. There was no change in cortical bone density but total body BMD increased significantly as well. As compared with placebo,

PTH reduced the risk of one or more new vertebral fractures by 65 and 69%, at the two doses respectively. New total nonvertebral fractures were reduced by 35 and 40%, respectively. When only fragility fractures were considered (not total nonvertebral fractures), the reduction in new nonvertebral fractures was 53% and 54%, respectively. Among the women with new vertebral fractures, mean loss in height was greater in the placebo group (−1.1 cm) than in the 20 μg and 40 μg PTH groups (−0.2 and −0.3 cm, respectively; p=0.002). Back pain was significantly reduced in the PTH group. Adverse events were uncommon. Nausea and headache occurred only in the higher 40 μg dose. Sustained increases in serum calcium above the normal range were significant only in the 40-μg dose (11%). The only adverse event that was greater than placebo in the approved 20 μg dose was leg cramping (not thrombophlebitis). There was no increase in the incidence of hypercalciuria or urolithiasis at either dose.

This pivotal trial was followed by an observational, follow-up period in which study subjects were given the option of switching to a bisphosphonate or not taking any further medications. Of the original cohort in the Neer *et al* study [92], 77% of the women were followed. A majority (60%) were treated with antiresorptive therapy after discontinuation of PTH. The effect of previous therapy with teriparatide and/or subsequent therapy with bisphosphonate to prevent fractures persisted for as long as 31 months after the discontinuation of treatment [113]. Non-vertebral fragility fractures were reported by proportionally fewer women previously treated with PTH (with or without a bisphosphonate) as compared with those treated with placebo (p < 0.03). Similarly, changes from baseline lumbar spine bone density remained significantly higher in the original PTH-treated groups. The data, however, do not indicate whether the administration of bisphosphonate was important in the subsequent maintenance of bone mass. In studies in the men treated with teriparatide (summarized later), the use of an antiresorptive after teriparatide would seem to be a key factor.

E. Combination Therapy with Teriparatide and an Antiresorptive Agent

The rationale for combination therapy with an antiresorptive is to control the increased remodeling space created by PTH exposure and thus provide even more impressive net gains in bone formation. Combined therapy with PTH and estrogen was studied by Lindsay *et al* in a 3-year randomized controlled trial of 52 postmenopausal osteoporotic women who were on at least 1 year of hormone replacement therapy [84]. The group receiving PTH had significant increases in bone density of 13% at the spine, 4.4% at the hip, and 3.7% in the total body (Fig. 92-3). It is noteworthy that bone density in the vertebral spine continued to increase in a linear fashion for the entire 3-year study. At the distal radius, there was neither bone gain nor bone loss. Although the numbers were small, teriparatide significantly reduced the percentage of women who had a vertebral fracture, based on a reduction in loss of vertebral height. Bone formation markers (osteocalcin) rose before bone resorption markers (N-telopeptide) during the first 6 months, followed by a return of both indices to baseline values within 2.5 years of initiation of treatment. It is of interest that the

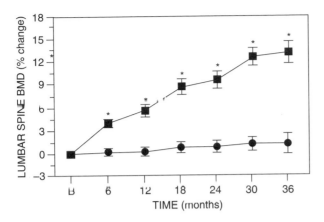

Fig. 92-3 The effect of parathyroid hormone (PTH) in women being treated with estrogen. Changes in lumbar spine bone mass when estrogen was given with (■) or without (●) PTH over 3 years to postmenopausal osteoporotic women. (From Cosman F, Nieves J, Woelfert L *et al.* [2001]. Parathyroid hormone added to established hormone therapy: Effects on vertebral fracture and maintenance of bone mass after parathyroid hormone withdrawal. *J Bone Miner Res.* 16:925–931, with permission.)

return of bone markers to baseline values was not associated with a reduction in the rate of bone gain in the vertebral spine, which continued for the entire 3-year period. Increases in bone density at the cortical skeleton were also observed, albeit at a more modest pace, reaching statistical significance.

Roe *et al* have obtained data from a study in postmenopausal women that was similar in design to the study of Lindsay *et al*. Women who were all on estrogen replacement therapy received teriparatide or no therapy except estrogen. The placebo group did not receive an injection. Using QCT, a technology that measures rather specifically cancellous bone of the lumbar spine, increases in vertebral BMD approached 80% after 2 years [85].

Recently, preliminary results of PTH administered with alendronate for 12 months to 93 postmenopausal women were presented [86]. Although the addition of alendronate limited the PTH-induced increases in bone formation, the effects of PTH on vertebral BMD were not compromised. In addition, alendronate seemed to minimize PTH-induced cortical bone loss.

F. Combination Therapy with Teriparatide and an Antiresorptive Agent in Glucocorticoid-induced Osteoporosis

Glucocorticoid-induced osteoporosis is characterized by prolonged suppression of bone formation and transient increases in bone resorption. A secondary increase in PTH is no longer considered by many to be of major pathophysiologic importance in GIO [87]. Hence, the use of PTH in combination with an antiresorptive to treat GIO has an appealing rationale. Lane *et al* conducted a 12-month, randomized, controlled trial of 51 postmenopausal women on hormone replacement therapy and glucocorticoids (>5 mg/day prednisone), who were randomized to hPTH (1–34) for 1 year or not (placebo injections were not used). By QCT, vertebral bone density increased 35% and by DXA 11%. Total hip bone density increased by 2% in the PTH group, whereas there was no difference in forearm BMD between groups. Bone markers showed an increase of bone

formation in the first 3 months, whereas resorption peaked later at 6 months [88].

G. Teriparatide in Men with Osteoporosis

The first randomized, controlled trial of PTH in men with idiopathic osteoporosis was carried out by Kurland *et al* [89]; 23 men, 30 to 68 years old, with idiopathic osteoporosis as defined by z-scores less than −2.0 at the lumbar spine or femoral neck and no definable cause for bone loss, were randomized to hPTH (1–34) 400 U/day or placebo in a double-blind experimental design for 18 months. The men who received PTH demonstrated an impressive increase in lumbar spine bone density from the beginning to the end of the 18-month trial, culminating in a 13.5% increase of lumbar spine bone density (Fig. 92-4). Hip bone density increased, but the changes were slower and not as robust, although significant. Cortical bone density did not increase in comparison to placebo. Bone turnover markers increased quickly and substantially in the men treated with PTH, with the bone formation markers rising and peaking earlier than the bone resorption markers. Both sets of bone markers returned to or toward baseline by 18 months. A baseline resorption marker (pyridinoline) and a 3-month post-treatment bone formation marker (osteocalcin) were the best predictors of the ultimate densitometric response to PTH [90].

More recently, results from a larger randomized, controlled trial of PTH in men have confirmed the findings of Kurland and colleagues [89]. Four hundred thirty-seven men with idiopathic or hypogonadal osteoporosis were randomized to either placebo or hPTH (1–34) 20 µg daily or 40 µg daily for a mean of 11 months [91]. Bone mineral density increased significantly at the lumbar spine in the treatment groups by 6% and 9%, respectively, regardless of gonadal status. The increase in bone density at the lumbar spine and the hip mirrored the increased in bone density at those sites in women from the study of identical experimental design reported earlier by Neer *et al* [92]. When the study was discontinued, the men were given the option to switch to a bisphosphonate in an open-label extension. When the group was considered together, irrespective of whether they did or did not take bisphosphonate, there was a 50% reduction in vertebral fracture risk 18 months after PTH was discontinued [91].

Parathyroid hormone has also been administered in combination with alendronate in men [93]. Eighty-three men with osteoporosis were treated for 18 months with alendronate, PTH, or both; PTH was begun at month 6. Parathyroid hormone and alendronate were superior to PTH alone for total body BMD, but, as observed in women treated with PTH and alendronate [86], alendronate may diminish the anabolic effect of PTH on spine BMD.

H. Mechanisms of the Anabolic Actions of Teriparatide

Earlier in this chapter, effects of bone density and bone turnover markers were considered in the light of antiresorptive agents. For PTH, clearly changes in bone density are important, as is the temporal discordance between bone formation and bone resorption markers. In this section, we concentrate on specific mechanisms by which PTH appears to provide its efficacious actions.

A

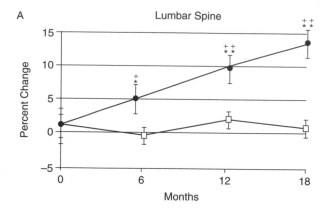

B

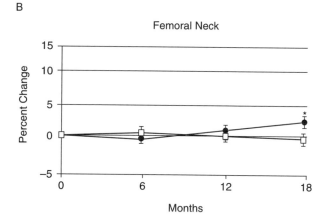

C

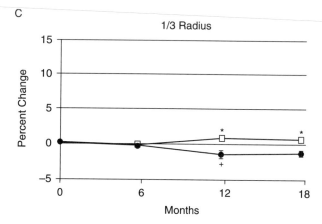

Fig. 92-4 Changes in bone density after parathyroid hormone (PTH) (1–34) treatment in men with idiopathic osteoporosis. Bone density at lumbar spine (A), femoral neck (B), and one-third site of the distal radius (C) in men receiving PTH (●) and in controls (□). The data are shown as percent changes from baseline ± standard error of measurement (SEM) for lumbar spine, FN, and ⅓ radius. *, $p < 0.05$ for repeated measures analysis of between-group comparisons; **, $p < 0.005$ for repeated measures analysis of between-group comparisons; +, $p < 0.05$ for repeated measures analysis of within-group comparisons between baseline and 6, 12, or 18 months; ++, $p < 0.005$ for repeated measures analysis of within-group comparisons between baseline and 6, 12, or 18 months. (From Kurland ES, Cosman F, McMahon D *et al.* [2000]. Parathyroid hormone as a therapy for idiopathic osteoporosis in men: Effects on bone mineral density and bone markers. *J Clin Endocrinol Metab.* 85:3069–3076, with permission.)

1. Bone Turnover and Teriparatide

An important characteristic of intermittent PTH therapy is stimulation of bone turnover, which marks an important distinction from the antiresorptives in which inhibition of bone turnover is the rule. The data suggest that there is a temporal uncoupling between bone turnover markers. Initially, bone formation markers rise rapidly, as early as 1 week after therapy with intermittent teriparatide has been initiated. Several months thereafter bone resorption markers increase. These kinetics provide a specific period of time when PTH is maximally anabolic and can be viewed as an "anabolic window," the time period between the increase in bone formation markers and the increase in bone resorption markers. Data suggest that the resorptive phase of the remodeling cycle is essentially bypassed for the first 6 months of therapy [84]. This allows for a substantial gain in bone mass before the number of resorption cavities, or stress-risers, begins to increase. Histomorphometric data confirm that PTH increases the bone formation rate within a few weeks on the periosteal and the endocortical and cancellous surfaces [94]. In time, both formation and resorption markers decline toward or to baseline levels [84,95].

2. Microarchitecture and Teriparatide

Histomorphometric analysis of paired biopsies before and after treatment with PTH are available for men and women from the studies of Lindsay *et al* and Kurland *et al*. Using standard two-dimensional static and dynamic histomorphometry and three-dimensional microcomputed tomographic analysis in tetracycline-labeled samples, it was possible to show not only quantitative improvements in cancellous bone indices but also major improvements in indices of connectivity (Fig. 92-5) [94]. Trabecular elements that were separated by short distances seemed to become connected or reconnected, because the increase in connectivity density was associated with improvements in trabecular number and thickness. Connectivity was actually augmented, as documented by a shortening of the marrow star volume, which measures the distance from central bone elements to the outer struts [96]. Parathyroid hormone, therefore, not only helped to remineralize the skeleton but also helped to re-establish deficits in trabecular microarchitecture. Equally important were the results at the cortical skeleton. Instead of an increase in cortical porosity, impressive increases in bone were apparent on the endocortical surface. The gains appeared to be based on positive bone balance during remodeling; a decrease in the eroded perimeter was consistent with a reduction in resorption at the endocortical surface [94]. The microarchitectural improvements in connectivity and in cortical bone density have also been reported by Jiang and Genant in a study of biopsies from the pivotal trial of Neer *et al* [80].

3. Periosteal Growth and Teriparatide

The initial increase in bone formation with PTH occurs as a direct stimulation of osteoblasts. Parathyroid hormone increases the osteoblast birth rate [97] and inhibits osteoblast apoptosis [69]. It has been postulated that osteoblastic recruitment with PTH occurs specifically from local periosteal connective tissue precursors [98,99]. Ensuing bone formation is thus manifested as periosteal growth. This concept was recently confirmed in

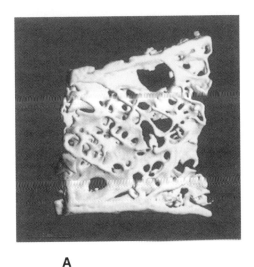

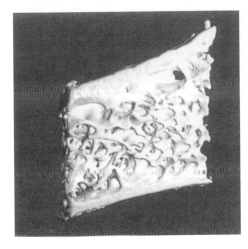

A   **B**

Fig. 92-5 Bone structure by scanning electron microscopy of bone biopsies before (A) and after (B) parathyroid hormone (PTH) treatment in one patient. Note the marked improvement in trabecular architecture and increase in cortical thickness following PTH treatment. (From Dempster DW, Cosman F, Kurland ES *et al.* [2001]. Effects of daily treatment with parathyroid hormone on bone microarchitecture and turnover in patients with osteoporosis: A paired biopsy study. *J Bone Miner Res.* 16:1846–1853, with permission.)

human subjects, when 101 postmenopausal women treated with PTH underwent peripheral quantitative computed tomography (pQCT) of the proximal radius after a median 18 months of treatment to assess specific changes in cortical bone density undetectable by DXA [100]. Similar to the primate model, PTH treatment resulted in significantly greater periosteal and endocortical circumferences and cortical area [100]. These differences resulted in greater polar and axial moments of inertia and torsional bone strength index, architectural indicators of the bone's resistance to bending and torsional loading. Cross-sectional diameter thus increased, so that the ratio of outer bone to inner bone increased with consequent increased biomechanical strength [101,102]. These microarchitectural changes contrast with those seen with primary hyperparathyroidism, in which both an expansion of inner and outer diameter occurs. Here, intermittent PTH therapy increased the outer diameter and decreased the inner diameter. The greater periosteal distribution of cortical bone, reflected in the moments of inertia, may contribute to the reduction in nonvertebral fractures that is not explained by changes in DXA in BMD alone. The resultant larger vertebral size likely contributes to fracture risk reduction [103]. An increase in cortical thickness was similarly found in 40 PTH-treated women who underwent digital x-ray radiogrametry, a technology that also measures subtle changes in cortical thickness of the radius that are undetectable by DXA [104].

These observations help to substantiate the densitometric observations at a structural level, suggesting that PTH may be improving the skeleton in ways that are distinctly different from the antiresorptives, and help to allay concerns that PTH may have adverse effects on the cortical skeleton. Recent data in PTH-treated mice suggest that the anabolic actions of PTH can occur at the long bones, possibly because they constitute areas of greater mechanical stress in mice [68]. These observations provide evidence that PTH is anabolic for cortical bone.

Furthermore, fracture data from the study of Neer *et al* [92] clearly indicate a substantial reduction in fractures of the nonvertebral skeleton.

4. Changes in Mineralization and Teriparatide

How can it be that PTH causes a decrease in cortical bone density yet a simultaneous increase in cortical strength? This seeming paradox can be explained by studying the actual distribution of bone mineral under the influence of PTH. Undoubtedly, PTH is stimulating the erosion of fully mineralized endocortical bone. The compensatory increase in periosteal bone is likely to be young and undermineralized, at least initially. A dynamic is thus created that would tend to change bone density as measured by DXA in opposite directions. The increase in bone size would tend to increase bone density while the increase in undermineralized bone would tend to decrease it. The dynamic is also set up with respect to bone strength, one tending to increase it (bone size), and the other tending to decrease it (undermineralized bone). It appears that the DXA measurement is dominated by the change in bone mineralization, whereas bone strength characteristics are dominated by the change in bone size. Of course, bone strength is also favorably influenced by the microarchitectural improvements in bone qualities. Animal data show that PTH treatment causes a decrease in lowest and highest density bone volume and a substantial increase in bone volume at mid-volumetric BMD (vBMD) levels [105].

5. Cortical Effects of Teriparatide

With PTH-driven increases in bone turnover, reductions in tissue mineralization, and increases in cortical porosity [74], expectations of negative effects on cortical bone deserve specific consideration. As noted earlier, however, the histomorphometric analysis of bone biopsy specimens before and after PTH therapy clearly show a net anabolic effect on cortical bone [44]. Cortical width was maintained in the men and significantly increased in the women. There was no increase in cortical porosity. A distinct anabolic effect on cortical bone was observed at the endosteal surface, with significant increases in the width of bone packets. This was accompanied by a significant decrease in eroded perimeter on this surface in both groups. The positive effects of increased endocortical wall width and cortical thickness may have been enhanced by a reduction in resorption on that surface because of a marked decrease in eroded perimeter. Anabolic action may have additionally occurred at the subperiosteal surface, but it was not possible to assess the wall width of newly formed bone units there.

Similar salutary effects on cortical bone strength are corroborated by animal data. A study in ovariectomized cynomolgus monkeys has shown that even when PTH administration increased intracortical porosity, there was no detrimental effect on the mechanical properties of bone [74]. The increased cortical porosity did not translate into decreased strength because it occurred in the inner one third of the bone, where the mechanical effect was small, and was offset by increases in cortical area and cortical thickness [74]. The consequent increase in cross-sectional diameter would be expected to increase bone strength. In a similar recent study, PTH was found to have beneficial effects on trabecular and cortical bone in ovariectomized cynomolgus monkeys, despite increasing cortical porosity [76]. Porosity did not adversely affect mechanical properties, because enhanced trabecular bone volume more than compensated for the porosity, resulting in increased strength. After PTH withdrawal, cortical porosity decreased during the remodeling phase, while strength remained elevated [76]. Any negative effects of increased cortical remodeling appear to be offset by the increase in cortical thickness [44,74,106]. The data are thus consistent with the clinical observations that nonvertebral fracture incidence falls significantly with PTH.

6. Osteocytes and Teriparatide

Parathyroid hormone appears to modulate the response of osteocytes to mechanical shear and strain forces [107,108]. Parathyroid hormone preserves osteocyte viability through inhibition of apoptosis [69]. This most likely represents another mechanism by which PTH protects against fractures.

I. Withdrawal of Teriparatide in Women and Men: The Post-Parathyroid Hormone Period

The effect of PTH followed by alendronate in postmenopausal women has been assessed in a randomized, controlled trial [82]. After treatment, those who had received the highest dose of PTH had impressive spinal bone density increases of up to 14.6%. It is unclear, however, how much of the bone density improvement occurred solely as a result of a continued anabolic effect after PTH withdrawal, because there was no placebo group that did not receive alendronate. In addition, what is not known is whether PTH administered concomitantly with a bisphosphonate is preferable to sequential therapy. A randomized trial sponsored by the National Institutes of Health (NIH) is currently underway to test that hypothesis [109,110].

In patients treated with PTH, there is evidence that the new bone matrix is not yet fully mineralized because of the high rate of bone turnover [54]. Using the technique of quantitative back-scattered electron imaging (qBEI), Roschger et al have shown that a greater than normal amount of matrix is found at lower mineralization densities because of the higher amounts of newly formed bone that have not yet had time to undergo complete secondary mineralization [111]. This observation is exactly opposite to mineralization density using the same technique applied to an antiresorptive agent such as alendronate. This is further illustrated by the resolution of cortical porosity that occurs after PTH withdrawal in ovariectomized cynomolgus monkeys [76]. This delay provides an explanation for the observation that apparent bone density, as measured by DXA, increases following parathyroidectomy [112]. As the bone turnover rate is decreased, more time is available for secondary mineralization, thereby resulting in an increase in apparent bone density.

In therapeutic regimens, the data give mixed results. When an antiresorptive is used or maintained after the period of PTH therapy, gains in bone density tend to be maintained or improved further. In the pivotal clinical trial reported by Neer et al in which postmenopausal women were followed up for 31 months after PTH withdrawal, the protective effect on fracture rate and lumbar spine bone density persisted [113]. During this follow-up period, however, 60% of the women switched to an antiresorptive agent. Without separating the women who took an antiresorptive from those who did not, it is not possible to know to what extent the antiresorptive was a key determinant in the post-PTH maintenance of bone mass. When these two groups were considered separately, the women who received an antiresorptive agent after teriparatide maintained bone density, whereas those who did not showed substantial reductions [113]. The importance of an antiresorptive agent following PTH is supported further by the studies of Lindsay et al and Lane et al. In both clinical trials, estrogen therapy was maintained after PTH was discontinued. In both studies, bone density was maintained [113–115]. These two studies did not have an arm in which estrogen was discontinued. Nevertheless, the continued presence of an antiresorptive or institution of an antiresorptive appear to maintain the gains achieved by PTH therapy [112,116].

As noted previously, the data suggest that when PTH therapy is not followed by an antiresorptive, bone density will fall. Kurland et al showed that when men were given a choice between following their PTH therapy with or without an antiresorptive, those who chose the bisphosphonate showed further increases of 3% in the lumbar spine. When a bisphosphonate was not taken, bone density fell rapidly, by as much as 6% in the lumbar spine [95,117]. Animal data suggest that administering a bisphosphonate after PTH is as effective as continuing PTH [118]. The results of further clinical trials to address these points are awaited [109].

J. PTH and Osteosarcoma

Long-term studies with high-dose rhPTH (1–34) administered to 6-week-old Fisher rats for 18 to 24 months have demonstrated a dose-related appearance of osteogenic sarcoma.

This effect is related not only to dose but also to duration of use, consistent with lifetime exposure in a growing rodent to about 75 human year equivalents. There is uncertainty, however, about whether this toxicity study in a rodent model has relevance to human physiology. Recently, Vahle *et al* [76] have reported the details of the experimental protocol and Tashjian and Chabner [119] have provided a comprehensive commentary on issues related to human safety of this drug. They point out that the rat responds to PTH with an exaggerated anabolic response, perhaps because the rat does not have an osteon remodeling system.

All primate studies to-date have failed to find an association between intermittent administration of PTH and osteogenic sarcoma. Moreover, among the millions of individuals who have been exposed to chronically elevated levels of PTH, there has been only one well-documented report of osteogenic sarcoma among patients with primary, secondary, or tertiary hyperparathyroidism [120]. Considering the millions of individuals worldwide who have primary hyperparathyroidism, it is surprising that so few cases have been reported. One might have expected more, simply on chance association. Furthermore, there have been no reports of osteogenic sarcoma among any of the patient cohorts in any of the clinical trials with PTH, amounting to more than 2500 patients [121]. Finally, in a second toxicity study in rats, a "no effect" dose is now defined, still larger and with greater exposure than any human being will experience. Further safety data are needed to evaluate these points. However, it is reasonable to assume that PTH is safe in humans in those most likely to benefit (i.e., postmenopausal women and men with fragility fractures and established osteoporosis). The benefits of PTH are likely also to extend to individuals with severe osteoporosis before fractures occur. In view of these rat toxicity data, approval of teriparatide as a therapy for osteoporosis is associated in the United States with a "black box" warning in which the rat toxicity data are summarized [122].

K. Other Anabolic Agents

1. Fluoride

Fluoride directly stimulates osteoblasts to form new bone, while having little effect on osteoclasts. Early studies of fluoride administration in postmenopausal women revealed impressive increases in bone mass both radiographically and by determination of BMD. However, subsequent, randomized, placebo-controlled trials with sodium fluoride at relatively high doses (75 mg daily) in postmenopausal women failed to show a significant benefit [124]. Despite marked increases in spine BMD, fluoride was not associated with a reduction in vertebral fracture incidence. A possible increase in nonvertebral fracture risk was also worrisome. Furthermore, severe gastrointestinal side effects and a disturbing lower extremity pain syndrome were reported as common adverse events. Subsequent clinical trials with a lower dose, slow-release formulation of fluoride in postmenopausal women have been more promising. Increases in bone mass and significant reductions in vertebral fractures were observed [125–130,132,133]. More recent data on the effects of fluoride in men suggest a similar salutary effect as in women [129]. Ringe and Rivati [134] reported preliminary results of a pilot study combining fluoride and the bisphosphonate etidronate.

2. Growth Hormone and Insulin-like Growth Factor-1

The rationale for considering growth hormone (GH) and IGF-1 as potential anabolic agents is that both are critical for the acquisition and maintenance of bone mass. In men in particular, GH and IGF-1 stimulate periosteal apposition, so it is logical to expect that both would be efficacious treatments. An added theoretical advantage is salutary effects on muscle strength and coordination, potentially leading to a reduction in falls and fracture rates. Insulin-like growth factor-1 promotes chondrocyte and osteoblast differentiation and growth [135]. It is also a pivotal factor in the coupling of bone turnover, because it is stored in the skeletal matrix and released during bone resorption [135]. When the IGF-1 receptor in bone is knocked out, decreased bone formation and suppressed mineralization ensue [136]. Two prospective studies have suggested that low levels of IGF-1 are linked with a greater risk of spine and hip fractures [137,138].

Most of the studies using GH in either gender, however, have been disappointing. Changes in bone mass are minimal in men [139] and women [140]. The lack of a beneficial effect with GH on bone mass could be due to the concomitant activation of bone resorption along with formation [142], so that a net gain does not occur. Another explanation for a lack of effect could be the relatively short, 1-year duration of many of these studies. Recent evidence has suggested a delayed and positive effect of GH on bone. In a double blind, randomized, placebo-controlled trial, 80 postmenopausal women with osteoporosis on estrogen replacement therapy were administered placebo, GH 1.0 U/day or GH 2.5 U/day for 18 months [143]. The women in both GH groups continued on treatment with GH for an additional 18 months. Although there was no difference between the groups after 3 years, at 4 years, the higher dose of GH resulted in a 14% increase in lumbar spine bone mineral content. These results are quite unexpected and conflict with most of the data on effective osteoporosis therapies in which the major increments in bone mass are typically limited to the first 3 years of therapy. One possible explanation for the "catch-up" bone gain after GH withdrawal might be that the drop in IGF-1 halts GH-stimulated resorption but allows osteoblastic stimulation to persist [144].

3. Insulin-like Growth Factor-1

Data on IGF-1 therapy exist for postmenopausal and young women. Insulin-like growth factor-1 is theoretically more appealing than GH, because it stimulates bone formation more directly and does not demonstrate many of the adverse effects related to GH, such as diabetes mellitus or carpal tunnel syndrome. When elderly women were administered low doses of rhIGF-1, markers of bone formation were differentially stimulated with only a minimal increase in bone resorption [145]. Similarly, markers of bone formation increased in short-term trials of young women with anorexia nervosa administered IGF-1 alone [146]. There is also evidence that IGF-1 might be more effective if administered together with its major binding protein IGFBP-3 [148]. A major drawback to the development of IGF-1 as a therapy for osteoporosis is its ubiquitous effect on many organ systems. Similar to GH, therefore, potential serious adverse effects could surface with chronic use of this agent.

4. Strontium

Strontium ranelate is a novel anabolic agent that has been studied in postmenopausal women; no data are yet available on its use in men. Strontium is a divalent cation that chemically resembles calcium and appears to participate in bone mineralization [149]. Anabolic properties include both an increase in bone formation and an uncoupling of bone formation from bone resorption. The mechanism appears to be stimulation of osteoblast proliferation and inhibition of osteoclast formation, possibly through regulation of bone cell differentiation [150]. An alternative mechanism might be activation of signaling pathways through a putative cation-sensing receptor (CaSR), believed to be specifically expressed in bone cells [151,152]. The CaSR appears to be activated by strontium ranelate in rats and mice, although the degree of activation probably depends on variations in the local calcium concentration [153].

Clinical trials support the use of strontium ranelate as a treatment for postmenopausal osteoporosis [50,123,154,155]. Recently, the results of a phase II, dose-ranging, randomized, placebo-controlled double-blind trial have corroborated the anabolic potential of strontium ranelate [155]. Three hundred fifty-three osteoporotic women with at least one vertebral fracture were randomized to receive placebo, 0.5 g, 1 g, or 2 g of strontium ranelate daily for 2 years. In the group receiving the highest dose, lumbar BMD increased significantly by 3.0%, after adjustment for the presence of strontium in bone. The rate of increase in BMD was virtually identical during the second year of treatment as during the first year, in contrast to antiresorptive treatments with which most of the gain occurs during the first year [156,157]. New vertebral deformities were also reduced significantly (relative risk 0.56) [155]. An increase in the bone formation marker, bone-specific alkaline phosphatase (BSAP), was observed in the group receiving the highest dose of strontium ranelate, along with a reduction in the bone resorption marker urinary N-telopeptide. Strontium ranelate was well tolerated at all doses. Results of the phase III clinical trial of 2 g daily of strontium ranelate have also been recently reported [158]. In a double-blind, randomized, placebo-controlled trial, 1649 postmenopausal women with at least one vertebral fracture were administered strontium ranelate daily or placebo for 3 years. A 41% reduction in relative risk of a new vertebral fracture was observed. Lumbar BMD also increased in the treatment group by 11.4% (uncorrected for the presence of strontium in bone), along with increases in BSAP and decreases in serum C-telopeptide [158].

5. Statins

Recent data in both men and women, mostly epidemiologic and cross-sectional, have suggested that the use of 3-hydroxy-3-methylglutaryl (HMG) coenzyme A reductase inhibitors (statins) is associated with a modest increase in BMD and a significant fracture risk reduction [159–164]. An anabolic effect of statins has been inferred from several intriguing observations. New bone formation was observed when statins were injected into the calvariae of mice [165]. This growth was associated with an increase in bone morphogenic protein-2 (BMP-2), a protein which plays an important role in osteoblast differentiation and bone formation. Statins probably enhance BMP-2 through a reduction in the prenylation of Rho and a

subsequent increase in endothelial nitric oxide synthase [166]. The increase in BMP-2 is inhibited by mevalonate, a downstream metabolite of HMG coenzyme A reductase, the rate-limiting step in cholesterol production [167–169]. Recently, lovastatin was found to increase cortical bone by single, local administration to the bone marrow cavity of young male rats [170]. In a small clinical trial, 17 hypercholesterolemic subjects who were administered simvastatin 20 mg daily for 4 weeks had a significant increase in the bone formation marker osteocalcin, although other markers including bone specific alkaline phosphatase did not change [171].

Important questions still remain unresolved about the beneficial skeletal effects of statins in both women and men. First, because the bisphosphonates also use the cholesterol biosynthetic pathway by inhibiting a downstream step, it is unclear how statins could stimulate bone formation while bisphosphonates, working in the same path, inhibit bone resorption. Second, when administered orally, statins do not localize preferentially to bone. They are almost exclusively cleared via first-pass hepatic metabolism, so it is not easily apparent how they could affect bone turnover. Third, no randomized, placebo-controlled trials to assess fracture risk reduction with statin administration have been reported yet. The existing observational trials may be prone to ascertainment bias. Statin users might have fewer fractures because of a higher baseline bone mass [172], possibly associated with a higher body mass index (BMI). Moreover, fracture risk reduction has not been found uniformly in all statin studies to date [173,174]. Two large scale cross-sectional surveys failed to show an association between statin use and fracture risk [175,176]. It is therefore premature to conclude that statins have antifracture potential and, if so, whether they can be classified as anabolic.

6. Androgens

Androgens are potential anabolic agents in both the male and female skeleton. In men, androgens are pivotal for the acquisition of peak bone mass [177]. Administration of androgens to men stimulates bone formation [178] by increasing periosteal bone apposition and thus cortical thickness [7]. This increase in areal (gm/cm^2), although not volumetric (gm/cm^3), bone density contributes to the decreased fracture risk in men. Certain of the beneficial effects of androgens result from an antiresorptive effect, probably mediated through aromatization to estrogen. However, it does appear that androgens, even when not aromatized, have an important salutary effect in the male skeleton [179]. In women, there is evidence that testosterone added to estrogen elicits greater increases in bone density than estrogen alone [180–182], through an increase in bone formation. However, undesirable androgenic effects must be considered. These include prostate growth in men, virilization in women, and potentially adverse lipid effects in both genders.

VI. Conclusions

The advent of anabolic therapy in the form of teriparatide, the first approved agent in the United States, is revolutionizing our approach to osteoporosis therapy. For the first time, a drug is available that significantly improves microarchitectural and geometric qualities of bone along with favorable changes in bone density and in bone turnover dynamics. Because the antiresorptives and anabolic agents clearly work by completely distinct mechanisms of action, it is possible that the combination of agents could be significantly more potent than either agent alone. This possibility, however, remains to be tested. In the future, PTH may be modified for easier and more targeted delivery. Oral or transdermal delivery systems may become available. A recent study [183] demonstrated that PTH can be formulated to provide systemic exposure following oral administration in rats and cynomolgus monkeys, although variations in interpatient bioavailability could be a potential problem. A bioactive recombinant PTH analog was also recently presented as a potential future oral agent [184]. Gowen *et al* [185] have described an oral calcilytic molecule that antagonizes the parathyroid cell calcium receptor, thus stimulating the endogenous release of PTH. This approach could represent a novel endogenous delivery system for intermittent PTH administration, although, if the rise in PTH is sustained, bone resorption might increase. Less frequent administration of PTH, such as once weekly, might also be an effective treatment option [110]. Clearly, we are on the threshold of a new paradigm in the treatment of osteoporosis. For women and for men, we can look forward to a period of unprecedented further advances in our approach to a disease that is surely to affect us all, if we live long enough.

VII. Suggestions for Further Investigations

The information summarized in this chapter defines a number of avenues for further investigation including: determining how anabolic therapy can be used in combination with antiresorptive therapy for maximal benefit. More data are needed on antiresorptives before, during, and after PTH. It is possible that different antiresorptives will give different results when used together with PTH. Can PTH be used in a cyclical mode? It is possible that subjects can be retreated with PTH after a single 2-year course. Other anabolic agents being developed are also going to provide further investigative opportunities as we seek to determine how best to reconstruct the osteoporotic skeleton.

References

1. (1993). Consensus Development Conference on Osteoporosis. Hong Kong, April 1–2, 1993. *Am J Med*. 95(5A):1S–78S.
2. Orwoll ES, Klein RF. (1995). Osteoporosis in men. *Endocr Rev*. 16:87–116.
3. National Osteoporosis Foundation. (2002). *Advocacy—The State of Osteoporosis and Low Bone Mass in the US*. Washington, DC: National Osteoporosis Foundation.
4. Riggs BL, Khosla S, Melton LJ 3rd. (1998). A unitary model for involutional osteoporosis: Estrogen deficiency causes both type I and type II osteoporosis in postmenopausal women and contributes to bone loss in aging men [see comments]. *J Bone Miner Res*. 13:763–773.
5. Falahati-Nini A, Riggs BL, Atkinson EJ *et al*. (2000). Relative contributions of testosterone and estrogen in regulating bone resorption and formation in normal elderly men. *J Clin Invest*. 106:1553–1560.
6. Kanis JA, Johnell O, Oden A *et al*. (2000). Long-term risk of osteoporotic fracture in Malm inverted question mark. *Osteoporos Int*. 11:669–674.
7. Turner RT, Wakley GK, Hannon KS. (1990). Differential effects of androgens on cortical bone histomorphometry in gonadectomized male and female rats. *J Orthop Res*. 8:612–67.
8. Seeman E. (2001). Clinical review 137: Sexual dimorphism in skeletal size, density, and strength. *J Clin Endocrinol Metab*. 86:4576–4584.
9. Parfitt AM. (1979). Quantum concept of bone remodeling and turnover: Implications for the pathogenesis of osteoporosis. *Calcif Tissue Int*. 28:1–5.
10. Meier DE, Orwoll ES, Jones JM. (1984). Marked disparity between trabecular and cortical bone loss with age in healthy men. Measurement by vertebral computed tomography and radial photon absorptiometry. *Ann Intern Med*. 101:605–612.
11. Ruff CB, Hayes WC. (1988). Sex differences in age-related remodeling of the femur and tibia. *J Orthop Res*. 6:886–896.
12. Duan Y, Turner CH, Kim BT, Seeman E. (2001). Sexual dimorphism in vertebral fragility is more the result of gender differences in age-related bone gain than bone loss. *J Bone Miner Res*. 16:2267–2275.
13. Melton LJ 3rd, Atkinson EJ, O'Fallon WM *et al*. (1993). Long-term fracture prediction by bone mineral assessed at different skeletal sites. *J Bone Miner Res*. 8:1227–1233.
14. Faulkner KG. (2000). Bone matters: Are density increases necessary to reduce fracture risk? *J Bone Miner Res*. 15:183–187.
15. Marshall D, Johnell O, Wedel H. (1996). Meta-analysis of how well measures of bone mineral density predict occurrence of osteoporotic fractures. *BMJ*. 312:1254–1259.
16. Cheng XU, Nicholson PH, Boonen S *et al*. (1997). Prediction of vertebral strength *in vitro* by spinal bone densitometry and calcaneal ultrasound. *J Bone Miner Res*. 12:1721–1728.
17. Hui SL, Slemenda CW, Johnston CC Jr. (1988). Age and bone mass as predictors of fracture in a prospective study. *J Clin Invest*. 81:1804–1809.
18. Orwoll E. (2000). Assessing bone density in men. *J Bone Miner Res*. 15:1867–1870.
19. Cooley H, Jones G. (2001). A population-based study of fracture incidence in southern Tasmania: Lifetime fracture risk and evidence for geographic variations within the same country. *Osteoporos Int*. 12:124–130.
20. (1996). Effects of hormone therapy on bone mineral density: Results from the postmenopausal estrogen/progestin interventions (PEPI) trial. The Writing Group for the PEPI [see comments]. *JAMA*. 276:1389–1396.
21. Chesnut CH 3rd, Silverman S, Andriano K *et al*. (2000). A randomized trial of nasal spray salmon calcitonin in postmenopausal women with established osteoporosis: The prevent recurrence of osteoporotic fractures study. PROOF Study Group. *Am J Med*. 109:267–276.
22. Ettinger B, Black DM, Mitlak BH *et al*. (1999). Reduction of vertebral fracture risk in postmenopausal women with osteoporosis treated with raloxifene: Results from a 3-year randomized clinical trial. Multiple Outcomes of Raloxifene Evaluation (MORE) Investigators. *JAMA*. 282:637–645.
23. Lindsay R, Cosman F. (1996). The Pharmacology of Estrogens in Osteoporosis. In *Principles of Bone Biology* (Bilezikian JP, Raisz LG, Rodan GA, eds.), pp. 1063–1068. Sand Diego, CA: Academic Press.
24. Fleisch H. (1996). Bisphosphonates: Mechanisms of Action and Clinical Use. In *Principles of Bone Biology* (Bilezikian JP, Raisz LG, Rodan GA, eds.), pp. 1037–1052. Sand Diego, CA: Academic Press.
25. Azria M, Avioli L. (1996). Calcitonin. In *Principles of Bone Biology* (Bilezikian JP, Raisz LG, Rodan GA, eds.), pp. 1083–1098. San Diego, CA: Academic Press.
26. Fogelman I, Ribot C, Smith R *et al*. (2000). Risedronate reverses bone loss in postmenopausal women with low bone mass: Results from a multinational, double-blind, placebo-controlled trial. BMD-MN Study Group. *J Clin Endocrinol Metab*. 85:1895–1900.
27. Kurland ES, Rosen CJ, Cosman F *et al*. (1997). Insulin-like growth factor-I in men with idiopathic osteoporosis [see comments]. *J Clin Endocrinol Metab*. 82:2799–2805.
28. Greenspan SL, Parker RA, Ferguson L *et al*. (1998). Early changes in biochemical markers of bone turnover predict the long-term response to alendronate therapy in representative elderly women: A randomized clinical trial. *J Bone Miner Res*. 13:1431–1438.
29. Liberman UA, Weiss SR, Broll J *et al*. (1995). Effect of oral alendronate on bone mineral density and the incidence of fractures in postmenopausal osteoporosis. The Alendronate Phase III Osteoporosis Treatment Study Group [see comments]. *N Engl J Med*. 333:1437–1443.
30. Liberman UA, Weiss SR, Broll J *et al*. (1995). Effect of oral alendronate on bone mineral density and the incidence of fractures in postmenopausal osteoporosis. The Alendronate Phase III Osteoporosis Treatment Study Group. *N Engl J Med*. 333:1437–1443.
31. Wasnich RD, Miller PD. (2000). Antifracture efficacy of antiresorptive agents are related to changes in bone density. *J Clin Endocrinol Metab*. 85:231–236.

32. Cummings SR, Karpf DB, Harris F *et al*. (2002). Improvement in spine bone density and reduction in risk of vertebral fractures during treatment with antiresorptive drugs. *Am J Med*. 112:281–289.

33. Miller PD, Bonnick SL, Rosen CJ. (1996). Consensus of an international panel on the clinical utility of bone mass measurements in the detection of low bone mass in the adult population. *Calcif Tissue Int*. 58:207–214.

34. Marcus R, Wong M, Heath H 3rd, Stock JL. (2002). Antiresorptive treatment of postmenopausal osteoporosis: Comparison of study designs and outcomes in large clinical trials with fracture as an endpoint. *Endocr Rev*. 23:16–37.

35. Black DM, Cummings SR, Karpf DB *et al*. (1996). Randomised trial of effect of alendronate on risk of fracture in women with existing vertebral fractures. Fracture Intervention Trial Research Group [see comments]. *Lancet*. 348:1535–1541.

36. Seeman E, McLung M, Zippel H *et al*. (2000). Rapid and sustained effect of risedronate in reducing hip fracture risk. *J Bone Miner Metab*. 15(Suppl 1):S149.

37. Watts N, Adami S, Chesnut CH 3rd. (2001). Risedronate reduces the risk of clinical vertebral fractures in just 6 months. *J Bone Miner Metab*. 16(S1):S407.

38. Parfitt AM. (1991). Use of bisphosphonates in the prevention of bone loss and fractures. *Am J Med*. 91(5B):42S–46S.

39. Garnero P, Hausherr E, Chapuy MC *et al*. (1996). Markers of bone resorption predict hip fracture in elderly women: The EPIDOS Prospective Study. *J Bone Miner Res*. 11:1531–1538.

40. Melton LJ 3rd, Khosla S, Atkinson EJ *et al*. (1997). Relationship of bone turnover to bone density and fractures. *J Bone Miner Res*. 12:1083–1091.

41. Riggs BL, Melton LJ 3rd. (2002). Bone turnover matters: The raloxifene treatment paradox of dramatic decreases in vertebral fractures without commensurate increases in bone density. *J Bone Miner Res*. 17:11–14.

42. Ito M, Amizuka N, Nakajima T, Ozawa H. (1999). Ultrastructural and cytochemical studies on cell death of osteoclasts induced by bisphosphonate treatment. *Bone*. 25:447–452.

43. Hochberg MC, Greenspan S, Wasnich RD *et al*. (2002). Changes in bone density and turnover explain the reductions in incidence of nonvertebral fractures that occur during treatment with antiresorptive agents. *J Clin Endocrinol Metab*. 87:1586–1592.

44. Dempster DW, Cosman F, Kurland ES *et al*. (2001). Effects of daily treatment with parathyroid hormone on bone microarchitecture and turnover in patients with osteoporosis: A paired biopsy study. *J Bone Miner Res*. 16:1846–1853.

45. Parfitt AM, Mathews CH, Villanueva AR *et al*. (1983). Relationships between surface, volume, and thickness of iliac trabecular bone in aging and in osteoporosis. Implications for the microanatomic and cellular mechanisms of bone loss. *J Clin Invest*. 72:1396–1409.

46. Silva MJ, Gibson LJ. (1997). Modeling the mechanical behavior of vertebral trabecular bone: Effects of age-related changes in microstructure. *Bone*. 21:191–199.

47. Mosekilde, L. (1988). Age-related changes in vertebral trabecular bone architecture—Assessed by a new method. *Bone*. 9:247–250.

48. Borah B, Dufresne TE, Chmielewski PA *et al*. (2002). Risedronate preserves trabecular architecture and increases bone strength in vertebra of ovariectomized minipigs as measured by three-dimensional microcomputed tomography. *J Bone Miner Res*. 17:1139–1147.

49. Bell GH, Dunbar O, Beck JS, Gibb A. (1967). Variations in strength of vertebrae with age and their relation to osteoporosis. *Calcif Tissue Res*. 1:75–86.

50. Meunier PJ, Boivin G. (1997). Bone mineral density reflects bone mass but also the degree of mineralization of bone: Therapeutic implications. *Bone*. 21:373–377.

51. Boivin GY, Chavassieux PM, Santora AC *et al*. (2000). Alendronate increases bone strength by increasing the mean degree of mineralization of bone tissue in osteoporotic women. *Bone*. 27:687–694.

52. Boivin G, Meunier PJ. (2002). Changes in bone remodeling rate influence the degree of mineralization of bone. *Connect Tissue Res*. 43:535–537.

53. Hernandez CJ, Beaupre GS, Keller TS, Carter DR. (2001). The influence of bone volume fraction and ash fraction on bone strength and modulus. *Bone*. 29:74–78.

54. Roschger P, Grabner BM, Messer P *et al*. (2001). Influence of intermittent PTH treatment on mineral distribution in the human ilium: A paired biopsy study before and after treatment. *J Bone Miner Res*. 16(Suppl 1):S179.

55. Noble BS, Reeve J. (2000). Osteocyte function, osteocyte death and bone fracture resistance. *Mol Cell Endocrinol*. 159:7–13.

56. Plotkin LI, Weinstein RS, Parfitt AM *et al*. (1999). Prevention of osteocyte and osteoblast apoptosis by bisphosphonates and calcitonin. *J Clin Invest*. 104:1363–1374.

57. Albright F, Aub JC, Bauer W. (1934). Hyperparathyroidism: A common and polymorphic condition as illustrated by seventeen proven cases from one clinic. *JAMA*. 102:1276–1287.

58. Albright F, Reifenstein EC. (1948). *The Parathyroid Glands and Metabolic Bone Disease*. Baltimore: Williams & Wilkins.

59. Juppner H, Kronenberg HM. (1996). PTH: Mechanism of Action. In *Primer on Metabolic Bone Diseases* (Favus M, ed.), pp. 117–124. Washington, DC: ASBMR.

60. Morley P, Whitfield JF, Willick GE. (1997). Anabolic effects of PTH on bone. *Trends Endocrinol Metab*. 8:225–231.

61. Abou-Samra AB, Jueppner H, Westerberg D *et al*. (1989). Parathyroid hormone causes translocation of protein kinase-C from cytosol to membranes in rat osteosarcoma cells. *Endocrinology*. 124:1107–1113.

62. Fraher LJ, Avram R, Watson PH *et al*. (1999). Comparison of the biochemical responses to human parathyroid hormone-(1–31)NH2 and hPTH-(1–34) in healthy humans. *J Clin Endocrinol Metab*. 84:2739–2743.

63. Canalis E, Centrella M, Burch W, McCarthy TL. (1989). Insulin-like growth factor I mediates selective anabolic effects of parathyroid hormone in bone cultures. *J Clin Invest*. 83:60–65.

64. Hock JM, Gera I, Fonseca J, Raisz LG. (1988). Human parathyroid hormone-(1–34) increases bone mass in ovariectomized and orchidectomized rats. *Endocrinology*. 122:2899–2904.

65. Linkhart TA, Mohan S. (1989). Parathyroid hormone stimulates release of insulin-like growth factor-I (IGF-I) and IGF-II from neonatal mouse calvaria in organ culture. *Endocrinology*. 125:1484–1491.

66. Watson PH, Lazowski DA, Han V *et al*. (1995). PTH restores bone mass and enhances osteoblast IGF-1 gene expression in ovariectomized rats. *Bone*. 16:1–9.

67. Ma YL, Cain RL, Halladay DL *et al*. (2001). Catabolic effects of continuous human PTH (1–38) *in vivo* is associated with sustained stimulation of RANKL and inhibition of osteoprotegerin and gene-associated bone formation. *Endocrinology*. 142:4047–4054.

68. Ilda-Klein A, Zhou H, Lu SS *et al*. (2002). Anabolic action of parathyroid hormone is skeletal site specific at the tissue and cellular levels in mice. *J Bone Miner Res*. 17:808–816.

69. Jilka RL, Weinstein RS, Bellido T *et al*. (1999). Increased bone formation by prevention of osteoblast apoptosis with parathyroid hormone. *J Clin Invest*. 104:439–446.

70. Baumann AP, Grasser W, Petras S *et al*. (2001). Inhibition of osteoclast formation by statins. *J Bone Miner Res*. 16(Suppl 1):M309.

71. Locklin RM, Khosla S, Riggs BL. (2001). Mechanisms of biphasic anabolic and catabolic effects of parathyroid hormone (PTH) on bone cells. *Bone Suppl*. 28:s80.

72. Baumann BD, Wronski TJ. (1995). Response of cortical bone to antiresorptive agents and parathyroid hormone in aged ovariectomized rats. *Bone*. 16:247–253.

73. Cheng PT, Chan C, Muller K. (1995). Cyclical treatment of osteopenic ovariectomized adult rats with PTH(1–34) and pamidronate. *J Bone Miner Res*. 10:119–126.

74. Burr DB, Hirano T, Turner CH *et al*. (2001). Intermittently administered human parathyroid hormone(1–34) treatment increases intracortical bone turnover and porosity without reducing bone strength in the humerus of ovariectomized cynomolgus monkeys. *J Bone Miner Res*. 16:157–165.

75. Kneissel M, Boyde A, Gasser JA. (2001). Bone tissue and its mineralization in aged estrogen-depleted rats after long-term intermittent treatment with parathyroid hormone (PTH) analog SDZ PTS 893 or human PTH(1–34). *Bone*. 28:237–250.

76. Vahle JL, Sato M, Long GG *et al*. (2002). Skeletal changes in rats given daily subcutaneous injections of recombinant human parathyroid hormone (1–34) for 2 years and relevance to human safety. *Toxicol Pathol*. 30:312–321.

77. Hurley MM, Okada Y, Sobue T *et al*. (2002). The anabolic effect of parathyroid hormone is impaired in bones of Fgf2 null mice. *J Bone Miner Metab*. 17(Suppl 1):1061.

78. Li J, Duncan RL, Burr DB, Turner CH. (2002). L-type calcium channels mediate mechanically induced bone formation *in vivo*. *J Bone Miner Res*. 17:1795–1800.

79. Lane N, Yao W, Arnaud CD. (2002). The association of serum RANKL and OPG levels with other biochemical markers of bone turnover in glucocorticoid induced osteoporosis patients treated with hPTH (1–34). *J Bone Miner Res*. 17(suppl 1):p. F366.

80. Jiang Y, Zhao JJ, Mitlak BH *et al*. (2003). Recombinant human parathyroid hormone (1-34) [teriparatide] improves both cortical and cancellous bone structure. *J Bone Miner Res*. 18(11):1932–1941.

81. Cosman F, Lindsay R. (1998). Is parathyroid hormone a therapeutic option for osteoporosis? A review of the clinical evidence. *Calcif Tissue Int.* 62:475–480.

82. Rittmaster RS, Bolognese M, Ettinger MP *et al.* (2000). Enhancement of bone mass in osteoporotic women with parathyroid hormone followed by alendronate [see comments]. *J Clin Endocrinol Metab.* 85:2129–2134.

83. Chesnut CH 3rd, Rose CJ. (2001). Reconsidering the effects of antiresorptive therapies in reducing osteoporotic fracture. *J Bone Miner Res.* 16:2163–2172.

84. Cosman F, Nieves J, Woelfert L *et al.* (2001). Parathyroid hormone added to established hormone therapy: Effects on vertebral fracture and maintenance of bone mass after parathyroid hormone withdrawal. *J Bone Miner Res.* 16:925–931.

85. Gori F, Hofbauer LC, Conover CA, Khosla S. (1999). Effects of androgens on the insulin-like growth factor system in an androgen-responsive human osteoblastic cell line. *Endocrinology.* 140:5579–5586.

86. Neer R, Hayes A, Rao A, Finkelstein J. (2002). Effects of parathyroid hormone, alendronate, or both on bone density in osteoporotic postmenopausal women. *J Bone Miner Metab.* 17(Suppl 1):1039.

87. Rubin MR, Bilezikian JP. (2002). Clinical review 151: The role of parathyroid hormone in the pathogenesis of glucocorticoid-induced osteoporosis: A re-examination of the evidence. *J Clin Endocrinol Metab.* 87:4033–4041.

88. Lacey DL, Timms E, Tan HL *et al.* (1998). Osteoprotegerin ligand is a cytokine that regulates osteoclast differentiation and activation. *Cell.* 93:165–176.

89. Kurland ES, Cosman F, McMahon D *et al.* (2000). Parathyroid hormone as a therapy for idiopathic osteoporosis in men: Effects on bone mineral density and bone markers. *J Clin Endocrinol Metab.* 85:3069–3076.

90. Kurland E, Cosman F, McMahon DJ *et al.* (1998). Parathyroid hormone (PTH 1–34) increases cancellous bone mass markedly in men with idiopathic osteoporosis (abstract). *Bone.* 23(Suppl 5):S158.

91. Orwoll ES, Scheele WH, Paul S *et al.* (2003). The effect of teriparatide (human parathyroid hormone [1-34]) therapy on bone density in men with osteoporosis. *J Bone Miner Res.* 18(1):9–17.

92. Neer RM, Arnaud CD, Zanchetta JR *et al.* (2001). Effect of parathyroid hormone (1–34) on fractures and bone mineral density in postmenopausal women with osteoporosis. *N Engl J Med.* 344:1434–1441.

93. Finkelstein J, Hayes A, Rao A, Neer R. (2002). Effects of parathyroid hormone, alendronate, or both on bone density in osteoporotic men. *J Bone Miner Metab.* 17(Suppl 1):1007.

94. Dempster D, Zhou H, Cosman F *et al.* (2001). PTH treatment directly stimulates bone formation in cancellous and cortical bone in humans. *J Bone Miner Res.* 16(suppl 1):1171.

95. Kurland ES, Cosman F, Rosen CJ *et al.* (2000). Parathyroid hormone (PTH 1–34) as a treatment for idiopathic osteoporosis in men: Changes in bone mineral density, bone markers and optimal duration of therapy. *J Bone Miner Res.* 15(suppl 1):F435.

96. Eriksen EF. (2002). Primary hyperparathyroidism: Lessons from bone histomorphometry. *J Bone Miner Res.* 17(Suppl 2)N95–97.

97. Nishida S, Yamaguchi A, Tanizawa T *et al.* (1994). Increased bone formation by intermittent parathyroid hormone administration is due to the stimulation of proliferation and differentiation of osteoprogenitor cells in bone marrow. *Bone.* 15:717–723.

98. Uchida A, Kikuchi T, Shimomura Y. (1988). Osteogenic capacity of cultured human periosteal cells. *Acta Orthop Scand.* 59:29–33.

99. Parfitt AM. (2002). Parathyroid hormone and periosteal bone expansion. *J Bone Miner Res.* 17:1741–1743.

100. Zanchetta JR, Bogado CE, Ferretti JL *et al.* (2003). Effects of teriparatide [recombinant human parathyroid hormone (1–34)] on cortical bone in postmenopausal women with osteoporosis. *J Bone Miner Res.* 18:539–543.

101. Hirano T, Burr DB, Turner CH *et al.* (1999). Anabolic effects of human biosynthetic parathyroid hormone fragment (1–34), LY333334, on remodeling and mechanical properties of cortical bone in rabbits. *J Bone Miner Res.* 14:536–545.

102. Ejersted C, Andreassen T, Oxlund H *et al.* (1993). Human parathyroid hormone (1–34) and (1–84) increase the mechanical strength and thickness of cortical bone in rats. *J Bone Miner Res.* 8:1097–101.

103. Mosekilde L. (1990). Sex differences in age-related changes in vertebral body size, density and biomechanical competence in normal individuals. *Bone.* 11:67–73.

104. Hyldstrup L, Jorgensen JT, Gaich GA. (2001). Assessment of effects of LY333334 [recombinant human parathyroid hormone (1–34)] on cortical bone using digital X-ray radiogrametry. First Joint Meeting of the International Bone and Mineral Society and the European Calcified Tissue Society, Madrid: IBMS, p. SC33 S.

105. Sato M, Westmore M, Clendenon J *et al.* (2000). Three-dimensional modeling of the effects of parathyroid hormone on bone distribution in lumbar vertebrae of ovariectomized cynomolgus macaques. *Osteoporos Int.* 11;871–880.

106. Mashiba T, Burr DB, Turner CH *et al.* (2001). Effects of human parathyroid hormone (1–34), LY333334, on bone mass, remodeling, and mechanical properties of cortical bone during the first remodeling cycle in rabbits. *Bone.* 28:538–547.

107. Fermor B, Skerry TM. (1995). PTH/PTHrP receptor expression on osteoblasts and osteocytes but not resorbing bone surfaces in growing rats. *J Bone Miner Res.* 10;1935–1943.

108. van der Plas A, Aarden EM, Feijen JM *et al.* (1994). Characteristics and properties of osteocytes in culture. *J Bone Miner Res.* 9:1697–1704.

109. Black DM, Rosen CJ, Greenspan SL *et al.* (2001). PTH and bisphosphonates in the treatment of osteoporosis: Design of the PTH and alendronate (PaTH) trial (abstract). ASBMR 23rd Annual Meeting.

110. Black DM, Rosen CJ. (2002). Parsimony with PTH: Is a single weekly injection of PTH superior to a larger cumulative dose given daily? *J Bone Miner Res.* 17(Suppl 1):SA367.

111. Misof BM, Roschger P, Cosman F *et al.* (2003). Effects of intermittent parathyroid hormone administration on bone mineralization density in iliac crest biopsies from patients with osteoporosis: A paired study before and after treatment. *J Clin Endocrinol Metab.* 88:1150–1166.

112. Dempster DW, Parisien M, Silverberg SJ *et al.* On the mechanism of cancellous bone preservation in postmenopausal women with mild primary hyperparathyroidism. *J Clin Endocrinol Metab.* 84:1562–1566.

113. Lindsay R, Scheele WH, Clancy AD *et al.* Reduction in nonvertebral fragility fractures and increase in spinal bone density is maintained 31 months after discontinuation of recombinant human parathyroid hormone (1–34) in postmenopausal women with osteoporosis. Eight-fourth Annual Meeting of the Endocrine Society, Bethesda, MD: Endocrine Society, pp. OR35–36.

114. Lindsay R, Nieves J, Formica C *et al.* (1997). Randomised controlled study of effect of parathyroid hormone on vertebral-bone mass and fracture incidence among postmenopausal women on oestrogen with osteoporosis. *Lancet,* 350:550–555.

115. Lane NE, Sanchez S, Modin GW *et al.* (2000). Bone mass continues to increase at the hip after parathyroid hormone treatment is discontinued in glucocorticoid-induced osteoporosis: Results of a randomized controlled clinical trial. *J Bone Miner Res.* 15:944–951.

116. Christiansen P, Steiniche T, Mosekilde L *et al.* (1990). Primary hyperparathyroidism: Changes in trabecular bone remodeling following surgical treatment—Evaluated by histomorphometric methods. *Bone.* 11:75–79.

117. Kurland ES, Heller SL, Cosman F *et al.* (2001). The post-PTH experience in men with idiopathic osteoporosis: Bisphosphonates vs. non-pharmacologic therapy. *J Bone Miner Res.* 16(suppl 1).

118. Rhee Y, Kim S, Nangung R *et al.* (2002). Maintenance of increased bone mass after rhPTH (1–84) with zoledronate treatment in ovariectomized rats. *J Bone Miner Metab.* 17(Suppl 1):SA 337.

119. Tashjian AH Jr, Chabner BA. (2002). Commentary on clinical safety of recombinant human parathyroid hormone 1–34 in the treatment of osteoporosis in men and postmenopausal women. *J Bone Miner Res.* 17:1151–1161.

120. Betancourt M, Wirfel KL, Raymond AK *et al.* (2003). Osteosarcoma of bone in a patient with primary hyperparathyroidism: A case report. *J Bone Miner Res.* 18:163–166.

121. Palmer M, Adami HO, Krusemo UB, Ljunghall S. (1988). Increased risk of malignant diseases after surgery for primary hyperparathyroidism. A nationwide cohort study. *Am J Epidemiol.* 127:1031–1040.

122. Eli Lilly. (2002). FORTEO (teriparatide [rDNA origin] injection). p. 1, package insert.

123. Meunier PJ, Roux C, Seeman E *et al.* (2004). The effects of strontium ranelate on the risk of vertebral fracture in women with postmenopausal osteoporosis. *N Engl J Med.* 350(5):459–468.

124. Kleerekoper M, Peterson EL, Nelson DA *et al.* (1991). A randomized trial of sodium fluoride as a treatment for postmenopausal osteoporosis. *Osteoporos Int.* 1:155–161.

125. Pak CY, Sakhaee K, Zerwekh JE *et al.* (1989). Safe and effective treatment of osteoporosis with intermittent slow release sodium fluoride: Augmentation of vertebral bone mass and inhibition of fractures. *J Clin Endocrinol Metab.* 68:150–159.

126. Pak CY, Sakhaee K, Adams-Huet B *et al.* (1995). Treatment of postmenopausal osteoporosis with slow-release sodium fluoride. Final report of a randomized controlled trial. *Ann Intern Med.* 123:401–408.

127. Pak CY, Zerwekh JE, Antich PP *et al.* (1996). Slow-release sodium fluoride in osteoporosis. *J Bone Miner Res.* 11:561–564.

128. Riggs BL, O'Fallon WM, Lane A *et al.* (1994). Clinical trial of fluoride therapy in postmenopausal osteoporotic women: Extended observations and additional analysis. *J Bone Miner Res.* 9:265–275.

129. Ringe JD. (1998). What is proven about hip fracture and fluoride treatment? *Osteologie.* 7:151–156.

130. Peiche P, Zamani O, Kupman W. (1995). Antiosteoporotic therapy with monofluorophosphate and calcium increases cortical and trabecular bone density. *Osteologie.* 4:87–98.

131. Fujita T, Inoue T, Morii H *et al.* (1999). Effect of an intermittent weekly dose of human parathyroid hormone (1–34) on osteoporosis: A randomized double-masked prospective study using three dose levels. *Osteoporos Int.* 9:296–306.

132. Meunier PJ, Sebert JL, Reginster JY *et al.* (1998). Fluoride salts are no better at preventing new vertebral fractures than calcium-vitamin D in postmenopausal osteoporosis: The FAVO Study. *Osteoporos Int.* 8:4–12.

133. Alexandersen P, Riis BJ, Christiansen C. (1999). Monofluorophosphate combined with hormone replacement therapy induces a synergistic effect on bone mass by dissociating bone formation and resorption in postmenopausal women: A randomized study. *J Clin Endocrinol Metab.* 84:3013–3020.

134. Ringe JD, Rovati LC. (2001). Treatment of osteoporosis in men with fluoride alone or in combination with bisphosphonates. *Calcif Tissue Int.* 69:252–255.

135. Donahue L, Rosen CJ. (1998). IGFs and bone. The osteoporosis connection revisited. *Proc Soc Exp Biol Med.* 219:1–7.

136. Zhao G, Monier-Faugere MC, Langub MC *et al.* (2000). Targeted overexpression of insulin-like growth factor I to osteoblasts of transgenic mice: Increased trabecular bone volume without increased osteoblast proliferation. *Endocrinology.* 141:2674–2682.

137. Sugimoto T, Nakaoka D, Nasu M *et al.* (1999). Effect of recombinant human growth hormone in elderly osteoporotic women. *Clin Endocrinol (Oxf).* 51:715–724.

138. Bauer DC, Rosen CJ, Cauley J, Cummings SR. (1998). Low serum IGF-1 but not IGFBP-3 predicts hip and spine fracture: The study of osteoporotic fracture. *J Bone Miner Res.* 23:S561.

139. Rudman D, Feller AG, Nagraj HS *et al.* (1990). Effects of human growth hormone in men over 60 years old. *N Engl J Med.* 323:1–6.

140. Holloway L, Butterfield G, Hintz RL *et al.* (1994). Effects of recombinant human growth hormone on metabolic indices, body composition, and bone turnover in healthy elderly women. *J Clin Endocrinol Metab.* 79:470–479.

141. Hodsman AB, Fraher LJ, Watson PH. (1999). Parathyroid Hormone. In *The Aging Skeleton* (Rosen CJ, Glowacki J, Bilezikian JP, eds.), pp. 563–578. Sand Diego, CA: Academic Press.

142. Ackert-Bicknell C, Rubin J, Zhu L *et al.* (2002). IGF-I acts as a coupling factor for bone remodeling by regulating osteoprotegerin and RANK ligand in vitro and osteoprotegerin in vivo. Eight-fourth Annual Meeting of the Endocrine Society, Bethesda, MD: Endocrine Society, p. P3–366.

143. Landin-Wilhelmsen K, Nilsson A, Bosaeus I, Bengtsson BA. (2003). Growth hormone increases bone mineral content in postmenopausal osteoporosis: A randomized placebo-controlled trial. *J Bone Miner Res.* 18:393–405.

144. Rosen CJ, Wuster C. (2003). Growth hormone rising: Did we quit too quickly? *J Bone Miner Res.* 18:406–409.

145. Ghiron LJ, Thompson JL, Holloway L *et al.* (1995). Effects of recombinant insulin-like growth factor-I and growth hormone on bone turnover in elderly women. *J Bone Miner Res.* 10:1844–1852.

146. Grinspoon S, Baum H, Lee K *et al.* (1996). Effects of short-term recombinant human insulin-like growth factor I administration on bone turnover in osteopenic women with anorexia nervosa. *J Clin Endocrinol Metab.* 81:3864–3870.

147. Body JJ, Gaich GA, Scheele WH *et al.* (2002). A randomized double-blind trial to compare the efficacy of teriparatide [recombinant human parathyroid hormone (1–34)] with alendronate in postmenopausal women with osteoporosis. *J Clin Endocrinol Metab.* 87:4528–4535.

148. Geusens P, Bouillon R, Broos P. (1998). Musculoskeletal effects of rhIGF-I/IGFBP-3 in hip fracture patients: Results from a double-blind, placebo controlled phase II study. *Bone.* 23:S157.

149. Johnson AR, Armstrong WD, Singer L. (1968). The incorporation and removal of large amounts of strontium by physiologic mechanisms in mineralized tissues. *Calcif Tissue Res.* 2:242–252.

150. Marie PJ, Amman P, Boivin G *et al.* (2001). Mechanisms of action and therapeutic potential of strontium in bone. *Calcif Tissue Int.* 69:121–129.

151. Quarles LD. (1997). Cation sensing receptors in bone: A novel paradigm for regulating bone remodeling? *J Bone Miner Res.* 12:1971–1974.

152. Brown EM, MacLeod RJ. (2001). Extracellular calcium sensing and extracellular calcium signaling. *Physiol Rev.* 81:239–297.

153. Coulombe J, Faure H, Robin B *et al.* (2002). Activation of the rat and mouse cation-sensing receptor by strontium ranelate and its modulation by extracellular calcium. *Osteoporos Int.* 13(Suppl 1):S25.

154. Reginster JY, Halkin V, Henrotin Y, Gosset C. (1999). Treatment of osteoporosis: Role of bone-forming agents. *Osteoporos Int.* 9(Suppl 2):S91–96.

155. Meunier PJ, Slosman DO, Delmas PD *et al.* (2002). Strontium ranelate: Dose-dependent effects in established postmenopausal vertebral osteoporosis—A 2-year randomized placebo controlled trial. *J Clin Endocrinol Metab.* 87:2060–2066.

156. Cranney A, Guyatt G, Krolicki N *et al.* (2001). A meta-analysis of etidronate for the treatment of postmenopausal osteoporosis. *Osteoporos Int.* 12:140–151.

157. Lees B, Stevenson JC. (2001). The prevention of osteoporosis using sequential low-dose hormone replacement therapy with estradiol-17 beta and dydrogesterone. *Osteoporos Int.* 12:251–258.

158. Meunier PJ, Roux C, Ortolani S *et al.* (2002). Strontium ranelate reduces the vertebral fracture risk in women with postmenopausal osteoporosis. *Osteoporos Int.* 13(Suppl 1):045.

159. Chung YS, Lee MD, Lee SK *et al.* (2000). HMG-CoA reductase inhibitors increase BMD in type 2 diabetes mellitus patients. *J Clin Endocrinol Metab.* 85:1137–1142.

160. Edwards CJ, Hart DJ, Spector TD. (2000). Oral statins and increased bone-mineral density in postmenopausal women. *Lancet.* 355:2218–2219.

161. Chan KA, Andrade SE, Boles M *et al.* (2000). Inhibitors of hydroxymethylglutaryl-coenzyme A reductase and risk of fracture among older women. *Lancet.* 355:2185–2188.

162. Meier CR, Schlienger RG, Kraenzlin ME *et al.* (2000). HMG-CoA reductase inhibitors and the risk of fractures. *JAMA.* 283:3205–3210.

163. Wang PS, Solomon DH, Mogun H, Avorn J. (2000). HMG-CoA reductase inhibitors and the risk of hip fractures in elderly patients. *JAMA.* 283:3211–3216.

164. Pasco JA, Kotowicz MA, Henry MJ *et al.* (2000). Statin use, bone mineral density, and fracture risk: Geelong Osteoporosis Study. *Arch Intern Med.* 162:537–540.

165. Mundy G, Garrett R, Harris S *et al.* (1999). Stimulation of bone formation *in vitro* and in rodents by statins. *Science.* 286:1946–1949.

166. Garrett IR, Gutierrez G, Chen D. (2001). Statins stimulate bone formation by enhancing eNOS expression. *J Bone Miner Res.* 16(Suppl 1):1018.

167. Coxon FP, Benford HL, Russell RG, Rogers MJ. (1998). Protein synthesis is required for caspase activation and induction of apoptosis by bisphosphonate drugs. *Mol Pharmacol.* 54:631–638.

168. Sugiyama M, Kodama T, Konishi K *et al.* (2000). Compactin and simvastatin, but not pravastatin, induce bone morphogenetic protein-2 in human osteosarcoma cells. *Biochem Biophys Res Commun.* 271:688–692.

169. Maeda T, Matsunuma A, Kawane T, Horiuchi N. (2001). Simvastatin promotes osteoblast differentiation and mineralization in MC3T3-E1 cells. *Biochem Biophys Res Commun.* 280:874–877.

170. Crawford DT, Qi, H Chidsey-Frink KL *et al.* (2001). Statin increases cortical bone in young male rats by single, local administration but fails to restore bone in ovariectomized rats by daily systemic administration. *J Bone Miner Res.* 16(Suppl 1):SA410.

171. Chan MH, Mak TW, Chiu RW *et al.* (2001). Simvastatin increases serum osteocalcin concentration in patients treated for hypercholesterolaemia. *J Clin Endocrinol Metab.* 86:4556–4559.

172. Braga V, Gatti D, Rossini M, Adami S. (2001). Association between lipid profile and bone mass in healthy men. *J Bone Miner Res.* 16(Suppl 1):F307.

173. Solomon DH, Finkelstein JS, Wang PS, Avorn J. (2001). Statin lipid-lowering drugs and bone density. *J Bone Miner Res.* 16(Suppl 1):SA399.

174. Reid IR, Hague W, Emberson J *et al.* (2001). Effect of pravastatin on frequency of fracture in the LIPID study: Secondary analysis of a randomised controlled trial. Long-term Intervention with Pravastatin in Ischaemic Disease. *Lancet.* 357:509–512.

175. van Staa TP, Wegman S, de Vries F *et al.* (2001). Use of statins and risk of fractures. *JAMA.* 285:1850–1855.

176. LaCroix AZ, Cauley J, Jackson R *et al*. (2000). Does statin use reduce risk of fracture in postmenopausal women? Results from the Women's Health Initiative Observational Study (WHI-OS). *J Bone Miner Res.* 15(Suppl 1):1066.

177. Finkelstein JS, Neer RM, Biller BM *et al*. (1992). Osteopenia in men with a history of delayed puberty. *N Engl J Med.* 326:600–604.

178. Katznelson L, Finkelstein JS, Schoenfeld DA *et al*. (1996). Increase in bone density and lean body mass during testosterone administration in men with acquired hypogonadism. *J Clin Endocrinol Metab.* 81:4358–4365.

179. Leder BZ, Schoenfeld DA, LeBlanc K, Finkelstein JS. (2001). Both estradiol and testosterone play fundamental roles in the maintenance of normal bone turnover in men. *J Bone Miner Res.* 16(suppl 1):1140.

180. Davis SR, McCloud P, Strauss BJ, Burger H. (1995). Testosterone enhances estradiol's effects on postmenopausal bone density and sexuality. *Maturitas.* 21:227–236.

181. Watts NB, Notelovitz M, Timmons MC *et al*. (1995). Comparison of oral estrogens and estrogens plus androgen on bone mineral density, menopausal symptoms, and lipid-lipoprotein profiles in surgical menopause. *Obstet Gynecol.* 85:529–537.

182. Barrett-Connor E, Young R, Notelovitz M *et al*. (1999). A two-year, double-blind comparison of estrogen-androgen and conjugated estrogens in surgically menopausal women. Effects on bone mineral density, symptoms and lipid profiles. *J Reprod Med.* 44:1012–1020.

183. Leone-Bay A, Sato M, Paton D *et al*. (2001). Oral delivery of biologically active parathyroid hormone. *Pharm Res.* 18:964–970.

184. Mehta NM, Gilligan JP, Stern B *et al*. (2002). Biological activity of recombinant PTH analog 7841. *J Bone Miner Metab.* 17(Suppl 1):SA362.

185. Gowen M, Stroup GB, Dodds RA *et al*. (2000). Antagonizing the parathyroid calcium receptor stimulates parathyroid hormone secretion and bone formation in osteopenic rats. *J Clin Invest.* 105:1595–1604.

93

Antiresorptive Therapies for Osteoporosis in Women and Men

CAROLYN BECKER, MD

Associate Clinical Professor of Medicine, Metabolic Bone Diseases Unit, Division of Endocrinology;
Associate Director, Toni Stabile Osteoporosis Center, College of Physicians and Surgeons,
Columbia University, New York, NY

Abstract

Over the past 15 years, management of postmenopausal osteoporosis has been facilitated by the introduction of the bisphosphonates, calcitonin, and raloxifene. These antiresorptive agents, along with estrogen, have provided postmenopausal women with a variety of therapeutic options for both the prevention and treatment of osteoporosis. Men with osteoporosis, on the other hand, have suffered from a delayed recognition of the disorder and inadequate inclusion in clinical trials. This chapter reviews the antifracture efficacy of the bisphosphonates, calcitonin, and raloxifene in postmenopausal women with osteoporosis, focusing on large, prospective, randomized, placebo-controlled clinical trials. Whenever possible, trials in men are also reviewed and compared with the results found in the female studies. Studies with drugs that are not yet approved for osteoporosis in the United States and clinical trials for glucocorticoid-induced osteoporosis (GIO) are included. The bisphosphonates, which have been investigated most extensively in women and men, appear to have similar beneficial effects on the skeleton, irrespective of gender. Calcitonin may have favorable effects on bone density for men with high turnover osteoporosis but the studies are too small to be conclusive. Finally, raloxifene has shown some surprising and intriguing gender-specific effects in a handful of studies in men. It appears that the efficacy of antiresorptive therapies for osteoporosis varies not only by class but by gender. Clearly, there is a pressing need for more research in the area of gender-specific responses to osteoporosis therapies.

I. Introduction

More than 60 years ago, Fuller Albright first linked estrogen deficiency at menopause with rapid bone loss in women [1]. For the next five decades, estrogen remained the only therapeutic option for this "women's disease." In the past 20 years, however, there has been an explosion of research in the field that has resulted in the introduction of several novel therapies for osteoporosis and recognition that osteoporosis in men is also a major public health problem. Unquestionably, osteoporosis is much more common among women than men. Reasons for this gender difference include women's achievement of lower peak bone mass, smaller bone size, accelerated bone loss at menopause, and greater longevity [2]. In men, the pathophysiology of osteoporosis is more obscure but hypogonadism, glucocorticoid use, and alcoholism are major causes. In addition, it now appears that estrogen may be a major factor for accrual and maintenance of bone mass in the male skeleton [3], an observation that has intriguing therapeutic implications.

In both sexes, osteoporosis occurs whenever there is an absolute or relative increase in bone resorption as compared with bone formation. The result is progressive bone loss. In women, bone loss accelerates after menopause, whereas, in men, bone loss occurs more gradually with aging. Among the elderly of both sexes, rates of bone loss are quite similar [4,5] so that, by the end of life, men experience up to two thirds of the bone loss of women [5–7]. Moreover, older men and women demonstrate elevated levels of bone turnover markers and parathyroid hormone compared with their younger counterparts [8]. Finally, histomorphometric abnormalities on bone biopsies in patients with age-related osteoporosis are indistinguishable by gender [9,10]. Thus, with regard to age-related bone loss, women and men may share common pathophysiologic changes associated with osteoporosis. By inference, they may respond similarly to therapeutic agents.

Currently, four types of pharmacologic agents are approved for either the treatment and/or the prevention of postmenopausal osteoporosis. These include estrogen, bisphosphonates, calcitonin, and raloxifene. Only one agent (alendronate) is approved for treatment of male osteoporosis, but both alendronate and risedronate are approved for use in GIO (Table 93-1). All of these agents are antiresorptives, which means that they function by decreasing the rate of bone resorption. In contrast, anabolic agents stimulate processes associated with bone formation. This chapter explores gender-specific responses to osteoporosis treatment by focusing on three of these antiresorptive therapies: the bisphosphonates, calcitonin, and the selective estrogen receptor modulator (SERM) raloxifene. Each section begins with a summary of the major studies in postmenopausal women followed by those in men (if available). Given the extensive literature on the effects of these agents in postmenopausal women, only large, randomized, placebo-controlled trials with fracture endpoints are reviewed here. There are no comparable large-scale clinical trials evaluating antiresorptive therapies in the management of male osteoporosis, but those studies that do exist are reviewed in detail (Tables 93-2 and 93-3).

II. Antiresorptive Therapies for Osteoporosis

A. Bisphosphonates

Bisphosphonates are stable pyrophosphate analogues that bind with high affinity to hydroxyapatite in bone. They inhibit bone resorption by decreasing the number, activity, and lifespan

Table 93-1

Approved Antiresorptive Therapies for Osteoporosis

Drug	Dose	Route	Prevention	Treatment
Postmenopausal women				
Alendronate	10 mg/day; 70 mg/wk	Oral	Yes	Yes
Risedronate	5 mg/day; 35 mg/wk	Oral	Yes	Yes
Calcitonin	200 IU/day	Intranasal	No	Yes
Raloxifene	60 mg/day	Oral	Yes	Yes
Estrogen	Variable	Oral/transdermal	Yes	
Men				
Alendronate	10 mg/day	Oral	No	Yes
Glucocorticoid-induced osteoporosis				
Alendronate	10 mg/day	Oral	No	Yes
Risedronate	5 mg/day	Oral	Yes	Yes

Table 93-2

Effects of Antiresorptive Therapies in Women and Men

Reference	Gender	Drug	Spine BMD	FN BMD	Resorption
Liberman *et al* [12]	F	ALN	8.8%↑	5.9%↑	—
Black *et al* [13]	F	ALN	6.2%↑	4.1%↑	39%↓
Cummings *et al* [14]	F	ALN	6.6%↑	4.6%↑	—
Pols *et al* [16]	F	ALN	4.9%↑	2.4%↑	53%↓
Harris *et al* [22]	F	RIS	4.3%↑	2.8%↑	30%↓
Reginster *et al* [23]	F	RIS	5.9%↑	3.1%↑	37%↓
Chesnut *et al* [54]	F	CAL	NS	NS	—
Ettinger *et al* [62]	F	RAL	2.6%↑	2.1%↑	—
Orwoll *et al* [17]	M	ALN	7.1%↑	2.5%↑	59%↓
Ringe *et al* [18]	M	ALN	10.1%↑	5.2%↑	—

ALN, alendronate; BMD, bone mineral density; CAL, nasal calcitonin; FN, femoral neck; NS, not statistically significant; RAL, raloxifene; resorption, markers of bone resorption; RIS, risedronate.

Table 93-3

Antiresorptive Therapies and Fracture Reduction

Reference	N	Prev Fxs	Dur (years)	VF Dec	NVF Dec	Hip Fx Dec
Liberman *et al* [12]	994	20%	3	48%	NS	—
Black *et al* [13]	2027	100%	3	47%	NS	51%
Cummings *et al* [14]	4432	0%	4.2	44%	NS	NS**
Pols *et al* [16]	1908	—	1	—	47%	—
Harris *et al* [22]	2458	80%	3	41%	39%	NS
Reginster *et al* [23]	1226	98%	3	49%	NS	NS
McClung *et al* [25]	5445	39%	3	—	20%	30%
McClung *et al* [25]	3886	—	3	—	NS	NS
Chesnut *et al* [54]	1255	79%	5	33%	NS	NS
Ettinger *et al* [62]	7705	—	3	55%*, 30%†	NS	NS
Orwoll *et al* [17]	241	50%	2	90%	NS	—
Ringe *et al* [18]	134	54%	2	NS	NS	—

Dur, duration of trial in years; Hip Fx Dec, hip fracture decrease; NS, not statistically significant; NVF Dec, nonvertebral fracture decrease; Prev Fxs, prevalent vertebral fractures; VF Dec, vertebral fracture decrease.

*Vertebral fracture reduction in patients without prevalent vertebral fractures.

**Women with femoral neck T-score ≤−2.5 had significant 36% decrease in clinical fractures and 56% decrease in hip fractures.

†Vertebral fracture reduction in patients with prevalent vertebral fractures.

of osteoclasts [11]. Currently, two oral bisphosphonates are approved in the United States for the prevention and treatment of postmenopausal osteoporosis: alendronate and risedronate. Alendronate is also approved for the treatment of male osteoporosis and GIO. Risedronate is approved for both prevention and treatment of GIO but not yet for male osteoporosis. All oral bisphosphonates are poorly absorbed (0.5 to 1%) and are taken with plain water on an empty stomach. Both alendronate and risedronate may be given daily (10 mg/day and 5 mg/day, respectively) or weekly (70 mg/week and 35 mg/week, respectively). Side effects are generally limited to the gastrointestinal (GI) tract with the daily dosing regimens being associated with a somewhat higher frequency of adverse upper GI events than weekly dosing. Rarely, patients may also complain of muscle aches and pains. A first-generation bisphosphonate etidronate is not approved for osteoporosis but has been studied in trials with both men and women in the United States and is prescribed widely throughout the world for management of osteoporosis. Other bisphosphonates that have been studied but not approved for osteoporosis include pamidronate and zoledronate, administered by intravenous infusion.

1. Alendronate in Women with Postmenopausal Osteoporosis

Four randomized, controlled clinical trials have examined the efficacy of alendronate in fracture reduction in postmenopausal women with osteoporosis. The first study reported by Liberman et al [12] evaluated three different doses of alendronate (5,10, or 20 mg/day) versus placebo in 994 postmenopausal women with osteoporosis. All patients received 500 mg of elemental calcium daily. Twenty percent of these women had prevalent (pre-existing) vertebral fractures at the start of the trial. After 3 years, the alendronate-treated women experienced a significant 48% reduction in new morphometric vertebral fractures compared with the placebo group. Symptomatic nonvertebral fractures were not significantly reduced in this study [12]. In the Fracture Intervention Trial, 6459 women (aged 55 to 80) were enrolled with femoral neck bone mineral density (BMD) ≤ 0.68 g/cm^2 (Hologic QDR-2000), corresponding to a T-score ≤ -2.0. After enrollment was completed, results from the Third National Health and Nutritional Examination Survey (NHANES) showed that this BMD corresponded to a T-score of -1.6. Thus, only one third of women in the FIT trials had femoral neck T-scores < -2.5. In the FIT-I, 2027 postmenopausal women (mean age 71 years) were treated with alendronate 5 mg/day for 2 years then 10 mg/day for the next 9 months or placebo [13]. All women received 500 mg of elemental calcium daily, and 82% also received vitamin D 250 IU/day. One hundred percent of the women had prevalent vertebral fractures. In this group, alendronate reduced the risk of new morphometric vertebral fractures by 47% and also reduced new, clinically symptomatic, vertebral fractures by 55%. The incidence of multiple (two or more) new vertebral fractures was reduced even more dramatically, by 90% [13]. Although alendronate did not significantly reduce total nonvertebral fractures in FIT-I, it did reduce hip fracture risk by a significant 51%. In the third trial, known as FIT-II, 4432 postmenopausal women (mean age 68 years) with low BMD at the femoral neck but *without* prevalent vertebral fractures were followed for an average of 4.2 years [14].

Women were randomized to alendronate 5 mg/day for 2 years then 10 mg/day for the duration of the study versus placebo. Again, alendronate significantly reduced the risk of new morphometric vertebral fractures by 44% compared with placebo, but it did not significantly reduce the risk of total clinically symptomatic fractures, including clinically symptomatic vertebral fractures. Moreover, alendronate did not reduce the incidence of multiple vertebral fractures, nonvertebral fractures, or hip fractures in FIT-2. A post hoc analysis of the data from FIT-2 revealed that women treated with alendronate who had osteoporosis of the femoral neck (T-score ≤ -2.5) did experience a significant 36% reduction in the risk of any clinical fracture, whereas those with higher femoral neck T-scores did not [14]. Another post hoc analysis found a significant 56% decrease in hip fracture risk in alendronate-treated women with baseline femoral neck BMD T-scores in the osteoporotic range (≤ -2.5) [14]. Combining women from both arms of the FIT who either had prevalent vertebral fractures or osteoporosis at the femoral neck, the risk of nonvertebral fractures was significantly decreased by 27% and the risk of hip fractures was reduced by 53% [15]. These results suggest that alendronate has its greatest antifracture efficacy in those subgroups of women at highest risk of fracture (those with BMD in the osteoporotic range and/ or those with prevalent vertebral fractures). However, the lack of demonstrated efficacy in those women with T-scores greater than -2.5 may reflect the reduced power of the study when patients were reclassified, rather than a true lack of efficacy. In the fourth trial, a multinational study (FOSIT) by Pols et al [16], 1908 postmenopausal women (mean age 63 years) received alendronate 10 mg/day or placebo for 1 year. All women received 500 mg elemental calcium/day. In this study, alendronate significantly reduced new clinical nonvertebral fractures by 47%.

In addition to reducing fracture incidence, alendronate was significantly more protective against progressive spinal deformity and loss of height than placebo in two trials [12,13]. In alendronate-treated patients, BMD increased significantly at the lumbar spine by 8.8% at 3 years [12], 6.2 to 6.6% at 2.9 to 4.2 years [13,14], and 4.9% at 1 year [16]. Corresponding BMD increases at the femoral neck were 5.9% [12], 4.1 to 4.6% [13,14], and 2.4% [16] compared with placebo. In keeping with its antiresorptive actions, alendronate significantly reduced markers of bone resorption by 39% [13], 49% [12], and 53% [16].

2. Alendronate in Men with Osteoporosis

To date, there are only two prospective, controlled studies of alendronate in men with osteoporosis. In 2000, Orwoll et al [17] reported results of a 2-year multinational, randomized, double-blind, placebo-controlled trial of 241 men with osteoporosis. All patients received 500 mg/day of elemental calcium and 400 IU/day of vitamin D. Alendronate administered orally at 10 mg daily was given to 146 men; 95 men received placebo. The patients, ranging in age from 31 to 87 years (mean age 63 years), were included in the trial if they met bone density criteria (femoral neck T-score ≤ -2.0 and lumbar spine T-score ≤ -1.0) or had a history of osteoporotic fracture and femoral neck T-score ≤ -1.0. The mean T-scores were -2.2 for the femoral neck and -2.0

for the lumbar spine. Hypogonadal men constituted 36% of the study population with the rest of the study subjects classified as having idiopathic osteoporosis. Men with history of peptic ulcer or esophageal disease within the previous year were excluded, but those on nonsteroidal anti-inflammatory drugs (NSAIDs) were not. One half of the men in the treatment and placebo groups had a radiologically confirmed vertebral fracture at baseline. The groups were well matched for other baseline parameters. After 2 years, the alendronate group demonstrated a significant increase from baseline in lumbar spine BMD of 7.1%, whereas the increase in the placebo group was only 1.8%, for a between-group difference of 5.3%. Smaller increases over baseline in the alendronate group were seen at the femoral neck (2.5%), trochanter (4.4%), total hip (3.1%), and total body (2.0%), but all were statistically significantly higher relative to both baseline and to placebo. Positive effects of alendronate on spinal BMD were independent of baseline free testosterone levels, estradiol levels, and age. At the end of the study, urinary excretion of N-telopeptides (NTX), a marker of bone resorption, had declined 9% in the placebo group and 59% in the alendronate group (p < 0.001), whereas serum bone-specific alkaline phosphatase, a marker of bone formation, declined 5% in the placebo group and 38% in the alendronate-treated group (p < 0.001). The rate of nonvertebral fractures did not differ between the two groups. Vertebral fractures, however, were decreased among the men taking alendronate. Overall, using semiquantitative analysis, there were seven new vertebral fractures in the placebo group (8.1%) and four in the alendronate group (3.1%) for an odds ratio of 0.36 (p = 0.119) favoring the alendronate-treated patients. Using more quantitative morphometric analysis, seven patients had a new fracture in the placebo group but only one in the alendronate group for an odds ratio of 0.10, which was statistically significant (p = 0.017). Men who received alendronate also showed significantly less height loss compared with men on placebo (0.6 mm vs 2.4 mm, respectively, p = 0.022) [17]. Similar to trials of alendronate in women, there were no differences between the groups in terms of safety or adverse events. In contrast to the studies with postmenopausal women, however, this trial included men with histories of digestive disorders and did not exclude those using NSAIDs or aspirin. Approximately 60% of the total study population took these medications during the trial.

A second trial of alendronate in male osteoporosis was reported by Ringe in 2001 [18]. In contrast to the Orwoll study, this 2-year trial was open label. However, it was randomized and prospective, comparing alendronate 10 mg/day versus 1-alfacalcidol 1 μg/day in 134 men with osteoporosis (baseline T-score at the lumbar spine < − 2.5). All men received 500 mg/day of elemental calcium. Patients with hypogonadism, major upper GI diseases, renal insufficiency, or abnormal calcium levels were excluded. Mean age of the patients was 53 years and mean T-scores were −3.4 at the lumbar spine and −2.5 at the femoral neck. Thus, despite younger average age, these patients had substantially lower bone densities than the men in the Orwoll study [17]. Slightly more than half the men (54%) had a pre-existing vertebral fracture, comparable to the Orwoll study. After 2 years, the alendronate group demonstrated a significant 10.1% increase in lumbar spine BMD over baseline,

whereas the alfacalcidol group increased by only 2.8%. At the femoral neck, BMD increased 5.2% and 2.2% in the alendronate and alfacalcidol groups, respectively. Thus, the increases in BMD in both the spine and femoral neck were higher among these men with more severe osteoporosis than in the Orwoll trial. Nonvertebral fractures rates were similar between the two treatment groups. Vertebral fractures were more common overall in this study than in the Orwoll study, but the men on alendronate (with a 7.4% vertebral fracture rate) showed a lower rate of incident fractures compared with those on placebo (18.2% vertebral fracture rate) for a difference that approached statistical significance (p 0.071). The total number of vertebral fractures in the alendronate group (n = 5) was reduced compared with the number of fractures in the alfacalcidol group (n = 14), a difference that reached statistical significance (p = 0.046). As in the Orwoll trial, height loss was significantly reduced in alendronate-treated men (1.4 mm loss) compared with placebo (8.3 mm loss; p < 0.05) [18]. Despite the lack of conclusive antifracture efficacy and the small numbers of fractures in these trials, alendronate has been approved for treatment of male osteoporosis in the United States.

3. Summary of Alendronate Effects in Men Compared with Women

Alendronate increases lumbar spine BMD in men and postmenopausal women to a very similar degree [19]. A small, open-label trial that actually included both men (n = 23) and postmenopausal women (n = 18) with osteoporosis demonstrated comparable spinal increases of 7% in the men and 5.4% in the women who received 10 mg/day of alendronate for 1 year [20]. Reductions in bone turnover markers with alendronate therapy appear consistent between the sexes. In the Orwoll study [17], urinary NTX declined 59% with alendronate treatment, which is almost identical to values reported in the trials with postmenopausal women [12,16,21]. The changes in stature reported in the male alendronate studies also compare favorably to those found in trials with postmenopausal women [12,13], suggesting consistent effects of alendronate on vertebral deformity and vertebral fracture risk in both sexes [19]. With respect to fractures, the studies in men infer that alendronate significantly reduces vertebral fractures in men. Data from the two male trials [17,18] show vertebral fracture odds ratios below 1 for alendronate-treated men, comparable to rate reductions seen in postmenopausal women [12–14]. However, because of the much smaller numbers of men included in these trials and the even smaller numbers of fractures, the confidence intervals are very wide. Thus, statements regarding alendronate and vertebral fracture risk in men remain inconclusive at this time.

4. Risedronate for Women with Postmenopausal Osteoporosis

There have been three, large, randomized, placebo-controlled trials examining effects of risedronate on fractures in postmenopausal women. The first two of these trials actually consist of the same trial carried out in two different sites: the *Vertebral Efficacy with Risedronate Therapy* (VERT) trial conducted in North America [22] and the multinational VERT trial conducted in Europe and Australia [23]. The North American VERT (VERT-NA) trial enrolled 2458 postmenopausal women (mean age 69 years), whereas the multinational VERT (VERT-MN) trial included 1226 postmenopausal women (mean age 71 years). Randomization was to risedronate 2.5 mg/day (note that this was changed to 5 mg/day after 1 year), 5 mg/day, or placebo for 3 years. All women received elemental calcium 1000 mg/day, whereas 9% (in VERT-NA) and 35% (in VERT-MN) received up to 500 IU of vitamin D per day. Eighty percent of the women in the North American trial and 98% of those in the multinational trial had prevalent vertebral fractures on entry. Subjects in VERT-NA had fewer prevalent vertebral fractures per patient (2.3 to 2.7) compared with those in VERT-MN (3 to 4 vertebral fractures per patient). Women with recent peptic ulcers, ulcers requiring hospitalization, or chronic dyspepsia requiring medication were included in the VERT trials, in contrast to the alendronate trials. New morphometric vertebral fractures were significantly reduced by 61–65% after 1 year and by 41 to 49% after 3 years of risedronate treatment [22,23]. In the multinational trial, those on risedronate had less height loss than the placebo group [23]. Nonvertebral fractures were significantly reduced by 39% in the North American study after 3 years on risedronate [22]. In the multinational arm, however, the 33% reduction in nonvertebral fractures seen with risedronate was not statistically different from placebo. The smaller size of the Multinational study coupled with the high dropout rate of 42% might have affected these results [24]. Neither trial demonstrated significant fracture reduction at any individual nonvertebral sites, such as the hip. In terms of effects on BMD, risedronate increased lumbar spine BMD by 4.3 to 5.9% and femoral neck BMD by 2.8 to 3.1% after 3 years, compared with placebo. Markers of bone resorption decreased by 30% [22] and 37% [23], respectively. These effects on BMD and bone resorption markers are somewhat less than those seen in the alendronate trials in women [12–14,16].

The third risedronate trial was a unique attempt to directly assess hip fracture risk reduction as the primary outcome of therapy [25]. One arm of this very large study enrolled 5445 women (aged 70 to 79 years) with osteoporosis defined by low femoral neck BMD (HIP I). The other arm included 3886 elderly women (age 80 or older) who had at least one "clinical risk factor" for hip fracture (HIP II). There was no BMD requirement. Only 31% of patients in the very elderly group had BMD measurements. A clinical risk factor was defined as low femoral neck BMD, difficulty standing, poor gait, smoking, previous hip fracture, maternal history of hip fracture, previous fall-related injury, or long hip axis length. Patients were treated with risedronate 2.5 mg/day, 5 mg/day, or placebo for 3 years. All women received elemental calcium 1000 mg/day, and those with low vitamin D levels (<16 ng/mL) received up to 500 IU/day of vitamin D. Similar to the other risedronate studies, this one was associated with a high attrition rate of 50% by the end of the trial. Nevertheless, among the HIP I women (70 to 79 years old) with femoral neck osteoporosis, risedronate significantly decreased hip fracture risk by 30%. At least 39% of these women had at least one vertebral fracture at baseline. When the data were analyzed according to prevalent vertebral fractures, those with vertebral fractures *and* femoral neck osteoporosis had a 60% reduction in hip fracture risk with risedronate. In those *without* a prevalent vertebral fracture, hip fracture was not significantly reduced. This is probably due to the low incidence of

hip fractures and small numbers of women in this group. In the second arm of the trial assessing elderly women with clinical risk factors for hip fracture (HIP II), risedronate did not significantly reduce hip fracture risk [25]. There are many possible explanations for this null effect. First, the women who discontinued treatment early were older, thinner, and more likely to smoke than those who completed the treatment and thus were at higher risk for hip fracture. Early discontinuation in this high-risk group would tend to limit the magnitude of the treatment effect. Also, the majority of the older women in HIP II did not have BMD measurements and may not have had osteoporosis. Only 941 of the 3886 women (24%) were known to have osteoporosis (T≤− 2.5). A subgroup of patients in HIP II had serial measurements of BMD and bone turnover markers and demonstrated treatment effects similar to those seen in HIP I patients, namely, increases in BMD and decreases in bone turnover. These effects, however, did not translate into lower hip fracture risk, emphasizing the importance of nonskeletal factors in the cause of hip fracture. With advancing age, nonskeletal risk factors assume a greater role in the etiology of hip fractures compared with skeletal risk factors such as BMD. Therapies that address skeletal issues only (e.g., antiresorptive agents) may be less effective in reducing hip fractures in the elderly.

Thus, in postmenopausal osteoporosis, both alendronate and risedronate increase BMD at the spine and hip, reduce markers of bone turnover, and significantly decrease vertebral and hip fractures in selected subgroups of women. Although no head-to-head studies of these two bisphosphonates have been carried out, alendronate therapy appears to increase BMD at the spine and hip and decrease bone resorption markers to a somewhat greater degree than risedronate. It is not clear whether these differences have clinical relevance. In terms of antifracture efficacy, both drugs appear effective in reducing vertebral fractures. Hip fractures, on the other hand, were significantly reduced by risedronate only among elderly women with prevalent vertebral fractures and femoral neck osteoporosis [25]. In contrast, alendronate significantly reduced hip fractures in women with [13] and without [14] prevalent vertebral fractures who had osteoporosis at the femoral neck. As mentioned previously, the number of women in the risedronate trial who did not have prevalent vertebral fractures may have been too small to show a significant effect in hip fracture reduction.

5. Etidronate in Women with Postmenopausal Osteoporosis

Etidronate, a first-generation bisphosphonate, is not approved for treatment of osteoporosis in the United States. Historically, the pivotal trials with etidronate were initiated before the Food and Drug Administration (FDA) required antifracture efficacy to be demonstrated. A recent meta-analysis of 13 clinical trials using etidronate in the treatment of postmenopausal osteoporosis found a significant reduction in vertebral fractures (pooled relative risk 0.63) in etidronate-treated patients [26]. However, this is not sufficient to meet FDA requirements. In addition, long-term use is associated with mineralization defects (osteomalacia) [27]. Nevertheless, etidronate is prescribed widely throughout the world for osteoporosis. It is still used in the United States because of its excellent tolerability and relative low cost [27]. In 1990, Watts *et al* [28] published results from a 2-year, randomized clinical trial of cyclical etidronate (400 mg/day in 2-week cycles every 91 days) in 423 postmenopausal women with one to four prevalent vertebral fractures [28]. After 2 years, vertebral fractures were significantly reduced in the etidronate-treated women, but, following a 1-year extension of the trial, there was no longer a significant difference compared with placebo [29]. Etidronate increased lumbar spine BMD by 3 to 4% after 2 years but did not significantly increase femoral neck or forearm BMD [28]. A number of smaller trials of etidronate demonstrated BMD increases but not significant vertebral fracture reductions [30,31]. Thus, although etidronate still has a role in osteoporosis management (it is used widely in Canada), the later-generation bisphosphonates alendronate and risedronate have replaced etidronate in many parts of the world.

6. Etidronate in Men with Osteoporosis

Several small trials using etidronate have been conducted in men with osteoporosis [32–35]. There is one large epidemiologic study [36]. The clinical trials generally show small increases in lumbar spine BMD and no improvement in femoral neck BMD after 12 to 31 months of etidronate [32–35]. In a large population-based study that included women and men, data on 7977 subjects in the United Kingdom taking cyclical etidronate and 7977 age-, sex-, and practice-matched osteoporotic controls not taking etidronate were analyzed. Those on etidronate had a 20% lower risk of nonvertebral fracture and a 34% lower risk of hip fracture, both statistically significant. There were no significant gender differences. This study supports the possible antifracture efficacy of cyclical etidronate in both sexes [36] but is limited by its epidemiologic nature.

7. Other Nonapproved Bisphosphonates for Osteoporosis

a. PAMIDRONATE. Pamidronate (also known as APD) is a potent bisphosphonate approved for treatment of malignant hypercalcemia, osteolytic bone metastases from multiple myeloma or breast cancer, and Paget's disease of bone. Pamidronate has been used in both oral and intravenous forms for prevention [37] and treatment [38] of postmenopausal osteoporosis. Because of major upper GI toxicity, it is usually given as an intravenous infusion. A standard intravenous regimen is 90 mg for the first dose followed by 30 mg every third month [39]. In men with osteoporosis treated with APD, an early study found beneficial effects on lumbar spine BMD and calcium balance [40].

A more recent application of this drug has been for men receiving androgen-ablation therapy for prostate cancer. Treatment of prostate cancer with gonadotropin-releasing hormone (GnRH) agonists, such as leuprolide, can lead to rapid decreases in bone density, increased bone turnover, and higher risk of fractures [41]. In a 48-week, open-label trial, 47 men with advanced or recurrent prostate cancer were randomly assigned to leuprolide alone or leuprolide and pamidronate (60 mg IV q 12 weeks). Men treated with leuprolide alone had significant BMD losses at the lumbar spine, trochanter, and total hip, whereas those who received pamidronate along with the leuprolide had no significant loss of BMD at any site [42]. In another study, 21 men with metastatic prostate cancer treated with combined androgen blockage (a long-acting GnRH agonist and an androgen

receptor antagonist) were randomly assigned to receive either placebo or 90 mg of intravenous pamidronate at baseline with a crossover at 6 months. A single dose of intravenous pamidronate totally prevented the rapid loss of bone from the spine and femoral neck and the accelerated bone turnover associated with hypogonadism for at least 6 months [43].

b. ZOLEDRONIC ACID (ZOLEDRONATE). Zoledronic acid is the most potent bisphosphonate currently available. It is approved for the treatment of malignant hypercalcemia and is also used to treat osteolytic metastases from lung and breast cancer and multiple myeloma. A recent clinical trial investigated the efficacy of intravenous zoledronic acid in the treatment of postmenopausal osteoporosis [44]. Five different dosing regimens were administered to 351 postmenopausal women with osteoporosis in a 1-year, randomized, double-blind, placebo-controlled trial. At the end of 1 year, all of the groups treated with intravenous zoledronic acid, in doses ranging from 0.25 mg every 3 months to 4 mg given once at the beginning of the trial, showed equivalently significant increases in lumbar spine BMD (4.3 to 5.1% above placebo) and femoral neck BMD (3.1 to 3.5% above placebo). Biochemical markers of bone turnover were suppressed equally for all active treatment regimens and remained suppressed at 1 year. Side effects from zoledronic acid included myalgias and fever, but dropout rates were not different from placebo [44]. Currently, there are no fracture data in patients treated with zoledronic acid and the drug is not approved for osteoporosis. Long-term safety issues are not resolved. Moreover, the clinical trial did not establish an optimal dose (all doses and administration regimens gave the same results) nor did it indicate how long the effects of single-dosing regimens will persist. It is not yet clear whether zoledronic acid will provide an alternative for women and men with severe osteoporosis for whom other therapies are either contraindicated or not well tolerated.

8. Bisphosphonate Therapy in Patients on Glucocorticoids

a. ALENDRONATE IN PATIENTS ON GLUCOCORTICOIDS. Alendronate has been studied for the prevention and treatment of GIO in both men and women but it is approved only for treatment of GIO. In 1998, Saag et al [45] reported results from two 48-week randomized, placebo-controlled studies using two doses of alendronate in 477 women and men who were receiving at least 7.5 mg/day of prednisone or its equivalent (median dose 10 mg/day). All patients received 800 to 1000 mg of elemental calcium and 250 to 500 IU of vitamin D daily. Subjects had an average age of 55 years and men comprised 28 to 33% of each treatment group. Interestingly, both premenopausal and postmenopausal women were included. There were no reports of any pregnancies among the premenopausal women taking alendronate. Overall, both doses of alendronate (5 mg/day and 10 mg/day) resulted in significant increases in spinal and femoral neck BMD and significant decreases in markers of bone turnover after 48 weeks. The average increase in lumbar spine BMD was 2.1% and 2.9% for the 5 mg/day and 10 mg/day doses, respectively. Corresponding values for femoral neck BMD were 1.2% and 1.0%, respectively. Urinary excretion of NTX, a marker of bone resorption, decreased by 60%, whereas serum bone-specific alkaline phosphatase, a marker of bone formation, decreased by

27% in alendronate-treated subjects. Vertebral fracture rates were very low. There were fewer vertebral fractures in the alendronate group but the difference from placebo was not statistically significant. Eighty-two percent of vertebral fractures occurred in postmenopausal women and the remainder in men. Beneficial effects of alendronate on BMD and markers of bone resorption were not related to the age or sex of the subjects, the underlying disease, or the dose of glucocorticoid [45].

b. RISEDRONATE IN PATIENTS ON GLUCOCORTICOIDS. Risedronate therapy was studied in 224 men and women, ages 18 to 85 years, who had begun taking long-term glucocorticoid treatment with a mean initial prednisone dose 21 mg/day within the previous 3 months. This was a multicenter, randomized, double-blind, placebo-controlled trial [46]. All patients received 500 mg/day of elemental calcium in addition to risedronate 2.5 mg/day, 5.0 mg/day, or placebo for 1 year. A total of 150 patients completed 12 months of the study. The mean age varied from 57.2 years among placebo-treated patients to 61.9 years among those receiving 5 mg/day of alendronate. Approximately one third of all patients were men, and two thirds of women were postmenopausal. The average lumbar spine T-score was in the normal range although 26 to 36% of patients in each treatment group had vertebral fractures at baseline. Lumbar spine BMD remained unchanged in the risedronate-treated groups but decreased significantly, by 2.8%, in the placebo group. The mean differences between risedronate 5 mg/day and placebo were 3.8% at the lumbar spine, 4.1% at the femoral neck, and 4.6% at the trochanter. Men and postmenopausal women had very similar BMD effects from the 5 mg/day dose of risedronate. In contrast, BMD changes among premenopausal women treated with risedronate did not differ from placebo. Although not powered to show fracture reduction, a trend toward reduction of vertebral fractures was noted in the 5-mg risedronate group compared with placebo (5.7% vs 17.3%, p = 0.072). As in the alendronate trial [45], vertebral fractures occurred only in postmenopausal women and men not in premenopausal women [46]. Risedronate therapy reduced bone turnover markers early in the trial. At 12 months, however, there were no statistically significant differences between treatment groups in either bone resorption or formation markers.

Another clinical trial of risedronate was conducted in parallel to that of Cohen *et al* and with a similar protocol [47]. In this second trial, 290 patients who had received moderate-to-high dose glucocorticoid therapy for at least 6 months before enrollment were included [47]. Results of the two trials were quite similar. In a post hoc analysis combining these two trials, risedronate 5 mg/day significantly reduced vertebral fractures by 70% compared with placebo (p = 0.01) [48]. Among men, the 5 mg/day risedronate dose lowered vertebral fractures by 66%, but this was not statistically significant (p = 0.12). In postmenopausal women, there was a significant 73% reduction (p = 0.05) in vertebral fractures with risedronate 5 mg/day [48]. There were no vertebral fractures in the premenopausal group. Risedronate is approved for both the prevention and treatment of GIO.

c. ETIDRONATE IN PATIENTS ON GLUCOCORTICOIDS. The first-generation bisphosphonate etidronate has also been studied in the prevention and treatment of GIO in men and women. Pitt

et al [49], investigated 49 patients (30 women, 19 men) who were randomized to 104 weeks of intermittent cyclical etidronate versus placebo. All patients had been on chronic glucocorticoids for at least 6 months at an average dose of prednisone 7.5 mg/day. After 104 weeks, patients treated with etidronate showed a 4.5% significant increase in the lumbar spine BMD compared with placebo. However, there were no significant differences observed at the hip or in markers of bone turnover [49]. In another study, 18 male and 21 female patients with established GIO on chronic prednisone therapy (≥10 mg/day) were enrolled in a prospective 12-month, open-label study [50]. Treatment with intermittent cyclic etidronate for 12 months resulted in significant increases of 5.7% and 6.8% in BMD of the spine and proximal femur, respectively, compared with a calcium-only group. This trial was unusual in that it demonstrated significant positive effects of etidronate on BMD at the hip [50].

In 1997, Adachi *et al* [51] published results of a 12-month, randomized, placebo-controlled prevention study of intermittent etidronate or 500 mg elemental calcium in 141 men and women. All had recently begun high-dose glucocorticoid therapy (average dose of prednisone 22 mg/day). At the end of 1 year, mean lumbar BMD change with etidronate was +0.6% versus −3.2% in the calcium group. Bone densities at the femoral neck and radius were similar between the groups. Postmenopausal women on etidronate showed a significant 85% reduction in new vertebral fractures compared with the placebo group (1 of 31 vs 7 of 32 patients fractured, respectively). However, men on etidronate actually had slightly more fractures than controls [51]. Etidronate is not currently approved for prevention or treatment of GIO.

d. CONCLUSIONS ABOUT BISPHOSPHONATES AND GIO. In the three largest studies described previously [45,46,51], only postmenopausal women benefited from bisphosphonate therapy in terms of vertebral fracture risk reduction. In 4 trials comprising 251 years of patient exposure, there were no vertebral fractures in premenopausal women on glucocorticoids [45,46,51,52]. In contrast, vertebral fracture rates in male control groups in these studies varied greatly from 2.1 to 23.5%, implying that a subgroup of male patients treated with glucocorticoids, most likely older men with low BMD, have a fracture risk approaching that of postmenopausal women [53]. These data suggest that prophylactic antiresorptive therapy against GIO is imperative in postmenopausal women and probably in older men with low BMD or other risk factors for osteoporosis. In younger men and premenopausal women on glucocorticoids, the presence of prevalent vertebral fractures, markedly low BMD, accelerated bone loss, or other major risk factors would argue for prophylactic bisphosphonate use. One should note that because of the long skeletal half-life of bisphosphonates and passage of the drug across the placenta, bisphosphonates must be used with great caution in premenopausal women.

B. Calcitonin

Calcitonin is an antiresorptive agent approved for the treatment of osteoporosis in women who are at least 5 years beyond the menopause. It is available in both injectable (subcutaneous) and intranasal formulations.

1. Calcitonin in Women with Postmenopausal Osteoporosis

In the *Prevent Recurrence of Osteoporotic Fracture* (PROOF) trial, three different doses of nasal spray calcitonin (100, 200, and 400 IU/day) were evaluated in 1255 postmenopausal women with osteoporosis of the lumbar spine and one to five prevalent vertebral fractures [54]. Subsequent analysis, however, revealed that 21% of the women enrolled did not have prevalent vertebral fractures and another 65 women had more than five fractures [24]. At the end of 5 years, the 200 IU/day dose of nasal calcitonin significantly reduced the cumulative risk of new morphometric vertebral fractures by 33%. Neither of the other two doses significantly reduced vertebral fractures. Moreover, calcitonin did not significantly reduce multiple vertebral fractures at any dose. In terms of total nonvertebral and hip fractures, only the 100 IU/day group showed significant risk reductions. At all doses, lumbar spine BMD increased significantly above placebo only during the first 2 years of the trial (and during the third year for the 400 IU/day dose) so that, by the end of the trial, there were no differences between calcitonin-treated groups and placebo in terms of lumbar spine BMD. None of the calcitonin doses significantly increased femoral neck or trochanter BMD [54]. Nasal calcitonin 200 IU/day significantly decreased serum C-telopeptide, a marker of bone resorption, compared with baseline during all 5 years of the trial. However, the reduction of C-telopeptide was only 12%, an effect that encompasses the least significant change of the measurement technology. Although this was statistically significant, such a modest reduction would not appear to have clinical significance in individual patients. The PROOF trial was weakened by a 59% dropout rate, by lack of clear dose-responses, and by various other flaws in the design and conduct of the trial. For these reasons, it is not possible to draw any definitive conclusions about the antifracture efficacy of nasal calcitonin in postmenopausal women [24].

2. Calcitonin for Men with Osteoporosis

There are very few trials using calcitonin in men. One early, small randomized study of men with osteoporosis found that treatment with calcitonin for 2 years reduced the incidence of vertebral fractures compared with calcium or multivitamin therapy [55]. Another small study in nine castrated young men (mean age 28 years) with high bone resorption and rapid bone loss from the lumbar spine showed that intranasal calcitonin could partially normalize markers of bone turnover [56]. A more recent study evaluated nine men aged 20 to 73 years with vertebral osteoporosis [57]. The patients were treated with salmon calcitonin 100 units injected subcutaneously three times per week for 3 months, then 3 months off medication, followed by another 3 months of calcitonin injections. All patients received 1000 mg of elemental calcium daily throughout the trial. After 1 year, BMD increased by 2 to 3% at both the spine and femoral neck compared with baseline. Because there was no placebo arm, however, it is not clear whether the gains were from calcitonin, calcium, or both [57]. Most recently, Trovas *et al* [58] evaluated effects of intranasal salmon calcitonin on BMD and biochemical markers of bone turnover in 28 men with idiopathic osteoporosis, aged 27 to 74 years. Patients were randomized to 200 IU nasal calcitonin or a nasal placebo daily

for 1 year along with 500 mg of elemental calcium daily. Spinal BMD increased significantly in the men who received nasal calcitonin compared with the placebo group (7.1% increase vs 2.4% increase, respectively, p < 0.05). There were no significant changes in hip, midshaft, or distal radius BMD in the treated group compared with either placebo or baseline. Various markers of bone resorption decreased significantly from baseline by 37 to 48% in the calcitonin-treated group, whereas no changes occurred in the placebo group. Men with the highest baseline levels of bone resorption showed the greatest BMD response to calcitonin [58]. Nasal calcitonin is not currently approved for treatment of osteoporosis in men. However, this recent study suggests that certain men with high-turnover spinal osteoporosis may benefit from short-term therapy with nasal calcitonin.

C. Raloxifene

The SERM raloxifene is approved for both prevention and treatment of postmenopausal osteoporosis. Raloxifene, a benzothiophene, has estrogen-agonist effects on bone but estrogen-antagonist effects on other tissues such as breast and endometrium. Unlike bisphosphonates and calcitonin that are bone-specific antiresorptive agents, raloxifene has a number of important nonskeletal targets including the liver, breast, and brain. Raloxifene lowers low-density lipoprotein (LDL) cholesterol and fibrinogen [59], may reduce cardiovascular events in high-risk women [60], and appears to lower the risk of estrogen-receptor positive breast cancer in women with osteoporosis [61]. Raloxifene may also induce hot flashes and is associated with an increased risk of thrombophlebitis [62].

1. Raloxifene for Women with Postmenopausal Osteoporosis

The *Multiple Outcomes of Raloxifene Evaluation* (MORE) trial considered the effects of two doses of raloxifene (60 or 120 mg/day) on the risk of fractures in postmenopausal women with osteoporosis [62]. Osteoporosis was defined as a femoral neck or lumbar spine T-score ≤ -2.5 or by the presence of one or more radiographically apparent prevalent vertebral fractures. In this large clinical trial (N = 7705) raloxifene significantly increased bone density at both the spine and femoral neck, decreased bone resorption, and reduced vertebral fractures in postmenopausal women compared with placebo [62]. After 3 years, 60 mg/day of raloxifene significantly decreased new morphometric vertebral fractures by 55% in women who did not have prevalent vertebral fractures and by 30% in women with prevalent vertebral fractures. The incidence of multiple vertebral fractures was reduced by 50 to 80% and painful clinical vertebral fractures by 60% in the pooled raloxifene-treated groups compared with placebo. The cumulative risk of nonvertebral fractures was not significantly different in the raloxifene groups compared with placebo at 3 years, but the MORE study was not statistically powered to detect reductions in nonvertebral fracture risk. Specifically, the trial was not powered to reach conclusions regarding hip fracture risk. Raloxifene modestly increased BMD at the spine and femoral neck and reduced bone resorption by 25% [62].

Data from the MORE trial suggest that raloxifene is a less potent antiresorptive agent than the two approved oral bisphosphonates and thus may not be the ideal agent for an elderly woman with severe osteoporosis or one at very high risk for a hip fracture. Moreover, combination therapy in which raloxifene is added to a potent antiresorptive such as alendronate does not appear to offer much benefit in terms of bone density [63]. In contrast, addition of alendronate to raloxifene can lead to further increases in BMD [63] although effects on fracture risk from combined therapy are unknown. The ideal candidate for raloxifene therapy may be the younger postmenopausal woman who wants to maintain bone density, reduce her risk of spinal fractures, and derive important nonskeletal benefits. If ongoing clinical trials confirm the effectiveness of raloxifene to reduce cardiovascular risk (the *R*aloxifene *U*se for *the H*eart or RUTH trial) and/or breast cancer (the *S*tudy of *T*amoxifen *a*nd *R*aloxifene or STAR trial) then the role of this drug in the care of postmenopausal women may be substantially enhanced.

2. Raloxifene for Men

As a tissue-specific estrogen receptor modulator that lacks feminizing properties [64], raloxifene may be an ideal agent for treatment of men with osteoporosis, assuming that declining levels of estrogen or estrogen action are involved, at least in part, in the pathogenesis of this disorder.

In 2000, Uebelhart *et al* [65] published an abstract regarding effects of raloxifene on the pituitary-gonadal axis and showed that raloxifene actions may be gender-specific. In postmenopausal women, raloxifene is associated with decreased follicle stimulating hormone (FSH) levels without effects on luteinizing hormone (LH) or prolactin [66]. In contrast, in 43 healthy males (mean age 56 years) treated with raloxifene 120 mg/day versus placebo in a cross-over trial, raloxifene caused statistically significant increases in FSH, LH, cortisol, total testosterone, free prostate specific antigen (PSA), and sex-hormone binding globulin (SHBG) compared with placebo, whereas prolactin and insulin-like growth factor-1 (IGF-1) showed significant declines. Lipids and renal function did not change [65]. This suggests that raloxifene has significant influences on the pituitary, gonadal, and adrenal axes in healthy men and that several of these changes are discordant with those seen in women. In 2001, Doran *et al* [67] published results of a study in 50 elderly men (mean age 69 years) randomized to daily raloxifene 60 mg/day or placebo. After 6 months, there were no significant differences in markers of bone turnover, serum sex steroid, or lipid levels with treatment. However, changes in one of the bone turnover markers, urinary cross-linked NTX excretion, decreased significantly in the subgroup of raloxifene-treated men whose baseline estradiol levels were lower (mean estradiol 22 pg/ml). In men with higher baseline estradiol levels (mean 30 pg/ml), urinary NTX excretion did not change or, in some cases, increased following raloxifene therapy. The authors concluded that raloxifene may be useful as an agonist in men with low baseline estradiol levels and osteoporosis [67]. In men with higher estrogen levels, it could function negatively as an antagonist. This is consistent with the work of Khosla *et al* [68] who evaluated cross-sectional studies of men and looked for a relationship between BMD and bioavailable estradiol level. Above a certain threshold, there was no significant relationship between estradiol

level and bone density in men. Below that threshold (in estrogen-deficient men), estradiol was directly related to BMD in males [68]. In another study, Uebelhart *et al* [69] reported on the effect of raloxifene versus placebo on biochemical markers of bone turnover and on renal handling of phosphate and calcium in 43 healthy men (average age 56 years). Men were randomly assigned to raloxifene 120 mg/day or placebo for 6 weeks followed by an 8-week washout period then crossed over to placebo or raloxifene 120 mg/day for the next 6 weeks followed by a final 8-week washout period. Raloxifene decreased markers of bone formation (serum osteocalcin and total alkaline phosphatase) without affecting markers of bone resorption (fasting urinary calcium/creatinine ratio and urinary deoxypyridinoline). Raloxifene was also associated with decreased levels of serum phosphate, renal phosphate transport, calcitriol, and IGF-1. Parathyroid hormone levels did not change. Calcium loading suggested a decrease in intestinal calcium absorption with raloxifene as well [69]. Although bone density was not measured here, these biochemical results in healthy young men without osteoporosis suggest that raloxifene may have quite different and potentially negative effects on bone metabolism in healthy young men or in men with adequate estrogen levels, in contrast to the generally positive effects seen in postmenopausal women and possibly in estrogen-deficient men.

III. Conclusions

The antiresorptive drugs have revolutionized our approach to postmenopausal osteoporosis and offer valuable options in our treatment of male osteoporosis. For postmenopausal women with low bone mass, there are a variety of therapeutic options including estrogen, bisphosphonates, and raloxifene for the prevention of osteoporosis, and bisphosphonates, calcitonin, and raloxifene for the treatment of established osteoporosis. Only one drug, alendronate, has been approved for treatment of male osteoporosis, but other bisphosphonates appear to be safe and efficacious as well. Unfortunately, any recommendation regarding drug therapy for male osteoporosis is hampered by the absence of large clinical trials with fracture endpoints. In general, bisphosphonates are the most potent antiresorptive agents for osteoporosis, irrespective of gender. Calcitonin is a relatively weak antiresorptive agent for women with postmenopausal osteoporosis, but, in men, there are simply not enough data to allow any definitive conclusions. Raloxifene is an important antiresorptive agent for women, with proven antifracture efficacy. The role of raloxifene in the management of male osteoporosis awaits further studies.

In the future, much larger clinical trials in men with osteoporosis are needed to define the role of current antiresorptive agents in our care of these patients. Another critical need is to elucidate the pathophysiology of male osteoporosis so that more rational treatments can be developed. Some men may respond well to antiresorptive agents, whereas others may require anabolic therapies to stimulate new bone formation and reverse low turnover states. Meanwhile, new advances in genetic research will allow us to direct osteoporosis therapies based on genome and gender. Within the next 10 to 15 years, the scope of osteoporosis therapy should expand widely to the benefit of both women and men.

IV. Suggestions for Further Investigations

- Larger trials in men with antiresorptive agents and fracture endpoints.
- New therapeutic interventions for men including low-dose estrogen for men with low estrodiol levels and use of selective androgen receptor modulators (SARMs).
- Trials in postmenopausal women and men using combination therapies (two antiresorptives or antiresorptive plus anabolic) with fracture endpoints.

References

1. Albright F, Smith PH, Richardson AM. (1941). Postmenopausal osteoporosis. *JAMA*. 116:2465–2474.
2. Scane AC, Sutcliffe AM, Francis RM. (1993). Osteoporosis in men. *Clin Rheumatol*. 7:589–601.
3. Riggs BL, Khosla S, Melton LJ III. (1998). A unitary model for involutional osteoporosis: Estrogen deficiency causes both type I and type II osteoporosis in postmenopausal women and contributes to bone loss in aging men. *J Bone Miner Res*. 13:763–773.
4. Hannan MT, Felson DR, Anderson JJ. (1992). Bone mineral density in elderly men and women: Results from the Framingham Osteoporosis Study. *J Bone Miner Res*. 7:547–553.
5. Jones G, Nguyen T, Sambrook P *et al*. (1994). Progressive loss of bone in the femoral neck in elderly people: Longitudinal findings from the Dubbo Osteoporosis Epidemiology Study. *BMJ*. 309:691–695.
6. Orwoll ES, Klein RF. (1995). Osteoporosis in men. *Endocr Rev*. 16:87–116.
7. Riggs BL, Wahner HW, Dunn WL *et al*. (1981). Differential changes in bone mineral density of the appendicular skeleton with aging: Relationship to spinal osteoporosis. *J Clin Invest*. 67:328–335.
8. Khosla S, Melton LJ III, Atkinson EJ *et al*. (1998). Relationship of serum sex steroid levels and bone turnover markers with bone mineral density in men and women: A key role for bioavailable estrogen. *J Clin Endocrinol Metab*. 83:2266 2274.
9. Kelepouris N, Harper KD, Gannon F *et al*. (1995). Severe osteoporosis in men. *Ann Intern Med*. 123:452–460.
10. Legrand E, Chappard D, Pascaretti C *et al*. (2000). Trabecular bone microarchitecture, bone mineral density, and vertebral fractures in male osteoporosis. *J Bone Miner Res*. 15:13–19.
11. Fleisch H. (1998). Bisphosphonates: Mechanism of action. *Endocr Rev*. 19:80–100.
12. Liberman UA, Weiss SR, Broll J *et al*. (1995). Effect of oral alendronate on bone mineral density and the incidence of fractures in postmenopausal osteoporosis. *N Engl J Med*. 333:1437–1443.
13. Black DM, Cummings SR, Karpf DB *et al*. (1996). Randomised trial of effect of alendronate on risk of fracture in women with existing vertebral fractures. *Lancet*. 348:1535–1541.
14. Cummings SR, Black DM, Thompson DE *et al*. (1998). Effect of alendronate on risk of fracture in women with low bone density but without vertebral fractures: Results from the Fracture Intervention Trial. *JAMA*. 280:2077–2082.
15. Black DM, Thompson DE, Bauer D *et al*. (2000). Fracture risk reduction with alendronate in women with osteoporosis: The Fracture Intervention Trial. *J Clin Endocrinol Metab*. 85:4118–4124.
16. Pols HA, Felsenberg D, Hanley DA *et al*. (1999). Multinational, placebo-controlled, randomized trial of the effects of alendronate on bone density and fracture risk in postmenopausal women with low bone mass: Results of the FOSIT study. *Osteoporos Int*. 9:461–468.
17. Orwoll E, Ettinger M, Weiss S *et al*. (2000). Alendronate for the treatment of osteoporosis in men. *N Engl J Med*. 343:604–610.
18. Ringe JD, Faber H, Dorst A. (2001). Alendronate treatment of established primary osteoporosis in men: Results of a 2-year prospective study. *J Clin Endocrinol Metab*. 86:5252–5255.
19. Ringe JD, Orwoll E, Daifotis A *et al*. (2002). Treatment of male osteoporosis: Recent advances with alendronate. *Osteoporos Int*. 13:195–199.
20. Ho YV, Frauman AG, Thomson W *et al*. (2000). Effects of alendronate on bone density in men with primary and secondary osteoporosis. *Osteoporos Int*. 11:98–101.
21. Karpf DB, Shapiro DR, Seeman E *et al*. (1997). Prevention of nonvertebral fractures by alendronate. A meta-analysis. *JAMA*. 277:1159–1164.
22. Harris ST, Watts NB, Genant HK *et al*. (1999). Effects of risedronate treatment on vertebral and nonvertebral fractures in women with postmenopausal osteoporosis: A randomized controlled trial. Vertebral Efficacy With Risedronate Therapy (VERT) Study Group. *JAMA*. 282:1344–1352.
23. Reginster J, Minne HW, Sorensen OH *et al*. (2000). Randomized trial of the effects of risedronate on vertebral fractures in women with established postmenopausal osteoporosis. *Osteoporos Int*. 11:83–91.
24. Marcus R, Wong M, Heath H III *et al*. (2002). Antiresorptive treatment of postmenopausal osteoporosis: Comparison of study designs and outcomes in large clinical trials with fracture as an endpoint. *Endocr Rev*. 23:16–37.
25. McClung M, Geusens P, Miller PD *et al*. (2001). Effect of risedronate on the risk of hip fracture in elderly women. *N Engl J Med*. 344:333–340.
26. Cranney A, Guyatt G, Krolicki N *et al*. (2001). A meta-analysis of etidronate for the treatment of postmenopausal osteoporosis. *Osteoporos Int*. 12:140–151.
27. Rosen CJ. (1997). A tale of two worlds in prescribing etidronate for osteoporosis. *Lancet*. 350:1340.
28. Watts NB, Harris ST, Genant HK *et al*. (1990). Intermittent cyclical etidronate treatment of postmenopausal osteoporosis. *N Engl J Med*. 323:73–79.
29. Harris ST, Watts NB, Jackson RD *et al*. (1993). Four-year study of intermittent cyclic etidronate treatment of postmenopausal osteoporosis: Three years of blinded therapy followed by one year of open therapy. *Am J Med*. 95:557–567.
30. Montessori ML, Scheele WH, Netelenbos JC *et al*. (1997). The use of etidronate and calcium versus calcium alone in the treatment of postmenopausal osteopenia: Results of three years of treatment. *Osteoporos Int*. 7:52–58.
31. Storm T, Thamsborg G, Steiniche T *et al*. (1990). Effect of intermittent cyclical etidronate therapy on bone mass and fracture rate in women with postmenopausal osteoporosis. *N Engl J Med*. 322:1265–1271.
32. Anderson FH, Francis RM, Bishop JC *et al*. (1997). Effect of intermittent cyclical disodium etidronate therapy on bone mineral density in men with vertebral fractures. *Age Ageing*. 26:359–365.
33. Heilberg IP, Martini LA, Teixeira SH *et al*. (1998). Effect of etidronate treatment on bone mass of male nephrolithiasis patients with idiopathic hypercalciuria and osteopenia. *Nephron*. 79:430–437.
34. Ringe JD, Rovati LC. (2001). Treatment of osteoporosis in men with fluoride alone or in combination with bisphosphonates. *Calcif Tissue Int*. 69:252–255.
35. Cortet B, Vasseur J, Grardel B *et al*. (2001). Management of male osteoporosis. *Joint Bone Spine*. 68:252–256.
36. Van Staa TP, Abenhaim L, Cooper C. (1998). Use of cyclical etidronate and prevention of non-vertebral fractures. *Br J Rheumatol*. 37:87–94.
37. Lees B, Garland SW, Walton C *et al*. (1996). Role of oral pamidronate in preventing bone loss in postmenopausal women. *Osteoporos Int*. 6:480–485.
38. Peretz A, Body JJ, Dumon JC *et al*. (1996). Cyclical pamidronate infusions in postmenopausal osteoporosis. *Maturitas*. 25:69–75.
39. Watts NB. (2001). Treatment of osteoporosis with bisphosphonates. *Rheum Dis Clin North Am*. 27:197–214.
40. Valkema R, Vismans F-JFE, Papapoulos SE *et al*. (1989). Maintained improvement in calcium balance and bone mineral content in patients with osteoporosis treated with the bisphosphonate APD. *J Bone Miner Res*. 5:183–192.
41. Stoch SA, Parker RA, Chen L *et al*. (2001). Bone loss in men with prostate cancer treated with gonadotropin-releasing hormone agonists. *J Clin Endocrinol Metab*. 86:2787–2791.
42. Smith MR, McGovern FJ, Zietman AL *et al*. (2001). Pamidronate to prevent bone loss during androgen-deprivation therapy for prostate cancer. *N Engl J Med*. 345:948–955.
43. Diamond TH, Winters J, Smith A *et al*. (2001). The antiosteoporotic efficacy of intravenous pamidronate in men with prostate carcinoma receiving combined androgen blockade: A double blind, randomized, placebo-controlled crossover study. *Cancer*. 92:1444–1450.
44. Reid I, Brown JP, Burckhardt P *et al*. (2002). Intravenous zoledronic acid in postmenopausal women with low bone mineral density. *N Engl J Med*. 346:653–661.
45. Saag KG, Emkey R, Schnitzer TJ *et al*. Alendronate for the prevention and treatment of glucocorticoid-induced osteoporosis. *N Engl J Med*. 339:292–299.
46. Cohen S, Levy RM, Keller M *et al*. (1999). Risedronate therapy prevents corticosteroid-induced bone loss: A twelve-month, multicenter, randomized, double-blind, placebo-controlled, parallel-group study. *Arthritis Rheum*. 42:2309–2318.
47. Reid DM, Hughes RA, Laan R *et al*. (2000). Efficacy and safety of daily risedronate in the treatment of corticosteroid-induced osteoporosis in men and women: A randomized trial. *J Bone Miner Res*. 15:1006–1013.

48. Wallach S, Cohen S, Reid DM *et al.* (2000). Effects of risedronate treatment on bone density and vertebral fracture in patients on corticosteroid therapy. *Calcif Tissue Int.* 67:277–285.

49. Pitt P, Li F, Todd P *et al.* (1998). A double blind placebo controlled study to determine the effects of intermittent cyclical etidronate on bone mineral density in patients on long-term oral corticosteroid treatment. *Thorax.* 53:351–356.

50. Struys A, Snelder AA, Mulder H. (1995). Cyclical etidronate reverses bone loss of the spine and proximal femur in patients with established corticosteroid-induced osteoporosis. *Am J Med.* 99:235–242.

51. Adachi JD, Bensen WG, Brown J *et al.* (1997). Intermittent etidronate therapy to prevent corticosteroid-induced osteoporosis. *N Engl J Med.* 337:382–387.

52. Sambrook PN, Birmingham J, Kelly PJ *et al.* (1993). Prevention of corticosteroid osteoporosis: A comparison of calcium, calcitriol and calcitonin. *N Engl J Med.* 337:382–387.

53. Sambrook PN. (2000). Corticosteroid osteoporosis: Practical implication of recent trials. *J Bone Miner Res.* 15:1645–1649.

54. Chesnut CH III, Silverman SL, Andriano K *et al.* (2000). A randomized trial of nasal spray salmon calcitonin in postmenopausal women with established osteoporosis: The Prevent Recurrence of Osteoporosis Fractures study. *Am J Med.* 109:267–276.

55. Agarwal R, Wallach S, Cohn S *et al.* (1981). Calcitonin Treatment of Osteoporosis. In *Calcitonin* (Pecile A, ed.), pp. 237–246. Amsterdam: Excerpta Medica.

56. Stepan JJ, Lachman M, Zverina J *et al.* (1989). Castrated men exhibit bone loss: Effect of calcitonin treatment on biochemical indices of bone remodeling. *J Clin Endocrinol Metab.* 69:523–527.

57. Erlacher L, Kettenback J, Kiener H *et al.* (1997). Salmon calcitonin and calcium in the treatment of male osteoporosis: The effect on bone mineral density. *Wien Klin Wochenschr.* 109:270–274.

58. Trovas GP, Lyritis GP, Galanos A *et al.* (2002). A randomized trial of nasal spray salmon calcitonin in men with idiopathic osteoporosis: Effects on bone mineral density and bone markers. *J Bone Miner Res.* 17:521–527.

59. Walsh BW, Kuller LH, Wild RA *et al.* (1998). Effects of raloxifene on serum lipids and coagulation factors in healthy postmenopausal women. *JAMA.* 279:1445–1451.

60. Barrett-Connor E, Grady D, Sashegyi A *et al.* (2002). Raloxifene and cardiovascular events in osteoporotic postmenopausal women: Four-year results from the MORE (Multiple Outcomes of Raloxifene Evaluation) randomized trial. *JAMA.* 287:847–857.

61. Cauley JA, Norton L, Lippman ME *et al.* (2001). Continued breast cancer risk reduction in postmenopausal women treated with raloxifene: Four-year results from the MORE trial. *Breast Cancer Res Treat.* 65:125–134.

62. Ettinger B, Black DM, Mitlak BH *et al.* (1999). Reduction of vertebral fracture risk in postmenopausal women with osteoporosis treated with raloxifene: Results from a 3-year randomized clinical trial. *JAMA.* 282:637–645.

63. Johnell O, Scheele WH, Lu Y *et al.* (2002). Additive effects of raloxifene and alendronate on bone density and biochemical markers of bone remodeling in postmenopausal women with osteoporosis. *J Clin Endocrinol Metab.* 87:985–992.

64. Sadovsky Y, Adler S. (1998). Selective modulation of estrogen receptor action. *Clin Endocrinol Metab.* 83:3–5 (editorial).

65. Uebelhart B, Bonjour JP, Draper MW *et al.* (2000). Effects of the selective estrogen receptor modulator raloxifene (RLX) on the pituitary gonadal axis in healthy males. *J Bone Miner Res.* 15(Suppl 1):S453.

66. Plouffe L Jr, Siddhanti S. (2001). The effect of selective estrogen receptors modulators on parameters of the hypothalamic-pituitary-gonadal axis. *Ann N Y Acad Sci.* 949:251–258.

67. Doran PM, Riggs BL, Atkinson AJ *et al.* (2001). Effects of raloxifene, a selective estrogen receptor modulator, on bone turnover markers and serum sex steroid and lipid levels in elderly men. *J Bone Miner Res.* 16:2118–2125.

68. Khosla S, Melton LJ III, Riggs BL. (2002). Clinical review 144: Estrogen and the male skeleton. *J Clin Endocrinol Metab.* 87:1443–1450.

69. Uebelhart B, Bonjour JP, Draper MW *et al.* (2000). Effects of the selective estrogen receptor modulator raloxifene (RLX) on bone metabolism in healthy males. *J Bone Miner Res.* 15(Suppl 1):S229.

94

The Role of Androgens and Estrogens in the Male Skeleton

SUNDEEP KHOSLA, MD* AND JOHN P. BILEZIKIAN, MD**

*Professor of Medicine and Research Chair, Division of Endocrinology, Metabolism,
and Nutrition Mayo Clinic and Foundation, Rochester, MN
**Professor of Medicine and of Pharmacology and Chief, Division of Endocrinology,
College of Physicians and Surgeons, Columbia University, New York, NY

Abstract

The sex steroids have for years been considered to be sex specific with regard to bone metabolism: estrogens as the key determinant of bone metabolism in women; testosterone (T) as the key determinant in men. New evidence with regard to the effect of sex steroids on each sex's bone has led to a revision of this earlier belief. With respect to men, convincing new evidence from multiple lines of investigation shows clearly that estrogen (E) is an important, if not the dominant, sex steroid in regulating male bone metabolism. Insights from the studies on the skeletal effects of E in men may also help reshape our thinking on the role of E in other aspects of men's health.

I. Introduction

Estrogen deficiency at the time of menopause has important clinical manifestations, including the onset of accelerated bone loss that can lead to severe osteoporosis in many women [1]. Estrogen is unequivocally important in regulating female skeletal metabolism. In contrast, because men lack a physiologic equivalent of a menopause (i.e., a period of abrupt loss of testicular function), the role of sex steroids in regulating the male skeleton has, until recently, been much less well defined. The assumption has been that, because T is the dominant male sex steroid, it should regulate male skeletal metabolism in a manner analogous to the central role of E in the female skeleton. The past several years, however, have witnessed a major paradigm shift in our thinking about the role of androgens versus E in the male skeleton. The accumulating evidence that forms the focus of this chapter is that, although T is important for bone metabolism in males, it appears that E plays a critical, and perhaps dominant, in the male skeleton [2]. This surprising emergence of E as a major regulator of bone metabolism in males, as well as females, has important implications for our understanding of bone loss in men and may also force us to rethink the role of E in other areas of male health, including cardiovascular disease, dementia, and prostate cancer.

II. Historical Views of Sex Steroids in the Male: Circa 1994

The conventional view that T regulates male skeletal metabolism was given a major impetus with the studies of Stepan *et al* [3] in which changes in bone mineral density (BMD) and bone turnover markers were examined in a group of Czech prisoners following orchidectomy for sexual crimes. Following castration, these young men demonstrated a pattern and rate of bone loss very similar to that found in women following natural or surgical menopause (Fig. 94-1). Increases in bone markers also were consistent with an accelerated period of bone turnover. Consistent with this set of observations, a number of other studies found that hypogonadism in men (as seen in patients with hypothalamic dysfunction, hyperprolactinemia, anorexia nervosa, Klinefelter syndrome, and castration) [reviewed in 4] was clearly a risk factor for osteoporosis. However, it was not appreciated then that these earlier studies in which androgen deficiency was implicated as the etiologic factor in bone loss were also invariably associated with E deficiency. On reflection, this point is obvious because the only way that the human can produce E is from aromatization of androgen. In any androgen deficiency state resulting from endogenous loss there must also be an associated E deficiency state. It remained possible, therefore, that the bone loss attributed to loss of androgen might have been due, at least in part, to loss of E.

III. The Human Experiments of Nature

A. Alpha-Estrogen Receptor Deficiency in the Male

This conventional view by which sex steroids regulated bone metabolism along strict gender lines was literally shattered in

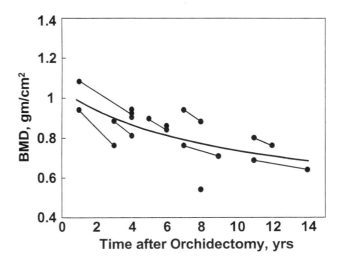

Fig. 94-1 Scattergram of lumbar spine bone mineral density (BMD) as a function of time after orchidectomy in 12 men. In 8 patients the measurement was repeated after 1 to 3 years. (Adapted from Stepan JJ, Lachman M, Zverina J *et al*. [1989]. Castrated men exhibit bone loss: Effect of calcitonin treatment on biochemical indices of bone remodeling. *J Clin Endocrinol Metab*. 69:523–527, with permission.)

men when the first male with an abnormal estrogen receptor (ER) gene was described. In 1994, Smith et al [5] described a 28-year-old man with a mutation in the alpha-ER gene. He was the product of a consanguineous marriage in which both parents carried a single copy of the abnormal alpha-ER gene. The point mutation was located at codon 157, where thymidine had replaced cytosine. The resulting stop codon was associated with a severely truncated ER unable to bind E. As expected, the subject's baseline estradiol (E_2) (119 pg/ml) and estrone (145 pg/ml) levels were markedly above normal. Although bound and free T and dihydrotestosterone concentrations were normal, the concentrations of luteinizing hormone (LH) (37 mIU/ml) and follicle stimulating hormone (FSH) (33 mIU/ml) were in the mildly castrate range. He was extremely tall (204 cm) with eunuchoid proportions. The epiphyses were still open (bone age, 15 years) and he was still growing. Genu valgum was prominent in the lower extremities. There were no features of acromegaly. The growth curve was steady and continuous, without evidence for a pubertal growth spurt. As measured by dual energy x-ray absorptiometry (DXA), bone density of the lumbar spine was 0.745 g/cm^2, corresponding to 2 standard deviations below average for a 15-year-old boy. Not unexpectedly, large doses of exogenous E (transdermal ethinyl E_2) with serum concentrations of E_2 reaching 10-fold higher than the typical male, 270 pg/ml (normal: 10 to 50), were unsuccessful. At this time, there does not appear to be any way to overcome the molecular defect in this disorder.

B. Aromatase Deficiency in the Male

Theoretically, males can also be rendered E deficient if the aromatase enzyme responsible for the conversion of androgens to estrogens is defective or absent. Four males have been reported with aromatase deficiency resulting from a genetic defect in the aromatase gene. Each male, the product of a consanguineous marriage [6–9] shows a point mutation in exon IX [6,7] or at exon V [8] or, in the most recent case [9] in intron V of the aromatase gene. Morishima et al [6] described a 24-year-old man with a cytosine to thymidine base pair change in exon IX at position 1123 and a resultant amino acid substitution at R375, adjacent to the heme binding site. Similarly, Carani et al [7] described a 31-year-old man with a single base pair change in exon IX at position 1094 (guanine to adenine) with the amino acid substitution at R365. In the newborn male, reported by Deladoey et al [8], the mutation was found in exon V, causing a frame shift mutation with an ensuing premature stop codon. In the case reported by Herrmann et al [9] a similar, premature stop codon was induced but through a substitution in intron V, at position −3 of the splicing acceptor site before exon VI. In each of these four cases, the gene product is completely inactive and thus E levels were not detectable.

The three adult men reported by Morishima et al [6], Carani et al [7], and Herrmann et al [9] were very tall with unfused epiphyses, a bone age consistent with a growing teenage boy, eunuchoid features (upper segment/lower segment = 0.85 to 0.88) and genu valgum. They were still growing. The patients of Morishima et al [6] and Herrmann et al [9] had elevated androgen levels. The complete biochemical profile of the patient described by Morishima et al [6] is shown in Tables 94-1 and

Table 94-1

Biochemical Parameters in a Man with Aromatase Deficiency

		Normal Range
Calcium	9.9	8.7–10.7 mg/dl
Phosphorus	3.3	2.5–4.5 mg/dl
Parathyroid hormone (PTH)	26	10–65 pg /ml
25-hydroxyvitamin D	36	9–52 ng/ml
1,25-dihydroxyvitamin D	55	15–60 pg /ml
Alkaline phosphatase	241	39–117 IU/L
Urinary calcium	185	150–300 mg/24 hours
Deoxypyridinoline	25.3	4–19 nmol/mmol Cr

(Adapted from Morishima A, Grumbach MM, Simpson ER et al. [1995]. Aromatase deficiency in male and female siblings caused by a novel mutation and the physiological role of estrogens. *J Clin Endocrinol Metab*. 80:3689–3698.)

94-2. The growth curve of that patient, similar to the man with the alpha-ER defect, did not give evidence for a pubertal growth spurt although in all other respects puberty was not delayed (Fig. 94-2). All three adult men with aromatase deficiency had reduced bone mass. The BMD of the patient described by Morishima et al [6] is shown in Figure 94-3. Because of his enlarged areal density, a correction had to be applied to determine the bone mineral apparent density. Even more impressive reductions became evident when areal size was taken into account with T-scores of −1.99 (spine), −2.12 (femoral neck), and −7.75 (forearm). Similarly, the male described by Herrmann et al had a T-score of −2.24 in the lumbar spine.

The men with aromatase deficiency responded to the administration of E [7,9–11]. The 5-year follow-up data on the patient described by Morishima, Bilezikian, and their colleagues provide instructive commentary on the potential anabolic qualities of estrogens in the setting of the growing male skeleton [12]. For most of the 5-year period of therapy, the dose of conjugated E was 0.75 mg daily. On this dosage, E_2 levels were maintained within normal limits for men. Concomitant with return of E levels to normal, androgen levels fell from markedly elevated levels to normal. The gonadotropins LH and FSH also returned to normal, illustrating the point that estrogens play an important role in controlling gonadotropin production in the male (Fig. 94-4). Within 6 months of beginning E therapy, the patient

Table 94-2

Sex Steroids and Gonadotropin Concentrations in a Man with Aromatase Deficiency

		Normal Range
Estradiol	<7	10–50 pg /ml
Estrone	<7	10–50 pg/ml
Testosterone	2015	200–1200 ng/dl
5α-dihydrotestosterone	125	30–85 ng/dl
Follicle stimulating hormone (FSH)	28.3	5–9.9 mIU/ml
Luteinizing hormone (LH)	26.1	2.0–9.9 mIU/ml

(Adapted from Simpson ER, Zhao Y, Agarwal VR et al. [1997]. Aromatase expression in health and disease. *Recent Prog Horm Res*. 52:185–214.)

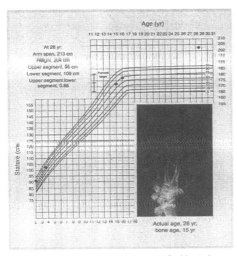

Smith et al,
N Eng J Med 331:1056-1061,199

Fig. 94-2 Growth curve and bone age before and after 5 years of estrogen therapy in a man with aromatase deficiency. After conjugated estrogen therapy was begun (bar), linear growth ceased promptly. Height has remained at 204 cm since therapy. All epiphyses were closed within 6 months (insets). The curves + and − numbers represent the mean and standard deviations for normal young men. (Reproduced from Bilezikian JP, Khosla S, Riggs BL. [2002]. Estrogen Effects on Bone in the Male Skeleton. In *Principles of Bone Biology* [Bilezikian JP, Raisz LG, Rodan GA, eds.], pp. 1467–1476. San Diego, CA: Academic Press, with permission.)

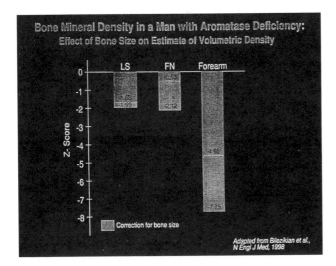

Fig. 94-3 Bone mineral density at baseline in a man with aromatase deficiency. For each site, the bone mass is shown as a two-dimensional value (g/cm^2) and as bone mineral apparent density using correction factors for body size. For each site, estimated true bone density (g/cc) is substantially lower than the direct measurement, as shown in the shaded area of each bar. (Reproduced from Bilezikian JP, Khosla S, Riggs BL. [2002]. Estrogen Effects on Bone in the Male Skeleton. In *Principles of Bone Biology* [Bilezikian JP, Raisz LG, Rodan GA, eds.], pp. 1467–1476. San Diego, CA: Academic Press, with permission.)

reported by Bilezikian, Morishima *et al*, showed no further longitudinal growth and the epiphyses closed (see Fig. 94-2). Bone mineral density increased dramatically. During the first 3 years, lumbar spine, femoral neck, and forearm improved by 20.7%, 15.7%, and 12.9% respectively. In years 4 and 5 of E therapy, the gains in the lumbar spine and femoral neck were maintained with further marked increases in the forearm bone density, now totaling 26% (Fig. 94-5). In the patient with aromatase deficiency described by Herrmann *et al* [9] impressive gains in bone density at the lumbar spine were seen with the T-score improving from −2.24 to −1.64 in 1 year. By quantitative computed tomography (QCT), the distal radius showed an improvement from 52 to 83 mg/cm^3 in the same period of time.

The effect of E to improve bone mass in this setting is best described as anabolic because of the magnitude of the change and also because further bone growth did not occur. In addition, osteocalcin, a marker of bone formation has been shown in some cases to increase dramatically [9]. Without further bone growth, the change in BMD is more likely to reflect improved mineralization per unit area. This property of E to stimulate the acquisition of bone mass is quite different from its effects in the postmenopausal woman, in whom the E effect is more accurately described as antiresorptive.

In the syndromes of E deficiency or resistance, height and inexorable growth, continuing well into adulthood, was not accompanied with a pubertal growth spurt. If estrogens are important for the pubertal growth spurt, syndromes of E excess might be expected to be linked to a premature growth spurt. Indeed, in the syndrome of aromatase excess, resulting from an activating mutation of the aromatase gene and elevated E levels, puberty does occur prematurely [13–16]. In the testicular feminization syndrome, XY males do not respond to androgens because of a mutation in the androgen receptor (AR) but they respond normally to estrogens. Again, confirming an important role for estrogens in the male, the pubertal growth spurt is seen in these XY males [17,18]. Finally, premature skeletal maturation has been reported in E-secreting tumors [19–21]. In the aggregate, these observations make a compelling point that in the male, as in the female, the pubertal growth spurt is a function of estrogens not androgens.

C. Aromatase Deficiency in the Female

Aromatase deficiency in the female is a more straightforward diagnosis because in the cases that have been reported [6,21–24] an anatomic abnormality is often detected at the time of birth. These girls have ambiguous genitalia resulting from the overexposure to androgens *in utero*. Hypogonadotropic hypogonadism, pseudohermaphrodism, and polycystic ovaries have also been described. Therapy is also much more straightforward and occurs earlier. As soon as the diagnosis is made, these girls are treated with estrogens in physiologic replacement doses.

D. Polymorphisms of the Aromatase Gene

The few cases of aromatase deficiency reported in the literature in males and females suggest that this rare disorder is unlikely to be a common cause of reduced bone mass. However, a polymorphism of this gene has recently been studied in women with

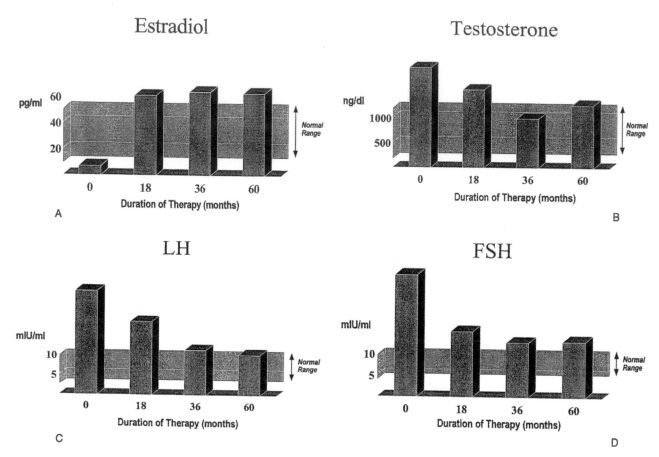

Fig. 94-4 Changes in sex steroids and in gonadotrophins with estrogen therapy in a man with aromatase deficiency. The data are shown for estradiol (A), testosterone (B), follicle stimulating hormone (FSH) (C), and luteinizing hormone (LH) (D). Over 5 years, estradiol levels initially rose and then were maintained in the normal range for males when administered at 0.75 mg/day. Testosterone levels fell into the normal range as did FSH and LH levels. (Reproduced from Bilezikian JP, Khosla S, Riggs BL. [2002]. Estrogen Effects on Bone in the Male Skeleton. In *Principles of Bone Biology* [Bilezikian JP, Raisz LG, Rodan GA, eds.], pp. 1467–1476. San Diego, CA: Academic Press, with permission.)

Change in BMD with Therapy

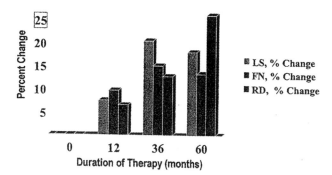

Fig. 94-5 Changes in bone mineral density with estrogen therapy in a man with aromatase deficiency. Percentage and T-score changes are shown for lumbar spine, femoral neck, and distal radius. The data shown are not corrected for bone size. (Reproduced from Bilezikian JP, Khosla S, Riggs BL. [2002]. Estrogen Effects on Bone in the Male Skeleton. In *Principles of Bone Biology* [Bilezikian JP, Raisz LG, Rodan GA, eds.], pp. 1467–1476. San Diego, CA: Academic Press., with permission.)

respect to it being a risk factor for low bone mass and fractures in women. A simple tetranucleotide tandem repeat polymorphism in intron 4 (TTTA) was shown to be related to low bone density and to an increase incidence of fractures. Women whose allele demonstrated a genotype with greater than 11 repeat sequences (NN genotype) had greater bone density and fewer fractures than those whose genotype consisted of alleles with fewer than 11 repeat sequences [25]. Although Salmen *et al* [26] have not confirmed these observations in a study of Finnish women, similar observations have been made in preliminary studies with men of African ancestry [27]. Masi *et al* [28] demonstrated that fibroblasts obtained from women with the high repeat genotype (NN) are able to convert more androgen to E_2 when compared with women with the low repeat genotype (CC). In the first large-scale prospective study of men, Van Pottelbergh *et al* [29] evaluated the same aromatase gene polymorphism. In 214 community dwelling men, 71 to 86 years old, followed for 4 years, they were able to confirm an association of higher bioavailable E levels with higher baseline bone mass and with a reduced rate of bone loss at the forearm and at the hip. Although the CYP19 gene (TTTA)n polymorphism was not associated with E_2 levels or with baseline BMD, those with the shorter number of TTTA repeat sequences had the highest rate of bone loss at the forearm. They also noted that the shortest (TTTA)n-repeat length polymorphism was overly represented in men with a positive personal history of fracture and among first-degree relatives.

IV. Animal Knockouts of the Estrogen Receptor and Aromatase Genes

Genetic models in which specific genes for the alpha ER or the beta ER are knocked out singly or together, as well as models in which the aromatase gene has been knocked out, have been helpful in elucidating further aspects of the role of estrogens in male skeletal development [30–32]. In the chapter by Vanderschueren and Bouillon, these animal models are considered in some detail. They are, therefore, only discussed briefly here. It should be noted that there are discrepancies between the genetic mouse models and the human gene knockout experiments of nature described previously [33]. Mouse models are not as clean as human models. The phenotypes of mice rendered deficient in the alpha or beta ER or deficient in aromatase activity do not invariably mirror accurately overt human phenotypes. For example, the lack of the alpha ER or the aromatase gene in human subjects is associated with continuous longitudinal bone growth. In the animal models, on the other hand, defects in these same genes are associated with reduced long bone growth. Moreover, it is not clear whether E deficiency in the animal models is associated with high or low bone turnover, whereas in the human subjects with these gene defects, high bone turnover is consistently observed. Nevertheless, the animal gene knockouts have been instructive in furthering our understanding of the role of estrogens in male skeletal development.

The alpha-ER knockout mouse displays a 20 to 25% reduction in bone density [30,34,35], consistent with the human patient described by Smith et al [5]. In contrast, the beta-ER knockout male mouse shows no skeletal abnormalities [36]. It is of interest that the same beta-ER defect in the adult female mouse, however, does show changes with an increase in bone mineral content resulting from an increase in cross-sectional cortical area.

Vidal et al [37] characterized male mice deficient in the alpha ER (ERKO) or the beta ER (BERKO) or both (DERKO), helping to establish further a role for specific ERs in the acquisition of skeletal mass in the male. The importance of the alpha ER in a number of skeletal characteristics of the male was clearly shown. Foreshortened long bone growth was seen only in the ERKO and DERKO mice but not in the BERKO animals, clearly attributing this estrogenic function to the alpha ER, not the beta ER. In addition, significant reductions in mice lacking the alpha ER, not the beta receptor, were observed in total body mineral content, femoral bone mineral content, and spine bone mineral content. The abnormalities persisted in the ERKO and DERKO mice when animal weight and skeletal length were accounted for. On the other hand, cancellous bone density as analyzed by peripheral quantitative tomography (pQCT) and by bone histomorphometry was unchanged in all animals. Cortical bone mineral content by pQCT was diminished in ERKO and DERKO animals as compared with wild type. The reduction in cortical bone mineral content was due to reduced cross-sectional area primarily because of smaller periosteal and endosteal circumferences. Similar to cancellous bone density, cortical volumetric density was unchanged. Mechanical strength was diminished in the ERKO animals with a tendency for a similar decline in the DERKO animals.

Observations with these knockout mice clearly established differences in the alpha and beta ERs, with all abnormalities observed being clearly a function of the alpha receptor not the beta receptor. However, in a number of key respects, the knockout animals did not confirm expectations that cancellous or cortical bone density would be diminished in the alpha-ER deficient knockout animal. These points are important but not clearly understood. It could be that the ERs are just not important in these aspects of the male mouse skeleton. Alternatively, it is possible that compensatory mechanisms were induced to adjust for the receptor deficiency. E and T levels are elevated in these animals. Elevated levels could have accounted for the lack of some of these expected changes. It is even possible that the elevated estrogens in these knockout animals were somehow activating a truncated version of the alpha receptor that has been shown to be present in alpha-receptor knockout animals [38]. Consistent with this point, Gentile et al [39] showed that in DERKO animals, estrogens can rescue the loss in bone density after ovariectomy when very high levels of estrogens are employed.

Sims et al [40] recently addressed this issue by creating male (and female) mice in which the gene knockouts are full and therefore do not express a truncated form of the receptor that theoretically could bind E. Consistent with the report of Vidal et al [37] only the alpha ER was shown to regulate bone remodeling in the male mouse.

Lindberg et al [41] continued their study of the relative importance of the alpha and beta ER on the male mouse skeleton by taking a different tact. Recognizing that the compensatory adjustments in sex steroids resulting from ER deficiency may have masked observations that might otherwise have been made, they subjected wild-type and the same knockout animals, ERKO, BERKO, and DERKO, to orchidectomy at 7 months of age. Their experimental premise was that elimination of all sex steroids by orchidectomy would permit assignment of a specific role for estrogens when 17β-E_2 was used subsequently to prevent the abnormalities induced by the abrupt loss of androgens.

After orchidectomy, total body areal BMD fell significantly in all groups. However, only in the animals with an intact alpha ER (WT, BERKO) could estrogens maintain bone density at baseline, preorchidectomy levels. It would appear valid to conclude that the lack of a beta ER did not impair the effect of E on the alpha ER and that the alpha receptor alone was sufficient to prevent the loss in total body BMD resulting from orchidectomy. Similarly, animals with an intact alpha ER (WT, BERKO) were able to respond to E such that femoral areal BMD and femoral bone mineral content were maintained. When femoral areal BMD and femoral bone mineral content were examined directly after orchidectomy and E replacement, again only the mice with intact alpha ERs (WT and BERKO) showed levels that were higher than postorchidectomy levels. It appears that E was not able to completely protect against some loss in femoral areal BMD and femoral bone mineral content.

The results of these elegant experiments clearly provide further confirmation of the importance of estrogens acting through the alpha ERs in developing and maintaining the male skeleton.

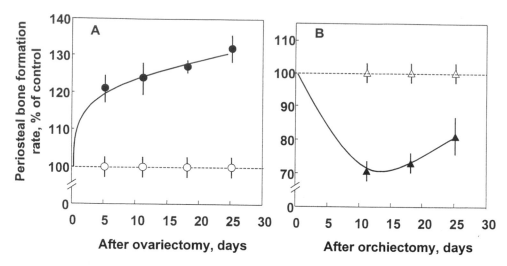

Fig. 94-6   The effect of ovariectomy (A) and orchidectomy (B) on periosteal bone formation rate. Open circles and triangles, intact controls; filled circles and triangles, ovariectomized and orchidectomized animals, respectively. $p < 0.01$ for all ovariectomy and orchidectomy time points compared with intact controls. (Adapted from Turner RT, Wakley GK, Hannon KS. [1990]. Differential effects of androgens on cortical bone histomorphometry in gonadectomized male and female rats. *J Orthop Res*. 8:612–617, with permission.)

The data would seem to argue that the beta ER has little if any role to play in male skeletal metabolism. In female animals, however, age-related reductions in cancellous bone volume seem to be diminished in animals lacking the beta ER. These observations suggest that the beta ER may play a permissive role in age-related bone loss or that by virtue of its absence, sensitivity to the protective effects of the alpha receptor is enhanced [31,42]. Sims *et al* [40] recently provided additional evidence to support a role for the beta ER in female (but not male) skeletal metabolism. Finally, in support of the dominant role of the alpha ER in male skeletal physiology, the man with the alpha ER mutation is osteoporotic [5], a telling comment on its importance in the acquisition of peak bone mass. Thus, at least in the human, the beta ER does not have an important role to play in the acquisition of peak bone mass.

Knockout of the aromatase gene has also been instructive as demonstrated by Oz *et al* [32] and first reported by Fisher *et al* [43]. The male mice show radiographic evidence for reduced BMD. Histologically, the mice show significant reductions in trabecular bone volume and in trabecular thickness. By histomorphometry, male knockout (but not female counterparts) show reductions in both osteoblastic and osteoclastic surfaces. Female mice showed a picture more consistent with high bone turnover. This sexual dimorphism with respect to these histomorphometric features has no ready explanation at this time. Nevertheless, these animal knockout experiments provide general confirmation of the human gene knockout disorders, documenting further the important role of estrogens in male skeletal development.

A. Other Studies in Experimental Animals

A number of additional studies in experimental animals, primarily rodents, have also dissected the roles of androgens and estrogens in the male skeleton. The animal counterpart to the testicular feminization patients, the testicular feminized rat,

has reduced bone size (compared with wild-type male rats) [44], but cancellous bone appears to be relatively preserved in these animals. These findings would suggest that, at least in the rodent (and perhaps also in humans), the lack of androgen action has minimal, if any, effects on cancellous bone. By contrast, the reduction in bone size is consistent with the most obvious skeletal difference between males and females in many species, including humans: males have bigger bones than females. The most likely explanation for this is that perhaps the major action of androgens is to increase bone size by effects on the deposition of bone on the outside surface of cortical bones, so-called periosteal apposition. That this is the case was directly demonstrated by Turner and colleagues [45], who found that ovariectomy in female rats resulted in an increase in periosteal bone formation, whereas orchidectomy in male rats resulted in a decrease in this parameter (Fig. 94-6). This effect of androgens on the periosteum may be mediated, at least in part, by insulin-like growth factor-1 (IGF-I), because IGF-I has been shown to have similar effects on the periosteum [46], and androgens do stimulate the production of IGF-I by osteoblastic cells [47]. Other studies indicate, however, that androgens likely have important effects not just on the periosteum but also in other parts of the skeleton. Thus, Vanderschueren *et al* [48] demonstrated that aromatizable and nonaromatizable androgens are effective in preventing bone loss in aged male rats following orchiectomy.

There have also now been a number of studies examining the possible role of E in the male rat and mouse skeleton. Thus, treatment with an aromatase inhibitor decreased BMD and bone size in growing rats [49], and aged male rats treated with an aromatase inhibitor were found to have reductions in BMD and increased indices of bone resorption [50].

V. Studies in Adult Humans

With the description of the ER and aromatase deficient males, along with the accumulating evidence from animal studies that both T and E were important for bone metabolism in males, attention then focused on dissecting the relative contributions of T and E toward bone metabolism in normal adult men. The rationale for this was that, although the human experiments of nature clearly indicated an important role for E in the growth and development of the male skeleton during puberty, these findings could not necessarily be extrapolated to adult men with mature skeletons.

The first approach to this question involved relating sex steroids to BMD and to bone turnover markers in cross-sectional observational studies. There have now been a number of such studies published [51–58], and the findings of these studies are remarkably consistent: serum E_2 levels are much better predictors of BMD and of bone resorption markers in men than are T levels. The results of these studies are perhaps best illustrated by the data of Amin *et al* [57], who studied a group of elderly men from the Framingham cohort (mean age 75.7 years) specifically selected for having borderline or low serum T levels [<10.4 nmol/L (300 ng/dl)]. Even in these men with modest hypogonadism, serum E_2 levels were much more predictive of BMD than were serum T levels. As shown in Figure 94-7A, there was no difference in BMD at the proximal femur between men in different quartiles of serum T, whereas there was a clear relationship between proximal femur BMD and the quartile of serum E_2 (Fig. 94-7B). Moreover, other studies have found that the fraction of E_2 not bound to sex hormone binding globulin (i.e., bioavailable E_2) is perhaps an even better predictor of BMD and of bone turnover in men than the total E_2 level [52,53,56,58].

Convincing as these cross-sectional data are, they can still be criticized for not being able to truly dissociate the effects of E on the acquisition of bone mass in males during puberty from its possible effects on the maintenance of bone mass in adult men with mature skeletons. If, for example, a given individual tracked for E_2 levels (relative to his peers) throughout life, BMD later in life could simply reflect the acquisition of bone mass related to that individual's E_2 level during growth. To try to dissociate the effects of E on bone in men during young adulthood from its possible effects in aging, Khosla *et al* [59] reported on the results of a longitudinal study in which the acquisition of bone mass in young adulthood (age 22 to 39 years) and the loss of bone mass in aging (age 60 to 90 years) over 4 years was related to T and E levels. The most significant associations in this study were found at the forearm sites (distal radius and ulna), perhaps because of the greater precision of the peripheral site measurements as compared with central sites such as the spine or hip. The young men had increases in BMD at the forearm sites of 0.42 to 0.43% per year, whereas the elderly men had decreases in BMD at these sites of 0.49 to 0.66% per year. Both the increase in BMD in the young men and the decrease in BMD in the elderly men were more closely associated with serum bioavailable E_2 levels than with T (total or bioavailable) levels (Table 94-3). Moreover, further analysis of the data suggested that there may be a threshold bioavailable E_2 level of approximately 40 pmol/L (11 pg/ml) below which the rate of bone loss in the elderly men was clearly associated with bioavailable E_2 levels, whereas above this level there did not appear to be any relationship between the rate of bone loss and bioavailable E_2 levels (Fig. 94-8). In these older men, a bioavailable E_2 level of 40 pmol/L (11 pg/ml) corresponded to a total E_2 level of approximately 114 pmol/L (31 pg/ml), which is close to the middle of the reported normal range for E_2 levels in men (10 to 50 pg/ml). These findings also suggested that relatively low E levels may well contribute to the processes associated

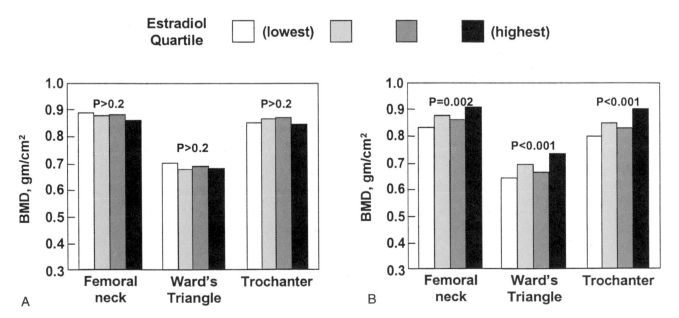

Fig. 94-7 (A) Mean bone mineral density (BMD) at the measured sites of the proximal femur, by testosterone quartile, in a group of elderly men (age 68 to 96 years) from the Framingham cohort. (B) Mean BMD at the measured sites of the proximal femur, by estradiol quartile. (Adapted from Amin S, Zhang Y, Sawin CT *et al.* [2000]. Association of hypogonadism and estradiol levels with bone mineral density in elderly men from the Framingham study. *Ann Intern Med.* 133:951–963, with permission.)

with age-related bone loss in men. This point is underscored further by the finding that bioavailable E$_2$ levels tend to decline fairly substantially with aging in men, resulting in large part to a marked increase in sex hormone binding globulin levels with increasing age [53]. Finally, these results suggest that there may be a difference between the reference range for E2 in men (10 to 50 pg/ml) and a physiologic normal range in men (>30 pg/ml).

These longitudinal findings have now been independently confirmed by two other studies. Thus, in a cohort of 200 elderly men (age range 55 to 85 years), Gennari et al [60] found that men with a free E$_2$ index (molar ratio of E$_2$ to sex hormone binding globulin) below the median had higher rates of bone loss at the femoral neck and Ward's triangle and a greater decrease in the speed of ultrasound measured at the calcaneus and higher markers of bone turnover as compared with men

with a free E$_2$ index above the median. By contrast, there were no differences in these parameters between men below or above the median value for the free androgen index. Similarly, Van Pottelbergh et al [29] found that in a population of 214 community-dwelling men aged 71 to 86 years, the serum bioavailable E$_2$ (but not bioavailable T) level was associated with bone loss at the forearm and femoral neck.

These longitudinal data, therefore, provide reasonably convincing evidence that E plays an important role in bone metabolism not just in the developing but also in the mature male skeleton. Nonetheless, all of these findings (cross-sectional and longitudinal) are correlative, and, to prove causality, interventional studies were needed.

In the first such study, Falahati-Nini et al [61] suppressed endogenous T and E production in a group (n = 59) of older men (mean age, 68 years) using a combination of a gonadotropin-releasing hormone (GnRH) agonist and an aromatase inhibitor. Physiologic E$_2$ and T levels were maintained by placing the men on the respective patches. After baseline measurements of bone turnover markers, the men were then randomized to one of four groups to rigorously delineate the relative contributions of E and T toward regulating bone resorption and formation. Group A (–T,–E) had both patches withdrawn; Group B (–T,+E) had the T patch withdrawn but continued the E patch; Group C (+T,–E) had the E patch withdrawn, but continued the T patch; and Group D (+T,+E) continued both patches. All subjects were continued on GnRH and the aromatase inhibitor.

Figure 94-9A shows the changes in the bone resorption markers, urine deoxypyridinoline (Dpd) and N-telopeptide of type I collagen (NTX), after the subjects had been on the variable treatments for a period of 3 weeks. As is evident, significant increases in both urinary Dpd and NTX excretion, Group A (–T,–E), were prevented completely by continuing T and E

Table 94-3

Spearman Correlation Coefficients Relating Rates of Change in BMD at the Radius and Ulna to Serum Sex Steroid Levels Among a Sample of Rochester, Minnesota Men Stratified by Age

	Young		Middle-Aged		Elderly	
	Radius	Ulna	Radius	Ulna	Radius	Ulna
T	−0.02	−0.19	−0.18	−0.25*	0.13	0.14
E$_2$	0.33**	0.22*	0.03	0.07	0.21*	0.18*
E$_1$	0.35†	0.34**	0.17	0.23*	0.16	0.14
Bio T	0.13	−0.04	0.07	0.01	0.23**	0.27**
Bio E$_2$	0.30**	0.20	0.14	0.21*	0.29**	0.33†

Bio, bioavailable; BMD, bone mineral density; E$_1$, estrone; E$_2$, estradiol; T, testosterone.

*, $p<0.05$; **, $p<0.01$; †, $p<0.001$.

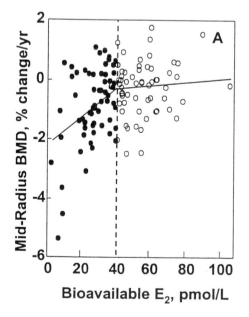 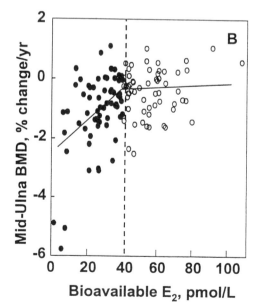

Fig. 94-8 Rate of change in midradius bone mineral density (BMD) (A) and midulna BMD (B) as a function of bioavailable estradiol (E$_2$) levels in elderly men. Model R^2 values were 0.20 and 0.25 for the radius and ulna, respectively, both <0.001 for comparison with a one-slope model. Solid circles correspond to subjects with bioavailable E$_2$ levels below 40 pmol/L (11 pg/mL) and open circles those with values above 40 pmol/L. (Reproduced from Khosla S, Melton LJ III, Atkinson EJ, O'Fallon WM. [2001]. Relationship of serum sex steroid levels to longitudinal changes in bone density in young versus elderly men. *J Clin Endocrinol Metab*. 86:3555–3561, with permission.)

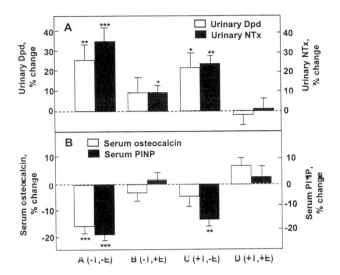

Fig. 94-9 Percent changes in (A) bone resorption markers (urinary deoxypyridinoline [Dpd] and N-telopeptide of type I collagen [NTX]) and (B) bone formation markers (serum osteocalcin and N-terminal extension peptide of type I collagen [PINP]) in a group of elderly men (mean age 68 years) made acutely hypogonadal and treated with an aromatase inhibitor (Group A), treated with estrogen (E) alone (Group B), testosterone (T) alone (Group C), or both (Group D). See text for details. Asterisks indicate significance for change from baseline: *, $p < 0.05$; **, $p < 0.01$; ***, $p < 0.001$. The estrogen and testosterone effects were analyzed using two-factor analysis of variance (ANOVA) models: Dpd: E effect, $p = 0.005$, T effect, $p = 0.232$; NTX: E effect, $p = 0.0002$, T effect, $p = 0.085$; osteocalcin, E effect, $p = 0.002$, T effect, $p = 0.013$; PINP: E effect, $p = 0.0001$, T effect, $p = 0.452$. (Adapted from Falahati-Nini A, Riggs BL, Atkinson EJ et al. [2000]. Relative contributions of testosterone and estrogen in regulating bone resorption and formation in normal elderly men. *J Clin Invest*. 106:1553–1560, with permission.)

replacement [Group D (+T,+E)]. E alone (Group B) was almost completely able to prevent the increase in bone resorption, whereas T alone (Group C) was much less effective. Using a two-factor analysis of variance (ANOVA) model, the effects of E on urinary Dpd and NTX excretion were highly significant ($p = 0.005$ and 0.0002, respectively). E accounted for 70% or more of the total effect of sex steroids on bone resorption in these older men, whereas T could account for no more than 30% of the effect. Using a somewhat different design, Leder et al [62] confirmed an independent effect of T on bone resorption, although the data in the aggregate clearly favor a more prominent effect of E on the control of bone resorption in men.

Figure 94-9B shows the corresponding changes in the bone formation markers, serum osteocalcin, and aminoterminal propeptide 7 type I collagen (PINP). The reductions in both osteocalcin and PINP levels with the induction of sex steroid deficiency (Group A) were prevented with continued E and T replacement (Group D). Interestingly, serum osteocalcin, which is a marker of function of the mature osteoblast and osteocyte [63], was maintained by either E or T (ANOVA p values of 0.002 and 0.013, respectively). By contrast, serum PINP, which represents type I collagen synthesis throughout the various stages of osteoblast differentiation [63], was maintained by E (ANOVA p value 0.0001) but not T.

Collectively, these findings provided conclusive proof of an important and dominant role for E in bone metabolism in the mature skeleton of adult men. Similar findings were subsequently reported by Taxel et al [64] in a study of 15 elderly men treated with an aromatase inhibitor for 9 weeks, in which suppression of E production resulted in significant increases in bone resorption markers and a suppression of bone formation markers.

The dominant role played by E in regulating bone resorption in men is perhaps somewhat surprising, because *in vitro* both E and T inhibit osteoclast development [65–67], enhance osteoclast apoptosis [68,69], and suppress production of the important proresorptive cytokine interleukin 6 [70–73]. These findings suggest that E and T may regulate some other key regulator of bone resorption in opposite directions. Recently, Khosla et al [74] reported that this may be the case for E versus T regulation of osteoprotegerin (OPG), which blocks the final effector molecule for osteoclast development, receptor activator of nuclear factor-κ ligand (RANKL) [75]. Thus, both *in vitro* [76,77] and *in vivo* [74], E stimulates OPG production whereas T tends to inhibit it [74,78]. Although these findings do not exclude the possibility that E and T may have differential effects on other molecules regulating osteoclastogenesis, they do suggest that OPG may be a candidate factor accounting for the differential effects of E and T on bone resorption.

These observations suggest a certain rationale regarding the use of E in men to maintain bone mass. Because E2, however, is associated with a relatively narrow therapeutic window in terms of possible feminizing effects, a selective estrogen receptor modulator (SERM) is a more attractive option. In a short-term (6 month) proof-of-concept study, Doran et al [79] treated 50 elderly men with either placebo or the SERM raloxifene (60 mg/day) and assessed bone turnover markers. Overall, raloxifene had no significant impact on urinary NTX excretion. However, the data did suggest that raloxifene may reduce bone resorption in the subset of elderly men with low E2 levels (below approximately 26 pg/ml). Clearly, further studies are needed in men with low E2 levels to test whether SERMs may have a role in preventing or treating osteoporosis in men.

Collectively, therefore, the data in adult men are consistent with the findings from the human experiments of nature. Estrogen does appear to be a major, and perhaps dominant, regulator of bone metabolism in men. It is the more potent regulator of bone resorption, although it is likely that T also has some antiresorptive effects. Both E and T appear to be important for the maintenance of bone formation. Testosterone also likely contributes to the sexual dimorphism of the skeleton by increasing periosteal bone formation. Finally, T serves as the precursor to E synthesis by the aromatase enzyme, both in the testes and in peripheral tissues including bone [80].

VI. Cross-talk Between Estrogen and Testosterone at the Molecular Level

The clinical observations that E plays a major role in bone metabolism in males are paralleled by intriguing *in vitro* observations of unexpected cross-talk at the receptor level between E and T. Thus, although it is clear that the traditional, transcriptional effects of E and T are likely mediated via the ER and AR, respectively, Kousteni et al [81] found that the effects of sex steroids on preventing osteoblast apoptosis, which are mediated via nongenomic actions involving activation of a Src/Shc/ERK signaling pathway, appear to be relatively gender-nonspecific. These effects are mediated by the ligand (rather than DNA) binding domain of ER-α, ER-β, or AR and can be transmitted with similar efficiency irrespective of whether the ligand is E or an androgen. Moreover, the ER antagonist ICI 182,780 can block either E_2 or T actions on preventing apoptosis, and the AR antagonist hydroxyflutamide can also block both E_2 and T effects (Fig. 94-10).

Further evidence for this molecular cross-talk comes from studies in the mouse prostate demonstrating that the T metabolite, 5α-androstane-3β,17β-diol, can bind ER-β and thereby reduce prostatic AR levels [82]. This, in turn, results in reduced proliferation of the epithelial cells of the prostate. Whether androgen metabolites have similar effects via ER-β in other tissues, such as bone, is at present unclear but certainly is an intriguing possibility.

VII. Summary and Conclusions

It is clear that the past several years have witnessed a dramatic shift in our thinking regarding sex steroid regulation of the male skeleton. Androgens are clearly important for bone metabolism in males; what has been unexpected is the major role played by E. Moreover, although age-related bone loss in men had generally been assumed to be independent of sex steroids, it appears that the observed decreases in circulating bioavailable E and T levels may well be contributing to the development of involutional osteoporosis in men. These findings also suggest the possibility that other disorders associated with aging in men, such as cardiovascular disease, dementia, and prostate cancer, may also be related to these changes in sex steroid and in particular E levels. Whether or not this turns out to be the case remains to be seen, but it is clear that the observations made on the regulation of bone metabolism by sex steroids in men should lead to additional studies not only in this area but also in other aspects of men's health.

VIII. Suggestions for Further Investigations

- Potential use of SERMs in men with lower estrogen levels and osteoporosis.
- Development and clinical assessment of selective androgen receptor modulators (SARMs) for their skeletal effects.
- Possible role of declining bioavailable sex steroid levels with aging in other aspects of men's health (i.e., cardiovascular disease, dementia, prostate cancer).

Acknowledgement

This work was supported by Grants AG04875 and AR27065 from the National Institutes of Health (SK) and the FDA grant 001024.

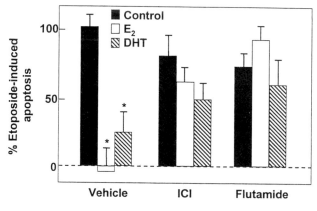

Fig. 94-10 Antiapoptotic effects of estrogen (E) and 5α-dihydrotestosterone (DHT) on osteoblastic cells and evidence for sex-nonspecific signaling. Mouse calvarial osteoblasts were pretreated with the estrogen receptor (ER) antagonist ICI 182,780 (10^{-7} M) or with the androgen receptor (AR) antagonist flutamide (10^{-7} M) for 30 minutes, followed by incubation with 10^{-8} M E2 or DHT for 1 hour. Subsequently, the apoptosis inducer etoposide was added and apoptotic cells were quantified after 6 hr. *, $p < 0.05$ versus vehicle, by analysis of variance (ANOVA). (Adapted from Kousteni S, Bellido T, Plotkin LI *et al.* [2001]. Nongenotropic, sex-nonspecific signaling through the estrogen or androgen receptors: Dissociation from transcriptional activity. *Cell.* 104:1–20, with permission.)

References

1. Riggs BL, Khosla S, Melton LJ III. (2002). Sex steroids and the construction and conservation of the adult skeleton. *Endocr Rev.* 23:279–302.
2. Khosla S, Melton LJ III, Riggs BL. (2002). Estrogen and the male skeleton. *J Clin Endocrinol Metab.* 87:1443–1450.
3. Stepan JJ, Lachman M, Zverina J *et al.* (1989). Castrated men exhibit bone loss: Effect of calcitonin treatment on biochemical indices of bone remodeling. *J Clin Endocrinol Metab.* 69:523–527.
4. Swerdloff RS, Wang C. (1993). Androgen and aging in men. *Exp Gerontol.* 28:435–446.
5. Smith EP, Boyd J, Frank GR *et al.* (1994). Estrogen resistance caused by a mutation in the estrogen-receptor gene in a man. *N Engl J Med.* 331: 1056–1061.
6. Morishima A, Grumbach MM, Simpson ER *et al.* (1995). Aromatase deficiency in male and female siblings caused by a novel mutation and the physiological role of estrogens. *J Clin Endocrinol Metab.* 80:3689–3698.
7. Carani C, Qin K, Simoni M *et al.* (1997). Effect of testosterone and estradiol in a man with aromatase deficiency. *N Engl J Med.* 337:91–95.
8. Deladoey J, Fluck C, Bex M *et al.* (1999). Aromatase deficiency caused by a novel P450 aromatase gene mutation: Impact of absent estrogen production on serum gonadotropin concentration in a boy. *J Clin Endocrinol Metab.* 84:4050–4054.
9. Herrmann BL, Saller B, Janssen OE *et al.* (2002). Impact of estrogen replacement therapy in a male with congenital aromatase deficiency caused by a novel mutation in the CYP gene. *J Clin Endocrinol Metab.* 87:5476–5484.
10. Bilezikian JP, Morishima A, Bell J, Grumbach MM. (1998). Increased bone mass as a result of estrogen therapy in a man with aromatase deficiency. *N Engl J Med.* 339:599–603.
11. Rochira V, Balestieri A, Faustini-Fustini M *et al.* (2002). Pituitary function in a man with congenital aromatase deficiency: Effect of different doses of transdermal E2 on basal and stimulated pituitary hormones. *J Clin Endocrinol Metab.* 87:2857–2862.
12. Bilezikian JP, Khosla S, Riggs BL. (2002). Estrogen Effects on Bone in the Male Skeleton. In *Principles of Bone Biology* (Bilezikian JP, Raisz LG, Rodan GA, eds.), pp. 1467–1476. San Diego, CA: Academic Press.
13. Hemsell DL, Edman CD, Marks JF *et al.* (1977). Massive extraglandular aromatization of plasma androstenedione resulting in feminization of a prepubertal boy. *J Clin Invest.* 60:455–464.
14. Bulun SE, Noble LS, Takayama K *et al.* (1999). Endocrine disorders associated with inappropriately high aromatase expression. *J Steroid Biochem Mol Biol.* 61:133–139.

15. Stratakis CA, Vottero A, Brodie A *et al.* (1998). The aromatase excess syndrome is associated with feminization of both sexes and autosomal dominant transmission of aberrant P450 aromatase gene transcription. *J Clin Endocrinol Metab.* 83:1348–1357.

16. Shozu M, Takayam K, Bulun SE. (1998). Mutation in 5'-flanking region of CYP19 gene causes excessive peripheral aromatase expression in boy with gynecomastia. *Proceedings of the 80th Annual Meeting of the Endocrine Society, New Orleans, LA.* Bethesda, MD: Endocrine Society Press.

17. Grumbach MM, Auchus RJ. (1999). Estrogen: Consequences and implications of human mutations in synthesis and action. *J Clin Endocrinol Metab.* 84:4677–4694.

18. Zachmann M, Prader A, Sobel EH *et al.* (1986). Pubertal growth in patients with androgen insensitivity: Indirect evidence for the importance of estrogen in pubertal growth of girls. *J Pediatr.* 108:694–697.

19. Coen P, Kuhn H, Ballantine T *et al.* (1991). An aromatase producing sex cord tumor resulting in prepubertal gynecomastia. *N Engl J Med.* 324:317–322.

20. Simpson ER, Mahendroo MS, Means GD *et al.* (1994). Aromatase cytochrome P450, the enzyme responsible for estrogen biosynthesis. *Endocr Rev.* 15:342–355.

21. Grumbach MM, Styne DM. (1998). Puberty: Ontogeny, Neuroendocrinology, Physiology, and Disorders. In *Williams Textbook of Endocrinology,* 9th Edition (Wilson JD, Foster DW, Kronenberg HM, Larsen PR, eds.), pp. 1509–1625. Philadelphia: WB Saunders.

22. Conte FA, Grumbach MM, Ito Y *et al.* (1994). A syndrome of female pseudohermaphrodism, hypergonadotropic hypogonadism, and multicystic ovaries associated with missense mutations in the gene encoding aromatase (P450arom). *J Clin Endocrinol Metab.* 78:1287–1292.

23. Ito Y, Fisher CR, Conte FA *et al.* (1993). Molecular basis of aromatase deficiency in an adult female with sexual infantilism and polycystic ovaries. *Proc Natl Acad Sci U S A.* 90:11673–11677.

24. Mullis PE, Yoshimura N, Kuhlmann B *et al.* (1997). Aromatase deficiency in a female who is compound heterozygote for two point mutations in the P450arom gene: Impact of estrogens on hypergonadotropic hypogonadism, multicystic ovaries, and bone densitometry in childhood. *J Clin Endocrinol Metab.* 82:1739–1745.

25. Masi L, Becherini L, Gennari L *et al.* (2002). Polymorphism of the aromatase gene in postmenopausal Italian women: Distribution and correlation with bone mass and fracture risk. *J Clin Endocrinol Metab.* 86:2263–2269.

26. Salmen T, Heikkinen A, Mahonen A *et al.* (2001). Relation of aromatase gene polymorphism and hormone replacement therapy to serum estradiol values, bone mineral density values, and fracture risk in early postmenopausal women. *J Bone Miner Res.* 16(Suppl 1):S474.

27. Zmuda JM, Cauley JA, Bunker CH *et al.* (2001). Genetic variants of aromatase (CYP19): Association with bone density among men of African ancestry. *J Bone Miner Res.* 16(Suppl 1):S476.

28. Masi L, Picariello L, Becherini L *et al.* (2001). Aromatase gene polymorphism: Role of the various genotypes in the estrogen production. *J Bone Miner Res.* 16(Suppl 1):S352.

29. Van Pottelbergh IV, Goemaere S, Kaufman JM. (2003). Bioavailable estradiol and an aromatase gene polymorphism are determinants of bone mineral density changes in men over 70 years of age. *J Clin Endocrinol Metab.* 88:3075–3087.

30. Couse JF, Korach KS. (1999). Estrogen receptor null mice: What have we learned and where will they lead us. *Endocr Rev.* 20:358–3417.

31. Windahl SH, Hollberg K, Vidal O *et al.* (2001). Female estrogen receptor B-/-mice are partially protected against age-related trabecular bone loss. *J Bone Miner Res.* 16:1388–1398.

32. Oz OK, Zerwekh JE, Fisher C *et al.* (2000). Bone has a sexually dimorphic response to aromatase deficiency. *J Bone Miner Res.* 15:507–514.

33. Bilezikian JP. (2002). Sex steroids, mice and men: When androgens and estrogens get very close to each other. *J Bone Miner Res.* 17:563–566.

34. Lubahn DB, Moyer JS, Golding TS *et al.* (1993). Alteration of reproductive function but not prenatal sexual development after insertional disruption of the mouse estrogen receptor gene. *Proc Natl Acad Sci U S A.* 90:11162–11166.

35. Korach KS, Couse JF, Curtis SW *et al.* (1996). Estrogen receptor gene disruption: Molecular characterization and experimental and clinical phenotypes. *Recent Prog Horm Res.* 51:159–186.

36. Windahl SH, Vidal O, Andersson G *et al.* (1999). Increased cortical bone mineral content but unchanged trabecular bone mineral density in female ER B-/-mice. *J Clin Invest.* 104:895–901.

37. Vidal O, Lindberg MK, Hollberg K *et al.* (2000). Estrogen receptor specificity in the regulation of skeletal growth and maturation in male mice. *Proc Natl Acad Sci U S A.* 97:5474–5479.

38. Denger S, Reid G, Kos M *et al.* (2001). ER-α gene expression in human primary osteoblasts: Evidence for the expression of two receptor proteins. *Mol Endocrinol.* 15:2064–2077.

39. Gentile MA, Zhang H, Harada S *et al.* (2001). Bone response to estrogen replacement in OVX double estrogen receptor- (α and β) knockout mice. *J Bone Miner Res.* 16(Suppl 1):S146.

40. Sims NA, Dupont S, Krust A *et al.* (2002). Deletion of estrogen receptors reveals a regulatory role for estrogen receptors-β in bone remodeling in females but not in males. *Bone.* 30:18–25.

41. Lindberg MK, Moverare SE, Skrtic S *et al.* (2002). Two different pathways for maintenance of trabecular bone in adult mice. *J Bone Miner Res.* 17: 555–562.

42. Ke HZ, Chidsey-Frink KL, Qi H *et al.* (2001). The role of estrogen receptor-β (ER-β) in the early age-related bone gain and later age-related bone loss. *J Bone Miner Res.* 16(Suppl 1):S160.

43. Fisher CR, Graves KH, Parlow AF, Simpson ER. (1998). Characterization of mice deficient in aromatase (ArKO) because of targeted disruption of the cyp19 gene. *Proc Natl Acad Sci U S A.* 95:6965–6970.

44. Vanderschueren D, Van Herck E, Suiker AMH *et al.* (1993). Bone and mineral metabolism in the androgen-resistant (testicular feminized) male rat. *J Bone Miner Res.* 8:801–809.

45. Turner RT, Wakley GK, Hannon KS. (1990). Differential effects of androgens on cortical bone histomorphometry in gonadectomized male and female rats. *J Orthop Res.* 8:612–617.

46. Bateman TA, Zimmerman RJ, Ayers RA *et al.* (1998). Histomorphometric, physical, and mechanical effects of spaceflight and insulin-like growth factor-I on rat long bones. *Bone.* 23:527–535.

47. Gori F, Hofbauer L, Conover CA, Khosla S. (1999). Effects of androgens on the insulin-like growth factor system in an androgen-responsive human osteoblastic cell line. *Endocrinology.* 140:5579–5586.

48. Vanderschueren D, Van Herck E, Suiker AMH *et al.* (1992). Bone and mineral metabolism in aged male rats: Short and long term effects of androgen deficiency. *Endocrinology.* 130:2906–2916.

49. Vanderschueren D, Van Herck E, Nijs J *et al.* (1997). Aromatase inhibition impairs skeletal modeling and decreases bone mineral density in growing male rats. *Endocrinology.* 138:2301–2307.

50. Vanderschueren D, Van Herck E, De Coster R, Bouillon R. (1996). Aromatization of androgens is important for skeletal maintenance of male rats. *Calcif Tissue Int.* 59:179–183.

51. Slemenda CW, Longcope C, Zhou L *et al.* (1997). Sex steroids and bone mass in older men: Positive associations with serum estrogens and negative associations with androgens. *J Clin Invest.* 100:1755–1759.

52. Greendale GA, Edelstein S, Barrett-Connor E. (1997). Endogenous sex steroids and bone mineral density in older women and men: The Rancho Bernardo study. *J Bone Miner Res.* 12:1833–1843.

53. Khosla S, Melton LJ III, Atkinson EJ *et al.* (1998). Relationship of serum sex steroid levels and bone turnover markers with bone mineral density in men and women: A key role for bioavailable estrogen. *J Clin Endocrinol Metab.* 83:2266–2274.

54. Center JR, Nguyen TV, Sambrook PN, Eisman JA. (1999). Hormonal and biochemical parameters in the determination of osteoporosis in elderly men. *J Clin Endocrinol Metab.* 84:3626–3635.

55. Ongphiphadhanakul B, Rajatanavin R, Chanprasertyothin S *et al.* (1998). Serum oestradiol and oestrogen-receptor gene polymorphism are associated with bone mineral density independently of serum testosterone in normal males. *Clin Endocrinol.* 49:803–809.

56. Van den Beld AW, de Jong FH, Grobbee DE *et al.* (2000). Measures of bioavailable serum testosterone and estradiol and their relationships with muscle strength, bone density, and body composition in elderly men. *J Clin Endocrinol Metab.* 85:3276–3282.

57. Amin S, Zhang Y, Sawin CT *et al.* (2000). Association of hypogonadism and estradiol levels with bone mineral density in elderly men from the Framingham study. *Ann Intern Med.* 133:951–963.

58. Szulc P, Munoz F, Claustrat B *et al.* (2001). Bioavailable estradiol may be an important determinant of osteoporosis in men: The MINOS study. *J Clin Endocrinol Metab.* 86:192–199.

59. Khosla S, Melton LJ III, Atkinson EJ, O'Fallon WM. (2001). Relationship of serum sex steroid levels to longitudinal changes in bone density in young versus elderly men. *J Clin Endocrinol Metab.* 86:3555–3561.

60. Gennari L, Merlotti D, Martini G *et al.* (2003). Longitudinal association between sex hormone levels, bone loss, and bone turnover in elderly men. *J Clin Endocrinol Metab.* 88:5327–5333.

61. Falahati-Nini A, Riggs BL, Atkinson EJ *et al.* (2000). Relative contributions of testosterone and estrogen in regulating bone resorption and formation in normal elderly men. *J Clin Invest.* 106:1553–1560.

62. Leder BZ, LeBlanc KM, Schoenfeld DA *et al.* (2003). Differential effects of androgens and estrogens on bone turnover in normal men. *J Clin Endocrinol Metab.* 88:204–210.

63. Lian JB, Stein GS, Canalis E *et al.* (1999). Bone Formation: Osteoblast Lineage Cells, Growth Factors, Matrix Proteins, and the Mineralization Process. In *Primer on the Metabolic Bone Diseases and Disorders of Mineral Metabolism*, 4th Edition (Favus MF, ed.), pp. 14–38. Philadelphia: Lippincott Williams & Wilkins.

64. Taxel P, Kennedy DG, Fall PM *et al.* (2001). The effect of aromatase inhibition on sex steroids, gonadotropins, and markers of bone turnover in older men. *J Clin Endocrinol Metab.* 86:2869–2874.

65. Shevde NK, Bendixen AC, Dienger KM, Pike JW. (2000). Estrogens suppress RANK ligand-induced osteoclast differentiation via a stromal cell independent mechanism involving c-Jun repression. *Proc Natl Acad Sci U S A.* 97:7829–7834.

66. Srivastava S, Toraldo G, Weitzmann MN *et al.* (2001). Estrogen decreases osteoclast formation by down-regulating receptor activator of NF-κ B ligand (RANKL)-induced JNK activation. *J Biol Chem.* 276:8836–8840.

67. Huber DM, Bendixen AC, Pathrose P *et al.* (2001). Androgens suppress osteoclast formation induced by RANKL and macrophage-colony stimulating factor. *Endocrinology.* 142:3800–3808.

68. Hughes DE, Dai A, Tiffee JC *et al.* (1996). Estrogen promotes apoptosis of murine osteoclasts mediated by TGF-β. *Nat Med.* 2:1132–1136.

69. Chen JR, Kousteni S, Bellido T *et al.* (2001). Gender-independent induction of murine osteoclast apoptosis *in vitro* by either estrogen or non-aromatizable androgens. *J Bone Miner Res.* 16(Suppl 1):S159.

70. Jilka RL, Hangoc G, Girasole G *et al.* (1992). Increased osteoclast development after estrogen loss: Mediation by interleukin-6. *Science.* 257:88–91.

71. Kassem M, Harris SA, Spelsberg TC, Riggs BL. (1996). Estrogen inhibits interleukin-6 production and gene expression in a human osteoblastic lineage cell line with high levels of estrogen receptors. *J Bone Miner Res.* 11:193–199.

72. Bellido T, Jilka RL, Boyce BF *et al.* (1995). Regulation of interleukin-6, osteoclastogenesis, and bone mass by androgens. *J Clin Invest.* 95:2886–2895.

73. Hofbauer LC, Ten RM, Khosla S. (1999). The anti-androgen hydroxyfluta-mide and androgens inhibit interleukin-6 production by an androgen-responsive human osteoblastic cell line. *J Bone Miner Res.* 14:1330–1337.

74. Khosla S, Atkinson EJ, Dunstan CR, O'Fallon WM. (2002). Effect of estrogen versus testosterone on circulating osteoprotegerin and other cytokine levels in normal elderly men. *J Clin Endocrinol Metab.* 87:1550–1554.

75. Khosla S. (2001). Minireview: The OPG/RANKL/RANK system. *Endocrinology.* 142:5050–5055.

76. Hofbauer LC, Khosla S, Dunstan CR *et al.* (1999). Estrogen stimulates gene expression and protein production of osteoprotegerin in human osteoblastic cells. *Endocrinology.* 140:4367–4370.

77. Saika M, Inoue D, Kido S, Matsumoto T. (2001). 17β-Estradiol stimulates expression of osteoprotegerin by a mouse stromal cell line, ST-2, via estrogen receptor-α. *Endocrinology.* 142:2205–2212.

78. Hofbauer LC, Hicok KC, Chen D, Khosla S. (2001). Regulation of osteoprotegerin gene expression and protein production by androgens and anti-androgens in human osteoblastic lineage cells. *Eur J Endocrinol.* 147:269–273.

79. Doran PM, Riggs BL, Atkinson EJ, Khosla S. (2001). Effects of raloxifene, a selective estrogen receptor modulator, on bone turnover markers and serum sex steroid and lipid levels in elderly men. *J Bone Miner Res.* 16:2118–2125.

80. Simpson E, Rubin G, Clyne C *et al.* (2000). The role of local estrogen biosynthesis in males and females. *Trends Endocrinol Metab.* 11:184–188.

81. Kousteni S, Bellido T, Plotkin LI *et al.* (2001). Nongenotropic, sex-nonspecific signaling through the estrogen or androgen receptors: Dissociation from transcriptional activity. *Cell.* 104:1–20.

82. Weihua Z, Makela S, Andersson LC *et al.* (2001). A role for estrogen receptor β in the regulation of growth of the ventral prostate. *Proc Natl Acad Sci.* 98:6330–6335.

83. Simpson ER, Zhao Y, Agarwal VR *et al.* (1997). Aromatase expression in health and disease. *Recent Prog Horm Res.* 52:185–214.

95

The Clinical Application of Gender-Based Databases for the Diagnosis of Osteoporosis and Fracture Risk Prediction

PAUL D. MILLER, MD

Clinical Professor of Medicine, University of Colorado Health Sciences Center Medical Director,
Colorado Center for Bone Research, Lakewood, CO

I. Introduction

Osteoporosis occurs in both men and women, and the incidence is increasing in both genders worldwide, predominately because of increased longevity of humans.

The rising incidence of osteoporotic-related fractures and their associated increased morbidity and mortality in both genders and the availability of proven effective therapeutic agents to reduce fracture risk in both genders will lead to increasing use of bone densitometry in clinical management of women and men (Figs. 95-1 to 95-3) [1–4]. Bone densitometry has proven to be a valuable tool in making the diagnosis of osteoporosis in women before the first fracture occurs and in the prediction of fracture risk in nonfractured patients. As more men are tested, the questions arise whether or not the same bone mineral density (BMD) criteria for the diagnosis of osteoporosis and use of BMD for fracture risk prediction that are well established in Caucasian postmenopausal women can also be applied to men. Although the Medicare Bone Mass Measurement Act (BMMA)

established in 1998 to expand the indications for reimbursement for bone densitometry in the Medicare population includes indications for either gender, there are some glaring deficiencies that could preclude specific coverage for men. For example, men with hip fractures could be denied coverage. Hypogonadal men also have no gender-specific coverage, although the BMMA coverage for "estrogen-deficient individuals" could apply to men as well because there is increasing data to strongly suggest that age-related bone loss in men, as in women, may be a common estrogen-deficient pathway [5]. This latter issue is an important one because a growing male population in whom bone loss occurs is the group of men with prostate cancer. Prostate cancer patients are intentionally made hypogonadal to treat the prostate cancer cell growth. This hypogonadal state is either induced by castration, leutinizing hormone releasing hormone (LHRH) agonists, or testosterone-receptor binding antagonists. In addition, there is evidence that bisphosphonates can prevent the loss of BMD in these patients [6,7]. Because alendronate and intermittent parathyroid hormone are also Food and Drug Administration

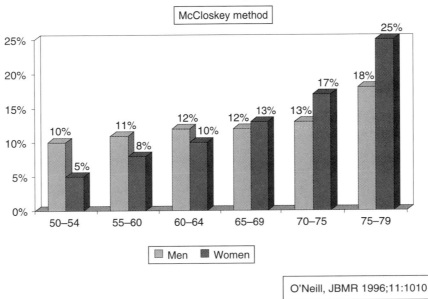

Fig. 95-1 The nearly comparable prevalence of vertebral fractures between Caucasian men and women as a function of age. (From O'Neill TW, Felsenberg D, Varlow J *et al.* [1996]. The prevalence of vertebral deformity in European women and men: The European Vertebral Osteoporosis Study [EVOS]. *J Bone Miner Res.* 11:1010–1017, with permission.)

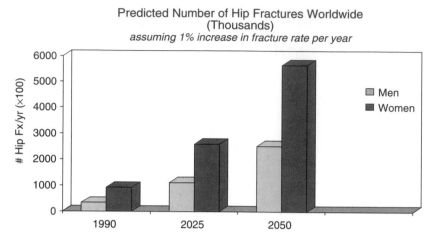

Fig. 95-2 The projected prevalence of hip fractures in Caucasian men and women over time. (From Gullberg B, Johnell O, Kanis JA. [1997]. World-wide projections for hip fracture. *Osteoporos Int.* 7:407–413, with permission.)

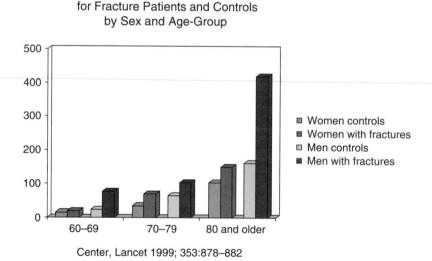

Fig. 95-3 Age-adjusted mortality after hip fracture in men versus women. (From Center JR, Nguyen TV, Schneider D *et al.* [1999]. Mortality after all major types of osteoporotic fracture in men and women: an observational study. *Lancet.* 353:878–882, with permission.)

(FDA)-registered for male osteoporosis, expanding the indications for this gender is also the right thing to do [4,8]. In fact, the positive effect of alendronate to increase BMD and mitigate height loss and morphometric vertebral fractures that was seen in treated men 60 years of age and older with T-scores <−2.0 calculated from a male young-normal reference population database is a reason to ensure that males have expanded coverage for BMD testing. Table 95-1 suggests when to do BMD in males. It also includes the testing of males without any additional risk factors at age 70 years, consistent with the male BMD screening recommendations of the International Society for Clinical

Table 95-1

Males Who Should Have Bone Mineral Density (BMD) Testing

Men with fragility fractures (vertebral and nonvertebral)
Men on chronic glucocorticoids
Hypogonadal men (androgen or estrogen)
Men with known secondary conditions
Screening at 70 years

(From Miller P. [2002]. Colorado Center for Bone Research.)

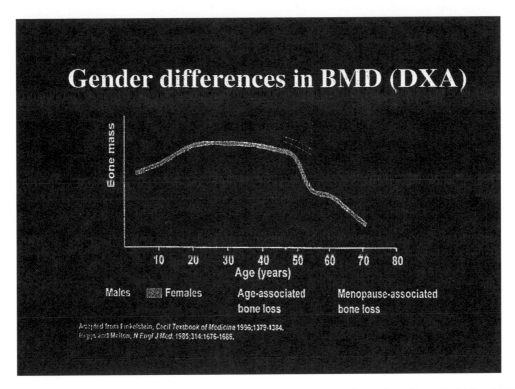

Fig. 95-4 Bone mineral density (BMD) changes in Caucasian men and women as a function of age. (From Riggs LB, Melton LJ III. [1985]. BMD differences between genders over age. *N Engl J Med.* 314:1676–1684, with permission.)

Densitometry (ISCD) [9]. This seems justified based on the observations that age-related bone loss begins in males in groups of patients around the age of 65 years regardless of their gonadal status (Fig. 95-4) [10].

II. World Health Organization Definitions

In 1994 the World Health Organization (WHO) Working Group on Osteoporosis published their technical report, which was intended to advise health economic and policy makers of the anticipated burden that osteoporotic fractures may be expected to become in the future in the Caucasian postmenopausal population [11]. The specific population that provided the data for establishing a BMD threshold for the diagnosis of osteoporosis in the postmenopausal population was derived from Sheffield, England and Rochester, Minnesota. What was observed was that, in Caucasian postmenopausal women 50 years of age and older, the prevalence with BMD defined as 2.5 standard deviations (SD) below the young-normal adult mean for healthy Caucasian means (20 to 29 years of age) at the femoral neck was 16%. The lifetime fracture risk for hip fractures in this population, if left untreated, was also 16%. Hence, the prevalence matched the risk. Thus, a −2.5 SD (T-score) was chosen as the BMD cut-off point to provide health care providers with what was felt to be a BMD level of unacceptable risk, and, therefore, to provide a diagnosis of osteoporosis based on a BMD level per se. A SD level rather than an absolute BMD level was chosen for this cut-off point because the WHO group were cognizant that various BMD devices, both central and peripheral dual-energy x-ray absortiometries (DXAs), had different absolute BMD values

(gm/cm²) because of different calibrations between device manufacturers even at the same region of interest (ROI) of measured bone. A SD score mitigates much of the differences between manufacturers. The osteopenia SD score (<− 1.0 to −2.5 SD) was also a separate classification included in the WHO classifications because fracture risk, as a function of low BMD, is not a threshold but a gradient risk. Thus, patients may develop fragility fractures in the osteopenic range if they also have additional independent risk factors for fragility fractures. As the number of risk factors increase, so does the risk (Fig. 95-5) [12]. In fact, in the most recent prospective fracture trial and the largest fracture trial ever done in postmenopausal women—National Osteoporosis Risk Assessment (NORA)—most of the fractures in the postmenopausal Caucasian population occurred in the osteopenic range (Fig. 95-6) [13,14]. Furthermore, in additional analysis recently completed from the NORA data set using multilogistic regression analysis of 32 possible independent risk factors, four risk factors stand out as the most important: low T score (<− 1.8), prevalent fragility fracture, poor mobility, and poor self-reported health status [15].

A. Pros and Cons of the Use of Standard Deviation Scores

Thus, it appears that the use of SD scores in bone densitometry is solidified in clinical practice, although there are pros and cons with regard to the use of SD scores. The greatest problem with SD scores is the influence that variable SD from the mean BMD of the reference population database, from which the T-scores or Z-scores are calculated, have on the T-score (from young-normals) or Z-score (from age-matched) calculations

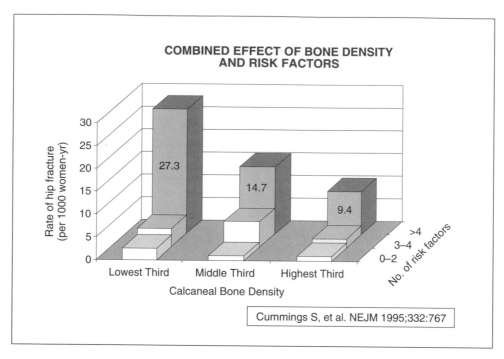

Fig. 95-5 Influence of bone mineral density (BMD) and additional risk factors on hip fracture risk. (From Cummings SR, Nevitt MC, Browner WS *et al.* [1995]. Risk factors for hip fracture in white women. *N Engl J Med.* 332:767–773, with permission.)

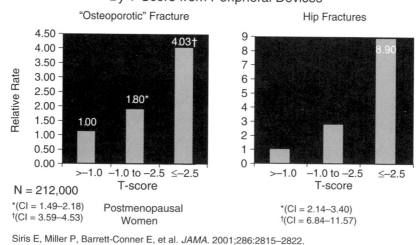

Fig. 95-6 Risk for fracture in the National Osteoporosis Risk Assessment (NORA) in postmenopausal women as a function of T-score. (From Siris ES, Miller PD, Barrett-Conner E *et al.* [2001]. Identification and fracture outcomes of undiagnosed low bone mineral density in post-menopausal women: Results from the National Osteoporosis Risk Assessment [NORA]. *JAMA.* 286:2815–2822, with permission.)

Table 95-2

Influence of Variable Population Standard Deviation (SD) on T-Score at Constant Bone Mineral Density (BMD)

SD = 10%	SD = 15%	SD = 20%	T-Score Difference
(0.90–1.00)/0.10 = T: –1.0	(0.90–1.00)/0.15 = T: –0.7	(0.90–1.00)/0.20 = T: –0.5	0.5 SD
(0.80–1.00)/0.10 = T: –2.0	(0.80–1.00)/0.15 = T: –1.3	(0.80–1.00)/0.20 = T: –1.0	1.0 SD
(0.70–1.00)/0.10 = T: –3.0	(0.70–1.00)/0.15 = T: –2.0	(0.70–1.00)/0.20 = T: –1.5	1.5 SD

(From Faulkner KG, VonStetten E, Miler PD. [1999]. Discordance in patient classification using T scores. *J Clin Densitom.* 2:343–350, with permission.)

(Table 95-2) [16]. When one examines the equation for T- or Z-scores, it becomes quite obvious how inconsistent reference population databases can profoundly influence the calculated value. The equation for T-score calculation is shown in Table 95-3.

Small differences in the SD of the reference population can have substantial affect on the calculated T- or Z-score (see Table 95-2). For example, for T-score calculations using young-normal reference populations, if two different young-normal groups are used to calculate the T-score, the same patients tested on the same DXA machine at the same skeletal site may have very different T-scores because the two healthy young-normal reference populations will invariably not have the same SD of the mean BMD (Table 95-4) [17].

Hence, defining the terms *prevalence* (WHO diagnosis) as opposed to *fracture risk prediction* become important both for their distinctions and their similarities because both are linked to SD scores. Thus, if the T-score calculated from one database underestimates the prevalence, it will accordingly also underestimate the risk.

Prevalence represents the percent of a population (women, men, or ethnic-specific) that are above or below a specific SD cut point, for example, –2.0 or –2.5 SD. It is apparent from the preceding equation for T- or Z-score calculation that the

Table 95-3

Equation for T-Score Calculation

Patient BMD – Mean BMD of young normals
SD of young normal population

BMD, bone mineral density; SD, standard deviation.

Table 95-4

Prevalence of WHO Osteoporosis at FN in Same 2500 Elderly PM Women with VCFs Using Same DXA Machine

	Institution YN FN Reference Database	Manufacturer YN FN Reference Database
	0.787 ± 0.119	0.805 ± 0.100
Percent with WHO <– 2.5	3%	23%

(From Ahmed AIH, Blake GM, Rymer JM, Fogleman I. [1997]. Screening for osteopoenia and osteoporosis: Do the accepted normal ranges lead to overdiagnosis? *Osteoporos Int.* 7:432–438, with permission.)
DXA, dual-energy x-ray absorptiometry; FN, femoral neck; PM, postmenopausal; VCFs, vertebrae compression fractures; WHO, World Health Organization; YN, young normal.

percentage of a specific gender or race that falls into a specific WHO classification will be affected by the T (or Z) score being calculated from a gender (or race) other than the gender (or race) of the measured patient. This again is a fundamental effect of the different SD values from two separate reference populations, which will not only differ between two young-normal groups of the same gender but also will differ if the T-score of one gender is calculated from the young-normal reference population of the opposite gender. For example, it has been shown that the prevalence of WHO classified osteoporosis is lower in men than in women when the T-score is calculated from a female young-normal reference population database as opposed to a male young-normal reference population database (Fig. 95-7) [18–20]. Hence, for this reason of diagnosis (and, subsequently for deciding on risk calculations and then therapeutic decisions), the ISCD Consensus Panel recommends T-score calculation in men from a male reference population database [9]. An editorial by Faulkner and Orwoll attempting to examine the relationship between prevalence and risk analogous to the methodology used by the WHO working group to arrive at a cut point of T-score that approximates the prevalence and risk concluded that not only does using a female reference population database to calculate prevalence in males underestimate the prevalence but it also underestimates the risk for lifetime fracture events [21]. In fact, based on the comparative methodology (albeit much more limited) to define the relationship between prevalence and risk in men used by the WHO working group to define the cut point for the diagnosis of osteoporosis in women, Faulkner and Orwoll suggest that for men the T-score for the diagnosis of osteoporosis in men should be –2.3 when calculated from a male database and –1.7 when calculated from a female database (Table 95-5).

Even within the Caucasian postmenopausal population the prevalence not only differs as a function of the reference population database being used for T-score calculation but the prevalence differ according to the T-score cut-off level. Hence, Professor Melton's [22] article in the *Journal of Bone and Mineral Research*, written just before the WHO selected a cut point of <–2.5 for the diagnosis of osteoporosis and had earlier suggested a T-score of –2.0 SD for the cut-point diagnosis of osteoporosis, was titled "How Many Women Have Osteoporosis?" Then in 1994 when the –2.5 cut point was the WHO working groups agreed cut point, Professor Melton's [23] next editorial in the same journal was entitled "How Many Women Have Osteoporosis, Now?" Thus, the prevalence (percentage of the population with a defined "disease") is also effected by the cut point that is selected to represent the disease.

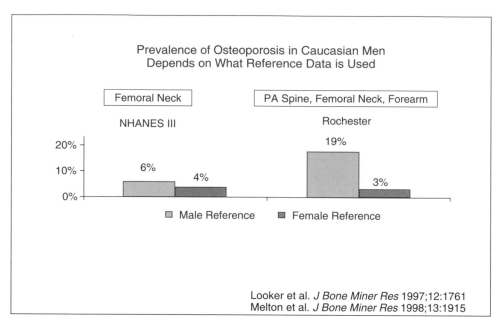

Fig. 95-7   Effect of gender-specific young-normal reference population database on the prevalence of osteoporosis. (From Ref. 18–20, with permission.)

Table 95-5

T-Scores at the Femoral Neck in Men that Best Approximate Lifetime Fracture Risk for Hip Fractures

T-score Threshold	T-score
Male norms	−2.3
Female norms	−1.7

(From Faulkner K, Orwoll E. [2002]. Implications in the use of T-scores for the diagnosis of osteoporosis in men. *J Clin Densitom.* 5:87–93, with permission.) These data are calculated from manufacturer-specific (hologic) young-normal (male vs female) reference population database.

III. Gender Differences in Fracture Risk

What about fracture risk differences and their densitometer reporting between the genders? The lifetime fracture risk for Caucasian men and women is best validated for hip fractures. Data indicate that the risk for a hip fracture in untreated Caucasian men is ~8% and is 16% for untreated Caucasian women, although the age-adjusted mortality in men is far greater than that of women (see Fig. 95-3) [3].The lower lifetime hip fracture risk in men may have several explanations including a higher BMD at peak bone mass, greater muscle mass, fewer frailty falls, and larger bone geometric diameter. However, lifetime fracture risk as it relates to any specific level of BMD at the time of life when BMD begins to decline has not been validated in either women or men. Fracture risk according to specific levels of BMD

have been validated over 1 year and 5 to 10 years following the BMD measurement for both women and men [11,24,25]. The reason why lifetime fracture risk models have never been validated in women from the menopause (age 50 years) and men from a mean age of 65 years when age-related bone loss begins in men, and probably never will be, is that bone densitometry has been around for only ~10 years, and, now with approved osteoporosis pharmacologic therapies, it would be unethical to follow patients, who have low BMD and are losing BMD, over a lifetime. The lifetime fracture models that have been developed and predict lifetime risk as a function of the BMD level at the menopause have been mathematical models. These models in essence take the directly validated 1- to 5-year fracture risk observed in older people as a function of their BMD assessed in many longitudinal population-based fracture trials, such as the study of osteoporotic fracture (SOF) and extrapolate backwards to the average age of menopause (50 years) assuming an average rate of bone loss of 1% per year to predict what the BMD probably would have been had BMD been measured earlier [24,25]. Intuitively these models predict that the lower the BMD at the time of life when BMD predictably begins to decline (menopause for women and age 65 years in men) the greater the lifetime fracture risk in untreated patients. Because women have lower peak adult bone mass than men and begin to lose BMD earlier in life, their lifetime risk for all fractures is greater.

Current (1-year, 5- to 10-year) fracture risk in both women and men has been directly validated as the risk relates to densitometric values both from population-based epidemiologic trials and from the pharmacologic clinical trials in the placebo arms of clinical trials [26–28]. Gender-comparative data have predicted risk either from the absolute BMD or SD scores from both female and male reference population databases. These data suggest that the absolute hip fracture risk is the same in both genders whether the risk is calculated from the absolute BMD (in gm/cm²) (Fig. 95-8) or T-scores that calculated from the female reference population database (Table 95-6) [29,30].

Each central BMD-DXA manufacturer uses gender-specific reference population databases to calculate both T-scores and Z-scores. Physicians and their technologists should, therefore, enter into the computer the specific gender of the patient on the DXA table for these SD score calculations. All of the ultrasound devices measuring ultrasound parameters, speed of sound (SOS) and broadband ultrasound attenuation (BUA), calculate their SD scores all from female Caucasian reference databases. Hence, if measuring a male on an ultrasound device, one has no choice other than to have the SD score calculated from a female database. There is very little fracture risk predictive data in men from ultrasound devices. What data are available suggests, as expected, that the prevalence of osteoporosis is lower measuring males on ultrasound devices when using a female reference population database [31,32]. However, heel ultrasound parameters of BUA are highly correlated to BMD of the heel measured by both single x-ray absorptiometry (SXA) and heel DXA. In this regard, heel SXA absolute BMD values do predict vertebral fracture risk at the same absolute BMD between men and women (see Fig. 95-9) [33,34].

Other data have also suggested that in men and women (Caucasian) absolute hip fracture risk is the same at the same absolute BMD (gm/cm²) of the hip (see Fig. 95-8) [29]. In addition, the 10-year prospective hip fracture data derived from the Caucasian Swedish population has suggested that the absolute risk is the same between genders at the same age when the SD (T-score) is calculated from the female reference population database (see Table 95-5) [30] Finally, data from Melton suggest that although the relative risk (RR) for fracture per SD reduction from the T-score is higher in women than in men (2.4/SD vs 1.3/SD), it is the same between genders whether the RR for fracture is calculated from the male or the female database (i.e., for men RR/SD is 1.3 calculated from a female or male young normal reference population and RR 2.2 in women is calculated from either a young-normal female or young-normal male reference population database) [35]. Thus, there has been discussion that

Table 95-6
10-year Absolute Hip Fracture Risk
from Sweden

	Males	Females
T-score	−2.5	−2.5
Age 75	24%	24%
Age 85	28%	28%

(From Kanis JA, Johnell O, Oden A *et al.* [2002]. Ten year risk of osteoporotic fracture and the effect of risk factors on screening strategies. *Bone*. 30:251–258, with permission.)
Data are calculated from the National Health and Nutrition Examination Survey (NHANES III) female YN database.

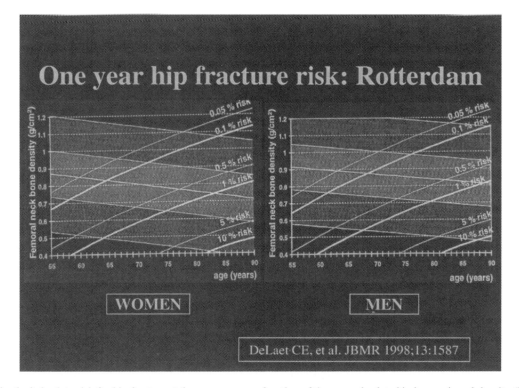

Fig. 95-8 Identical absolute risk for hip fracture at the same age as a function of the same absolute hip bone mineral density (BMD). (From De Laet CEDH, Van Hout BA, Burger H *et al.* [1998]. Hip fracture prediction in the elderly men and women: Validation in the Rotterdam study. *J Bone Miner Res*. 13:1587–1593, with permission.)

when a male is on the DXA table that the technologists enter into the computer for T-score calculation "female." This concept is not yet widely accepted nor should it be until we define the effect of bone size, greater in men than in women, on fracture risk independent of BMD or databases [36–38]. In addition to the previously cited study suggesting that males may fracture at male-derived T-scores better than females, another editorial examining the incident vertebral fractures between men and women from non head-to-head clinical trials suggests that men may also fracture vertebrae at absolute BMD values greater than that of women (see Fig. 95-10) [38]. Although the prevalence data suggest that vertebral fracture prevalence is similar between genders over the age of 60 years, the incident data suggest that incident vertebral fractures are greater in women than in men (Fig. 95-11) [40]. Not until two prospective studies are completed comparing both prevalence and incident risk from both areal and volumetric BMD determinations will we have the answer to the question about the influence of bone geometry on fracture risk. Professor Orwoll, who is the overall principle investigator of the prospective National Institutes of Health (NIH) funded male osteoporosis study (Mr Os), and Professor Bilezikian, who is the principle investigator of the NIH funded trial examining the effect of alendronate versus placebo in both men and women with asymptomatic primary hyperparathyroidism where bone mineral density (BMD) will be measured by both dual energy x-ray absorptiometry (DXA) and quantitative computerized tomography (QCT), will ultimately provide insights into the effect of bone size that is adjusted for areal BMD on fracture risk within genders and between genders. This type of head-to-head data is the only means to define the effect of bone size on fracture risk between genders. Although there are distinctions between genders in periosteal as opposed to endocortical bone apposition versus expansion as each gender ages (Fig. 95-11) [41], it is unknown to what degree these differences may contribute of differences in fracture events in the aging population. It is certain

that abundant investigation is being done to try to explain gender differences in fracture events that may be adjusted for BMD alone.

IV. Summary

In summary, both genders experience a high risk for osteoporotic-related fractures as a function of increased longevity. Diagnostic criteria for men, although not strictly defined, seem comparable to that of women, as might risk for fracture at the same absolute BMD or T-scores calculated from female reference population databases. However, until the issues of the effects of differential bone size between genders on fracture risk differences are defined, it seems more appropriate to calculate T-score in men from male databases, because the percentage of males defined as having low T-scores will be underestimated using a female reference population database, as might the lifetime risk for fracture. Bisphosphonates seem to be effective in men and should be considered in men 60 years of age and older who are either hypogonadal, have fragility fractures, have secondary conditions that can lead to bone loss (steroids, celiac disease, etc.), or have male-derived T-scores <− 2.0. The BMMA must have expanded indications for Medicare coverage for BMD testing in men. Low BMD in both genders is underdiagnosed and undertreated. Physicians need standardized BMD reporting and standardized databases from which to both calculate T-scores and to interpret data for both prevalence (diagnosis) and fracture risk. As more data evolve, we will be better able to determine if different databases should be used between genders.

All these challenges are conquerable, and, for both genders, osteoporosis should no longer be an acceptable process of aging.

V. Suggestions for Further Investigations

- Defining broader indications for BMD testing in men.
- Defining the effect on differences in bone size on fracture risk between genders.

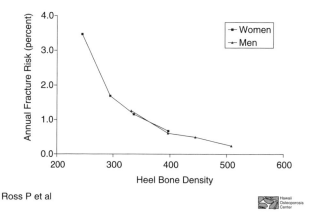

Ross P et al

Fig. 95-9 Identical risk for vertebral fracture in women and men at the same absolute bone mineral density (BMD). (From Ross PD, Yhee Y-K, Davis JW, Wasnich RD. [1993]. Bone Density Predicts Fracture Incidence Among Elderly Men. In *Proceedings and Consensus Development Conference*, Hong Kong, 27 March–2 April 1993, Handelstrykkeriet Aalborg ApS, Aalborg, Denmark [Christiansen C, Riis B, eds.], with permission.)

Relationship Between Baseline
BMD and Vertebral Fracture Incidence

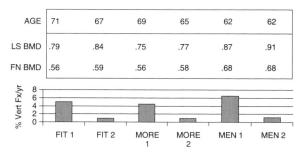

Orwoll, JBMR Oct 2000

Fig. 95-10 Data (non head-to-head) suggesting that men may fracture at higher bone mineral density (BMD) than women. (From Orwoll E. [2000]. Assessing bone density in men. *J Bone Miner Res.* 15:1867–1870, with permission.)

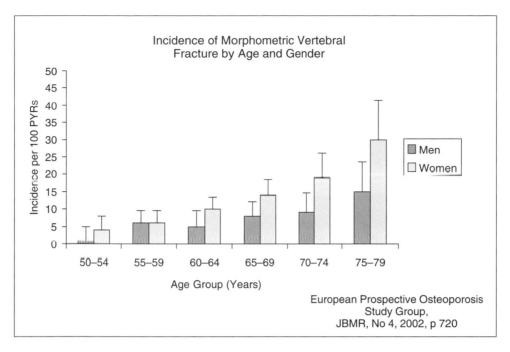

Fig. 95-11   Incident vertebral fractures between genders as a function of age. (From [2002]. Incidence of vertebral fracture in Europe: results from the European Prospective Osteoporosis Study Group. *J Bone Miner Res.* 4:716–724, with permission.)

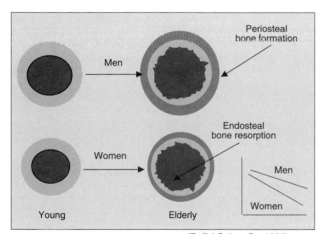

Fig. 95-12   Differential effects of aging on periosteal and endocortical bone between genders. (From Ruff CB, Hayes WC. [1988]. Sex differences in age-related remodeling of the femur and tibia. *J Orthop Res.* 6:886–896, with permission.)

References

1. O'Neill TW, Felsenberg D, Varlow J *et al.* (1996). The prevalence of vertebral deformity in European women and men: The European Vertebral Osteoporosis Study (EVOS). *J Bone Miner Res.* 11:1010–1017.

2. Gullberg B, Johnell O, Kanis JA. (1997). World-wide projections for hip fracture. *Osteoporos Int.* 7:407–413.

3. Center JR, Nguyen TV, Schneider D *et al.* (1999). Mortality after all major types of osteoporotic fracture in men and women: an observational study. *Lancet.* 353:878–882.

4. Orwoll E, Ettinger M, Weiss S *et al.* (2000). Alendronate for the treatment of osteoporosis in men. *N Engl J Med.* 343:604–610.

5. Khosla S, Riggs BL. (2003). Androgens, estrogens, and bone turnover in men. *J Clin Endocrinol Metab.* 88:2352–2353.

6. Smith MR, McGovern FJ, Zeitman AL *et al.* (2001). Pamidronate to prevent bone loss during androgen-deprivation therapy for prostate cancer. *N Engl J Med.* 345:948–955.

7. Mittan D, Lee S, Miller E *et al.* (2002). Bone loss following Hypogonadism in men with prostate cancer treated with GnRH analogs. *J Clin Endocrinol Metab.* 87:3656–3661.

8. Kurland E, Cosman F, McMahon D *et al.* (2000). Parathyroid hormone as a therapy for idiopathic osteoporosis in men: Effects on bone mineral density and bone markers. *J Clin Endocrinol Metab.* 85:3069–3076.

9. Binkley NC, Schmeer P, Wasnich RD, Lenchik L. (2002). What are the criteria by which a densitometric diagnosis of osteoporosis can be made in males and non-Caucasians? *J Clin Densitom.* 5:519–527.

10. Riggs LB, Melton LJ III. (1985). BMD differences between genders over age. *N Engl J Med.* 314:1676–1684.

11. Kanis JA, Gleur CC. (2000). An update on the diagnosis and assessment of osteoporosis with densitometry. *Osteoporos Int.* 11:192–202.

12. Cummings SR, Nevitt MC, Browner WS *et al.* (1995). Risk factors for hip fracture in white women. *N Engl J Med.* 332:767–773.

13. Siris ES, Miller PD, Barrett-Conner E *et al.* (2001). Identification and fracture outcomes of undiagnosed low bone mineral density in post-menopausal women: Results from the National Osteoporosis Risk Assessment (NORA). *JAMA.* 286:2815–2822.

14. Miller PD, Siris ES, Barrett-Conner E *et al.* (2002). Prediction of fracture risk in post-menopausal Caucasian women with peripheral bone density testing: Evidence from the National Osteoporosis Risk Assessment (NORA). *J Bone Miner Res.* 17:2222–2230.

15. Miller PD, Barlas S, Brenneman SK *et al.* (2004). An approach to identifying osteopenic women at increased short-term risk of fracture. *Arch Int Med.* 164:1–8.

16. Faulkner KG, VonStetten E, Miler PD. (1999). Discordance in patient classification using T scores. *J Clin Densitom.* 2:343–350.

17. Ahmed AIH, Blake GM, Rymer JM, Fogleman I. (1997). Screening for osteopoenia and osteoporosis: Do the accepted normal ranges lead to over-diagnosis? *Osteoporos Int.* 7:432–438.

18. Looker AC, Wahner HW, Dunn WL *et al.* (1995). Proximal femur bone mineral levels of US adults. *Osteoporos Int.* 5:389–409.

19. Looker AC, Wahner HW, Dunn WL *et al*. (1998). Updated data on proximal femur bone mineral density levels in US adults. *Osteoporos Int*. 8:468–469.

20. Melton LJ III, Atkinson EJ, O'Conner MK *et al*. (1998). Bone densitometry and fracture risk in men. *J Bone Miner Res*. 13:1915–1923.

21. Faulkner K, Orwoll E. (2002). Implications in the use of T-scores for the diagnosis of osteoporosis in men. *J Clin Densitom*. 5:87–93.

22. Melton LJ, 3rd, Chrischilles EA, Cooper C *et al*. (1992). Perspective. How many women have osteoporosis? *J Bone Miner Res*. 7:1005–1010.

23. Melton LJ, 3rd. (1995). How many women have osteoporosis now? *J Bone Miner Res*. 10:175–177.

24. Black DM, Steinbuch M, Palmero L *et al*. (2001). An assessment tool for predicting fracture risk in postmenopausal women. *Osteoporos Int*. 12:519–528.

25. Oden A, Dawson A, Dere W *et al*. (1999). Lifetime risk of hip fracture is underestimated. *Osteoporos Int*. 8:599–603.

26. Cummings S, Black D, Nevitt M *et al*. (1993). Bone density at various sites for prediction of hip fractures. The study of osteoporotic fractures research group. *Lancet*. 341:72–75.

27. Dargent-Molina P, Favier F, Grandjean H *et al*. for the EPIDOS Group. (1996). Fall-related factors and risk of hip fracture: The EPIDOS prospective study. *Lancet*. 348:145–149.

28. Singer BR, McLauchlan CJ, Robinson CM, Christie J. (1994). Epidemiology of fracture in 15,000 adults: The influence of age and gender. *J Bone Joint Surg Br*. 80:234–238.

29. De Laet CEDH, Van Hout BA, Burger H *et al*. (1998). Hip fracture prediction in the elderly men and women: Validation in the Rotterdam study. *J Bone Miner Res*. 13:1587–1593.

30. Kanis JA, Johnell O, Oden A *et al*. (2002). Ten year risk of osteoporotic fracture and the effect of risk factors on screening strategies. *Bone*. 30:251–258.

31. Adler RA, Funkhouser HL, Holt CM. (2001). Utility of heel ultrasound bone density in men. *J Clin Densitom*. 4(3):225–230.

32. Mulleman D, Legroux-Gerot I, Duquesnoy B *et al*. (2002). Quantitative ultrasound of bone in male osteoporosis. *Osteoporos Int*. 13:388–393.

33. Ross PD, Yhee Y-K, Davis JW, Wasnich RD. (1993). Bone Density Predicts Fracture Incidence Among Elderly Men. In *Proceedings and Consensus Development Conference*, Hong Kong, 27 March–2 April 1993, Handelstrykkeriet Aalborg ApS, Aalborg, Denmark (Christiansen C, Riis B, eds.), pp. 71–74.

34. Cheng S, Suomien H, Era P, Heikkinen E. (1994). Bone density of the calcaneus and fractures in 75- and 80-year old men and women. *Bone*. 11:229–352.

35. Melton JL III, Atkinson EJ, O'Connor MK *et al*. (1998). Bone density and fracture risk in men. *J Bone Miner Res*. 13:1915–1923.

36. Seeman E. (1999). Osteoporosis in men. *Osteoporos Int*. 2(Suppl):S97–S110.

37. Gilsanz V, Boechat MI, Gilsanz R *et al*. (1994). Gender differences in vertebral size in adults: Biomechanical implications. *Radiology*. 190:678–682.

38. Eastell R, Boyle IT, Compston J *et al*. (1998). Management of male osteoporosis: Report of the UK Consensus Group. *Q J Med*. 91:71–92.

39. Orwoll E. (2000). Assessing bone density in men. *J Bone Miner Res*. 15:1867–1870.

40. European Prospective Osteoporosis Study Group. (2002). Incidence of morphometric vertebral fracture by age and gender. *J Bone Miner Res*. 4:720.

41. Ruff CB, Hayes WC. (1988). Sex differences in age-related remodeling of the femur and tibia. *J Orthop Res*. 6:886–896.

96

Animal Models for Gender-Based Skeletal Differences

DIRK VANDERSCHUEREN, MD, PhD, KATRIEN VENKEN, AND ROGER BOUILLON, MD, PhD

Laboratory for Experimental Medicine and Endocrinology, Katholieke Universiteit Leuven, Leuven, Belgium

I. Introduction: Sexual Dimorphism of the Skeleton

Males have more bone than females across species. Such skeletal sexual dimorphism is characterized by (1) greater length, (2) greater outer and inner bone perimeter, and (3) greater cortical mass. Volumetric bone mineral density (BMD divided by volume) is not different from female bones in both laboratory animals and humans [1]. Because purely technical artefact of areal bone density measurements (g/cm^2 projected area instead of volumetric g/cm^3) the BMD may appear to be higher. Indeed, any bigger three-dimensional bone looks denser when projected on a two-dimensional surface [1,2]. Thus, measurement of a greater areal BMD in males is not due to a more dense bone but to a greater bone size. In other words, the male skeleton differs from female more in size than in composition.

Therefore, sex-related skeletal differences are to a large extent limited to cortical bone size. Cortical bone size starts to increase in male relative to female at the start of puberty in laboratory rats. Although rodents, unlike humans, do not experience epiphyseal closure at the end of puberty, relative gender difference in size usually does not further increase at mature age. Therefore, although rodents continue to grow throughout their entire lifespan, gender differences of the skeleton are established during a relative short period of pubertal growth. In this respect, sexual skeletal dimorphism is similar in humans and laboratory animals.

In all these species the underlying mechanism of these sex differences is probably similar. The principal regulators of bone growth are genetic or environmental and mechanical. Laboratory animals, therefore, offer an unique opportunity to study both regulatory mechanisms with respect to gender-based differences of the skeleton.

II. Regulation of Skeletal Gender Differences by Mechanical Strain

A. Regulation of Bone Mass by Mechanical Strain

Mechanical strain is continuously generated by body weight and more especially by muscle attached to the skeleton. To adapt to changes in body weight and muscle, the skeleton must be highly responsive to mechanical stress. In fact, no tissue other than bone compensates to a similar extent to mechanical force. According to the mechanostat theory elaborated by Harold Frost [3], skeletal growth is indeed fully regulated by a dominant feedback system (the "mechanostat") that both senses mechanical strain and adapts to it by remodeling bone. In healthy bone this feedback system adjusts bone mass to keep peak mechanical strains in bone within an acceptable range [4]. Bone

Table 96-1
Comparison of the Percentage of Bone Mineral Content (BMC) in Humans Versus Laboratory Animals

	Males		Females	
	Body Weight (kg)	%BMC	Body Weight (kg)	%BMC
Rat	0.564 ± 0.040	3.1 ± 0.1	$0.311 \pm 0.024*$	$3.6 \pm 0.3*$
Mouse	0.024 ± 0.0013	2.1 ± 0.2	$0.020 \pm 0.009*$	$2.5 \pm 0.2*$
Human	76.4 ± 13	3.5 ± 0.5	$63.0 \pm 14.1*$	$3.4 \pm 0.5**$

Data obtained from women and men aged 20–40 years, from 10-week-old male and female Balb/c mice, and from male Wistar rats aged 12 months and female Wistar rats aged 9 months.

$*p < 0.001$ and $**p < 0.05$ versus male.

Personal unpublished observations.

in disuse undergoes bone loss, bone in overuse adds new bone on existing bone surfaces. The setpoint of the bone mechanostat is thought to be modified by different endocrine and metabolic factors. Thus, when mechanical strain exceeds a certain limit, osteocytes might sense this (setpoint) and send out signals that may lead to adaptations in bone mass and architecture. Greater weight and more muscle, therefore, translates as more bone both across and among species. Bone mass indeed correlates with body weight and even better with muscle (often determined by its lean body mass surrogate). However, interspecies differences in bone mineral relative to body weight are small (Table 96-1). Humans and rats have similar bone mineral content (BMC) relative to body weight. Mice have relatively less bone. Therefore, mice appear to have a higher mechanical setpoint than rats and humans. Moreover, not only between but even within species the setpoint of mechanical strain, which is determined genetically, may be different. Such differences of mechanical setpoint may lead to significant strain differences of bone volume in appendicular versus axial bone [5,6].

B. Skeletal Modeling and Remodeling

The basic processes of skeletal adaptation to mechanical loading/unloading are respectively skeletal modeling during growth and remodeling after growth. Skeletal modeling (Fig. 96-1) is a highly synchronized process of both removal and addition of bone during skeletal growth in order to adapt to the very variable but constantly high mechanical strain induced by growth rate.

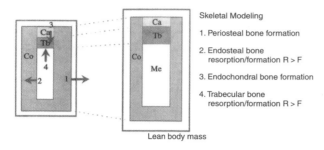

Fig. 96-1 Skeletal modeling. Ca, cartilaginous growth plate; Co, cortex; Me, medulla; Tb, trabeculae.

Skeletal modeling synchronizes transversal and longitudinal bone drifts creating new bone in three dimensions:

1. "Cortical drift," which consists of both periosteal bone formation and medullary expansion. Medullary expansion is a combination of endosteal bone resorption and formation, the former dominating the latter leading to expansion of the marrow cavity.
2. Longitudinal (endochondral) bone formation versus trabecular resorption/formation.

The volume of the cancellous bone compartment at maturity ultimately depends on the sum of new bone created by endochondral bone formation at the upper end and bone added by the combined trabecular resorption and formation at the lower end. The peak cortical thickness is the end result of the periosteal bone formation at the outer site minus the combined endosteal bone resorption and formation at the inner site.

Skeletal modeling is not species specific. Humans, in contrast with rodents, stop growing after puberty. Growth plates close and modeling stops. Mechanical strain decreases as result of growth arrest. The human skeleton reacts to mechanical strain by remodeling after epiphyseal closure. Bone remodeling is a coupled process consisting of removal and addition of new bone at localized "activated" bone sites (basic multicellular units) throughout the adult nongrowing skeleton. Bone resorption always precedes formation (coupling) and the amount of bone resorbed and formed are quantitatively similar. Although mice and rats continue to grow continuously and do not experience epiphyseal closure, growth slows down considerably in the aged animal. Their skeleton, therefore, depends more on remodeling than on modeling.

C. Sex and Mechanical Loading

Males are bigger than females. Males indeed not only have higher body weight and length but also grow faster than females; as a result, mechanical strain is greater in males. This extra gender-related mechanical strain during a period of fast growth maximally stimulates skeletal modeling. In accordance, strategies, such as exercise, that increase maximal strain have maximal effect when implemented during a period of fast skeletal growth, and this occurs well before peak bone mass and maturity are reached. The previously described skeletal gender differences between sexes are, therefore, predictable and, to a large extent, are explained by the mechanostat theory.

A similar extra mechanical loading applied to both male and female rats results in greater skeletal response in males than in females [7]. However, when corrected for body weight and growth rate, the corresponding response is not different between males and females. Therefore, skeletal response to mechanical loading does not appear gender-specific.

D. Interaction of Sex with the Mechanostat

If there were absolutely no interaction of sex with the mechanostat, BMC relative to body weight would be the same in males and females. However, Table 96-1 indicates that this is not the case. Female rats have more bone than male rats relative to body weight over a wide range of body weights representing large differences in mechanical load [8]. Relative to body weight, females have greater bone volume but similar leg muscle mass. Therefore, the mechanical setpoint in females must be lower. In other words, females add more bone during growth relative to mechanical load. According to an Argentine study [9,10] a similar evolution is observed during puberty in adolescents; as expected, bone mass increases along with lean body mass in both boys and girls. However, the slope of this increase is significantly higher in girls indicating that puberty lowers their mechanical setpoint.

Therefore, the mechanostat seems to favor females or discriminate males. Accordingly, even when adult males have a larger bone size than females, they should have even larger sizes if sex did not interfere with the mechanostat. As shown in Table 96-1, the %BMC is either slightly different between sexes (human) or even higher (rats and mice) in the female despite increased mechanical loading in males of all species.

The question remains how female sex interferes with the mechanostat. More and more data support the concept that estrogen via estrogen receptor α (ERα) interacts with mechanical signaling. Damien and colleagues showed that mechanical strain stimulates osteoblast proliferation through ERα [11,12]. Therefore, both estrogen and mechanical loading may stimulate osteoblast proliferation via common pathways. Such action may compensate to some extent for the lower mechanical loading during growth in the female. As a result, females store more bone during puberty in anticipation of future demands of pregnancy and lactation.

III. Regulation of Skeletal Gender Differences by Hormones

A. Animal Models

Overall growth rate also regulates skeletal growth. Therefore, hormones that interact with growth rate also affect skeletal gender differences. Animals offer the opportunity to study the effect of manipulation of hormone action on sexual skeletal dimorphism in detail. Genetic models such as transgenic and natural mutants evaluate hormone action during the entire lifespan, whereas experimental procedures such as castration, sex steroid replacement, and pharmacologic administration of hormone agonist/antagonist or enzyme inhibitors interfering with hormone metabolism evaluate hormone action only during a well-defined experimental period. Conditional knockout (KO) or transgenic experiments may add a new dimension by regulatory time and tissue-selective gene expression, but such experiments have only begun to be introduced in the bone field. The major growth regulatory hormones are growth hormone–insulin-like growth factor-1 (GH-IGF-1) and sex steroids. As discussed later, both sex steroids and GH-IGF-1, however, closely interact not only in the neonatal but also in pubertal and even postpubertal life.

B. Castration with or without Sex Steroid Replacement and Gender Differences

Castration with or without sex steroid replacement clearly demonstrates the interaction of hormones with both growth rate and skeletal gender differences. In aged slowly growing rats, however, both growth rate and related skeletal gender differences are much less affected by castration than in growing rats of both sexes (Table 96-2).

Orchidectomy (orx) of growing male rats decreases growth rate [8,13–16]. As a result, skeletal modeling is also impaired: Periosteal bone formation (outer perimeter) [17–19] and endochondral bone formation (length) [15,20–22] decrease (Table 96-3, Fig. 96-2).

Ovariectomy (ovx) in the female on the other hand (temporarily) increases growth rate [23,24]. Accordingly, skeletal modeling also

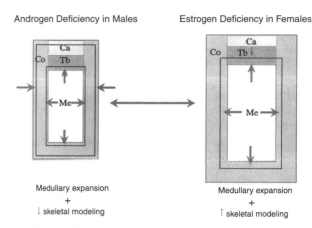

Fig. 96-2 Effects of androgen deficiency versus estrogen deficiency in male and female rats, respectively. Ca, cartilaginous growth plate; Co, cortex; Me, medulla; Tb, trabeculae.

increases periosteal bone formation (outer perimeter) [13] and longitudinal bone formation (length) [25,26] (see Table 96-3, Fig. 96-2).

The end results are opposite cortical phenotypical changes in the castrated female versus male rat. A more female-like cortical bone in the orx male and a more male-like cortical bone in the ovx female.

A similar female-like cortical bone size is observed in androgen-resistant testicular feminized male (Tfm) rats, suggesting that the androgen response via androgen receptor (AR) is involved in the regulation of both growth rate and skeletal gender differences [19,35].

Although longitudinal growth increases in ovx females, chondrocyte differentiation into osteoblasts also decreases. Such mechanism may further contribute to the net loss of trabecular bone in ovx females [13,23,26]. Indeed, in both sexes and in all species, castration accelerates medullary expansion induced by greater endosteal and trabecular resorption (rather than formation) during both fast and slow skeletal growth. Therefore, the sexual dimorphism of response to castration in cortical bone, characterized by high versus low turnover in ovx female and orx male, respectively, is not observed in trabecular bone. Castration of both genders increases trabecular bone turnover [13,17,19, 23,24,26,27,30,33].

Table 96-2

Effects of Castration with or without Sex Steroid Replacement in Aged Male and Female Rats

	Growth Rate	Bone Size	Cortical Bone Area	Trabecular Bone Volume
Males				
Orx	= [30,31]	= [30,31]	↓ [30–32]	↓ [30,33]
Orx + androgen replacement	= [30,32]	= [30]	↑[30,32]	↑ [30,32]
Females				
Ovx	↑ [24]	= [24]	↓ [24]	↓ [24]
Ovx + estrogen replacement	↓ [34]	NA	↑ [34]	↑ [34]

Effects of castration are compared with sham-operated animals, effects of castration plus replacement are compared with castration alone. NA, not available; Orx, orchidectomy; ovx, ovariectomy.

Table 96-3

Effects of Castration with or without Sex Steroid Replacement in Growing Male and Female Rats

	Growth Rate	Bone Size	Cortical Bone Area	Trabecular Bone Volume
Males				
Orx	↓ [8,13–16]	↓[15,20–22]	↓ [17–19]	↓[13,17,19]
Orx + androgen replacement	↑ [28]	= [28]	↑ [18]	↑ [28]
Females				
Ovx	↑ [23]	↑ [25,26]	= [13]	↓[13,23,26]
Ovx + estrogen replacement	↓[25,26,29]	↓[25,26,29]	↓ [18]	↑ [25,26,29]

Effects of castration are compared with sham-operated animals, effects of castration plus replacement are compared with castration alone. Orx, orchidectomy; ovx, ovariectomy.

Both androgens and estrogens restore the opposite cortical phenotypical changes induced by orx in the male and by ovx in the female, respectively [18,30,32]. Estrogens inhibit growth in the female, whereas androgens promote growth in the male. The response of growth rate and cortical bone size to respectively androgens and estrogens may, however, be gender-specific [18]. Androgens may stimulate growth in the orx male but inhibit growth in the ovx female. However, the effect of estrogens may also depend on dose. Low-dose estrogen may stimulate growth, whereas higher dose may be inhibitory in both sexes [36,37]. The cortical response to estrogen however may be to large extent GH-dependent [21]. Zhang *et al* [21] showed that the increase of growth rate does not occur in the GH-deficient female suggesting that estrogens inhibit growth in the female via GH.

The response of trabecular bone does not appear gender-specific in many species, including human. Estrogens and androgens seem to have similar effects on trabecular bone via both ERα/ß and AR [30,38]. Both sex steroids slow down bone resorption and marrow expansion probably via interaction through similar mechanisms in the bone marrow. The bone-sparing effects of sex steroids in the trabecular compartment also are independent of growth and mechanical loading. Conditions of unloading, such as space flight, reduce cancellous bone formation in male gonad-intact rats without affecting cancellous bone resorption [39]. On the contrary, additional bone loss is seen in ovx female rats resulting from an increase in bone resorption above that caused by ovx alone [40]. This may indicate that the cellular mechanism for skeletal adaptation to changes in mechanical use is influenced by gonadal hormones.

C. Growth Hormone–Insulin-like Growth Factor-1 Axis and Sexual Dimorphism

Postnatal growth is primarily regulated by the GH-IGF-1 axis. Exclusion of IGF-1 action either directly [41–43] or indirectly [44,45] via disruption of the GHR (the receptor that translates GH stimulation) dramatically decreases growth rate in both male and female mice. As indicated in Table 96-4, such decrease in growth rate, however, only affects cortical [41,45] but not trabecular bone [45,46], which may be even increased in insulin-like growth factor-1 knockout (IGF-1 KO) mice [41].

A functional GH-IGF-1 axis is also essential for skeletal sexual dimorphism. Both growth hormone receptor knockout (GHRKO) mice and IGF-1 KO mice abolishes not only gender differences in growth rate but also gender differences in skeletal (again only cortical) size.

Therefore, the male cortical phenotype requires a functional and more active GH-IGF-1 axis. The GH-IGF-1 axis is already differentially imprinted in males compared with females neonatally [47]. Such imprinting depends on neonatal androgen secretion. Absence of neonatal androgen secretion in androgen-resistant Tfm rats clearly demonstrates the importance of androgen programming of the GH-IGF-1 system for male growth. Androgen-resistant Tfm rats not only have more female-like GH profiles but also female-like growth rates and bone size [48].

During puberty, a rise in GH-IGF-1 activity occurs in both males and females. After puberty, serum IGF-1 levels tend to be higher in men and male rats compared with females [49,50], but no gender difference is observed in mice [41,51,52].

Table 96-4

Effects of GH-IGF-1 Action in Male and Female Knockout (KO) Mice

	Growth Rate	Serum IGF-1	Bone Size	Cortical Bone Area	Trabecular Bone Volume
GHRKO					
Males	↓[44,46]	↓[44,46]	↓[45]	↓[45,46]	=[45,46]
Females	↓[44,46]	↓[44,46]	↓[46]	↓[45,46]	=[45,46]
IGF-1 KO					
Males	↓[41]	↓[41]	↓[41]	↓[41]	↑[41]
Females	↓[41]	↓[41]	↓[41]	↓[41]	↑[41]

Effects are compared with wild-type male and female mice.
GH-IGF-1, growth hormone–insulin-like growth factor-1; GHRKO, growth hormone receptor knockout; IGF-1, insulin-like growth factor-1; IGF-1 KO, insulin-like growth factor-1 knockout.

Table 96-5

Effects of Estrogen Action in Male Knockout (KO) Mice

	Growth Rate	Serum IGF-1	Bone Size	Cortical Bone Area	Trabecular Bone Volume
ERαKO	↓ [2]/= [58,59]	↓ [2]	↓ [2,58]/= [59]	↓ [2,58,59]	↑ [58,59]/= [2]
ERβKO	= [2,59]	= [2]	= [2,59]	= [2,59]	= [2,59]
ERα/βKO	↓ [2,59]	↓ [2]	↓ [2,59]	↓ [2,59]	= [2]/↑ [59]
ArKO	↓ [53]	NA	↓ [53]	↓ [53,54]	↓ [53,54]

Effects are compared with wild-type male mice.
ArKO, aromatase knockout; ERαKO, estrogen receptor α knockout; ERβKO, estrogen receptor β knockout; IGF-1, insulin-like growth factor-1; NA, not available.

Table 96-6

Effects of Estrogen Action in Male Rats

	Growth Rate	Serum IGF-1	Bone Size	Cortical Bone Area	Trabecular Bone Volume
Inhibition of aromatase	↓ [20]	↓ [20,55,56]	↓ [20,55]	↓ [20,55]	↓ [20,55,56]
ICI 182,780	= [62,63]	– [63]	– [62,63]	– [62,63]	= [62,63]

Effects are compared with control male rats.

IGF-1, insulin-like growth factor-1.

D. Estrogen Action in Males

Models (Tables 96-5 and 96-6) that interfere with estrogen action show that estrogens stimulate not only the GH-IGF-1 axis but also growth rate and bone size during puberty, in females and in males. Estrogen action on growth rate depends on aromatization of androgens into estrogens as shown by models that manipulate the aromatase enzyme (this enzyme converts androgens into estrogens). Knockout of the aromatase enzyme in mice (ArKO) [53,54] and administration of an inhibitor of the aromatase enzyme in rats [20,55,56] tend to decrease growth rate, serum IGF-1, and cortical bone size. Moreover, estrogen action may also be involved in body composition, which may interfere with mechanical strain. Indeed, ArKO mice accumulate more fat [57]; more fat and less muscle may lead to less mechanical loading and, therefore, less bone.

Also, males that lack ERα grow more slowly according to some [2] but not all studies [58,59], whereas ERβKO male mice grow normally [2,59]. Therefore, ERα and not ERβ appears to stimulate growth in males. Such growth stimulatory action of low concentrations of estrogen via ERα seems mediated via the GH-IGF-1 axis. In accordance, the ER antagonist ICI 182,780 that does not cross the blood-brain-barrier and, therefore, does not affect GH-IGF-1, has no effect on growth rate. It seems that androgens promote male periosteal bone growth before via aromatization into estrogens. These estrogens derived from androgens then centrally stimulate GH via ERα.

In conclusion, the higher growth rate and resulting bone size in males may, at least partly, be explained by estrogen and not androgen. In addition, both inhibition or disruption of the aromatase enzyme causes trabecular bone loss in rodents [20,53–56]. In contrast, according to some studies, disruption of either ERβ [2,59] or ERα [2] or both [2] does not induce trabecular bone loss. ERαKO and ERα/βKO mice may even have more trabecular bone [58,59]. Moreover, the trabecular compartment of ERαKO

mice remains responsive to both orx and testosterone replacement [58]. Therefore, according to some [46,60] but not all authors [61], androgens and estrogens may be interchangeable sex steroids. In addition, recent data indicate that the trabecular bone compartment may be "promiscuously" influenced by non-genomic activation of sex steroid hormone receptors by several hormones [60].

E. Direct Effects of Androgens in Males and Sexual Dimorphism

From the previous chapters it is now clear that, at least part of the androgen growth promoting effect is mediated via ERα and the GH-IGF-1 axis. Therefore, the question remains to what extent androgens directly interfere with growth rates independently of ER or IGF-1. The Tfm rat model is confounded, as discussed earlier, by the female type of GH profile and high estrogen levels [35]. Therefore, it is very difficult to extrapolate from this model to what extent the observed female type of bone structure directly depends on AR-mediated androgen action or alternatively is mediated via estrogen and/or GH-IGF-1.

Growth rates and accordingly skeletal modeling decrease in GH-deficient rats compared with GH-wild types following castration [21], suggesting that androgens stimulate growth rate and skeletal modeling also independently from GH. Unfortunately, androgen replacement was not evaluated in this model. Whether androgens must be aromatized into estrogen and stimulate the ERα or directly stimulate the AR to promote pubertal growth independently of the IGF-1 axis remains unknown.

Male rodents treated with an antiandrogen (Casodex) or a 5-α-reductase inhibitor (Finasteride) seem to grow normally and do not have a bone phenotype [14,64]. Human data, however, suggest that DHT stimulates growth in adolescents suffering from delayed puberty without corresponding increase in serum IGF-1 [65].

Table 96-7

Effects of Androgen Action in Male Rats and Mice

	Growth Rate	Serum IGF-1	Bone Size	Cortical Bone Area	Trabecular Bone Volume
Rat					
Tfm	↓ [19,35]	↓ [19,35]	↓ [19,35]	↓ [19,35]	= [19,35]
5-α-reductase inhibitor	= [14]	NA	= [14]	= [14]	= [14]
Mouse					
Antiandrogen	= [64]	NA	NA	= [64]	= [64]

Effects are compared with wild-types or controls, respectively.

IGF-1, insulin-like growth factor-1; NA, not available; Tfm, testicular feminized male.

Androgens may however promote skeletal growth indirectly via their action on body composition independently of changes in growth rate. Androgen secretion changes male body composition during puberty in favor of more muscle and less fat [66]. It is not known to what extent such extra muscle contributes to extra male skeletal modeling. However, extra mechanical loading in rats induced by exercise is able to prevent to some extent skeletal effects induced by orx [67]. In this experiment the orx-induced muscle loss was also significantly reduced by extra mechanical loading. Therefore, it is tempting to speculate that anabolic properties of androgens interact with skeletal homeostasis.

F. Estrogen Action in the Female

As discussed earlier, ovx and estrogen replacement increases and decreases, respectively, bone size in the female. Such growth inhibitory action of estrogen is not observed in ovx GH-deficient female rats and is, therefore, GH-dependent [21]. Accordingly, the antiestrogen ICI 182,780 that does not cross the blood-brain-barrier (and therefore does not inhibit GH) does not affect growth rate [68–70] nor bone size in female rats [68,69]. However, ICI 182,780 does induce trabecular bone loss in females [68,69], indicating again that estrogen action on trabecular bone may occur independent of growth rate and GH.

The role of the ERα and ERβ has recently also been studied extensively in transgenic models with KO of one or both ERs. The effects of disruption of these receptors on the female skeleton resulted in puzzling and often contradictory phenotypes that are summarized as follows (Table 96-8):

- Growth rate is not affected by the disruption of ERα in some [59] but not all studies [52,71].
- Percentage fat increases in ERαKO mice [52].
- Opposing effects of ERα versus ERβ on longitudinal growth rate of appendicular but not axial skeleton were reported with decreased [52,71] and increased [52] femur length, respectively, according to one study, whereas in another study neither receptor affected skeletal growth [51,59].

The decrease of femoral length reported in the former study was related to lower GH-IGF-1 secretion [52,71].
- Trabecular bone mass is not decreased by either ERα or ERβ disruption and may be even increased [51,52,59] in contrast with ovx models. The double KO, however, does have, in analogy with ovx, less trabecular bone [59]. In contrast with ovx, bone turnover (and especially formation) is decreased and not increased. Ovx-induced bone loss in ERα/ß KO mice is prevented by a high dose of estradiol. This suggests that estradiol may act via a non-ER mediated mechanism [72].
- Cortical bone size, again in contrast with ovx, can be increased [52] in both ERαKO and the double KO, but others report a decrease in ERαKO mice [59].

Several explanations are given for the unexpected bone phenotypes of these transgenic mice: These include confounding compensatory increases of estrogen and/or androgen that may to some extent rescue the phenotype and/or incomplete disruption of the receptor that in turn may explain incomplete penetration of the phenotype. Recently, in addition to the 66-kDa ERα isoform, an alternative 46-kDa ERα isoform was described [73]. The expression of two ERα protein isoforms may account, in part, for the differential action of estrogens. This may indicate that the present KO models are not selective and should, therefore, be reconsidered to take account of the presence of these two ERα protein isoforms in bone.

G. Androgen Action in Female

Antiandrogens decrease the longitudinal growth rate of the female bone according to some [75] but not all studies [76,77]. Cancellous and periosteal bone formation rate is also significantly reduced in intact female rats treated with the antiandrogen Casodex [75]. Lea et al [75], however, found no reduction in cancellous bone volume or reduced trabecular thickness in antiandrogen-treated rats, but this was only evaluated during a rather short experimental period. The androgen androstenedione

Table 96-8

Effects of Estrogen Action in Female Mice

	Growth Rate	Serum IGF-1	Bone Size	Cortical Bone Area	Trabecular Bone Volume
ERαKO	= [59]/↑ [52,71]	↓ [52,71]	↓ [52,71]/= [59]	↑ [52]/↓ [59]	↑ [52,59]
ERβKO	= [51,52,59,71]	= [51]/↑ [52]	↑ [52]/= [51,59]	= [59]/↑ [51,52,74]	↑ [51,52,59]
ERα/βKO	= [59]/↑ [52]	↓ [52]	↓ [52]/= [59]	↑ [52]/↓ [59]	↓ [59]
ICI 182,780	= [68–70]	NA	= [68,69]	= [68]	↓ [68,69]
ArKO	= [54]	NA	= [53]	↓ [53,54]	↓ [53,54]

Effects are compared with wild-type female mice.
ArKO, aromatase knockout; ERαKO, estrogen receptor α knockout; ERβKO, estrogen receptor β knockout; IGF-1, insulin-like growth factor-1; NA, not available.

Table 96-9

Effects of Estrogen Action in Female Rats

	Growth Rate	Serum IGF-1	Bone Size	Cortical Bone Area	Trabecular Bone Volume
ICI 182,780	= [68–70]	NA	= [68,69]	= [68]	↓ [68,69]

Effects are compared with control female rats.
IGF-1, insulin-like growth factor-1; NA, not available.

Table 96-10
Androgen Action in Female Rats

	Growth Rate	Serum IGF-1	Bone Size	Cortical Bone Area	Trabecular Bone Volume
Antiandrogen (Casodex/ flutamide)	↓ [75]/= [76,77]	NA	NA	= [75]	= [75]/↓ [76,77]
Ovx + androstenedione	↓ [78]	NA	NA	NA	↑ [78]
Ovx + androstenedione + aromatase inhibitor	= [78]	NA	NA	NA	↑ [78]
Ovx + androstenedione + antiandrogen	↓ [78]	NA	NA	NA	= [78]

Antiandrogen action is compared with wild-type female rats; androstenedione, androstenedione plus aromatase inhibitor, androstenedione plus antiandrogen action are compared with ovx female rats.

IGF-1, insulin-like growth factor-1; NA, not available; Ovx, ovariectomy.

has bone-sparing effects in ovx female rats [78]. Cancellous bone loss is reduced in ovx rats treated with androstenedione. This protective effect of androstenedione on cancellous bone is completely prevented by antiandrogen treatment but not by an aromatase-inhibitor, indicating that androstenedione action on bone is mediated via the AR and not the ER.

II. Sex Steroids and Epiphyseal Closure

Estrogens and androgens promote growth closure at the end of puberty. However, androgens (for reviews see ref. [79]) must be aromatized in estrogens and stimulate ERα in both men and women to promote epiphyseal fusion. Estrogen action on growth plate does not appear species-specific because high-dose estrogens also close growth plates in both sexes of rats (which normally close spontaneously at very advanced age).

IV. Summary and Conclusion

Gender-based skeletal differences are mainly differences in cortical bone size that are generated during a period of active skeletal modeling. Gender-based differences depend on differences in growth rate (length and width). Males, therefore, accumulate more (cortical) bone because of higher body weight and (relative to fat) muscle gain. Gender differences do not exist in animals that have severely impaired growth rates resulting from disruption of the GH-IGF-1 axis, indicating that this axis contributes to or mediates the gender differences. Sex steroids interact with the GH-IGF-1 axis both during the neonatal period and after puberty. The extent to which sex steroids affect gender-based differences independently of GH is not well defined. Castration and sex steroid replacement have opposite effects on growth rate and cortical bone size in males and females but similar effects on trabecular bone (which appears as a non–gender-related or less gender-related bone compartment).

Estrogen appears to interact via ERα with the GH-IGF-1 axis and affects growth rate and size in males and is responsible for epiphyseal closure in both genders. The role of the ERs in either males or females based on transgenic mice data remains unsettled at present mainly because inconsistency of the bone phenotypes in the female. However, estrogen may be responsible for a lower mechanical threshold (presumably via ERα) and accumulation of more bone in the female during puberty.

V. Suggestions for Further Investigations

Future studies with more selective and bone-specific KO of steroid or IGF-1 receptors are needed to better define the role of steroid action and its interaction with the GH-IGF-1 axis with respect to gender-based skeletal differences.

Therefore, relevant future research topics with respect to the regulation of gender-based skeletal differences include the following:

- The interaction of mechanical stimuli with sex steroids
- The interaction of sex steroids with body composition
- The investigation of the specific role of sex steroids versus the GH-IGF-1 axis
- The role of organ-specific sex steroid receptors

Acknowledgements

This study was supported by F.W.O. grant G.0221.99 and O.T. grant OT/01/39 (A6401). Dr. D. Vanderschueren is a Senior Clinical Investigator of the Fund for Scientific Research-Flanders, Belgium (F.W.O.-Vlaanderen).

References

1. Seeman E. (2001). Clinical review 137: Sexual dimorphism in skeletal size, density, and strength. *J Clin Endocrinol Metab*. 86:4576–4584.
2. Vidal O, Lindberg MK, Hollberg K et al. (2000). Estrogen receptor specificity in the regulation of skeletal growth and maturation in male mice. *Proc Natl Acad Sci U S A*. 97:5474–5479.
3. Frost HM. (1987). Bone "mass" and the "mechanostat": A proposal. *Anat Rec*. 219:1–9.
4. Frost HM. (1983). A determinant of bone architecture. The minimum effective strain. *Clin Orthop*. 175:286–292.
5. Sheng MH, Baylink DJ, Beamer WG et al. (1999). Histomorphometric studies show that bone formation and bone mineral apposition rates are greater in C3H/HeJ (high-density) than C57BL/6J (low-density) mice during growth. *Bone*. 25:421–429.
6. Sheng MH, Baylink DJ, Beamer WG et al. (2002). Regulation of bone volume is different in the metaphyses of the femur and vertebra of C3H/HeJ and C57BL/6J mice. *Bone*. 30:486–491.
7. Mosley JR, Lanyon LE. (2002). Growth rate rather than gender determines the size of the adaptive response of the growing skeleton to mechanical strain. *Bone*. 30:314–319.
8. Saville PD. (1969). Changes in skeletal mass and fragility with castration in the rat; a model of osteoporosis. *J Am Geriatr Soc*. 17:155–166.
9. Zanchetta JR, Plotkin H, Alvarez Filgueira ML. (1995). Bone mass in children: Normative values for the 2-20-year-old population. *Bone*. 16:393S–399S.

10. Schiessl H, Frost HM, Jee WS. (1998). Estrogen and bone-muscle strength and mass relationships. *Bone.* 22:1–6.

11. Damien E, Price JS, Lanyon LE. (1998). The estrogen receptor's involvement in osteoblasts' adaptive response to mechanical strain. *J Bone Miner Res.* 13:1275–1282.

12. Damien E, Price JS, Lanyon LE. (2000). Mechanical strain stimulates osteoblast proliferation through the estrogen receptor in males as well as females. *J Bone Miner Res.* 15:2169–2177.

13. Turner RT, Hannon KS, Demers LM *et al.* (1989). Differential effects of gonadal function on bone histomorphometry in male and female rats. *J Bone Miner Res.* 4:557–563.

14. Rosen HN, Tollin S, Balena R *et al.* (1995). Bone density is normal in male rats treated with finasteride. *Endocrinology.* 136:1381–1387.

15. Schoutens A, Verhas M, L'hermite-Baleriaux M *et al.* (1984). Growth and bone haemodynamic responses to castration in male rats. Reversibility by testosterone. *Acta Endocrinol (Copenh).* 107:428–432.

16. Wink CS, Felts WJ. (1980). Effects of castration on the bone structure of male rats: A model of osteoporosis. *Calcif Tissue Int.* 32:77–82.

17. Gunness M, Orwoll E. (1995). Early induction of alterations in cancellous and cortical bone histology after orchiectomy in mature rats. *J Bone Miner Res.* 10:1735–1744.

18. Turner RT, Wakley GK, Hannon KS. (1990). Differential effects of androgens on cortical bone histomorphometry in gonadectomized male and female rats. *J Orthop Res.* 8:612–617.

19. Vanderschueren D, Van Herck E, Geusens P *et al.* (1994). Androgen resistance and deficiency have different effects on the growing skeleton of the rat. *Calcif Tissue Int.* 55:198–203.

20. Vanderschueren D, Van Herck E, Nijs J *et al.* (1997). Aromatase inhibition impairs skeletal modeling and decreases bone mineral density in growing male rats. *Endocrinology.* 138:2301–2307.

21. Zhang XZ, Kalu DN, Erbas B *et al.* (1999). The effects of gonadectomy on bone size, mass, and volumetric density in growing rats are gender-, site-, and growth hormone-specific. *J Bone Miner Res.* 14:802–809.

22. Gaumet-Meunier N, Coxam V, Robins S *et al.* (2000). Gonadal steroids and bone metabolism in young castrated male rats. *Calcif Tissue Int.* 66:470–475.

23. Wronski TJ, Dann LM, Horner SL. (1989). Time course of vertebral osteopenia in ovariectomized rats. *Bone.* 10:295–301.

24. Kalu DN, Liu CC, Hardin RR, Hollis BW. (1989). The aged rat model of ovarian hormone deficiency bone loss. *Endocrinology.* 124:7–16.

25. Wronski TJ, Dann LM, Scott KS, Crooke LR. (1989). Endocrine and pharmacological suppressors of bone turnover protect against osteopenia in ovariectomized rats. *Endocrinology.* 125:810–816.

26. Wronski TJ, Lowry PL, Walsh CC, Ignaszewski LA. (1985). Skeletal alterations in ovariectomized rats. *Calcif Tissue Int.* 37:324–328.

27. Wronski TJ, Dann LM, Scott KS, Crooke LR. (1989). Endocrine and pharmacological suppressors of bone turnover protect against osteopenia in ovariectomized rats. *Endocrinology.* 125:810–816.

28. Wakley GK, Schutte HD Jr, Hannon KS, Turner RT. (1991). Androgen treatment prevents loss of cancellous bone in the orchidectomized rat. *J Bone Miner Res.* 6:325–330.

29. Wronski TJ, Cintron M, Doherty AL, Dann LM. (1988). Estrogen treatment prevents osteopenia and depresses bone turnover in ovariectomized rats. *Endocrinology.* 123:681–686.

30. Vanderschueren D, Van Herck E, Suiker AM *et al.* (1992). Bone and mineral metabolism in aged male rats: Short and long term effects of androgen deficiency. *Endocrinology.* 130:2906–2916.

31. Verhas M, Schoutens A, L'hermite-Baleriaux M *et al.* (1986). The effect of orchidectomy on bone metabolism in aging rats. *Calcif Tissue Int.* 39:74–77.

32. Vanderschueren D, Van Herck E, Schot P *et al.* (1993). The aged male rat as a model for human osteoporosis: Evaluation by nondestructive measurements and biomechanical testing. *Calcif Tissue Int.* 53:342–347.

33. Erben RG, Eberle J, Stahr K, Goldberg M. (2000). Androgen deficiency induces high turnover osteopenia in aged male rats: A sequential histomorphometric study. *J Bone Miner Res.* 15:1085–1098.

34. Verhaeghe J, van Bree R, Van Herck E *et al.* (1996). Effects of recombinant human growth hormone and insulin-like growth factor-I, with or without 17 beta-estradiol, on bone and mineral homeostasis of aged ovariectomized rats. *J Bone Miner Res.* 11:1723–1735.

35. Vanderschueren D, Van Herck E, Suiker AM *et al.* (1993). Bone and mineral metabolism in the androgen-resistant (testicular feminized) male rat. *J Bone Miner Res.* 8:801–809.

36. Lindberg MK, Moverare S, Skrtic S *et al.* (2002). Two different pathways for the maintenance of trabecular bone in adult male mice. *J Bone Miner Res.* 17:555–562.

37. Cutler GB Jr. (1997). The role of estrogen in bone growth and maturation during childhood and adolescence. *J Steroid Biochem Mol Biol.* 61:141–44.

38. Turner RT, Lifrak ET, Beckner M *et al.* (1990). Dehydroepiandrosterone reduces cancellous bone osteopenia in ovariectomized rats. *Am J Physiol.* 258:E673–677.

39. Turner RT, Evans GL, Wakley GK. (1995). Spaceflight results in depressed cancellous bone formation in rat humeri. *Aviat Space Environ Med.* 66:770–774.

40. Cavolina JM, Evans GL, Harris SA *et al.* (1997). The effects of orbital spaceflight on bone histomorphometry and messenger ribonucleic acid levels for bone matrix proteins and skeletal signaling peptides in ovariectomized growing rats. *Endocrinology.* 138:1567–1576.

41. Bikle D, Majumdar S, Laib A *et al.* (2001). The skeletal structure of insulin-like growth factor I-deficient mice. *J Bone Miner Res.* 16:2320–2329.

42. Liu JP, Baker J, Perkins AS *et al.* (1993). Mice carrying null mutations of the genes encoding insulin-like growth factor I (Igf-1) and type 1 IGF receptor (Igf1r). *Cell.* 75:59–72.

43. Powell-Braxton L, Hollingshead P, Warburton C *et al.* (1993). IGF-I is required for normal embryonic growth in mice. *Genes Dev.* 7:2609–2617.

44. Zhou Y, Xu BC, Maheshwari HG *et al.* (1997). A mammalian model for Laron syndrome produced by targeted disruption of the mouse growth hormone receptor/binding protein gene (the Laron mouse). *Proc Natl Acad Sci U S A.* 94:13215–13220.

45. Sjogren K, Bohlooly YM, Olsson B *et al.* (2000). Disproportional skeletal growth and markedly decreased bone mineral content in growth hormone receptor -/- mice. *Biochem Biophys Res Commun.* 267:603–608.

46. Sims NA, Clement-Lacroix P, Da Ponte F *et al.* (2000). Bone homeostasis in growth hormone receptor-null mice is restored by IGF-I but independent of Stat5. *J Clin Invest.* 106:1095–1103.

47. Jansson JO, Ekberg S, Isaksson OG, Eden S. (1984). Influence of gonadal steroids on age- and sex-related secretory patterns of growth hormone in the rat. *Endocrinology.* 114:1287–1294.

48. Jansson JO, Eden S, Isaksson O. (1985). Sexual dimorphism in the control of growth hormone secretion. *Endocr Rev.* 6:128–150.

49. Bouillon R, Bex M, Van Herck E *et al.* (1995). Influence of age, sex, and insulin on osteoblast function: Osteoblast dysfunction in diabetes mellitus. *J Clin Endocrinol Metab.* 80:1194–1202.

50. Handelsman DJ, Spaliviero JA, Scott CD, Baxter RC. (1987). Hormonal regulation of the peripubertal surge of insulin-like growth factor-I in the rat. *Endocrinology.* 120:491–496.

51. Windahl SH, Hollberg K, Vidal O *et al.* (2001). Female estrogen receptor beta-/- mice are partially protected against age-related trabecular bone loss. *J Bone Miner Res.* 16:1388–1398.

52. Lindberg MK, Alatalo SL, Halleen JM *et al.* (2001). Estrogen receptor specificity in the regulation of the skeleton in female mice. *J Endocrinol.* 171:229–236.

53. Oz OK, Zerwekh JE, Fisher C *et al.* (2000). Bone has a sexually dimorphic response to aromatase deficiency. *J Bone Miner Res.* 15:507–514.

54. Miyaura C, Toda K, Inada M *et al.* (2001). Sex- and age-related response to aromatase deficiency in bone. *Biochem Biophys Res Commun.* 280:1062–1068.

55. Vanderschueren D, Van Herck E, De Coster R, Bouillon R. (1996). Aromatization of androgens is important for skeletal maintenance of aged male rats. *Calcif Tissue Int.* 59:179–183.

56. Vanderschueren D, Boonen S, Ederveen AG *et al.* (2000). Skeletal effects of estrogen deficiency as induced by an aromatase inhibitor in an aged male rat model. *Bone.* 27:611–617.

57. Jones MEE, Thorburn AW, Britt KL *et al.* (2000). Aromatase-deficient (ArKO) mice have a phenotype of increased adiposity. *Proc Natl Acad Sci U S A.* 97:12735–12740.

58. Vandenput L, Ederveen AG, Erben RG *et al.* (2001). Testosterone prevents orchidectomy-induced bone loss in estrogen receptor-alpha knockout mice. *Biochem Biophys Res Commun.* 285:70–76.

59. Sims NA, Dupont S, Krust A *et al.* (2002). Deletion of estrogen receptors reveals a regulatory role for estrogen receptors-beta in bone remodeling in females but not in males. *Bone.* 30:18–25.

60. Kousteni S, Bellido T, Plotkin LI *et al.* (2001). Nongenotropic, sex-nonspecific signaling through the estrogen or androgen receptors: Dissociation from transcriptional activity. *Cell.* 104:719–730.

61. Bilezikian JP. (2002) Sex steroids, mice, and men: When androgens and estrogens get very close to each other. *J Bone Miner Res.* 17:563–566.

62. Turner RT, Evans GL, Dobnig H. (2000). The high-affinity estrogen receptor antagonist ICI 182,780 has no effect on bone growth in young male rats. *Calcif Tissue Int.* 66:461–464.

63. Vandenput L, Swinnen JV, Van Herck E *et al.* (2002). The estrogen receptor ligand ICI 182,780 does not impair the bone-sparing effects of testosterone in the young orchidectomized rat model. *Calcif Tissue Int.* 70:170–175.

64. Broulik PD, Starka L. (1997). Effect of antiandrogens Casodex and epitestosterone on bone composition in mice. *Bone.* 20:473–475.

65. Keenan BS, Richards GE, Ponder SW *et al.* (1993). Androgen-stimulated pubertal growth: The effects of testosterone and dihydrotestosterone on growth hormone and insulin-like growth factor-I in the treatment of short stature and delayed puberty. *J Clin Endocrinol Metab* 76:996–1001.

66. Kaplowitz HJ, Wild KA, Mueller WH *et al.* (1988). Serial and parent-child changes in components of body fat distribution and fatness in children from the London Longitudinal Growth Study, ages two to eighteen years. *Hum Biol.* 60:739–758.

67. Yao W, Jee WS, Chen J *et al.* (2000). Making rats rise to erect bipedal stance for feeding partially prevented orchidectomy-induced bone loss and added bone to intact rats. *J Bone Miner Res.* 15:1158–1168.

68. Gallagher A, Chambers TJ, Tobias JH. (1993). The estrogen antagonist ICI 182,780 reduces cancellous bone volume in female rats. *Endocrinology.* 133:2787–2791.

69. Sibonga JD, Dobnig H, Harden RM, Turner RT. (1998). Effect of the high-affinity estrogen receptor ligand ICI 182,780 on the rat tibia. *Endocrinology.* 139:3736–3742.

70. Lea CK, Flanagan AM. (1999). Ovarian androgens protect against bone loss in rats made oestrogen deficient by treatment with ICI 182,780. *J Endocrinol.* 160:111–117.

71. Vidal O, Lindberg M, Savendahl L *et al.* (1999). Disproportional body growth in female estrogen receptor-alpha-inactivated mice. *Biochem Biophys Res Commun.* 265:569–571.

72. Gentile MA, Zhang H, Harada S *et al.* (2001). Bone response to estrogen replacement in ovx double estrogen receptor-(alpha and beta) knockout mice. *J Bone Miner Res.* 16:S146.

73. Denger S, Reid G, Kos M *et al.* (2001). ERalpha gene expression in human primary osteoblasts: Evidence for the expression of two receptor proteins. *Mol Endocrinol.* 15:2064–2077.

74. Windahl SH, Vidal O, Andersson G *et al.* (1999). Increased cortical bone mineral content but unchanged trabecular bone mineral density in female ERbeta(-/-) mice. *J Clin Invest.* 104:895–901.

75. Lea C, Kendall N, Flanagan AM. (1996). Casodex (a nonsteroidal antiandrogen) reduces cancellous, endosteal, and periosteal bone formation in estrogen-replete female rats. *Calcif Tissue Int.* 58:268–272.

76. Goulding A, Gold E. (1993). Flutamide-mediated androgen blockade evokes osteopenia in the female rat. *J Bone Miner Res.* 8:763–769.

77. Gallagher A, Chambers TJ, Tobias JH. (1996). Androgens contribute to the stimulation of cancellous bone formation by ovarian hormones in female rats. *Am J Physiol.* 270:E407–E412.

78. Lea CK, Flanagan AM. (1998). Physiological plasma levels of androgens reduce bone loss in the ovariectomized rat. *Am J Physiol.* 274:E328–E335.

79. Grumbach MM, Auchus RJ. (1999). Estrogen: Consequences and implications of human mutations in synthesis and action. *J Clin Endocrinol Metab.* 84:4677–4694.

97

Epidemiology of Osteoporosis and Fracture in Men and Women

ANNE C. LOOKER, PhD

Division of Health Examination Statistics, National Center for Health Statistics, Centers for Disease
Control and Prevention, Hyattsville, MD

I. Introduction

Osteoporosis is a skeletal disorder defined by loss of bone mass and strength with a concomitant increased fracture risk [1]. Osteoporosis is not a single disease with a single cause [2]. In some instances it arises secondarily as a consequence of other conditions or treatments, such as hypogonadism or glucocorticoid use. However, osteoporosis is often primary in nature. Possible mechanisms underlying primary osteoporosis include failure to adapt to mechanical loading; genetic defects; deficiencies of estrogen, calcium, and vitamin D; and alterations in various systemic or cellular factors [2].

Until recently, osteoporosis was considered to be a disease found almost exclusively in white women, but it is now recognized that men and nonwhite women are affected as well. The traditional view that osteoporotic fractures occur primarily at the hip, wrist, and spine has also been revised to acknowledge that almost all fractures in older persons are osteoporotic [3].

Fractures occur when the bone has insufficient strength to withstand the mechanical forces it encounters. Bone strength depends on the amount of bone material and its quality, which is determined by architecture, turnover, damage accumulation, and mineralization [1]. At present, only the amount of bone material, measured as bone mineral density (BMD), can be easily determined in most clinical settings. Bone mineral density levels are higher in men than in women at all ages; the magnitude varies with age, being greater among young adults than in the elderly,

but on average the difference is roughly 10% [4]. Bone mineral density has been shown to predict fracture risk in several prospective studies, with risk generally doubling for each standard deviation decline in BMD [5]. The ability of BMD to predict hip fracture is approximately equal to that of blood pressure to predict stroke and superior to that of serum cholesterol to predict coronary heart disease [6].

In 1994, an expert panel convened by the World Health Organization (WHO) developed operational definitions of osteoporosis and low bone density for white women based on BMD alone [6]. These definitions, which are shown in Table 97-1, represented an important advance for the study of the epidemiology of this disease because the prevalence of the population at risk of fracture before its occurrence can be assessed. These definitions are also often used as diagnostic criteria in clinical practice.

However, the WHO definitions also suffer from some important limitations. For example, it is not clear how to apply these definitions to men, nonwhite women, or children [1]. In addition, discrepancies in the magnitude of the population prevalence or in diagnosis of an individual patient can occur when different skeletal sites are assessed or different types of densitometry techniques are used [7,8]. There is currently considerable discussion underway to develop an optimal approach to overcome these limitations [7,8]. Definitions based on absolute fracture risk could circumvent many of the problems, and efforts are currently underway to develop them. However, practical difficulties in obtaining accurate estimates of absolute

Table 97-1
WHO Diagnostic Criteria for Osteoporosis and Low Bone Density [6]

Diagnostic Category	Hip BMD Value
Normal	No more than 1 SD below the young adult female reference mean (T-score* of −1 or more positive)
Low bone mass (Osteopenia)	More than 1 SD below reference mean but less than 2.5 SD below this value (T-score between −1 and −2.4)
Osteoporosis	2.5 SD or more below reference mean (T score of −2.5 or more negative)
Severe osteoporosis (Established osteoporosis)	BMD 2.5 SD or more below reference mean plus one or more fragility fractures

*T-score = number of SDs above or below reference group mean.
BMD, bone mineral density; SD, standard deviation.

fracture risk in different groups and in achieving consensus on a clinically significant level of risk exist, so it is unclear how soon WHO definitions might be replaced by absolute fracture risk definitions [8]. In the meantime, the WHO definitions continue to be widely used.

II. Burden of Osteoporosis and Fracture

A. Prevalence of Osteoporosis

According to the third National Health and Nutrition Examination Survey (NHANES III), approximately 6 million (18%) noninstitutionalized women ages 50 years and older in the United States had osteoporosis of the femoral neck in the early 1990s, and estimates for men ranged from 1 to 2 million (4 to 6%) [9]. Osteopenia, the milder reduction in BMD, was much more common: approximately 17 million (50%) older women in the United States and 9 to 13 million (33 to 47%) older men in the United States had reduced bone mass in the femur neck [9]. Estimates of both conditions tend to increase with age, as illustrated in Figure 97-1.

It is important to note that these estimates, although substantial, likely do not completely capture the full magnitude of the osteoporosis burden. For example, they do not include institutionalized individuals, among whom the prevalence of osteoporosis is high [10]. In addition, the number of individuals has likely increased since the early 1990s because of the growing number of older persons in the U.S population. For example, recent estimates from the National Osteoporosis Foundation suggest that the number with osteoporosis increased to 8 million women and 2.3 million men in 2002 and that these values will reach 10 million and 3 million for women and men, respectively, by 2020 [11]. Finally, these estimates are based on a single skeletal site, but prevalence estimates based on more than one skeletal site are also likely to be higher. For example, the prevalence of osteoporosis in older women in Rochester Minnesota at the hip, wrist, or lumbar spine was ~16 to 17% when these sites were considered separately, but it rose to 30% when those with osteoporosis at any one of the three were considered [12].

B. Osteoporotic Fractures

Osteoporotic fractures are a common occurrence among older individuals. At age 50 years, the risk of experiencing any fracture at some point before death (e.g., the lifetime risk) has been estimated to be as high as 75% for white women [13]. Generally osteoporotic fractures show a steep increase in incidence with age and incidence also tends to be higher in women than in men. For example, the lifetime risk of hip, spine, or forearm fracture among white women aged 50 years and older is 40%, compared with 13% for white men [12]. Risk varies by race and ethnicity as well, with nonwhites generally having lower rates of fractures at most skeletal sites [14–16]. Although these patterns hold true in general, fractures at different skeletal sites follow them to a different degree, as summarized in the following sections.

1. Hip Fracture

Hip fracture occurrence varies noticeably by sex. According to the National Hospital Discharge Survey, there were 380,000 discharges for fracture of the femur neck in the United States in 1999 [17]. Of these 73% occurred in women and 27% occurred in men. Patterns of hip fracture occurrence by age differ somewhat between the sexes, as illustrated in Figure 97-2. Specifically, hip fracture rates in women begin to increase at approximately age 50, whereas in men, the increase begins roughly 10 years later. Rates in both sexes increase noticeably after age 70. By age 85 years, the annual incidence of hip fracture is approximately 3% in white women and 1.9% in white men [18]. Interestingly, the female-to-male hip fracture ratio tends to vary by race and ethnicity, with rates being more similar between genders in blacks than in whites [19].

The lifetime risk of a hip fracture for a 50 year-old white woman in the United States has been estimated to be 15 to 18%, whereas for a white man of that age, it is estimated to be 5% [8,20]. The lifetime risk of hip fracture in women exceeds the lifetime risk of breast cancer (~10%) and approaches that of stroke (~20%) [21]. Lifetime hip fracture risk remains relatively constant with age. This is because it couples risk of fracture, which increases with age, with length of remaining lifespan, which decreases with age [20]. Thus, an 80-year-old white woman with an expected remaining life expectancy of 9 years still has roughly a 15% risk of suffering a hip fracture before death.

2. Vertebral Fracture

Vertebral fractures are more common than hip fracture, but their epidemiology is less well established, in part because roughly 70% are asymptomatic [22]. In addition, no universally accepted definition of vertebral fracture currently exists [23]. Prevalence estimates of vertebral fracture can differ by a factor of three depending on the definition used [24]. When based on radiographic evaluation of morphometry (as opposed to clinically evident fracture), an estimated 20 to 25% of older women suffer from vertebral fractures [25].

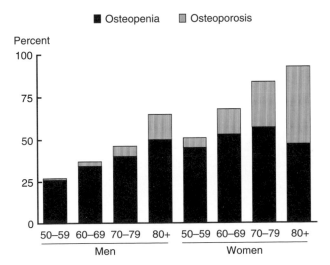

Fig. 97-1 Prevalence of osteoporosis and low bone density (osteopenia) at the femur neck by age and gender in noninstitutionalized U.S. adults from NHANES III. (From CDC/NCHS, third National Health and Nutrition Examination Survey, 1988–1994.)

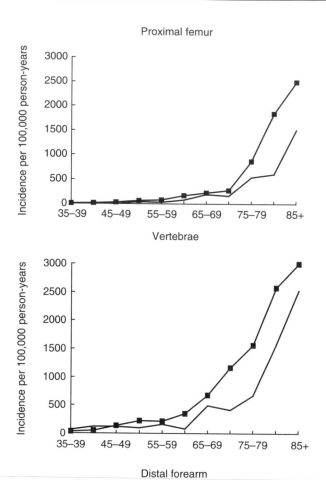

Proximal femur

Vertebrae

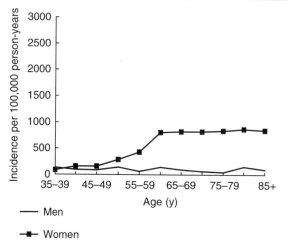

Distal forearm

—— Men

—■— Women

Fig. 97-2 Incidence of fractures of the proximal femur, vertebrae, and distal forearm by sex among residents of Olmsted County, Minnesota in 1989 to 1991. (Adapted from Melton LJ III, Crowson CS, O'Fallon WM. [1999]. Fracture incidence in Olmsted County, Minnesota: Comparisons of urban with rural rates and changes in urban rates over time. *Osteoporos Int.* 9:29–37.)

The incidence of radiographically evident vertebral fracture rises with age in both men and women (see Fig. 97-2). The extent to which vertebral fracture rates differ by gender is somewhat unresolved. Some studies have suggested a much higher

prevalence in women than men, whereas others report more similar rates by gender overall [22,25–27]. More recent data suggest that gender differences may depend on age: rates may be similar, or even greater, in middle-aged men than women, whereas after age 60 years, rates in women are two to three times higher [1,26,28]. The gender similarity at younger ages has been attributed to the likelihood that men experience more sports- and work-related trauma than women [26]. Lifetime risk of vertebral fracture at age 50 years is 16% in white women but only 5% in white men [25].

3. Wrist Fracture and Other Fractures

Fractures of the distal radius, or Colles' fractures, are also considered to be classic osteoporotic fractures, but their epidemiology differs somewhat from fractures at the hip or spine. In specific, these fractures show the classic pattern of being more common in women than men but do not show the same exponential increase with age [29]. As illustrated in Figure 97-2, rates increase in women between 40 to 65 years of age and then stabilize. In contrast, among men rates are constant across the adult lifespan. Lifetime risk of wrist fracture has been estimated to be 15% for white women at age 50, compared with 2% for white men at the same age [20].

Less is known about the epidemiology of osteoporotic fractures at skeletal sites other than the hip, spine, and wrist. Among the elderly, the highest incidence of peripheral fractures occurs at the most proximal and most distal ends of the limbs [14]. In specific, proximal humerus and distal forearm fractures are most common in the upper limb, whereas hip and ankle fractures are most common in the lower limb. Patterns of upper and lower limb fracture by age are complex. Fractures at the most proximal sites on both the upper and lower limb display the classic osteoporotic pattern of large increases with age. However, these patterns are weaker at sites farther down the limbs, especially in the lower limb. Ankle fracture, in particular, does not appear to be strongly associated with osteoporosis [3].

4. Morbidity, Mortality, and Cost of Osteoporotic Fractures

Hip fractures result in significant morbidity. For example, of those living independently before the fracture, approximately 50% require long-term care or need assistance with daily living a year after the fracture [23]. Likewise, of those who could walk before the fracture, approximately half cannot walk without assistance afterwards [23]. Although not as debilitating as hip fracture, vertebral fractures also result in increased morbidity, including hospitalization [30], back pain, bed rest and associated limitations in activity, and other functional limitations [31]. The height loss and kyphosis associated with vertebral fractures may affect self-esteem, mood, and body image [23,32]. Some studies suggest that vertebral deformities result in greater morbidity in men than women [33,34]; the reason for this difference is not known. Wrist fractures do not carry a high risk of disability, although some activities, such as meal preparation, can be affected [35].

Of greater concern than morbidity is the increased mortality observed after various osteoporotic fractures. For example, hip fractures are associated with a 12 to 35% increase in mortality [36], most of which occurs within the first year following the fracture, although risk can remain elevated for up to 5 years [37]. Mortality following hip fracture is higher in men than in women [38–40]. Some studies have attributed the excess mortality associated with hip fractures almost entirely to the presence of co-morbid conditions [41,42], whereas others have found evidence for a direct effect of hip fracture [37,40], which may be greater in men than in women [40].

Accumulating evidence indicates mortality increases after fractures at other skeletal sites as well. For example, mortality rates are modestly increased among those with vertebral fractures and radiographic vertebral deformities [30,39,43,44]. Mortality after vertebral fracture is higher in men than in women [39]. The pathophysiology of the excess mortality associated with vertebral fracture is not clear at present [45]. Other fractures associated with an increase in mortality include pelvis, rib, and humerus [39,41].

The costs associated with osteoporotic fractures are enormous. The total direct cost in the United States has been estimated at $17 billion in 2001 dollars [23]. The majority is associated with inpatient hospitalization, followed by nursing home care and outpatient services [46]. The exact proportion of the economic burden that is attributable to hip fracture ranges from approximately 33 to 60%, depending on whether total medical expenditures or incremental costs of osteoporotic fractures are considered [46,47]. In 1995, medical expenditures related to osteoporosis in men and nonwhite women were approximately $3.4 billion [46]; this substantial amount, although only one fourth of the total cost, underscores the need to consider prevention in these groups as well.

Despite the high cost of osteoporotic fractures economically and in terms of morbidity and mortality, osteoporosis often goes unrecognized or undertreated in health care settings. Data from the National Ambulatory Medical Care Survey indicated that less than 2% of white women ages 60 years and older received a diagnosis of osteoporosis or vertebral fracture during visits to primary care physicians in 1993 to 1997, even though the expected prevalence was 20 to 30% for these conditions [48]. In addition, appropriate drug treatment was offered to only 36% of diagnosed patients. Women with multiple risk factors for osteoporosis may also not be receiving preventive counseling or BMD testing [49].

5. Clustering of Fractures in Individuals

The undertreatment of men or women who have already sustained fractures [50–52] is of particular concern because fractures tend to cluster within individuals. Perimenopausal and postmenopausal women with a previous fracture have roughly twice the risk of future fractures [53]. This risk is even greater at the spine: women with one previous vertebral fracture are roughly four times more likely to sustain a subsequent vertebral fracture than are women without vertebral fractures, and the risk increases by two to four times for each additional fracture present [53]. Data are more limited for men but suggest that similar relationships exist [53].

The relationship between prior and subsequent fracture appears to be independent of current bone density, suggesting that prior

fractures may reflect other non-BMD mechanisms that increase fracture risk, such as defects in bone microarchitecture or the presence of factors related to falls [53]. However, low bone density and prior low-trauma fractures tend to co-exist, and their combination results in a very high risk of future fractures [53,54].

6. Secular Trends and Future Projections

The number of osteoporotic fractures will almost certainly increase in the future simply because life expectancy and the number of elderly individuals are increasing in all regions of the world [23]. Increases in the incidence rate of fractures could further exacerbate the problem. However, there is a varying amount of data regarding secular trends in fracture incidence at different skeletal sites, and in some cases, the evidence conflicts.

Secular trends in incidence of hip fracture have been the most intensely studied. Incidence rates in some countries, such as Hong Kong [55], showed strong evidence of an increase in the latter half of the 20th century, whereas data for other countries are conflicting. For example, data from Rochester, Minnesota, suggest that hip fracture incidence plateaued in women around 1950 and in men around 1980 [56], but data from the National Hospital Discharge Survey suggest that incidence increased during the 1990s in some population subgroups [57]. Data suggesting an increased risk of hip fracture for successive birth cohorts in the Framingham cohort are also consistent with an increase in hip fracture rates in the United States over time [58]. Uncertainty about the magnitude of secular trends in hip fracture incidence complicates the estimation of the future hip fracture burden. To overcome this difficulty, Gullberg et al [59] used different assumptions about the presence and magnitude of these trends in different countries when projecting the future worldwide burden. Their calculations resulted in projections that were staggering: estimates ranged from 8.2 million to more than 21 million hip fractures in 2050.

Data on secular trends at other skeletal sites are much more scanty. Data from Rochester, Minnesota, indicate no secular increase in vertebral fracture overall between 1950 to 1989 [60]. There was also no evidence of an increase in distal forearm fracture resulting from moderate trauma between 1945 to 1994 in Rochester [61] or in fractures of the proximal humerus between 1969 to 1971 and 1989 to 1991 [62]. An increased incidence of fractures of the tibia and ankle was observed, however [62].

7. Geographic Variation in Fracture

Osteoporosis and fracture occurrence vary in different populations around the world. The bulk of the data available are for hip fracture, which has been found not only to vary between countries [19] but within individual countries as well [63,64]. For example, there is a north-south gradient in hip fracture incidence in the United States, with rates being highest in the South [65,66]. This gradient is observed in both femoral neck and trochanteric hip fractures [66]. There is some suggestion that this relationship may reflect the effect of residence early in life more than current residence [67].

Data on fracture at other skeletal sites are more limited. There appears to be less geographic variation in vertebral fracture

Table 97-2
Examples of Risk Factors for Hip Fracture in Older White Women

Measurement (Comparison or Unit)	% Approximate Increase in Hip Fracture Risk
Age (per 5 yr)	40
History of maternal hip fracture (vs none)	80
Increase in weight since age 25 (per 20%)	−20
Height at age 25 (per 6 cm)	30
Self-rated health (per 1-point decrease)	60
Previous hyperthyroidism (vs none)	70
Current use of long-acting benzodiazepines (vs no current use)	60
Current use of anticonvulsant drugs (vs no current use)	100
Current caffeine intake (per 190 mg/day)	20
Walking for exercise (vs not walking for exercise)	−30
On feet ≤4 hr/day (vs >4 hr/day)	70
Inability to rise from chair (vs no inability)	70
Lowest quartile for distant depth perception (vs other three)	40
Low-frequency contrast sensitivity (per 1 SD decrease)	20
Resting pulse >80 beats/min (vs ≤80 beats/min)	70
Any fracture since age 50 (vs none)	50
Calcaneal BMD (per 1 SD decrease)	60

(From Black DM, Cooper C. [2000]. Epidemiology of fractures and assessment of fracture risk, *Clin Lab Med*. 20:439–453, as adapted from Cummings SR, Nevitt MC, Browner WS *et al*. [1995]. Risk factors for hip fracture in white women. *N Engl J Med*. 332:767–763, with permission.)
BMD, bone mineral density; SD, standard deviation.

between countries than in hip fracture. Studies performed in Europe using standardized methods to assess vertebral fracture suggest that rates in northern Europe are somewhat greater than elsewhere in Europe [26]. However, variation within countries was almost as great as that between countries [26].

Within the United States, geographic variation has been observed in distal forearm and proximal humerus fracture among elderly persons; interestingly, these fractures showed an east-west gradient (higher in east) rather than the north-south gradient observed for hip fracture. In contrast, no geographic pattern was observed for ankle fracture [65].

8. Risk Factors for Fracture

Many environmental and genetic factors affect fracture risk, either via low bone density or independently of BMD [1,68,69]. No single study has evaluated all risk factors and outcomes of interest simultaneously, and thus although there is usually general concordance between studies, there is not always complete agreement regarding the importance or ranking of risk factors [1,70–72]. In addition, most of the studies have focused on white women, although the number of studies in men and nonwhite women is growing. The number of risk factors evaluated in these other groups is more limited to date, but, in general, the factors identified have been similar to those seen in white women [73–76]. Obvious exceptions by gender are related to differences in gonadal and reproductive factors. However, even some of these factors may play a more similar role in both genders than previously realized: for example,

recent data indicate that estrogen plays a much more important, and possibly dominant, role in skeletal health among men than testosterone [77].

Most studies on risk factors for fracture have focused on hip fracture. Examples of the scope and diversity of risk factors that have been identified for hip fracture [71] are shown in Table 97-2. These factors include some which affect risk via bone density and some that affect risk of falling. More importantly, these risk factors have been found to act additively to increase risk, as illustrated in Figure 97-3. This effect was observed at all levels of BMD, but it was particularly striking in the lowest BMD tertile: women with five or more of these risk factors had an annual rate of hip fracture that was 10 times higher than in women with zero to two risk factors [71].

Risk factors for other osteoporotic fractures are less well characterized. All osteoporotic fractures share common risk factors to a large extent, but the differences between fractures in patterns by demographic characteristics and geography suggest that some differences in pathophysiology or in contribution from different risk factors also exist. For example, the cause of cervical and trochanteric hip fractures appears to differ somewhat in women [78]. Risk factors may contribute differently to different fractures as well. For example, falls play a more important role in risk of hip and limb fractures than in risk of vertebral fracture [22,79,80]. Furthermore, the orientation of the fall (e.g., forward vs sideways) is also associated with fracture risk differently (e.g., falls to the side are more likely to result in hip fractures, whereas falling forward raises the risk of wrist fracture) [81,82]. Finally, some risk factors may need to co-exist for fracture to occur. For example, although 90% of hip fractures are the result of falls [80], only 1% of falls result in hip fracture. This indicates that other factors, such as reduced soft tissue padding over the hip and low bone density, must also be present for fracture to occur [81,82].

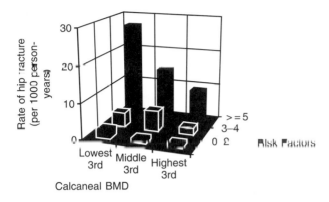

Fig. 97-3 Additive nature of risk factors and bone density on rate of hip fracture among elderly Caucasian women. (Data from Cummings SR, Nevitt MC, Browner WS *et al.* [1995]. Risk factors for hip fracture in white women. *N Engl J Med.* 332:767–773.)

III. Clinical Applications

Many of the findings from epidemiologic studies described previously have important clinical applications. Among the more important is the clarification that, although most of the burden of osteoporosis and fracture occurs in women, the number and cost in men is not trivial. Furthermore, although fewer men suffer fractures, their prognosis may be worse, because both hip and vertebral fracture are associated with a higher mortality rate in men than in women. Thus, the possibility that osteoporosis occurs in male patients should no longer necessarily be viewed as remote.

Another important application results from the development of definitions of osteoporosis based on BMD alone, because individuals can be identified before fracture and before considerable loss of bone density has already occurred. Recommendations for BMD testing have been published by several clinical and health organizations [83–86]. At present, there is consensus that screening of perimenopausal and early menopausal women is not warranted unless other risk factors are present, indicating that an individualized approach is necessary [1]. Most screening recommendations support screening of all women older than 65 years. A summary of recent recommendations for women is shown in Table 97-3. Unfortunately there are presently no recommendations regarding BMD testing in men.

Table 97-3

Summary of Recent BMD Screening Recommendations from Selected Clinical and Health Organizations

Characteristic	Organization, Date			
	American Association of Clinical Endocrinologists 2001 [83]	American College of Obstetricians and Gynecologists 2002 [84]	National Osteoporosis Foundation 1998 [85]	North American Menopause Society 2002 [86]
Women ages 65+ years	✓	✓	✓	✓
Postmenopausal women with fracture	✓ (Ages 40+ years)	✓	✓	✓ (Also premenopausal women with low trauma fracture)
Perimenopausal and postmenopausal women considering or starting osteoporosis interventions	✓		✓	✓
Premenopausal and postmenopausal women with certain diseases, medical conditions, or use of medications associated with bone loss or risk of osteoporosis*	✓	✓		✓
Perimenopausal and early postmenopausal (<65 years) with risk factors**	✓	✓	✓	✓

*Examples include glucocorticoid therapy, symptomatic hyperparathyroidism, hypogonadism, malabsorption syndromes, and other causes of secondary osteoporosis.

**Risk factors include personal history of fracture as an adult/nonvertebral fracture after menopause, Caucasian race, impaired eyesight, history of alcoholism, low body weight (<127 lb), family history (first-degree relative) of hip or vertebral fracture. See specific guidelines for more details.

However, there is considerable discussion underway on this topic, including how to resolve the uncertainty regarding the application of the WHO criteria for low bone density to men, as discussed in Chapter 4 on use of gender-based databases.

Finally, another important application stems from the findings that almost all fractures in older individuals are osteoporotic and that previous fractures are strong risk factors for subsequent fracture in both men and women. Thus, a history of previous fracture provides an important clinical opportunity to identify individuals who are at significant risk of further fractures. Once identified, there may be some urgency to initiate effective interventions, because the risk of subsequent fractures appears to be particularly high in the year following the initial fracture [54,87]. Fortunately, several effective pharmacologic interventions now exist to address osteoporosis in both men and women, as discussed in subsequent chapters.

IV. Suggestions for Further Investigations

Although considerable progress has been made in understanding the epidemiology of osteoporosis and fracture, additional work is sorely needed to expand our knowledge of this important chronic disease, especially in men and nonwhite women. In specific, future questions to be answered include the following:

- What is the best approach to identify individuals at risk of fracture, especially in men and nonwhite women?
- What is the epidemiology of osteoporotic fractures at skeletal sites other than the hip, wrist, and spine?
- What factors account for the differences in the epidemiology of different osteoporotic fractures?

References

1. NIH Consensus Development Panel on Osteoporosis Prevention, Diagnosis, and Therapy. (2001). Osteoporosis prevention, diagnosis, and therapy. *JAMA*. 285:785–795.
2. Raisz LG, Seeman E. (2001). Causes of age-related bone loss and fragility: An alternative view. *J Bone Miner Res*. 16:1948–1952.
3. Seeley DG, Browner WS, Nevitt MC *et al*. (1991). Which fractures are associated with low appendicular bone mass in elderly women? *Ann Intern Med*. 115:837–842.
4. Looker AC, Wahner HW, Dunn WL *et al*. (1998). Updated data on proximal femur bone mineral levels of US adults. *Osteoporos Int*. 8:468–489.
5. Marshall D, Johnell O, Wedel H. (1996). Meta-analysis of how well measures of bone mineral density predict occurrence of osteoporotic fractures. *BMJ*. 312:1254–1259.
6. World Health Organization. (1994). *Assessment of Fracture Risk and its Application to Screening for Postmenopausal Osteoporosis*. Technical Report Series 843. Geneva Switzerland: World Health Organization.
7. Delmas PD. (2000). Do we need to change the WHO definition of osteoporosis? *Osteoporos Int*. 11:189–191.
8. Melton LJ III. (2000). Who has osteoporosis? A conflict between clinical and public health perspectives. *J Bone Miner Res*. 15:2309–2314.
9. Looker AC, Orwoll ES, Johnston CC *et al*. (1997). Prevalence of low femoral bone density in older U.S. adults from NHANES III. *J Bone Miner Res*. 12:1761–1768.
10. Zimmerman SI, Girman CJ, Buie VC *et al*. (1999). The prevalence of osteoporosis in nursing home residents. *Osteoporos Int*. 9:151–157.
11. National Osteoporosis Foundation. (2002). *America's Bone Health: The State of Osteoporosis and Low Bone Mass in Our Nation*. Washington DC: National Osteoporosis Foundation. Available at http://www.nof.org (accessed February 27, 2004).
12. Melton LJ III. (1995). How many women have osteoporosis now? *J Bone Miner Res*. 10:175–177.
13. Eddy D, Johnston C, Cummings SR *et al*. (1998). Osteoporosis: Review of the evidence for prevention, diagnosis, and treatment and cost-effectiveness analysis. *Osteoporos Int*. 8(Suppl 4):1–86.
14. Baron JA, Karagas M, Barrett J *et al*. (1996). Basic epidemiology of fractures of the upper and lower limb among Americans over 65 years of age. *Epidemiology*. 7:612–618.
15. Lauderdale DS, Jacobsen SJ, Furner SE *et al*. (1998). Hip fracture incidence among elderly Hispanics. *Am J Public Health*. 88:1245–1247.
16. Lauderdale DS, Jacobsen SJ, Furner SE *et al*. (1997). Hip fracture incidence among elderly Asian-American populations. *Am J Epidemiol*. 146:502–509.
17. Popovic JR. (2001). 1999 National Hospital Discharge Survey: annual summary with detailed diagnosis and procedure data. *Vital Health Stat* 13(151). Hyattsville MD: National Center for Health Statistics. Available at http://www.cdc.gov/nchs/data/series/sr_13/sr13_151.pdf (accessed February 27, 2004).
18. Cooper C, Melton LJ III. (2001). Magnitude and Impact of Osteoporosis and Fractures. In *Osteoporosis*, 2nd Edition (Marcus R, Feldman D, Kelsey J, eds.), pp. 419–431. San Diego, CA: Academic Press.
19. Maggi S, Kelsey JL, Litvak J, Heyse SP. (1991). Incidence of hip fractures in the elderly: A cross-national study. *Osteoporos Int*. 1:232–241.
20. Cummings SR, Black DM, Rubin SM. (1989). Lifetime risks of hip, Colles' or vertebral fracture and coronary heart disease among white postmenopausal women. *Arch Intern Med*. 149:2445–2448.
21. Grady D, Rubin SM, Petitti DB *et al*. (1992). Hormone therapy to prevent disease and prolong life in postmenopausal women. *Ann Intern Med*. 117:1016–1037.
22. Cooper C, Atkinson EJ, O'Fallon WM, Melton LJ III. (1992). Incidence of clinically diagnosed vertebral fractures: A population-based study in Rochester, Minnesota, 1985–1989. *J Bone Miner Res*. 7:221–227.
23. Cummings SR, Melton LJ III. (2002). Epidemiology and outcomes of osteoporotic fractures. *Lancet*. 359:1761–1767.
24. Black DM, Palermo L, Nevitt MC *et al*. for the Study of Osteoporotic Fractures Research Group. (1995). Comparison of methods for defining prevalent vertebral deformities: The Study of Osteoporotic Fracture. *J Bone Miner Res*. 10:890–902.
25. Melton LJ III. (1997). Epidemiology of spinal osteoporosis. *Spine*. 22(24 Suppl):2S–11S.
26. O'Neill TW, Felsenberg D, Varlow J *et al*. and the European Vertebral Osteoporosis Study Group. (1996). The prevalence of vertebral deformity in European men and women: The European Vertebral Osteoporosis Study. *J Bone Miner Res*. 11:1010–1018.
27. Van der Klift J, De Laet CEDH, McCloskey EV *et al*. (2002). The incidence of vertebral fractures in men and women: The Rotterdam study. *J Bone Miner Res*. 17:1051–1056.
28. The European Prospective Osteoporosis Study Group. (2002). Incidence of vertebral fracture in Europe: Results from the European Prospective Osteoporosis Study (EPOS). *J Bone Miner Res*. 17:716–724.
29. Owen RA, Melton LJ III, Johnson KA *et al*. (1982). Incidence of Colles' fracture in a north American community. *Am J Public Health*. 72:605–607.
30. Ensrud KE, Thompson DE, Cauely JA *et al*. for the Fracture Intervention Trial Research Group. (2000). Prevalent vertebral deformities predict mortality and hospitalization in older women with low bone mass. *J Am Geriatr Soc*. 48:241–249.
31. Nevitt MC, Ettinger B, Black DM *et al*. (1998). The association of radiographically detected vertebral fractures with back pain and function: A prospective study. *Ann Intern Med*. 128:793–800.
32. Gold DT, Lyles KW, Shipp KM, Drezner MK. (2001). Osteoporosis and Its Nonskeletal Consequences: Their Impact on Treatment Decisions. In *Osteoporosis*, 2nd Edition (Marcus R, Feldman D, Kelsey J, eds.), pp. 479–484. San Diego, CA: Academic Press.
33. Burger H, Van Daele PLA, Grashuis K *et al*. (1997). Vertebral deformities and functional impairment in men and women. *J Bone Miner Res*. 12:152–157.
34. Matthis C, Weber U, O'Neill TW, Raspe H. (1998). Health impact associated with vertebral deformities: Results from the European Vertebral Osteoporosis Study (EVOS). *Osteoporos Int*. 8:364–372.
35. Chrischilles E, Butler CD, Davis CS, Wallace RB. (1991). A model of lifetime osteoporosis impact. *Arch Intern Med*. 151:2026–2032.
36. Keene GS, Parker JM, Pryor GA. (1993). Morbidity and mortality after hip fractures. *BMJ*. 307:1248–1250.
37. Magaziner J, Lydick E, Hawkes W *et al*. (1997). Excess mortality attributable to hip fractures in white women aged 70 years and older. *Am J Public Health*. 87:1630–1636.
38. Jacobsen SJ, Goldberg J, Miles TP *et al*. (1992). Race and sex difference in mortality following a fracture of the hip. *Am J Publ Health*. 82:1147–1150.

39. Center JR, Nguyen TV, Schneider D et al. (1999). Mortality after all major types of osteoporotic fracture in men and women: An observational study. Lancet. 353:878–882.

40. Fransen M, Woodward M, Norton R et al. (2002). Excess mortality or institutionalization after hip fracture: Men are at greater risk than women. J Am Geriatr Soc. 50:685–690.

41. Browner WS, Pressman AR, Nevitt MC, Cummings SR. (1996). Mortality following fractures in older women. The Study of Osteoporotic Fractures. Arch Intern Med. 156:1521–1525.

42. Meyer HE, Tverdal A, Falch JA, Pedersen JI. (2000). Factors associated with mortality after hip fracture. Osteoporos Int. 11:228–232.

43. Kado DM, Browner WS, Palermo L et al. (1999). Vertebral fractures and mortality in older women: A prospective study. Arch Intern Med. 159:1215–1220.

44. Cooper C, Atkinson EJ, Jacobsen SJ et al. (1993). Population-based study of survival after osteoporotic fractures. Am J Epidemiol. 137:1001–1005.

45. Melton LJ III. (2000). Excess mortality following vertebral fracture. J Am Geriatr Soc. 48:338–339.

46. Ray NF, Chan JK, Thamer M, Melton LJ III. (1997). Medical expenditures for the treatment of osteoporotic fracture in the United States in 1995: Report from the National Osteoporosis Foundation. J Bone Miner Res. 12:24–35.

47. Gabriel SE, Tosteson ANA, Leibson CL et al. (2002). Direct medical costs attributable to osteoporotic fractures. Osteoporos Int. 13:323–330.

48. Gehlbach SH, Fournier M, Bigelow C. (2002). Recognition of osteoporosis by primary care physicians. Am J Public Health. 92:271–273.

49. Gallagher TC, Geling O, Comite F. (2002). Missed opportunities for prevention of osteoporotic fracture. Arch Intern Med. 162:450–456.

50. Cuddihy MT, Gabriel SE, Crowson CS et al. (2002). Osteoporosis intervention following distal forearm fractures. A missed opportunity? Arch Intern Med. 162:421–426.

51. Juby AG, De Geus-Wenceslau CM. (2002). Evaluation of osteoporosis treatment in seniors after hip fracture. Osteoporos Int. 13:205–210.

52. Riley RL, Carnes RL, Gudmundsson A, Elliott ME. (2002). Outcomes and secondary prevention strategies for male hip fractures. Ann Pharmacother. 36:17–23.

53. Klotzbuecher CM, Ross PD, Landsman PB et al. (2000). Patients with prior fractures have an increased risk of future fractures: A summary of the literature and statistical synthesis. J Bone Miner Res. 15:721–739.

54. Lindsay R, Silverman SL, Cooper C et al. (2001). Risk of new vertebral fracture in the year following a fracture. JAMA. 285:320–323.

55. Lau EMC, Cooper C, Wickham C et al. (1990). Hip fractures in Hong Kong and Britain. Int J Epidemiol. 19:1119–1121.

56. Melton LJ III, Atkinson EJ, Madhok R. (1996). Downturn in hip fracture incidence. Public Health Rep. 111:146–150.

57. Bacon WE. (1996). Secular trends in hip fracture occurrence and survival: Age and sex differences. J Aging Health. 8:538–553.

58. Samelson EJ, Zhang Y, Kiel DP et al. (2002). Effect of birth cohort on risk of hip fracture: Age-specific incidence rates in the Framingham Study. Am J Public Health. 92:858–862.

59. Gullberg B, Johnell O, Kanis JA. (1997). World-wide projections for hip fracture. Osteoporos Int. 7:407–413.

60. Cooper C, Atkinson EJ, Kotowicz M et al. (1992). Secular trends in the incidence of postmenopausal vertebral fractures. Calcif Tissue Int. 51:100–104.

61. Melton LJ III, Amadio PC, Crowson CS, O'Fallon WM. (1998). Long-term trends in the incidence of distal forearm fractures. Osteoporos Int. 8:341–348.

62. Melton LJ 3rd, Crowson CS, O'Fallon WM. (1999). Fracture incidence in Olmsted County, Minnesota: Comparison of urban with rural rates and changes in urban rates over time. Osteoporos Int. 9:29–37.

63. Elffors I, Allander E, Kanis JA et al. (1994). The variable incidence of hip fracture in southern Europe: The MEDOS study. Osteoporos Int. 4:253–263.

64. Jacobsen SJ, Goldberg J, Miles TP et al. (1990). Regional variation in the incidence of hip fracture. U.S. white women aged 65 years and older. JAMA. 264:500–502.

65. Karagas MR, Baron JA, Barrett JA, Jacobsen SJ. (1996). Patterns of fracture among the United States elderly: Geographic and fluoride effects. Ann Epidemiol. 6:209–216.

66. Karagas MR, Lu-Yao GL, Barrett JA et al. (1996). Heterogeneity of hip fracture: Age, race, sex, and geographic patterns of femoral neck and trochanteric fractures among the US elderly. Am J Epidemiol. 143:677–682.

67. Lauderdale DS, Thisted RA, Goldberg J. (1998). Is geographic variation in hip fracture rates related to current or former region of residence? Epidemiology. 9:574–577.

68. Ralston SH. (2002). Genetic control of susceptibility to osteoporosis. J Clin Endocrinol Metab. 87:2460–2466.

69. Nelson HD, Morris CD, Kraemer DF et al. (2001). Osteoporosis in Postmenopausal Women: Diagnosis and Monitoring. Evidence Report/Technology Assessment No. 28 (Prepared by the Oregon Health & Science University Evidence-based Practice Center under Contract No. 290-97-0018). AHRQ Publication No. 01-E032. Rockville, MD: Agency for Healthcare Research and Quality. Available at http://www.ahrq.gov/clinic/epcix.htm (accessed February 27, 2004).

70. Espallargues M, Sampietro-Colom L, Estrada MD et al. (2001). Identifying bone-mass-related risk factors for fracture to guide bone densitometry measurements. A systematic review of the literature. Osteoporos Int. 12:811–822.

71. Cummings SR, Nevitt MC, Browner WS et al. (1995). Risk factors for hip fracture in white women. Study of Osteoporotic Fractures Research Group. N Engl J Med. 332:767–773.

72. Johnell O, Gullberg B, Kanis JA et al. (1995). Risk factors for hip fracture in European women: The MEDOS study. J Bone Miner Res. 10:1802–1815.

73. Orwoll ES, Bevan L, Phipps KR. (2000). Determinants of bone mineral density in older men. Osteoporos Int. 11:815–821.

74. Mussolino ME, Looker AC, Madans JH et al. (1998). Risk factors hip fracture in white men: The NHANES I Epidemiological Follow-Up Study. J Bone Miner Res. 13:918–924.

75. Grisso JA, Kelsey JL, Strom BL et al. (1994). Risk factors for hip fracture in black women: The Northeast Hip Fracture Study Group. N Engl J Med. 330:1555–1559.

76. Fujiwara S, Kasagi F, Yamada M, Kodama K. (1997). Risk factors for hip fracture in a Japanese cohort. J Bone Miner Res. 12:998–1004.

77. Khosla S, Melton LJ III, Riggs BL. (2002). Clinical review 144: Estrogen and the male skeleton. J Clin Endocrinol Metab. 87:1443–1450.

78. Mautalen CA, Vega EM, Einhorn TA. (1996). Are the etiologies of cervical and trochanteric hip fractures different? Bone. 18:133S–137S.

79. Grisso JA, Capezuti E, Schwartz A. (1996). Falls as Risk Factors for Fractures. In Osteoporosis (Marcus R, Feldman D, Kelsey J, eds.), pp. 599–611. San Diego, CA: Academic Press.

80. Youm T, Koval KJ, Kummer FJ, Zuckerman JK. (1999). Do all hip fractures result from a fall? Am J Orthop. 28:190–194.

81. Nevitt MC, Cummings SR. (1993). Type of fall and risk of hip and wrist fractures: The Study of Osteoporotic Fractures. J Am Geriatr Soc. 41:1226–1234.

82. Greenspan SL, Myers ER, Maitland LA et al. (1994). Fall severity and bone mineral density as risk factors for hip fracture in ambulatory elderly. JAMA. 271:128–133.

83. Osteoporosis Task Force, American Association of Clinical Endocrinologists. (2001). 2001 Medical guidelines for clinical practice for the prevention and management of postmenopausal osteoporosis. Endocr Pract. 7:293–312.

84. Committee on Gynecologic Practice, American College of Obstetricians and Gynecologists. (2002). ACOG Committee opinion #270. Bone density screening for osteoporosis. American College of Obstetricians and Gynecologists. Obstet Gynecol. 99:523–525.

85. National Osteoporosis Foundation. (1998). Physician's Guide to Prevention and Treatment of Osteoporosis. Washington DC: National Osteoporosis Foundation. Available at http://www.nof.org/physguide/index.htm (accessed February 27, 2004).

86. North American Menopause Society. (2002). Management of postmenopausal osteoporosis: Position statement of the North American Menopause Society. Menopause. 9:84–101.

87. Colon-Emeric CS, Sloane R, Hawkes WG et al. (2000). The risk of subsequent fractures in community-dwelling men and male veterans with hip fracture. Am J Med. 109:324–326.

98

Gender and Sports Medicine in the Adult Athlete

CLAUDIA L. GINSBERG, MD* AND JORDAN D. METZL, MD**

*Private practice at Tri-County Orthopaedics and Sports Medicine, Morristown, NJ
**Medical Director of The Sports Medicine Institute for Young Athletes; Assistant Professor, Department of Pediatrics,
Hospital for Special Surgery, Cornell Medical College; Assistant Attending Physician,
Hospital for Special Surgery, New York, NY

I. Introduction

The last hundred years have seen an exponential rise in the number of women participating in sports at every level. Some of this growth may be attributed to a handful of women athlete pioneers who excelled in their sport, breaking cultural stereotypes of their day and gaining public attention. Perhaps the biggest boost to women's sports, however, came in 1972 with Title IX of the Education Amendments.

"No person in the United States shall, on the basis of sex, be excluded from participation in, be denied the benefits of, or be subject to discrimination under any educational program or activity receiving Federal financial assistance."
(Title IX of the Educational Amendments of 1972 to the 1964 Civil Rights Act)

This antidiscrimination law requires educational institutions receiving Federal funding to maintain policies, practices, and programs that do not discriminate on the basis of gender. Even private institutions, which may not directly receive federal assistance, fall under the Title IX umbrella because a portion of their student body is supported by federal financial aid programs. Although Title IX applies to all aspects of education, curricular and extracurricular, its most noticeable impact has been on athletics. Specifically, Title IX requires that women and men be provided equitable opportunities to participate in sports and receive scholarships proportional to their participation. Equal treatment with respect to equipment, supplies, facilities, games, practice time, coaching, housing, and support services is also included under the law [1].

With increasingly flexible gender roles and greater opportunities through Title IX, the number of women who participate in sports has proportionately increased since the 1970s. According to the National Federation of State High School Associations Participation Study there were more than 3.6 million male high school athletic participants in 1971 and only 294,015 female athletes. By 2001 these numbers had only inched up to 3.9 million for boys but had grown 9-fold for girls to 2.7 million [2]. The National Collegiate Athletic Association Sports Sponsorship and Participation Report shows that in 1982 just over 70,000 young women participated in college athletics. By 2001, women athletes numbered more than 150,000, accounting for 40% of college athletes [3].

Today women of every age are more active than ever before, and along with this growth has been a rise in the number of sports injuries. Muscle strains and ligament sprains are the most common musculoskeletal injuries in both sexes [4]. However, there is a growing awareness that some sports injuries may have different characteristics in men and women. Injuries in general are more sport-specific than gender-specific [5,6]. Swimmers are more prone to shoulder injuries and basketball players are more prone to ankle injuries. Furthermore, contact sports are known to put both sexes at higher injury risk than noncontact sports. However, some patterns of injury fall along gender lines. Much investigation and speculation has surrounded the cause of these observed differences. Studying these patterns provides the impetus for improving injury prevention, recognition, and treatment for all athletes.

This chapter reviews basic anatomic and physiologic differences between men and women and highlights a handful of medical and orthopedic topics that affect men and women differently. Medical topics include the female athlete triad, exercise during pregnancy, and breast injuries. The musculoskeletal focus is on anterior cruciate ligament (ACL) tears, stress fractures, and patellofemoral stress syndrome.

II. Sex Differences in Athletes

A. Anatomic Differences

Despite the fact that men and women are much more similar than they are different, there are many notable sex differences. How these differences affect dynamic motion, sports performance, and injury rates is unclear and is an active area of research. This section underlines some of the important anatomic and physiologic differences between men and women.

Children's sizes and shapes before puberty are rather uniform. This also holds true for heart rate, strength, and aerobic power [7]. During puberty, when sex steroids have varying effects on body tissues and metabolic processes, anatomic sex differences become more pronounced. Under the influence of estrogen, a girl's hips broaden relative to her shoulders and waist, but her muscle mass does not undergo significant change. In contrast, a boy's shoulders broaden relative to his hips and his muscle mass increases dramatically under testosterone's influence [8]. In the United States, men become an average of 13 cm taller and 18 kg heavier than women. Men develop approximately 20 kg more lean body mass and 5 kg less fat. Females typically accumulate fat in the hips and thighs, whereas men concentrate fat around the abdomen [9].

In general, an adult woman's pelvis is wider and more shallow than a man's. From this wider position, a woman's femur has a greater slant inward toward the knee, causing a greater tibio-femoral angle. This angle and the placement of the tibial tubercle contribute to a women's larger quadriceps angle (Q-angle). The characteristic female skeleton is also associated with femoral anteversion, external tibial torsion, foot pronation, and less developed thigh musculature (Fig. 98-1).

In terms of extremities, a woman's limbs are generally shorter than a man's. Her arm is not as long as her forearm, whereas

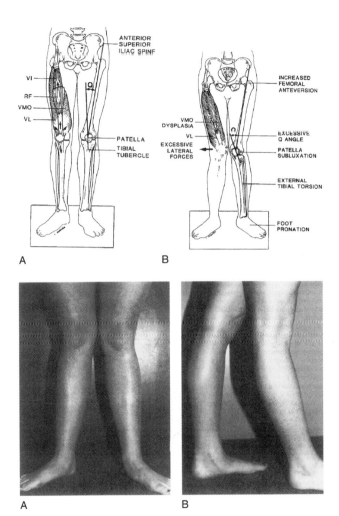

Fig. 98-1 Drawings: Patellofemoral disorders are common in women. A, Normal alignment with normal Q angle measured from anterosuperior iliac spine central portion of the patella, patella to tibial tubercle of less than 15 degrees, and normal musculature of developed vastus medialis obliquus create forces that centralize the patella, resulting in normal patellofemoral tracking. B, Miserable malalignment syndrome consists of increased femoral anteversion, excessive Q angle, external tibial torsion, and foot pronation. All of these factors cause lateral patellar subluxation. Photographs: This miserable malalignment syndrome is frequently seen in women. Clinical example of collegiate swimmer from the front, (A) showing 20 degrees of genu valgum, external tibial torsion, hypoplastic vastus medialis obliquus, heel valgus, and pes planus with forefoot pronation. B, Hyperflexibility of 20 degrees of hyperextension is seen from the side in a clinical view. (From Fu FH, Stone DA eds. [1994]. *Sports Injuries: Mechanism, Prevention and Treatment,* 2nd Edition. Baltimore: Williams & Wilkins, p. 159, with permission.)

the opposite is true for a man. This, in addition to women's increased "carrying angle" at the elbow, confers disadvantage in throwing [10]. Women's legs are shorter in absolute terms, and, when indexed to height, the result is a lower center of gravity in women, which may have an advantage for balance, although not for power in throwing and kicking [11]. Men's feet tend to pronate less than women's, which means men place more pressure on their lateral midfoot and forefoot. The result is a more rigid foot [12]. Women's foot pronation also adds to their knee valgus, further altering forces through the knee [13].

A man's greater power is not only related to a larger frame, which provides a mechanical lever advantage, but also to greater overall muscle mass. A woman's strength potential is generally about two thirds of man's [14]. This difference is more pronounced in the upper extremities than the lower. Women have 60 to 85% of the number of muscle fibers and total cross-sectional area of men [15]. Muscle fiber composition, however, is much the same with equal relative proportions of slow twitch fibers, for aerobic activity, and fast twitch fibers, used more for anaerobic activity [16]. Muscle fiber differences are more related to type of training than sex. Women can make significant gains in muscle mass and strength with weight training, but not to the same extent as men, who have testosterone working in their favor [17]. Testosterone levels among women vary greatly; although on average women have one tenth the amount of a man (Table 98-1) [18].

B. Physiologic Differences

Women have smaller hearts with smaller stroke volumes as a consequence [19]. Less blood can be pumped out to a woman's muscles with each beat, and some women adjust for this with faster heart rates. With 6% fewer red blood cells and 15% less hemoglobin per red cell, women possess a lower oxygen-carrying capacity [20]. Less total lung capacity and less vital capacity means less air can be moved through the lungs in one maximal breath [21]. These differences contribute to men's greater aerobic ability, which is commonly expressed as VO_{2max} [22]. Absolute VO_{2max} values are on average 40% higher in men; however, this difference is drastically cut when expressed per kilogram of body weight and relative to fat-free weight [23]. Both sexes peak their VO_{2max} between ages 16 to 20 [24]. Adaptation to physical training is more similar than different in men and women with respect to decrease in heart rate, blood pressure, and percent body fat and increases in muscle strength and endurance [25].

Men and women are more alike than different, however, sex differences are often implicated when gender differences in acute or overuse injuries are discovered. Much research has attempted to uncover causal relationships to observed characteristics, but few have been conclusive. Lower extremity malalignment, for example, although seen in both sexes is more commonly found in women. This malalignment predisposes to knee problems, especially patellar dislocations and patellofemoral syndrome [26,27]. That many women with malalignment do not have any knee problems or pain implies that other factors must be at play. More specifics are discussed under each musculoskeletal topic.

Table 98-1
Anatomic and Physiologic Differences Between Men and Women

Anatomic Differences

Factor	Women	Men	Impact
Height	64.5″	68.5″	
Weight	56.8 kg	70.0 kg	
Limb Length	Shorter	Longer	Men can achieve a greater force for hitting or kicking
Articular Surface	Smaller	Larger	May provide men with greater joint stability; men have greater surface area to dissipate impact force
Body Shape	Narrower shoulders	Wider shoulders	Women have lower center of gravity and therefore greater balance ability; women have an increased valgus angle at the knee which increases knee injuries; women and men have different running gaits
	Wider hips	Narrower hips	
	Legs 51.2% of height	Legs 52% of height	
	More fat in lower body	More fat in upper body	
% Muscle/TBW*	~36%	~44.8%	Men have greater strength and greater speed
% Fat/TBW†	~22%–26%	~13%–16%	Women are more buoyant and better insulated; they may be able to convert to fatty acid metabolism more rapidly
Age at Skeletal Maturation	17–19 yr	21–22 yr	Women develop adult body shape/form sooner than men

Physiologic Differences

System/Factor	Women	Men	Impact
Cardiovascular			
Heart size	Smaller	Larger	Women's stoke volume is less, necessitating an increased heart rate for a given submaximal cardiac output; cardiac output in women is ~30% less than men; women may be less at risk of developing hypertension
Heart volume	Smaller	Larger	
Systolic blood pressure	Lower	Higher	
Hemopoietic			
Hemoglobin		10–15%> per 100 mL blood	Men's blood has a greater oxygen-carrying capacity
Pulmonary			
Chest size	Smaller	Larger	Total lung capacity in men is greater than in women
Lung size	Smaller	Larger	
Vital capacity	Smaller	Larger	
Residual volume	Smaller	Larger	
Efficiency of Cardiorespiratory System			
Oxygen pulse	Lower	Higher	Higher oxygen pulse provides men an advantage in aerobic activity
Level of Aerobic Fitness (reflects performance of cardiorespiratory and muscular systems)			
VO$_{2max}$	Lower	Higher	Men have greater aerobic ability
Metabolism (BMR)	~6%–10% lower (when related to body surface area)	~6%–10% higher (when related to body surface area)	Women need fewer calories to sustain same activity level as men
Thermoregulation	Female=Male	Female=Male	Both sexes can adequately sweat in hot weather to decrease core body temperature

*Comparisons are made for "average" postpubertal male and female.
†Varies somewhat with age, sport, and level of conditioning.
BMR, basal metabolic rate; TBW, total body weight.
(From Yurko–Griffin L, Harris SS. [1999]. Female athletes. In Sullivan JA, Anderson SJ [eds]: Care of the Young Athlete. Rosemont, III, American Academy of Orthopaedic Surgeons, pp. 137–148.)

III. Medical Issues and Gender in the Adult Athlete

A. Female Athlete Triad

1. Eating Disorders

Many female athletes feel significant pressure to keep an ultrathin physique largely because of perceived advantages in athletic performance and appearance. This is especially true in activities such as crew, cheerleading, and gymnastics where appearance is integral to success in sport and being slender is an asset. When disordered eating in exercising individuals is accompanied by amenorrhea, osteoporosis is one of the feared consequences. The dangerous combination of disordered eating, amenorrhea, and osteoporosis is termed the Female Athlete Triad and was first made widely known by Yeager in 1993 [28]. The triad is not only a diagnosis of elite competitive athletes, but also of active young women [29]. Contrary to the intentions of many athletes, the triad has a negative effect on athletic performance [30].

Disordered eating habits are widespread in our weight-focused society and athletes are at particular risk. Studies estimate disordered eating among female college athletes to be between 15 and 62% [31,32]. Habits include ritualistic food restriction; food binges; self-induced vomiting; and use of diuretics, laxatives, and diet pills. It is important to note that the diagnoses anorexia nervosa and bulimia nervosa, as defined by the *Diagnostic and Statistical Manual of Mental Disorders*, 4th ed. (DSM-IV), are merely endpoints on a continuum of disordered eating habits. Disordered eating, which is more pervasive and inconspicuous, includes many inappropriate and dangerous behaviors that often fail to meet strict diagnostic criteria. Such behaviors are independently dangerous and put women at risk for developing more serious eating disorders, such as anorexia nervosa. The gravity of the situation is underlined by complications of anorexia, which include electrolyte imbalances, cardiac dysfunction, and even death. The crude mortality rate for anorexia nervosa is estimated at 5.9% [33].

Men are also affected by pressures imposed by sports and society to control their weight and physique. Rates of anorexia and bulimia in men are thought to be one tenth that of women [34]. The rate of disordered eating among male athletes is even less clear, although the most dangerous practices are often seen in wrestlers and men's lightweight rowers, attempting to fit into particular weight categories [35].

2. Athletic Amenorrhea

Vigorous exercise can have both harmful and beneficial effects on menses. Exercise can lessen the abdominal pain, back pain, headaches, and analgesic use associated with menses [36]. Unfortunately, menstrual dysfunction is another common side effect. Menstrual dysfunction can have has many causes, and athletic amenorrhea should be considered a diagnosis of exclusion. Athletes are more likely to experience irregular menses than nonathletes with numbers ranging from 1 to 66% for athletes and 2 to 5% for women in general [37]. Some studies show menstrual irregularities to be 20 times more common in exercising women [38]. Leading theories to explain the amenorrhea of exercise are inhibition of hypothalamic gonadotropin-releasing hormone (GnRH) production and "energy drain" from a negative caloric balance [39]. Although studies are still lacking, research is focused on the complex interplay of nutrition, exercise intensity, exercise volume, percentage body fat, hormonal alterations, and psychologic stressors. Regardless of the cause, amenorrhea has the potential to devastate bone health.

Athletes often do not report amenorrhea to trainers and health professionals. Many athletes, parents, and coaches consider missing periods to be a normal part of intense training. Some women find it desirable, convenient, and even advantageous to their performance to skip their menses and any accompanying symptoms [40]. It should be noted that studies have not conclusively demonstrated any phase of the menstrual cycle to have appreciable effects on athletic performance [41], and women have won gold medals and set records during all menstrual phases [42].

3. Osteopenia/Osteoporosis

Although many athletes are not concerned, menstrual dysfunction largely as a reflection of a low estrogen state can have disastrous effects on bone health [43]. Duration and severity of menstrual dysfunction is proportionate with bone density [44,45] and is the most accurate predictor of fracture risk [46,47]. The positive effects exercise can have on bone health are often offset by the associated low estrogen state. Amenorrheic hypoestrogenic athletes further increase their risk of osteoporosis when menstrual irregularities are combined with nutritional deficiencies from disordered eating—the female athlete triad. Because maximum bone density is achieved around age 30, young women have a finite window to lay down new healthy bone. Good nutrition, sufficient vitamin D and calcium, regular menses, and a balanced exercise program are the key elements of achieving peak bone mass and preventing fractures throughout the lifespan. Thus, bone loss in this young population is particularly concerning.

The secretive nature of eating disorders and the fear of losing athletic advantage through even minimal weight gains make the triad and its components a challenge to treat. A multidisciplinary team approach, involving doctors, trainers, mental health professionals, nutritionists, and coaches, is paramount to treating these complex issues. Early detection is imperative and systematic screenings should begin at preparticipation physicals. Some studies indicate that with treatment of disordered eating, athletes can regain some of the bony losses [48]; however, there is also evidence that these athletes will never attain the peak bone mass that would have been expected [49].

B. Exercise and Pregnancy

1. Safety

Before research data was available, there were many concerns about potentially harmful effects of exercise during pregnancy. Early recommendations warned about infertility, abortion, hemorrhage, congenital deformities, premature and difficult labor, fetal brain damage, and others. Surprisingly, it was not until 1994 that the American College of Obstetrics and Gynecology (ACOG) published its first recommendations on exercise during pregnancy.

In 2002 the guidelines were updated using the expanded body of knowledge related to exercise and pregnancy. The research on exercise in pregnancy fails to support many of the early concerns [50,51]. Healthy expectant mothers without medical or obstetrical complications are encouraged to engage in 30 minutes or more of moderate intensity physical activity on most days of the week. This recommendation holds even if the expectant mother has never exercised before becoming pregnant [52]. Women should discuss their sporting activities with their physicians but, in general, exercise is recommended throughout the pregnancy even in the third trimester [53,54].

There are many medical and psychologic benefits that can be derived for both the fetus and the expectant mother from low to moderate regular exercise in pregnancy. Moderate activity is usually defined as 3 to 4 METS, the equivalent of brisk walking. Cardiovascular benefits, limited weight gain, less postpartum depression, and more rapid labor and recovery with fewer complications are all reported advantages for expectant mothers who exercise [55,56]. The most notable benefit is in the prevention of gestational diabetes [57,58].

For the fetus, concerns have centered on birth weight and premature labor. Some studies show that children of mothers who exercise in pregnancy have lower birth weights than children of sedentary mothers. Importantly, all birth weights in the exercising group remained within the normal range [59]. In contrast to very arduous occupational work [60], moderate exercise does not harbor an association with preterm delivery or spontaneous abortion [61,62]. Some studies demonstrate the babies of mothers exercising have higher stress tolerance, less baby fat, and advanced neurobehavioral maturation [63].

2. Recommendations

Although a wide range of physical activities are deemed safe in pregnancy, there are a few notable exceptions. High contact sports and activities with increased falls risk, such as gymnastics and downhill skiing, are discouraged especially after the first trimester. The complete supine position is also to be avoided during exercise after the first trimester because of the potential for compromising venous return and lowering cardiac output. Exertion at high altitudes and scuba diving are thought to be harmful to a pregnancy, because diving places the fetus at high risk for compression sickness [64]. Table 98-2 lists the absolute contraindications to exercise during pregnancy.

There are a number of relative contraindications as well, which include poor control of medical conditions, extremes of weight, and orthopedic limitations. These are listed in Table 98-3. This list highlights the fact that under a doctor's care, exercise can even be safe for pregnant women with medical issues. Patients

Table 98-2
Absolute Contraindications to Exercise in Pregnancy

Hemodynamically significant heart disease
Restrictive lung disease
Incompetent cervix/cerclage
Multiple gestation at risk for premature labor
Persistent second or third trimester bleeding
Placenta previa after 26 weeks of gestation
Premature labor during the current pregnancy
Ruptured membranes
Preeclampsia/pregnancy-induced hypertension

(From ACOG Committee Opinion No. 267. [2002]. Exercise during pregnancy and the postpartum period. *Obstet Gynecol*. 99:171–173, with permission.)

Table 98-3
Relative Contraindications to Exercise in Pregnancy

Severe anemia
Unevaluated maternal cardiac arrhythmias
Chronic bronchitis
Poorly controlled type 1 diabetes
Extreme morbid obesity
Extreme underweight (BMI <12)
History of extremely sedentary lifestyle
Intrauterine growth restriction in current pregnancy
Poorly controlled hypertension
Orthopedic limitations
Poorly controlled seizure disorder
Poorly controlled hyperthyroidism
Heavy smoker

(From ACOG Committee Opinion No. 267. [2002]. Exercise during pregnancy and the postpartum period. *Obstet Gynecol*. 99:171–173, with permission.) BMI, body mass index.

should know their limits, use caution, and consult their doctors regularly.

C. Breast Injuries

1. Breast

The breast, as a prominent structure on the chest wall in both women and men, is vulnerable to multiple types of trauma. The nipple is the most commonly injured part of the breast. The true number of breast injuries in sports is unknown, likely secondary to under-reporting [65].

The breast can be injured in a variety of ways. Acute trauma, such as lacerations and contusions, can lead to hematomas and thrombophlebitis. Hematomas should be monitored because they can result in secondary induration, scarring, and calcification that can last for years. Mondor's disease is a trauma-induced superficial thrombophlebitis of the breast, which most often resolves with supportive care [66].

The breast may also suffer repetitive trauma, such as from excess bounce or vigorous abrasions. The breast has little in the way of natural supports [67]. Breasts are composed mainly of adipose tissue and are suspended by skin and deep fascia. (Cooper's ligaments separate glands but do not support the breast [68].) Excessive motion can strain breast myofascial attachments and the pectoralis muscle itself. Sports bras are designed to help with these issues. A properly fitted sports bra should lift and separate breasts, thereby limiting motion. Sometimes sports bras themselves may generate minor trauma from wires, hooks, straps, or general pressure. Padded shoulder straps may provide extra comfort in women with larger breasts. A woman with significant asymmetry in breast size may require extra cup padding to secure a proper fit.

2. Nipple

The nipple is particularly vulnerable to the environment. Nipple abrasions, caused by close fitting or coarse clothing, are commonly termed "jogger's nipple" [69]. Although breast injuries are often thought of as a female issue, one study of marathon runners found a male-to-female nipple injury rate of 20:1 [70]. Nipple abrasions can be prevented by application of protective bandages or petroleum jelly [71]. "Bicyclist's nipple" is a cold-induced thermal injury to the nipple, which can result in a bleeding painful nipple [72]. The combination of evaporating perspiration and wind chill can damage the nipple. Although exercise is strongly associated with decreased breast cancer risk in women [73,74], cancer should at least be considered in the differential diagnosis of any woman or man with what appears to be a bloody nipple discharge.

IV. Musculoskeletal Issues and Gender

A. Anterior Cruciate Ligament Injury

The anterior cruciate ligament (ACL) of the knee is the primary restraint to rotation and anterior translation of the tibia relative to the femur. Anterior cruciate ligament rupture can result from a direct blow to the knee or a noncontact injury. Noncontact ACL tears in sports are typically incurred during a deceleration from a jump, sudden stop, or rapid change of direction. This is often termed a "plant and twist" injury. Both contact and noncontact mechanisms are commonly seen in sports. Regardless of mechanism, once an ACL ruptures it will not regenerate, leaving many individuals with symptomatic knee instability. The natural progression of an unstable knee involves cartilage injury and premature arthritis [75]. Therefore, many individuals wishing to continue an active lifestyle choose to have their ACLs reconstructed.

The literature on ACL injuries demonstrates that women incur noncontact ACL tears 3 to 10 times the rate of their male counterparts in similar activities. The difference is seen most dramatically for women in jumping and pivoting sports such as soccer and basketball [76,77]. There has been much speculation as to the cause of this observed difference. Anatomic, hormonal, and physiologic differences have all been implicated, but the cause remains elusive.

How an athlete's nonmodifiable (intrinsic) and modifiable (extrinsic) risk factors affect ACL injury rates has been a topic of intense research. To date, none of the suspected intrinsic, nonmodifiable features have been shown to be solely responsible for higher ACL tear rates in women, including limb alignment, intercondylar notch size and shape, and ligament size and laxity [78]. A good portion of this debate has centered on laxity and notch size. Early research suggested ligamentous laxity predisposed all athletes to ACL tears [79]. Studies implied that women possessed increased laxity compared with men [80], and subsequently laxity was used to explain sex differences in tear rates. More rigorous studies have questioned this causal relationship and the premise of sex differences in laxity [81,82]. Another theory proposes the smaller distance between femoral condyles in women could increase sheering forces on ACL and thereby predispose to injury [83,84]. No firm consensus has been reached on sex differences in intercondylar notch size and the relationship to ACL injury [85].

A female athlete's potentially modifiable features may also be partially to blame for the predisposition to ACL injury. These factors include type of sport, fitness and skill level, muscle strength, neuromuscular recruitment patterns, environment, and equipment. Many studies fault a lower baseline conditioning level for a variety of women's sports injuries [86,87]. However, training alone has not been shown to increase women's

predisposition to ACL injury [88]. A high shoe-surface friction and a rough playing surface are thought to increase an athlete's ACL tear risk [89]. However, this holds true for both sexes.

Sex differences in posture, joint position, and movement patterns hold potential in uncovering reasons for the ACL tear discrepancy. Women tend to assume a more erect posture on jump landings, with more knee valgus and less knee flexion [90,91]. These motor patterns, may jeopardize the ACL on decelerations and landings. Prevention programs developed to teach safer body positioning during athletic activity have met with some success [92,93]. As a consequence many clinicians and coaches recommend preventative training programs focusing on safer sport specific movement patterns, especially more linear knee movements and low body positioning. Although women's susceptibility to ACL injury is likely to be multifactorial, women's neuromuscular lower extremity control seems to be the most promising area of research to date [94].

Potential hormonal contributions to ACL injury have not been overlooked. Estrogen has relaxing properties on many soft tissues and helps regulate metalloproteinases and their inhibitors [95]. Because estrogen has receptors on the ACL [96], its influence on type I collagen integrity might affect the ACL's composition and mechanical properties. Accordingly, researchers are investigating a possible inverse relationship between estrogen levels and ACL strength and ACL tear susceptibility during the menstrual cycle [97,98]. Such research could have important implications for injury prevention. Because oral contraceptives typically expose women to less hormonal fluctuation and less estrogen than women cycling naturally, investigators are also examining a possible protective role for oral contraceptives. A clear relationship has yet to be established [99].

Research in the area of gender differences in ACL injuries has proven to be very challenging. When future research refines our understanding of predisposition to ACL injuries, risk factors might be modified to reduce both men's and women's risk of rupture.

B. Stress Fractures

Stress fractures were originally described in the 1800s in the feet of marching soldiers. Formerly called march fractures, stress fractures are an overuse injury of the bone. Bones can fatigue and develop microfractures in response to prolonged repetitive loads. Stress fractures can occur when these forces override the bone's ability to remodel and repair. Today, stress fractures are common diagnoses. They can be seen in participants of any sporting activity, although most commonly in runners, in whom they account for 5 to 15% of all running injuries [100]. Symptoms include sharp, localized pain that increases with activity. Pain may improve with rest, but in severe cases rest pain may also be present. On physical examination, point tenderness is found. Palpation may reveal an irregular bone surface and pain referred back to the fracture area on percussion of a more distant site.

For both men and women, stress fractures most often occur in the weight-bearing bones of the lower extremity, with the lower third of the tibia being the most typical location [101]. However, stress fracture rates in women are higher than in men. Studies of women in organized and recreational sports demonstrate about 3.5 times a man's risk [102–104]. In data from military recruits, women have been reported to have up to 12 times greater risk [105,106]. Inadequate conditioning was initially blamed for this discrepancy. Further research has shown that stress fracture cause is dependent on the numerous factors that shift the dynamic between bone reabsorption and regeneration [107].

An athlete's genetics, bone density, internal hormonal environment, biomechanics, nutritional status, and training program are the key players in this dynamic. When muscles fatigue, they alter the way forces load bones. Weak muscles are less able to absorb or divert forces away from neighboring bones. Biomechanical factors such as leg length discrepancies, tibial torsion, external rotation at the hip, and excessive foot pronation or supination can predispose to stress fracture by asymmetrically loading forces to the lower extremity. Other mitigating issues arise from dietary insufficiencies and errors with training and equipment. A new activity or a sudden increase in intensity, duration, or frequency of an activity can have a major impact on stress fracture development [108]. Infrequent changes in footwear and unforgiving activity surfaces add more stress to bone, and insufficient rest time between workouts thwarts the body's reparative efforts. Although Wolff's law teaches that bone has the ability to actively remodel in response to stress, subclinical bone injuries can become symptomatic with insufficient recovery periods.

Women's status as a high-risk population for stress fractures is in part secondary to the prevalence of irregular menses and disordered eating [109]. In one study, athletes who had had oligomenorrhea were six times as likely to have a history of a stress fracture, whereas those who said they watched their weight were eight times as likely [110]. Treatment in such individuals involves addressing disordered eating and menstrual irregularities in addition to significant reductions in activities or substitution of sports. Return to sports is made on an individual basis, usually after evidence of clinical and radiographic healing is present.

C. Patellofemoral Stress Syndrome

The patella, a sesamoid bone within the quadriceps tendon, articulates with the trochlear groove of the distal femur at the patellofemoral joint. This complex joint is the source of many knee complaints especially in active individuals. Patellofemoral stress syndrome (PFSS) is a general name for poorly localized anterior knee pain arising from the knee extensor mechanism, without another concrete diagnosis such as patellar instability or patellar tendonitis. It is one of the leading causes of anterior knee pain and is more common in women [111,112].

The anterior knee pain of PFSS is characteristically increased with activities that increase patellofemoral compressive and rotational forces such as stair climbing and squatting. Prolonged periods of knee flexion, such as long car rides or movies, can exacerbate knee pain and stiffness. The pain is usually bilateral, associated with activity, and minimal at rest. The physical examination frequently finds hamstring inflexibility, underdeveloped quadriceps musculature, tender patellar facets, and pain with forced patellar compression.

The cause of this vague anterior knee pain is poorly understood and may have multiple origins. Because women incur PFSS more commonly than men, there has been much speculation as to which female predominant anatomic or biologic factors cause patellofemoral pain. Pes planus (flat feet), large Q-angles, femoral anteversion, global hip weakness, and tightness of the iliotibial band and hamstring are all implicated because of their tendency to create lateral and rotational forces on the patella [113]. Interestingly, many patients with malpositioned knees do not experience any pain. To date, no single biomechanical factor has been shown to be a primary cause of PFSS, and studies have not consistently shown biomechanical or alignment differences between patients with and without PFSS [114]. Leading hypotheses suggest that symptoms stem from abnormal joint loading produced by the combination of factors related to joint alignment, surrounding soft tissues, neuromuscular control, and functional demands [115,116].

Patellofemoral stress syndrome may present with or without lower extremity and patellar malalignment. X-rays can be helpful in demonstrating if the patella is tilted or subluxed relative to the femur's trochlear groove, but they are most often normal. X-rays show static relationships but are of limited value as they fail to assess the dynamic relationship of anatomic and neuromuscular factors affecting the knee [117]. When PFSS is accompanied by significant malalignment, patients are often described as having "miserable malalignment syndrome." This well-known combination of femoral anteversion, increased Q-angle, tibio-femoral valgus, external tibial torsion, and subtalar pronation (see Fig. 98-1) is thought to add joint stress from the foot to the hip and contribute to lower extremity injury [118]. The constellation of issues also predisposes to lateral patellar subluxation [119]. It seems that athletes of either sex whose joints show straighter alignment tend to sustain fewer injuries [120].

Neuromuscular rehabilitation is the cornerstone of treatment for PFS. Hamstring and iliotibial band stretching and quadriceps strengthening are central to the therapy. These practices are designed help with patellar tracking by decreasing the forces directing the patella laterally and increasing the medial pull [121]. Patellar taping, knee sleeves, and orthotics can be helpful adjuncts. Surgery is rarely indicated, and most patients with PFSS respond to nonoperative treatment.

V. Conclusion

In general, sports injuries are more closely tied to sporting activity than one's sex. However, there are certain patterns of illness and injury in athletic individuals that seem to have a gender-specific predisposition. Practitioners should strive to appreciate these issues to improve their knowledge base and skills related to injury diagnosis, treatment, and prevention of sports injuries for both men and women.

VI. Suggestions for Further Investigations

- Current lawsuits are challenging Title IX as effectively discriminating against men. What does the future hold for Title IX?
- What is the effect of the menstrual cycle on athletic injuries?
- Could a hormone pill be created to enhance ACL strength?

References

1. www.ncaa.org (accessed 4/16/03).
2. www.ncaa.org/library/research (accessed 4/16/03).
3. www.ncaa.org/library/research (accessed 4/16/03).
4. DeHaven KE, Lintner DM. (1986). Athletic injuries: Comparison by age, sport, and gender. Am J Sport Med. 14:218–224.

5. Clarke KS, Buckley WE. (1980). Women's injuries in collegiate sports: A preliminary comparative overview of three seasons. *Am J Sports Med.* 8:187–191.

6. DeHaven KE, Lintner DM. (1986). Athletic injuries: Comparison by age, sport, and gender. *Am J Sport Med.* 14:218–224.

7. Greydanus DE, Patel D. (2002). The female athlete. Before and beyond puberty. *Pediatr Clin North Am.* 49:553–580.

8. Carbon RJ. (1992). The Female Athlete. In *Textbook of Science and Sports Medicine* (Bloomfield J, Fricker PA, Fitch KD, eds.), pp. 467–487. Champaign, IL: Human Kinetics Books.

9. Sanborn CF, Jankowski CM. (1994). Gender Specific Physiology. In *Medical and Orthopaedic Issues of the Active and Athletic Woman* (Agostini R, ed.), pp. 23–27. Philadelphia: Hanley and Belfus.

10. Carbon RJ. (1992). The Female Athlete. In *Textbook of Science and Sports Medicine* (Bloomfield J, Fricker PA, Fitch KD, eds.), pp. 467–487. Champaign, IL: Human Kinetics Books.

11. Arnheim D. (1989). *Modern Principles of Athletic Training*, 7th Edition. San Diego, CA: Mosby.

12. Pink MM, Jobe FW. (1997). The Foot Shoe Interface. In *Running Injuries* (Guten GN, ed.), pp. 20–29. Philadelphia: WB Saunders.

13. Griffin LY. (1994). Orthopedic Concerns. In *Women and Exercise: Physiology and Sports Medicine* (Shangold MM, Mirkin G, eds.), pp. 234–260. Philadelphia: FA Davis.

14. Holloway JB. (1994). Individual Differences and Their Implications for Resistance Training. In *Essentials of Strength Training and Conditioning* (Baechle TR, ed.), pp. 151–162. Champaign, IL: Human Kinetics.

15. Cureton KJ, Collins MA, Hill DW *et al.* (1988). Muscle hypertrophy in men and women. *Med Sci Sports Exerc.* 20:338–344.

16. Cureton KJ, Collins MA, Hill DW *et al.* (1988). Muscle hypertrophy in men and women. *Med Sci Sports Exerc.* 20:338–344.

17. Carbon RJ. (1992). The Female Athlete. In *Textbook of Science and Sports Medicine* (Bloomfield J, Fricker PA, Fitch KD, eds.), pp. 467–487. Champaign, IL: Human Kinetics Books.

18. Hakkinen K, Pakarinen A, Kyrolainen H *et al.* (1990). Neuromuscular adaptations and serum hormones in females during prolonged power training. *Int J Sport Med.* 11(2):91–98.

19. Wells CL. (1991). *Women, Sport and Performance*, 2nd Edition, pp. 3–34. Champaign, IL: Human Kinetics.

20. Sanborn CF, Jankowski CM. (1994). Gender Specific Physiology. In *Medical and Orthopaedic Issues of the Active and Athletic Woman* (Agostini R, ed.), pp. 23–27. Philadelphia: Hanley and Belfus.

21. Wells CL. (1991). *Women, Sport and Performance*, 2nd Edition, pp. 3–34. Champaign, IL: Human Kinetics.

22. Wells CL. (1991). *Women, Sport and Performance*, 2nd Edition, pp. 3–34. Champaign, IL: Human Kinetics.

23. Lebrun CM. (1994). Effects of Menstrual Cycle and Birth Control Pills on Athletic Performance. In *Medical and Orthopaedic Issues of the Active and Athletic Woman* (Agostini R, ed.), pp. 78–91. Philadelphia: Hanley and Belfus.

24. Sanborn CF, Jankowski CM. (1994). Gender Specific Physiology. In *Medical and Orthopaedic Issues of the Active and Athletic Woman* (Agostini R, ed.), pp. 23–27. Philadelphia: Hanley and Belfus.

25. Baechle TR. (1984). Women in resistance training. *Clin Sport Med.* 3:791–880.

26. Sanborn CF, Jankowski CM. (1994). Gender Specific Physiology. In *Medical and Orthopaedic Issues of the Active and Athletic Woman* (Agostini R, ed.), pp. 23–27. Philadelphia: Hanley and Belfus.

27. Griffin LY. (1994). Orthopedic Concerns. In *Women and Exercise: Physiology and Sports Medicine* (Shangold MM, Mirkin G, eds.), pp. 234–260. Philadelphia: FA Davis.

28. Yeager KK, Agostini R, Nattiv A *et al.* (1993). The female athlete triad: Disordered eating, amenorrhea, osteoporosis. *Med Sci Sports Exerc.* 25:775–777.

29. Ise CL. (2002). Amenorrhea in the Adolescent Athlete. In *Pediatric Sports Medicine for Primary Care* (Birrer RB, Griesemer BA, Cataletto MB, eds.), pp. 160–170. Philadelphia: Lippincott Williams & Wilkins.

30. Otis CL, Drinkwater B, Johnson M *et al.* (1997). American College of Sports Medicine position stand. The female athlete triad. *Med Sci Sports Exerc.* 19:I–IX.

31. Hobart JA. (2000). The female athlete triad. *Am Fam Physician.* 61:3357–3364.

32. Nattiv A, Lynch L. (1994). The female athlete triad. *Phys Sports Med.* 22:60–68.

33. Sullivan PF. (1995). Mortality in anorexia nervosa. *Am J Psychiatry.* 152:1073–1074.

34. Johnson MD. (1994). Disordered Eating. In *Medical and Orthopaedic Issues of the Active and Athletic Woman* (Agostini R, ed.), pp. 141–151. Philadelphia: Hanley and Belfus.

35. Dale KS, Landers DM. (1999). Weight control in wrestling: Eating disorders or disordered eating. *Med Sci Sports Exerc.* 31:1382–1389.

36. Lebrun CM. (1994). Effects of Menstrual Cycle and Birth Control Pills on Athletic Performance. In *Medical and Orthopaedic Issues of the Active and Athletic Woman* (Agostini R, ed.), pp. 78–91. Philadelphia: Hanley and Belfus.

37. Burrows M, Bird S. (2000). The physiology of the highly trained female endurance runner. *Sports Med.* 30:281–300.

38. DeCree C. (1998) Sex steroid metabolism and menstrual irregularities in the exercising female: A review. *Sports Med.* 25:369–406.

39. Loucks AB, Callister R. (1993). Induction and prevention of low-T3 syndrome in exercising women. *Am J Physiol.* 264:R924–30.

40. Ise CL. (2002). Amenorrhea in the Adolescent Athlete. In *Pediatric Sports Medicine for Primary Care* (Birrer RB, Griesemer BA, Cataletto MB, eds.), pp. 160–170. Philadelphia: Lippincott Williams & Wilkins.

41. Frankovich RJ, Lebrun CM. (2000). Menstrual cycle, contraception and performance. *Clin Sports Med.* 19:251–271.

42. Lebrun CM. (1994). Effects of Menstrual Cycle and Birth Control Pills on Athletic Performance. In *Medical and Orthopaedic Issues of the Active and Athletic Woman* (Agostini R, ed.), pp. 78–91. Philadelphia: Hanley and Belfus.

43. Drinkwater BL, Nilson K, Chestnut CH III *et al.* (1994). Bone mineral content of amenorrheic and eumenorrheic athletes. *N Engl J Med.* 311:277–281.

44. Otis CL, Drinkwater B, Johnson M *et al.* (1997). American College of Sports Medicine position stand. The female athlete triad. *Med Sci Sports Exerc.* 19:I–IX.

45. Drinkwater BL, Bruemner B, Chesnut CH III. (1996). Menstrual history a determinant of current bone density in young athletes. *JAMA.* 276:238–240.

46. Melton LJ 3rd. (1997). Epidemiology of spinal osteoporosis. *Spine.* 22(Suppl 24): 2S–11S.

47. Yeager KK, Agostini R, Nattiv A *et al.* (1993). The female athlete triad: Disordered eating, amenorrhea, osteoporosis. *Med Sci Sports Exerc.* 25: 775–777.

48. Hergenroeder AC, Smith EO, Shypailo R *et al.* (1997). Bone mineral changes in young women with hypothalamic amenorrhea treated with oral contraceptives, medroxyprogesterone, or placebo over 12 months. *Am J Obstet Gynecol.* 176:1017–1025.

49. Jonnavithula S, Warren MP, Fox RP *et al.* (1993). Bone density is compromised in amenorrheic women despite return of menses: A 2-year study. *Obstet Gynecol.* 81:669–674.

50. ACOG Committee on Obstetric Practice. (2002). Exercise during pregnancy and the postpartum period, Committee Opinion No. 267. *Int J Gynaecol Obstet.* 77:79–81.

51. Clapp JF 3rd. (2000). Exercise during pregnancy: A clinical update. *Clin Sport Med.* 19:273–286.

52. Clapp JF 3rd. (2000). Beginning regular exercise in early pregnancy: Effect on fetoplacental growth. *Am J Obstet Gynecol.* 183:1484–1488.

53. Bell RJ, Palma SM, Lumley JM. (1995). The effect of vigorous exercise during pregnancy on birth weight. *Aust N Z J Obstet Gynaecol.* 35:46–51.

54. Kardel KR, Kase T. (1998). Training in pregnant women: Effects on fetal development and birth. *Am J Obstet Gynecol.* 178:280–286.

55. Clapp JF 3rd, Dickstein S. (1984). Endurance exercise and pregnancy outcome. *Med Sci Sports Exerc.* 16:556–562.

56. Artel R, O'Toole M. (2003). Guidelines of ACOG for exercise during pregnancy and the postpartum period. *Br J Sport Med.* 37:6–12.

57. ACOG Committee on Obstetric Practice. (2002). Exercise during pregnancy and the postpartum period, Committee Opinion No. 267. *Int J Gynaecol Obstet.* 77:79–81.

58. Dye TD, Knox KL, Artal R *et al.* (1997). Physical activity, obesity and diabetes in pregnancy. *Am J Epidemiology.* 146:961–965.

59. Lokey EA, Tran ZV, Wells CL *et al.* (1991). Effects of physical exercise on pregnancy outcomes: A meta-analytic review. *Med Sci Sports Exerc.* 23:1234–1239.

60. Henriksen TB, Hedegaard M, Secher NJ, Wilkcox AJ. (1995). Standing at work and preterm delivery. *Br J Obstet Gynaecol.* 102:198–206.

61. Clapp JF 3rd. (1990). The course of labor after endurance exercise during pregnancy. *Am J Obstet Gynecol.* 163:1799–1805.

62. Clapp JF 3rd. (1989). The effects of maternal exercise on early pregnancy outcome. *Am J Obstet Gynecol.* 161:1453–1457.

63. Clapp JF 3rd, Lopez B, Harcar-Sevcik R. (1999). Neonatal behavioral profile of the offspring of women who continued to exercise regularly throughout pregnancy. *Am J Obstet Gynecol.* 180:91–94.

64. Camporesi EM. (1996). Diving and pregnancy. *Semin Perinatol.* 20:292–302.

65. Haycock CE. (1994). The Breast. In *Women and Exercise*: *Physiology and Sports Medicine* (Shangold MM, Mirkin G, eds.) pp. 217–222. Philadelphia: FA Davis.

66. Loud KJ, Micheli LJ. (2001). Common athletic injuries in adolescent girls. *Curr Opin Pediatr*. 13:317–322.

67. Haycock CE. (1994). The Breast. In *Women and Exercise*: *Physiology and Sports Medicine* (Shangold MM, Mirkin G, eds.) pp. 217–222. Philadelphia: FA Davis.

68. Haycock CE. (1994). The Breast. In *Women and Exercise*: *Physiology and Sports Medicine* (Shangold MM, Mirkin G, eds.) pp. 217–222. Philadelphia: FA Davis.

69. Greydanus DE, Patel DR, Baxter TL. (1998). The breast and sports: Issues for the clinician. *Adolesc Med State Art Rev*. 9:533–550.

70. Nequin ND. (1978). More on jogger's ailments. *N Engl J Med*. 298:405–406.

71. Greydanus DE, Patel DR, Baxter TL. (1998). The breast and sports: Issues for the clinician. *Adolesc Med State Art Rev*. 9:533–550.

72. Powell B. (1983). Bicyclist's nipples. *JAMA*. 249:2457.

73. Thune I, Brenn T, Lund E *et al*. (1997). Physical activity and the risk of breast cancer. *N Engl J Med*. 336:269–275.

74. Friedenreich CM, Rohan TE. (1995). A review of physical activity and breast cancer. *Epidemiology*. 6:311–317.

75. Sherman MF, Warren RF, Marshall JL, Savatsky GJ. (1988). A clinical and radiographic analysis of 127 ACL insufficient knees. *Clin Orthop*. 227:229–237.

76. Ardent E, Dick R. (1995). Knee injury patterns among men and women in collegiate basketball and soccer: Data and review of the literature. *Am J Sports Med*. 23:694–701.

77. Malone T, Hardaker W, Garrett W *et al*. (1992). Relationship of gender to anterior cruciate ligament injuries in intercollegiate basketball players. *J South Orthop Assoc*. 2:36–39.

78. Griffin LY, Agel J, Albohm MJ *et al*. (2000). Noncontact anterior cruciate ligament injuries: Risk factors and prevention strategies. *JAAOS*. 8(3):141–150.

79. Nicholas JA. (1970). Injuries to knee ligaments: Relationship to looseness and tightness in football players. *JAMA*. 212:2236–2239.

80. Lars-Goran L, Baum J, Mudholkar GS. (1987). Hypermobility: Features and differential incidence between the sexes. *Arthritis Rheum*. 30:1426–1430.

81. Daniel D, Malcom L, Losse G *et al*. (1983). Instrumented measurement of ACL disruption. *Orthop Trans*. 7:585–586.

82. Weesner CL, Albolim MJ, Ritter MA. (1986). A comparison of anterior and posterior cruciate ligament laxity between female and male basketball players. *Phys Sports Med*. 14(5):149–154.

83. Harner CD, Paulos LE, Greenwald AE *et al*. (1994). Detailed analysis of patients with bilateral anterior cruciate ligament injuries. *Am J Sports Med*. 22:37–43.

84. Norwood LA Jr, Cross MJ. (1977). The intercondylar shelf and the anterior cruciate ligament. *Am J Sports Med*. 5:171–176.

85. Griffin LY, Agel J, Albohm MJ *et al*. (2000). Noncontact anterior cruciate ligament injuries: Risk factors and prevention strategies. *JAAOS*. 8(3):141–150.

86. Ardent E, Dick R. (1995). Knee injury patterns among men and women in collegiate basketball and soccer: Data and review of the literature. *Am J Sports Med*. 23:694–701.

87. Hutchinson M, Ireland ML. (1985). Knee injuries in female athletes. *Sports Med*. 19:288–302.

88. Gray JE, Tauton DC. (1985). A survey of injuries to the anterior cruciate ligament of the knee in female basketball players. *Int J Sports Med*. 6:314–316.

89. Lambson RB, Barnhill BS, Higgins RW. (1996). Football cleat design and its effect on anterior cruciate ligament injuries: A three-year prospective study. *Am J Sports Med*. 24:155–159.

90. Huston LJ, Wojtys EM. (1996). Neuromuscular performance characteristics in elite female athletes. *Am J Sports Med*. 24:427–436.

91. Putnam CA. (1993). Sequential motions of body segments in striking and throwing skills: Descriptions and explanations. *J Biomech*. 26:125–135.

92. Hewett TE, Stroupe AL, Nance TA *et al*. (1996). Plyometric training in female athletes: Decreased impact forces and increased hamstring torques. *Am J Sports Med*. 24:765–773.

93. Hewett TE, Lindenfeld TN, Riccobene JV, Noyes FR. (1996). The effect of neuromuscular training on the incidence of knee injury in female athletes: A prospective study. *Am J Sports Med*. 27:699–706.

94. Griffin LY, Agel J, Albohm MJ *et al*. (2000). Noncontact anterior cruciate ligament injuries: Risk factors and prevention strategies. *JAAOS*. 8(3):141–150.

95. Liu SH, A1-Shaikh RA, Panossian V *et al*. (1997). Estrogen affects the cellular metabolism of the anterior cruciate ligament: A potential explanation for female athletic injury. *Am J Sports Med*. 25:704–709.

96. Liu SH, A1-Shaikh RA, Panossian V *et al*. (1997). Estrogen affects the cellular metabolism of the anterior cruciate ligament: A potential explanation for female athletic injury. *Am J Sports Med*. 25:704–709.

97. Heitz NA, Eisenman PA, Beck CL, Walker JA. (1999). Hormonal changes throughout the menstrual cycle and increased anterior cruciate ligament laxity in females. *J Athletic Training*. 34:144–149.

98. Slauterbeck, JR, Hardy DM. (2001). Sex hormones and knee ligament injuries in female athletes. *Am J Med Sci*. 322:196–199.

99. Toth AP, Cordasco FA. (2001). Anterior cruciate ligament injuries in the female athlete. 4(4):25–34.

100. Burr DB. (1997). Bone, exercise and stress fractures. *Exerc Sport Sci Rev*. 25:171–194.

101. Leach RE, Zecher SB. (1997). Stress Fractures. In *Running Injuries* (Guten GN, ed.), pp. 30–46. Philadelphia: WB Saunders.

102. Nattiv A, Armsey TD Jr. (1997). Stress injury to bone in the female athlete. *Clin Sports Med*. 16:197–224.

103. Matheson GO, Clement DB, McKenzie DC *et al*. (1987). Stress fractures in athletes. *Am J Sports Med*. 15:46–58.

104. Burr DB. (1997). Bone, exercise and stress fractures. *Exerc Sport Sci Rev*. 25:171–194.

105. Milgrom C, Giladi M, Stein M *et al*. (1985). Stress fractures in military recruits: A prospective study showing an unusually high incidence. *J Bone Joint Surg (Br)*. 67:732–735.

106. Greaney RB, Gerber FH, Laughlin RL *et al*. (1983). Distribution and natural history of stress fractures in U.S. Marine recruits. *Radiology*. 146:339–346.

107. Griffin LY. (2003). The Female Athlete. In *DeLee and Drez's Orthopaedic Sports Medicine*: *Principles and Practice*, 2nd Edition (DeLee JC, ed.), pp. 505–520. Philadelphia: Elsevier Science.

108. Arendt EA. (2000). Stress fractures and the female athlete. *Clin Orthop*. 372:131–138.

109. Myburgh K, Hutchins J, Fataar AB *et al*. (1990). Low bone density is an etiologic factor for stress factors in athletes. *Ann Intern Med*. 113:754–759.

110. Bennell KL, Malcolm SA, Thomas SA *et al*. (1995). Risk factors for stress fractures in female track-and-field athletes: A retrospective analysis. *Clin J Sport Med*. 5:229–235.

111. Yates C, Grana WA. (1986). Patellofemoral pain: A prospective study. *Orthopedics*. 9:663–667.

112. Griffin LY. (1994). Orthopedic Concerns. In *Women and Exercise*: *Physiology and Sports Medicine* (Shangold MM, Mirkin G, eds.), pp. 234–260. Philadelphia: FA Davis.

113. Natri A, Kannus P, Jarvinen, M. (1998). Which factors predict the long-term outcome in chronic patellofemoral pain syndrome? A 7-yr prospective follow-up study. *Med Sci Sports Exerc*. 30:1572–1577.

114. Thomee R, Renstrom P, Karlsson J, Grimby G. (1995). Patellofemoral pain syndrome in young women. I. A clinical analysis of alignment, pain parameters, common symptoms and functional activity level. *Scand J Med Sci Sports*. 5:237–44.

115. Post WR, Teitge R, Amis A. (2002). Patellofemoral malalignment: Looking beyond the viewbox. *Clin Sports Med*. 21:521–546.

116. Fredericson M, Powers CM. (2002). Practical management of patellofemoral pain. *Clin J Sports Med*. 12:36–38.

117. Fredericson M, Powers CM. (2002). Practical management of patellofemoral pain. *Clin J Sports Med*. 12:36–38.

118. Arendt E. (1994). Knee Injuries. In *Medical and Orthopaedic Issues of the Active and Athletic Woman* (Agostini R, ed.), pp. 307–315. Philadelphia: Hanley and Belfus.

119. Theut PC, Fulkerson JP. (2003). Anterior Knee Pain and Patellar Subluxation in the Adult. In *DeLee and Drez's Orthopaedic Sports Medicine: Principles and Practice*, 2nd Edition (DeLee JC, ed.), pp. 1772–1815. Philadelphia: Elsevier Science.

120. Guten GN. (1997). Overview of leg injuries in running. In *Running Injuries* (Guten GN, ed.), pp. 61–92. Philadelphia: WB Saunders.

121. Theut PC, Fulkerson JP. (2003). Anterior Knee Pain and Patellar Subluxation in the Adult. In *DeLee and Drez's Orthopaedic Sports Medicine: Principles and Practice*, 2nd Edition (DeLee JC, ed.), pp. 1772–1815. Philadelphia: Elsevier Science.

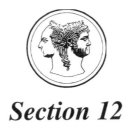

Section 12

IMMUNOLOGY/RHEUMATOLOGY

Robert G. Lahita, MD, PhD

Chairman of Medicine, Jersey City Medical Center; Professor of Medicine, Mount Sinai School of Medicine, Jersey City, NJ

I. Gender and the Immune System

Sex steroids play an important role in the maturation of organ systems that affect animals throughout life and therefore important to the health of most vertebrates. Although the most obvious effects occur at puberty in the development of secondary sexual characteristics, hormones affect major developmental changes even before parturition. Diverse biologic functions including behavior, intelligence, sexual preference, physical stature, and the immune system are likely targets for these hormones. The effects of sex steroids on the immune system are profound and longlasting because they control the maturation of various cell systems and may influence susceptibility to disease through modulation of immune cell populations throughout the life of the animal. This might happen through alteration of cytokine levels, control of cell populations through processes such as apoptosis, or alteration of very basic molecular mechanisms. Lupus is one disease that is very affected by hormones because the skew toward females is so great.

Most of the autoimmune diseases have a predilection for women. The reason for this predilection is not known. A variety of theories have been proposed and some are related to the metabolism of sex hormones, which have been studied in diseases such as systemic lupus erythematosus (SLE) or rheumatoid arthritis. Molecular ideas for this predilection as well as the current views about sexual dimorphism are given throughout this section.

This section will deal with the effects of sex on the immune system. These effects are anything but subtle. The molecular mechanisms likely to be involved in the work of sex steroids on immune function are delivered in Chapter 100 by Gary Kammer. Although no specific anomaly can be responsible for all effects on immune disease, you will see that sex has a significant effect on basic molecular mechanisms. In Chapter 99, Virginia Rider

and Nabih Abdou discuss the dimorphic sexual nature of the immune response, a topic not readily understood. Topics such as the synthesis of immunoglobulin, the varying classes of immune cells, and the response to antigens for different genders are discussed. Gender and tissue transplantation is a particularly interesting chapter. The issue of liver failure provides one example of the importance of gender and transplantation. Hilary Sanfey provokes our interest in this different approach to gender and the immune system in Chapter 103. The influence of male and female metabolism and the various changes of sex steroid metabolism in diseased patients are reported here in the hope that they might explain the change of activity within a disease. The primary observation—that there are metabolic differences within certain autoimmune diseases—is important. The etiologies of these diseases are unknown but are affected by sex hormones. Pregnancy is discussed by Anne Parke in Chapter 102. This is a special time for women with immune disease and in many instances is a time of remission. This is certainly the case for many women with rheumatoid arthritis and multiple sclerosis. We get insight into the possible mechanisms from her writing. The immune system is affected by gonadotrophins as well as sex steroids and is also covered in a brilliant chapter by Sara Walker (Chapter 104). The overall prevalence and incidence of the autoimmune diseases may be affected by gender or genetically influenced factors that have little to do with sex hormones.

Sex steroids are potent modulators of immunity in all animal systems. They are very important in patients with SLE and might help to explain the fluctuant activity in the disease lupus. Their role in the maturation of the immune system and their effect on the development of organs such as the brain could explain some of the abnormalities found in these systems.

99

Sexual Dimorphism and the Immune System

VIRGINIA RIDER, PhD* AND NABIH I. ABDOU, MD, PhD**

*Department of Biology, Pittsburg State University, Pittsburg, KS
**Center of Rheumatic Diseases, Allergy-Immunology, Kansas City, MO

Abstract

Evidence suggests that sex differences extend beyond the reproductive system and include sex-dependent differences in the cardiovascular, neural, and immune systems. This chapter reviews some differences in immune responses between males and females. In particular, this chapter focuses on the role of hormones as modulators of the immune response and their possible role in autoimmunity. Sex steroid hormone receptors have been identified in most cells comprising the immune system. However, the function of sex hormone receptors, working through their specific immune system gene targets, has not been widely explored. Systemic lupus erythematosus (SLE) is a gender-biased autoimmune disease with female predominance. The evidence for sex hormone influence on this disease is compelling, and new studies provide clues about the underlying mechanisms by which sex hormones may influence the development or progression of this prototypic autoimmune disease. Sex steroids have been shown to regulate the expression of genes that play critical roles in the adaptive immune response, including programmed cell death, cell proliferation, and signal transduction. Moreover, the evidence now emerging suggests that sex hormones can affect both lymphocyte development and influence mature lymphocytes in circulation. Sex differences that are relevant to human health and disease are not only dependent on sex but also are influenced by complex interactions between genetics and the environment. The future challenge is to develop a better understanding of the nature of these interactions and to identify the differences between the sexes that are consequential for human health.

I. Introduction

Differences between the sexes in the prevalence and severity of diseases and disorders have long been suspected but not well-documented. Humans are considered to be dimorphic with regard to sex because an individual can be chromosomally XX and female or XY and male. Gender, however, is more of a continuum, and a person's sense of gender may change during the individual's lifetime [1]. In 2001 a panel of experts determined that understanding sex differences in health and disease is important because the sex-based differences that are known seriously affect human health [1]. Moreover, the panel anticipated that additional differences remain to be uncovered. The purpose of this chapter is to review the current knowledge of sex hormones and their effects on the immune system.

This chapter highlights some differences in the immune system between the sexes; however, there is increasing evidence that sexual dimorphism could play a major role in cardiovascular, neurologic, and psychologic disorders [1]. The epidemiology of sex-discrepant illnesses [2], and most notably autoimmune diseases [3], arises from complex interactions between biology and behavior. In 1994, the average life expectancy at birth was 79 years for females and 72.3 years for males. This sex difference in mortality that favored women over men increased steadily from the 1900s until the 1970s. However, despite the advantage for sex-based longevity, women generally perceive themselves to be less healthy and report higher rates of most acute and chronic conditions than men [2]. Women report more problems with major depressive disorders, anxiety, musculoskeletal function disorders, eating disorders [2], and autoimmune diseases [3]. Men, however, report higher rates of alcohol and drug abuse and antisocial personality. These gender differences persist across race and different levels of income, education, and occupation [2].

We highlight the major differences between males and females with respect to the normal immune system and suggest how sex hormones may contribute to the induction or progression of autoimmune diseases. To maintain the focus on human health we have emphasized human-related studies, although pertinent animal data are mentioned briefly. It will be apparent from the literature that evaluating differences in the levels of sex steroids in circulation in health and disease has not clarified the potential mechanisms by which sex hormones influence the immune system. Moreover, difficulties in understanding the influence of sex hormones on the immune system are complicated by studies that have not considered menstrual cycle–dependent hormonal fluctuations and have not taken into account that study participants may use sex hormones for prevention of osteoporosis, for sexual dysfunction, or for infertility in the form of "over-the-counter supplements." Despite these limitations, however, understanding the gene targets of hormones and their receptors on the immune system and assessing how endocrine-immune interactions function in health and disease may provide new insight into the pathogenesis of some diseases. As will become evident in this chapter, steroid hormone receptors have been identified in most of the cells mediating the immune response. Localization of hormone receptors to immunomodulatory cells has opened new opportunities to identify the gene targets in these cells and to assess the molecular mechanisms by which sex hormones participate in stimulating or suppressing specific immune responses. Importantly, increased understanding about the differences of sex hormone action on the immune system between men and women may lead to the development of novel and specific interventions in the treatment of a variety of human disorders.

Innate and immune-specific responses are sexually dimorphic regarding both the magnitude and the type of response [4]. Females in general mount a greater immune response to antigens and display more vigorous cell-mediated immunity than males. In animal models, and in humans, females are more likely to develop T-helper type 1 (Th1-type) proinflammatory responses except during pregnancy, where the Th2 antiinflammatory response is the predominant arm of the immune system [5,6]. Although studies suggest that sex-based differences in the synthesis and secretion of a variety of hormones, including the sex steroids, may contribute to biologic differences between the sexes, it is still not clear how sex steroids, pituitary hormones, prolactin, or growth hormone exert these sex-based effects on the immune response [4,7].

II. Sexual Dimorphism and the Immune Response

A. Sexual Dimorphism and Innate Immunity

The ability of the host to resist microbial infection is dependent on many mechanisms including an appropriate physical barrier, phagocytosis, effector killer cells, and various humoral effector factors including the complement system. Innate immunity is an important first line of defense when microbial exposure occurs because it does not require prior sensitization. The innate immune system shows specificity by discriminating between self and non-self and between classes of pathogens. This discrimination is mediated through a class of pattern-recognition receptors (PRRs) that bind conserved pathogen-associated molecular patterns (PAMPs) that are shared by broad classes of microorganisms [8,9]. Adaptive or specific immunity, however, requires prior sensitization, and the response is delayed by a few days after the first exposure of the host to the invading organism. Adaptive immunity is specific in nature, and both cellular factors and immunoglobulins play a role in this type of immune response [10].

The major histocompatability complex (MHC) is a contiguous region of DNA containing multiple loci whose gene products function in discrimination of self versus non-self. The tumor necrosis factor genes (TNF-α, TNF-ß) are located within a cluster of loci that produce complement proteins and are collectively called class III genes. The effect of sex and the human major histocompatability complex (HLA) on innate immunity was recently investigated by an *in vitro* assay in which lipopolysaccharide (LPS)-stimulated whole blood cultures were examined for the production of TNF in culture supernatants. In the LPS assay, females showed a 30% lower innate immune response than males [10]. Moreover, the differences were independent of the HLA region of the TNF locus and the response was independent of plasma estrogen levels. These data suggest that LPS-stimulated TNF production shows substantial sex-related variation, although the factors responsible are not known. Although specific responses, such as LPS-stimulation show sexual dimorphism, males and females do not differ in their response to infection regardless of whether the invading organism is a virus, bacterium, or parasite [1].

B. Sexual Dimorphism and the Adaptive Immune Response

Differences in the adaptive response of the normal immune system, however, exist between males and females [11–13]. Some of these differences include increased serum immunoglobulins, cytokine profiles, and ratio of T-cell subclasses. Women have more immunoglobulin M (IgM) and IgG in their sera, and the ratio of CD4+ to CD8+ T cells is higher in females than in males [13]. In addition, the relative number of circulating CD8+ T cells is lower in some females [13]. These sex-based differences that favor an increase in CD4+ cells in females may provide a partial explanation for the more vigorous antibody response to exogenous antigens that is characteristic of women and ultimately play an important role in either the expression and/or the severity of several autoimmune diseases [7,14,15].

III. Sexual Dimorphism and Autoimmunity

Autoimmune diseases affect a large number of individuals, particularly women, and are an important cause of morbidity [3,11]. Many of these diseases share common mechanisms of pathogenesis arising from abnormal function of T cells, B cells, or T–B cell interactions. These diseases can be classified as organ specific, which includes such disorders as insulin-dependent diabetes mellitus or Hashimoto's thyroiditis, or they can be considered systemic, such as SLE, in which multiple organ systems are affected [16]. Some autoimmune diseases, particularly those involving rheumatic, hepatic, and thyroid disorders, are more prevalent in females [3,4]. The acquisition of some autoimmune diseases differs by sex, and the clinical phenotype of several autoimmune diseases can be sex influenced. For example, female subjects with rheumatoid arthritis have lower incidences of erosive disease and rheumatoid nodules than their male counterparts. Understanding the molecular basis for the predominance of diseases that occur more frequently in one sex, and delineating the underlying molecular basis for sex-specific disease expression, may provide new insights into unsuspected biologic differences between males and females [1]. The most compelling evidence for a link between sex hormones and disease has been established for SLE [7,11,14,15]. SLE is a female-predominant autoimmune disease that affects women more frequently than men. Because the molecular basis for interactions between the endocrine and immune system are emerging, we will highlight studies of SLE as the prototypic human autoimmune disease with female predominance.

A. Genetics, Sexual Dimorphism, and Autoimmunity

Research over the last several years points to the complexity involved in the acquisition of autoimmune diseases [17–23]. Although autoimmune diseases often require a genetic predisposition [23], the disease may not develop, even in genetically susceptible individuals, in the absence of exposure to environmental triggers [24]. Our understanding of the underlying genetic susceptibility in people with SLE has been advanced by analysis of specific genes in animals using transgenic and "knockout" mouse models [21]. Perhaps the most significant findings from such studies is that systemic autoimmunity can be induced by multiple abnormalities, most of which involve genes coding for proteins that control central immune functions including apoptosis, cytokine production, and signal transduction. Although a similar approach cannot be used for the genetic analysis of human autoimmune diseases, the available evidence suggests that SLE disease susceptibility in humans is polygenic, and certain susceptibility genes will be more important in some racial groups than in others [22,23]. The complex interplay between genetics and environmental factors is exemplified by the weak linkage that most of the loci identified in humans show to SLE [23] and the genetic differences in susceptibility among races for this prototypic autoimmune disease [22]. In addition, there does not seem to be a single external trigger for disease onset because a wide variety of seemingly unrelated environmental agents ranging from dietary factors, infectious organisms, and certain drugs and toxins [24] can activate SLE in genetically susceptible individuals.

Despite the limited information gained from characterizing the genes involved in the pathogenesis of human SLE, studies suggest some role for the sex chromosomes in SLE susceptibility. Young males affected with Klinefelter syndrome (XXY genotype) and SLE display a female rather than male estrogen and androgen metabolic pattern [25]. These same patients benefited by treatment with synthetic androgens. Such observations are consistent with the possibility that differential inactivation of the X chromosome may contribute to gender-biased autoimmunity because random X-chromosome inactivation could enhance or diminish the expression of susceptibility gene loci. However, preliminary evidence suggests that X chromosome inactivation, *per se*, does not predispose females to develop SLE [26]. In a small study using five monozygotic twin pairs [26], the pattern of DNA methylation was compared at the CpG region in exon 1 of the androgen receptor gene. The patterns of X-chromosome inactivation were similar between affected and nonaffected twins, suggesting that differences in X-chromosome inactivation (as assessed by DNA methylation) could not account for the development of SLE in one twin versus another [26].

Endocrine influence on the sexual dimorphism of the immune system may arise from a genetic basis for an individual's response to sex hormones. In classical target tissues such as the pituitary gland and female reproductive tract, phenotypic variation in estrogen responsiveness is well established [27–29]. These variations occur in a diverse range of target cell types and include responses that range from the number of eosinophils that infiltrate the uterus [28] to the estrogen-dependent growth of the pituitary [29] and increase in uterine wet weight [27]. Phenotypic variation that is dependent on the genotype of the individual, suggests that the cellular responses to estrogen could be genetically modified. Recent evidence indicates that genetics play a role in the magnitude of the response. By the use of genome exclusion mapping [27], loci have been identified that control the intensity of a target cell's response to the estrogen. Quantitative trait loci that mediate estrogen-dependent responses in classical target cells have been identified by several investigators [27–29]. Although similar loci have yet to be mapped in humans, the possibility that a genetic basis for estrogen responsiveness exists is intriguing and warrants further investigation in humans, particularly in the context of gender-biased autoimmune diseases.

B. Sex Hormones

Sex hormones produced by the ovaries (estrogen, progesterone) and the testes (testosterone, dihydrotestosterone) travel through the bloodstream to affect a variety of target organs. For cells to respond to sex steroids the cells must express specific hormone receptors. Cells that express these receptors have the capacity to respond to the specific ligand (hormone) in circulation. When sex steroids cross the plasma membrane of target cells and bind to their receptor proteins, a conformational change is induced in the hormone-receptor complex. This change, termed transformation, allows the ligand bound receptor to interact with specific regulatory regions along the DNA of target genes and alter the rates of transcription [30]. Although the details of transcriptional regulation vary among the different hormone receptors, the underlying mechanisms that control gene transcription are shared among the members of this supergene family. The androgen [31] and progesterone [32] receptors each arise from a single gene, whereas there are two distinct genes for the estrogen receptor [33] termed estrogen receptor (ER)-α and ER-ß. Estrogens are generally implicated as enhancers of the immune response, whereas androgens and progesterone are considered natural immune suppressors [34,35].

C. Estrogens and the Immune System

Although the targets for estrogen action on immune system function are still under investigation, estrogens could theoretically enhance the immune response by several different mechanisms. Increased levels of hormone in circulation would be expected to enhance estrogenic effects on the immune system. However, in general, levels of estradiol 17-ß are within the normal range between women without and with gender-biased autoimmune diseases, although increased plasma estradiol has been reported in some patients with SLE [36,37]. Most cells involved in the immune response express messenger RNA (mRNA) for both subtypes of the ER; therefore, the absence of one receptor subtype does not seem to be involved in enhancing estrogen influence on the immune system. Peripheral blood mononuclear cells from females [38–41] and males [40] express ER-α and ER-ß transcripts. Our research has shown [38] that ER-α transcripts are found in peripheral blood mononuclear cells from patients with SLE and normal individuals. Furthermore, our data [38] suggest that the peripheral blood T cells and monocytes and B-cell lines obtained from patients with SLE express ER-α transcripts similar to those of normal cells. These findings have been confirmed by Kassi *et al* [41], who found that peripheral blood mononuclear cells of SLE patients with SLE expressed wild-type ER-α, ER-ß, and the same ER-α variants as normal individuals. The identification of both ER subtype transcripts in human T cells suggests that differential sensitivity in response to estrogen could arise by altered action of either ER-α, ER-ß, or in the ratio of the two subtypes (ER-α/ER-ß) in SLE versus normal T cells (Fig. 99-1). This possibility requires further testing. We initially found the concept of alternative splicing of the ER primary transcripts an attractive explanation for increased sensitivity to estrogen action in female SLE T cells. However, our data [38] do not support the postulate that any alternatively spliced variant is preferentially associated with SLE. Moreover,

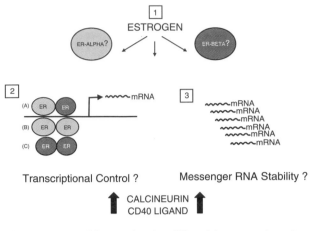

Fig. 99-1 A model proposing that differential estrogen-dependent regulation of T-cell activation markers (calcineurin, CD40 ligand) in systemic lupus erythematosus (SLE) T cells could occur by transcriptional control [panel 2] or messenger RNA (mRNA) stability [panel 3] mechanisms. We have shown [40,102,103,105] that estrogen, acting through the estrogen receptor (ER), increases expression of calcineurin and CD40 ligand in female SLE T cells. Human T cells express both forms (ER-α, ER-ß) of the receptor [38,40]. Differential gene expression of T-cell activation markers could arise by altered ER binding in the form of heterodimers (2A) or homodimers of ER-α (2B) or ER-ß (2C) at the promoter of target genes. Alternatively, estrogen may stabilize calcineurin and CD40 ligand mRNA, thereby prolonging expression of these T-cell activation markers. Both types of regulation may operate to some degree, and further experiments are necessary to resolve the mechanisms involved.

the binding affinity, activity, and quantity of ER-α was not altered in women with lupus [38,39].

The efficacy of estrogen action in target cells is also dependent on the metabolism and turnover of the ligand receptor complex. Estrogen (estradiol 17-ß) metabolism in patients with SLE is disordered, with a skewing toward biologically active metabolites [34,36]. Specifically, the hydroxylation of estrone is favored such that the 16-hydroxylated compounds are more abundant metabolites than the catechol estrogens. The consequence of this altered metabolism could have important consequences because biologically active metabolites may prolong estrogen action on target tissues. Estriol is elevated in women with SLE and men with Klinefelter syndrome, whereas patients of both sexes have increased amounts of 16-α hydroxyestrone. As mentioned earlier, most studies have not found significant differences in the levels of estrogen in circulation in the form of estradiol 17-ß.

Although controversy about the role of estradiol in moderating immune responses exists, several reports [42–44] indicate that flares of SLE may be associated with certain phases of the menstrual cycle and occur more frequently during pregnancy when sex steroid levels in circulation are high. Ovulation induction and *in vitro* fertilization procedures increase estradiol levels and are associated with *de novo* SLE and flares [45]. After menopause, flares of lupus tend to subside and the number of new cases substantially decreases [46]. The safety of oral contraceptives and hormone replacement therapy (HRT) for women with stable or moderate SLE disease is being tested

by The Safety of Estrogens in Lupus Erythematosus-National Assessment [47]. The results from that trial are important because other studies [48] have suggested postmenopausal HRT increases the risk of developing SLE. Furthermore, the latter study [48] suggested that in addition to age- and dose-dependent considerations, the duration of treatment may be a critical factor for women taking exogenous estrogen in the form of HRT.

Because SLE is a systemic disease with different organ involvement, there may be inherent differences among the patients in terms of their response to estrogen. If the molecular basis of estrogen action on the immune system was known, it would be easier to predict an individual's response to exogenous hormone administration. Additional complications in predicting outcomes may arise from inherent differences in the nature of the sex hormone abnormality associated with the individual. As mentioned earlier in this chapter, there could be alterations in steroid metabolism, the dominance of one ER receptor subtype over another (see Fig. 99-1), or changes in other hormones such as prolactin or progesterone that alter and sustain estrogen action on target cells. If these alterations only occur after chronic exposure to the steroid, diagnosis will be further complicated. It seems imperative that increased understanding about regulatory mechanisms, particularly those that alter normal signal transduction events, is necessary to assess inherent differences within complex gender-biased autoimmune diseases. Such an approach is expected to eventually lead to more individualized treatments for patients depending on the nature of the inherent defects.

In animal models, sex differences have been reported [49] in the estrogen-dependent expression of proinflammatory cytokines such as interferon gamma and interleukin-2 (IL-2) in the splenocytes from normal C57BL/6 mice. Increased expression was enhanced in females compared with their male counterparts. In one SLE mouse model, NZB × NZW F1 female mice develop lupus and die at an earlier age than their male counterparts. Administration of exogenous estrogen to those mice enhanced lupus disease pathology and increased anti-DNA antibody levels [50]. Castrated male mice treated with estrogen died at an earlier age than untreated males, whereas survival was prolonged in ovariectomized female mice treated with androgens [50]. Strain-dependent differences in the binding properties of the ER have been reported in the spleen and lymph nodes of adult autoimmune MRL/lpr/lpr (Fas-deficient) mice compared with immature mice. These differences were not detected in non-autoimmune BALB/c mice [51].

It is interesting that the liver tissue in the lupus-prone NZB × NZW F1 female mice contained more ER than liver tissue from males [52]. Although the function of the liver is not known to contribute to autoimmunity, there are changes in the double-negative T-cell (CD4/CD8) populations in the liver. Cytokine changes correlated with autoimmune disease progression and aging in certain mouse models for autoimmune disease [53]. Autoimmune-prone lpr and wild-type mice expressed ER-α in their lymphocytes, whereas ER-ß was predominantly expressed in CD4/CD8 double-negative T cells in the lymph nodes of lpr mice. Both ER subtypes were detected in immature thymic T cells [54]. Although spontaneous and induced autoantibody production was higher in female lpr mice compared with their male counterparts [54], it was unclear if the autoantibody response was estrogen-dependent. Several studies have utilized ER antagonists to investigate if estrogen action is mediated through its receptor protein. Perhaps it is not surprising that the antiestrogens tamoxifen [55] and raloxifene [56] delayed disease progression in both NZB×NZW F1 and MRL lpr/lpr mice, respectively.

Taken together, these data indicate that peripheral blood mononuclear cells and immature T cells express transcripts for both subtypes of the ER. Estrogen enhances disease activity and progression in some human studies as well as in SLE mouse models. Furthermore, the effects of estrogen on peripheral blood mononuclear cells and immature T cells are blocked by the use of ER antagonists. These findings therefore suggest that estrogen, working through its receptor protein, is biologically active in human and rodent T cells and may be an important moderator of the immune response.

B cells are central to the development of lupus in lpr mice [57,58]. Human B-cell lines and murine B cells express ER-α [38,59] and ER-ß [60]. Treatment of transgenic mice carrying an immunoglobulin heavy chain of a pathogenic anti-DNA antibody with estradiol abrogates B-cell tolerance by altering the maturation of splenic B-cell precursors. In addition, estradiol stimulates the expansion of marginal zone B cells in both transgenic and nontransgenic BALB/c mice [61]. The importance of estrogen in B-cell maturation is not limited to females. Male mice lacking ER-α by targeted mutagenesis have smaller thymuses than males with intact receptor [62]. The number of B-lymphocyte subpopulations in male mice lacking the ER is reduced [59], suggesting an important role for the ER in B-cell maturation.

Some of the actions of estradiol on B-cell maturation may be mediated through the peptide hormone prolactin [63]. Prolactin receptors have been identified on T and B lymphocytes [64,65], and increased levels of prolactin in circulation correlate with SLE activity [66–68]. Blocking the secretion of prolactin using bromocriptine, an agent that inhibits prolactin secretion from the pituitary, improved disease in some patients with SLE [69,70] and in female NZB/W mice [71]. Because estradiol acts synergistically with the transcription factor Pit-1 to stimulate the synthesis of prolactin [72], it was possible that the estrogen-dependent effects on B cells could be mediated through prolactin. To explore this possibility, Peeva et al [63] used a transgenic mouse model in which the transgenic mice carried the heavy immunoglobulin chain of a pathogenic anti-DNA antibody. Autoreactive B cells in these transgenic mice did not undergo activation after treatment with estrogen and bromocriptine. However, when the mice were exposed to estrogen alone the B cells were activated, suggesting that bromocriptine could block estrogen-dependent activation, presumably by inhibiting prolactin secretion. IgG deposits in the kidneys of mice treated with both estrogen and bromocriptine were reduced compared with mice treated with estrogen alone, again suggesting that prolactin was at least, in part, mediating the estrogenic effects. There were other estrogen-dependent changes, however, that were not inhibited by bromocriptine and therefore did not involve prolactin. In the same transgenic mice, the enhanced expression of Bcl-2 and the expansion of marginal zone B cells was not blocked by bromocriptine. Thus, it appears that estrogen exerts multiple

effects on B-cell maturation and development, some of which act through prolactin, whereas other effects are prolactin independent [63].

Taken together, the data indicate that lymphocytes express ER-α and ER-ß. The absence of ER by targeted mutagenesis and the use of transgenic mouse models have shown that estrogen exerts biologic effects on the development of T and B cells and on mature lymphocytes in circulation. Although there are no clear and consistent data regarding the mechanisms of estrogen action, ligand-bound sex hormone receptors act as transcription factors. It is reasonable to hypothesize, therefore, that estrogen will alter the regulation of some genes that are involved in the immune response and, thereby, have the potential to contribute to sex differences in the immune system (see Fig. 99-1).

D. Progesterone and the Immune System

Progesterone is credited with being immunosuppressive [73]. Progesterone levels in the circulation of women with SLE may be lower than normal control women [74], and this could potentially lead to more potent estrogen action on target cells. Autoimmune MRL/MP-lpr/lpr mice have an apparent defect in the action of estradiol on progesterone receptor synthesis that was not observed in the nonautoimmune BALB/c mice. It is not clear if that lowered response is characteristic of all autoimmune mouse models or simply reflects strain differences in the mice [51].

During pregnancy, the number of gamma/delta TCR+ cells increase in the peripheral blood of pregnant women [75]. The number of these TCR+ cells is greater in healthy women than in women who have recurrent problems with spontaneous abortions. Most (97%) of the TCR+ lymphocytes express progesterone receptors [75]. The gamma/delta TCR+ cells may play a critical role in the immune response because these cells take up progesterone, which binds to the progesterone receptor and activates the synthesis of a protein called progesterone-induced blocking factor (PIBF). PIBF interferes with the action of phospholipase A2 in the production of arachidonic acid. It is proposed that the inhibition of arachidonic acid through the action of the progesterone receptor leads to the Th2 switch in the immune response that is characteristic of pregnancy [76]. An imbalance, therefore, in the ratio of estrogen and progesterone during pregnancy or the menstrual cycle could contribute to abnormal estrogen action and perhaps a loss of the immunosuppressive effects of progesterone.

Mice lacking the progesterone receptor by targeted mutagenesis display a wide range of abnormalities including sexual behavior, mammary gland development, ovulation, and implantation [77]. More recently, an unsuspected role for progesterone in the development of pre-T cells has been shown [78]. Progesterone action on the stromal cells in the thymus blocked pre-T–cell (CD3-CD44+CD25+) development. Moreover, in the absence of active progesterone receptor, the thymus did not undergo involution. Progesterone receptor expression in the thymus was required for normal fertility because transplants of progesterone receptor negative thymuses to wild-type mice inhibited fertility [78].

Taken together, these studies suggest that female sex hormones (estrogen and progesterone) can influence the development of early lymphocytes as well as their maturation into specific T-cell [78] and B-cell [59,60] subsets in adult animals. These data thus raise the possibility that abnormalities in sex hormone levels or metabolism could alter the developmental lineage of specific T and B cells. The consequences of these alterations could result in either an amplification or downregulation of the immune response.

E. Androgens and the Immune System

Androgens are generally thought to be immunoprotective. Their mechanism of action is similar to estrogen and progesterone in that the two most common androgens, testosterone and dihydrotestosterone, bind to the androgen receptor activating the hormone-receptor complex and altering the rates of transcription of target genes. Although the number of men afflicted with SLE is substantially less than women, men are susceptible to the disease. The levels of testosterone in male patients with SLE range from normal [79] to low [80]. In addition, male patients often have increased levels of gonadotropins [79,80]. It is of interest that gonadotropin-releasing hormone (GnRH) exacerbates SLE in the SWR×NZB F1 lupus mouse model [70]. However, worsening of disease was limited to female mice. The potential involvement of GnRH in human SLE remains to be explored.

The role of androgens in the normal immune system has not been widely studied; therefore the gene targets for this hormone are not known. Androgen receptors are expressed in the lymphoid and nonlymphoid cells of the thymus and bone marrow of mice [81]. Furthermore, androgens, working through the receptor, exert important effects on both T and B lymphocyte development [82]. Both estrogen and androgens influence lymphoid development in male and female mice. The number of B lymphocytes is altered in mice treated with estrogen and dihydrotestosterone [60,83,84]. Antagonism of the ER using ICI 182,780, an ER antagonist that abrogates estrogen action, blocked the estrogen-dependent inhibition of B-cell precursor expansion in culture [60]. Moreover, male mice lacking ER-α by targeted mutagenesis showed fewer cells in all bone marrow B-lymphocyte subpopulations [59]. Chimeric mice, engineered to contain androgen receptor–defective populations of lymphoid or epithelial/stromal cells, showed that it was the thymic epithelial cells and the bone marrow stromal cells that influenced the response to androgens. Androgens, working through the receptor, affected the number of immature B lymphocytes [81]. Furthermore, immature B cells from normal mouse bone marrow were not able to act alone and required marrow stromal cells in culture to respond to androgens [81]. Subsequent analysis revealed that cultured marrow stromal cells produced transforming growth factor-beta (TGF-ß) in response to androgen. Neutralization of TGF-ß with an antibody blocked the suppressive effects of androgen on B-cell number, suggesting that the inhibition of expansion of the bone marrow B-cell population by androgens was controlled by TGF-ß. These data now indicate that at least one candidate gene for androgen action in the immune system is TGF-ß. TGF-ß is known to be immunosuppressive [85,86], and if the regulation of TGF-ß is controlled by the action of the androgen receptor, as suggested from these studies, it could account for the immunoprotective effects accorded to androgens [34,35].

In summary, these studies suggest that sex steroids, acting through their cognate receptors, can exert important effects on the development and maturation of lymphocytes. The evidence—now emerging—suggests that sex hormones not only effect the development of lymphocytes but also can exert influence on mature lymphocytes in circulation. These findings are very exciting because they provide novel opportunities to explore potential differences between the sexes that may be very consequential for human health and disease.

F. Other Hormones and Autoimmunity

We have focused this review specifically on the sex hormones estrogen, progesterone, and androgens as potential candidates for mediating differences between male and female immune systems. However, other hormones besides the gonadal steroids are known to influence the progression of some autoimmune diseases. Prolactin levels increase in about 20% of lupus patients who are younger than age 50 years. However, there has been no consistent finding that increased levels of prolactin positively correlated with disease activity [70]. Bromocriptine, a dopamine agonist that prevents the secretion of prolactin by the anterior pituitary, was shown to have beneficial effects in the NZB/W lupus mouse model [71] and in some patients with lupus whose disease activity is mild or moderate [70]. Although we only mention prolactin briefly, interested readers are referred to excellent reviews on this hormone [70,87,88].

The adrenal steroid hormone dehydroepiandrosterone (DHEA) is beneficial in the treatment of some patients with SLE [47,89]. Although DHEA is a precursor for sex hormone synthesis, it also acts as an anabolic steroid [90]. DHEA levels are low in patients with SLE regardless of sex [90–92]. DHEA supplementation may reduce the catabolic effects of chronic glucocorticoid administration, particularly in females, because they lack testes, which are the major source of anabolic androgens in males [90].

IV. Molecular Mechanisms of Hormone Action and Autoimmunity

Multiple aberrations within the intracellular milieu of both T cells [93–98] and B cells [99,100] have been reported in patients with autoimmune diseases. In humans, the binding of antigen to the T-cell receptor (TCR) initiates a signal transduction cascade that transmits signals from the plasma membrane to the nucleus [101]. This signal transduction pathway is calcium-dependent, includes changes in the phosphorylation status of regulatory proteins, and leads to new protein synthesis and secretion, many of which are cytokines. T cells stimulated through the TCR complex are activated and therefore interact with B cells to help stimulate the production of antibody and autoantibody.

A. Signal Transduction

Because the binding of antigen initiates the signaling cascade, it is reasonable to assume that abnormalities in the TCR complex could account, in part, for the aberrant signal transduction in SLE. Abnormalities in both the protein and mRNA of the zeta chain protein in the TCR complex have been reported in SLE

T cells [98]. Altered cell signaling in response to antigen binding at the TCR complex owing to structural polymorphism could contribute to functional differences in autoimmune T cells. This possibility is further suggested by the report of Vassilopoulos et al [93] showing that activated SLE T cells sustained their release of free calcium compared with normal T cells in response to TCR activation. Sustainment of increased levels of intracellular calcium would be expected to activate calcineurin, a calcium/calmodulin-dependent protein phosphatase.

Consistent with this postulate, we reported that T cells from women with SLE cultured in medium containing physiologic amounts of estradiol showed increased calcineurin mRNA and phosphatase activity compared with normal T cells and T cells from males with SLE [102]. More recently, we found that the expression of one of the downstream targets for calcineurin activity, CD40 ligand, increased on the surface of SLE T cells in response to estrogen [103]. CD40 ligand is a transmembrane protein that is transiently expressed on activated T cells during the contact-dependent help for antibody production [104]. We proposed that increased CD40 ligand on the surface of SLE T cells could lead to increased or sustained T–B cell interactions and thereby amplify the production of autoantibody [40,105]. The amplification mechanism does not seem to be mediated simply by estrogen acting on calcineurin. SLE T cells cultured in estradiol and treated with ionomycin to stimulate a release in free calcium and activate calcineurin did not show the expected increase in CD40 ligand mRNA. SLE T cells activated through the TCR, however, did show an increase in CD40 ligand mRNA. Whereas those results relate specifically to the estrogen-dependent increase in CD40 ligand expression, the work of Yi et al [96] showed that cyclosporin A could block CD40 ligand expression in SLE T-cell lines during their initial activation by anti-CD3. However, when the drug was added later, it was not as effective, suggesting that the calcium-calcineurin-NFAT pathway was not the only one involved in regulating CD40 ligand expression. Subsequent analysis revealed that one of the mitogen-activated protein kinases, extracellular signal-related kinase (ERK), was maintained in a phosphorylated state, which prevented the SLE T cells responding to anergy inducing protocols [96]. Together, these findings are consistent with genetic studies that suggest development or sustainment of some autoimmune diseases will involve proteins that mediate cell signaling events. In addition, our findings [102,103,105] suggest that some of the key signaling proteins in SLE T cells are sensitive to estrogen in culture, whereas those same genes in normal T cells are not responsive.

B. Cell-Cycle Regulation

The role of sex hormones in regulating proteins that act directly in the cell cycle has been clearly established in nonimmune target cells [106,107]. In response to the appropriate signals, cells can exit the proliferative pathway and enter into apoptosis. There is some evidence that sex hormones can influence both of these processes in human T and B cells [108,109]. At pharmacologic levels, sex steroids altered normal cell-cycle progression of transformed human T and B cell lines, in part, by decreasing the expression of cyclin A [108]. Both estrogen and testosterone inhibited proliferation of T-cell lines by inhibiting cell-cycle progression and increasing the apoptosis of T cells [109].

Progesterone also inhibited T-cell proliferation, but its effects on T-cell lines in culture were cytostatic without an accompanying increase in apoptosis [109]. We reported that estrogen, at physiologic levels, increased apoptosis of human SLE blood mononuclear cells in culture. The increase in the number of apoptotic cells correlated with a decrease in TNF-α production by these cells [110].

Estrogen can increase apoptosis in cultured T-cell lines by increasing the levels of Bcl-2 protein [109]. Furthermore, there may be complex interactions between estrogen and progesterone in this process because progesterone antagonized the estrogen-dependent increase in Bcl-2. Although caution is always warranted when pharmacologic levels of steroids are used, these observations suggest that female sex steroids can differentially regulate cell-cycle transit and apoptosis in both T and B lymphocytes. Moreover, the data provide initial support for the idea that at least some of the sex hormone–dependent effects on the immune system may be exerted on genes that control cell proliferation and programmed cell death. Additional studies are now required to determine if endocrine-regulated cell-cycle control and apoptosis are involved in the immune dysregulation associated with gender-biased autoimmune diseases.

Female mice lacking the cyclin kinase inhibitor p21 by targeted mutagenesis develop antibodies against double-stranded DNA, lymphadenopathy, and glomerulonephritis with earlier mortality than their male counterparts [111]. Most interestingly, the female sex hormone environment exacerbated these defects in the p21 null mice because the female mice developed lupuslike syndromes before the first year, unlike their male counterparts [111]. However, results from a study using a different strain of mice [112] did not show sex differences among p21 null mice. In addition, the p21 mice in that latter report [112] displayed only mild manifestations characteristic of autoimmune disease. Further studies are now necessary to identify if the female hormonal microenvironment could exacerbate autoimmune disease perhaps by exacerbating tolerance defects that lead to aberrant T–B cell interactions and autoimmune disease.

C. Cytokines

Interleukin-10 (IL-10) is a cytokine with pleiotropic effects in inflammation and immunoregulation [113–116]. Patients with SLE are high producers of IL-10, and this heightened expression is the result, in part, of polymorphisms in the IL-10 promoter [115]. Single nucleotide polymorphisms in the distal IL-10 promoter affect production of this cytokine, and certain polymorphisms are associated with increased risk of developing SLE [113,115]. Estrogen increases the expression of IL-10 and anti-double-stranded DNA and IgG secretion in peripheral blood mononuclear cells from patients with SLE [116]. In a small clinical trial comprised of five females and one male [117], administration of an anti-IL-10 murine monoclonal antibody improved disease in all patients and allowed for a concurrent reduction in corticosteroid treatment. The mechanisms by which IL-10 expression is enhanced by estrogen is not known. There is a Pit-1 transcription factor binding site in the distal promoter of the IL-10 gene. Because estrogen is known to upregulate expression of Pit-1 transcription factors, it is possible that control of IL-10 expression is through Pit-1 regulation. Alternatively,

IL-10 could be upregulated by direct binding of the ER at repeat sequences that serve as a canonical ER binding site at the promoter [114].

A number of other cytokines including IL-1 [118,119], IL-4 [120], and interferon gamma [49,121] are influenced by sex hormones and are therefore differentially expressed in females and males. Some of these cytokines, if abnormally expressed, may influence either the development or progression of autoimmune diseases. For example, C3H mice congenic for transgenic expression of IL-4 develop B-cell hyperactivity that resulted from apparent IL-4–induced B-cell polyclonal activation [120]. Overexpression of an interferon-gamma transgene in the epidermis of CBA×B10 F1 mice lead to anti-double-stranded DNA antibodies as well as immune complex glomerulonephritis. It is interesting that the glomerulonephritis was more prevalent in females than in their male counterparts [121]. Although differences in cytokine profiles between males and females exist [122], there is no single abnormality in cytokine gene expression that consistently correlates with gender-biased autoimmune diseases. Until the molecular switches involved in disease development are known, it will be difficult to assess if altered expression of cytokine genes reflects a primary cause for immune dysregulation or is simply the result of upstream events.

Sex hormones, at pharmacologic doses, can also repress the production of certain cytokine genes. McMurray et al [123] showed that estradiol 17-ß suppressed IL-2 and IL-2 receptors. Estrogen suppressed the transcription of IL-2 in activated peripheral blood T cells and CD4+ T-cell lines. Transcriptional repression was associated with decreased binding in nuclear extracts of both NFκB and AP1 to the IL-2 promoter. The decreased binding of NFκB was associated with estrogen-induced increases in IκBα protein levels, which inhibit NFκB nuclear translocation. Estradiol also inhibited IL-2 receptor expression in activated peripheral blood T cells. The suppressive effects of the estrogen were expected to direct the immune system from the Th1 to the Th2 type response [123].

V. Perspectives

Silverstein and Rose [124] present a compelling argument for the idea that some immune responses will be primarily protective whereas others will be harmful. Regardless of the immunogen involved, both components of the immune response could occur. Recent data suggest that the survival of naive T cells [125], and B cells [126], requires continuous exposure to autoantigens. This emerging concept—that autoreactivity is an important component for normal immune function [124]— suggests that small or subtle changes in the normal microenvironment could account for the unbridled autoreactivity that is characteristic of autoimmune diseases. In view of the complexities discussed earlier in this chapter, it seems likely that several types of defects can lead to autoimmune disease. As highlighted by studies in transgenic and knockout mice, changes in gene expression that alter signal transduction pathways, apoptotic mechanisms, and/or cytokine production can lead to symptoms characteristic of autoimmunity including increased autoantibody production. How then, might steroid sex hormones exert influences on these parameters and thereby contribute to gender bias in some autoimmune diseases? An attractive hypothesis that

requires further testing is that small or subtle changes in the microenvironment contribute to the acquisition of autoimmune disease by lowering activation thresholds. Lowered thresholds of activation may lead to alterations in the magnitude of cell signals that could impart deviations along the normal signal transduction pathway required for activation or tolerance to lymphocytes. Thus, genes that control the immune response are likely affected by changes in the cellular milieu, and emerging data reviewed in this chapter suggest that some of these genes may be modulated by sex hormones.

A key question posed by our own studies [40,102,103] is as follows: "What is the molecular basis for the differential sensitivity of some female SLE patients' T cells to estrogen?" There are several possibilities that require further investigation. We speculate that T cells from men with SLE do not respond in the same way as do T cells from women with SLE because the number of ERs is lower in men than in women. However, we have not measured the number of receptors in male vs female T cells, and to our knowledge those data do not exist. Alternatively, it is possible that the ratio of ER-α to ER-ß differs in women with SLE compared with men and normal controls (see Fig. 99-1). Although these experiments are technically difficult, quantitative information of the different receptor subtypes and their gene targets will provide essential information about estrogen action in the T cells of men and women.

ER can regulate gene transcription directly by binding to the promoter region of target genes or indirectly by interacting with other transcription factors such as SP1 and AP1. ER-dependent transcription is associated with the recruitment of coactivators such as steroid receptor coactivator 1 (SRC-1) and its related factors TIF2 and RAC-3 to the promoter regions of active genes. These co-activator proteins couple hormone receptors to other transcriptional regulators such as CREB-binding protein (CBP), p300, and PCAF, all of which are capable of acetylating histones and increasing the rate of transcription [127–129]. Changes in the immune response that alter the cellular milieu and increase generic transcriptions factors, such as SP1 and AP1, could trip the threshold response in favor of ER interaction with these proteins, thereby facilitating the transcription of genes (calcineurin, CD40 ligand, IL-10) that are not normally regulated by ER. The technology now exists to experimentally test this possibility [130,131]. Alternatively, sex hormones are known to stabilize the mRNA of a variety of gene transcripts [132]. Increased stability of calcineurin and CD40 ligand mRNAs would allow for sustained function of these proteins and contribute to prolonged T-cell activation and aberrant T–B cell interactions. It is therefore important to explore the mechanisms of estrogen action in controlling the expression of genes that are established regulators of the immune response. Furthermore, the universality of these findings for other strongly gender-biased autoimmune diseases, such as Hashimoto's thyroiditis, should be tested.

As our understanding about the complex genetic and environmental components that stimulate the onset of autoimmune diseases increases, it is likely that new, more specific drugs to treat these disorders will emerge. Current treatments usually involve a combination of corticosteroids in combination with antiproliferative agents [133]. Delivery of inflammatory cytokine inhibitors such as interferon gamma receptor, soluble TNF-α receptor monoclonal anti-TNF antibodies, and IL-1 receptor antagonists ameliorate a variety of autoimmune diseases in mice and some human autoimmune diseases [134]. In female mice, ER antagonists have also been effective in reducing disease progression [55,56]. Testing of antiestrogens in women with SLE now seems warranted. As the underlying molecular basis for diseases are unraveled, it should be possible to provide more specific treatments, perhaps using "cocktails," that block specific targets and produce less undesirable side effects.

In conclusion, it seems that at least some of the interesting biologic differences between the immune systems of males and females will be influenced by sex hormones. As pointed out earlier, the development of autoimmune diseases is complex and undoubtedly entails a variety of interacting events. Polymerase chain reaction technology has led to the discovery of persistent fetal cells in the circulation of women decades after their pregnancies [135–137]. It has been suggested that this phenomenon, termed fetal microchimerism, may contribute to the development of autoimmunity [138]. This proposal is attractive because it is consistent with the more frequent occurrence of some autoimmune diseases in women compared with men. However, the relevance of microchimerism to the pathogenesis of autoimmune disease requires further investigation because microchimerism is detected in healthy individuals and women who have not been pregnant can develop autoimmune disease [138]. As we explore the differences between the sexes, it seems prudent to consider relevant endocrine-immune interactions in the context of the genetic and behavioral differences between men and women. Identification of sex hormone receptors in cells mediating the immune response has been a major step forward. It is now important to extend these findings by identifying their gene targets in normal immune processes and in disease. The real challenge for the future will be to determine those differences between males and females that significantly affect human health and disease. There seems to be no dispute that sex matters. The question is how does it matter?

VI. Suggestions for Further Investigations

- Further investigation is necessary to fully characterize estrogen receptor subtypes and their down-stream targets in normal and SLE T cells.
- Studies of gene susceptibility loci coupled with sex hormone levels and metabolism in families with autoimmune diseases are necessary to clarify the role of sex steroids and their metabolites on gene regulatory mechanisms that induce various pathogenic markers in autoimmune diseases.
- Additional research is necessary to correlate clinical and molecular data with specific sex hormone receptor antagonism and test if there are therapeutic benefits by blocking specific hormone receptors in female predominant autoimmune diseases.

Acknowledgements

Supported in part by NIH grants AI49272 and RR-16475 from the BRIN Program of the National Center for Research Resources. We thank Dr. Lindsey Hutt-Fletcher (UMKC) for critical review of this chapter. We are grateful to Hope Schreck for secretarial assistance.

References

1. Sex affects health. (2001). In: Wizeman TM, Pardue ML, eds. *Exploring the Biological Contributions to Human Health. Does Sex Matter?* Washington, DC: National Academy Press. 117–172.
2. Gabriel SE. (1999). The epidemiology of gender-discrepant illness. *Lupus.* 8:339–345.
3. Jacobson DL, Gange SJ, Rose NR, *et al.* (1997). Epidemiology and estimated population burden of selected autoimmune diseases in the United States. *Clin Immunol Immunopath.* 84:223–243.
4. Whitacre CC, Reingold SC, O'Looney PA. (1999). A gender gap in autoimmunity. *Science.* 283:1277–1278.
5. Dudley DJ, Chen CL, Mitchell MD, *et al.* (1993). Adaptive immune responses during murine pregnancy: pregnancy-induced regulation of lymphokine production by activated T lymphocytes. *Am J Obstet Gynecol* 168:1155–1164.
6. Hill JA, Polgar K, Anderson DJ. (1995). T-helper 1-type immunity to trophoblast in women with recurrent spontaneous abortion. *JAMA.* 273:1933–1936.
7. Olsen NJ, Kovacs WJ. (1996). Gonadal steroids and immunity. *Endocrin. Rev.* 17:367–84.
8. Medzhitov R, Janeway CA Jr. (2002). Decoding the patterns of self and nonself by the innate immune system. *Science.* 296:298–300.
9. Fujita T. (2002). Evolution of the lectin-complement pathway and its role in innate immunity. *Nature Rev.* 2:346–353.
10. Moxley G, Posthuma D, Carlson P, *et al.* (2002). Sexual dimorphism in innate immunity. *Arthritis Rheum.* 46:250–258.
11. Beeson PB. (1994). Age and sex associations of 40 autoimmune diseases. *Am J Med.* 96:457–462.
12. Miller L, Hunt JS. (1996). Sex steroids, hormones and macrophage function. *Life Sci.* 59:1–14.
13. Lisse IM, Aaby P, Whittle H, *et al.* (1997). T-lymphocyte subsets in West African children: impact of age, sex, and season. *J Pediatr.* 130:77–85.
14. Homo-Delarche F, Fitzpatrick F, Christeff N, *et al.* (1991). Sex steroids, glucocorticoids, stress and autoimmunity. *J Steroid Biochem Mol Biol.* 40: 619–637.
15. Cutulo M, Sulli A, Villaggio B, *et al.* (1998). Relations between steroid hormones and cytokines in rheumatoid arthritis and systemic lupus erythematosus. *Ann Rheum Dis.* 57:573–577.
16. Sakaguchi S, Sakaguchi N. (2000). Role of genetic factors in organ-specific autoimmune diseases induced by manipulating the thymus or T cells, and not self-antigens. *Rev Immunogenet.* 2:147–153.
17. Theofilopoulos AN, Dummer W, Kono DH. (2001). T cell homeostasis and systemic autoimmunity. *J Clin Invest.* 108:335–340.
18. Whitacre CC. (2001). Sex differences in autoimmune disease. *Nature Immunol.* 2: 777–780.
19. Davidson A, Diamond B. (2001). Autoimmune diseases. *N Engl J Med.* 345:340–350.
20. Diamond B, Bluestone J, Wofsy D. (2001). The immune tolerance network and rheumatic disease. *Arthritis Rheum.* 44:1730–1735.
21. Theofilopoulos AN, Kono DH. (1999). The genes of systemic autoimmunity. *Proc Assoc Am Phys.* 111:228–240.
22. Moser KL, Neas BR, Salmon JE, *et al.* (1998). Genome scan of human systemic lupus erythematosus. Evidence for linkage on chromosome 1q in African-American pedigrees. *Proc Natl Acad Sci U S A.* 95:14869–14874.
23. Arnett FC. (2000). Genetic studies of human lupus in families. *Int Rev Immunol.* 19:297–317.
24. Mongey AB, Hess EV. (1997). The role of environment in systemic lupus erythematosus and associated disorders. In: Wallace DJ, Hahn BH, eds. *Dubois' Lupus Erythematosus.* Baltimore: Williams and Wilkins. 31–37.
25. Lahita RG, Bradlow HL. (1987). Klinefelter's syndrome: Hormone metabolism in hypogonadal males with systemic lupus erythematosus. *J Rheumatol.* 14:154–157.
26. Huang Q, Parfitt A, Grennan DM, *et al.* (1997). X-chromosome inactivation in monozygotic twins with systemic lupus erythematosus. *Autoimmunity.* 26:85–93.
27. Roper RJ, Griffith JS, Lyttle CR, *et al.* (1999). Interacting quantitative trait loci control phenotypic variation in murine estradiol-regulated responses. *Endocrinology.* 140:556–561.
28. Griffith JS, Jensen SM, Lunceford JK, *et al.* (1997). Evidence for the genetic control of estradiol-regulated responses. Implications for variation in normal and pathological hormone-dependent phenotypes. *Am J Pathol.* 150:2223–2230.
29. Wendell DL, Gorski J. (1997). Quantitative trait loci for estrogen-dependent pituitary tumor growth in the rat. *Mamm. Genome.* 8:823–829.
30. Tsai MJ, O'Malley BW. (1994). Molecular mechanisms of action of steroid/thyroid receptor superfamily members. *Annu Rev Biochem.* 63:451–486.

31. Zhou ZX, Wong CI, Sar M, *et al*. (1994). The androgen receptor: an overview. *Recent Prog Horm Res*. 49:249–274.

32. Misrahi M, Loosfelt H, Atger M, *et al*. (1990). Structural and functional studies of mammalian progesterone receptors. *Horm Res*. 33:95–98.

33. Kuiper GG, Enmark E, Pelto-Huikko M, *et al*. (1996). Cloning of a novel receptor expressed in rat prostate and ovary. *Proc Natl Acad Sci U S A*. 93:5925–5930.

34. Lahita RG. (2000). Sex hormones and systemic lupus erythematosus. *Rheum Dis Clin North Am*. 26:951–968.

35. Cutolo M, Wilder RL. (2000). Different roles for androgens and estrogens in the susceptibility to autoimmune rheumatic diseases. *Rheum Dis Clin North Am*. 26:825–839.

36. Lahita RG, Bradlow HL, Kunkel HG, *et al*. (1981). Increased 16 alpha hydroxylation of estradiol in systemic lupus erythematosus. *J Clin Endocrinol Metab*. 53:174–178.

37. Verthelyi D, Petri M, Tlamus M, *et al*. (2001). Disassociation of sex hormone levels and cytokine production in SLE patients. *Lupus*. 10:352–358.

38. Suenaga R, Rider V, Evans M, *et al*. (1998). Peripheral blood T cells and monocytes and B cell lines derived from patients with lupus express estrogen receptor transcripts similar to those of normal cells. *J Rheumatol*. 25:1305–1312.

39. Suenaga R, Rider V, Evans MJ, *et al*. (2001). *In vitro*-activated human lupus T cells express normal estrogen receptor proteins which bind to the estrogen response element. *Lupus*. 10:116–122.

40. Rider V, Jones SR, Evans M, *et al*. (2000). Molecular mechanisms involved in the estrogen-dependent regulation of calcineurin in systemic lupus erythematosus T cells. *Clin Immunol*. 95:124–134.

41. Kassi EN, Vlachoyiannopoulos PG, Moutsopoulos HM, *et al*. (2001). Molecular analysis of estrogen receptor alpha and beta in lupus patients. *Eur J Clin Invest*. 31:86–93.

42. Garovich M, Agudelo C, Pisko E. (1980). Oral contraceptives and systemic lupus erythematosus. *Arthritis Rheum*. 23:1396–1398.

43. Cooper GS, Dooley MA, Treadwell EL, *et al*. (1998). Hormonal, environmental, and infectious risk factors for developing systemic lupus erythematosus. *Arthritis Rheum*. 41:1714–1724.

44. Mund AJ, Simson J, Rothfield N. (1963). Effect of pregnancy on course of systemic lupus erythematosus. *JAMA*. 183:109–112.

45. Casoli P, Tumiati B, LaSala G. (1997). Fatal exacerbation of systemic lupus erythematosus after induction of ovulation. *J Rheumatol*. 24:1639–1640.

46. Font J, Pallares L, Cervera R, *et al*. (1991). Systemic lupus erythematosus in the elderly: clinical and immunological characteristics. *Ann Rheum Dis*. 50:702–705.

47. Buyon JP. (2000). Clinical trials in systemic lupus erythematosus. *Curr Rheumatol*. Rep. 2:11–12.

48. Sanchez-Guerrero J, Liang MH, Karlson EW, *et al*. (1995). Post-menopausal estrogen therapy and the risk for developing systemic lupus erythematosus. *Ann Intern Med*. 122:430–433.

49. Karpuzoglu-Sahin E, Zhi-Jun Y, Lengi A, *et al*. (2001). Effects of long-term estrogen treatment on IFN-gamma, IL-2 and IL-4 gene expression and protein synthesis in spleen and thymus of normal C57BL/6 mice. *Cytokine*. 14:208–217.

50. Roubinian JR, Talal N, Greenspan JS, *et al*. (1978). Effect of castration and sex hormone treatment on survival, anti-nucleic acid antibodies, and glomerulonephritis in NZB/NZW F1 mice. *J Exp Med*. 147:1568–1583.

51. Dhaher YY, Chan K, Greenstein BD, *et al*. (2000). Impaired estrogen priming of progesterone receptors in uterus of MRL/Mp-lpr/lpr mice, a model of systemic lupus erythematosus (SLE). *Int J Immunopharmacol*. 22:537–547.

52. Roa R, Greenstein BD. (2000). Evidence for pleomorphism of estrogen receptor capacity and affinity in liver and thymus of immature BALC/c and (NZBxNZW) F1 mice, a model of systemic lupus erythematosus. *Int J Immunopharmacol*. 22:897–903.

53. Tang B, Matsuda T, Akira S, *et al*. (1991). Age-associated increase in interleukin 6 in MRL/lpr mice. *Int Immunol*. 3:273–278.

54. Törnwall J, Carey AB, Fox RI, *et al*. (1999). Estrogen in autoimmunity: expression of estrogen receptors in thymic and autoimmune T cells. *J Gend Specif Med*. 2:33–40.

55. Wu WM, Lin BF, Su YC, *et al*. (2000). Tamoxifen decreases renal inflammation and alleviates disease severity in autoimmune NZB/W F1 mice. *Scan J Immunol*. 52:393–400.

56. Apelgren LD, Bailey DL, Fouts RL, *et al*. (1996). The effect of a selective estrogen receptor modulator on the progression of spontaneous autoimmune disease in MRL lpr/lpr mice. *Cell Immunol*. 173:55–63.

57. Chan OT, Madaio MP, Shlomchik MJ. (1999). B cells are required for lupus nephritis in the polygenic, Fas-intact MRL model of systemic autoimmunity. *J Immunol*. 163:3592–3596.

58. Chan OT, Shlomchik MJ. (2000). Cutting edge: B cells promote CD8+ T cell activation in MRL-Fas(lpr) mice independently of MHC class I antigen presentation. *J Immunol*. 164:1658–1662.

59. Thurmond TS, Murante FG, Staples JE, *et al*. (2000). Role of estrogen receptor alpha in hematopoietic stem cell development and B lymphocyte maturation in the male mouse. *Endocrinology*. 141:2309–2318.

60. Smithson G, Couse JF, Lubahn DB, *et al*. (1998). The role of estrogen receptors and androgen receptors in sex steroid regulation of B lymphopoiesis. *J Immunol*. 161:27–34.

61. Grimaldi CM, Michael DJ, Diamond B. (2001). Cutting Edge: Expansion and activation of A population of autoreactive marginal zone B cells in a model of estrogen-induced lupus. *J Immunol*. 167:1886–1890.

62. Staples JE, Gasiewicz TA, Fiore NC, *et al*. (1999). Estrogen receptor alpha is necessary in thymic development and estradiol-induced thymic alterations. *J Immunol*. 163:4168–4174.

63. Peeva E, Grimaldi C, Spatz L, *et al*. (2000). Bromocriptine restores tolerance in estrogen-treated mice. *J Clin Invest*. 106:1373–1379.

64. Pellegrini I, Lebrun J, Ali S, *et al*. (1992). Expression of prolactin and its receptor in human lymphoid cells. *Mol Endocrinol*. 6:1023–1031.

65. Gagnerault MC, Touraine P, Savino W, *et al*. (1993). Expression of prolactin receptors in murine lymphoid cells in normal and autoimmune situations. *J Immunol*. 150:5673–5681.

66. Folomeev M, Prokaeva T, Nassonova V, *et al*. (1990). Prolactin levels in men with SLE and RA. *J Rheumatol*. 17:1569–1570.

67. Neidhart M. (1996). Elevated serum prolactin or elevated prolactin/cortisol ratio are associated with autoimmune processes in systemic lupus erythematosus and other connective tissue diseases. *Br J Rheumatol*. 23:476–481.

68. Miranda JM, Prieto RE, Paniagua R, *et al*. (1998). Clinical significance of serum and urine prolactin levels in lupus glomerulonephritis. *Lupus*. 7:387–391.

69. Alvarez–Nemegyei J, Cobarrubias-Cobos A, Escalante-Triay F, *et al*. (1998). Bromocriptine in systemic lupus erythematosus: a double-blind, randomized, placebo-controlled study. *Lupus*. 7:414–419.

70. Walker SE, Jacobson JD. (2000). Roles of prolactin and gonadotropin-releasing hormone in rheumatic diseases. *Rheum Dis Clin North Am*. 26:713–736.

71. McMurray R, Keisler D, Kanuckel K, *et al*. (1991). Prolactin influences autoimmune disease activity in the female NZB/W mouse. *J Immunol*. 147:3780–3787.

72. Simmons DM, Voss JW, Ingraham HA, *et al*. (1990). Pituitary cell phenotypes involve cell-specific Pit-1 mRNA translation and synergistic interactions with other classes of transcription factors. *Genes Dev*. 4:695–711.

73. Sites DP, Siiteri PK. (1983). Steroids as immunosuppressants in pregnancy. *Immunol Rev*. 75:117–138.

74. Arnalich F, Benito-Urbina S, Gonzalez-Gancedo P, *et al*. (1992). Inadequate production of progesterone in women with systemic lupus erythematosus. *Br J Rheumatol*. 31:247–251.

75. Polgar B, Barakonyi A, Xynos I, *et al*. (1999). The role of gamma/delta T cell receptor positive cells in pregnancy. *Am J Reprod Immunol*. 41:239–244.

76. Szekeres-Bartho J, Barakonyi A, Par G, *et al*. (2002). Progesterone as an immunomodulatory molecule. *Int Immunopharmacol*. 1:1037–1048.

77. Lyndon JP, DeMayo FJ, Funk CR, *et al*. (1995). Mice lacking progesterone receptor exhibit pleiotropic reproductive abnormalities. *Genes Dev*. 9:2266–2278.

78. Tibbetts TA, DeMayo F, Rich S, *et al*. (1999). Progesterone receptors in the thymus are required for thymic involution during pregnancy and for normal fertility. *Proc Natl Acad Sci U S A*. 96:12021–12026.

79. Mok CC, Lau CS. (2000). Profile of sex hormones in male patients with systemic lupus erythematosus. *Lupus*. 9:252–257.

80. Sequeira JF, Keser G, Greenstein B, *et al*. (1993). Systemic lupus erythematosus: sex hormones in male patients. *Lupus*. 2:315–317.

81. Olsen NJ, Gu X, Kovacs WJ. (2001). Bone marrow stromal cells mediate androgenic suppression of B lymphocyte development. *J Clin Invest*. 108:1697–1704.

82. Olsen NJ, Kovacs WJ. (2001). Effects of androgens on T and B lymphocyte development. *Immunol Res*. 23:281–288.

83. Medina KL, Kincade PW. (1994). Pregnancy-related steroids are potential negative regulators of B lymphopoiesis. *Proc Natl Acad Sci U S A*. 91: 5382–5386.

84. Frey-Wettstein M, Craddock CG. (1970). Testosterone-induced depletion of thymus and marrow lymphocytes as related to lymphopoiesis and hematopoiesis. *Blood*. 35:257–271.

85. Nakamura K, Kitani A, Strober W. (2001). Cell contact-dependent immunosuppression by CD4(+)CD25(+) regulatory T cells is mediated by cell surface-bound transforming growth factor beta. *J Exp Med*. 194:629–644.

86. Valujskikh A, VanVuskirk AM, Orosz CG, *et al.* (2001). A role for TGFbeta and B cells in immunologic tolerance after intravenous injection of soluble antigen. *Transplantation.* 72:685–693.

87. Walker SE, Allen SH, McMurray RW. (1993). Prolactin and autoimmune disease. *Trends Endocrinol Metab.* 4:147–151.

88. Walker SE, McMurray RW, Houri JM, *et al.* (1998). Effects of prolactin in stimulating disease activity in systemic lupus erythematosus. *Ann NY Acad Sci.* 840:762–772.

89. Van Vollenhoven RF. (2002). Dehydroepiandrosterone for the treatment of systemic lupus erythematosus. *Expert Opin Pharmacother.* 3:23–31.

90. Robinzon B, Cutolo M. (1999). Should dehydroepiandrosterone replacement therapy be provided with glucocorticoids? *Rheumatology* 38:488–495.

91. Lahita RG, Bradlow HL, Ginzler E, *et al.* (1987). Low plasma androgens in women with systemic lupus erythematosus. *Arthritis Rheum.* 30: 241 248.

92. Straub RH, Zeuner M, Anoniou E, *et al.* (1996). Dehydroepiandrosterone sulfate is positively correlated with soluble interleukin-2 receptor and soluble intercellular adhesion molecule in systemic lupus erythematosus. *J Rheumatol.* 23:856–861.

93. Vassilopoulos D, Dovacs B, Tsokos GC. (1995). TCR/CD3 complex-mediated signal transduction pathway in T cells and T cell lines from patients with systemic lupus erythematosus. *J Immunol.* 155:2269–2281.

94. Blasini AM, Alonzo E, Chacon R, *et al.* (1998). Abnormal pattern of tyrosine phosphorylation in unstimulated peripheral blood T lymphocytes from patients with systemic lupus erythematosus. *Lupus.* 7:515–523.

95. Wu J, Edberg JC, Gibson AW, *et al.* (1999). Single-nucleotide polymorphisms of T cell receptor zeta chain in patients with systemic lupus erythematosus. *Arthritis Rheum.* 42:2601–2605.

96. Yi Y, NcNerney M, Datta SK. (2000). Regulatory defects in Cbl and mitogen-activated protein kinase (extracellular signal-related kinase) pathways cause persistent hyperexpression of CD40 ligand in human lupus T cells. *J Immunol.* 165:6627–6634.

97. Tsokos GC, Kammer GM. (2000). Molecular aberrations in human systemic lupus erythematosus. *Mol Med Today.* 6:418–424.

98. Nambiar MP, Enydey EJ, Warke VG, *et al.* (2001). T cell signaling abnormalities in systemic lupus erythematosus are associated with increased mutations/polymorphisms and splice variants of T cell receptor zeta chain messenger RNA. *Arthritis Rheum.* 44:1336–1350.

99. Odendahl M, Jacobi A, Hansen A, *et al.* (2000). Disturbed peripheral B lymphocyte homeostasis in systemic lupus erythematosus. *J Immunol.* 165:5970–5979.

100. Arce E, Jackson DG, Gill MA, *et al.* (2001). Increased frequency of pre-germinal center B cells and plasma cell precursors in the blood of children with systemic lupus erythematosus. *J Immunol.* 167:2361–2369.

101. Weiss A, Littman DR. (1994). Signal transduction by lymphocyte antigen receptors. *Cell.* 76:263–274.

102. Rider V, Foster RT, Evans M, *et al.* (1998). Gender differences in autoimmune diseases: estrogen increases calcineurin expression in systemic lupus erythematosus. *Clin Immunol Immunopath.* 89:171–180.

103. Rider V, Jones S, Evans M, *et al.* (2001). Estrogen increases CD40 ligand expression in T cells from women with systemic lupus erythematosus. *J Rheumatol.* 28:2644–2649.

104. Grewal IS, Flavell RA. (1998). CD40 and CD154 in cell-mediated immunity. *Ann Rev Immunol.* 16:111–132.

105. Rider V, Abdou NI. (2001). Gender differences in autoimmunity: Molecular basis for estrogen effects in systemic lupus erythematosus. *Int Immunopharmacol.* 1:1009–1024.

106. Musgrove EA, Sutherland RL. (1994). Cell cycle control by steroid hormones. *Cancer Biol.* 5:381–389.

107. Rider V. (2002). Progesterone and the control of uterine cell proliferation and differentiation. *Front Biosci.* 7:d1545–1555.

108. Jenkins JK, Suwannaroj S, Elbourne KB, *et al.* (2001). 17-ß-estradiol alters Jurkat lymphocyte cell cycling and induces apoptosis through suppression of Bcl-2 and cyclin A. *Int Immunopharmacol.* 1:1897–1911.

109. McMurray RW, Suwannaroj S, Ndebele K, *et al.* (2001). Differential effects of sex steroids on T and B cells: modulation of cell cycle phase distribution apoptosis and Bcl-2 protein levels. *Pathobio.* 69:44–58.

110. Evans M, MacLaughlin S, Marvin RD, *et al.* (1997). Estrogen decreases *in vitro* apoptosis of peripheral blood mononuclear cells from women with normal menstrual cycles and decreases TNF-α production in SLE but not in normal cultures. *Clin Immunol Immunopath.* 82:258–262.

111. Balomenos D, Martin-Caballero J, Garcia MI, *et al.* (2000). The cell cycle inhibitor p21 controls T cell proliferation and sex-linked lupus development. *Nature Med.* 6:171–176.

112. Santiago-Raber ML, Lawson BR, Dummer W, *et al.* (2001). Role of cyclin kinase inhibitor p21 in systemic autoimmunity. *J Immunol.* 167: 4067–4074.

113. Eskdale J, Gallagher G. (1995). A polymorphic dinucleotide repeat in the human IL-10 promoter. *Immunogenet.* 42:444–445.

114. Kube D, Rieth H, Eskdale J, *et al.* (2001). Structural characterisation of the distal 5' flanking region of the human interleukin-10 gene. *Genes Immun.* 2:181–190.

115. Gibson AW, Edberg JC, Wu J, *et al.* (2001). Novel single nucleotide polymorphisms in the distal IL-10 promoter affect IL-10 production and enhance the risk of systemic lupus erythematosus. *J Immunol.* 166: 3915–3922.

116. Kanda N, Tsuchida T, Tamaki K. (1999). Estrogen enhancement of anti-double stranded DNA antibody and immunoglobulin G production in peripheral blood mononuclear cells from patients with systemic lupus erythematosus. *Arthritis Rheum.* 42:328–337.

117. Llorente L, Richaud-Patin Y, Garcia-Padilla C, *et al.* (2000). Clinical and biologic effects of anti-interleukin-10 monoclonal antibody administration in systemic lupus erythematosus. *Arthritis Rheum.* 43:1790–1800.

118. Da Silva JA, Peers SH, Perretti M, *et al.* (1993). Sex steroids affect glucocorticoid response to chronic inflammation and to interleukin-1. *J Endocrinol.* 136:389–397.

119. Rivier C. (1994). Stimulatory effect of interleukin-1 beta on the hypothalamic-pituitary-adrenal axis of the rat: influence of age, gender and circulating sex steroids. *J Endocrinol.* 140:365–372.

120. Erb KJ, Ruger B, von Brevern M, *et al.* (1997). Constitutive expression of interleukin (IL)-4 in vivo causes autoimmune-type disorders in mice. *J Exp Med.* 185:329–339.

121. Seery JP, Carroll JM, Cattell V, *et al.* (1997). Antinuclear autoantibodies and lupus nephritis in transgenic mice expressing interferon γ in the epidermis. *J Exp Med.* 186:1451–1459.

122. Giron-Gonzalez JA, Moral FJ, Elvira J, *et al.* (2000). Consistent production of a higher TH1:TH2 cytokine ratio by stimulated T cells in men compared with women. *Eur J Endocrinol.* 143:31–36.

123. McMurray RW, Ndebele K, Hardy KJ, *et al.* (2001). 17-beta-estradiol suppresses IL-2 and IL-2 receptor. *Cytokine.* 14:324–333.

124. Silverstein AM, Rose NR. (2000). There is only one immune system! The view from immunopathology. *Immunol.* 12:173–178

125. Goldrath AW, Bevan MJ. (1999). Selecting and maintaining a diverse T-cell repertoire. *Nature.* 402:255–262.

126. Gu H, Tarlinton D, Muller W, *et al.* (1991). Most peripheral B cells in mice are ligand selected. *J Exp Med.* 173:1357–1371.

127. DiRenzo J, Shang Y, Phelan M, *et al.* (2000). BRG-1 is recruited to estrogen-responsive promoters and cooperates with factors involved in histone acetylation. *Mol Cell Biol.* 20:7541–7549.

128. Shang Y, Myers M, Brown M. (2002). Formation of the androgen receptor transcription complex. *Cell.* 9:601–610.

129. Shang Y, Brown M. (2002). Molecular determinants for the tissue specificity of SERMs. *Science.* 295:2465–2468.

130. Ren B, Cam H, Takahashi Y, *et al.* (2002). E2F integrates cell cycle progression with DNA repair, replication, and G(2)/M checkpoints. *Genes Dev.* 16:245–256.

131. Weinmann AS, Yan PS, Oberley MJ, *et al.* (2002). Isolating human transcription factor targets by coupling chromatin immunoprecipitation and CpG island microarray analysis. *Genes Dev.* 16:235–244.

132. Ing NH, Ott TL. (1999). Estradiol up-regulates estrogen receptor-alpha messenger ribonucleic acid in sheep endometrium by increasing its stability. *Biol Reprod.* 60:134–139.

133. Moroni G, Della Casa Alberighi O, Ponticelli C. (2001). Combination treatment in autoimmune disease: systemic lupus erythematosus. *Springer Semin Immunopathol.* 23:75–89.

134. Prud'home GJ, Lawson BR, Theofilopoulos AN. (2001). Immunotherapeutic gene transfer into muscle. *Trends Immunol.* 22:149–155.

135. Johnson KL, Nelson JL, Furst DE, *et al.* (2001). Fetal cell microchimerism in tissue from multiple sites in women with systemic sclerosis. *Arthritis Rheum.* 44:1848–1854.

136. Tanaka A, Lindor K, Ansari A, *et al.* (2000). Fetal microchimerism in the mother: immunologic implications. *Liver Transpl.* 6:138–143.

137. Nelson JL. (1996). Maternal-fetal immunology and autoimmune disease. Is some autoimmune disease auto-alloimmune or allo-autoimmune. *Arthritis Rheum.* 39:191–194.

138. Nelson JL. (2001). HLA relationships of pregnancy, microchimerism and autoimmune disease. *J Reprod Immunol.* 52:77–84.

100

Estrogen, Signal Transduction, and Systemic Lupus Erythematosus: Molecular Mechanisms

GARY M. KAMMER, MD

Department of Internal Medicine, Department of Microbiology & Immunology,
Wake Forest University School of Medicine, Winston-Salem, NC

I. Introduction

The fundamental pathophysiology of systemic lupus erythematosus (SLE) is a product of an abnormal cellular and humoral immune response [1]. However, a gender bias in autoimmune disorders, such as SLE, has long been appreciated [2–4]. Experimental evidence has gradually accumulated over the past several decades implicating sex hormones, including estrogen and prolactin [5,6]. Despite remarkable advances in our understanding of how hormones regulate gene transcription and translation, however, the molecular basis for this gender predilection in SLE still remains obscure.

Because of the relevance of sex hormones to immune functions in general [7–9] and the pathophysiology of SLE [4,6,10,11] in particular, this chapter will focus on the known molecular mechanisms by which 17β-estradiol (E_2) regulates gene transactivation to modify cellular functions. Because SLE is a product of T- and B-cell dysfunctions [12], it is germane to first briefly review our current understanding of these cellular abnormalities and how they are believed to contribute to abnormal immunity in SLE. Within this context, I will also discuss the hypothesis that a fundamental abnormality in SLE is the existence of a primary T-cell disorder as a result of aberrant signal transduction [13,14]. Finally, to provide a perspective for the molecular mechanisms of estrogen action, I will briefly review the existing evidence implicating estrogen in the aberrant immune response in SLE. Because limited information is available regarding the effects of estrogen and prolactin on T- and B-cell functions, this discussion of hormone action will largely focus on estrogen and T cells and briefly review what is known about estrogen and prolactin effects on T and B cells.

II. Abnormal Immunity in Systemic Lupus Erythematosus

The fundamental abnormality of immunity in SLE is the production of autoantibodies directed against diverse intracellular and extracellular autoantigens. These autoantigens are believed to derive largely from apoptotic cells [15] and, in the appropriate immunogenetic setting, are processed in and presented by antigen-presenting cells (APCs) to naïve T cells in a process that results in the generation of autoreactive T-cell clones. It is currently held that continuous, exaggerated T-cell help to abnormal B-cell clones initiates and drives the production of these autoantibodies. This production of autoantibodies is a component of the polyclonal hypergammaglobulinemia often observed in SLE that is composed of natural antibodies and pathologic autoantibodies. Indeed, it is this production of autoantibodies that defines SLE as an autoimmune disorder.

Exaggerated T-cell help is the product of an imbalance between CD4+ T helper (Th) and CD8+ T cytotoxic/suppressor (Tc) functions [14,16]. Enhanced CD4+ Th function and diminished CD8+ Tc activity are associated with augmented expression of cell surface CD11a, CD154, and HLA-DR molecules [17–19]. Although definitive evidence is lacking, current theory proposes that presentation of autoantigens by APCs to autoreactive Th clones results in clonal proliferation, chronic activation, and upregulation of these cell-surface molecules. Of particular interest is the finding *in vitro* and *in vivo* that T-cell overexpression of the adhesion molecule, CD11a, appears to enhance T-cell binding to activated APCs in the absence of specific antigen, resulting in spontaneous activation of these autoreactive T cells [17,20,21]. Although the proportion of activated T cells is relatively small [22,23], several mechanisms may contribute to the persistent activation of T cells in SLE.

One potential outcome of activated T-cell clones is skewed cytokine and chemokine production. Indeed, there is reduced production of Th1 cytokines (IL-2,IFN-γ) and increased generation of Th2 cytokines (IL-6, IL-10) by SLE T cells [24]. Similarly, there is an imbalance in β-chemokine production characterized by reduced levels of RANTES (regulated on activation, normal T-cell exposed, CCL-5 and secreted.) and increased amounts of MCP-1 (monocyte chemoattractant protein-1, CCl-2) [25]. In the presence of Th2 cytokines, enhanced interaction between CD4+ CD154+ Th cells and CD40+ B cells is believed to provide a strong, enduring signal [18,26] resulting in clonal B-cell proliferation, maturation, and hypergammaglobulinemia. Formation of antigen-antibody complexes and their subsequent fixation of complement often results in their deposition in and binding to tissue-associated receptors, initiating a destructive, end-organ inflammatory response that can culminate in organ failure. Anti-double-stranded DNA and anti-C1q are two autoantibodies that have been implicated in the immunopathogenesis of lupus glomerulonephritis [27,28].

Although the presence of abnormal T-cell effector functions has long been known [29], the mechanism(s) underlying these dysfunctions has remained uncertain. Recognition of a relationship between impaired CD8+ Tc function and altered cyclic adenosine monophosphate/protein kinase A (cAMP/PKA) pathway function [30] raised the possibility that abnormal signal transduction might contribute to T-cell effector dysfunctions. Accumulating evidence now supports the concept of a primary T-cell disorder in SLE [14,16]. This primary T-cell disorder is defined by abnormal signal transduction that is intrinsic to the T cell. To date, more than 10 discrete abnormalities of signal transduction and gene regulation have been identified [16]. Together, these are responsible for reduced (T-cell receptor ζ chain, PKA type I regulatory β-subunit) or increased (double-stranded RNA-dependent protein kinase R [PKR]) expression of signaling molecules; increased concentrations of a second messenger (Ca^{++}); augmented mitochondrial transmembrane potential; decreased concentrations of adenosine triphosphate (ATP); and abnormal PKA-, PKR-, and extracellular receptor kinases (ERK) $\frac{1}{2}$-catalyzed protein phosphorylation [31–38]. It is currently proposed that in toto these discrete signaling defects lead to faulty function of the cell's signaling apparatus, contributing to such endpoints as increased apoptosis and loss of tolerance. Moreover, it is likely that exogenous factors, such as cytokines, chemokines and hormones, bind to T-cell receptors and activate intrinsically defective signaling pathways, potentially enhancing skewed gene expression. Such aberrant gene expression may lead to abnormal T-cell effector functions.

III. Estrogen Receptors

Having briefly considered the known molecular mechanisms underlying abnormal T-cell function in SLE, we can now turn our attention to the role of hormones, such as estrogen, in lupus pathogenesis. Because it has long been appreciated that there is a disproportionate occurrence of autoimmunity in females, there has been a historical emphasis on the role of estrogens in the predilection for autoimmunity. This has not been to the exclusion of other hormones, such as progesterone and prolactin or even testosterone; still, the emphasis continues to be on estrogen. Therefore, this chapter will focus on E_2-ER (estrogen receptor) interactions in various cell types and, where information is available, will highlight what is known about these interactions in T cells.

A. ERα and ERβ

It has been 42 years since the uterine ER that binds E_2 was initially identified [39]. Thereafter, it took more than two decades until the first ER was cloned and sequenced [40–42]. It is now termed ERα. The second ER, termed ERβ, was identified in rat prostate and subsequently cloned and sequenced [43].

ERs are widely distributed in tissues. Both ER subtypes have been identified in the central nervous system, cardiovascular system, breast, urogenital tract, bone, and immune cells [44–47]. By contrast, only ERα is found in liver and only ERβ is identified in the gastrointestinal tract to date. Although there has been longstanding functional evidence of ERs in CD8$^+$ T cells [48,49], recent analyses have identified transcripts for both ERα and ERβ in murine thymocytes [50,51] and human peripheral blood CD4$^+$ and CD8$^+$ T-cell subsets [46,47]. However, only ERα protein has been unambiguously identified in human T-cell lysates to date [52]. More comprehensive analyses are warranted to quantify the ratio of ER subtypes in each T-cell subset as well as their role in specific T-cell effector functions.

Of particular interest is the recent discovery of ERβ isoforms [53–55]. ERβ transcripts exhibit other open reading frames upstream of the initially identified sequence and two translation start sites. The ERβ isoforms vary from 485 to 548 amino acids and express differential NH$_2$ or COOH-terminal sequences [54]. Functionally, ERβ2, which has an 18-amino acid insert in the ligand binding domain (LBD) of ERβ1 [56,57], binds E_2 poorly but can form ERβ2-ERβ or ERβ2-ERα heterodimers. Notwithstanding, these heterodimers are transcriptionally silent, suggesting that ERβ2 acts as a dominant-negative isoform.

ERs are nuclear transcription factors that bind to *cis*-regulatory estrogen response elements (EREs) with a palindromic consensus sequence of 5'-AGGTCAnnnTGACCT-3' in the promoter of target genes (Fig. 100-1). Because of their homology with other nuclear receptors, ERs have been categorized as type I nuclear steroid receptors (Table 100-1). ERs possess five domains, A–F [58,59]. AF-1 (or A/B) is the activation function-1 domain that contributes to transcriptional regulation. It is the most N-terminal domain and is the least conserved between the two ER species. By contrast, the DNA-binding domain (DBD or C domain) is the most conserved. This sequence, comprised of two zinc finger motifs, possesses a dimerization site that mediates DNA binding. The hinge domain (D domain), located in the mid-segment of the molecule, and the F domain, the most COOH-terminal domain, exhibit only 30% and 17.9% homology between the two ER subtypes, respectively. It is interesting that the hinge region is one of two domains that interact with the chaperonin, heat shock protein 90 (HSP90). Just NH$_2$-terminal to the F domain is the ligand-binding or AF-2 domain (LBD or E domain), which possesses nearly 60% homology between the ER species. Together with the AF-1 domain, these sites are required in ligand-driven transactivation [60]. This site supports binding of receptor agonists and antagonists, cofactor binding, dimerization, and transactivation. This domain also mediates nuclear localization and may also be another region for HSP90 binding. The molecular sequence of these domains and their homology between the ER subtypes are shown in Fig. 100-1.

Following ligand binding, ERs form homodimers (i.e., α-α or β-β) or heterodimers (α-β) that bind to EREs [61] and either upregulate or downregulate transcriptional activity depending on the concomitant binding of coactivators or corepressors (see Fig. 100-1). Indeed, ER transactivation depends on its dimerization [62], although the extent of heterodimerization and its physiologic activity *in vivo* are still uncertain. Nevertheless, transactivation requires a functional AF-2 domain of each component ER, which confirms earlier observations using dominant-negative constructs [62,63]. In some genes, repeated half palindromes (i.e., 5'-TGACC-3') also function as EREs [64]. Ligand-ER complexes function as nuclear transcription factors that activate or inhibit specific target genes, thus modifying their expression based on estrogen binding to its receptors. Although both ER subtypes bind to the consensus ERE shown earlier, this complete sequence has only been identified in the *vitellogenin* promoter. To date, several partial ERE sequences have been sequenced in other E_2-responsive genes, the most common of which are half-sites with variable nucleotide structures. Although both ERα and ERβ can bind these EREs, differing affinities for these EREs suggest that activation of individual genes may vary [65]. In the mouse, for example, ERβ has a modestly lower affinity for E_2 ($K_d = 0.5$ nM) compared to ERα ($K_d = 0.2$ nM) [66].

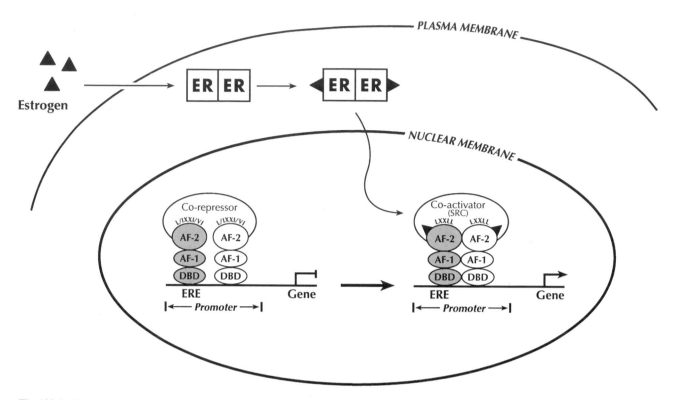

Fig. 100-1 Estradiol-estrogen receptor (E_2-ER)-dependent on–off movement of corepressors and coactivators, which bind to the L/IXXI/VI and LXXLL motifs, respectively [76], of helix 12 within the AF-2 region of the ligand binding domain. (Adapted with permission from Kato S, Masuhiro Y, Watanabe M *et al*. [2000]. Molecular mechanisms of a cross-talk between oestrogen and growth factor signaling pathways. *Genes to Cells*. 593–601.)

Table 100-1

Type I Steroid Receptors

Androgen receptor (AR)
Estrogen receptor (ER)
Glucocorticoid receptor (GR)
Mineralocorticoid receptor (MR)
Progesterone receptor (PR)

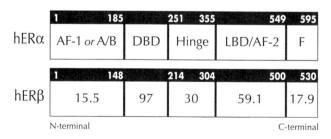

hERα	1	185	251	355	549	595
	AF-1 *or* A/B		DBD	Hinge	LBD/AF-2	F

hERβ	1	148	214	304	500	530
	15.5		97	30	59.1	17.9

N-terminal   C-terminal

Fig. 100-2 Sequence of domains A through F and their homology between the estrogen receptor (ER) subtypes. (Reproduced by permission of the Society for Endocrinology: Gustaffson JA. [1999]. Estrogen receptor β—a new dimension in estrogen mechanism of action. *J Endocrinol*. 163:379–383.)

B. Interdependence between AF-1 and AF-2

AF-1 and AF-2 are the two domains that mediate transactivation. As shown in Fig. 100-2, AF-1 is localized within the N-terminal A/B domain, whereas AF-2 is found in the more C-terminal E domain. Evidence suggests that these domains function synergistically in a tissue- and promoter-specific manner [67]. However, AF-1 function is ligand-independent, whereas AF-2 is entirely ligand-dependent. Thus, following binding of AF-2 by ligand, the E_2-ER complex translocates to the nucleus and AF-1 binds to the coactivator p300 [68]. It may be that the combination of ligand binding to the AF-2 domain and p300 binding derepresses AF-1, leading to functional synergism between AF-1 and AF-2 *(vide infra)*. The E_2-ER complex can then initiate transcription once bound to an ERE.

C. The DNA-Binding Domain

The DBDs of ERα and ERβ are 97% homologous (see Fig. 100-2). Both ER subtypes possess two canonical zinc finger motifs that mediate DNA-binding. Figure 100-3 shows the presence of nine cysteine residues and several functional subdomains within this region. One subdomain, the P-box, specifically mediates DNA-binding capacity, although it is not the only motif involved in this function. As shown in the diagram, two of the conserved cysteines are contained within this motif. Its sequence, CEGCKA (see Fig. 100-3), recognizes the DNA motif, AGGTCA. Of particular interest is the crystal structure revealing how the DBD contacts DNA [69,70]. Here, a second subdomain, the D-box, mediates dimerization between two ERs. The D-box possesses a dimerization interface that is localized in the N-terminal portion of the second zinc finger (see Fig. 100-3). Because dimerization significantly enhances DNA-binding by further stabilizing the interaction between the nuclear receptor and the ERE [71], this site is important for efficient transactivation [72]. Homodimerization takes on further significance when it is

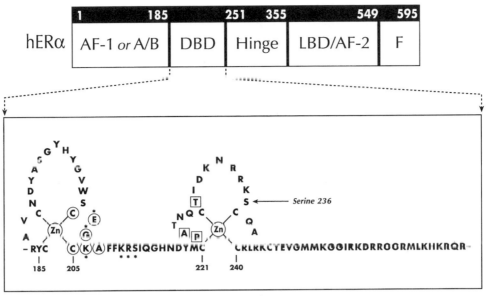

Zinc fingers within the core DBD

Fig. 100-3   Zinc fingers containing the P- and D-box subdomains of the DNA binding domain. Nine conserved cysteine residues are present within this region. The P-box mediates DNA-binding capacity. Two of the conserved cysteines are contained within this motif. Its sequence, CEGCKA, recognizes the DNA motif, AGGTCA. The D-box mediates dimerization between two estrogen receptors. The D-box possesses a dimerization interface that is localized in the NH_2-terminal portion of the second zinc finger. Asterisks denote residues that interact with basepairs of ERE. (Adapted with permission from Pettersson K, Gustafsson JA. [2001]. Role of estrogen receptor beta in estrogen action. *Annu Rev Physiol.* 63:165–192.)

recognized that ERs often bind to ERE variants, which are found in the majority of estrogen-responsive genes [71].

D. The Ligand-Binding Domain

The LBDs of ERα and ERβ, localized in the more COOH-terminal portion of the ER between the D and F domains, are 59% homologous (see Fig. 100-2). Following ligand binding, this domain undergoes a conformational modification [73,74]. Twelve α-helices in the LBD (annotated as H1–12) form a pocket to bind and hold the estrogen ligand [75]. Crystallographic analyses revealed that diethylstilbestrol (ligand)-bound ERα in the presence of a glucocorticoid receptor interacting protein-1 (GRIP1) coactivator peptide results in a conformational change by the binding of the peptide as a short alpha helix to a hydrophobic groove on the LBD surface. More specifically, H12 of the LBD undergoes the shift, thereby resulting in AF-2 activity and its subsequent synergistic interaction with AF-1 [74]. By contrast, binding of the antiestrogens, tamoxifen and raloxifene, causes H12 to be translocated to a position that obstructs the coactivator contact site, preventing coactivator attachment and inhibiting ER-dependent transactivation [73,74]. Thus, the shift in helix 12 is integral to the dissociation of corepressors and association of coactivators [74] and, ultimately, transactivation.

Although in general the binding specificities of the two ER subtypes are similar, there is an interesting difference in ligand affinity for certain agonists and antagonists. The well-known antiestrogen receptor agent, tamoxifen, used as an adjunct in breast cancer therapy, has a tissue- and cell-specific dual binding

affinity for ERα, whereas it is an antagonist for ERβ [77,78]. This differential binding affinity may in part be accounted for by the variable sequences of the AF-1 domain between the two receptor subtypes. From a therapeutic standpoint, differential binding between the LBDs raises the possibility that specific pharmaceuticals having higher specificities for each receptor could be synthesized [78].

E. Plasma Membrane Estrogen Receptors

ERs are classically defined as nuclear receptors. Recently, however, compelling functional, biochemical, and immuno-histocytochemical data have suggested the presence of ERs in the plasma membrane of diverse cell types [79].

To demonstrate the presence of a surface ER(s), four criteria have been established. First, cells exhibit a rapid physiologic response following E_2 binding. For instance, E_2 binding to human monocytes stimulates a rapid increase in $[Ca^{++}]_i$, resulting in nitric oxide (NO) production in less than a minute [80]. Second, both cell-permeable E_2 and impermeable E_2-BSA (bovine serum albumin) bind to endothelial cells and stimulate (a) a rapid increase in cyclic guanine monophosphate (cGMP); (b) activation of p38 mitogen activated protein kinase (MAPK), MAP kinase-protein kinase 2 (MAPKAP2), and ERKs; (c) production of NO; and, (d) phosphorylation of heat shock protein 27 (HSP27) [81–83]. In pulmonary artery endothelium, E_2 binding stimulates the MAPK pathway and activation of NO synthase in less than five minutes, leading to vascular relaxation [82]. Third, binding of E_2-BSA to the cell surface of various cell types, such as T cells, has been identified by confocal immuno-fluorescent microscopy as well as other immunocytochemical techniques [83–85]. Finally, within the central nervous system of animals that lack both ERα and ERβ or whose ERs have been knocked out, hypothalamic and hippocampal neurons exhibit rapid downstream signaling, including activation of PKA and protein kinase C (PKC), on E_2 binding. Taken together, these results support the existence of a surface ER(s) on some cell types that can initiate signal transduction.

The concept that a surface ER(s) exists and can activate downstream signaling pathways is still an evolving concept. Of particular interest is that these receptors interact with G-proteins, much the way that adenosine, adrenergic, and prostaglandin receptors do. In various tissues, for instance, membrane ER(s) can activate $G\alpha_s$- and $G\alpha_q$- proteins [86–88], resulting in (a) activation of phospholipase C-β (PLC-β) [88]; (b) rapid intra-cellular calcium (Ca^{++}_i) fluxes [80,83,88,89] and entry of Ca^{++} via store-operated Ca^{++} channels [89]; and (c) activation of PKC and PKA isozymes [86,90]. Not unexpectedly, specific signaling cascades are preferentially utilized in particular cell types, resulting in, for example, activation of PLC-β or PKC-δ.

Despite evidence for the existence of a membrane ER(s), intense controversy exists about the nature of these receptors. The GH3/B6/F10 pituitary tumor cell is a case in point. E_2 binding to these cells produces (a) a rapid influx of Ca^{++} via voltage-gated Ca^{++} channels; (b) intracellular Ca^{++} fluxes; and (c) subsequent prolactin production [84,85]. Moreover, binding of impermeable E_2-BSA has been identified by confocal immunofluorescence microscopy. Yet, questions about the fundamental biology and chemistry of the ER arise. Is the ER a transmembrane protein or a glycophosphatidylinositol (GPI)-anchored structure? If the ER is a GPI-anchored structure, is it linked to another transmembrane receptor? What is the ER isoform? Is the ER expressed on the cell surface or is it harbored within a membrane structure, such as caveolae [79]? These and other questions remain to be investigated.

F. Coregulators of Estrogen Receptor-Dependent Transactivation

ER coregulators are cofactors recruited by the AF-1 and AF-2 domains to modify transcriptional control of promoters possessing EREs. These cofactors are defined functionally as coactivators, corepressors, and cointegrators [91,92]. Because more than 30 such cofactors have been identified to date, this chapter will focus on the SRC/p160 family of coactivators, the CBP/p300 cointegrator, and the repressor of estrogen receptor activity (REA) corepressor and their relationship to ERs.

1. The SRC Family of Coactivators

Estrogen receptor-associated proteins (ERAP) were initially identified as cofactors that promote ER-dependent transactivation [93]. The 160-kD ERAP was found to interact with E_2-ER and to enhance its capacity to transcribe genes whose promoters possess an ERE. Mutant ER incapable of mediating transcription failed to bind ERAP-160. Of particular interest was that the estrogen antagonists 4-hydroxytamoxifen and ICI 164384 dissociated ERAP-160 from the ER. The discovery of ERAPs

led to the cloning and identification of ERAPs as components of the SRC/p160 family [94]. Table 100-2 summarizes the current nomenclature of the SRC/p160 family [91,92,95], although these designations have not yet been universally adopted.

The identification of ERAP-160 led to the cloning and sequencing of the first transcriptional cofactor for nuclear receptors, steroid receptor-coactivator-1 (SRC-1/human SRC-1). Thus, ERAP-160 is now termed SRC-1 [94]. Not restricted to a specific nuclear receptor, SRC-1 coactivates liganded ER, glucocorticoid receptor (GR), progesterone receptor (PR), and thyroid receptor (TR), among others. SRC-1 exhibits several diverse functions. First, it prevents PR transcriptional squelching by activated ER. That is, binding of PR to a promoter in the presence of SRC-1 prevents inhibition of transactivation by another activated nuclear receptor (NR). Second, SRC-1 can coactivate other transcription factors, including AP-1 and NF-κB [96,97]. Third, SRC-1 facilitates synergistic interaction of the NH_2-terminal AF-1 region with the COOH-terminal AF-2 motif of the LBD to promote recruitment of the preinitiation complex [98]. This is mediated by an α-helical LXXLL motif termed a NR box [76], which is common to many coactivators and may be present in one or more copies (see Fig. 100-1) (see the section on phosphorylation in this chapter). NR boxes form amphipathic α helices with leucine residues to create a hydro-phobic surface on one side of the helix. Finally, by interacting with other cofactors, such as p300/CBP and p300/CBP-associated factor (PCAF), SRC-1 exhibits acetyltransferase activity that targets histone tails of nucleosomes and facilitates transactivation (see Histone Acetylation/Deacetylation later in this chapter). Indeed, both CBP/p300 and PCAF possess intrinsic acetyl-transferase activity [99,100].

SRC-2 is the second member of the SRC family; this desig-nation is synonymous with nuclear receptor coactivator-2 (NCoA-2), GRIP1, and transcription intermediary factor 2 (TIF2) (see Table 100-2). GRIP1, the murine SRC-2, and TIF1, the human SRC-2, bind to the LBD of liganded NRs, including the ER [101–103], thereby promoting transactivation. Moreover, like SRC-1, SRC-2 appears to be able to obviate ER squelching [101]. Although SRC-2 was initially identified as a coactivator, it can also mediate corepressor activity at the collagenase-3

Table 100-2
Steroid Receptor Coactivator (SRC) Family Nomenclature

Current	Initial/Previous Designation	Reference
SRC-1	human SRC-1 (hSRC-1)* [94]	
mSRC-1*	NCoA-1	[112]
SRC-2	hSRC-2, TIF2	[101]
mSRC-2	GRIP1, NCoA-2	[102,114]
SRC-3	hSRC-3, RAC3, ACTR,	[101,152]
	TRAM-1, AIB1	[105,153]
		[106,154]
mSRC-3	p/CIP	[114]

*h, human; m, mouse.
(From Li H, Chen JD. [1998]. The receptor-associated coactivator 3 activates transcription through CREB-binding protein recruitment and autoregulation. *J Biol Chem.* 273:5948–5954.)

promoter [104]. This unexpected finding suggests that cofactors may be able to mediate either coactivator or corepressor activity, perhaps depending on the particular promoter, concurrent binding of other cofactors, and local conditions.

SCR-3 is the third member of the SRC/p160 family. As shown in Table 100-2, it is a polymorphic protein that has been variously identified as p300/CBP cointegrator-associated protein (p/CIP), activator of thyroid receptor (ACTR), amplified in breast cancer-1 (AIB-1), receptor-associated coactivator-3 (RAC-3), thyroid receptor activator molecule-1 (TRAM-1), and SRC-3. Like other SRC members, SRC-3 is capable of coactivating multiple NRs, including the ER [105]. It is interesting that SRC-3 preferentially enhances the transcriptional function of ERα compared to ERβ, which may reflect its LBD-binding capacity to the α isoform [106]. In addition to its coactivator function for NRs, SRC-3 may contribute to NF-κB-mediated gene expression [107]. Tumor necrosis factor-alpha (TNF-α) stimulates IκB kinase (IKK)-catalyzed phosphorylation of SRC-3, resulting in its subsequent nuclear translocation from the cytoplasm. Simultaneously, IKK phosphorylates IκB, resulting in its release, degradation, and subsequent nuclear translocation of NF-κB. In the nucleus, phosphorylated SRC-3 appears to augment NF-κB-mediated gene expression. Based on these data, one might anticipate that SRC-3 could also function in immune cells, where it would mediate both immune and inflammatory responses that are dependent on NF-κB transactivation.

Although three principal isoforms of the SRC/p160 family have been identified, their capacity to associate in complexes with multiple NRs raises the possibility of some overlap in their functions. In part, this may reflect their NH$_2$-terminal sequence homology in the tandem basic helix-loop-helix (bHLH) and Per/ Arnt/Sim (PAS) regions. Because these domains mediate homo-dimerization and heterodimerization [108], SRC members may form dimers that facilitate assembly of preinitiation complexes [109].

2. CBP/p300 Cointegrators

CREB-binding protein (CBP) was initially identified as a coactivator for the nuclear transcription factor, CREB [110,111]. However, subsequent analyses have revealed that CBP coactivates diverse transcription factors, including the ER [112]. Like other NR coactivators, CBP possesses a NR box in its NH$_2$-terminus that mediates binding to the ER [76]. Similarly, p300 coactivates several transcription factors, including NRs [113].

In addition to its binding to the ER, CBP and p300 can specifically bind to principal SRC isoforms [101,112,114–116]. These interactions between CBP/p300, ER, and SRC may create a multiprotein complex that integrates incoming signals from the cytosol and directs the transactivation of multiple genes possessing cis-acting EREs in their promoters. However, despite the synergistic interaction of CBP/P300 and ER, in vitro differences between CBP and p300 and their interaction with the ER have been observed [117]. Notwithstanding, the capacity of CBP/p300 to efficiently integrate diverse afferent signals accounts for its designation as a nuclear cointegrator [112].

3. Corepressors

Silencing mediator of retinoic acid and thyroid hormone receptor (SMRT) and nuclear receptor corepressor (NCoR) are the two classic corepressors that interact with type II NRs, such as TR. As corepressors, their action represses transcription of the type II NRs. Several mechanisms appear to operate coordinately to mediate repression of basal transcription by the type II NRs. First, unliganded NRs can generate a steric hindrance that inhibits DNA binding and, apparently, prevents coactivator interaction with NR [118]. This passive repression is the result of competition for DNA-binding or dimerization targets [119]. Second, unliganded NRs can interact with inactive heterodimers to repress transcription [120]. A third process occurs when an unliganded receptor, such as the TR, interacts with the basal transcription factor TFIIB, sequestering it and resulting in transcriptional repression [121]. A fourth mechanism, transrepression, is the process by which an unliganded NR complexes with other factors that prevent recruitment and assembly of a preinitiation complex. One of the earliest examples of this mechanism was the reciprocal antagonistic effect of NRs and AP-1 by the GR [122]. Here, liganded GR diminishes the response of an AP-1-mediated promoter to a Ras-dependent stimulus.

To date, three corepressors of ER-mediated transactivation have been identified. SMRT corepresses ERα only in the presence of its cognate partial agonist, 4-hydroxytamoxifen (4HT) [123]. That SMRT interacts with 4HT-ERα complexes suggests that ERα may harbor an undetected motif(s) that becomes exposed as a result of a conformational change on antagonist binding. Whether interaction of SMRT with ERα occurs in vivo in the absence of an antiestrogen remains uncertain.

REA is a 37-kDa selective ER corepressor that was initially identified by its inhibitory capacity for dominant-negative ERs and antiestrogens [124]. By competing with SRC-1 for binding to the ER AF-2 domain, REA blocks SRC-1 coactivator activity. Because REA has no intrinsic corepressor activity of its own, does not prevent nuclear import of ER, and does not impede ER binding to EREs, REA appears to function as an anticoactivator by competitively inhibiting SRC-1 interaction with ERα and ERβ. Parenthetically, it is germane to point out that REA has no sequence homology with SMRT or NCoR. REA selectively binds to liganded ER; by contrast, unliganded ER is inactive and exhibits no repressor activity. Only when wild-type (wt) ER binds to an antiestrogen can it function as a repressor.

Short heterodimer partner (SHP) is an atypical member of the NR family that possesses a LBD but lacks a conserved DBD [125]. SHP interacts with liganded ERα and ERβ to repress transactivation [126,127]. It is surprising that the mechanism by which SHP interacts with ERs is via LXXLL-like motifs [128]. As noted earlier, LXXLL motifs comprise the NR box that mediates coactivator binding to the LBD within AF-2 of NRs. This new evidence suggests that the NR box can mediate coactivation or corepression, depending on the cofactor. Together with dimeric ERs, SHP is thought to mediate repression via a ternary complex at the ERE [128].

Although antiestrogens have been regarded as the principal mechanism for repression of ER-dependent transactivation, accumulating evidence suggests that natural corepressors exist that interact with either unliganded or liganded ER to repress transactivation. Future investigation is likely to identify other corepressors whose mode of action may or may not be analogous to that of SMRT, REA, and SHP.

IV. Mechanisms that Mediate E_2-ERE Transactivation

From the previous discussion, it is evident that transactivation or repression of E_2-dependent ERE gene expression depends on complex interactions with multiprotein complexes. Several concomitant posttranslational processes regulate these events. Of these, histone acetylation/deacetylation and phosphorylation will be further discussed.

A. Histone Acetylation and Deacetylation

Acetylation of histone tail lysine residues within the nucleosome modifies the relationship between the ERE and nucleosome by disrupting higher-order chromatin structure. This event promotes transcriptional activation by permitting access of transcription factors to the promoter region [99]. Several coactivators within multiprotein complexes possess histone acetylase activity, including P300/CBP, P/CAF (p300/CBP-associated factor), and SRC-1 and -3 [129]. P300/CBP interacts with helix 12 in the LBD via LXXLL motifs (see Fig. 100-1). By contrast, histone deacetylases (HDAC) remove lysine residues, altering charge–charge interactions between histones and nucleosomes and inhibiting access of transcription factors [99]. Multiprotein corepressors possess HDAC activity, which interacts with Mad, NCoR, SMRT, and mSIN3, to restructure chromatin into an inactive status, repressing transactivation [130,131].

B. Phosphorylation

Phosphorylation of ERs on serine and/or tyrosine residues is a pivotal posttranslational regulatory event that regulates their transactivational activity. Both ERα and ERβ become phosphorylated on tyrosine (try)[537] in the LBD by src tyrosine kinases independent of E_2, but this posttranslational modification alone does not initiate transactivation [132]. However, mutational analyses indicate that substitution of asparagine (asn) for tyr results in an E_2-independent, constitutively-active ER that exhibits transactivational function [133]. Because tyr[537] is localized in the LBD that also mediates dimerization and transcription, it has been suggested that tyr[537] phosphorylation may be necessary for ligand binding to the ER [133].

ERα is also phosphorylated on ser[118] in the A/B domain via the MAP kinase pathway [134,135]. Like phosphorylation of tyr[537] by src tyrosine kinases, MAP kinase-catalyzed phosphorylation of ser[118] is independent of E_2 binding to ERα and triggers its transactivational function. Moreover, growth factors, such as epidermal growth factor (EGF), can also stimulate MAP kinase-catalyzed ser[118] phosphorylation that augments ER-dependent transactivation [136,137]. However, ERα can also be phosphorylated via MAP kinase-independent pathways [138,139]. For instance, PKA phosphorylates ser[236], preventing dimerization and thereby inhibiting DNA binding [140]. Moreover, E_2 induces both casein kinase II- and pp90rsk1-catalyzed phosphorylation of ser[167] [141,142].

In contrast to ERα, murine ERβ is phosphorylated on ser[106] and ser[124] in the AF-1 region by the MAP kinase pathway in a ligand- and AF-2-independent manner [66,143]. Phosphorylation of these sites promotes the recruitment of the coactivator SRC-1 and its interaction with and ligand-independent transactivation

of ERβ [143]. Because binding of growth factors, such as EGF and insulin growth factor-1 (IGF-1), to their surface receptors activates downstream MAP kinase pathways and enhances recruitment of SRC-1, this may further augment ERβ transactivational efficiency. In the presence of E_2, ser[124] phosphorylation synergistically enhances the transactivational activity of ERβ. Indeed, SRC-1 induces ERβ transactivation in the absence or presence of ligand [66].

In addition to its phosphorylation of ERs, MAP kinase also phosphorylates ser[884] of the thyroid receptor binding protein (TRBP), a residue just -3 from the single LXXLL motif through which it interacts with nuclear receptors [144]. In this flanking position, ser[884] may influence nuclear receptor selectivity. Indeed, phosphorylation of this residue appears to regulate the specificity with which TRBP binds to ERβ vs ERα as well as TR and RXR.

Taken together, phosphorylation is a pivotal posttranslational mechanism regulating the transactivational activity of ERs. That factors other than the natural ligand for ERs can transactivate genes possessing EREs [145] and that SRC-1 can be recruited via phosphorylation of nuclear receptors [143] further underscores the central importance of this mechanism. Of potential pertinence to ER transactivation function is the recognition that phosphorylation of discrete ser/thr residues in the AF-1 domain of other nuclear receptors can upregulate or downregulate their functions [146,147]. For instance, MAP kinase-dependent phosphorylation of the A/B domain of PPARγ diminishes its transcriptional activity [146] by altering LBD affinity for its ligand through domain–domain interactions [148]. Such an effect may also occur on AF-1 phosphorylation of ERβ.

V. Sex Hormones and Predisposition to Systemic Lupus Erythematosus

Although there is consensus about the gender diathesis for SLE [4], considerable debate centers on the relative roles of estrogen and prolactin in the pathogenesis of SLE [6,149]. Whereas current immunoendocrinologic evidence suggests that both estrogen and prolactin modulate the immune response, prolactin may promote a Th2 response that contributes to autoantibody production [6]. Notwithstanding, the mechanisms by which estrogen and prolactin modify cellular and humoral immune responses is still largely unexplored. Recent work has begun to delve further into the relative roles of the estrogen, progesterone, glucocorticoid, and prolactin in lupus immunopathogenesis [7,150].

Consistent with the concept of regulatory roles for both estrogen and prolactin in immune cell function, E_2 was found to regulate survival and activation of anti-DNA-specific B cells in nonautoimmune mice transgenic for the heavy chain of a pathogenic anti-DNA autoantibody [11]. E_2 stimulated an increased frequency of high-affinity anti-DNA autoantibody-secreting B cells and increased anti-DNA autoantibody serum titers, eventuating in deposition of immune complexes in renal glomeruli. This was associated with immunohistologic evidence of increased Bcl-2 in splenic B cells, although it is unclear whether these were anti-DNA-secreting B cells. These data were interpreted as consistent with the capacity of E_2 to break tolerance in a nonautoimmune mouse.

However, when these animals were treated with both E_2 and bromocriptine, an increased frequency of high-affinity anti-DNA autoantibody-secreting B cells and intracellular Bcl-2 persisted, but the titers of anti-DNA autoantibodies in the serum declined and reduced immune complex-mediated glomerular deposits were observed compared to animals treated with E_2 alone. It was concluded that reduced anti-DNA autoantibody serum titers reflect a subpopulation of anergic, high-affinity anti-DNA B cells, and that anergy may be the result of inhibition of prolactin secretion by bromocriptine.

Studies such as these provide important information about the role of sex hormones in tolerance and anergy. Nevertheless, the molecular mechanism by which E_2 breaks tolerance in transgenic B cells has yet to be identified. Moreover, it remains uncertain whether E_2 would have a similar effect in wt non-autoimmune mice.

Because both ERα and ERβ are expressed in T cells, efforts were also undertaken to determine if ER structure and function are altered in murine and human lupus. In human lupus, initial work identified the presence of both a wt and an exon 5-deficient ER isoform (presumably ERα isoforms) in normal and SLE peripheral blood mononuclear cells (PBMC) [151]. Whereas normal cells expressed both wt and exon 5-deleted isoforms, SLE cells apparently expressed either the wt or deleted isoforms. In follow-up work from the same group, however, cells were found to have wt ERα as well as exon 5 and 7 deletion isoforms, but there were no differences between normal and SLE subjects [46] compared to the previous analysis [151]. By contrast, another group's analysis revealed that ERα and ERβ exhibit splice variants resulting in deletions of exons 2, 5, and 7 in comparable frequencies between normal subjects and subjects with SLE. In particular, no relationship between polymorphisms of ERα exons 1 and 2 was linked to SLE [47]. Because the results of these analyses are incongruous, further work should be pursued to clarify this fundamental issue.

In conclusion, accumulating evidence supports the concept of abnormal signaling and skewed gene expression in immune cells from subjects with SLE. Although initial analyses have not identified abnormalities of ER structure in SLE immune cells, additional efforts are clearly warranted to determine whether physiologic E_2-ERα/β interactions occur and the outcome of their regulation of ERE-containing genes.

VI. Suggestions for Further Investigations

Goals to enhance our understanding of molecular mechanisms of estrogen effects on T cell functions:

- Delineate the molecular mechanisms by which estrogen contributes to regulation of effector functions, including help and cytotoxicity.
- Delineate the molecular mechanisms by which estrogen may modify or alter T cell tolerance.

Acknowledgements

This work was partially supported by NIH grants RO1 AR39501, RO1 AI46526, and RO1 AI42269.

References

1. Kammer GM, Tsokos GC. (1999). *Lupus: Molecular and Cellular Pathogenesis.* Totowa, NJ: Humana Press.
2. Harvey AM, Shulman LE, Tumulty PA. (1954). Systemic lupus erythematosus: review of the literature and clinical analysis of 138 cases. *Medicine.* 33:291–437.
3. Hochberg MC. (1992). Epidemiology of systemic lupus erythematosus. In: Lahita RG, ed. *Systemic Lupus Erythematosus.* New York: Churchill Livingstone. 103–117.
4. Lahita RG. (1996). The connective tissue diseases and the overall influence of gender. *Int J Fertil Menopausal Stud.* 41:156–165.
5. Lahita RG. (1992). The importance of estrogens in systemic lupus erythematosus. *Clin Immunol Immunopathol.* 63:17–18.
6. McMurray RW. (2001). Sex hormones in the pathogenesis of systemic lupus erythematosus. *Frontiers Biosci.* 6:193–206.
7. Watson CS, Gametchu B. (2001). Membrane estrogen and glucocorticoid receptors—implications for hormonal control of immune function and autoimmunity. *Int Immunopharmacol.* 1:1049–1063.
8. Okasha SA, Ryu S, Do Y, *et al.* (2001). Evidence for estradiol-induced apoptosis and dysregulated T cell maturation in the thymus. *Toxicology.* 163:49–62.
9. Jenkins JK, Suwannaroj S, Elbourne KB, *et al.* (2001). 17-β-Estradiol alters Jurkat lymphocyte cell cycling and induces apoptosis through suppression of Bcl-2 and cyclin A. *Int Immunopharmacol.* 1:1897–1911.
10. Rider V, Abdou NI. (2001). Gender differences in autoimmunity: molecular basis for estrogen effects in systemic lupus erythematosus. *Int Immunopharmacol.* 1:1009–1024.
11. Bynoe MS, Grimaldi CM, Diamond B. (2000). Estrogen up-regulates Bcl-2 and blocks tolerance induction of naïve B cells. *Proc Natl Acad Sci U S A.* 97:2703–2708.
12. Tsokos GC. (1999). Overview of cellular immune function in systemic lupus erythematosus. In: Lahita RG, ed. *Systemic Lupus Erythematosus.* New York: Academic Press. 17–54.
13. Dayal AK, Kammer GM. (1996). The T cell enigma in lupus. *Arthritis Rheum.* 39:23–33.
14. Tsokos GC, Kammer GM. (2000). Molecular aberrations in human systemic lupus erythematosus. *Mol Med Today.* 6:418–424.
15. Casciola-Rosen LA, Anhalt G, Rosen A. (1994). Autoantigens targeted in systemic lupus erythematosus are clustered in two populations of surface structures on apoptotic keratinocytes. *J Exp Med.* 179:1317–1330.
16. Kammer GM, Perl A, Richardson BC, *et al.* (2002). Abnormal T cell signal transduction in systemic lupus erythematosus. *Arthritis Rheum.* 46:1139–1154.
17. Richardson BC. (1986). Effect of an inhibitor of DNA methylation on T cells. II. 5-Azacytidine induces self-reactivity in antigen-specific T-4+ cells. *Hum Immunol.* 17:456–470.
18. Koshy M, Berger D, Crow MK. (1996). Increased expression of CD40 ligand on systemic lupus erythematosus lymphocytes. *J Clin Invest.* 98:826–837.
19. Utermohlen V, Winfield JB, Zabriskie JB, *et al.* (1974). A depression of cell-mediated immunity to measles antigen in patients with systemic lupus erythematosus. *J Exp Med.* 139:1019–1024.
20. Richardson BC, Strahler JR, Pivirotto TS, *et al.* (1992). Phenotypic and functional similarities between 5-azacytidine-treated T cells and a T cell subset in patients with active systemic lupus erythematosus. *Arthritis Rheum.* 35:647–662.
21. Richardson BC, Powers D, Hooper F, *et al.* (1994). Lymphocyte function-associated antigen 1 overexpression and T cell autoreactivity. *Arthritis Rheum.* 37:1363–1372.
22. Inghirami G, Simon J, Balow JE, *et al.* (1988). Activated T lymphocytes in the peripheral blood of patients with systemic lupus erythematosus induce B cells to produce immunoglobulin. *Clin Exp Rheumatol.* 6:269–276.
23. Kammer GM. (1999). High prevalence of T cell type I protein kinase A deficiency in systemic lupus erythematosus. *Arthritis Rheum.* 42:1458–1465.
24. Froncek MJ, Horwitz DA. (2002). Cytokines in the pathogenesis of systemic lupus erythematosus. In: Wallace DJ, Hahn BH, eds. *Dubois' Lupus Erythematosus.* Philadelphia: Lippincott Williams & Wilkins. 187–204.
25. Kaneko H, Ogasawara H, Naito T, *et al.* (1999). Circulating levels of β-chemokines in systemic lupus erythematosus. *J Rheumatol.* 26:568–573.
26. Desai-Mehta A, Lu LJ, Ramsey-Goldman R, *et al.* (1996). Hyperexpression of CD40 ligand by B and T cells in human lupus and its role in pathogenic autoantibody production. *J Clin Invest.* 97:2063–2073.
27. Wener MH. (2000). Immune complexes. In: Tsokos GC, ed. *Principles of Molecular Rheumatology.* Totowa, NJ: Humana Press. 127–144.
28. Hahn BH. (1998). Antibodies to DNA. *N Engl J Med.* 338:1359–1368.

29. Kammer GM, Stein RL. (1990). T lymphocyte immune dysfunctions in systemic lupus erythematosus. *J Lab Clin Med*. 115:273–282.

30. Mandler R, Birch RE, Polmar S, *et al*. (1982). Abnormal adenosine-induced immunosuppression and cAMP metabolism in T lymphocytes of patients with systemic lupus erythematosus. *Proc Natl Acad Sci U S A*. 79:7542–7546.

31. Liossis SNC, Ding XZ, Dennis GJ, *et al*. (1998). Altered pattern of TCR/CD3-mediated protein-tyrosyl phosphorylation in T cells from patients with systemic lupus erythematosus—Deficient expression of the T cell receptor zeta chain. *J Clin Invest*. 101:1448–1457.

32. Takeuchi T, Tsuzaka K, Pang M, *et al*. (1998). TCRβ chain lacking exon 7 in two patients with systemic lupus erythematosus. *Int Immunol*. 10:911–921.

33. Brundula V, Rivas LJ, Blasini AM, *et al*. (1999). Diminished levels of T cell receptor zeta chains in peripheral blood T lymphocytes from patients with systemic lupus erythematosus. *Arthritis Rheum*. 42:1908–1916.

34. Laxminarayana D, Khan IU, Mishra N, *et al*. (1999). Diminished levels of protein kinase A RIα and RIβ transcripts and proteins in systemic lupus erythematosus T lymphocytes. *J Immunol*. 162:5639–5648.

35. Grolleau A, Kaplan MJ, Hanash SM, *et al*. (2000). Impaired translational response and increased protein kinase PKR expression in T cells from lupus patients. *J Clin Invest*. 106:1561–1568.

36. Vassilopoulos D, Kovacs B, Tsokos GC. (1995). TCR/CD3 complex-mediated signal transduction pathway in T cells and T cell lines from patients with systemic lupus erythematosus. *J Immunol*. 155:2269–2281.

37. Gergely P Jr, Grossman C, Niland B, *et al*. (2002). Mitochondrial hyperpolarization and ATP depletion in patients with systemic lupus erythematosus. *Arthritis Rheum*. 46:175–190.

38. Deng C, Kaplan MJ, Yang J, *et al*. (2001). Decreased ras-mitogen-activated protein kinase signaling may cause DNA hypomethylation in T lymphocytes from lupus patients. *Arthritis Rheum*. 44:397–407.

39. Jensen EV, Jacobson HI. (1962). Basic guides to the mechanism of estrogen action. *Recent Prog Horm Res*. 18:387–414.

40. Walter P, Green S, Greene G, *et al*. (1985). Cloning of the human estrogen receptor cDNA. *Proc Natl Acad Sci U S A*. 82:7889–7893.

41. Green S, Walter P, Kumar V, *et al*. (1986). Human oestrogen receptor cDNA: sequence, expression and homology to v-erb-A. *Nature*. 320:134–139.

42. Greene GL, Gilna P, Waterfield M, *et al*. (1986). Sequence and expression of human estrogen receptor complementary DNA. *Science*. 231:1150–1154.

43. Kuiper GGJM, Enmark E, Pelto-Huikko M, *et al*. (1996). Cloning of a novel estrogen receptor expressed in rat prostate and ovary. *Proc Natl Acad Sci U S A*. 93:5925–5930.

44. Gustafsson JA. (1999). Estrogen receptor β—a new dimension in estrogen mechanism of action. *J Endocrinol*. 163:379–383.

45. Mosselman S, Polman J, Dijkema R. (1996). ER beta: identification and characterization of a novel human estrogen receptor. *FEBS Lett*. 392:49–53.

46. Suenaga R, Evans MJ, Mitamura K, *et al*. (1998). Peripheral blood T cells and monocytes and B cell lines derived from patients with lupus express estrogen receptor transcripts similar to those of normal cells. *J Rheumatol*. 25:1305–1312.

47. Kassi EN, Vlachoyiannopoulos PG, Moutsopoulos HM, *et al*. (2001). Molecular analysis of estrogen receptor alpha and beta in lupus patients. *Eur J Clin Invest*. 31:86–93.

48. Cohen JHM, Danel L, Cordier G, *et al*. (1983). Sex steroid receptors in peripheral T cells: absence of androgen receptors and restriction of estrogen receptors to OKT8-positive cells. *J Immunol*. 131:2767–2771.

49. Stimson WH. (1988). Oestrogen and human T lymphocytes: Presence of specific receptors in the T-suppressor/cytotoxic subset. *Scand J Immunol*. 28:345–350.

50. Tornwall J, Carey AB, Fox RI, *et al*. (1999). Estrogen in autoimmunity: expression of estrogen receptors in thymic and autoimmune T cells. *J Gend Specif Med*. 2:33–40.

51. Mor G, Munoz A, Redlinger Jr R, *et al*. (2001). The role of the Fas/Fas ligand system in estrogen-induced thymic alteration. *Am J Reprod Immunol*. 46:298–307.

52. Suenaga R, Rider V, Evans MJ, *et al*. (2001). *In vitro*-activated human lupus T cells express normal estrogen receptor proteins which bind to the estrogen response element. *Lupus*. 10:116–122.

53. Ogawa S, Inoue S, Watanabe T, *et al*. (1998). The complete primary structure of human estrogen receptor beta (hERbeta) and its heterodimerization with ER alpha *in vivo* and *in vitro*. *Biochem Biophys Res Commun*. 243:122–126.

54. Moore JT, McKee DD, Slentz-Kesler K, *et al*. (1998). Cloning and characterization of human estrogen receptor beta isoforms. *Biochem Biophys Res Commun*. 247:75–78.

55. Bhat RA, Harnish DC, Stevis PE, *et al*. (1998). A novel human estrogen receptor beta: identification and functional analysis of additional N-terminal amino acids. *J Steroid Biochem Mol Biol*. 67:233–240.

56. Maruyama K, Endoh H, Sasaki-Iwaoka H, *et al*. (1998). A novel isoform of rat estrogen receptor beta with 18 amino acid insertion in the ligand binding domain as a putative dominant negative regulator of estrogen action. *Biochem Biophys Res Commun*. 246:142–147.

57. Petersen DN, Tkalcevic GT, Koza-Taylor PH, *et al*. (1998). Identification of estrogen receptor beta2, a functional variant of estrogen receptor beta expressed in normal rat tissues. *Endocrinology*. 139:1082–1092.

58. Parker MG. (1995). Structure and function of estrogen receptors. *Vitam Horm*. 51:267–287.

59. Enmark E, Gustafsson JA. (1999). Oestrogen receptors—an overview. *J Int Med*. 246:133–138.

60. Nagpal S, Friant S, Nakshatri H, *et al*. (1993). RARs and RXRs: evidence for two autonomous transactivation functions (AF-1 and AF-2) and heterodimerization *in vivo*. *EMBO J*. 12:2349–2360.

61. Martinez E, Wahli W. (1989). Cooperative binding of estrogen receptor in imperfect estrogen-responsive DNA elements correlates with their synergistic hormone-dependent enhancer activity. *EMBO J*. 8:3781–3791.

62. Tremblay GB, Tremblay A, Labrie F, *et al*. (1999). Dominant activity of activation function 1 (AF-1) and differential stoichiometric requirements for AF-1 and -2 in the estrogen receptor alpha-beta heterodimeric complex. *Mol Cell Biol*. 19:1919–1927.

63. Ogawa S, Inoue S, Orimo A, *et al*. (1998). Cross-inhibition of both estrogen receptor alpha and beta pathways by each dominant-negative mutant. *FEBS Lett*. 423:129–132.

64. Kato S, Tora L, Yamauchi J, *et al*. (1992). A far upstream estrogen response element of the ovalbumin gene contains several half-palindromic 5′-TGACC-3′ motifs acting synergistically. *Cell*. 68:731–742.

65. Hyder SM, Chiappetta C, Stancel GM. (1999). Interaction of human estrogen receptors α and β with the same naturally occurring estrogen response elements. *Biochem Pharmacol*. 57:597–601.

66. Tremblay GB, Tremblay A, Copeland NG, *et al*. (1997). Cloning, chromosomal localization, and functional analysis of the murine estrogen receptor beta. *Mol Endocrinol*. 11:353–365.

67. Tora L, White J, Brou C, *et al*. (1989). The human estrogen receptor has two independent nonacidic transcriptional activation functions. *Cell*. 59:477–487.

68. Kobayashi Y, Kitamoto T, Masuhiro Y, *et al*. (2000). p300 mediates functional synergism between AF-1 and AF-2 of estrogen receptor α and β by interacting directly with the N-terminal A/B domains. *J Biol Chem*. 275:15645–15651.

69. Schwabe JW, Neuhaus D, Rhodes D. (1990). Solution structure of the DNA-binding domain of the oestrogen receptor. *Nature*. 348:458–461.

70. Schwabe JW, Chapman L, Finch JT, *et al*. (1993). The crystal structure of the estrogen receptor DNA-binding domain bound to DNA: how receptors discriminate between their response elements. *Cell*. 75:567–578.

71. Kuntz MA, Shapiro DJ. (1997). Dimerizing the estrogen receptor DNA binding domain enhances binding to estrogen response elements. *J Biol Chem*. 272:27949–27956.

72. Glass CK. (1994). Differential recognition of target genes by nuclear receptor monomers, dimers, and heterodimers. *Endocr Rev*. 15:391–407.

73. Brzozowski AM, Pike AC, Dauter Z, *et al*. (1997). Molecular basis of agonism and antagonism in the oestrogen receptor. *Nature*. 389:753–758.

74. Shiau AK, Barstad D, Loria PM, *et al*. (1998). The structural basis of estrogen receptor/coactivator recognition and the antagonism of this interaction by tamoxifen. *Cell*. 95:927–937.

75. Wurtz JM, Bourguet W, Renaud JP, *et al*. (1996). A canonical structure for the ligand-binding domain of nuclear receptors. *Nat Struc Biol*. 3:206.

76. Heery M, Kalkhoven E, Hoare S, *et al*. (1997). A signature motif in transcriptional co-activators mediates binding to nuclear receptors. *Nature*. 387:733–736.

77. Watanabe T, Inoue S, Ogawa S, *et al*. (1997). Agonistic effect of tamoxifen is dependent on the cell type, ERE-promoter context, and estrogen subtype: Functional difference between estrogen receptors α and β. *Biochem Biophys Res Commun*. 236:140–145.

78. Barkhem T, Carlsson B, Nilsson Y, *et al*. (1998). Differential response of estrogen receptor alpha and estrogen receptor beta to partial estrogen agonists/antagonists. *Mol Pharmacol*. 54:105–112.

79. Kelly MJ, Levin ER. (2001). Rapid actions of plasma membrane estrogen receptors. *Trends Endocrinol Metab*. 12:152–156.

80. Stefano GB, Prevot V, Beauvillain JC, *et al*. (1999). Estradiol coupling to human monocyte nitric oxide release is dependent on intracellular calcium transients: evidence for an estrogen surface receptor. *J Immunol*. 163:3758–3763.

81. Razandi M, Pedram A, Levin ER. (2000). Estrogen signals to the preservation of endothelial cell form and function. *J Biol Chem.* 275:38540–38546.

82. Chen Z, Yuhanna IS, Galcheva-Gargova Z, et al. (1999). Estrogen receptor α mediates the nongenomic activation of endothelial nitric oxide synthase by estrogen. *J Clin Invest.* 103:401–406.

83. Benten WP, Lieberherr M, Giese G, et al. (1998). Estradiol binding to cell surface raises cytosolic free calcium in T cells. *FEBS Lett.* 422:349–353.

84. Norfleet AM, Thomas ML, Gametchu B, et al. (1999). Estrogen receptor-alpha detected on the plasma membrane of aldehyde-fixed GH3/B6/F10 rat pituitary tumor cells by enzyme linked immunocytochemistry. *Endocrinology.* 140:3805–3814.

85. Norfleet AM, Clarke CH, Gametchu B, et al. (2000). Antibodies to the estrogen receptor-alpha modulate rapid prolactin release from rat pituitary tumor cells through plasma membrane estrogen receptors. *FASEB J.* 14:157–165.

86. Lagrange AH, Ronnekleiv OK, Kelly MJ. (1997). Modulation of G protein-coupled receptors by an estrogen receptor that activates protein kinase A. *Mol Pharmacol.* 51:605–612.

87. Razandi M, Pedram A, Greene GL, et al. (1999). Cell membrane and nuclear estrogen receptors derive from a single transcript: studies of ERα and ERβ expressed in CHO cells. *Mol Endocrinol.* 13:307–319.

88. Le Mellay V, Grosse B, Lieberherr M. (1997). Phospholipase C beta and membrane action of calcitriol and estradiol. *J Biol Chem.* 272: 11902–11907.

89. Picotto G, Vazquez G, Boland R. (1999). 17β-oestradiol increases intracellular Ca^{2+} concentration in enterocytes. Potential role of phospholipase C-dependent store-operated Ca^{2+} influxes. *Biochem J.* 339:71–77.

90. Doolan CM, Condliffe SB, Harvey BJ. (2000). Rapid non-genomic activation of cytosolic cyclic AMP-dependent protein kinase activity and $[Ca^{2+}]$ by 17β-oestradiol in rat distal colon. *Br J Pharmacol.* 129:1375–1386.

91. McKenna NJ, O'Malley BW. (2002). Combinatorial control of gene expression by nuclear receptors and coregulators. *Cell.* 108:465–474.

92. Hermanson O, Glass CK, Rosenfeld MG. (2002). Nuclear receptor coregulators: multiple modes of modification. *Trends Endocrinol Metab.* 13:55–60.

93. Halachmi S, Marden E, Martin G, et al. (1994). Estrogen receptor-associated proteins: possible mediators of hormone-induced transcription. *Science.* 264:1455–1458.

94. Onate SA, Tsai SY, Tsai MJ, et al. (1996). Sequence and characterization of a coactivator for the steroid hormone receptor superfamily. *Science.* 270:1354–1357.

95. Li H, Chen JD. (1998). The receptor-associated coactivator 3 activates transcription through CREB-binding protein recruitment and autoregulation. *J Biol Chem.* 273:5948–5954.

96. Lee SK, Kim HJ, Na SY, et al. (1998). Steroid receptor coactivator-1 coactivates activating protein-1-mediated transactivations through interaction with the c-Jun and c-Fos subunits. *J Biol Chem.* 273:16651–16654.

97. Na SY, Lee SK, Han SJ, et al. (1998). Steroid receptor coactivator-1 interacts with the p50 subunit and coactivates NF-kB-mediated transactivation. *J Biol Chem.* 273:10831–10834.

98. Onate SA, Boonyaratanakornkit V, Spencer TE, et al. (1998). The steroid receptor coactivator-1 contains multiple receptor interacting and activation domains that cooperatively enhance the activation function 1 (AF-1) and AF-2 domains of steroid receptors. *J Biol Chem.* 273:12101–12108.

99. Kouzarides T. (1999). Histone acetylases and deacetylases in cell proliferation. *Curr Opin Genet Dev.* 9:40–48.

100. Yang XJ, Ogryzko VV, Nishikawa J, et al. (1996). A p300/CBP-associated factor that competes with the adenoviral oncoprotein E1A. *Nature.* 382:319–324.

101. Voegel JJ, Heine MJ, Zechel C, et al. (1996). TIF2, a 160-kDa transcriptional mediator for the ligand-dependent activation function AF-2 of nuclear receptors. *EMBO J.* 15:3667–3675.

102. Hong H, Kohli K, Trivedi A, et al. (1996). GRIP1, a novel mouse protein that serves as a transcriptional coactivator in yeast for the hormone binding domains of steroid receptors. *Proc Natl Acad Sci U S A.* 93: 4948–4952.

103. Hong H, Kohli K, Garabedian MJ, et al. (1997). GRIP1, a transcriptional coactivator for the AF-2 transactivation domain of steroid, thyroid, retinoid, and vitamin D receptors. *Mol Cell Biol.* 17:2735–2744.

104. Rogatsky I, Zarember KA, Yamamoto KR. (2001). Factor recruitment and TIF2/GRIP1 corepressor activity at a collagenase-3 response element that mediates regulation by phorbol esters and hormones. *EMBO J.* 20:6071–6083.

105. Anzick SL, Kononen J, Walker RL, et al. (1997). AIB1, a steroid receptor coactivator amplified in breast and ovarian cancer. *Science.* 277:965–968.

106. Suen CS, Berrodin TJ, Mastroeni R, et al. (1998). A transcriptional coactivator, steroid receptor coactivqator-3, selectively augments steroid receptor transcriptional activity. *J Biol Chem.* 273:27645–27653.

107. Wu RC, Qin J, Hashimoto Y, et al. (2002). Regulation of SRC-3 (pCIP/ACTR/AIB1/RAC3/TRAM-1) coactivator activity by IkB kinase. *Mol Cell Biol.* 22:3549–3561.

108. Hankinson O. (1995). The aryl hydrocarbon receptor complex. *Ann Rev Pharmacol Toxicol.* 35:307–340.

109. McKenna NJ, Nawaz Z, Tsai SY, et al. (1998). Distinct steady-state nuclear receptor coregulator complexes exist in vivo. *Proc Natl Acad Sci U S A.* 95:11697–11702.

110. Chrivia JC, Kwok RSP, Lamb N, et al. (1993). Phosphorylated CREB binds specifically to the nuclear protein CBP. *Nature.* 365:855–859.

111. Kwok RSP, Lundblad JR, Chrivia JC, et al. (1994). Nuclear protein CBP is a coactivator for the transcription factor CREB. *Nature.* 370:223–226.

112. Kamei Y, Xu L, Heinzel T, et al. (1996). A CBP integrator complex mediates transcriptional activation and AP-1 inhibition by nuclear receptors. *Cell.* 85:403–414.

113. Chakravarti D, LaMorte VJ, Nelson MC, et al. (1996). Role of CBP/p300 in nuclear receptor signalling. *Nature.* 383:99–103.

114. Torchia J, Rose DW, Inostroza J, et al. (1997). The transcriptional co-activator p/CIP binds CBP and mediates nuclear-receptor function. *Nature.* 387:677–684.

115. Yao TP, Ku G, Zhou N, et al. (1996). The nuclear hormone receptor coactivator SRC-1 is a specific target of p300. *Proc Natl Acad Sci U S A.* 93:10626–10631.

116. Hanstein B, Eckner R, DiRenzo J, et al. (1996). p300 is a component of an estrogen receptor coactivator complex. *Proc Natl Acad Sci U S A.* 93: 11540–11545.

117. Kraus WL, Kadonaga JT. (1998). p300 and estrogen receptor cooperatively activate transcription via differential enhancement of initiation and reinitiation. *Genes Dev.* 12:331–342.

118. Hudson LG, Santon JB, Glass CK, et al. (1990). Ligand-activated thyroid hormone and retinoic acid receptors inhibit growth factor receptor promoter expression. *Cell.* 62:1165–1175.

119. Glass CK, Rosenfeld MG. (2000). The coregulator exchange in transcriptional functions of nuclear receptors. *Genes Dev.* 14:121–141.

120. Forman BM, Samuels HH. (1990). Dimerization among nuclear hormone receptors. *New Biol.* 2:587–594.

121. Baniahmad A, Ha I, Reinberg D, et al. (1993). Interaction of human thyroid hormone receptor beta with transcription factor TFIIB may mediate target gene derepression and activation by thyroid hormone. *Proc Natl Acad Sci U S A.* 90:8832–8836.

122. Jonat C, Rahmsdorf HJ, Park KK, et al. (1990). Antitumor promotion and antiinflammation: down-modulation of AP-1 (Fos/Jun) activity by glucocorticoid hormone. *Cell.* 62:1189–1204.

123. Smith CL, Nawaz Z, O'Malley BW. (1998). Coactivator and corepressor regulation of the agonist/antagonist activity of the mixed antiestrogen, 4-hydroxytamoxifen. *Mol Endocrinol.* 11:657–666.

124. Montano MM, Ekena K, Delage-Mourroux R, et al. (1999). An estrogen receptor-selective coregulator that potentiates the effectiveness of antiestrogens and represses the activity of estrogens. *Proc Natl Acad Sci U S A.* 96:6947–6952.

125. Seol W, Choi HS, Moore DD. (1996). An orphan nuclear hormone receptor that lacks a DNA binding domain and heterodimerizes with other receptors. *Science.* 272:1336–1339.

126. Seol W, Hanstein B, Brown M, et al. (1998). Inhibition of estrogen receptor action by the orphan receptor SHP (short heterodimer partner). *Mol Endocrinol.* 12:1551–1557.

127. Johansson L, Thomsen JS, Damdimopoulos AE, et al. (2002). The orphan nuclear receptor SHP inhibits agonist-dependent transcriptional activity of estrogen receptors ERα and ERβ. *J Biol Chem.* 274:345–353.

128. Johansson L, Bavner A, Thomsen JS, et al. (2000). The orphan nuclear receptor SHP utilizes conserved LXXLL-related motifs for interactions with ligand-activated estrogen receptors. *Mol Cell Biol.* 20:1124–1133.

129. Korzus E, Torchia J, Rose DW, et al. (1998). Transcription factor-specific requirements for coactivators and their acetyltransferase functions. *Science.* 279:703–707.

130. Nagy L, Kao HY, Chakravarti D, et al. (1997). Nuclear receptor repression mediated by a complex containing SMRT, mSin3A, and histone deacetylase. *Cell.* 89:373–380.

131. Knoepfler PS, Eisenman RN. (1999). Sin meets NuRD and other tails of repression. *Cell.* 99:447–450.

132. Arnold SF, Vorojeikina DP, Notides AC. (1995). Phosphorylation of tyrosine 537 on the human estrogen receptor is required for binding to an estrogen response element. *J Biol Chem*. 270:30205–30212.

133. Zhang QX, Borg A, Wolf DM, *et al*. (1997). An estrogen receptor mutant with strong hormone-independent activity from a metastatic breast cancer. *Cancer Res*. 57:1244–1249.

134. Ali S, Metzger D, Bornert JM, *et al*. (1993). Modulation of transcriptional activation by ligand-dependent phosphorylation of the human oestrogen receptor A/B region. *EMBO J*. 12:1153–1160.

135. Arnold SF, Obourn JD, Jaffe H, *et al*. (1995). Phosphorylation of the human estrogen receptor by mitogen-activated protein kinase and casein kinase II: Consequence on DNA binding. *J Steroid Biochem Mol Biol*. 55:163–172.

136. Kato S, Endoh H, Masuhiro Y, *et al*. (1995). Activation of the estrogen receptor through phosphorylation by mitogen-activated protein kinase. *Science*. 270:1491–1494.

137. Bunone G, Briand PA, Miksicek RJ, *et al*. (1996). Activation of the unliganded estrogen receptor by EGF involves the MAP kinase pathway and direct phosphorylation. *EMBO J*. 15:2174–2183.

138. Aronica SM, Katzenellenbogen BS. (1993). Stimulation of estrogen receptor-mediated transcription and alteration in the phosphorylation state of the rat uterine estrogen receptor by estrogen, cyclic adenosine monophosphate, and insulin-like growth factor-1. *Mol Endocrinol*. 7:743–752.

139. Joel PB, Traish AM, Lannigan DA. (1998). Estradiol-induced phosphorylation of serine 118 in the estrogen receptor is independent of p42/p44 mitogen-activated protein kinase. *J Biol Chem*. 273:13317–13323.

140. Chen DS, Pace PE, Coombes RC, *et al*. (1999). Phosphorylation of human estrogen receptor α by protein kinase A regulates dimerization. *Mol Cell Biol*. 19:1002–1015.

141. Arnold SF, Obourn JD, Jaffe H, *et al*. (1994). Serine 167 is the major estradiol-induced phosphorylation site on the human estrogen receptor. *Mol Endocrinol*. 8:1208–1214.

142. Joel PB, Smith J, Sturgill TW, *et al*. (1998). pp90rsk1 regulates estrogen receptor-mediated transcription through phosphorylation of Ser-167. *Mol Cell Biol*. 18:1978–1984.

143. Tremblay A, Tremblay GB, Labrie F, *et al*. (1999). Ligand-independent recruitment of SRC-1 to estrogen receptor beta through phosphorylation of activation function AF-1. *Mol Cell* 3:513–519.

144. Ko L, Cardona GR, Iwasaki T, *et al*. (2002). Ser-884 adjacent to the LXXLL motif of coactivator TRBP defines selectivity for ERs and TRs. *Mol Endocrinol*. 16:128–140.

145. Weigel NL, Zhang Y. (1998). Ligand-independent activation of steroid hormone receptors. *J Mol Med*. 76:469–479.

146. Hu E, Kim JB, Sarraf P, *et al*. (1996). Inhibition of adipogenesis through MAP kinase-mediated phosphorylation of PPARγ. *Science*. 274:2100–2103.

147. Taneja R, Rochette-Egly C, Plassat JL, *et al*. (1997). Phosphorylation of activation functions AF-1 and AF-2 of RARα and RARγ is indispensable for differentiation of F9 cells upon retinoic acid and cAMP treatment. *EMBO J*. 16:6452–6465.

148. Shao D, Rangwata SM, Bailey ST, *et al*. (1998). Interdomain communication regulation ligand binding by PPAR-γ. *Nature*. 396:377–380.

149. Walker SE, Allen SH, McMurray RW. (1993). Prolactin and autoimmune disease. *Trends Endocrinol Metab*. 4:147–151.

150. Greenstein B, Roa R, Dhaher Y, *et al*. (2001). Estrogen and progesterone receptors in murine models of systemic lupus erythematosus. *Int Immunopharmacol*. 1:1025–1035.

151. Wilson KB, Evans M, Abdou NI. (1996). Presence of a variant form of the estrogen receptor in peripheral blood mononuclear cells from normal individuals and lupus patients. *J Reprod Immunol*. 31:199–208.

152. Li H, Gomes PJ, Chen JD. (1997). RAC3, a steroid/nuclear receptor-associated coactivator that is related to SRC-1 and TIF2. *Proc Natl Acad Sci U S A*. 94:8479–8484.

153. Chen H, Lin RJ, Schiltz RL, *et al*. (1997). Nuclear receptor coactivator ACTR is a novel histone acetyltransferase and forms a multimeric activation complex with P/CAF and CBP/p300. *Cell*. 90:569–580.

154. Takeshita A, Cardona GR, Koibuchi N, *et al*. (1997). TRAM-1, a novel 160-kDa thyroid hormone receptor activator molecule exhibits distinct properties from steroid receptor coactivator-1. *J Biol Chem*. 272: 27629–27634.

101

Sex Hormone Metabolism, Immune Function, and the Effect of Sex Hormones on Various Rheumatic Diseases

ROBERT G. LAHITA, MD, PhD

Chairman of Medicine, Jersey City Medical Center; Professor of Medicine, Mount Sinai School of Medicine, Jersey City, NJ

I. Introduction

The entire area of steroid biochemistry and metabolism remains one of the most controversial areas in both endocrinology and immunology. The convergence of these two disciplines can be difficult because there is little known about the effects that phenomena in one specialized area have on the other. In this chapter, the metabolic changes found in a variety of autoimmune diseases are described. The full importance of these changes, where they occur, and their effects on the immune system are not fully known. This discipline—called immunoendocrinology—is very young. In the study of immunoendocrinology the results of the hormonal changes may be more significant to disease than expected, but the endocrine system is complex and the outcome of elevated levels of a sex steroid might not be immediate in biology. As an example, various changes of cytokines in response to shifting levels of sex steroids are known to occur, but at the level of a particular organ like the ovary or the liver such responses may only be apparent over long periods. Such changes at the "local" level have effects on the host, but the complexity of these effects and careful study of the initial stimulus is the material of future research.

II. Androgens

Androgens have many effects on immune function. They are considered immunosuppressive hormones because of in vitro observations on their effects in normal lymphocytes and because of their effects on the disease manifestations of inbred autoimmune mice [1]. Testosterone suppresses anti-DNA antibody production in peripheral blood mononuclear cells from patients with systemic lupus erythematosus (SLE) [2] and also inhibits pokeweed mitogen stimulation of B-cell differentiation. This occurs through the downregulation of interleukin-6 (IL-6) and the inhibition of B-cell activity. Graft rejection in rodents is delayed by the injection of testosterone. Resistance to certain viral infections can be reduced, and in some cases enhanced, when androgens are given at certain doses [3,4]. A consistent effect of androgens in one animal is the immunosuppression of chickens through the retardation of the function and development of the bursa of fabricius [5–8]. Androgens also have an effect on the pluripotential stem cells of the bone marrow: namely, the accelerated proliferation and differentiation of such stem cells into compartments of cells that include lymphoid elements. The important effects of androgens on immune maturation are reflected by the discovery of receptors for estrogen and dihydrotestosterone, a 5α reduced metabolite of testosterone in the thymus [9–11], and these receptors are on thymocytes [8,9]. Androgen receptors

are also found on lymphocytes (specifically CD8 cells), but the data are inconsistent [12,13]. Androgens inhibit B- and T-cell maturation, reduce B-cell synthesis of immunoglobulins, and suppress the phytohemagglutinin-induced blast transformation of lymphocytes [14,15]. The androgens are implicated as modifiers of regulatory genes that influence the function of structural genes [16]. For example, guinea pig mammary epithelial Ia antigens are increased in number through the effects of estrogens and prolactin and are decreased by testosterone [17]. The wide range of effects that this steroid has on immune function might be the result of variable androgen sensitivity of certain cell groups and the in vivo conversion of androgens to estrogens through well-recognized pathways.

III. Estrogens

Female mice make more antibodies to foreign antigens than do males, and this difference is reported for a variety of antigens [18]. Estrogens, depending on dose and condition, are both immunosuppressors and immunostimulants. The steroid 17β-estradiol prolongs first and second set skin grafts in mice after X-irradiation and inhibits corneal graft acceptance in preimmunized rabbits [19]. In general, however, skin allograft rejection is naturally better in females than in males [20]. Estrogens regulate immunity by way of the thymus in rodents [21] and decrease the overall thymic population of small lymphocytes. Estrogen given prior to bone marrow Transplantation, results in increased graft failure. Estradiol and diethylstilbestrol (in concentrations of 10–50 mgm/ml) are known to reduce the phytohemagglutinin and concanavalin-A response of lymphocytes in vitro [22]. The mixed lymphocyte reaction is enhanced by estradiol. Enhanced lymphocyte activity is observed at 200 ng/ml, whereas the effects are inhibited at 2000 ng/ml (thymidine incorporation). Fluctuant lymphocyte responses are observed during normal menses [4], during pregnancy, and during the use of oral contraceptives [23]. Castrated male and certain female mice display hyperplastic spleens and thymuses after challenge with thymic-dependent antigens, indicating an effect of the estrogens on thymic cell activity [8,24–26]. Moreover, castration of males leads to accelerated allograft rejection. Syngeneic grafts of ovaries in males and grafts of testes in females have no significant effect on allograft rejection [27]. Sustained levels of estrogens in mice leads to a marked reduction in natural killer cell activity. In other studies, estrogens have been found to depress cell-mediated immunity, natural killer cell function, and cancer cell immune surveillance. Estrogens also deplete thymic hormones and are known to produce a relative lymphopenia when given in excessive amounts.

Estrogens are detrimental to all animals with SLE, and both mice and dogs are adversely affected. In fact, tamoxifen and antiestradiol antibody have beneficial effects on experimental SLE, and this benefit occurs via cytokine regulation [28]. Men with prostatic cancer who are given diethylstilbestrol have markedly depressed cell-mediated immunity. Using normal lymphocytes, estradiol treatment of pokeweed-mitogen–treated B cells show an increase in plaque-forming cells (in vitro) [26,29,30]. Estrogen receptors are found on CD8+ and CD4+ T lymphocytes in some studies from mice and men [12,31,32]. In that regard, there are studies to show that CD4+ T helper cells increase after estrogen therapy [33], whereas other studies show estrogens as an inhibitor of CD8+ suppressor T cells. Consequently, helper T cells would be enhanced with resulting polyclonal B-cell immunoglobulin production. An exciting new direction is the inhibition of apoptosis in vitro using peripheral blood mononuclear cells from women with normal menses. Estradiol decreases tumor necrosis factor (TNF)-α in SLE cells but not those from normal people [34].

IV. Progestogens

Other sex steroids such as progesterone have been considered as therapeutic agents in diseases such as SLE. That is because progesterone is an immunosuppressive agent [26,35] and levels of this substance increase during pregnancy when the placenta assumes an active role in its synthesis and secretion. This steroid at concentrations of 10–15 mgm/ml reduces lymphocyte responses to phytohemagglutinin and to concanavalin A in vitro. Other analogues such as 20α-hydroxyprogesterone have similar effects [36]. Progesterone has been known to increase the relative amounts of CD8+ suppressor cells in humans and to decrease them in mice. In addition, progesterone has been invoked to explain many of the suppressive effects found in the sera of pregnant females.

V. Normal Estrogen and Androgen Metabolism

A. Estrogens

It is important to know the nuances of sex hormone metabolism before one can truly understand the implications of changes. Estradiol is quickly converted to estrone that can be metabolized in one of two ways. Estrone can be hydroxylated either to a very feminizing pathway, or to 16-alpha hydroxyestrone or estriol, or the estrone can be shifted toward one of the catechol estrogens, 2-hydroxy or 2–methoxy estrone, which are less feminizing hormones (Fig. 101-1). The change appears to have some importance to the normal physiology of the individual, and the magnitude of the products depends on the substrate amounts of estradiol. In the female the metabolism is likely to have profound effects, whereas in the male the overall effects of the lesser amounts of estradiol are unknown. An elevation of the 16 hydroxylated estrogens in the male results in adverse effects on the male such as gynecomastia or decreased libido. Any significant switch of estrone hydroxylation toward the catechol estrogens in the female will have effects related to less feminizing hormones such as oligomenorrhea or osteoporosis. Factors affect the direction of estrone metabolism; these include smoking,

diet, and normal physiologic changes such as pregnancy. Whereas smoking and dietary change might increase the metabolism of estrone toward the 2-hydroxylated compounds, pregnancy shifts the hydroxylation of estrone toward the very feminizing compounds (Fig. 101-2).

One estrogen, 16α-hydroxyestrone, is feminizing, highly uterotropic, and modestly bound to cytosol receptors and

Estrogens

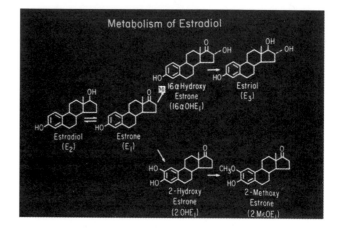

Fig. 101-1 The metabolism of estradiol is reversible towards estrone. Estrone can be metabolized in the direction of either the very feminine 16 hydroxylated compounds or the less feminizing 2 hydroxylated compounds. In the disease lupus erythematosus, the metabolism is directed primarily toward the 16 metabolites.

Estrogen Metabolism

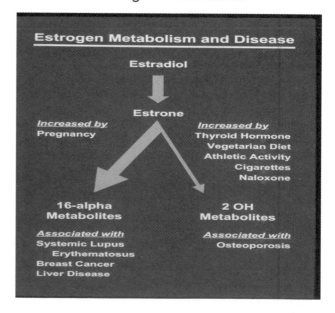

Fig. 101-2 The overall metabolism of estrogen. In diseases like lupus, the hydroxylation of estrone is directed toward the 16-alpha metabolites. There are many factors which increase the hydroxylation toward the 2 hydroxyl metabolites, which are less feminizing.

testosterone-estradiol-binding globulin (TEBG), which is in contradistinction to compounds such as 17β-estradiol [37] (Fig. 101-3). A radioimmunoassay, however, failed to show uniformly elevated levels of 16α-hydroxyestrone in all active patients with SLE [38]. This suggested either that a conjugated form of this steroid was active or that there are other metabolites of importance to SLE that are not apparent. Enzymatic systems in certain animals might favor the formation of such compounds, although nothing is known about lupus mice with regard to the metabolism of estrone.

Clinical studies on the steroid 16α-hydroxyestrone showed that it had interesting properties *in vivo* that might explain its possible role in disease; these include covalent binding of this steroid to erythrocytes and lymphocytes via a Heyn's rearrangement *in vivo* and the possibility that such covalent binding might occur at the level of the estrogen receptor or the T-cell receptor and result in alteration of immune function [39,40]. Studies of family members of patients with SLE indicated that elevated hydroxylation of estradiol was commonly observed in nonaffected first-degree relatives as well as patients [41].

Normal women ingesting oral contraceptives have enhanced binding of l6α-hydroxyestrone to various cell proteins. Specific antiestrogen–protein adduct immunoglobulins are isolated from normal patients and patients with SLE ingesting oral contraceptives, which means that these adducts are common. This finding suggested a common pathway to adduct formation in all women who ingest large amounts of estradiol or for one reason or another have an endogenous source of high estrogen level [42]. Males with SLE who had hormone protein adduct-specific immunoglobulin G (IgG) in their sera also were reported.

B. Androgens

Several studies of androgen levels in plasma of men and women with SLE and of androgen metabolism in men and women with SLE [43] are of interest. An early reason proposed for SLE in the male was that it was the result of too little androgen and too much estrogen [44,45] (Fig. 101-4). However, most studies indicate that young men with SLE are hormonally normal and that estrogen:androgen ratios are minimally elevated if at all. Furthermore, data from the studies of males with SLE do not help to explain the large numbers of females who predominate with the disease. Studies of androgen metabolism in females with SLE indicate that a difference in the overall metabolism of androgens can be found. The oxidation of testosterone at C17 in females with SLE is increased in comparison to males, who have both normal oxidation of testosterone and normal plasma androgen levels [46] (Figs. 101-5 and 101-6). Several studies of females with active SLE who never took corticosteroids show that the females had decreased plasma levels of androgen [32,47,48] (Fig. 101-7). This observation is found in patients with Klinefelter syndrome (XXY) as well as in women with lupus. Low plasma androgens in women with SLE form the basis for androgen replacement therapy in this disease. Clinical studies involving the use of dehydroepiandrosterone (DHEA) as a therapy for lupus are a result of this observation.

Evidence Suggesting That Androgen
Metabolism is Important to SLE in the
Human

• Low Male Incidence	After puberty (1:10 M:F)
• Low Androgens in Females with SLE	Low Plasma Androgens (Jungers *et al.*, 1982; Lahita *et al.*, 1986)
	Increased oxidation of testosterone in females with SLE (Lahita *et al.*, 1983)

Fig. 101-4 Evidence of a role for androgen in the disease SLE.

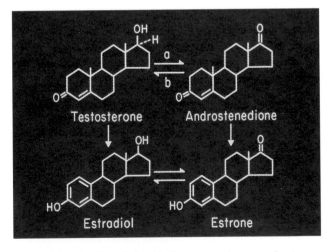

Fig. 101-5 The interrelationship between androgen and estrogen metabolism. Estrone is further metabolized towards the 16 or 2 hydroxyl pathways. Testosterone is oxidized to androstenedione, which then has an option to become dehydroepiandrosterone.

Differences in Biological Activities
of Estrogenic Metabolites

	2-Hydroxy *Catechols*	16-Hydroxy *Very feminizing*
Uterotropic Activity	Negative	Positive
TEBG Binding	Positive	Negative
Receptor Binding	Positive	Positive
LH Secretion	Up regulated	Down regulated
Prolactin Secretion	Down regulated	Up regulated

Fig. 101-3 The different biologic activities of both the feminizing estrogens and the nonfeminizing estrogens. TEBG, testosterone binding globulin; LH, leuteotrophic hormone.

Similar to estrogen, the end products of androgen metabolism in the normal individual, whether male or female, depend on the total amount. Testosterone is oxidized to androstenedione, converted to DHEA, and then sulfated [49]. Both testosterone and androstenedione can be metabolized to estrone and estradiol. After the male hormones are aromatized to estrogens they can then enter the pathways for estrone hydroxylation. Specific cytokine levels change with levels of the sex steroids. By this

mechanism, certain sex steroid levels affect the T-cell populations and determine antiinflammatory versus proinflammatory cytokine profiles [50].

VI. Sex Hormones and Systemic Lupus Erythematosus

In certain rheumatic diseases such as SLE these sex hormone pathways are important because they appear to change with the disease. Moreover, their subtle effects are of some importance to the overall well being of the female with autoimmune disease. In the case of lupus, these metabolites and their conversion have been studied. The metabolism of estrogen or androgens has not been applied to any other autoimmune illnesses because the data on the lupus changes appeared in the early 1980s. However, new urine assays and other means of measuring these metabolites have made the accrual of data on other conditions possible.

Sex steroids affect the severity of SLE [2,24,51]. As we can see from other conditions and emerging data, the effects of sex steroids on conditions such as fibromyalgia or Hashimoto's thyroiditis also are important. However, a direct relationship of both androgen and estrogen metabolites on the severity of the disease, the production of antibodies, or the appearance of certain clinical signs in SLE has never been established. The basic observations found in patients with lupus erythematosus involved the hydroxylation of estrone and the oxidation of testosterone.

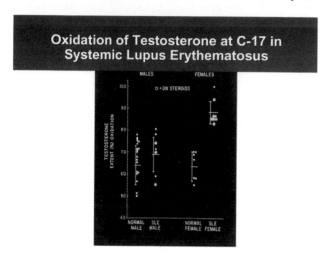

Fig. 101-6 The oxidation of testosterone at C-17 is increased in females with systemic lupus erythematosus (SLE), but not in males.

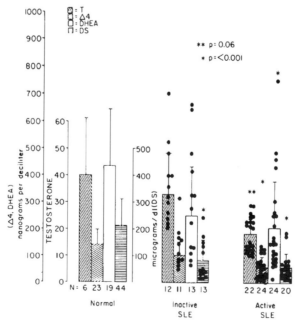

Fig. 101-7 The overall levels of plasma testosterone in women with systemic lupus erythematosus (SLE) decreases with clinical activity. These patients are not taking prednisone at the time of measurement.

VII. Sex Hormones and Rheumatoid Arthritis

Rheumatoid arthritis is also associated with hormone changes [52,53]. In many cases of rheumatoid arthritis low androgen levels have been described. Also, in many cases the signs and symptoms of disease coincide with the menstrual cycle, an observation that has also been made anecdotally in patients with lupus [54]. Several observations about rheumatoid arthritis are not clear, namely the remission of rheumatoid arthritis in the pregnant female and also the response of many patients and animal models to estrogen [55–57]. Exacerbations of rheumatoid arthritis occur during certain times in the menstrual cycle. This is one of the few diseases in which this observation is made.

VIII. Sjögren's Syndrome and Antiphospholipid Syndrome

There are data from Sjögren's syndrome to show that the levels of androgens in the tears of patients with the disease are low [58]. The significance of this finding is not known.

The antiphospholipid syndrome, an autoimmune disease that produces a procoagulant condition in most patients, has no apparent predilection for sex. The disease affects more women than men in its secondary form; however, the primary condition does not favor one sex over another.

IX. Gonadotropins

Prolactin is an immunomodulatory pituitary hormone and could be considered a cytokine itself. In the human, prolactin elevations have been observed in juveniles with SLE and correlated with both disease activity and central nervous system manifestations [59]. This finding is supported by *in vitro* work showing IgG- and IgM-induced anti-DNA antibodies by both normal and SLE lymphocytes in the presence of high levels of prolactin. Lectins did not produce this effect [60]. One study correlates elevated prolactin levels with elevated cortisol levels [61].

Women who are pregnant have higher serum prolactin levels if they have SLE [62]. Moreover, some investigators have associated the decline in serum testosterone during pregnancy in patients with to hyperprolactinemia. Perhaps, however, the most significant descriptions of hyperprolactinemia have been in men with SLE [63]. These descriptions of hyperprolactinemia are of particular interest because hyperprolactinemia is readily treated with bromocriptine. Studies using bromocriptine to treat SLE are routine in some clinics around the world [64,65].

Many studies refute the significance of prolactin in human SLE [66,67–69]. In a detailed study of a Chinese cohort of patients with SLE, Mok *et al* [68] found no correlation of clinical activity with levels of prolactin in 72 patients with lupus. A look at autoantibodies in patients with lupus found no association of prolactin levels with specific lupus autoantibodies [70]. One particular study suggests that prolactin is complexed with IgG but remains biologically active in the patient with lupus [71,72]. This binding of prolactin (a specific 23-kd nonglycosylated form) to IgG is not covalent. Delayed clearance of this complex as a result of its high molecular weight is the proposed reason for the activity of the prolactin in most patients with lupus.

Many investigators associate prolactin with disease activity [73]. In one study, 61.9% of patients with hyperprolactinemia had active disease. The Systemic Lupus Erythematosus Disease Activity Index (SLEDAI) correlated with the levels of prolactin in these patients as well when prolactin levels were measured by both tests of immunoradioactivity and biologic activity. Another series noted an association of hyperprolactinemia in the serum and urine of patients with severe renal disease [74]. The statistical power of most of these prolactin studies could explain the lack of consistency among research laboratories. One study suggests that the published results are contradictory because of the statistical power of the studies. In fact, the authors reviewed five studies and found that two of the studies did not have the statistical power to conclude an association with lupus activity and prolactin levels, whereas the other three studies did suggest an association [66]. High prolactin levels are found in 20–30% of patients with SLE in some clinics [75]. In addition to the suggestion that prolactin is itself a cytokine that provokes the synthesis of immunoglobulins by lymphocytes [76], German investigators, using lymphocytes from patients with SLE and measuring clinical activity with the European activity measure (ECLAM), found that, patients with SLE have lymphocytes that are sensitive to levels of prolactin and likely to be activated by physiologic concentrations [77]. These data are supported by the findings that T lymphocytes from patients with SLE secrete more prolactin than controls, suggesting a difference in regulation of genes responsible for control of this cytokine. In fact, single nucleotide polymorphisms in the upstream promoter regions of both pituitary and nonpituitary prolactin secretion exist. Such specific polymorphisms can affect prolactin transcription and possibly disease association in a cohort of lupus patients with lupus. This was the case in a study in which patients had an increased frequency of the prolactin-1149G allele when compared to control subjects [78]. Whether prolactin is a cytokine or is itself increased by cytokines common in certain patients with active lupus remains the subject of major investigation.

Finally, prolactin levels of mothers who were pregnant or breastfeeding and had lupus were studied as reproductive risk factors for the development of disease [79]. Surprisingly, breast-feeding was associated with a decreased risk of developing SLE. In addition, the numbers of pregnancies or live births with lupus activity showed no relationship to levels of prolactin. These authors found no association of elevated prolactin levels with an increased risk of lupus.

X. Males with Systemic Lupus Erythematosus

The age of onset of SLE is more evenly distributed in males because one-fourth are diagnosed after age 50 years [80]. The data from the hormonal metabolic studies suggest that an increase in feminizing 16-hydroxylated estrogenic metabolites are found in SLE males, although no phenotypic evidence of hyperestrogenism is found [41,81–84]. The BXSB mouse develops SLE-like disease in nonhormone–dependent fashion. The presence of the Y chromosome is most important in this strain. A group of human male relatives has been described who resemble the mouse strain BXSB in that "male-predominant" families exist in which SLE occurs in men in preference to females [85]. In one interesting study of males with lupus, it was found that females who have a male relative with lupus were more likely to have renal disease [86].

Males with SLE are in some series reported to be clinically different [2,51,87]. Whereas several male studies show no clinical difference in severity of disease between women and men, others have suggested that males have a more severe form of the disease [88]. For example, increased pleuropericardial disease and peripheral neuropathy are said to be more common in males. Men were found to have more discoid lupus erythematosus and papular nodular mucinosis [89]. In a Spanish series of 261 patients with SLE 11.5% were males, and they had less arthritis, more serositis, and a greater propensity for discoid rashes. A 1999 database on males from Malta also found more cardiorespiratory problems in males [90], and a Taiwan study suggested that males have a significantly lower FcγR distribution on monocytes and neutrophils and high prolactin levels that might have a role in the pathogenesis of lupus in this sex [91]. All of these data are collected from small numbers of men, and such things as statistical bias might be significant.

Sex hormone profiles indicate that men with lupus have significantly higher levels of gonadotropins (follicle-stimulating hormone [FSH] and luteinizing hormone [LH]) than controls. A small percentage of patients (14%) in one study had low testosterone levels and elevated LH levels [92]. The patients with the low androgens had more central nervous system disease and serositis when compared to controls. Finally, the prolactin to testosterone levels correlated with the SLEDAI scores in these men.

Studies of Russian male patients with lupus are perhaps the most insightful [93,94]. The investigators describe elevated LH and FSH in SLE males; a lower trochanteric index (1.89 vs 2.00 for normal men), which is indicative of a lack of androgen effect on bone growth; severe aortic insufficiency and sacroiliitis (12% of all men); and overall a greater incidence of severe vascular diseases such as Raynaud's phenomenon and digital vasculitis [93]. The Russian investigators found more severe disease in men, with 63% dying from end-stage renal disease. The only significant increases in Russian males with SLE are the incidences of nephritis, Raynaud's phenomenon, and malar rash.

Finally, the Russian study also includes male patients with SLE with profound impotence. The causes of such impotence in young males with SLE remain unknown. Elderly males who present with SLE are also found to have low androgen levels and are hypogonadal [95]. Such males might respond to androgen therapy.

XI. Hypogonadism

Patients with Klinefelter syndrome can also have a variety of rheumatic diseases, such as SLE and scleroderma [96–99]. Such males commonly have gynecomastia, infertility, a female fat phenotype, and the usual sequelae of hypogonadism. These males with Klinefelter syndrome have met the ACR criteria for SLE both serologically and clinically. The incidence of SLE or any other autoimmune disease is not increased in patients with Klinefelter syndrome, although this is frequently stated. Patients with SLE and Klinefelter syndrome together have the estrogen and androgen metabolism of females with SLE [100] but low

levels of both sex steroid classes. This is why the Klinefelter syndrome is a hypergonadotropin state. When SLE does occur in young males with Klinefelter syndrome, it can be treated with the synthetic androgens usually given to such males. Androgens such as methyl testosterone as tablet, androgen patch, or gel can alleviate the symptoms of the disease in males with Klinefelter syndrome but do not alter the amount or type of autoantibody. The male with Klinefelter syndrome and SLE oxidizes testosterone in exaggerated fashion like females with SLE. This increased oxidation is not found in the male with SLE with a normal XY karyotype. The hypergonadotropic state of men with Klinefelter syndrome and SLE has not been adequately investigated at this time and may have some role in the etiopathogenesis of the disease.

Patients with hypogonadism have manifested all of the metabolic abnormalities found in patients who do not have hypergonadotropin syndromes. Patients with Klinefelter syndrome described to have connective tissue diseases such as rheumatoid arthritis, lupus, and other conditions have the same hydroxylation profiles as females with the disease. Most patients with Klinefelter syndrome have an increase of estrone hydroxylation toward estriol and increased oxidation of testosterone at C17. In these patients there is neither elevated estrogen nor androgen and the gonadotropins are high. A principal clinical manifestation in these patients includes cardiopulmonary disease. At least two of these patients were known to have multiple estrogen-dependent illnesses such as porphyria, lupus, and chronic active liver disease.

XII. Use of Hormones to Alter Disease States

A. Oral Contraceptives and Postmenopausal Hormone Replacement in the Rheumatic Diseases

Data from the mouse and human have shown that unopposed estrogens exacerbate SLE. The data from human studies, however, are largely *in vitro* or derived from anecdotal studies of patients taking oral contraceptives. Most studies involving oral contraceptives and SLE or hormone replacement therapy (HRT) in postmenopausal women with SLE suggest that the disease worsens with these agents [79,101,102]. However, these studies are inconclusive and difficult because of the variability of the human illness, the designate endpoints of therapy, the steroids chosen, and the lack of a double-blinded study. Data from 1997 strongly suggest that the use of HRT predispose women to the development of SLE [103]. The results of the contraceptive/hormone replacement trial, a double-blinded control study to look at oral contraceptive use and HRT in women with lupus is in progress, and data should be available shortly. Current epidemiologic studies do not support the idea that female hormones increase the risk of developing SLE [56,79]. Sex steroids have been considered for use in inflammatory diseases such as gout and osteoarthritis because estrogens suppress neutrophil function and that is why gout is uncommon in the premenopausal female [104–106]. The overall gender-related mechanisms for the selectivity of one sex for a disease over another continues to evade explanation, and there is debate about this from some quarters [107]. Estrogens may be effective in the treatment of rheumatoid arthritis, and several clinical studies have argued both for [108,109] and against their use [110]. The mechanism of suppression of inflammation in cases of rheumatoid arthritis may give some significant insight into the pathogenesis of this common disease and is based on two observations: first is that patients improve when pregnant, and second is that oral contraceptives may have a protective effect.

Menopause is an interesting time for most patients with lupus. For many years, patients with SLE who reached menopause were known by most clinicians to improve. These conclusions were without data until 1999, when menopause conclusively was associated with remission of illness [111]. Most authors conclude that a "modest" decrease of activity occurs in those women reaching menopause [112].

B. Hyperestrogenism

Hyperestrogenic conditions are associated with autoantibodies in both normal males and females. In the human female periods of hormonal change such as pregnancy and the normal menses are associated with changes in immune function. These changes are also observed in mice. Clinical syndromes such as insulin-resistant diabetes mellitus, hirsutism, and cystic ovaries are found in patients with autoantibodies [113]. Polycystic ovary disease may be considered autoimmune, and autoantibodies could result from the unopposed actions of plasma estrogen [114]. More recently autoantibodies have been described in patients with endometriosis, and such patients have a lupuslike illness [115–117]. This may be of particular interest because the uterus and the ovaries of humans and animals are a source of cytokines [118].

C. Androgens as a Treatment for Lupus

The use of anabolic steroids such as danazol or cyproterone acetate is not effective therapy for either murine or human SLE [119,120]. However, the use of hormones such as danazol in idiopathic thrombocytopenic purpura increases platelet numbers and coagulation factors such as factor VIII. This suggests a role for androgen therapy in certain patients with SLE. Other androgens are under study, such as 19-nortestosterone, that also have had limited use in the treatment of SLE in women. Doses used were 100 mg/ml per week intramuscularly. The overall condition of female patients improved, and patients admitted increased energy, loss of joint pains, and resolution of systemic abnormalities such as skin rashes or anemia. We noted no significant change of serologies. Anti-DNA and ANA (antinuclear antibodies) titers remained elevated. Most curious in this treatment group was an overall worsening of lupus symptoms in male patients [121]. These findings in males taking 19-nortestosterone correlated with lowered endogenous testosterone levels and elevated estradiol levels.

Another steroid, cyproterone acetate, a potent antigonadotrophic agent [122], resulted in resolution of some systemic abnormalities such as oral ulcers after 50 mg daily for a mean of 63 months. As with other androgens, no improvement in serologic features was observed.

Another approach to the treatment of lupus involves the use of gonadotropin-releasing hormone agonists. These agents are used effectively to treat endometriosis and prostate carcinoma.

Data about their use in SLE are inconclusive because of small numbers studied [123,124].

One androgen, studied extensively in women, is DHEA [125,126]. This drug at doses of 200 mg/day in tablet form results in clinical improvement as measured by standard indices. It also is steroid sparing—that is to say that the total dose of prednisone might be lowered with its use (ref revise). DHEA suppresses cytokine levels such as IL-4, -5 and -6 and increases IL-2 during treatment. Natural killer cell activity also increases with this agent [127–129].

XIII. Sex Hormones, Behavior, and Autoimmune Diseases

Sex steroids are important to the development of various organs, and a major one is the brain. Recent attention has directed to cerebral development, cerebral dominance, and the incidence of autoimmune disease [130,131]. Some studies say that patients with autoimmune disease are predominantly left handed, indicating dominance of the right cerebral hemisphere. This variation is reported in patients with SLE [131–134] and other diseases of the immune system. Neuronal migration is under the influence of steroids such as testosterone, and new data suggest that SLE mice have aberrant neuronal migration patterns consistent with those observed in humans with learning disabilities such as dyslexia. Handedness in patients with SLE is more directed to the left than in the normal population. The finding of increased learning disabilities such as developmental dyslexia in patients with SLE, their unaffected male offspring, and unaffected male siblings has been confirmed by several groups and is a subject of considerable interest.

XIV. Fibromyalgia

There are other related conditions that are found almost exclusively in women [135–138]. Such symptoms do occur in men but with rarity. A link to sex hormone levels has not been established. Fibromyalgia is a chronic painful condition that is real. It is not associated with any abnormal serology or elevation of acute phase reactants. In fact, it is likely that fibromyalgia is an endocrine disorder regulated by sex steroids such as estrogen and testosterone, which each affect serotonin; this is a hypothesis, however. The ratio of men to women is not known, but it could be that women predominate at a ratio of 50 to 1. The condition is one that involves specific points of pain that are elicited on physical examination and are associated with a lack of sleep. The condition is often confused with the associated connective tissue disorder, and often patients are overtreated because of this confusion. For example, a patient who has normal serologic tests and a diagnosis of SLE might have her trigger points mistaken for a flare of her disease. A physician who fails to follow the serologic course of such a patient or fails to recognize the appropriate trigger points for fibromyalgia might increase the corticosteroid dose according to the patient's clinical complaints of pain. This would result in a patient who is ingesting large amounts of corticosteroid, with all of the attendant side effects of that drug, who really needs an analgesic and a pharmacologic aid to sleep.

Although the etiology of fibromyalgia is unknown, it is believed to include a disorder of stage 4 REM (rapid eye movement) sleep [137]. Once the patient is able to sleep, the symptoms and signs of fibromyalgia often abate. It is therefore important to give patients sleep testing to document the sleep disorder objectively. Once this is accomplished, the patient can be treated with agents that induce sleep, such as tricyclic antidepressants, gamma hydroxybutyric acid, or others, along with nonnarcotic analgesics. The use of the analgesics in non-prn form is very effective in the relief of pain. Aerobic exercise is also encouraged to gradually begin a normal sleep cycle.

There is no experience in the use of hormones to treat fibromyalgia; however, the observation that females who are postmenopausal, those who withdraw from estrogen replacement therapy, and those who have estrogen-dependent illnesses such as lupus get more fibromyalgia would suggest that these steroids might be useful [138,139]. Research into the effects on serotonin when estrogen or androgen is withdrawn would be important to an understanding of this illness.

XV. Murine Models of Autoimmunity and Sex Hormones

It is appropriate to briefly mention the background for the study of gender effects on experimental SLE. Several strains of mice are used as models of autoimmune disease [140–142]. The disease in some murine models predominates in females of the species; examples are the *New Zealand White/Black (NZW/NZB)Fl hybrid* and the *MRL lpr* strains, in which females die before males [23,24]. In one specific strain of mice the disease favors males, the *BXSB* (derived from the *C57Bl/6* and satin beige mouse), and this strain is unusual in that the males die of early SLE-like disease [143–145]. Unlike the female predisposed strains of mice, the disease manifestations in the *BXSB* mouse are not hormonally mediated because neither administration of sex steroids nor gonadal extirpation improves or changes the disease manifestations. One strain of mice bred because the mouse developed polyarteritis nodosa, called the *Palmerston North* (PN) mouse [146], also develops an SLE-like illness that predominates in the females. Gender is not solely responsible for the disease lupus in these inbred strains because all mice succumb to lupus, male and female; however, sex hormones affect both the severity and onset of the illness in both sexes of any species.

A. NZB/NZW Strains

The effects of gonadal hormones were first noted to play a regulatory role with regard to SLE in New Zealand (NZB/NZW). The F1 descendants of the parental strains were important to lupus because inbreeding resulted in accelerated disease, development of disease manifestations such as autoimmune hemolytic anemia [140,142], and diffuse proliferative glomerulonephritis. Circulating DNA-containing immune complexes and a variety of autoantibodies like those to native DNA and ssDNA also accompanied the clinical disease as in the human. Before the discovery of the NZB/W strain, the manifestations of autoimmune disease were unknown in any animal species except man. The gender difference is not amazingly large in the parent strains because a high percentage of the NZB females develop severe proliferative glomerulonephritis and die by

15 months of age, whereas the mortality for males is 17 months. When NZB mice are mated with NZW mice, the offspring (F1 hybrids) begin to develop kidney disease at 9 months, and again the most severe lesions are found in females. To re-emphasize gender, renal lesions are more common to the female (NZB×NZW) F1 in the cross of an NZB female and NZW male. In the F1 hybrids, 90% of the females develop dsDNA antibodies at age 8.5 months and more than 50% of the females die as a result of renal disease [147,148].

An explanation of various immune functions in these lupus mice has not revealed much. Thymic function in these mice, in particular T-cell-mediated responses, has been studied and is blunted [149]. After age 22 weeks, phytohemagglutinin responsiveness of circulating lymphocytes is lost, and this loss of function is more pronounced in females. This finding, one that is distinctly skewed toward the female, might be the result of the development of anti T-cell antibodies [150].

These murine observations are more commonly found in the females of the F1 generation and have an apparent B-cell abnormality that is present from birth that results in the overproduction of IgM [151]. Athymic NZB mice are known to have hyperactive B cells (consistent with polyclonal B-cell activation) [152]. Aberrant B-cell dysfunction in NZB mice is reflected by their resistance to the induction and maintenance of tolerance [153]. This last characteristic is part of the "female character" of most of the murine SLE strains. Sex hormones also influence the response of the NZB strain to thymus-dependent antigens because high-dose testosterone therapy decreases and orchidectomy increases plaque-forming colonies (PFC) in NZB males if the mice are irradiated sublethally after treatment with sex hormones [154].

Sex steroids also adversely affect the course of disease in F1 female hybrids of the NZB/NZW cross. As the mice age, the illness becomes more profound, but prepubertal castration of the NZB female mouse does not decrease the death rate. Early estrogen therapy accelerates the disease in females, whereas ovariectomy or testosterone therapy prolongs the life of the mouse. In males of this strain castration causes early death and estrogen produces a mortality rate that is similar to that of females [155,156]. Overall testosterone therapy of female mice prolongs life and decreases overall morbidity [2,154].

It is possible that sex steroids modulate the generation of antigen-specific suppressor cells and that true sex differences in the responses to T-cell and B-cell mitogens exist in this strain. Androgens increase suppressor cell activity in NZB/NZW mice, and it may do this by increasing levels of IL-2. Androgens also suppress the development of the thymocytotoxic antibody.

It is not rewarding to study sex hormone receptors on the lymphocytes of these mice because there are no differences. The thymus, a target of sex steroids, is of great physiologic significance, but estrogen and testosterone receptors are not located on mouse peripheral blood lymphocytes [157]. However, estrogen-induced receptor binding is observed in thymic tissues from male NZB/NZW mice and estrogens may act entirely on the thymus gland [21,149,158]. The role of sex steroids in the pathogenesis of lupuslike disease in the inbred mouse is based on simple observations that alteration of sex steroid levels or gonadectomy affects the progression of disease. It is important to note that the mouse will succumb to lupus whether male or female, but the sex steroids regulate disease activity.

B. MRL Strain

The MRL (lpr/lpr or n/n) strain of mice has a lupuslike disease that is closer serologically to the human disease for various reasons. This mouse produces a greater variety of antibodies to antigens like DNA, RNP, SM, and rheumatoid factor [159–162]. Because of rheumatoid factor, this strain is a useful model for the study of rheumatoid arthritis. These mice are also models of Sjögren's disease because of serologic characteristics and the development of signs such as lymphadenopathy. The mice are homozygous for the lymphoproliferative gene lpr, and a large number have profound lymphadenopathy. The congenic n/n or +/+ strain lacks the lpr gene.

Sex differences in these MRL mice are less marked than in the NZB/NZW strain. No lymphadenopathy is found in the +/+ mice, although necrotizing arteritis and glomerulonephritis are common and about 50% of the +/+ mice die with neoplasms. Again the female gender predominates, and consequently the mean ages for death are 17 months for females and 22 months for males.

Hormone therapy of these mice using high doses of the androgens testosterone and 5α-dihydrotestosterone delayed the occurrence of both lymphadenopathy and autoantibody production. Increased prolactin levels accelerate autoimmune diseases in NZB/W F1 mice.

C. BXSB Strain

BXSB mice are unique in that spontaneous autoimmune disease is more common in the males. This is distinctly different from the female predilection in most murine lupus strains. The males have a mean life span of 5 months, and the female life span averages 15 months. Examinations of cell populations of this strain have shown that both B- and T-cell functions are normal. The accelerated autoimmune disease in these mice is linked to the Y chromosome, and prepubertal castration will not alter the course of the disease. The transfer of bone marrow cells from diseased males to nondiseased males leads to the development of the autoimmune disease.

D. General Remarks about Murine Lupus and Sex Steroids

All of the evidence cited here indicates that sex hormones play a major role in the modulation of autoimmune diseases of some lupus mouse strains. There are certainly many other aspects to consider in the morbidity of murine SLE, and the major ones are genetics and possibly the presence of a transmissible agent. It is also apparent that sex steroids have an adverse effect on the disease, as in the human. The disease manifestations wax and wane in a fashion commensurate with fluctuating steroid levels, and these vary with the estrus cycle in females. Fundamental questions such as the susceptibility to SLE and the "window" if any during which sex steroids exert their most profound influence are the subjects of current investigation.

E. Sex Chromosomal Effects

Chromosomal effects are important because at least one murine strain, the BXSB, depends on the Y chromosome for the character of its immune responses. There are many other examples. Immune responses to DNA are linked to the presence of the X chromosome in the NZB/NZW mouse. NZB or NZW males mated to BXSB females result in female offspring that die of SLE nephritis at an early age. This suggests a role for the recessive X chromosome in the male parent [163].

F. Steroid Effects

Some researchers on the effects of androgens on immune function suggest that they act on immune tolerance [164]. Mice that develop autoimmune diseases have defective tolerance to a variety of antigens, and androgen levels could be at the heart of the problem. Graft vs host disease can induce an SLE-like syndrome in some mouse strains, and tolerance probably has a major position in the schema of autoimmunity. Because androgens modulate T-cell phenotype in transition from marrow to the thymus, the target of androgen action is likely to be the thymocytes. Using 20α-hydroxysteroid dehydrogenase as a T-cell marker, investigators noted a decrease in thymocytes and an increase in T suppressor cells after androgen administration. The hypothesis that androgens act in this manner is attractive because androgens afford a method of altering the absolute numbers of T cells.

G. Gonadotropin Effects

There is great interest in the effects of prolactin on immune function in mice and humans [66,79,165]. There are diverse effects of hyperprolactinemia in both male and female mice, and multiple studies show that prolactin stimulates the appearance of murine disease. Early on studies found that male NZW/NZB mouse autoimmune disease was accelerated and mortality worsened by prolactin. Murine lupus, as noted earlier, is similar to that found in the human in that prolactin has a role to play in the exacerbation and possibly the initiation of lupus in the human. Estrogens stimulate prolactin and may be the overriding mechanism. Bromocriptine inhibits the development of murine lupus. Murine studies even demonstrate that estrogen itself might depend on the stimulation of prolactin for activity.

XVI. Suggestions for Further Investigations

- In what organ are the oxidative enzymes involved in the conversion of steroids like estrone to the 16 or 2 metabolites located?
- What relationship do the enzymes of oxidation have on immune stimulation?
- Is the patient with autoimmune disease more likely to have rapid oxidative processes?
- How does local enzymatic metabolism—such as that found in the ovary—affect overall immune function?
- Are the estrogen or androgen metabolites graded in their degree of immune activity?

References

1. Ahmed SA, Dauphinee M, Talal N. (1985). Effects of short term administration of sex hormones on normal and autoimmune mice. *J Immunol.* 134:204–210.

2. Blank M, Mendlovic S, Fricke H, *et al.* (1990). Sex hormone involvement in the induction of experimental systemic lupus erythematosus by a pathogenic anti-DNA idiotype in naive mice. *J Rheumatol.* 17:311–317.

3. Yohn DS. (1973). Sex related resistance in hamsters to adenovirus oncogenesis. *Prog Exp Tumor Res.* 18:138.

4. Bjune G. (1979). *In vitro* lymphocyte responses to PHA show co-variation with the menstrual cycle. *Immunol Abstracts.* 51.

5. Verheul HA, Tittes EV, Kelder J, *et al.* (1986). Effects of steroids with different endocrine profiles on the development, morphology and function of the bursa of Fabricius in chickens. *J Steroid Biochem.* 25:665–675.

6. Hirota Y, Suzuki T, Bito Y. (1980). The B-cell development independent of bursa of Fabricius but dependent upon the thymus in chickens treated with testosterone propionate. *Immunology.* 39:37–46.

7. Meyer RK, Rao MA, Aspinall RL. (1959). Inhibition of the development of the bursa of Fabricius in the embryos of the common fowl by 19-nortestosterone. *Endo.* 64:890.

8. Stimson WH, Hunter IC. (1980). Estrogen induced immunoregulation mediated through the thymus. *J Clin Lab Immunol.* 4:27–33.

9. Grossman CJ, Sholitan LJ, Roselle G. (1982). Estradiol regulation of thymic lymphocyte function in the rat: mediation by serum thymic factors. *J Steroid Biochem.* 16:683–690.

10. Grossman CJ, Sholitan LJ, Blaha GC, *et al.* (1989). Rat thymic estrogen receptor II. Physiologic properties. *J Steroid Biochem.* 11:1241.

11. Sholitan LJ, Grossman CJ, Taylor BB. (1980). Rat thymic homogenates convert testosterone to androgenic metabolites. *J Steroid Biochem.* 13:1365.

12. Cohen JHM, Danel L, Cordier G, *et al.* (1983). Sex steroid receptors in peripheral T cells: absence of androgen receptors and restriction of estrogen receptors to OKT8 positive cells. *J Immunol.* 131:2767–2771.

13. Raveche ES, Vigersky RA, Rice MK, *et al.* (1980). Murine thymic androgen receptors. J *Immunopharmacol.* 2:425.

14. Dunkel L, Taino VM, Savilahti E, *et al.* (1985). Effect of endogenous androgens on lymphocyte subpopulations. *Lancet.* 440–441.

15. Weinstein Y, Isakov Y. (1983). Effects of testosterone metabolites and of anabolic androgens on the bone marrow and thymus in castrated female mice. *Immunopharmacol.* 5:229–237.

16. Lubahn DB, Joseph DR, Sar M, *et al.* (1988). The human androgen receptor: complementary deoxyribonucleic acid cloning, sequence analysis and gene expression in prostate. *Mol Endocrinol.* 2:1265–1275.

17. Klareskog L, Forsum U, Peterson PA. (1980). Hormonal regulation of the expression of Ia antigens on mammary gland epithelia. *Eur J Immunol.* 10:958–963.

18. Terres G, Morrison SL, Habicht GL. (1968). A quantitative difference in the immune response between male and female mice. *Proc Exp Biol Med.* 27:664.

19. Thompson JS, Crawford MK, Reilly R, *et al.* (1957). Estrogenic hormones in immune responses in normal and X irradiated mice. *J Immunol.* 98:331.

20. Waltman SR, Brude RM, Benios J. (1971). Prevention of corneal rejection by estrogens. *Transplantation.* 11:194.

21. Brodie JY, Hunter IC, Stimson WH, *et al.* (1980). Specific estradiol binding in cytosols from the thymus glands of normal and hormone-treated male rats. *Thymus.* 1:337.

22. Wyle FA, Kent JR. (1977). Immunosuppression by sex steroid hormones. I. The effect upon PHA- and PPD-stimulated lymphocytes. *Clin Exp Immunol.* 27:407–415.

23. Satoh PS, Fleming WE, Johnstone KA, *et al.* (1977). Active E rosette formation in women taking oral contraceptives. *N Engl J Med.* 296:54.

24. Golsteyn EJ, Fritzler MJ. (1987). The role of the thymus-hypothalamus-pituitary-gonadal axis in normal immune processes and autoimmunity. *J Rheumatol.* 14:982–990.

25. Olsen NJ, Watson MB, Henderson GS, *et al.* (1991). Androgen deprivation induces phenotypic and functional changes in the thymus of adult male mice. *Endo.* 129:2471–2476.

26. O'Hearn M, Stites DP. (1983). Inhibition of murine suppressor cell function by progesterone. *Cell Immunol.* 77:340–348.

27. Sasson S, Mayer M. (1981). Effect of androgenic steroids on rat thymus and thymocytes in suspension. *J Steroid Biochem.* 14:509–518.

28. Buskila D, Berezin M, Gur H, *et al.* (1995). Autoantibody profile in the sera of women with hyperprolactinemia. *J Autoimmun.* 8(3):415–424.

29. Paavonen T, Aronen H, Pyrhonen S, *et al.* (1991). The effects of anti-estrogen therapy on lymphocyte functions in breast cancer patients. *APMIS.* 99:163–170.

30. Sthoeger Z, Chiorazzi N, Lahita RG. (1988). Regulation of the immune response by sex steroids. *J Immunol.* 141:91–98.

31. Danel L, Sovweine G, Monier JC, *et al.* (1983). Specific estrogen binding sites in human lymphoid cells and thymic cells. *J Steroid Biochem.* 18:559.

32. Jungers P, Pelissier C, Bach JF, *et al.* (1980). Les androgenes plasmatiques chez les femmes atteintes de lupus erythemateux dissemine (LED). *Pathologie Biologie.* 28:391–392.

33. Stimson WH. (1988). Estrogen and human T lymphocytes: presence of specific receptors in the T-suppressor/cytotoxic subset. *Scand J Immunol.* 28:345–350.

34. Evans MJ, MacLaughlin S, Marvin RD, *et al.* (1997). Estrogen decreases *in vitro* apoptosis of peripheral blood mononuclear cells from women with normal menstrual cycles and decreases TNF-alpha production in SLE but not in normal cultures. *Clin Immunol Immunopathol.* 82(3):258–262.

35. Clemens LE, Siiteri PK, Stites DP. (1979). Mechanisms of immunosuppression of progesterone on maternal lymphocyte activation during pregnancy. *J Immunol.* 122:1978–1985.

36. Mori T, Kobayashi H, Nishimoto H. (1977). Inhibitory effect of progesterone and 20-hydroxy-pregn-4-en-3-one on the phytohemagglutinin-induced transformation of human lymphocytes. *Am J Obstet Gynecol.* 127:151.

37. Fishman J, Martucci C. (1980). Biological properties of 16-alpha hydroxy-estrone: implications in estrogen physiology and pathophysiology. *J Clin Endo Metab.* 51:611–615.

38. Ikegawa S, Lahita RG, Fishman J. (1983). Concentration of 16 alpha hydroxyestrone in human plasma as measured by a specific RIA. *J Steroid Biochem.* 18:329–332.

39. Bucala R, Fishman J, Cerami A. (1984). The reaction of 16-a hydroxyestrone with erythrocytes *in vitro* and *in vivo. Eur J Biochem.* 140:593–598.

40. Bucala R, Fishman J, Cerami A. (1982). Formation of co-valent adducts between cortisol and 16-alpha-hydroxyestrone and protein, possible role in pathogenesis of cortisol toxicity and SLE. *Proc Nat Acad Sci.* 79:3320.

41. Lahita RG, Bradlow HL, Fishman J, *et al.* (1982). Estrogen metabolism in systemic lupus erythematosus: patients and family members. *Arthritis Rheum.* 25:843–846.

42. Bucala R, Lahita RG, Fishman J, *et al.* (1987). Anti-estrogen antibodies in users of oral contraceptives and in patients with systemic lupus erythematosus. *Clin Exp Immunol.* 67, 167–175.

43. Lahita RG. (1992). Sex steroids and SLE: metabolism of androgens to estrogens [editorial]. *Lupus.* 1:125–127.

44. Inman RD. (1978). Immunologic sex differences and the female preponderance in systemic lupus erythematosus. *Arthritis Rheum.* 21:849–852.

45. Inman RD, Jovanovic L, Markenson JA. (1982). Systemic lupus erythematosus in men: genetic and endocrine features. *Arch Intern Med.* 142:1813–1815.

46. Lahita RG, Bradlow HL, Kunkel HG, *et al.* (1983). Increased oxidation of testosterone in systemic lupus erythematosus. *Arthritis Rheum.* 26:1517–1521.

47. Jungers P, Nahoul K, Pelissier C. (1982). Low plasma androgens in women with active or quiescent SLE. *Arthritis Rheum.* 25:454–457.

48. Lahita RG, Bradlow HL, Ginzler E, *et al.* (1987). Low plasma androgens in women with systemic lupus erythematosus. *Arthritis Rheum.* 30:241–248.

49. Spencer NFL, Poynter ME, Hennebold JD, *et al.* (1996). Does DHEAS restore immune competence in aged animals through its capacity to function as a natural modulator of peroxisome activities? In: Bellino FL, Daynes RD, Hornsby PJ, *et al.*, eds. *Dehydroepiandrosterone (DHEA) and Aging.* New York: New York Academy of Sciences. 200–216.

50. Zietz B, Reber T, Oertel M, *et al.* (2000). Altered function of the hypothalamic stress axes in patients with moderately active systemic lupus erythematosus. II. Dissociation between androstenedione, cortisol, or dehydroepiandrosterone and interleukin 6 or tumor necrosis factor. *J Rheumatol.* 27(4):911–918.

51. Ansar Ahmed S, Penhale WJ, Talal N. (1985). Sex hormones, immune responses, and autoimmune diseases. Mechanisms of sex hormone action. *Am J Pathol.* 121:531–551.

52. Cutolo M, Accardo S. (1991). Sex hormones and rheumatoid arthritis. *Clin Exp Rheum.* 9:641–646.

53. Rhodes K, Scott A, Markham RL, *et al.* (1969). Immunological sex differences. A study of patients with rheumatoid arthritis, their relatives and controls. *Ann Rheum Dis.* 28:104.

54. Latman N. (1983). Relation of menstrual cycle to the symptoms of rheumatoid arthritis. *Am J Med.* 74:957–960.

55. Bijllsma JWJ, Huber-Bruning O, Thijssen JHH. (1987). Effect of estrogen treatment on clinical and laboratory manifestation of rheumatoid arthritis. *Ann Rheum Dis.* 46:777–779.

56. Liang MH, Karlson EW. (1996). Female hormone therapy and the risk of developing or exacerbating systemic lupus erythematosus or rheumatoid arthritis. *Proc Assoc Am Phys.* 108(1):25–28.

57. Spector TD, Brennan P, Harris P, *et al.* (1991). Does estrogen replacement therapy protect against rheumatoid arthritis? *J Rheumatol.* 18:1473–1476.

58. Sullivan DA, Kelleher RS, Vaerman JP, *et al.* (1990). Androgen regulation of secretory component synthesis by lacrimal gland acinar cells in vitro. *J Immunol.* 145(12):4238–4244.

59. El-Garf A, Salah S, Shaarawy M, *et al.* (1996). Prolactin hormone in juvenile systemic lupus erythematosus: a possible relationship to disease activity and CNS manifestations. *J Rheumatol.* 23(2):374–377.

60. Gutierrez MA, Molina JF, Jara LJ, *et al.* (1996). Prolactin-induced immunoglobulin and autoantibody production by peripheral blood mononuclear cells from systemic lupus erythematosus and normal individuals. *Int Arch Allergy Immunol.* 109(3):229–235.

61. Folomeev M, Dougados M, Beaune J, *et al.* (1992). Plasma sex hormones and aromatase activity in tissues of patients with systemic lupus erythematosus. *Lupus.* 1(3):191–195.

62. Jara Quezada L, Graef A, Lavalle C. (1991). Prolactin and gonadal hormones during pregnancy in systemic lupus erythematosus. *J Rheumatol.* 18:349–353.

63. Lavalle C, Loyo E, Paniagua R, *et al.* (1987). Correlation study between prolactin and androgens in male patients with systemic lupus erythematosus. *J Rheumatol.* 14:268–272.

64. Blank M, Krause I, Buskila D, *et al.* (1995). Bromocriptine immunomodulation of experimental SLE and primary antiphospholipid syndrome via induction of nonspecific T suppressor cells. *Cell Immunol.* 162(1):114–122.

65. McMurray RW, Weidensaul D, Allen SH, *et al.* (1995). Efficacy of bromocriptine in an open label therapeutic trial for systemic lupus erythematosus. *J Rheumatol.* 22(11):2084–2091.

66. Blanco-Favela F, Quintal-Alvarez G, Leanos-Miranda A. (1999). Association between prolactin and disease activity in systemic lupus erythematosus. Influence of statistical power. *J Rheumatol.* 26(1):55–59.

67. Buskila D, Lorber M, Neumann L, *et al.* (1996). No correlation between prolactin levels and clinical activity in patients with systemic lupus erythematosus [see comments]. *J Rheumatol.* 23(4):629–632.

68. Mok CC, Lau CS. (1996). Lack of association between prolactin levels and clinical activity in patients with systemic lupus erythematosus [letter: comment]. *J Rheumatol.* 23(12):2185–2186.

69. Ostendorf B, Fischer R, Santen R, *et al.* (1996). Hyperprolactinemia in systemic lupus erythematosus? *Scand J Rheumatol.* 25(2):97–102.

70. Kozakova D, Rovensky J, Cebecauer L, *et al.* (2000). Prolactin levels and autoantibodies in female patients with systemic lupus erythematosus. *Z Rheumatol.* 59 Suppl 2:II/80–II/84.

71. Leanos-Miranda A, Pascoe-Lira D, Chavez-Rueda KA, *et al.* (2001). Antiprolactin autoantibodies in systemic lupus erythematosus: frequency and correlation with prolactinemia and disease activity. *J Rheumatol.* 28(7):1546–1553.

72. Leanos-Miranda A, Chavez-Rueda A, Blanco-Favela F. (2001). Biologic activity and plasma clearance of prolactin-IgG complex in patients with systemic lupus erythematosus. *Arthritis Rheum.* 44(4):866–875.

73. Pacilio M, Migliaresi S, Meli R, *et al.* (2001). Elevated bioactive prolactin levels in systemic lupus erythematosus—association with disease activity. *J Rheumatol.* 28(10):2216–2221.

74. Miranda JM, Prieto RE, Paniagua R, *et al.* (1998). Clinical significance of serum and urine prolactin levels in lupus glomerulonephritis. *Lupus.* 7(6):387–391.

75. Jara LJ, Vera-Lastra O, Miranda JM, *et al.* (2001). Prolactin in human systemic lupus erythematosus. *Lupus.* 10(10):748–756.

76. Jacobi AM, Rohde W, Volk HD, *et al.* (2001). Prolactin enhances the *in vitro* production of IgG in peripheral blood mononuclear cells from patients with systemic lupus erythematosus but not from healthy controls. *Ann Rheum Dis.* 60(3):242–247.

77. Jacobi AM, Rohde W, Ventz M, *et al.* (2001). Enhanced serum prolactin (PRL) in patients with systemic lupus erythematosus: PRL levels are related to the disease activity. *Lupus.* 10(8):554–561.

78. Stevens A, Ray DW, Worthington J, *et al.* (2001). Polymorphisms of the human prolactin gene—implications for production of lymphocyte prolactin and systemic lupus erythematosus. *Lupus.* 10(10):676–683.

79. Cooper GS, Dooley MA, Treadwell EL, *et al.* (2002). Hormonal and reproductive risk factors for development of systemic lupus erythematosus: results of a population-based, case-control study. *Arthritis Rheum.* 46(7):1830–1839.

80. Stahl N, Decker J. (1978). Androgenic status of males with SLE. *Arthritis Rheum.* 21:665–668.

81. Alarcon-Segovia D, Alarcon-Riquelme ME. (2002). Etiopathogenesis of Systemic Lupus Erythematosus: A tale of three troikas. In: Lahita RG, editor. *Systemic Lupus Erythematosus.* San Diego: Academic Press. 55–66.

82. Lahita RG, Bradlow HL, Kunkel HG, *et al.* (1981). Increased 16 alpha hydroxylation of estradiol in systemic lupus erythematosus. *J Clin Endo Metab.* 53:174–178.

83. Lahita RG, Bradlow HL, Kunkel HG, *et al.* (1979). Alterations of estrogen metabolism in SLE. *Arthritis Rheum.* 22:1195–1198.

84. Lahita RG, Bucala R, Bradlow HL, *et al.* (1985). Determination of 16-hydroxy-estrone by radioimmunoassay in systemic lupus erythematosus. *Arthritis Rheum.* 28:1122–1127.

85. Lahita RG, Chiorazzi N, Gibofsky A. (1983). Familial systemic lupus erythematosus in males. *Arthritis Rheum.* 26:39.

86. Stein CM, Olson JM, Gray-McGuire C, *et al.* (2002). Increased prevalence of renal disease in systemic lupus erythematosus families with affected male relatives. *Arthritis Rheum.* 46(2):428–435.

87. Hughes GR. (1984). Current understanding of systemic lupus erythematosus. *Inflammation* 8 Suppl:S75–S79.

88. Sthoeger ZM, Geltner D, Rider A, *et al.* (1987). Systemic lupus erythematosus in 49 Israeli males: a retrospective study. *Clin Exp Rheum.* 5:233–240.

89. Anisman H, Baines MG, Berczi I, *et al.* (1996). Neuroimmune mechanisms in health and disease: 2. Disease. *Can Med Assoc J.* 155(8):1075–1082.

90. Camilleri F, Mallia C. (1999). Male SLE patients in Malta. *Adv Exp Med Biol.* 455:173–179.

91. Chang DM, Chang CC, Kuo SY, *et al.* (1998). The clinical features and prognosis of male lupus in Taiwan. *Lupus.* 7(7):462–468.

92. Mok CC, Lau CS. (2000). Profile of sex hormones in male patients with systemic lupus erythematosus. *Lupus.* 9(4):252–257.

93. Alekberova Z, Kotelnikova G, Folomeev M. (1989). Aortic defects in systemic lupus erythematosus. (Rus). *Terapeuticheskii Arkhiv.* 61(5):35–38.

94. Alekberova ZS, Folomeev MI. (1985). [Sexual dimorphism in rheumatic diseases]. *Revmatologiia (Mosk).* 58–61.

95. Lahita RG. (1986). Sex and age in systemic lupus erythematosus. In: Lahita RG, editor. Systemic Lupus Erythematosus. New York: John Wiley and Sons. 523–539.

96. Aoki N. (1999). Klinefelter's syndrome, autoimmunity, and associated endocrinopathics. *Intern Med.* 38(11):838–839.

97. Fam A, Izsak M, Saiphoo C. (1980). SLE and Klinefelter's syndrome. *Arthritis Rheum.* 23:124.

98. French MAH, Hughes P. (1983). Systemic lupus erythematosus and Klinefelter's syndrome. *Ann Rheum Dis.* 42:471–473.

99. Kobayashi S, Shimamoto T, Taniguchi O, *et al.* (1991). Klinefelter's syndrome associated with progressive systemic sclerosis: report of a case and review of the literature. *Clin Rheumatol.* 10:84–86.

100. Lahita RG, Bradlow HL. (1987). Klinefelter's syndrome: hormone metabolism in hypogonadal males with systemic lupus erythematosus. *J Rheumatol.* 14 Suppl 13:154–157.

101. Asherson RA, Harris NE, Gharavi AE, *et al.* (1986). Systemic lupus erythematosus, antiphospholipid antibodies, chorea and oral contraceptives. *Arthritis Rheum.* 29:1535–1536.

102. Chapel TA, Burns RE. (1971). Oral contraceptives and exacerbations of SLE. *Am J Obstet Gynecol.* 110:366.

103. Sanchez-Guerrero J, Karlson E, Liang MH, *et al.* (1997). Past use of oral contraceptives and the risk of developing systemic lupus erythematosus. *Arthritis Rheum.* 40(5):804–808.

104. Buyon J, Korchack HM, Rutherford LE. (1984). Female hormones reduce neutrophil responsiveness *in vitro*. *Arthritis Rheum.* 27:623–630.

105. Bodel P, Dillard GM, Kaplan SS, *et al.* (1972). Antiinflammatory effects of estradiol on human blood leukocytes. *J Lab Clin Med.* 80:373–384.

106. Mikkelson WM, Dodge NJ, Vlakenberg H. (1965). The distribution of serum uric acid values in a population unselected as to gout or hyperuricemia. *Am J Med.* 39:242.

107. Lockshin MD. Invited review: sex ratio and rheumatic disease. (2001). *J Appl Physiol.* 91(5):2366–2373.

108. Linos A, Worthing JW, O'Fallon WM, *et al.* (1989). The epidemiology of rheumatoid arthritis in Rochester, Minnesota: a study of its incidence, prevalence, and mortality. *Am J Epidemiol.* 111:87–98.

109. Linos A, O'Fallon WM, Worthington JW, *et al.* (1983). Case control study of rheumatoid arthritis and prior use of oral contraceptives. *Lancet.* 1:1299.

110. Oka M, Vainio U. (1966). Effect of pregnancy on the prognosis and serology of rheumatoid arthritis. *Acta Rheum Scand.* 12:47.

111. Mok CC, Lau CS, Ho CT, *et al.* (1999). Do flares of systemic lupus erythematosus decline after menopause? *Scand J Rheumatol.* 28(6):357–362.

112. Sanchez-Guerrero J, Villegas A, Mendoza-Fuentes A, *et al.* (2001). Disease activity during the premenopausal and postmenopausal periods in women with systemic lupus erythematosus. *Am J Med.* 111(6):464–468.

113. DeClue TJ, Shah SC, Marchese M, *et al.* (1991). Insulin resistance and hyperinsulinemia induce hyperandrogenism in a young type B insulin resistant female. *J Clin Endocrinol Metab.* 72:1308–1311.

114. Harrison LC, Dean B, Peluso J, *et al.* (1985). Insulin resistance, acanthosis nigricans, and polycystic ovaries associated with a circulating inhibitor of postbinding insulin action. *J Clin Endo Metab.* 60:1047–1052.

115. Dmowski WP, Gebel HM, Rawlins RG. (1989). Immunological aspects of endometriosis. Obstetrics and Gynecology clinics of North America. Philadelphia: W.B. Saunders. 93–103.

116. Dmowski WP, Braun D, Gebel H, *et al.* (1990). Peripheral blood monocyte (PBM) and peritoneal macrophage (PM) cytotoxicity in women with endometriosis and the effect of Danazol. *Am Fert J.* Abstract.

117. Dmowski WP, Steele RW, Baker GF. (1981). Deficient cellular immunity in endometriosis. *Am J Obstet Gynecol.* 141:377.

118. Tung KSK, Smith S, Teuscher C. (1987). Murine autoimmune oophoritis, epididymoorchitis and gastritis induced by day 3 thymectomy: Immunopathology. *Am J Pathol.* 126:293.

119. Dmowski WP, Danazol. (1990). A synthetic steroid with diverse biologic effects. *J Reprod Med.* 35:69–74; discussion 74–75.

120. Olsen NJ, Kovacs WJ. (1995). Case report: testosterone treatment of systemic lupus erythematosus in a patient with Klinefelter's syndrome. *Am J Med Sci.* 310(4):158–160.

121. Lahita RG, Cheng CY, Monder C, *et al.* (1990). Experience with 19-nortestosterone in the therapy of systemic lupus erythematosus: worsened disease after treatment with 19-nortestosterone in men and lack of improvement in women. *J Rheumatol.* 19(4):547–555.

122. Jungers P, Kutten F, Liote F, *et al.* (1985). Hormonal modulation in systemic lupus erythematosus. Preliminary clinical and hormonal results with cyproterone acetate. *Arthritis Rheum.* 28(11):1243–1250.

123. Ivanova AV, Shardina LA, Benediktov II. (1989). [Gonadotropic and sex hormones in women with systemic lupus erythematosus]. *Revmatologiia (Mosk).* 3–8.

124. Vilarinho ST, Costallat LT. (1998). Evaluation of the hypothalamic-pituitary-gonadal axis in males with systemic lupus erythematosus. *J Rheumatol.* 25(6):1097–1103.

125. Van VR, Engleman EG, McGuire JL. (1995). Dehydroepiandrosterone in systemic lupus erythematosus. Results of a double-blind, placebo-controlled, randomized clinical trial. *Arthritis Rheum.* 38(12):1826–1831.

126. Van Vollenhoven RF, McGuire JL. (1996). Studies of dehydroepiandrosterone (DHEA) as a therapeutic agent in systemic lupus erythematosus. *Ann Med Intern. (Paris).* 147(4):290–296.

127. Araneo BA, Daynes RA. (1995). Dehydroepiandrosterone functions as more than an antiglucocorticoid in preserving immunocompetence after thermal injury. *Endo.* 136(2):393–401.

128. Daynes RA, Dudley DJ, Araneo BA. (1990). Regulation of murine lymphokine production *in vivo* II. Dehydroepiandrosterone is a natural enhancer of interleukin 2 synthesis by helper T cells. *J Immunol.* 20:793–802.

129. Daynes RA, Araneo BA. (1992). Programming of lymphocyte responses to activation: extrinsic factors, provided microenvironmentally, confer flexibility and compartmentalization to T cell function. *Chem Immunol.* 54:1–20.

130. Nandy K, Harbous L, Bennet D, *et al.* (1983). Correlation between learning disorder and elevated brain reactive antibodies in aged C57B1/6 and young NZB mice. *Life Sci.* 33:1499.

131. Sherman GF, Galaburda AM, Geschwind N. (1983). Ectopic neurons in the brain of the autoimmune mouse: a neuropathophysiologic model of dyslexia? *Neuropath Proc.* 275:6.

132. Lahita RG. (1988). Systemic lupus erythematosus: learning disability in the male offspring of female patients and relationship to laterality. *Psychoneuroendocrinology.* 13:385–396.

133. Wood LC, Cooper DS. (1989). Autoimmune thyroid disease, left-handedness, and developmental dyslexia. Unpublished work.

134. Wyckoff PM, Miller LC, Tucker LB, *et al.* (1995). Neuropsychological assessment of children and adolescents with systemic lupus erythematosus. *Lupus.* 4:217–220.

135. Alarcon GS. (1997). Arthralgias, myalgias, facial erythema, and a positive ANA: not necessarily SLE. *Cleve Clin J Med.* 64(7):361–364.

136. Bennet RM. (1995). Confounding features of the fibromyalgia syndrome: a current perspective of differential diagnosis. *J Rheumatol.* 19(Suppl.): 58–61.

137. Bennet RM, Clark SR, Campbell SM. (1992). Somatomedin-C levels in patients with the fibromyalgia syndrome: a possible link between sleep and muscle pain. *Arthritis Rheum.* 35:1113–1116.

138. Carette S, Dessureault M, Belanger A. (1992). Fibromyalgia and sex hormones. *J Rheumatol.* 19(5):831–832.

139. Ferraccioli G, Cavalieri F, Salaffi F. (1990). Neuroendocrinologic findings in primary fibromyalgia (soft tissue chronic pain syndrome) and in other chronic rheumatic conditions (rheumatoid arthritis, low back pain). *J Rheumatol.* 17:869–873.

140. Andrews BS, Eisenberg RA, Theofilopoulos AN. (1978). Spontaneous murine lupus-like syndromes. Clinical and immunopathological manifestations in several strains. *J Exp Med.* 148:1198.

141. Theofilopoulos AN, Dixon FJ. (1985). Murine models of systemic lupus erythematosus. *Adv Immunol.* 37:269–390.

142. Theofilopoulos AN, Kono DH. (1999). Murine lupus models: Gene Specific and Genome-Wide Studies. In: Lahita RG, ed. *Systemic Lupus Erythematosus.* San Diego: Academic Press. 145–182.

143. Ansar Ahmed S, Boone J, Verthelyi D. (1993). Anticardiolipin antibodies in autoimmune-prone BXSB and MRL/Lpr mice, and estrogen-treated normal C57BL/6J mice crossreact with other phospholipids. *Int J Immunopathol Pharmacol.* 6(3):135–147.

144. Eisenberg RA, Izui S, McConahey PJ. (1980). Male determined accelerated autoimmune disease in BXSB mice: transfer by bone marrow and spleen cells. *J Immunol.* 125:1032.

145. Murphy ED, Roths JB. (1979). A Y chromosome associated factor in strain BXSB producing accelerated autoimmunity and lymphoproliferation. *Arthritis Rheum.* 22:1188–1193.

146. Walker SE, Gray RH, Fulton M. (1978). Palmerston north mice, a new animal model of systemic lupus erythematosus. *J Lab Clin Med.* 92:932.

147. Howie JB, Helyer BJ. (1965). Autoimmune diseases in mice. *Ann N Y Acad Sci.* 124:167–177.

148. Howie JB, Helyer BJ. (1968). The immunology and pathology of NZB mice. *Adv Immunol.* 9:215–266.

149. Nabarra B, Dardenne M, Bach JF. (1990). Thymic reticulum of autoimmune mice. II: Ultrastructural studies of mice with lupus-like syndrome (NZB, BXSB, MRL/l). *J Autoimmun.* 3:25–36.

150. Shirai T, Yashiki T, Mellors RC. (1972). Age decrease of cells sensitive to an autoantibody-specific for thymocytes and thymus dependent lymphocytes in NZB mice. *Clin Exp Immunol.* 12:455.

151. Motsopoulos HM, Boehm-Truitt M, Kassan SS. (1977). Demonstration of activation of B lymphocytes in New Zealand black mice at birth by an immunoradioactive assay for murine IgM. *J Immunol.* 119:1639.

152. Ohsugi Y, Gershwin ME. (1979). Studies of congenitally immunologic mutant New Zealand mice III. Growth of B lymphocyte clones in congenitally athymic (nude) and hereditary asplenic (Dh/+)NZB mice: a primary B cell defect. *J Immunol.* 123:1260.

153. Staples PJ, Steinberg AD, Talal N. (1980). Induction of immunological tolerance in older New Zealand mice repopulated with young spleen, bone marrow, or thymus. *J Exp Med.* 131:1223.

154. Morton JI, Weyant DA, Seigel BV, *et al.* (1981). Androgen sensitivity and autoimmune disease I. Influence of sex and testosterone on the humoral immune responses of autoimmune and nonautoimmune mouse strains to SRBC. *Immunology.* 44:661.

155. Siiteri PK, Jones LA, Roubinian J, *et al.* (1980). Sex steroids and the immune system—I. Sex difference in autoimmune disease in NZB/NZW hybrid mice. *J Steroid Biochem.* 12:425–432.

156. Stites DP, Siiteri P. (1983). Steroids as immunosuppressants in pregnancy. *Immunol Rev.* 75:117–138.

157. Jacobson JD, Ansari MA, Kinealy M, *et al.* (1999). Gender-specific exacerbation of murine lupus by gonadotropin-releasing hormone: potential role of G alpha(q/11). *Endo.* 140(8):3429–3437.

158. Chiodi H. (1940). The relationship between the thymus and the sex organs. *Endo.* 26:107–135.

159. Cohen MG, Pollared KM, Schreiber L. (1988). Relationship of age and sex to autoantibody expression in MRL +/+ and MRL lpr mice. *Clin Exp Immunol.* 72:50–54.

160. Hang L, Theofilopoulos AN, Dixon FJ. (1982). A spontaneous rheumatoid arthritis-like disease in MRL/l mice. *J Exp Med.* 155:1690.

161. Jevnikar AM, Grusby MJ, Glimcher LH. (1994). Prevention of nephritis in major histocompatibility complex class II-deficient MRL-lpr mice. *J Exp Med.* 179:1137–1143.

162. Smith HR, Hansen CL, Rose R, *et al.* (1990). Autoimmune MRL-lpr/lpr mice are an animal model for the secondary antiphospholipid syndrome. *J Rheumatol.* 17:911–915.

163. Mazes E, Fuchs S. (1974). Linkage between immune response potential to DNA and X chromosome. *Nature.* 249:167–168.

164. Laskin CA, Taurog JD, Smathers PA, *et al.* (1981). Studies of defective tolerance on murine lupus. *J Immunol.* 127:1743.

165. Elbourne KB, Keisler D, McMurray RW. (1998). Differential effects of estrogen and prolactin on autoimmune disease in the NZB/NZW F1 mouse model of systemic lupus erythematosus. *Lupus.* 7(6):420–427.

102

Pregnancy—Success or Failure: The Influence of Autoimmune Diseases

ANN L. PARKE, MD

Professor of Medicine, University of Connecticut Health Center, Farmington, CT

Autoimmune disease is known to be associated with infertility; increased fetal wastage; and significant fetal and neonatal pathology, which may be a consequence of transplacental passage of maternal immunoglobulin (Table 102-1). Conversely, pregnancy may exacerbate or improve clinical autoimmune diseases and in some cases may even contribute to the pathogenesis of autoimmunity by permitting microchimerism, which may persist for years (Table 102-2). For us to understand more about the interrelationship of pregnancy and autoimmune disease, it is important to address the apparent paradox of normal pregnancy. Why is the fetal semiallograph allowed to persist and grow in what would normally be a hostile environment? This chapter will address the immunology of pregnancy and the short- and long-term consequences of the interrelationships between pregnancy and various autoimmune diseases.

I. The Immunology of Pregnancy

In normal pregnancy, the fetal semiallograph is tolerated by the maternal immune system, allowed to persist and even to thrive. This immune tolerance is still not completely understood, but it appears to arise as a consequence of several immune adaptations that all need to interact if pregnancy is to be successful. This topic is expertly reviewed in several recent articles [1–5]. Indeed, there is now considerable evidence to suggest that infertility, recurrent pregnancy loss, and preeclampsia may be the consequence of immunologic defects [6–9]. In 1953, Medawar proposed four potential immunologic mechanisms that could permit human pregnancy to proceed: (1) the fetus is not immunogenic, (2) maternal immunity is suppressed, (3) the uterus is an immune-privileged site, and (4) there is a barrier between the mother and the fetus [10]. It is now known that none of these hypothesized mechanisms is true, and Thellin *et al* proposed at least 10 mechanisms that may be vital to support the fetal placental graft [5]. Starting with protective mechanisms present in seminal fluid, it is known that spermatozoa do not express human leukocyte antigen (HLA) class I and II antigens, but many other cells in the ejaculate do express these antigens [11]. There is evidence that certain seminal proteins, in particular transforming growth factor-beta (TGF-β), play an essential role in suppressing the maternal immune response [12]. Animal studies have shown that TGF-β induces an endometrial inflammatory response, which may be responsible for immune modulation switching from T helper 1 (Th1) to Th2 cytokine production—vital if pregnancy is to succeed [13,14]. Human studies have also shown other benefits of exposure to seminal fluid in that *in vitro* fertilization (IVF) is more successful if couples have had intercourse prior to the IVF procedure [15].

To survive, the embryonic trophoblast has to invade and embed in the uterine wall, and in normal pregnancies the spiral arteries of the uterus undergo physiologic changes and dilate up to 30 times their normal size to support and nourish this invading graft. For this to happen the invading trophoblast must avoid the maternal immune system; this deception is helped by the fact that the trophoblast does not express major histocompatability

Table 102-1
Effect of Autoimmune Disease on Pregnancy

1. Infertility	Thyroid disease
2. Increased fetal wastage	Systemic lupus erythematosus
	Phospholipid antibody (aPL) syndrome
	Other Connective tissue disease (i.e., scleroderma)
	Primary Sjögren's syndrome
3. Fetal and/or neonatal disease	
a. Transient	Thyroid disease
	Myasthenia gravis
	Thrombocytopenia
	Cutaneous neonatal lupus syndrome
b. Permanent	Primary congenital complete heart block (neonatal lupus syndrome)
	Learning disorders
	Childhood malignancies

Table 102-2
Effect of Pregnancy on Maternal Clinical Autoimmune Diseases

Beneficial	Rheumatoid arthritis
	Multiple sclerosis
	Thyroid disease
Note: Flares of all of these diseases are usually seen in the postpartum period.	
Detrimental	Phospholipid syndrome
	Systemic lupus erythematosus
Contributory	Scleroderma
	Hashimoto's thyroiditis
	Multiple sclerosis

complex (MHC) class I or II molecules [6]. The trophoblast does, however, express a tissue-specific nonclassic MHC gene that encodes HLA-G antigen, essential for protecting the trophoblast [17,18]. The HLA-G binds to natural killer (NK) cells blocking their cytotoxic effects and thereby reduces susceptibility to attack by NK cells [19]. Moffet-King has shown that trophoblast invasion is accompanied by an influx of NK cells into the uterus, and it has been suggested that in normal pregnancy these cells may play a role in inducing the production of Th2 cytokines essential for trophoblast invasion [20]. Apoptosis of maternal immune cells may be crucial for normal pregnancy to proceed. Under the influence of Cortrophin releasing hormone (CRH), the trophoblast expresses Fas ligand (FAS-L) and thereby has the ability to induce apoptosis of the maternal Fas-positive T cells [21]. Mice that are deficient in functional Fas L have extensive leukocyte infiltration at the placental-decidual interface and small litter sizes [22]. Fas/FasL interaction and its induction of temporary maternal immune tolerance could also help to explain the improvement of some maternal autoimmune diseases during pregnancy. Similarly, inhibition of complement activation could limit the expression of maternal autoimmune disease, and the trophoblast expresses complement regulation proteins CD46, CD55, and CD59 that inhibit the activation of the complement system [23]. Mice that lack Crry a cell-surface protein that protects against C3 and C4 complement activation, experience fetal loss [24]. This fetal wastage can be prevented if the Crry-negative animals are crossbred with C3-negative mice, demonstrating that the fetal wastage in these animals is a direct consequence of complement activation [24]. Work by Holers *et al* has shown that complement activation is essential for the fetal loss that occurs in murine models of phospholipid antibody (aPL) syndrome. In a series of experiments, these authors demonstrated deposition of human immunoglobulin G (IgG) and C3 in the placentas of murine models of aPL syndrome. If Crry-Ig was also given at the time of administration of the antiphospholipid IgG, there was a lack of IgG and C3 deposition in the placentae of these animals. Also, C3-deficient mice were resistant to the fetal lethal effects of aPL syndrome [25].

Immune modulation through cytokine production is now known to have a dramatic influence on the outcome of pregnancy [13,14,26,27]. Although this cytokine modulation is not completely black and white, it appears that Th1 cytokines are detrimental to pregnancy. Tumor necrosis factor-alpha (TNF-α) inhibits trophoblast invasion and stimulates apoptosis of human trophoblast cells [28]. Th2 cytokines, however, promote trophoblast invasion, and studies have demonstrated that pregnancy loss is associated with reduced Th2 cytokine production [29,30]. Suppression of Th1 cytokine production by placental products (i.e., progesterone and prostaglandin E$_2$ [PGE$_2$]) may help to explain the clinical disease remission that is seen in about 80% of pregnant patients with rheumatoid arthritis [31] and has led some to consider the use of TNF inhibitors in patients with infertility and/or fetal wastage.

Another factor considered to provide vital protective roles for the successful completion of pregnancy is leukemia inhibitory factor (LIF), which is synthesized by the decidua and Th2 lymphocytes and is considered vital for blastocyst implantation [32]. Progesterone and other hormones play an important role in the synthesis of LIF by the endometrium [33].

The maternal immune system may also be disarmed through a variety of other mechanisms. Annexins are a family of glycoproteins, and it is known that an annexin V shield plays a vital role in protecting the invading trophoblast. This shield is disrupted in phospholipid antibody pregnancies [34]. Annexin II is also synthesized by the placenta and is known to inhibit immunoglobin secretion by maternal immune cells [35].

Indoleamine 2,3-dioxygenase (IDO) is an enzyme that breaks down tryptophan, an amino acid vital for T-cell nutrition; Mellor *et al* have shown that blocking IDO production causes a high rate of abortion in mice [36].

It would appear that many different mechanisms are working in concert to either sabotage or to fool the maternal immune system into tolerating the fetal–placental semiallograph. The precise role of each of these mechanisms, however, remains elusive.

II. Autoimmunity and Infertility

Infertility is defined as the failure to conceive and become pregnant after 1 year of unprotected sexual intercourse in a female with regular menstrual cycles [37]. Infertility occurs in 15% of couples attempting pregnancy [37]. There are numerous causes of infertility, both male and female, and many studies have suggested that autoimmune disease may be more prevalent in women who are infertile [38–42].

Autoimmune thyroid disease in particular has been incriminated in the pathogenesis of infertility and fetal wastage [40, 43–45]. Because thyroid disease is known to affect normal ovarian function [46], perhaps thyroid-induced infertility should not come as a surprise. One recent study of 438 infertile women determined that the prevalence of antibodies to thyroid peroxidase (TPO-Ab) was higher in infertile patients compared to normal controls, but this difference only reached statistical significance in the women with a female cause for the infertility (18% vs 8%) [45]. An even higher prevalence of these antibodies was found in women with endometriosis (29%) [45], confirming a previous study by Gerhard *et al* [47] and contributing to the evidence suggesting that autoimmunity may be involved in the pathogenesis of endometriosis [48–50]. Endometriosis *per se* is associated with infertility, but a review by Van Voorhis and Stovall concluded that there was no consistent evidence demonstrating a role of endometrial antibodies in the pathogenesis of endometriosis and/or infertility associated with endometriosis [6].

An increased prevalence of autoantibodies to smooth muscle, nuclear, and phospholipids antigens has been found in several studies of infertile women [38–40], but these associations have not been found consistently in other studies, except for a high prevalence of phospholipid antibodies found in women attending *in vitro* fertilization clinics [6]. The presence of phospholipid autoantibodies does not appear to adversely affect the rate of successful *in vitro* fertilization [6].

It is interesting to note that infertility is not a problem for women with nonorgan–specific autoimmune disease. In fact, patients with rheumatoid arthritis have no problems with pregnancy—becoming pregnant or completing pregnancy successfully [51]. Patients with systemic lupus erythematosus (SLE), however, are not infertile but have increased fetal wastage [52–54].

III. Autoimmunity and Fetal Loss

Fetal loss is increased in both organ and nonorgan–specific autoimmune disease including SLE, aPL syndrome, the neonatal lupus syndrome, and thyroid disease. Rheumatoid arthritis is one of the few autoimmune diseases that does not appear to have a detrimental effect on pregnancy [51], and previous reports suggesting an increase in fetal loss prior to the onset of disease [55] have not been substantiated in subsequent studies [56,57]. Increased fetal wastage in patients with SLE is well established, and lupus disease activity and the aPL syndrome clearly contributed to this fetal loss [52–54]. Recurrent fetal loss is now a clinical criterion for the aPL syndrome [58]. SLE and aPL pregnancies are also complicated by preeclampsia, intrauterine growth restriction, preterm delivery, and increased disease activity in the mother [59–61].

A. Phospholipid Antibody Syndrome

The recognition of the aPL syndrome and the neonatal syndrome has taught us that specific autoantibodies may predispose patients to develop specific clinical complaints. The neonatal syndrome is included in more detail under the section of fetal/neonatal injury but is considered to be a consequence of the transplacental passage of maternal antibodies to Ro and/or La [62]. Unlike the antibodies to Ro and La known to be associated with the neonatal lupus syndrome, phospholipid antibodies appear to have a detrimental effect on pregnancy outcome by interfering with the physiologic process of pregnancy [63,64], and the fetuses born to these mothers are invariably perfect. Although this syndrome is still called phospholipid antibody syndrome, it is now known that these antibodies are directed against a protein/phospholipids antibody complex [65,66]. The best-studied protein cofactor is $\beta 2$ glycoprotein 1 [65]. Antibodies to phospholipid/protein complexes predispose patients to develop recurrent clinical thrombosis [58,65]. Numerous studies have shown that more than 50% of patients who have previously demonstrated the clinical features of aPL syndrome are at risk for additional clinical thrombotic events if not aggressively anticoagulated [67,68], and more than 70% of patients rethrombose on the same side of the vascular tree [67,68].

Placental thrombosis and infarctions leading to placental insufficiency are some of the mechanisms for fetal wastage in patients with this syndrome [69,70], and it has been suggested that aPLs may interfere with the physiologic antithrombotic effects mediated by annexin V in the placenta [34,71].

The annexins are a family of proteins, and annexin V has a high affinity for anionic phospholipids and the ability to displace coagulation factors from phospholipid surfaces making it a potent anticoagulant [72]. Annexin V is expressed by placental trophoblasts and is necessary to maintain placental integrity [34]. Studies with aPL model animals have shown that annexin V antibodies result in fetal wastage [73]. Rand et al have determined that aPL placentas have reduced annexin V expression and that IgG fractions from patients with aPL syndrome reduce the quantity of annexin V on cultured trophoblasts [74].

More recent evidence has suggested that other mechanisms may also contribute to fetal wastage in this syndrome. Although the pathology of aPL syndrome is a bland thrombotic diathesis, not associated with inflammation [75], there is now evidence to suggest that complement activation is one mechanism contributing to aPL-mediated pregnancy loss [25,76]. Salmon et al have demonstrated that they could prevent fetal loss in animal aPL models by blocking complement activation with C3 convertase inhibitor Crry-Ig [25,76]. Mice that are C3 deficient are resistant to fetal loss induced by aPL antibodies [25]. Additional studies of the deciduas in mice injected with human aPL reveal immunoglobulin and C3 deposition, necrosis, apoptosis, and polymorphonuclear leucocyte infiltration in the deciduas, changes not seen in the control animals [25]. These authors suggest that complement activation is a requirement for thrombosis generation and for the fetal loss associated with aPL syndrome [76].

It is now known that up to 20% of women with recurrent fetal loss have aPL antibodies [77]. Treating pregnant patients who have aPL syndrome with anticoagulation throughout pregnancy improves the fetal wastage rate in some patients [78,79], but our studies of aPL placentas showed that there was still significant pathologic changes in these placentas even if the pregnancy produced a live infant [70]. Some patients never completed pregnancy despite a variety of treatments. If complement activation is a requirement for aPL fetal loss, then targeting complement may be an important therapeutic step forward in the management of these patients. Until specific complement targets are developed, it could be argued that antiinflammatory drugs may be useful, but corticosteroids are inadvisable in these patients because they are predisposed to develop hypertension, toxemia of pregnancy, and preeclampsia [78,79]

B. Systemic Lupus Erythematosus and Fetal Loss

Fetal wastage is increased in patients with SLE [52–54]. Many factors contribute to this increased fetal wastage, but as discussed earlier, aPL antibodies predispose women to recurrent fetal loss [77–79]; therefore patients with SLE who also have aPL (i.e., secondary aPL syndrome) have a double jeopardy when it comes to fetal outcome.

Other autoantibodies associated with SLE and primary Sjögren's syndrome may also influence fetal survival [62]. It is now known that the transplacental passage of antibodies to Ro and/or La may result in the development of neonatal lupus syndrome (see section on fetal outcome), which may cause fetal/neonatal death [81,82]. Other factors that contribute to fetal loss in patients with SLE include activity of the disease itself [83,84]. It has been our advice to patients with lupus who aspire for motherhood that their disease should be inactive for at least 6 months prior to attempting conception. We also monitor the patients carefully throughout pregnancy looking for clinical and laboratory changes that may suggest a flare in disease activity [85] and treat active disease usually with oral corticosteroids.

Previous studies have documented that discontinuing antimalarial drugs can result in flares of SLE [86–88], and because flares of disease are a known factor that adversely affects pregnancy outcome it really makes no sense to discontinue antimalarial drugs in a patient with SLE that becomes pregnant unexpectedly. Studies by us and others have suggested that the 4-amino quinolone drugs can be used safely throughout pregnancy [89–91], although animal studies have shown that they cross the placenta and can be deposited in pigmented tissues such as the eye [92].

C. Other Connective Tissue/Autoimmune Diseases and Fetal Loss

Although rheumatoid arthritis does not adversely affect pregnancy outcome, other rheumatic diseases may increase fetal wastage. The literature pertaining to systemic sclerosis and pregnancy has produced conflicting results [93–96]. Steen *et al* concluded that infertility and fetal wastage are not increased in patients with systemic sclerosis when compared to patients with rheumatoid arthritis [93]; however, both patients with scleroderma and rheumatoid arthritis produced more premature births when compared to normal controls [93]. Live birth occurred in 84% of patients with limited scleroderma and 77% of those with diffuse disease, not a significantly different outcome from mothers without this disease [96].

A retrospective case-control study determined that primary Sjögren's syndrome also adversely affects pregnancy outcome [97]. A comprehensive study addressing perinatal outcome in women residing in Norway with a variety of connective tissue disease and inflammatory rheumatic disease determined that the rate of preterm birth, small-for-gestation-date babies, and perinatal and postnatal deaths were increased in these patients [98]. Maternal Graves' disease, even if previously treated, may still cause problems for the fetus and/or neonate. Maternal thyroid-stimulating hormone (TSH) receptor antibodies may induce fetal hyperthyroidism, which can cause intrauterine growth restriction, cardiac failure, and fetal death [99].

IV. Other Fetal and/or Neonatal Disease, a Consequence of Maternal Autoimmune Disease

Transient fetal and/or neonatal disease may occur as a consequence of transplacental maternal antibody (see Table 102-1), but in some diseases the effects of this maternal autoantibody may have long-lasting consequences [100]. Maternal autoimmune disease may also contribute to significant pathology arising in the offspring of these mothers, and the mechanisms for this pathology are not so well understood.

A. Neonatal Lupus Syndrome

The neonatal lupus syndrome (NNL) is considered to be a result of the transplacental passage of maternal antibody to Ro and/or La ribonucleoproteins [62,82,83,101–103]. This may present as a transient disease with a rash that typically appears in the first few weeks of life and disappears by age 6 months, when maternal autoantibodies disappear from the baby [102]. Other transient manifestations include liver disease [104], hematologic problems including thrombocytopenia [105], and neurologic disease [106].

Unfortunately, not all features of NNL are transient, and the most severe and devastating consequence of this syndrome is heart disease, including congenital complete heart block [100,103,109]. This pathology is permanent. More than 85% of

mothers producing fetuses with primary congenital complete heart block have antibodies to Ro and/or La antigens even in the absence of clinical disease in these mothers themselves [101,110]. The risk of a mother with these antibodies producing a child with congenital heart block is about 2% [111] but the risk of subsequent pregnancies being affected after the birth of a child with congenital heart block is less than 20% [112], demonstrating that other fetal factors affect the development of the syndrome. These fetal factors remain unknown.

The research registry for the NNL has collected data from 186 families each of whom have a least one child affected by congenital heart block and the mother has been documented to have antibodies to either Ro and/or La antigens. This registry has produced interesting long-term follow-up data on these affected children. Previous reports had suggested that many of these children did not do well, with 60% requiring a pacemaker and approximately 20% dying during childhood [113]. The most recent data by this group would suggest that the long-term prognosis for these infants is even worse. Several children enrolled in the registry demonstrated progression of heart block after birth, prompting these authors to recommend that electrocardiograms should be performed on all infants born to mothers with Ro/La antibodies [114]. Data from the Toronto Registry group on 102 children with NNL presenting between 1965 and 1998 have shown that fetal presentation of isolated complete heart block is associated with a 43% mortality rate. A gestational age of less than 33 weeks was associated with a high mortality rate [115]. It is interesting that cardiac pathology of endocardial fibroelastosis (FFE) was reported in three children who did not have complete heart block [116] and cardiac disease continued to develop in children who had been previously treated with antiinflammatory drugs and pacemakers [117]. All of this evidence suggests that the cardiac pathology of NNL may be more varied than previously documented and that it may continue to proceed even after birth. It is also interesting that the maternal heart does not appear to be affected by the circulating antibody, and long-term follow up of these children suggests that they do not go on to develop systemic rheumatic diseases [118].

B. Thyroid Disease

Maternal thyroid disease may result in fetal hypothyroidism, and many studies have demonstrated that fetal hypothyroidism can impair neurocognitive function [119,120], similar to that seen in children originating from areas of the world that are iodine deficient. These neurocognitive and psychologic impairments emphasize the need for careful monitoring of women with known thyroid disease who become pregnant, especially because one study suggests that maternal thyroid replacement may be inadequate during pregnancy, resulting in elevated neonatal TSH levels and reduced birth weight and head circumference [121].

C. Diabetes

Similar studies have shown that tight control of blood sugar levels from the time of conception throughout pregnancy reduces the risk of fetal malformations and perinatal mortality [122]. Other studies addressing the risks of childhood malignancy in children born to parents with autoimmune diseases have produced conflicting results. A study of 4340 children born to mothers with diabetes between 1987 and 1997 revealed that the odds ratio for childhood cancer in these children was 2.25%, whereas 5842 children born to mothers with other autoimmune disease did not reveal any increased rise for developing a childhood malignancy [123], confirming a previous report by Mellemkjaer *et al* [124]. However, when specific types of malignancy were analyzed, the earlier study suggested that parental autoimmune disease was associated with an increased risk of childhood lymphoma and leukemia [124].

D. Systemic Lupus Erythematosus and Phospholipid Antibody Syndrome

Learning defects have also been documented in children, particularly sons, born to mothers with SLE. In a controlled study, Ross *et al* studied 58 children born to mothers with SLE and determined that sons born to mothers with SLE were more likely to have a learning disorder than daughters born to mothers with SLE or children of either sex in the control group. Factors that appeared to contribute to the learning disabilities were lupus disease activity during pregnancy in the presence of Ro/La antibodies [125].

At least 20% of children born to mothers with SLE and or aPL syndrome are small for gestational age or are delivered preterm (i.e., before 37 weeks gestation) [126–128]. Small for gestational age and/or preterm delivery are both known to predispose infants to a variety of medical problems including cerebral palsy, which occurs in between 5% and 8% of premature infants born less than 33 weeks gestation compared to 0.1–0.3% in normal population [129]. Insulin resistance, type 2 diabetes, hypertension, coronary artery disease, and cognitive deficits are also increased in these children [130].

V. Effect of Pregnancy on Clinical Expression of Maternal Autoimmune Disease

A. Beneficial Effects

1. Rheumatoid Arthritis

Approximately 80% of patients with rheumatoid arthritis can anticipate an improvement in clinical disease during pregnancy [31] that will be repeated in subsequent pregnancies; this benefit is almost certainly a consequence of the immune modulation that is essential for pregnancy to proceed [26,27]. Although there is literature suggesting that exogenous estrogens may be beneficial in preventing the development of rheumatoid arthritis [131], it is important to note that the benefits of pregnancy afforded the patients with rheumatoid arthritis extends beyond delivery into the postpartum period, a time when hormonal levels should be normal, suggesting that the benefits of pregnancy are more than a hormonal effect.

Hench's original observations have been confirmed by several subsequent studies [132,133,134]. Barrett *et al* followed 140 patients with rheumatoid arthritis through pregnancy and for 6 months postpartum and confirmed the benefits of pregnancy and the previously known risk of flare of disease in the postpartum period, with two-thirds of the patients reporting an increase in joint pain during the first 6 months postpartum [134]. The risk of developing rheumatoid arthritis *de novo* during pregnancy is also less than would be expected, but conversely, the postpartum period is a time of increased risk for developing the disease [135] as is breast-feeding [136].

2. Autoimmune Thyroid Disease

Like rheumatoid arthritis, Graves' disease may ameliorate during pregnancy but returns with a flare of disease postpartum [137,138]. Transient maternal hyperthyroidinemia may also occur during pregnancy; one cause of this is the TSH agonist effects of placental human chronic gonadotropin (HCG) [139]. This transient hyperthyroidinemia is seen in about 0.2% of pregnant women [140], and there is some evidence that this phenomenon contributes to the development of hyperemesis gravidarum [140,141].

Postpartum autoimmune thyroid disease may flare, and a condition known as postpartum thyroid disease (PPTD) may occur in up to 10% of unselected postpartum patients [143]. Patients with type I diabetes have a threefold incidence of PPTD [144]. Transient hyperthyroidism occurs, followed rapidly by hypothyroidism—a consequence of autoimmune thyroiditis [145]. PPTD occurs in 50% of patients positive for thyroid peroxidase (TPO) antibody, and the hypothyroidism is permanent in up to 30% [146].

3. Multiple Sclerosis

Multiple sclerosis is a chronic demyelinating disease of the central nervous system that is characterized by relapses and remissions, and like most "autoimmune" diseases multiple sclerosis occurs more frequently in young women [147]. The effect of pregnancy on multiple sclerosis has been studied extensively, and the consensus of opinion is that the relapse rate of multiple sclerosis is substantially lower during pregnancy [148,149] with flares of disease observed during the postpartum period [148,150]. The relapse rate was not found to correlate with breast-feeding [150,151] and may be reduced by the use of intravenous gamma globulin intravenous immune globulin (IVIG) [152]. This pattern of clinical disease during pregnancy and the postpartum period is very similar to that found in rheumatoid arthritis. It is therefore very interesting to note that the tremendous benefit of cytokine inhibitors afforded to patients with rheumatoid arthritis is not seen in patients with multiple sclerosis, and in some cases TNF inhibitors have been reported to exacerbate demyelinating syndromes [153,154]. This is particularly interesting because animal models for multiple sclerosis–like diseases have demonstrated that pregnant rats develop less severe experimental autoimmune encephalomyelitis (EAE) than nonpregnant rats with modulation of cytokine expression in the spinal cord inflammatory infiltrate [155]. Other studies have shown that the pregnancy hormone estriol can ameliorate EAE in mice with an increased production of the Th2 cytokine IL I0 [156], and human studies evaluating the use of estriol as a treatment for multiple sclerosis have initially produced encouraging results [157].

B. Detrimental Effects

1. Systemic Lupus Erythematosus

The debate over whether pregnancy causes flares of SLE continues, and some authors do not consider pregnancy to be detrimental to SLE [53,158–160]. It is important, however, to recognize that the best control for studying patients with SLE is the patient herself because all patients have a distinct pattern of disease expression. Petri *et al* studied patients with lupus when they were pregnant and compared flare rates with the same patients when they were no longer pregnant and determined that the flare rate per patient (0.136 per patient per month) was significantly higher during pregnancy [161], a finding confirmed by Ruiz-Irastorza *et al* [162]. Using similar self nonpregnant controls, Zulman concluded that flares of SLE are increased throughout pregnancy [163]. Most studies suggest that flares of SLE during pregnancy are no more severe than nonpregnant flares of disease [161,162]. Patients with preexisting renal disease appear to be at risk for hypertension and preeclampsia during pregnancy, but permanent deterioration in renal function is rare [164].

Diagnosing and managing flares of disease during pregnancy can be difficult because many of the complications of pregnancy can mimic flares of SLE. Complement levels increase during normal pregnancy so any decrease in complement levels (even if still within the so-called normal range) can signify disease activity [85]. Decreasing complement levels, increasing DNA levels, and an active urine sediment all indicate active disease, but the majority of disease flares do not develop major organ involvement and include a predominance of cutaneous and musculoskeletal manifestations [161].

Flares of disease are usually managed with prednisone because the transplacental passage of this drug is miniscule; however, reports appear to confirm that hydroxychloroquine can be used safely during pregnancy [89–91] It is our opinion that hydroxychloroquine should not be stopped just because of pregnancy [89]. Discontinuing this drug has been shown to produce flares of disease in these patients [86–88], and active disease is known to be detrimental for fetal outcome [83–84].

Patients with lupus desiring motherhood need to be counseled that pregnancy can be complicated by lupus disease. Not only is there a risk of flaring the disease in the mother necessitating treatment with corticosteroids, but also there is an increase in fetal wastage, preterm delivery, and preeclampsia, particularly in patients who have phospholipid antibodies. Recent advances in obstetrics and medical management have improved both maternal and fetal outcomes. The secret for success is close careful monitoring of the patient and her fetus and prompt action if complications arise.

2. Phospholipid Antibody Syndrome

The presence of phospholipid antibodies does not *per se* dictate a prothrombotic state, but those patients who have aPL and have declared themselves to be at risk for thrombosis are particularly at risk for clinical thrombotic episodes when they are pregnant, postpartum, or taking oral contraceptives or when they have flares of SLE, have infections, or undergo surgical procedures [165,166]. These physiologic and or pathologic triggers have been called the "second hit" phenomenon [165]. The pregnant patient with lupus who also has aPL is therefore at particular risk for a clinical thrombotic event during pregnancy or the postpartum period. We routinely anticoagulate all of our patients with SLE/aPL who have experienced a prior clinical thrombotic event throughout the entire pregnancy and for a minimum of 6 weeks postpartum because it is our experience, and that of others, that the prothrombotic disease state is still increased for several weeks postpartum [165,166].

VI. Pregnancy Contributing to the Pathogenesis of Autoimmune Disease?

A. Microchimerism and Autoimmune Disease

Microchimerism is the persistence of nonhost cells in a vulnerable host organism [167], a physiologic process known to occur during pregnancy [167,168] and also found in patients who have undergone bone marrow transplant [169]. It is now known that these nonhost cells may persist for years [170,171], and recent work has suggested that this immune aberration may result in significant pathology, suggesting that some so-called autoimmune diseases may in fact be alloimmune [172].

Bone marrow transplantation has been shown to be associated with exacerbation, induction *de novo*, or improvement of autoimmune disease states [173–175]. Animal studies of EAE have shown that bone marrow transplants from resistant rats to susceptible affected rats can induce remission in affected animals [176].

Scleroderma has many clinical features that are similar to graft vs host disease, and several reports have now shown that microchimerism occurs more frequently in patients with scleroderma than in normal individuals [177–179]. Studies of women known to have produced male offspring revealed persistence of the male DNA indicating persistent microchimerism occurred more frequently in women with scleroderma than in healthy controls [178]. Similar studies have suggested that as many as 47% of women with Hashimoto's thyroiditis may have microchimerism compared with 4% of control women with multinodular goiter [180]. Similar studies failed to detect microchimerism in patients with Sjögren's syndrome [181], which is interesting because sicca complaints may be a manifestation of graft vs host disease.

Transfer of fetal cells and maternal cells is known to occur during pregnancy, and it is now known that long-term persistence of maternal cells may occur even in immunocompetent offspring [171]. The fact that microchimerism is found in normal controls raises the question of the true significance of this phenomenon, but to date the evidence would suggest that this phenomenon may be an important factor in the pathogenesis of some so-called autoimmune diseases.

VII. Conclusion

This chapter details how maternal autoimmune disease can prevent or disrupt pregnancy. Autoimmune disease can also produce transient or permanent pathology in offspring, which sometimes is influenced by as-yet-unknown fetal and maternal factors. Pregnancy, however, may exacerbate or ameliorate maternal clinical autoimmune disease, but benefits are typically temporary with the disease flaring in the postpartum period. Reports suggest that we need to consider that pregnancy may even contribute to the pathogenesis of autoimmune disease, with studies suggesting that microchimerism may play a role in the pathogenesis of systemic sclerosis, autoimmune thyroid disease, and even multiple sclerosis.

VIII. Suggestions for Further Investigations

Clearly there is much to be learned from the study of pregnancy and autoimmune disease.

- Why do rheumatoid arthritis and multiple sclerosis get better, only to return?
- Why do patients with phospholipid antibodies fail to sustain pregnancy when their fetuses are usually perfect?
- Does complement activation play a major role in augmenting pregnancy loss in a disease in which the pathology is typically noninflammatory?

Hopefully, a better understanding of the immunology and physiology of pregnancy will help to resolve these questions and provide further insight into the relationships between pregnancy, sex hormones, and autoimmune disease.

References

1. Veenstra van Nieuwenhoven AL, Heineman MJ, Faas MM. (2003). The immunology of successful pregnancy. *Human Reprod Update.* 9(4):347–357.
2. Mellor AL, Munn DH. (2000). Immunology at the maternal–fetal interface. Lessons for T cell tolerance and suppression. *Ann Rev Immunol.* 18:367–391.
3. Sacks G, Sargent I, Redman C. (1999). An innate view of human pregnancy. *Immunol Today.* 20(3):114–118.
4. Weetman AP. (1999). The immunology of pregnancy. *Thyroid.* 9(7):643–646.
5. Thellin O, Coumans B, Zorzi W, *et al.* (2000). Tolerance to the foeto-placental "graft": ten ways to support a child for nine months. *Curr Opin Immunol.* 12(6):731–737.
6. Van Voorhis BJ, Stovall DW. (1997). Autoantibodies and infertility: a review of the literature. *J Reprod Immunol.* 33:239–256.
7. Rote NS, Stetzer BP. (2003). Autoimmune disease as a cause of reproductive failure. *Clin Lab Med.* 23:265–293.
8. Carp HJA, Toder VR, Mashiach S. (1992). Immunotherapy of habitual abortion. *Am. J Reprod Immunol.* 28:281–284.
9. Robillard PY, Hulsey TC, Derker GA, *et al.* (2003). Preeclampsia and human reproduction. An essay of long-term reflection. *J Reprod Immunol.* 59(2): 93–100.
10. Medawar PB. (1953). Some immunological and endocrinological problems raised by evolution of vivparity in vertebrates. *Symp Soc Exp Biol.* 7:320–328.
11. Johnson PM. (1993). *Reproductive and maternofetal relations. Clinical aspects of immunology.* Blackwell: Oxford. 755–767.
12. Robertson SA, Mau JA, Hudson SN, *et al.* (1997). Cytokine-leukocyte networks and the establishment of pregnancy. *Am J Reprod Immunol.* 37: 438–442.
13. Lim KJH, Odukoya OA, Ajjan RA, *et al.* (1998). Profile of cytokine mRNA expression in peri-implantation human endometrium. *Mol Human Reprod.* 4:77–81.
14. Raghupathy R. (1997). Th-1 type immunity is incompatible with successful pregnancy. *Immunol Today.* 18:478–482.
15. Tremellen KP, Valbuena D, Landeras J, *et al.* (2000). The effect of intercourse on pregnancy rates during assisted human reproduction. *Human Reprod.* 15:2653–2658.
16. Wood GW. (1994). Is restricted antigen presentation the explanation of fetal allograft survival. *Immunol Today.* 15:15–18.
17. Kovats S, Main EK, Librrack C, *et al.* (1990). Class I antigen HLA-G expressed in human trophoblasts. *Science.* 248:220–223.
18. Carosella ED, Dausset J, Kirzem B. (1996). HLA-G revisited. *Immunol Today.* 17:407–409.
19. Moreau P, Paul P, Rouas-Freiss N, *et al.* (1998). Molecular and immunologic aspects of the nonclassical HLA class I antigen HLA-G: evidence for an important role in the maternal tolerance of the fetal allograft. *Am J Reprod Immunol.* 40:136–146.
20. Moffett-King A. (2002). Natural killer cells and pregnancy. *Nature Rev Immunol.* 2:656–663.
21. Makrigiannakis A, Zoumakis E, Kalantaridou S, *et al.* (2001). Corticotropin–releasing hormone promotes blastocyst implantation and early maternal tolerance. *Nature Immunol.* 2:1018–1024.
22. Hunt JS, Vassmer D, Ferguson TA, *et al.* (1997). Fas ligand is positioned in mouse uterus and placenta to prevent trafficking of activated leukocytes between the mother and the conceptus. *J Immunol.* 158:4122–4128.
23. Holmes CH, Simpson KL. (1992). Complement and pregnancy. New insights into the immunobiology of the feto maternal relationship. *Ballieres Clin Ostet Gynaecol.* 6:439–460.
24. Xu C, Mao D, Holers VM, *et al.* (2000). A critical role for the murine complement regulator Crry in feto maternal tolerance. *Science.* 287:498–501.
25. Holers VM, Girardi G, Mo L, *et al.* (2001). Complement C3 activation is required for antiphospholipid antibody induced fetal loss. *J Exp Med.* 195:211–220.
26. Hill JA, Polgar K, Anderson DJ. (1995). T helper 1 type immunity to trophoblast in women with recurrent spontaneous abortion. *JAMA.* 273:1933–1937.
27. Marzi M, Vigano A, Trabattoni D, *et al.* (1996). Characterization of Type 1 and Type 2 cytokine production profile in physiologic and pathologic human pregnancy. *Clin Exp Immunol.* 106:127–133.
28. Yui J, Garcia Lloret M, Wegmann TG, *et al.* (1994). Cytotoxicity of tumour necrosis factor-alpha and gamma-interferon against primary human placental trophoblasts. *Placenta.* 15:819–835.
29. Chaouat G, Assa I, Malien IA, *et al.* (1995). IL-10 prevents naturally occurring fetal loss in the CBA × DBA/2 mating combination and local defect in IL-10 production in the abortion prone combination is corrected by *in vivo* injection of IFN-TAU. *J Immunol.* 154:4261–4268.
30. Piccinni MP, Maggie M, Romagnani S. (2000). Role of hormone controlled T cell cytokines in the maintenance of pregnancy. *Biochem Soc Trans.* 28:212–215.
31. Hench PS. (1938). The ameliorating effect of pregnancy on chronic atrophic (infectious rheumatoid) arthritis, fibrositis, and intermittent hydrarthrosis. *Mayo Clin Proc.* 13:161–167.
32. Piccinni MP, Beloni L, Livi C, *et al.* (1998). Defective production of both L.I.F. and Type 2 Helper cytokines by decidual T cells in unexplained recurrent abortions. *Nat Med.* 4:1020–1024.
33. Piccinni MP, Giudizi MG, Biagiotti R, *et al.* (1995). Progesterone favors the development of human T helper cells producing Th 2 type cytokines and promotes both IL-4 production and membrane CD 30 expressions in established Th1 cell clones. *J Immunol.* 155:128–133.
34. Rand JH. (2000). Antiphospholipid antibody mediated disruption of the annexin V antithrombotic shield: A thrombogenic mechanism for the aPL syndrome. *J Autoimmun.* 15:107–111
35. Aarli A, Matre R. (1998). Suppression of immuno globulin secretion by soluble annexin II. *Scand J Immunol.* 48:522–526.
36. Mellor AL, Sivakumar J, Chandler P. *et al.* (2001). Prevention of T cell-driven complement activation and inflammation by tryptophan catabolism during pregnancy. *Nature Immunol.* 2:64–68.
37. Healy DL, Trounson AO, Andersen AN. (1994). Female infertility: Causes and Treatment. *Lancet.* 18:1539–1544.
38. Wilson C, Eade OE, Elstein M, *et al.* (1975). Smooth muscle antibodies in infertility. *Lancet.* 1:238–239.
39. Taylor PV, Campbell JM, Scott JS. (1989). Presence of autoantibodies in women with unexplained infertility. *Am J Obstet Gynecol.* 161:377–379.
40. Roussex RG, Kaider BD, Price DE, *et al.* (1996). Laboratory evaluation of women experiencing reproductive failure. *Am J Reprod Immunol.* 35: 415–420.
41. Gleicher N, El-Roeiy A, Confino E, *et al.* (1989). Reproductive failure because of auto antibodies: unexplained infertility and pregnancy wastage. *Am J Obstet Gynecol.* 160:1376–1385.
42. Gleicher N. (1992). Autoantibodies in normal and abnormal pregnancy. *Am J Reprod Immunol.* 28:269–273.
43. Lejeunne B, Grun JP, Le Nayer P, *et al.* (1993). Antithyroid drugs, underlying thyroid abnormalities and miscarriage, or pregnancy induced hypertension. *Br J Obstet Gynecol.* 7:669–672.

44. Singh A, Dantas ZN, Stone SC, et al. (1995). Presence of thyroid autoantibodies in early reproductive failure: biochemical verses clinical pregnancies. Fertil Steril. 63:277–281.

45. Poppe K, Glinoer D, Stirtheghem A, et al. (2002). Thyroid dysfunction and auto immunity in infertile women. Thyroid. 12(11):997–1001.

46. Krassas GE. (2000). Thyroid disease and female reproduction. Fertil Steril. 74:1063–1070.

47. Gerhard I, Becker T, Eggert-Kruse W, et al. (1991). Thyroid and ovarian function in infertile women. Human Reprod. 6:338–345.

48. Odukoya OA, Wheatcroft N, Weetman AP, et al. (1995). The prevalence of endometrial immunoglobulin G antibodies in patients with endometriosis. Human Reprod. 10:1214–1219.

49. Wild RA, Podezaski E9, Hirigoye V, et al. (1991). Endometrial antibodies versus CA-125 for the detection of endometriosis. Fertil Steril. 55:90–96.

50. Gleicher N, El-Rociy A, Confino E et al. (1987). Is endometriosis an autoimmune disease? Obstet Gynecol. 70:115–122.

51. Nelson JL, Ostensen M. (1997). Pregnancy and rheumatoid arthritis. Rheum Dis Clin North Am. 23(1):195–211.

52. Fraga A, Mintz G, Orozco J, et al. (1974). Sterility and fertility rates, fetal wastage and maternal morbidity in SLE. J Rheum. 1:293–298.

53. Mintz G, Niz J, Quitierraz C, et al. (1986). Prospective study of pregnancy in SLE. Results of multidisciplinary approach. J Rheum. 13:732–739.

54. Petri M. (1997). Hopkins Lupus Pregnancy Center 1987–1996. Rheum Dis Clin North Am. Vol 23:1–13.

55. Kaplan J. (1986). Fetal wastage in patients with rheumatoid arthritis. J Rheum. 13:875–877.

56. Nelson JH, Voigt LF, Koepsell TD, et al. (1992). Pregnancy outcome in women with rheumatoid arthritis before disease onset. J Rheum. 19:18–21.

57. Spector TD, Silman AJ. (1990). Is poor pregnancy outcome a risk factor in rheumatoid arthritis. Ann Rheum Dis. 49:12–14.

58. Wilson A, Gharavi AE, Koike T. (1999). International consensus statement on preliminary classification criteria for definite antiphospholipid syndrome. Arthritis Rheum. 42:1309–1311.

59. Branch DW, Scott JR, Kochenour NK, et al. (1985). Obstetric complications associated with lupus anticoagulant. N Engl J Med. 313:1322–1326.

60. Branch DW, Silver RM, Blackwell JK, et al. (1992). Outcome of treated pregnancies in women with antiphospholipid syndrome; An update of the Utah experience. Obstet Gynecol. 80:614–620.

61. Lima F, Khamashta MA, Buchanan NM, et al. (1996). A study of sixty pregnancies in patients with antiphospholipid syndrome. Clin Exp Rheum. 14:131–136.

62. Reed BR, Lee LA, Harmon C. et al. (1983). Autoantibodies to SS-A/Ro in infants with congenital heart block. J. Pediatr. 103(6):889–991.

63. Di Somone N, Meroni PL, Delpapa N. (2000). Antiphospholipid antibodies affect trophoblasts gonadotrophin secretion and invasiveness by binding directly and through adhered B2 glycoprotein 1 (2000). Arthritis Rheum. 43:140–150.

64. Rand JH, Wu XX, Guller S, et al. (1994). Reduction of annexin V on placental villi of women with aPL and recurrent spontaneous abortions. Am J Obstet Gynecol. col. 171:1566–1579.

65. Galli M, Comfurius P, Maasen C, et al. (1990). Anticardiolipin (ACA) antibodies directed not to cardiolipin but to a plasma protein cofactor. Lancet. 336:1544–1547.

66. Bevers EM, Galli M, Barbui T, et al. (1991). Lupus anticoagulant IgG's (LA) are not directed to phospholipids only but to a complex of lipid-bound human prothrombin. Thromb Haemost. 66:629–632.

67. Rosove MH, Brewer PMC. (1992). Antiphospholipid thrombosis clinical course after the first thrombotic event in 70 patients. Ann Intern Med. 117:303–308.

68. Khamashta MA, Cuddrado MJ, Mujic F, et al. (1995). The management of thrombosis in the antiphospholipid antibody syndrome. N Engl J Med. 332:993–997.

69. Out HJ, Kooijman CP, Bruinse HW, et al. (1991). Histopathological findings in placentae from patients with intra-uterine fetal death and antiphospholipid antibodies. Eur J Obstet Gynecol Reprod Biol. 41:179–186.

70. Salafia CM, Parke AL. (1997). Placental pathology in SLE and phospholipid antibody syndrome. Rheum Dis Clin North Am. 23 1:85–97.

71. Rand JH, Wu XX, Andree HAM, et al. (1998). Antiphospholipid antibodies accelerate plasma coagulation by inhibiting annexin V binding to phospholipids: A lupus procoagulant phenomenon. Blood. 92:1652–1660.

72. Andree HAM, Hermens WT, Herker HC, et al. (1992). Displacement of Factor V and by annexin V in Phospholipid Binding and Anticoagulant Action of Annexin V. H.A.M. Andree ED Univeqsitaire per Maastricht. The Netherlands. 73–83.

73. Wang X, Campos B, Kaetzel MA, et al. (1999). Annexin V is critical in the maintenance of murine placental integrity. Am J Obstet Gynecol. col. 180:1008–1016.

74. Rand JH, Wu XX, Guller S, et al. (1997). Antiphospholipid immunoglobulin G antibodies reduce annexin V levels on syncytiotrophoblasts apical membranes and in culture media of placental villi. Am J Obstet Gynecol. 117:918–923.

75. Lie JR. (1996). Pathology of antiphospholipid syndrome. In: Asherson RA, Cervera R, Piette JC, et al., eds. The Antiphospholipid Syndrome. Boca Raton, FL: CRC Press. 89–104.

76. Salmon JE, Girardi G, Holers VM. (2002). Complement activation as a mediator of antiphospholipid antibody induced pregnancy loss and thrombosis. Ann Rheum Dis. 61(Suppl 11) 46–50.

77. Stephenson MD. (1996). Frequency of factors associated with habitual abortion in 197 couples. Fertil Steril. 66:24–29.

78. Lubbe WF, Palmer SJ, Butler WS, et al. (1983). Fetal survival after prednisone suppression of maternal lupus anticoagulant. Lancet. 1:1361–1363.

79. Kutteh WH. (1996). Antiphospholipid antibody associated recurrent pregnancy loss: treatment with heparin and low dose aspirin is superior to low dose aspirin alone. Am J Obstet Gynecol. 174:1584–1589.

80. Tincani A, Branch W, Levy RA, et al. (2003). Treatment of pregnant patients with antiphospholipid syndrome. Lupus. 12:524–529.

81. Jaeggi ET, Hamilton RM, Silverman ED, et al. (2002). Outcome of children with fetal neonatal or childhood diagnosis of isolated congenital atrio ventricular block. J Amer Coll Cardiol. 39:130–137.

82. Nield LE, Silverman ED, Taylor GP, et al. (2002). Maternal anti-Ro and anti-La antibody associated endocardial fibroelastosis. Circulation. 105:842–848.

83. Tozman ECS, Urowitz MB, Gladman DD. (1980). Systemic lupus erythematosus and pregnancy. J Rheum. 7:624–632.

84. Boumpas DT, Fessler BJ, Austin HA, et al. (1995). Systemic lupus erythematosus emerging concepts. Ann Intern Med. 123:42–53.

85. Buyon JP, Tamerius J, Orodrica S, et al. (1992). Activation of the alternative complement pathway accompanies disease flares in SLE during pregnancy. Arthritis Rheum. 35:55–61.

86. Rudnicki RD, Gresham GE, Rothfield NF. (1975). The efficacy of anti malarials in SLE. J Rheum. 2.323–330.

87. The Canadian Hydroxychloroquine Study Group. (1991). A randomized study of the effect of withdrawing hydroxychloroquine sulfate in SLE. New Engl J Med. 324:150–154.

88. Petri M, Howard D, Repke J, et al. (1992). The Hopkins Lupus Pregnancy Center 1987–1991. Update. Am J Reprod Immunol. 28:188–191.

89. Parke AL. (1993). Antimalarial drugs, pregnancy and lactation. Lupus. 2:21–23.

90. Parke AL, West B. (1996). Hydroxychloroquine in pregnant patients with SLE. J Rheum. 23:1715–1718.

91. Khamashta MA, Buchanan NM, Hughes GRV. (1996). The use of hydroxychloroquine in Lupus pregnancy. The British Experience. Lupus. 5(Suppl 1): 65–67.

92. Ullberg S, Lindquist NJ, Sjostrand SE. (1970). Accumulation of chorioretinotoxic drugs in the fetal eye. Nature. 227:1257–1258.

93. Steen VD, Conte C, Day N, et al. (1989). Pregnancy in women with systemic sclerosis. Arthritis Rheum. 32:151–157.

94. Silman AJ, Black CM. (1998). Increased incidence of spontaneous abortion and infertility in women with scleroderma before disease onset. A controlled study. Ann Rheum Dis. 47:6441–6444.

95. Slate WG, Graham AR. (1968). Scleroderma and pregnancy. Am J Obstet Gynecol. col. 101:335–340.

96. Steen VD, Brodeum M, Conte C. (1996). Prospective pregnancy study in women with systemic sclerosis (SSc) Arthritis Rheum. 39:5151.

97. Julkunen H, Kaaja R, Kurki P, et al. (1995). Fetal outcome in women with primary Sjögren's syndrome. A retrospective case control study. Clin Exp Rheum. 13:65–71.

98. Skomsvoll JF, Ostensen M, Irgens LM, et al. (1999). Perinatal outcome in pregnancies of women with connective tissue disease and inflammatory rheumatic disease in Norway. Scand J Rheum. 28:352–356.

99. Foley TP. (1991). Maternally transferred thyroid disease in the infant: Recognition and treatment advances in perinatal thyroidology. In: Bercu BB, Shulman DI. Advances in perinatal thyroidology. New York: Plenum Press. 209–226.

100. Chameides L, Truex RC, Vetter V, et al. (1977). Association of maternal SLE with congenital complete heart block. N Engl J Med. 297:1204–1207.

101. Scott JS, Maddison PJ, Taylor PV *et al.* (1983). Connective tissue disease, autoantibodies to nitronucleoprotein and congenital heart block. *N Engl J Med.* 309(4) 209–212.

102. Lee LA, Weston WL. (1998). Neonatal lupus erythematosus. *Semin Dermatol.* 7:66.

103. Reichlin M, Brucato A, Frank MB, *et al.* (1994). Concentration of autoantibodies to native 60 Kd Ro/SSA and denatured 52 KD Ro/SSA in eluates from the heart of a child who died with congenital complete heart block. *Arthritis Rheum.* 37:1698–1670.

104. Lee LA, Sokol RJ, Buyon JP. (2002). Hepatobiliary disease in neonatal lupus. Prevalence and clinical characteristics in cases enrolled in a national registry. *Pediatrics.* 109:E11.

105. Watson R, Kang JE, May M, *et al.* (1988). Thrombocytopenia in the neonatal lupus syndrome. *Arch Dermatol.* 124:560.

106. Wallace SA, Aron AM, Taff I. (1984). Neonatal lupus involving the central nervous system. *Ann Neurol.* 16:399.

107. Herreman G, Galezewski N. (1985). Maternal connective tissue disease and congenital heart block. *N Engl J Med.* 312–329.

108. Buyon JP, Waltuck J, Klein C, *et al.* (1995). *In utero* identification and therapy of CHB. *Lupus.* 4:116.

109. Tseng CE, Buyon JP. (1997). Neonatal lupus syndrome. *Rheum Dis Clin North Am.* 23 1:31–54.

110. Lee LA. (1993). Neonatal lupus erythematosus. *J Invest Dermatol.* 100:9s–13s.

111. Brucato A, Frass IM, Franceschin F, *et al.* (2001). Risk of congenital complete heart block in newborns of mother with anti Ro/SSA antibodies detected by counter immuno electrophoresis: A prospective study of 100 women. *Arthritis Rheum.* 44:1832–1835.

112. Buyon JP. (2003). Neonatal lupus syndrome in systemic lupus erythematosus. In *Lupus, 4th ed.,* Lahita R, ed. San Diego: Academic Press (in press).

113. Buyon JP, Gieber TR, Copel J, *et al.* (1998). Autoimmune associated congenital heart block. Morality, morbidity and recurrence rates obtained from a national neonatal lupus registry. *J Am Coll Cardiol.* 31:1658–1666.

114. Askanase AD, Friedman DM, Dischem MR, *et al.* (2002). Spectrum and progression of conduction abnormalities in infants born to mothers with anti SSA/Ro/SSB La antibodies. *Lupus.* 11:145–151.

115. Jaeggi ET, Hamilton RM, Silverman ED, *et al.* (2002). Outcome of children with fetal/neonatal or childhood diagnosis of isolated congenital atrio ventricular block. *J Am Coll Cardiol.* 39:130–137.

116. Nield LE, Silverman ED, Smallhorn JF, *et al.* (2002). Endocardial fibroelastosis associated with maternal anti-Ro and anti La antibodies in the absence of AV block. *J Am Coll Cardiol.* 40:796–802.

117. Neild LE, Silverman ED, Taylor GG, *et al.* (2002). Maternal anti Ro and anti La antibody associated endocardial fibroelastosis. *Circulation.* 105:843–848.

118. Martin V, Lee LA, Askanase AD, *et al.* (2002). Long term follow up of children with neonatal lupus and their unaffected siblings. *Arthritis Rheum.* 46:2377–2383.

119. Man EB, Brown JF, Serunian SA. (1991). Maternal hypothyroidinaeimia psycho-neurological deficits of pregnancy. *Ann Clin Lab Sci.* 19:83–86.

120. Haddow JE, Palomaki GE, Allan WC, *et al.* (1999). Maternal thyroid deficiency during pregnancy and subsequent neuropsychological development of the child. *N Engl J Med.* 341:549–555.

121. Blazer S, Moreh-Waterman Y, Miller-Lotan R, *et al.* (2003). Maternal hypothyroidism may affect fetal growth and neonatal thyroid function. *Obstet Gynecol.* 102:232–241.

122. Lepercq J. (2003). The diabetic pregnant woman. *Ann Endocrinol.* 64: Suppl 3 S7–11.

123. Westbom L, Aber GA, Kallen B. (2002). Childhood malignancy and maternal diabetes or other autoimmune disease during pregnancy. *Br J Cancer.* 86(7):1078–1080.

124. Mellemkjaer L, Alexander F, Olson JH. (2000). Cancer among children of parents with autoimmune diseases. *Br J Cancer.* 82:1353–1357.

125. Ross G, Sammaritano L, Nass R, *et al.* (2003). Effects of mothers autoimmune disease during pregnancy on learning disabilities and hand preference in their children. *Arch Pediatr Adol Med.* 157:(4)397–402.

126. Branch DW, Silver RM. Blackwell JL, *et al.* (1992). Outcome of treated pregnancies in women with antiphospholipid syndrome: An update of the Utah experience. *Obstet Gynecol.* 80:614–620.

127. Gimovsky M, Montoro M. (1991). SLE and other connective tissue diseases. *Clin Obstet Gynecol.* 34:35–50.

128. Pollard KK, Scott JR, Branch DW. (1992). Outcome of children born to women treated during pregnancy for antiphospholipid syndrome. *Obstet Gynecol.* 80:365–368.

129. Scott JR. (2002). Risk to children born to mothers with autoimmune diseases. *Lupus.* 11:655–660.

130. Robinson R. (2001). The fetal origins of adult disease. *BMJ.* 322:375–376.

131. Silman AJ, Hochberg MC. (1993). *Epidemiology of the rheumatic diseases.* Oxford, England: Oxford University Press. 37–42.

132. Ostensen M, Aune B, Husby G. (1983). Effect of pregnancy and hormonal changes on the activity of rheumatoid arthritis. *Scand J Rheumatol.* 12(2)69–72.

133. Neely NT, Persellin RH. (1977). Activity of rheumatoid arthritis during pregnancy. *Texas Med.* 73:59–63.

134. Barrett JH, Brennan P, Fiddler M, *et al.* (1999). Does rheumatoid arthritis remit during pregnancy and relapse postpartum. Results from a nationwide study in the United Kingdom performed prospectively from late pregnancy. *Arthritis Rheum.* 42(6) 1219–1227.

135. Silman AJ, Kay A, Brennan P. (1992). Timing of pregnancy in relation to the onset of rheumatoid arthritis. *Arthritis Rheum.* 35:152–155.

136. Brennan P, Silman A. (1994). Breast feeding and the onset of rheumatoid arthritis. *Arthritis Rheum.* 37:808–813.

137. Kung AWC, Jones BM. (1998). A change from stimulatory to blocking antibody activity in Graves disease during pregnancy. *J Clin Endocrin Metab.* 83:514–518.

138. Gonzalez-Jimenez A, Fernandez-Soto ML, Escobar-Jimenez F, *et al.* (1993). Thyroid function parameters and TSH receptor antibodies in healthy subjects and Graves disease patients: a sequential study before, during and after pregnancy. *Thyroidology.* 5:13–20.

139. Yoshimura M, Nishikania M, Yoskikania N, *et al.* (1991). Mechanism of thyroid stimulation by human chorionic gonadotrophin in sera of normal pregnant women. *Acta Endocrinol.* 124:173–178.

140. Tanaka S, Yamada H, Kato E, *et al.* (1998). Gestational transient hyperthyrotoxinaema (GTH) screening for thyroid function in 23,163 pregnant women using dried blood spots. *Clin Endocrinol.* 49:325–329.

141. Kimura M, Amino N, Tamaki H, *et al.* (1993). Gestational thyrotoxicosis and hyperemesis gravidarum: Possible role of HCG with higher stimulating activity. *Clin Endocrinol.* 38:345–351.

142. Goodwin TM, Montoro M, Mestman JH, *et al.* (1992). The role of chorionic gonadotrophin in transient hyperthyroidism of hyperemesis gravidarum. *J Clin Endocrinol Metab.* 75:1333–1337.

143. Hall R. (1995). Pregnancy and autoimmune endocrine disease. *Ballieres Clin Endocrinol Metab.* 9:137–155.

144. Weetman AP. (1994). Insulin dependent diabetes mellitus and post partum thyroiditis: an important association. *J Clin Endocrinol.* 79:7–9.

145. Creach FM, Parkes AB, Lee A, *et al.* (1994). The iodide perchlorate discharge test in women with previous post partum thyroiditis: relationship to sonograph appearance and thyroid function. *J Clin Endocrinol.* 40: 765–768.

146. Lazarus J, Kokandi A. (2000). Thyroid disease in relation to pregnancy, a decade of change. *J Clin Endocrinol.* 53:265–278.

147. Duquette P, Pleines J, Girard M, *et al.* (1992). The increased susceptibility of women to multiple sclerosis. *Can J Neurol Sci.* 19:466–471.

148. Poser S, Poser N. (1983). Multiple sclerosis and gestation. *Neurology.* 33:1422–1427.

149. Runmarker B, Anderson O. (1995). Pregnancy is associated with lower risk of onset and a better prognosis in multiple sclerosis. *Brain.* 118: 253–261.

150. Confavreux C, Hutchinson M, Hours M, *et al.* (1998). Rate of pregnancy related relapses in multiple sclerosis. *N Engl J Med.* 339:285–291.

151. Nelson L, Franklin GM, Jones MC. (1988). Risk of multiple sclerosis exacerbation during pregnancy and breast feeding. *JAMA.* 259:3441–3443.

152. Orvieto R, Achiron A, Rotstein A, *et al.* (1999). Pregnancy and multiple sclerosis: a two year study. *Eur J Obstet Gynecol Reprod Biol.* 82:191–194.

153. Anon. (1999). TNF neutralization in MS: results of a randomized placebo controlled multicenter study. The Lenercept MS. Study group and the University of British Columbia MS/MRI Analysis Group. *Neurology.* 53:457–465.

154. Mohan N, Edwards E, Cupps T, *et al.* (2001). Demyelination occurring during anti TNFα therapy for inflammatory arthritis. *Arthritis Rheum.* Vol 44 12:2862–2869.

155. Harness J, McCombe PA. (2002). The effects of pregnancy on myelin basic protein induced experimental autoimmune encephalomyelitis in Lewis rats: suppression of clinical disease modulation of cytokine expression in spinal cord inflammatory infiltrate and suppression of lymphocyte proliferation by pregnancy sera. *Am J Reprod Immunol.* 46(6) 405–412.

156. Kim S, Liva SM, Dalal MA, et al. (1999). Estriol ameliorates autoimmune demyelinating disease: implications for multiple sclerosis. *Neurology.* 52(6):1230–1238.

157. Sicotte NL, Liva SM, Klutch R, et al. (2002). Treatment of multiple sclerosis with the pregnancy hormone estriol. *Ann Neurol.* 52(4):421–428.

158. Lockshin MD, Reinitz E, Druzin ML, et al. (1984). Lupus pregnancy: case-control study demonstrating absence of lupus exacerbation during or after pregnancy. *Am J Med.* 77:893–898.

159. Lockshin MD. (1989). Pregnancy does not cause SLE to worsen. *Arthritis Rheum.* 32:665–670.

160. Cervera R, Font J, Carmona F, et al. (2002). Pregnancy outcome in SLE: good news for the new millennium. *Autoimmun Rev.* 1:354–359.

161. Petri M, Howard D, Repke J. (1991). Frequency of lupus flare in pregnancy. The Hopkins lupus pregnancy center experience. *Arthritis Rheum.* 34:1538–1545.

162. Ruiz-Irastorza G, Lima F, Alves J, et al. (1996). Increased rate of lupus flare during pregnancy and the puerperium. *Br J Rheumatol.* 35:133–138.

163. Zulman J, Talal N, Hoffman GS, et al. (1980). Problems associated with the management of pregnancy in patients with SLE. *J Rheumatol.* 7:37–49.

164. Huong DL, Wechsler B, Vauthier-Brouzel D, et al. (2001). Pregnancy in past or present lupus nephritis: a study of 32 pregnancies from a singer center. *Ann Rheum Dis.* 60 (6):599–604.

165. Lockshin MD. (1996). Pathogenesis of the antiphospholipid antibody syndrome. *Lupus.* 5:404–408.

166. Asherson RA, Cervera R, Piette JC, et al. (1998). Catastrophic antiphospholipid syndrome clinical and laboratory features of 50 patients. *Medicine.* 77:195–207.

167. Galliard MC, Ouvre E, Liegeois A, et al. (1978). The concentration of fetal cells in maternal heamatopoetic organs during pregnancy, an experimental study in mice. *J Gynecol Obstet Biol Reprod.* 7:1043–1050.

168. Lo YM, Lo ES, Watson N, et al. (1996). Two-way cell traffic between mother and fetus, biologic and clinical implications. *Blood.* 88:4390–4395.

169. Liegeois A, Escourrou J, Ouvre EI, et al. (1997). Microchimerism: A stable state of low ratio proliferation of allogenic bone marrow. *Transplant Proc.* 9:273–276.

170. Bianchi DW, Zickwolf GK, Weil GJ, et al. (1996). Male fetal progenitor cells persist in maternal blood for as long as 27 years post partum. *Proc Natl Acad Sci U S A.* 93:705–708

171. Maloney S, Smith A, Furst DE, et al. (1999). Microchimerism of maternal origin persist into adult life. *J Clin Invest.* 104:41–47.

172. Nelson JL. (1996). Maternal fetal immunology and autoimmune disease, is some autoimmune disease auto-alloimmune or allo-autoimmune? *Arthritis Rheum.* 39:191–194.

173. Alpouri MA, Ruggier R, Epstein O, et al. (1990). Adoptive transfer of hyperthyroidism following allergenic bone marrow transplantation for chronic myeloid leukemia. *Br J Haematol.* 74:118–119.

174. Holland FJ, McConnon JK, Volpe R, et al. (1991). Concordant Graves disease after bone marrow transplantation—implications for pathogenesis. *J Clin Endocrinol Metab.* 72:837–840.

175. Sherer Y, Shoenfeld Y. (1998). Autoimmune disease and autoimmunity post bone marrow transplantation. *Bone Marrow Transplant.* 22:873–881.

176. van Gelder, van Bekkum DW. (1995). Treatment of relapsing experimental autoimmune encephalomyelitis in rats with allogenic bone marrow transplantation from a resistant strain. *Bone Marrow Transplant.* 16:343–351.

177. Nelson JL, Furst DE, Maloney S, et al. (1998). Microchimerism and HLA compatible relationships of pregnancy in SSc. *Lancet.* 351:559–562.

178. Arlett CM, Smith JB, Jimenez SB. (1998). Identification of fetal DNA and cells in shin lesions from women with systemic sclerosis. *N Engl J Med.* 338:1186–1191.

179. Nelson JL. (1998). Microchimerism and autoimmune disease. *N Engl J Med.* 338:1224–1225.

180. Klintschar M, Schwaiger P, Mannweiler S. (2001). Evidence of fetal microchimerism in Hashimoto's thyroiditis. *J Clin Endocrinol Metab.* 86:2494–2498.

181. Toda I, Kumana M, Tsubotak K (2001). Lack of evidence for an increased microchimerism in the circulation of patients with Sjögren's syndrome. *Ann Rheum Dis.* 60:248–253.

103

Gender-Specific Issues in Organ Transplantation

HILARY SANFEY, FACS, FRCSI

Associate Professor, Department of Surgery and Transplant Division, University of Virginia Health Systems, Charlottesville, VA

The relationship between sex hormones and immunologic processes is well documented. Women are known to have higher immunoglobulin levels than men, a higher incidence of immunologically based illnesses, and the ability to mount a more vigorous immune response to infections. Both cell-mediated immunity and natural killer cell activity are diminished during pregnancy, and menopausal women have an increased release of interleukin-1 by monocytes, which is reversible by hormone replacement therapy (HRT) [1]. Depending on dose, estrogens may act as immunosuppressors or immunostimulants. Estrogen administered before bone marrow transplantation has been shown to result in increased graft failure. The mixed lymphocyte reaction is enhanced by estradiol, and fluctuating lymphocyte responses are observed during normal menses [2], pregnancy, and the use of oral contraceptives [3]. As might be expected, pregnancy and the menstrual cycle affect the severity of autoimmune disease [1]. Androgens also affect immune function. Testosterone has been shown to suppress anti-DNA antibody production in peripheral blood mononuclear cells from patients with systemic lupus erythematosus (SLE) [4], and graft rejection in rodents is delayed by injection of testosterone. Progesterone is an immunosuppressive agent [5,6] and may be the basis for the gender gap in the disease SLE [7]. It is possible that genes related to autoimmunity may be hormonally regulated, although there is no direct evidence for this. Given these data it is hardly surprising to find that many gender-related differences exist in the arena of organ transplantation. These differences will be discussed as they relate to organ failure, and liver, kidney, and pancreas transplantation.

I. Organ Failure

A. Liver Failure

Liver failure may be acute, occurring *de novo* in a previously healthy patient or chronic in a patient with established cirrhosis. Certain forms of liver disease such as primary biliary cirrhosis and autoimmune hepatitis are seen almost exclusively in women [8]. Oral contraceptives have been associated with several hepatobiliary diseases [9], and there is some controversy regarding the risk of liver injury associated with estrogen replacement therapy. Androgen therapy has been implicated in the pathogenesis of focal nodular hyperplasia of the liver. Because women with liver disease may not have the hepatic capacity to metabolize endogenous or exogenous estrogens, impaired liver function is a contraindication to HRT [10]. Nonoral estrogens may be safer in these patients because they do not undergo a first-pass effect. Progestins are not mediated through a direct effect on hepatic clearance or excretion of metabolites [11] and may be used safely in patients with chronic hepatobiliary disease [12]. Selective estrogen receptor modulators such as tamoxifen are metabolized in the liver and have been associated with cholestatic jaundice and hepatotoxicity. Menstrual irregularities resulting in anovulation and infertility may be the first clinical indication of liver dysfunction in a woman [13] and may improve following successful liver transplantation. Liver failure may occur as a result of pregnancy or may be exacerbated by pregnancy occurring in a patient with known liver dysfunction.

1. Liver Failure in Pregnancy

A number of clinical syndromes, resulting in liver failure and arising in pregnancy in previously healthy women, have been described. Acute fatty liver of pregnancy (AFLP) is characterized by mitochondrial dysfunction [14] and complicates between 1 in 7000 [15] and 1 in 13,000 pregnancies [16]. It is possible that hormonal changes augment the effects of an otherwise tolerable insult to the mitochondria [17]. AFLP occurs more frequently in primiparous women but can occur after several nonaffected pregnancies [18,19]. The only treatment is immediate delivery. After delivery, most patients improve slowly, but a full clinical and laboratory recovery may take from 1 to 4 weeks. Four cases of recurrent AFLP have been reported [20–22]. Intrahepatic cholestasis is characterized by disturbed enterohepatic circulation with a decreased hepatocyte capacity to transport bile acids possibly because of an inherited hypersensitivity to estrogen at the gene level [23]. Patients with increased estrogen levels or with a history of cholestatic hepatitis induced by oral contraceptive pills have an increased incidence. Treatment is directed at relieving the symptoms. The HELLP syndrome (hemolysis, elevated liver enzymes, and low platelets) complicates 0.1% of pregnancies and is observed in up to 10% of patients with preeclampsia [8,24]. This syndrome usually peaks 24 hours after delivery, followed by clinical improvement, with laboratory levels gradually returning to normal within 3–11 days. The lower the gestational age at onset of symptoms the higher the risk of eclampsia [25]. Women with nadir platelet counts <50,000 cells/μL have an increased risk for adverse maternal outcomes. Once a clinical diagnosis has been made, aggressive intervention and expeditious delivery is indicated. Budd-Chiari syndrome may present in either the pregnant or the postpartum patient [26]. Inherited thrombophilic states, particularly in women who use birth control pills, predispose pregnant patients to thrombotic events [27]. In addition, pregnancy is regarded as a hypercoagulable state [28]. Among women previously treated for Budd-Chiari syndrome, successful pregnancy and delivery is possible [29,30].

2. Pregnancy in Liver Failure

Pregnancy is associated with changes in maternal physiology that may adversely affect portal hypertension and increase the risks of variceal hemorrhage [24]. However, pregnancy is uncommon in patients with cirrhosis because of decreased fertility associated with advanced liver disease. The spontaneous abortion rate in patients with cirrhosis is about 15–20% [24]. Postpartum hemorrhage occurs in women with portal hypertension who become pregnant in 7–10% of cases and is more common in those with cirrhosis [31]. Pregnancy may induce a hypercoagulable state and cause portal hypertension in patients with or without cirrhosis, leading to portal vein thrombosis [32]. Hepatitis A infection is no more severe in pregnant women than in non-pregnant individuals [33]. Chronic hepatitis B (HBV) carriers usually have normal pregnancies unless there is also severe chronic hepatitis or secondary cirrhosis and associated complications [34]. The significance of HBV infection derives from its potential to be transmitted vertically. Of infants born to women with acute HBV infection during the first trimester of pregnancy, 10% are positive for hepatitis B surface antigen (HBsAg) at birth [35], and 80–90% become HBsAg-positive without prophylactic therapy if acute maternal infection develops during the third trimester of pregnancy [36]. Hepatitis B immunization has been shown to be feasible and effective in postpartum women [37]. Transmission of HCV is horizontal through parenteral exposure to blood and blood products and, rarely, vertical unless maternal viral titers are unusually high. There is no evidence that pregnancy alters the natural history of hepatitis C (HCV) or that HCV interferes with normal pregnancy, unless the patient has cirrhosis.

B. Kidney Failure

There are a number of gender-specific considerations unique to patients with end-stage renal disease. The rate of progression of many renal diseases is faster in men than women [38–41], and men show a standardized mortality rate twice that of women [42,43]. Sex hormones may cause this gender difference [44] by an effect on mesangial proliferation and extracellular matrix formation through the release of cytokines, vasoactive agents, and growth factors. Estrogens show potent antioxidant activity, unlike testosterone. Two prospective studies suggest that the protection afforded by female gender is only evident in premenopausal women [41,45]. Other investigators have shown that manipulation of the hormonal environment influences the progression of experimental models of chronic renal disease [46]. Gender plays a major role in the expression of SLE: most patients are female, SLE is exacerbated by estrogens and oral contraceptives [47,48], and activity may worsen during the menstrual cycle [49] and pregnancy. Male and female patients with SLE have normal levels of estrogen; however, the overall metabolism of such compounds is altered to favor more feminizing compounds [50]. Studies of androgen metabolism in women with active SLE demonstrate decreased plasma levels of androgen [51,52]. Early data [53] suggest that there are significant health benefits from the use of HRT in postmenopausal patients, but premenopausal use of estrogens in SLE should be avoided because hormone supplements induce a flare of disease in this group.

Kausz et al [54] noted that women and non-white people demonstrated significantly higher odds for late initiation of dialysis compared with men and white people. In addition, women are less likely to receive a renal transplant but are more likely to donate a kidney [55,56]. They postulated that this discrepancy may be the result of a lack of physician awareness of possible gender and race effects on the presentation and management of illnesses, inaccurate assessment of renal function leading to overestimation of residual renal function, inadequate recognition of and efforts to overcome cultural barriers to medical care, and lack of financial resources to pay for medical care. Whites and women have an increased rate of hospitalization [54]. Blacks and women have lower hematocrits than whites and men, and black people and men have poorer blood pressure control than white people and women. Blacks and women are less likely to have fistulas compared with whites and men [57]. A possible explanation for the gender difference in fistula placement is the technical difficulty in creating fistulas in women, who tend to be smaller than men and therefore have smaller blood vessels. This may be of significance since Sehgal noted that use of a catheter for vascular access is one of the more important barriers to adequate delivery of hemodialysis [57]. Thus, interventions that expedite placement of fistulas may lead to improved adequacy of dialysis. In a national sample males were about 10% more likely than women to be noncompliant with therapy [57]. As in the general population, male patients undergoing dialysis have a slightly higher mortality rate compared with female patients [58]. This gender difference is attributable to a higher risk of death among men from cardiac causes and malignancy [59]. Eliminating racial and gender differences requires that we become aware of such differences, determine barriers to optimal outcomes, and develop interventions to overcome these barriers.

1. Pregnancy and Renal Disease

Fertility is significantly reduced in women with renal failure. Only 10–42% [60,61] of women dialysis patients of childbearing age menstruate. Prematurity is the greatest cause of morbidity and mortality in the infants of women with renal disease who manage to become pregnant. The National Register of Pregnancy in Dialysis recorded 222 pregnancies in women who were receiving dialysis at the time of conception. Only 55% of pregnancies that reached the second trimester resulted in surviving infants, and 18% of the liveborn infants died in the neonatal period. Three maternal deaths have been reported [62]. The timing of delivery is a matter of debate, but most physicians are reluctant to prolong the pregnancy beyond 38 weeks of gestation. Physicians should regard childbearing as one of the goals of treatment for renal disease in women of childbearing age, rather than as an accident to be dealt with when it occurs. The problems of hypertension, increased proteinuria, and infection can be anticipated and managed appropriately. Transplant recipients and women with renal insufficiency face the possibility that pregnancy may adversely affect renal function. For the transplant recipient, pregnancy is further complicated by immunosuppression and the risk for opportunistic infection. There have been reports suggesting that disease progresses less rapidly in women with similar degrees of renal dysfunction who do not become pregnant [62]. In diabetic nephropathy, as in other renal diseases, the level of renal function at the time of conception is the most important determinant of the effect of pregnancy on the progression of the disease. There are a number of reasons to anticipate that pregnancy might have an adverse effect on the progression of renal disease. Normal pregnancy is accompanied by an increased glomerular filtration rate, but the increase is brought about by increased renal blood flow, not by increased intraglomerular pressure [62]. In addition pregnancy is frequently accompanied by hypertension, proteinuria, and urinary tract infections [63]. Women who start dialysis for progressive renal insufficiency usually require continued dialysis postpartum.

2. Sexual Function

Disturbances in sexual function are a common feature of chronic renal failure [64]. Approximately 50% of men with uremia complain of erectile dysfunction, and an even greater percentage of both men and women complain of decreased libido and a marked decline in the frequency of intercourse [65,66]. The causes are multifactorial and include uremia, peripheral neuropathy, autonomic insufficiency, and peripheral vascular disease. Psychologic and physical stresses also contribute. In men with chronic renal failure, disturbances in the pituitary–gonadal axis can be detected as the renal failure progresses [64,67]. These disorders rarely normalize with initiation of hemodialysis or peritoneal dialysis but may improve in patients with a well-functioning kidney transplant. Chronic renal failure is associated with impaired spermatogenesis and testicular damage, often leading to infertility [68]. Elevated plasma prolactin levels are commonly found in men who have undergone dialysis [69] and may be related in part to the development of secondary hyperparathyroidism. Extreme hyperprolactinemia is associated with infertility, loss of libido, low circulating testosterone levels, and inappropriately low luteinizing hormone (LH) levels in men with normal renal function. Controlling the degree of secondary hyperparathyroidism may be of benefit in lowering prolactin levels and improving sexual function in some patients [64].

Disturbances in menstruation and fertility are commonly encountered in women with chronic renal failure. The menstrual cycle typically remains irregular after the initiation of dialysis [70]. Many women with uremic are anovulatory, resulting in infertility [71]. Women receiving chronic dialysis also tend to complain of decreased libido and reduced ability to reach orgasm [66,72]. Women with chronic renal failure commonly have elevated circulating prolactin levels, and, as is the case in men, these elevated prolactin levels may impair hypothalamic–pituitary function and contribute to sexual dysfunction. The age at which menopause begins in chronic renal failure tends to be decreased when compared to healthy women [64].

C. Diabetes Mellitus

Type 1 diabetes mellitus is a disease in which beta cells within the islets of Langerhans are destroyed by an autoimmune process resulting from genetic and unknown environmental factors. The annual incidence is approximately 55 new cases per million of the population. Diabetes is the leading cause of blindness and renal failure in the United States. People with diabetes are four to seven times more likely to require an amputation and twice as likely to die of heart disease than the general population [73]. As with other medical conditions, gender-based differences have been noted in diabetes. Olivarius [74] found a relationship between body height and renal involvement in newly diagnosed patients with type 2 diabetes and noted that urinary albumin concentration increased with decreasing height for women but not men. An association between diabetes mellitus and central obesity with short stature is more common in women [75,76]. In experimental models, females are more prone to develop diabetes than males [77,78]. There are several indications that the islet itself can respond to sex hormones because androgens lower insulin sensitivity, whereas estrogens increase it [79,80]. Sex steroids also have recognized effects on leukocyte function, induce prediabetic islet abnormalities, and are known to modulate cytokine production by leukocytes, in particular by mononuclear phagocytes [81]. Bilbao noted that autoantibodies against insulin occur more frequently in female patients with diabetes and speculated that these differences could reflect the severity and specificity of the autoimmune attack against the endocrine pancreas and influence the rate of progression to type 1 diabetes [82]. Davis *et al* reasoned that a differential gender response to antecedent hypoglycemia may explain why women with type 1 diabetes do not suffer a greater prevalence of hypoglycemia despite inherently reduced counterregulatory responses [83]. Gender inequity in people with diabetes was explored in one study from Sweden. In this study Jonsson demonstrated that women with diabetes in Sweden report more frequent outpatient contacts, less patient satisfaction, and a lower health-related quality of life than men with diabetes. No gender differences were found in glucose control [84].

1. Pregnancy and Diabetes

Diabetes occurs during 3% of all pregnancies. Risk factors include obesity, age older than 35 years, family history of type 2 diabetes, and prior delivery of a large (>9 lb) infant. White's classification stratifies diabetes during pregnancy based on duration of diabetes, therapy, and the presence of retinopathy, nephropathy, or heart disease [85]. Those women in class D with secondary complications of diabetes have the greatest potential for complications during pregnancy. Organogenesis occurs early in the first trimester; therefore tight blood glucose control during this interval decreases congenital malformations and miscarriages. Oral hypoglycemic agents should be switched to insulin as soon as possible because these drugs cross the placenta and can cause prolonged fetal hyperinsulinemia. Most women with uncomplicated type I diabetes do well during pregnancy, although maternal risks and perinatal mortality are increased slightly. Risk factors for maternal morbidity and relative contraindications to pregnancy include established renal disease (creatinine >2.0 mg/dL or proteinuria >2 g/day), uncontrolled hypertension, and atherosclerotic vascular disease. Diabetic retinopathy progresses in 10–50% of cases; therefore patients should be examined by an ophthalmologist each trimester. Women with gestational diabetes usually normalize their blood glucose immediately postpartum, about two thirds will have gestational diabetes in subsequent pregnancies, and up to 50% will develop diabetes over the next 15 years [85].

II. Organ Donation

Boulware [86] performed a cross-sectional telephone survey of Maryland households to assess race and gender differences in willingness to donate blood and cadaveric organs and noted that before adjustment, black females were least willing to donate blood (41%) and black males were least willing to become cadaveric donors (19%). Adjustment for respondent concerns about mistrust of hospitals and discrimination in hospitals explained most differences in willingness to donate blood, whereas adjustment for respondents' beliefs regarding the importance of spirituality and religion explained most differences in willingness to donate cadaveric organs. Clearly donor recruitment efforts should focus on race-gender groups with the lowest levels of willingness. In 1972, Simmons and Fulton [87] compared individuals who had signed an organ donor card with neighbors who had not signed the card and identified being a young woman as one of the major determinants for willingness to be considered as a potential cadaveric donor.

It is generally agreed that living donor transplantation represents the single best form of therapy for end-stage renal disease [88,89]. Although the ethics of living donor transplantation have been debated, the gap between the supply of cadaveric donors and the demand for organs has encouraged an increasing use of living donors. Studies from the larger transplant registries and single-center experiences showed that in most subgroups, women predominated among living donors [90–94]. Bloembergen et al [91] reviewed the U.S. Renal Data System database from 1991 to 1993 and found women were 28% more likely to donate a kidney. Zimmerman et al [95] noted that 59% of the 198 living donor transplants in their institution were from women. The largest contributing factor to the overall excess of female donors is the overwhelming predominance of women among spousal donors. The United Network for Organ Sharing database [94] reported that 73% of the 360 spousal donations were wife to husband. Although immunologic issues are a real consideration in husband-to-wife allografts in cases in which a woman has borne her husband's child, such concerns did not explain the underrepresentation of husbands. All spousal donations occurred as a result of the donor volunteering. This observation would seem to contradict the hypothesis of some investigators [96,97] that women's greater tendency toward risk aversion accounts in part for their lower rate of access to such invasive procedures as angiography, cardiac bypass, and renal transplantation [95]. What is unclear from this study is why husbands do not appear to come forward under similar circumstances. In an early study [98] it was found that compared with men, women were more likely to perceive donation as an extension of their obligation to their family. Nearly equal proportions of male and female potential donors were excluded because of medical illness or ABO incompatibility.

III. Transplantation

A. Liver

The first human liver transplant was performed in Colorado in 1963. Since then the concept of liver transplantation has changed from a procedure once regarded as experimental in patients with no hope of surviving to a widely accepted therapy for people with end-stage liver disease. The number of transplants performed annually has increased to a point where demand for donor organs outstrips supply. This has resulted in considerable discussion in the transplant community about expanding the donor pool to include marginal donors and more recently the use of right or left lobes from living donors. A number of studies have correlated donor-recipient factors to identify risk factors that might lead to optimum organ utilization. Marino et al [99] found that graft failure was significantly associated with donor age greater than 45 years, donor gender, previous liver transplantation, and United Network for Organ Sharing (UNOS) status of the recipient. Livers from female donors yielded significantly poorer results, with 2-year graft survival of female to male being 55%; female to female, 64%; male to male, 72%; and male to female, 78%. Candinas et al [100] noted transplantation of a liver from a male donor into a female recipient was associated with an increased probability of chronic rejection. Sensitization to antigens expressed by bile-duct epithelium as in primary biliary cirrhosis or exposure to donor bile-duct minor histocompatibility antigens, such as the male sex-related H-Y antigen, may provide an explanation [100]. Francavilla [101] noted that donor and recipient gender also affect graft and patient survival after pediatric liver transplantation. There is possibly an increased incidence of lymphoproliferative disease in the gender-mismatched group [102]. It has been suggested that this difference in outcome may be hormone related [103]. Human liver displays gender-related differences, such as increased hepatic content of microsomal oxidative enzymes in males and different numbers of estrogen and androgen receptors on hepatocytes in males and females [104,105]. In a rat model, following partial hepatectomy serum estrogen levels and the number of estrogen hepatic receptors increase concomitantly with liver regeneration, and in a murine experiment, Kahn et al [106] demonstrated a reduction in the number of estrogen receptors in the livers of gender-mismatched recipients (male to female and female to male) 10 days after transplantation. Thus, it is possible that the worse outcome of the female to male gender combination in humans is the result of a reduced number of estrogen receptors in the male recipients of a female organ [103]. These data will not have an immediate effect on organ allocation because of the relative shortage of suitable grafts.

B. Kidney

Kidney transplantation remains the treatment of choice for most people with end-stage renal disease. Studies suggest that patients who undergo transplantation enjoy a more prolonged life and an improved quality of life in comparison with individuals who choose dialysis [107–109]. Although living-related and living-unrelated kidney transplant rates have increased steadily over the past several years, cadaveric transplantation rates have declined sharply as a result of increased organ demand and decreased supply. A gender effect similar to that seen in liver transplantation has also been observed in kidney transplantation. Neugarten et al [43] showed a particularly poor prognostic trend for kidneys from older female donors. It was suggested that gender-related kidney size and nephron count discordance were responsible for the different outcome. Kouli [110] retrospectively analyzed donor-recipient factors independent of rejection after kidney transplantation and noted that Cr clearance was 14.1 mL/min less in female recipients than in male recipients with female-to-female transplants having the lowest subsequent Cr clearance values.

C. Pancreas

The goals of pancreas transplantation are to provide physiologic insulin replacement and prevent secondary complications of diabetes [111]. Male patients with diabetes are more likely to be afflicted by end-stage renal disease than female patients with diabetes, and this is reflected in the number of men who require kidney pancreas transplantation [111]. However, this fact does not explain why female patients represent such a high proportion of pancreas transplant alone (PTA) recipients because the incidence of type 1 diabetes is equal in male and female patients [112]. It appears that female patients with diabetes who do not have uremia are more likely to seek pancreas transplantation as an alternative to treatment with exogenous insulin. Although it takes at least 5 years of normoglycemia, a pancreas transplant can reverse the lesions of diabetic nephropathy [111]. Such reversal does not guarantee normal function because independent damage to the kidney may occur from the calcineurin inhibitors needed to prevent graft rejection. Other groups have also shown that a successful pancreas transplant can ameliorate microvascular complications, including retinopathy, nephropathy, and neuropathy [111,113]. Recent successes with islet transplantation [114] suggest that the dream of eliminating the major surgery of pancreas transplantation may soon be achieved.

IV. Outcome: Post-Transplantation

A. Graft Function

The therapeutic effect and efficacy of many immunosuppressive drugs can be regulated by their rate of metabolism and elimination. Glucuronidation is an important metabolic process by which drugs are converted to a more readily excreted hydrophilic compound [115]. Gender-dependent differences in rates of glucuronidation are known to exist [116]. It is believed that mycophenolic acid (MPA) could compete for the same binding sites as estrogens and could explain the lower glucuronidation rate in females. Cotreatment with tacrolimus was also shown to affect MPA glucuronidation. Therefore gender differences and cotreatment with tacrolimus must be taken into consideration when the immunosuppressive drug mycophenolate mofetil (MMF) is being administered. Gasbarrini et al [117] demonstrated that isolated livers from female rats undergo greater oxidative injury during postischemia reperfusion than livers isolated from male animals. Other investigators have demonstrated that women are more sensitive to different kinds of liver injury, such as alcoholic liver disease [118] and that sex-specific liver diseases exist [119]. It has been demonstrated that in the basal condition, modulation of several enzyme activities is related to the influence of estrogens [120]. In particular, it has been shown by Ikejima et al [121] that the increased susceptibility of females to alcohol is related to estrogen activity that increases expression of CD14 in Kupffer cells, leading to increased production of toxic mediators, thus exacerbating liver injury [121]. Similarly, sex mismatch of donor and recipient after orthotopic liver transplantation (OLT) appears to be a main risk factor for chronic irreversible rejection [100,101]. One possible explanation is that the increased incidence of chronic rejection in women receiving a male liver is related to an immune attack against the Y chromosome antigen [100]. However, the association between HLA matching and the incidence of chronic rejection suggests that mechanisms other than the H-Y minor histocompatibility antigen may be involved [99]. It can be hypothesized that a greater sensitivity to ischemia-reperfusion injury may play an important role. It is still not clear why females are more sensitive than males to oxidative stress, but because gender markedly affects the extent of postischemic reperfusion injury in isolated rat liver it is possible that this may account for the poor outcome of female organs after liver transplantation [117].

Female renal transplant recipients have an increased relative risk for acute rejection compared with male renal transplant recipients [43,122]. In contrast women have a decreased relative risk for the development of chronic allograft failure. This decreased risk for chronic allograft failure is age dependent, with the younger patients demonstrating little difference between men and women. In contradistinction, patients older than 45 years of age demonstrate a marked difference in the risk for chronic allograft failure between men and women. Meier-Kriesche et al [122] noted that the increased risk of acute rejection in female renal transplant recipients is equal to their overall decreased risk for chronic allograft failure (10% for each), and this may help explain why it has been difficult to document any difference in outcome between women and men [123–127]. The relative protective status of female gender from chronic allograft failure may in large part explain the paradox of increased rejection yet equivalent long-term death censored graft survival seen in women. In men increasing age linearly increases the risk of developing chronic allograft failure, whereas in women only the oldest age group (age >65) shows evidence of an increased risk of developing chronic allograft failure [122]. It is possible that estrogen is in part responsible for the protective effect against chronic allograft failure that is seen in women. The increased risk of acute rejection seen in women may relate in some way to a general increase in immunoreactivity [128]. It is also possible that the increased risk of sensitizing events in women (i.e., pregnancy) may also predispose to a higher risk of acute rejection. The protective effect against chronic allograft failure noted for women is likely related to differences in estradiol and testosterone levels between the sexes, and this is supported by experimental studies [129–131]. The Meier-Kriesche study also demonstrated that MMF decreases the risk of developing chronic allograft failure to a significantly greater extent in women than in men. Therefore female renal transplant recipients compared with male transplant recipients have an increased risk of acute rejection and a decreased relative risk for the development of chronic allograft failure, particularly after the age of 45 years. The etiology of these differences is unclear but likely reflects hormonal, immunologic, and aging differences between the sexes [122].

B. Osteoporosis

Patients with cirrhosis are predisposed to develop osteopenia because of poor nutrition, alcohol consumption, prolonged bed rest, reduced muscle mass, hormonal imbalances, and reduced levels of vitamin D, all of which contribute to metabolic bone disease [132]. Chronic cholestasis results in decreased concentrations of bile acids in the intestine and subsequent malabsorption of vitamin D and calcium. After the initial posttransplant bone loss, bone density eventually stabilizes and subsequently improves to pretransplant values. Immunosuppressive therapy is strongly implicated in the rapid postoperative loss of bone mass after OLT. Even doses as low as 7.5 mg/day of prednisone may induce trabecular bone loss. Cyclosporine and tacrolimus can produce a high turnover osteopenia and accelerated bone resorption [132]; therefore transplant recipients are at increased risk for the development of fractures [133,134]. Estrogens are useful to prevent bone loss in normal postmenopausal patients, but, as with calcium supplementation, no controlled trials have been performed in OLT recipients. Most physicians are reluctant to prescribe estrogen because of concerns regarding hepatic toxicity.

Most patients undergoing renal transplantation have some evidence of renal osteodystrophy prior to surgery. Silkensen [135] demonstrated that female gender was associated with an elevated risk of fracture in a group of renal transplant recipients. Some investigators have demonstrated a decreased rate of vertebral fractures with calcitriol, although this drug should be used cautiously in patients with persistent hyperparathyroidism and a risk of hypercalcemia. In addition to the risk factors associated with renal transplantation, those undergoing kidney pancreas transplantation appear to be at even greater risk of fracture. Fractures occur in approximately 50% of recipients within the first 5 years after transplantation [136]. Factors that may be associated with increased osteopenia in diabetics include chronic hypocalcemia, insulin deficiency, relative hypoparathyroidism, decreased physical activity, impaired gonadal function, and metabolic acidosis. Sex steroid secretion is important in regard to outcome after transplantation. Shane [137] and others [133–136] have cited the contributing role of untreated hypogonadism to loss of bone density and increased fracture risk after solid organ transplantation. In one study 50% of patients had hypogonadism prepancreas transplant and 70% had hormone abnormalities posttransplant. In this small series reproductive hormone abnormalities were common in women but uncommon in men before and after pancreas transplantation [138]. The presence of longstanding untreated hypogonadism may have implications for bone loss and cardiovascular risk after pancreas transplantation, particularly in women. With correction of the metabolic abnormalities, normalization of gonadal function should then be expected. Prednisone use after transplantation can aggravate insulin resistance and increase adrenal and ovarian androgen production with aromatization to estrogen, as seen in the polycystic ovarian syndrome.

C. Pregnancy after Transplantation

Pregnancy has occurred less frequently in liver transplant recipients than renal transplant recipients. Scantlebury *et al*

[139] reported 20 pregnancies in 17 liver transplant recipients in whom the rate of hepatic allograft dysfunction was 37% during pregnancy and 53% in the postpartum period. Findings in another group of 37 liver transplant recipients included drug-treated hypertension (46%), eclampsia/preeclampsia (21%), allograft rejection (17%), and graft loss (5.7%) [140]. There was a high rate of prematurity and low birth weight among these infants. More recent data from the University of Pittsburgh have suggested that when managed by an experienced team of physicians, pregnancy after transplantation has a good outcome [141]. Breast-feeding does perpetuate exposure of the newborn to drugs with nephrotoxic and immunosuppressive side effects [142]. In addition maternal immunosuppression may increase the risk of infections with cytomegalovirus. Renal dysfunction is the primary cause of adverse pregnancy outcomes in liver transplant recipients [142].

Fertility is usually restored in women with successful renal transplants, and pregnancy is not unusual [62]. A report from the European Dialysis and Transplant Association that included 53 women who became pregnant found renal function unchanged in 67% and worse in 9% [143]. The evidence suggests that graft function is generally not adversely affected by pregnancy in women with serum creatinine levels less than 1.5 mg/dL. Acute rejection and graft loss have been reported in patients with preexisting graft dysfunction or unstable graft function [144]. Calcineurin inhibitor levels should be closely monitored during pregnancy, particularly in the third trimester, when fetal metabolism of cyclosporine or tacrolimus may account for increased overall clearance. Adrenal insufficiency is unlikely in the infants of transplant recipients if a woman's daily prednisone dose has been decreased to 15 mg [144,145]. Use of corticosteroids during pregnancy has been associated with fetal growth restriction [142]. Azathioprine crosses the placenta readily, but to be active, it must be converted to 6-mercaptopurine. The immature fetal liver lacks the enzyme inosinate pyrophosphorylase, which is needed for conversion. In high doses (6 mg/kg), azathioprine is teratogenic in animals, but it has been used in thousands of pregnant women with the suggestion of teratogenicity in only one small study [62,142,146]. Cyclosporine has not been associated with congenital anomalies but is associated with a higher risk for small-for-gestational-age babies and hypertension. Cyclosporine increases production of thromboxane and endothelin, both of which have been implicated in the pathogenesis of preeclampsia. There is one case report of severe growth restriction associated with exposure to tacrolimus during pregnancy [147], and hyperkalemia was noted in some infants [140,141]. There is virtually no experience with MMF in pregnancy. It is embryo toxic in animals and should be avoided until more is known about its effects. Delivery of preterm babies is more frequent in transplant recipients than in the normal population, but intervention for obstetric reasons is a contributing factor [148]. Major congenital malformations occur in 3% of deliveries in the nontransplant population and in 4% of transplant recipients taking corticosteroids, 7% with azathioprine, and 3–5% with cyclosporine [149–152]. The National Transplantation Pregnancy Registry has reported 26 pregnancies for 20 female pancreas-kidney transplant (PKT) recipients and 21 pregnancies fathered by 17 male PKT recipients as of August 1998. It is unknown how many men and women sought pregnancy but were unsuccessful and why they were unsuccessful [138].

Women of childbearing age awaiting renal transplantation should receive the rubella vaccine because live virus vaccines are contraindicated posttransplantation [62]. Women who are blood type Rhesus negative and receive organs from Rhesus-positive donors should be made aware of this. The data suggest that the frequency of prematurity is greater when pregnancy is undertaken earlier than 2 years posttransplantation. Therefore, because the risks of rejection and infection also decrease 2 years posttransplant, it is advisable for women to wait 2 years before actively seeking conception. Renal function should be stable, blood pressure should be normal or easily controlled with medication, and 24-hour urine protein levels should be less than 500 mg [62].

D. Infections

Women transplant recipients are at increased risk for bacterial infections, predominantly urinary tract infections, during pregnancy [62]. Maternal infection can cause infection in the fetus in 20–40% of the pregnant women who have primary cytomegalovirus (CMV) infections [153]. The efficacy of treatment of the mother with either ganciclovir or CMV hyperimmune globulin in preventing disease in the fetus has not been established. Herpes simplex is usually spread from mother to child during birth, rather than through intrauterine infection [154]. Infection with toxoplasmosis during pregnancy results in neonatal infection in 25–65% of the infants [155]. Hepatitis B and C have already been discussed in Section IA(2). The effect of gender on outcome of infection in hospitalized patients is unclear. Crabtree *et al* [156] evaluated a total of 892 patients in the surgical units of their hospital with 1470 consecutive infectious episodes. Among all infections, there was no significant difference in mortality based on gender: 11.1% for men compared with 14.2% for women. Mortality was higher in women for lung and soft-tissue infection, but for other infectious sites, it did not differ by gender. These authors also noted that despite similar severity of illness and length of treatment and a slightly younger age, infected men were hospitalized longer following initiation of treatment. They concluded that although gender may not be predictive of mortality among all infections, women appear to be at increased risk for death from hospital-acquired pneumonia, even after controlling for other comorbidities.

E. Risk of Malignancy

1. Women

The risk of developing cervical carcinoma has been estimated to be 3 to 16 times higher for renal transplant recipients than for the general population; however, 70% of these patients have *in situ* lesions [157,158]. The incidence appears to be particularly increased among premenopausal patients with functioning grafts [159]. Most cervical neoplasms in transplant recipients respond well to conventional therapy when treated at an early stage [160,161]; therefore immunosuppressed women should undergo annual pelvic examinations. A recent report on more than 23,000 female renal transplant recipients noted a breast cancer incidence of 0.3% during the first year after transplantation.

This represented a relative risk of 0.49, compared with the general population [162]. It has been suggested that immunosuppression during a premalignant phase in breast neoplasia may reduce the incidence of subsequent development of breast cancer [163]; however, it is possible that the lower incidence of breast cancer may be a direct consequence of increased examinations and screening before renal transplantation [162]. Women with family histories of premenopausal breast cancer warrant aggressive screening, although there are few data to substantiate this. Several organizations have made detailed recommendations regarding screening for breast cancer [164–166]. Applying these guidelines to the screening of women after renal transplantation seems to be prudent, although there have been no studies evaluating the effects of breast cancer screening in this population [167].

2. Men

The incidences of prostate cancer among renal transplant recipients range from 0.3% to 1.9% [168–170]. In renal transplant recipients radiation therapy could be associated with nephritis and damage to the renal allograft [169]. The prostate-specific antigen test appears to be valid for the early detection of prostate cancer after renal transplantation [171]. There have been insufficient data to conclusively demonstrate decreases in the mortality rate for prostate cancer as a result of screening, however [172,173], but it seems prudent to screen immunosuppressed patients yearly starting at age 50 years for men whose life expectancy is 10 years or longer. It is also reasonable to initiate screening at an earlier age (such as age 40 years) for men with special risk factors, such as black race and family histories of prostate cancer [162].

V. General Considerations

A. Quality of Life

Depending on the specific instrument used to assess quality of life, different conclusions can be reached about blacks and women compared with whites and men. One large study of 700 patients found no difference between blacks and whites with 10 instruments, higher quality-of-life scores for blacks with two instruments, and lower scores for blacks with seven instruments. Women had the same score as men with 15 instruments, higher scores with two instruments, and lower scores with two instruments. Two more recent studies found higher quality-of-life scores among blacks. A few studies with modest sample sizes have examined employment among patients undergoing dialysis. In the most recent national study 59% of men were employed compared with 41% of women [174–179]. Because patients receiving dialysis can decide to discontinue treatment at any time, a willingness to continue such treatment may also be viewed as a measure of patient quality of life. Among females, 21% of deaths were associated with withdrawal compared with 18% among males. Greater life satisfaction was most strongly associated with being in control of one's health and living a normally active life with satisfying emotional relationships [180]. Previous work has highlighted the importance of normality, functional status, and social support networks in kidney transplant recipients and patients with end-stage renal disease

[180–184]. Comorbidities are common, but their effect on life satisfaction differed. The relative importance placed on these comorbid conditions by patients may be different from that assumed by the physician. For example, hypertension was of greater concern to physicians but blurred vision had a greater impact on patients' perception of their quality of life. Significant sexual deficits are common and do not always improve after transplantation [89]. The few studies examining female sexuality in the posttransplantation setting suggested that this issue is at least as prevalent as in men [185,186]. In one study by Hricik *et al* [180], headaches had almost as strong an effect on quality of life as sexual dysfunction and a stronger effect than that of the more common adverse effects of altered body habitus, swelling of extremities, changes in hair growth, tremors, and easy bruising. Health-related worry such as fear of rejection and stress related to body image alteration are important factors in transplant recipients [180,187,188]. The length of time spent receiving dialysis before transplantation may be relevant to a patient's perception of change in quality of life. In a study looking at four types of solid organ transplant recipients from one center, Pinson *et al* [189] showed that patients receiving different types of transplants start at different levels of health-related quality of life. Lung and heart recipients start out the worst, liver recipients in the middle, and kidney recipients the best, perhaps because of dialysis support. Renal transplant recipients improve the least and retain their preoperative stratification during the first 2 postoperative years. The more limited improvement recorded in kidney recipients compared with the others may be explained by the much higher incidence of diabetes with secondary complications in this patient population [189].

B. Access to Transplantation

A number of studies have evaluated factors affecting access to renal transplantation and have identified such characteristics as female gender and black race as barriers to receipt of a renal allograft [107]. National data clearly show that substantial differences exist between age, race, and sex with regard to wait listing and time from wait listing to cadaveric renal transplantation. Many of these differences in access to transplantation are independent of panel reactive antibody (PRA) and geographic region [190]. Female patients have previously been found to have a lower probability of receiving a renal transplant than males [108,191,192]. Wolfe *et al* [190] found a 16% lower rate of wait listing after the diagnosis of end-stage renal disease for females than for males. Women were about 10% less likely than men to be placed on a waiting list and 10% less likely to be transplanted following wait listing [192,193]. A barrier to wait listing may exist for females because of patient preference, gender selection by health care personnel, concerns about steroid-induced osteoporosis, gender bias on the part of family and friends, and economic or other reasons [97,194,195]. Elevated PRA among women may be responsible for much of the difference in transplantation rates between males and females because transplantation rates are not significantly different for males and females after adjusting for PRA levels. To better understand these differences, Wolfe examined the relative importance of steps related to medical suitability, interest in transplantation, completion of the pretransplant work-up and moving up the

waiting list, and noted that women were slightly less likely than men to complete each step [97,190]. Blacks and women are also less likely to receive living-related transplants compared with whites and men. The rate among women is 1.6 compared with 2.0 among men [190]. Women in the general population are about 30% more likely than men to donate kidneys for living-related transplantation. Yet, female patients with renal failure are less likely than men to receive such transplants [194]. The relative importance of patient vs provider factors in explaining this gender difference is unclear. It is interesting to note that despite several poorer intermediate outcomes, blacks and women do better than whites and men in survival. Garg *et al* also noted that women are less likely to be placed on the waiting list than men [196]. An earlier study reported that women with new-onset end-stage renal disease were approximately 30% less likely than men to receive a kidney transplant, even after accounting for comorbid medical conditions [197]. Because men and women are referred to nephrologists at similar stages of renal failure [198], reduced wait-listing rates for women cannot be explained by delays in presentation that preclude early discussion. In fact, a recent study of renal transplant waiting-list registrants demonstrated that although men outnumbered women by nearly 50%, the wait-listed women were slightly more likely than corresponding men to have been activated before initiating dialysis [199]. Additionally, provider concerns about patient outcomes after transplantation are not likely to be explanatory because studies have shown comparable patient and graft survival for men and women after transplantation [200]. Lower rates of wait listing also may result if women are less aggressive about negotiating the multiple steps necessary for activation on the waiting list [201,202]. Finally, the possibility of a gender bias by providers, as shown in the use of cardiovascular procedures, should be considered. Recent data suggest that patients with end-stage renal disease receiving Medicare who lack private supplementary insurance may face financial barriers that limit their access to the waiting list [203]. Nevertheless, despite the inclusion of insurance information, women were less likely than men to be wait listed in that study as well.

Although equity in access to the transplant waiting list is desirable, it will not reduce waiting times. The likelihood of transplantation is not principally affected by how quickly one progresses through the system but by the availability of donor organs and, to a lesser extent, the efficiency with which those organs are allocated.

VI. Conclusions

As might be predicted given the relationship between sex hormones and immunologic processes, many gender-related differences exist in the arena of organ failure and transplantation. Certain forms of liver and kidney disease are more common in either men or women and appear to be subject to hormonal fluctuation. The physiologic changes associated with pregnancy present unique challenges to the transplant physician. Transplant recipients and women with renal insufficiency face the possibility that pregnancy may adversely affect renal function. For the transplant recipient, pregnancy is further complicated by immunosuppression and the risk for opportunistic infection. Donor and recipient gender affect graft and patient survival after transplantation and may contribute to an increased incidence of lymphoproliferative disease in the gender-mismatched group. In addition there is clearly some gender bias in organ donation and transplantation.

VII. Suggestions for Further Investigations

- Why are women more susceptible to acute rejection and less prone to chronic rejection?
- Why is liver graft survival inferior in males who receive female organs?
- Why are women less likely to receive a kidney transplant but more likely to donate an organ?

References

1. Legato MJ. (1997). Immunology. In: *Gender Specific Aspects of Human Biology for the Practising Physician*. Armonk, NY: Futura Publishing Company.
2. Lahita RG. (2000). Sex hormones and systemic lupus erythematosus. *Rheum Dis Clin North Am*. 26(4):951–968.
3. Sthoeger ZM, Chiorazzi N, Lahita RG. (1988). Regulation of the immune response by sex hormones. I. *In vivo* effects of estradiol and testosterone on pokeweed mitogen-induced B-cell differentiation. *J Immunol*. 141:91–98.
4. Kanda N, Tsuchida T, Tamaki K. (1997). Testosterone suppresses anti-DNA antibody production in peripheral blood mononuclear cells from patients with systemic lupus erythematosus. *Arthritis Rheum*. 40:1703–1711.
5. Jo T, Terada N, Saji F, et al. (1993). Inhibitory effects of estrogen, progesterone, androgen and glucocorticoid on death of neonatal mouse uterine epithelial cells induced to proliferate by estrogen. *J Steroid Biochem Mol Biol*. 46:25–32.
6. Van VR, McGuire JL. (1994). Estrogen, progesterone, and testosterone: Can they be used to treat autoimmune diseases? *Cleve Clin J Med*. 61:276–284.
7. Whiteacre C, Reingold SC, O'Looney PA, et al. (1999). A gender gap in autoimmunity. *Science*. 283:1277–1278.
8. George ED, Schluger LK. (2000). Special women's health issues in hepatobiliary diseases. *Clin Fam Prac*. 2(1):155–169.
9. Dourakis SP, Tolis G. (1998). Sex hormonal preparations and the liver. *Eur J Contracept Reprod Health Care*. 3:7–16.
10. American College of Obstetricians and Gynecologists. (1992). Technical Bulletin. *Hormone Replacement Therapy*. 166:1–8.
11. Tierney S, Nakeeb A, Wong O, et al. (1999). Progesterone alters biliary flow dynamics. *Ann Surg*. 229:205–209.
12. Connolly TJ, Zuckerman AL. (1998). Contraception in the patient with liver disease. *Semin Perinatol*. 22:178–182.
13. Brenner PF. (1996). Differential diagnosis of abnormal uterine bleeding. *Am J Obstet Gynecol*. 175:766–769.
14. Bacq Y, Zarka O, Brechot JF, et al. (1996). Liver function tests in normal pregnancy: A prospective study of 103 pregnant women and 103 matched controls. *Hepatology*. 23:1030–1034.
15. Castro MA, Fassett MJ, Reynolds TB, et al. (1999). Reversible peripartum liver failure: a new prospective on the diagnosis, treatment and cause of acute liver failure of pregnancy based on 28 consecutive cases. *Am J Obstet Gynecol*. 181:389–395.
16. Reyes Humberto. (1999). Acute Fatty Liver of Pregnancy. A cryptic disease threatening mother and child. *Clin Liver Dis*. 3(1):69–81.
17. Fromenty B, Pessayre D. (1995). Inhibition of mitochondrial beta-oxidation as a mechanism of hepatotoxicity. *Pharmacol Ther*. 67(1):101–154.
18. Burroughs AK, Seong NGH, Dojcinov DM, et al. (1982) Idiopathic acute fatty liver of pregnancy in 12 patients. *Quart J Med*. 204:481–497.
19. Reyes H, Sandoval L, Wainstein A, et al. (1994). Acute fatty liver of pregnancy: A clinical study of 12 episodes in 11 patients. *Gut*. 35:101.
20. Barton CH, Mirahmadi MK, Vaziri ND. (1982) Effects of long-term testosterone administration on pituitary-testicular axis in end-stage renal failure. *Nephron*. 31:61–64.
21. MacLean MA, Cameron AD, Cumming GP, et al. (1994). Recurrence of acute fatty liver of pregnancy. *Br J Obstet Gynaecol*. 101:453–454.
22. Visconti M, Manes G, Giannattasio F, et al. (1995). Recurrence of acute fatty liver of pregnancy. *J Clin Gastroenterol*. 21:243–245.
23. Davidson KM. (1998). Intrahepatic cholestasis of pregnancy. *Semin Perinatol*. 22:104–111.
24. Misra S, Sanyal AJ. (1999). Pregnancy in a patient with portal hypertension. *Clin Liver Dis*. 3(1):147–162.
25. Haddad B, Barton JR, Livingston JC, et al. (2000). Risk factors for adverse maternal outcomes among women with HELLP (hemolysis, elevated liver enzymes, and low platelet count) syndrome. *Am J Obstet Gynecol*. 183(2) 444–448.
26. Gordon Stuart C. (1999). Pregnancy and liver disease. Budd-Chiari and infarct in pregnancy. *Clin Liver Dis*. 3:97–113.
27. De Stefano V, Leone G, Mastrangelo S. (1994). Thrombosis during pregnancy and surgery in patients with congenital deficiency of antithrombin III, protein C and protein S. *Thromb Haemost*. 71:799.
28. De Boer K. (1991). *Haemostasis in normal and complicated pregnancy* [thesis]. Rodopi, Amsterdam: University of Amsterdam. 31–42.
29. Vons C, Smadja C, Franco D, et al. (1984). Successful pregnancy after Budd-Chiari syndrome. *Lancet*. 2:975.
30. Walcott WO, Derick DE, Jolley JJ, et al. (1978). Successful pregnancy in a liver transplant patient. *Am J Obstet Gynecol*. 132:340.
31. Cheng YS. (1977). Pregnancy in liver cirrhosis and/or portal hypertension. *Am J Obstet Gynecol*. 128:812–822.
32. Goodrich MA, James EM, Baldus WP, et al. (1993). Portal vein thrombosis associated with pregnancy. *J Reprod Med*. 38:969–972.
33. Reinus JF, Leikin EL. (1999). Pregnancy and Liver Disease. Viral Hepatitis in Pregnancy. *Clin Liver Dis*. 3(1):115–130.
34. Schweitzer IL, Peters RL. (1976). Pregnancy in hepatitis B antigen positive cirrhosis. *Obstet Gynecol*. 48:535.
35. Sweet RL. (1990). Hepatitis B infection in pregnancy. *Obstet Gynecol*. Report 2:128.
36. Arevalo JA. (1989). Hepatitis B in pregnancy. *West J Med*. 150:668.
37. Jurema MW, Polaneczky M, Ledger WJ. (2001). Hepatitis B Immunization in postpartum women. *Am J Obstet Gynecol*. 185(2)355–358.
38. Ishikawa I, Maeda K, Nakai S, et al. (2000). Gender differences in the mean age at the induction of hemodialysis in patients with autosomal dominant polycystic kidney disease. *Am J Kidney Dis*. 35(6):1072–1075.
39. Hannedouche T, Chauveau P, Kalou E, et al. (1993). Factors affecting progression in advanced chronic renal failure. *Clin Nephrol*. 39:312–320.
40. Tierney WM, McDonald CJ, Luft FC. (1989). Renal disease in hypertensive adults: Effect of race and type II diabetes mellitus. *Am J Kidney Dis*. 13:485–493.
41. Coggins CH, Lewis JB, Caggiula AW, et al. (1998). Differences between women and men with chronic renal disease. *Nephrol Dial Transplant*. 13:1430–1437.
42. Schrander-VD, Meer AM, van Saase JLCM, et al. (1995). Mortality in patients receiving renal replacement therapy, a single-center study. *Clin Nephrol*. 43:174–179.
43. Neugarten J, Silbiger SR. (1994). The impact of gender on renal transplantation. *Transplantation*. 58:1145.
44. Kochakian CD. (1977). Regulation of kidney growth by androgens. *Adv Steroid Biochem Pharmacol*. 6:1–34.
45. Simon P, Ramee MP, Autuly V, et al. (1994). Epidemiology of primary glomerular diseases in a French region: Variations according to period and age. *Kidney Int*. 46:1192–1198.
46. Silbiger SR, Neugarten J. (1995). The impact of gender on the progression of chronic renal disease. *Am J Kidney Dis*. 25:515–533.
47. Chapel TA, Burns RE. (1971). Oral contraceptives and exacerbations of SLE. *Am J Obstet Gynecol*. 110:366–369.
48. Petri M, Robinson C. (1997). Oral contraceptives and systemic lupus erythematosus. *Arthritis Rheum*. 40:797–803.
49. Rose E, Pillsbury DM. (1944). Lupus erythematosus (erythematodes) and ovarian function: Observations on a possible relationship with a report of six cases. *Ann Intern Med*. 21:1022–1032.
50. Lahita RG. (1992). Sex steroids and SLE: Metabolism of androgens to estrogens [editorial]. *Lupus*. 1:125–127.
51. Jungers P, Nahoul K, Pelissier C. (1982). Low plasma androgens in women with active or quiescent SLE. *Arthritis Rheum*. 25:454–457.
52. Jungers P, Pelissier C, Bach JF, et al. (1980). Les androgenes plasmatiques chez les femmes atteintes de lupus erythemateux dissemine (LED). *Pathol Biol (Paris)*. 28:391–392.
53. Buyon JP. (1998). Hormone replacement therapy in postmenopausal women with systemic lupus erythematosus. *J Am Med Womens Assoc*. 53:13–17.
54. Kausz AT, Obrador GT, Arora P, et al. (2000). Late initiation of dialysis among women and ethnic minorities in the United States. *J Am Soc Nephrol*. 11(12):2351–2357.

55. Delano B, Macey L, Friedman E. (1997). Gender and racial disparity in peritoneal dialysis patients undergoing kidney transplantation. *ASAIO J.* 43:M861–M864.

56. Bloembergen WE, Young EW, Woods JD, et al. (1997). Factors associated with late referral among new dialysis patients in the US. *J Am Soc Nephrol.* 8:186A (abstr).

57. Sehgal AR. (2000). Outcomes of renal replacement therapy among blacks and women. *Am J Kidney Dis.* 35(4 suppl 1):S148–S152.

58. US Renal Data System. (2000). USRDS 2000 Annual Data Report. The National Institutes of Health, National Institutes of Diabetes and Digestive and Kidney Diseases, Bethesda, MD.

59. Bloembergen WE, Port FK, Mauger EA, et al. (1994). Causes of death in dialysis patients. Racial and gender differences. *J Am Soc Nephrol.* 5:1231–1242.

60. Holley JL, Schmidt RJ, Bender FH, et al. (1997). Gynecologic and reproductive issues in women on dialysis. *Am J Kidney Dis.* 29:685–690.

61. Perez RJ, Lipner H, Abdulla N, et al. (1978). Menstrual dysfunction of patients undergoing hemodialysis. *Obstet Gynecol.* 51:552–555.

62. Hou S. (1999). Pregnancy in chronic renal insufficiency and end stage renal disease. *Am J Kidney Dis,* 33(2):235–252.

63. Jones DC, Hayslett JP. (1996). Outcome of pregnancy in women with moderate or severe renal insufficiency. *N Engl J Med.* 335(4):226–232.

64. Palmer BF. (1999). Sexual dysfunction in uremia. *J Am Soc Nephrol.* 10(6):1381–1388.

65. Procci WR, Goldstein DA, Adelstein J, et al. (1981). Sexual dysfunction in the male patient with uremia: A reappraisal. *Kidney Int.* 19:317–323.

66. Toorians AW, Janssen E, Laan E, et al. (1987). Chronic renal failure and sexual functioning: Clinical status *versus* objectively assessed sexual response. *Nephrol Dial Transplant.* 12:2654–2663.

67. Handelsman DJ. (1985). Hypothalamic-pituitary gonadal dysfunction in renal failure, dialysis and renal transplantation. *Endocrinol Rev* 6:151–182.

68. Prem AR, Punekar SV, Kalpana M, et al. (1996). Male reproductive function in uraemia: Efficacy of haemodialysis and renal transplantation. *Br J Urol.* 78:635–638.

69. Gomez F, de la Cueva R, Wauters JP, et al. (1980). Endocrine abnormalities in patients undergoing long-term hemodialysis: The role of prolactin. *Am J Med.* 68:522–530.

70. Holley JL, Schmidt RJ, Bender FH, et al. (1987). Gynecologic and reproductive issues in women on dialysis. *Am J Kidney Dis.* 29:685–690.

71. Ginsburg ES, Owen WF Jr. (1993). Reproductive endocrinology and pregnancy in women on hemodialysis. *Semin Dial.* 6:105–116.

72. Steele TE, Wuerth D, Finkelstein S, et al. (1996). Sexual experience of the chronic peritoneal dialysis patient. *J Am Soc Nephrol.* 7:1165–1168.

73. Peters C, Sutherland DE, Simmons RL, et al. (1981). Patient and graft survival in amputated versus nonamputated diabetic primary renal allograft recipients. *Transplantation.* 32(6):498–503.

74. Olivarius ND. (2001). Renal involvement is related to body height in newly diagnosed diabetic women aged 40 years or over. *Diabetes Metab.* 27(1):14–18.

75. Pan WH. (2001). Undiagnosed diabetes mellitus in Taiwanese subjects with impaired fasting glycemia: impact of female sex, central obesity and short stature. *Chin J Physiol.* 44(1):44–51.

76. Wong GW. (2000). Sex differences in the growth of diabetic children. *Diabetes Res Clin Pract.* 50(2):187–193.

77. Rosmalen JG. (2001). Sex steroids influence pancreatic islet hypertrophy and subsequent autoimmune infiltration in nonobese diabetic (NOD) and NOD scid mice. *Lab Invest.* 81(2):231–239.

78. Fitzpatrick F, Lepault F, Homo-Delarche F, et al. (1991). Influence of castration, alone or combined with thymectomy, on the development of diabetes in the nonobese diabetic mouse. *Endocrinology.* 129:1382–1390.

79. Kava RA, West DB, Lukasik VA, et al. (1989). Sexual dimorphism of hyperglycemia and glucose tolerance in Wistar fatty rats. *Diabetes.* 38:159–163.

80. Leiter EH (1989). The genetics of diabetes susceptibility in mice. *FASEB J.* 3:2231–2241.

81. Homo-Delarche F, Durant S. (1994). Hormones, neurotransmitters and neuropeptides as modulators of lymphocyte functions. In: Rola-Pleszczynski M, ed. *Immunopharmacology of lymphocytes. Handbook of immunopharmacology.* London: Academic Press.

82. Bilbao JR, Rica I, Vazquez JA, et al. (2000). Influence of sex and age of onset on autoantibodies against insulin, GAD 65, and IA2 in recent onset type 1 diabetics. *Horm Res.* 54(4):181–185.

83. Davis SN, Shavers C, Costa F. (2000). Gender related differences in counterregulatory responses to antecedent hypoglycemia in normal humans. *J Clin Endocrinol Metab.* 85(6):2148–2157.

84. Jonsson PM. (2000). Gender equity in health care: the case of Swedish diabetes care. *Health Care Women Int.* 21(5):413–431.

85. Elliot D. (2000). Pregnancy: hypertension and other common medical problems. In: Goldman L. Cecil Textbook of Medicine, 21st ed. Philadelphia: W. B. Saunders Company. 1355–1357.

86. Boulware LE. (2002). Understanding disparities in donor behavior: race and gender differences in willingness to donate blood and cadaveric organs. *Med Care.* 40(2):85–95.

87. Simmons RG, Fulton R. (1972). The prospective organ transplant donor: Problems and perspectives of medical innovations. *Omega.* 3:319–339.

88. Russell JD, Barcroft ML, Ludwin D, et al. (1985). The quality of life in renal transplantation – a prospective study. *Transplantation.* 54:656–660.

89. Laupacis A, Keown P, Pus N, et al. (1996). A study of the quality of life and cost-utility of renal transplantation. *Kidney Int.* 50(1):235–237.

90. Binet I, Bock AH, Vogelbach P, et al. (1997). Outcome in emotionally related living kidney donor transplantation. *Nephrol Dial Transplant.* 12:1940–1948.

91. Bloembergen WE, Port FK, Mauger EA, et al. (1996). Gender discrepancies in living related renal transplant donors and recipients. *J Am Soc Nephrol.* 7:1139–1144.

92. Pirsh JD, D'Alessandro AM, Sollinger HW, et al. (1990). Living-unrelated renal transplantation at the University of Wisconsin. *Clin Transplant.* 241–245.

93. Sesso R, Klag MJ, Ancao MS, et al. (1992). Kidney transplantation from living unrelated donors. *Ann Intern Med.* 117:983–989.

94. Terasaki PI, Cecka JM, Gjertson DW, et al. (1995). High survival rates of kidney transplants from spousal and living unrelated donors. *N Engl J Med.* 333:333–336.

95. Zimmerman D, Donnelly S, Miller J, et al. (2000). Gender disparity in living renal transplant donation. *Am J Kidney Dis.* 36(3):534–540.

96. Karlson EW, Daltroy LH, Liang MK, et al. (1997). Gender differences in patient preferences may underlie differential utilization of elective surgery. *Am J Med.* 102:524–530.

97. Aaronson KD, Schwartz JS, Goin JE, et al. (1995). Sex differences in patient acceptance of cardiac transplant candidacy. *Circulation.* 91:2753–2761.

98. Simmons RG, Klein SD. (1977). Gift of life: The social and psychological impact of organ transplantation. New York: Wiley.

99. Marino IR, Doyle HR, Aldrighetti L, et al. (1995). Effect of donor age and sex on the outcome of liver transplantation. *Hepatology.* 22:1754–1762.

100. Candinas D, Gunson BK, Nightingale P, et al. (1985). Sex mismatch as a risk factor for chronic rejection of liver allografts. *Lancet.* 346:1117.

101. Francavilla R, Hadzic N, Heaton N, et al. (1998). Gender matching and outcome after pediatric liver transplantation. *Transplantation.* 66(5):602–605.

102. Brooks BK, Levy MF, Jennings LW, et al. (1996). Influence of donor and recipient gender on the outcome of liver transplantation. *Transplantation.* 62:1784.

103. Kahn D, Gavaler JS, Makowka L, et al. (1993). Gender of donor influences outcome after orthotopic liver transplantation in adults. *Dig Dis Sci.* 38:148514.

104. Gustafsson JA, Mode A, Norstedt G, et al. (1983). Sex steroid induced changes in hepatic enzymes. *Annu Rev Physiol.* 45:51.

105. Roy AK, Chateterjee B. (1983). Sexual dimorphism in the liver. *Annu Rev Physiol.* 45:37.

106. Kahn D, Zeng Q, Makowka L, et al. (1989). Orthotopic liver transplantation and the cytosolic estrogen-androgen receptor status of the liver: the influence of the sex of the donor. *Hepatology.* 10:861.

107. Chertow GM, Zenios SA. (2001). Gridlock on the road to kidney transplantation. *Am J Kidney Dis.* 37(2):435–437.

108. Eggers PW. (1988). Effect of transplantation on the Medicare end-stage renal disease program. *N Engl J Med.* 318:223–229.

109. Wolfe RA, Ashby VB, Milford EL, et al. (2000). Differences in access to cadaveric renal transplantation in the United States. *Am J Kidney Dis.* 36(5):1025–1033.

110. Kouli F. (2001). Impact of donor/recipient traits independent of rejection on long term renal function. *Am J Kidney Dis.* 37(2):356–365.

111. Sutherland DE, Gruessner RW, Dunn DL et al. (2001). Lessons learned from more than 1000 pancreas transplants in a single institution. *Ann Surg.* 233(4):463–501.

112. Laporte RE, Matsushima M, Chang YF. (1995). Prevalence and incidence of insulin-dependent diabetes. In: Harris MI, ed. *Diabetes in America.* Bethesda, MD: National Institutes of Health, NIDDK. 37–46.

113. Navarro X, Sutherland DER, Kennedy WR. (1997). Long term effects of pancreatic transplantation on diabetic neuropathy. *Ann Neurol.* 42:727–736.

114. Shapiro AM, Lakey JR, Ryan EA *et al.* (2000). Islet transplantation in seven patients with type 1 diabetes mellitus I using a glucocorticoid free immunosuppressive regimen. *N Engl J Med.* 343:23–238.

115. Morissette P, Albert C, Busque S, *et al.* (2001). *In vivo* higher glucuronidation of mycophenolic acid in male than in female recipients of a cadaveric kidney allograft and under immunosuppressive therapy with mycophenolate mofetil. *Ther Drug Monit.* 23(5):520–525.

116. Mulder GJ. (1986). Sex differences in drug conjugations and their consequences for drug toxicity. Sulfation, glucuronidation and glutathione conjugation. *Chem Biol Interact.* 57:1–15.

117. Gasbarrini A, Adolorato G, Campli C, *et al.* (2001).Gender affects reperfusion injury in rat liver. *Dig Dis Sci.* 46(6):1305–1312.

118. Norton R, Batey R, Dwyer T, *et al.* (1987). Alcohol consumption and the risk of alcohol related cirrhosis in women. *Br Med J.* 295:80–82.

119. Guattery JM, Faloon WW. (1987). Effect of estradiol upon serum enzymes in primary liver cirrhosis. *Hepatology.* 7:737–742.

120. Becker U. (1993). The influence of ethanol and liver disease on sex hormones and hepatic estrogen receptors in women. *Dan Med Bull.* 40: 447–459.

121. Ikejima K, Enomoto N, Iimuro Y, *et al.* (1998). Estrogen increase sensitivity of Kupffer cells to endotoxin. *Am J Physiol.* 274:G669–G676.

122. Meier-Kriesche H, Ojo A, Leavey S, *et al.* (2001). Gender differences in the risk for chronic renal allograft failure. *Transplantation.* 71(3):429–432.

123. Cecka JM. (1986). The roles of sex, race, and ABO groups. *Clin Transpl.* 199–221.

124. Koka P, Cecka JM. (1990). Sex and age effects in renal transplantation. *Clin Transpl.* 437–446.

125. Shibue T, Kondo K, Iwaki Y, *et al.* (1987). Effect of sex on kidney transplants. *Clin Transpl.* 351–360.

126. Yuge J, Cecka JM. (1991). Sex and age effects in renal transplantation. *Clin Transpl.* 257–267.

127. Zhou YC, Cecka JM. (1989). Effect of sex on kidney transplants. *Clin Transpl.* 361–367.

128. Michet CJJ, McKenna CH, Elveback LR, *et al.* (1985). Epidemiology of systemic lupus erythematosus and other connective tissue diseases in Rochester, Minnesota, 1950 through 1979. *Mayo Clin Proc.* 60:105.

129. Kwan G, Neugarten J, Sherman M, et al. (1996). Effects of sex hormones on mesangial cell proliferation and collagen synthesis. *Kidney Int.* 50:1173.

130. Muller V, Szabo A, Viklicky O, et al. (1999). Sex hormones and gender-related differences: their influence on chronic renal allograft rejection. *Kidney Int.* 55:2011.

131. Zeier M, Schonherr R, Amann K, *et al.* (1998). Effects of testosterone after glomerular growth after uninephrectomy. *Nephrol Dial Transplant.* 13:2234.

132. Munoz SJ, Rothstein KD, Reich D, *et al.* (2000). Long term care of the liver transplant recipient. *Clin Liver Dis.* 4(3):691–710.

133. Epstein S, Shane E, Bilezikian JP. (1995). Organ transplantation and osteoporosis. *Curr Opin Rheumatol.* 7:255.

134. Ramsey-Goldman R, Dunn JE, Dunlop DD, *et al.* (1999). Increased risk of fracture in patients receiving solid organ transplants. *J Bone Miner Res.* 14:456.

135. Silkensen JR. (2000). Long-term complications in renal transplantation. *J Am Soc Nephrol.* 11(3):582–588.

136. Chiu MY, Sprague SM, Bruce DS, *et al.* (1998). Analysis of fracture prevalence in kidney-pancreas allograft recipients. *J Am Soc Nephrol.* 9:677.

137. Shane E, Silverberg S, Donovan D. (1996). Osteoporosis in lung transplantation candidates with end-stage pulmonary disease. *Am J Med.* 101:262.

138. Mack-Shipman LR, Ratanasuwan T, Leone JP, *et al.* (2000). Reproductive hormones after pancreas transplantation. *Transplantation.* 70(8): 1180–1183114.

139. Scantlebury V, Gordon R, Tzakis A, *et al.* (1990). Childbearing after liver transplantation. *Transplantation.* 49(2):317–321.

140. Radomski JS, Moritz MJ, Munoz SJ, *et al.* (1995). National transplantation registry: Analysis of pregnancy outcome in female liver transplant recipients. *Liver Transplant Surgery.* 1:281–284.

141. Jain A, Venkataramanan R, Fung JJ, *et al.* (1997). Pregnancy after liver transplantation under tacrolimus. *Transplantation.* 64:559–565.

142. Molmenti EP, Jain AB, Marino N, *et al.* (1999). Pregnancy and liver disease liver transplantation and pregnancy. *Clin Liver Dis.* 3(1): 163–174.

143. Rizzoni G, Ehrich JHH, Broyer M, *et al.* (1992). Successful pregnancies in women on renal replacement therapy: Report from the EDTA Registry. *Nephrol Dial Transplant.* 7:279–287.

144. Cohen D, Galbraith C. (2001). General health management and long term care of the renal transplant recipient. *Am J Kidney Dis.* 38(6):S10–24.

145. Penn I, Makowski EL, Harris P. (1980). Parenthood following renal transplantation. *Kidney Int.* 18(2):221–233.

146. Saarikoski S, Seppala M. (1973). Immunosuppression during pregnancy. Transmission of azathioprine and its metabolites from mother to fetus. *Am J Obstet Gynecol.* 115:1100–1106.

147. Ville Y, Fernandez H, Samuel D, *et al.* (1993). Pregnancy in liver transplant recipients: Course and outcome in 19 cases. *Am J Obstet Gynecol.* 168:896–902.

148. Kainz A. (2000). Analysis of 100 pregnancy outcomes in women treated systemically with Tacrolimus. *Transpl Int.* 13:S299–300.

149. Armenti VT, Moritz MJ, Davison JM. (1998). Drug safety issues in pregnancy following transplantation and immunosuppression: effects and outcomes. *Drug Safety.* 19:219.

150. Armenti VT, Coscia LA, McGrory CH, *et al.* (1998). National Transplantation Pregnancy Registry. Update on pregnancy and renal transplantation. *Nephrology News & Issues.* 12(8):19–23.

151. Lamarque V, Leleu MF, Monka C, *et al.* (1997). Analysis of 629 pregnancy outcomes in transplant recipients treated with Sandimmune. *Transplant Proc.* 29:2480.

152. Product Information Neoral 55. (1999). In: *Physicians' Desk Reference 55,* 53rd ed. Montvale, NJ: Medical Economics Company Inc. 2067.

153. Stagno S, Whitley RJ. (1985). Herpesvirus infections of pregnancy. Part I: Cytomegalovirus and Epstein-Barr virus infection. *N Engl J Med.* 313:1270–1274.

154. Hutto C, Arvin A, Jacobs R, *et al.* (1987). Intrauterine herpes simplex virus infections. *J Pediatr.* 110:97–101.

155. MacLeod CL, Lee RV. (1988). Parasitic infections. In: Burrow GN, Ferris TF, eds. *Medical Complications During Pregnancy.* Philadelphia: Saunders. 425–427.

156. Crabtree TD, Pelletier SJ, Gleason TG, *et al.* (1999). Gender-dependent differences in outcome after the treatment of infection in hospitalized patients. *JAMA.* 282(22):2143–2148.

157. Fairley CK, Sheil AGR, McNeil JJ, *et al.* (1994). The risk of ano-genital malignancies in dialysis and transplant patients. *Clin Nephrol.* 41:101–105.

158. Halpert R, Fruchter RG, Sedlis A, *et al.* (1986). Human papillomavirus and lower genital neoplasia in renal transplant patients. *Obstet Gynecol.* 68:251–258.

159. Brunner FP, Landais P, Selwood NH. (1995). Malignancies after renal transplantation: The EDTA-ERA Registry experience. *Nephrol Dial Transplant.* 10[Suppl 1]:74–80.

160. ter Haar-van Eck SA, Rischen-Vos J, Chadha-Ajwani S, *et al.* (1995). The incidence of cervical intraepithelial neoplasia among women with renal transplant in relation to cyclosporine. *Br J Obstet Gynaecol.* 102:58–61.

161. Porreco R, Penn I, Droegemueller W, *et al.* (1975). Gynecologic malignancies in immunosuppressed organ homograft recipients. *Obstet Gynecol.* 45: 359–364.

162. Weiss NS. (1995). Risk of breast cancer after renal or cardiac transplantation. *Lancet.* 346:1422.

163. Stewart T, Tsai S-CJ, Grayson H, *et al.* (1995). Incidence of de-novo breast cancer in women chronically immunosuppressed after organ transplantation. *Lancet.* 346:796–798.

164. National Cancer Institute. (1998). Screening for Breast Cancer [Pamphlet]. Bethesda, MD: National Institutes of Health.

165. United States Preventive Services Task Force. (1996). Screening for breast cancer. In: Di Guiseppi C, Atkins D, Woolf S, eds. *Guide to Clinical Preventive Services,* 2nd ed. Baltimore: Williams & Wilkins. 73–87.

166. Leitch AM, Dodd GD, Costanza M, *et al.* (1997). American Cancer Society guidelines for the early detection of breast cancer: Update 1997. *CA Cancer J Clin.* 47:150–153.

167. Kasiske BL, Vazquez MA, Harmon WE, *et al.* (2000). Recommendations for the outpatient surveillance of renal transplant recipients. *J Am Soc Nephrol.* 11 Suppl 15:S1–86.

168. Birkeland SA, Storm HH, Lamm LU, *et al.* (1995). Cancer risk after renal transplantation in the Nordic countries, 1964–1986. *Int J Cancer* 60: 183–189.

169. Konety BR, Tewari A, Howard RJ, *et al.* (1998). Prostate cancer in the post-transplant population. *Urology.* 52:428–432.

170. Reppeto L, Granetto C, Hall RR. (1998). Prostate cancer. *Crit Rev Oncol Hematol.* 27:145–146.

171. Morton JJ, Howe SF, Lowell JA, *et al.* (1995). Influence of end-stage renal disease and renal transplantation on serum prostate-specific antigen. *Br J Urol.* 75:498–501.

172. United States Preventive Services Task Force. (1996). Screening for prostate cancer. In: Di Guiseppi C, Atkins D, Woolf S, eds. *Guide to Clinical Preventive Services*, 2nd ed. Baltimore: Williams & Wilkins. 119–134.

173. National Cancer Institute: Screening for Prostate Cancer. (1998). [Pamphlet]. Bethesda, MD: National Institutes of Health.

174. Gross CR, Savik K, Bolman RM, et al. (1995). Long term health status and quality of life outcomes of lung transplant recipients. *Chest.* 108:1587–1593.

175. Jofre R, Lopez-Gomez JM, Moreno F, et al. (1998) Changes in quality of life after renal transplantation. *Am J Kidney Dis.* 32:93–100.

176. Painter PL, Luetkemeier MJ, Moore GE, et al. (1997). Health-related fitness and quality of life in organ transplant recipients. *Transplant.* 1997; 64:1795–1800.

177. Littlefield C, Abbey S, Fiducia D, et al. (1996). Quality of life following transplantation of the heart, liver, and lungs. *Gen Hosp Psych.* 18:36S–47S.

178. Grieco A, Long C. (1984). Investigation of the Karnofsky Performance Status is a measure of quality of life. *Health Psychol.* 3:129–142.

179. Testa MA, Simonson DC. (1996). Assessment of quality-of-life outcomes. *N Engl J Med.* 334.835–840.

180. Hricik DE, Halbert RJ, Barr ML, et al. (2001). Life satisfaction in renal transplant recipients: Preliminary results from the transplant Learning Center. *Am J Kidney Dis.* 38(3):580–587.

181. Fisher R, Gould D, Wainwright S, et al. (1998). Quality of life after renal transplantation. *J Clin Nurs.* 7:553–563.

182. King K. (2000). Patients' perspective of factors affecting modality selection: A National Kidney Foundation patient survey. *Adv Ren Replace Ther.* 7:261–268.

183. Manninen DL, Evans RW, Dugan MK. (1991). Work disability, functional limitations, and the health status of kidney transplantation recipients post transplant. In: Terasaki P, ed. *Clinical Transplants.* Los Angeles: UCLA Tissue Typing Laboratory. 193–203.

184. Shidler NR, Peterson RA, Kimmel PL. (1998). Quality of life and psychosocial relationships in patients with chronic renal insufficiency. *Am J Kidney Dis.* 32:557–566.

185. Schover LR, Novick AC, Steinmuller DR, et al. (1990). Sexuality, fertility, and renal transplantation: A survey of survivors. *J Sex Marital Ther.* 16:3–13.

186. Alleyne S, Dillard P, McGregor C, et al. (1989). Sexual function and mental distress status of patients with end-stage renal disease on hemodialysis. *Transplant Proc.* 21:3895–3898.

187. Sutton TD, Murphy SP. (1989). Stressors and patterns of coping in renal transplant patients. *Nurs Res.* 38:46–49.

188. Fallon M, Gould D, Wainwright SP. (1997). Stress and quality of life in the renal transplant patient: A preliminary investigation. *J Adv Nurs.* 25:562–570.

189. Pinson CW, Feurer ID, Payne JL, et al. (2000). Health related quality of life after different types of solid organ transplantation. 232(4):597–607.

190. Wolfe RA, Ashby VB, Milford EL, et al. (2000). Differences in access to cadaveric renal transplantation in the United States. *Am J Kidney Dis.* 36(5):1025–1033.

191. Kjellstrand KM. (1988). Age, sex and race inequality in renal transplantation. *Arch Intern Med.* 148:1305–1309.

192. Bloembergen WE, Mauger EA, Wolfe RA, et al. (1997). Association of gender and access to cadaveric renal transplantation. *Am J Kidney Dis.* 30:733–738.

193. Bloembergen WE, Young EW, Woods JD, et al. (1997). Factors associated with late referral among new dialysis patients in the US. *J Am Soc Nephrol.* 8:186A.

194. Soucie JM, Neylan JF, McClellan W. (1992). Race and sex differences in the identification of candidates for renal transplantation. *Am J Kidney Dis.* 19:414–419.

195. Healy B. The Yentl syndrome. (1991). *N Engl J Med.* 325:274–276.

196. Garg PP, Furth SL, Fivush BA, et al. (2000). Impact of gender on access to the renal transplant waiting list for pediatric and adult patients. *J Am Soc Nephrol.* 11:958–964.

197. Gaylin DS, Held PJ, Port FK, et al. (1993). The impact of comorbid and sociodemographic factors on access to renal transplantation. *JAMA.* 269(5):603–608.

198. Arora P, Obrador GT, Ruthazer R, et al. (1999). Prevalence, predictors, and consequences of late nephrology referral at a tertiary care center. *J Am Soc Nephrol.* 10:1281–1286.

199. Kasiske BL, London W, Ellison MD. (1998). Race and socioeconomic factors influencing early placement on the kidney transplant waiting list. *J Am Soc Nephrol.* 9:2142–2147.

200. Port F, Wolfe R, Mauger E, et al. (1993). Comparison of survival probabilities for dialysis patients vs cadaveric renal transplant recipients. *JAMA.* 270:1339–1343.

201. Alexander GC, Sehgal AR. (2001). Why hemodialysis patients fail to complete the transplantation process. *Am J Kidney Dis.* 37:321–328.

202. Alexander GC, Sehgal AR. (1998). Barriers to cadaveric renal transplantation among blacks, women, and the poor. *JAMA.* 280:1148–1152.

203. Garg P, Powe NR. (1999). The impact of Medicare supplementary insurance on access to the kidney transplant waiting list. *J Gen Int Med.* 14[suppl 2]:32.

104

Prolactin in Autoimmune Disease

SARA E. WALKER, MD, MACP

Professor of Internal Medicine, University of Missouri–Columbia, Columbia, MO

Abstract

Prolactin (PRL) has the potential to stimulate immune responses and is a cytokine. Circulating PRL is elevated above the norm in a number of autoimmune diseases, including systemic lupus erythematosus (SLE). Bromocriptine, which suppresses the pituitary secretion of PRL, has been used with success to treat autoimmune illness. Successful use of PRL-suppressive treatments in selected diseases supports the contention that PRL contributes to active autoimmunity and opens up the possibility of using these relatively nontoxic drugs as adjunct therapy for immune-mediated diseases.

I. Prolactin

PRL, a peptide hormone, is produced in the anterior pituitary gland and stimulates mammary growth and differentiation. Pituitary secretion of PRL is stimulated by suckling and stress and is restricted by hypothalamic dopamine [1]. It is now recognized that PRL is produced in a number of sites outside the pituitary, including lymphocytes [2]. PRL is important in maintaining immune competence [3,4], has cytokine activity in human leukocytes [5], and has a permissive effect on antigen presentation [6]. PRL therefore has the potential to stimulate autoimmunity [7–11]. PRL receptors are distributed throughout the immune system [3] and are included in a novel receptor family that includes receptors for interleukin (IL)-2 beta, IL-3, IL-4, IL-6, IL-7, growth hormone, and erythropoietin [12].

A. Prolactin and the Immune System

PRL can influence the immune system directly through the thymus [13,14] by inducing IL-2 receptors on lymphocytes [15] and by acting as a requisite lymphocyte growth factor. Lymphocytes synthesize and release a biologically active form of PRL [16] that cells use as an autocrine and paracrine growth factor. Mechanisms that control the production of lymphocyte PRL are not completely understood. It is not known if lymphocyte PRL is affected by circulating pituitary PRL or by dopamine agonists such as bromocriptine, which inhibit pituitary secretion of PRL.

It is not known if lymphocytes can produce enough PRL to cause an increase in serum PRL levels. A lymphoblastoid human B-cell line that produces prolactin has been identified [17], and hyperprolactinemia was found in patients with advanced multiple myeloma [18]. Immunoreactive PRL was detected by immunoblot in leukemic cells from a patient with acute myeloid leukemia who was hyperprolactinemic. It was postulated that the leukemic myeloblasts were a source of excessive PRL and that this PRL

was detected at high levels in the serum PRL assay [19]. The question of the ability of lymphoid cells to produce detectable circulating PRL becomes important when one considers the fact that hyperprolactinemia is present in a number of patients with autoimmune diseases.

Nagy and Berczi [20,21] showed the importance of PRL in maintaining normal immune function and sustaining life. Hypophysectomy suppressed cell-mediated immune responses in rats, and this suppression was abrogated by PRL injections and by implanted syngeneic pituitary glands. The pituitary transplants, separated from the inhibiting influence of the hypothalamus, produced excessive PRL in an uninhibited manner. When rats were deprived completely of PRL by hypophysectomy and treatment with anti-PRL antibody, they became anergic and anemic and died within 8 weeks. Replacement injections of either PRL or growth hormone stimulated expression of the *c-myc* growth-promoting gene and reversed spleen and thymus involution [22].

High levels of circulating PRL stimulate immune responses. Hyperprolactinemia that was created in mice, by either implanting one or two syngeneic pituitary glands or by injecting exogenous mouse PRL, increased primary humoral antibody responses to sheep red blood cells [23]. In contrast, low levels of PRL led to immune suppression. Cysteamine is a sulfhydryl reducing agent that lowers PRL through mechanisms independent of the pituitary. Mice treated with cysteamine developed severe immunosuppression, with thymic atrophy and depressed lymphocyte responses to T-cell mitogens and B-cell mitogens [24].

B. PRL and Transgenic BALB/c Mice with Estrogen-Induced Systemic Lupus Erythematosus

BALB/c mice that have been made transgenic for the heavy chain of a pathogenic anti-DNA antibody have lupuslike disease that is induced by treatment with estrogen, with expansion of B-cells producing anti-DNA antibody and immunoglobulin deposits in the renal glomeruli. Estradiol treatment leads to expansion and activation of a subset of autoreactive B cells that produce anti-DNA [25]. Estrogen is a potent stimulator of pituitary prolactin production in mice. Therefore, studies were performed to determine whether estrogen alone, or prolactin that was induced by the exogenous estrogen, induced growth of the autoreactive cells. Mice were treated with estradiol with the addition of bromocriptine, a potent inhibitor of prolactin secretion. Animals that received the combination treatment had milder disease with lower anti-DNA titers and diminished immunoglobulin (IgG) deposits in the glomeruli. They also had anergic high-affinity anti-DNA B cells, suggesting that bromocriptine had induced anergy in the autoreactive B cells [26]. The impression that prolactin, not estrogen, was the key factor in development of induced autoimmunity in this model was supported by additional experiments. When the transgenic BALB/c mice were treated directly with prolactin for 4 weeks, they had high-titer anti-DNA antibodies and increased glomerular deposits of immunoglobulin. Prolactin treatment led to increased mature follicular and marginal zone B cells, and the DNA-reactive B cells had a follicular cell phenotype [27].

C. Prolactin and NZB/NZW Mice with Spontaneous Systemic Lupus Erythematosus

The NZB/NZW mouse develops SLE spontaneously, and its disease closely resembles SLE in humans. The animals develop antibodies to double-stranded (ds) DNA and die with immune-mediated glomerulonephritis. Disease in females begins earlier and is more severe compared to males. Lupus in NZB/NZW mice is accelerated by estrogen and suppressed by testosterone [28].

T helper 1 (Th1) responses, which are traditionally thought to be involved in cell-mediated immunity, are key effectors in development of SLE in the NZB/NZW mouse [29]. PRL upgrades Th1 responses [30]. The transcription factor gene, interferon regulatory factor-1 (IRF-1), is an important regulator of T-cell and B-cell differentiation and maturation and is required for Th1 immune responses. PRL is a potent stimulator of interferon (IFN) gamma and IFN regulatory factor 1 (IRF-1) in T cells [4]. PRL therefore has the potential to increase production of IRF-1, which in turn regulates expression of Th1 cytokines. The potential of IRF-1 to promote autoimmunity was demonstrated when type II collagen-induced arthritis was induced in mice that were either IRF-1 deficient (−/−) or IRF-1 positive (+/−). Disease was reduced in the IRF-1 −/− mice compared to the +/− mice. It was concluded that absence of IRF-1 gene activity was protective in a model with induced autoimmune disease [31].

D. Hormonal Interactions and Pathogenesis of Disease in NZB/NZW Mice

Estrogen is a potent stimulus for production of pituitary PRL in rodents. Earlier studies of lupus in estrogen-treated NZB/NZW mice did not take this fact into account. Estrogen treatment of female NZB/NZW mice resulted in hyperplasia and functioning adenomas of the anterior pituitary gland. Serum PRL concentrations in estrogen-treated mice were 10–91 times greater than controls [32]. It has been widely reported that estrogen treatment accelerated autoimmune disease in NZB/NZW mice. In fact, secondary elevation of PRL may have contributed to the apparent stimulation of autoimmune disease in estrogen-treated mice [33].

In NZB/NZW mice, hyperprolactinemia resulted in premature death from autoimmune renal disease, but PRL-lowering therapy was beneficial. Female NZB/NZW mice were made chronically hyperprolactinemic (representative mean serum concentrations 127–182 ng/ml) by implantation of two syngeneic pituitary glands under the renal capsule of each mouse. Control females had serum PRL of 53–109 ng/ml. Pituitary transplantation resulted in premature glomerulonephritis and early mortality. In contrast, mice treated with bromocriptine had delayed anti ds DNA and significant prolongation of lifespans [34]. Another group of NZB/NZW females had four pituitary glands transplanted into each animal. Serum PRL concentrations (743–1643 ng/ml) were greater than in the mice that received two transplants. Twelve weeks after the pituitary glands were implanted, 80% of recipient mice had anti ds DNA and striking hypergammaglobulinemia [35]. Male NZB/NZW mice also responded to hyperprolactinemia. Their lupuslike disease, which is usually indolent, was accelerated following transplantation of either two or four pituitary glands [36]. Naturally occurring hyperprolactinemia was detrimental in parous NZB/NZW mice that had either whelped two litters and had the young removed shortly after birth, whelped and suckled two litters, or experienced prolonged pseudopregnancy [37].

Elbourne et al [38] found that PRL was required for estrogen to stimulate autoimmune disease in NZB/NZW mice. Groups of females that were manipulated to have either high or low circulating estrogen concentrations were implanted with pituitary glands to create concurrent hyperprolactinemia or treated with bromocriptine to create hypoprolactinemia. High circulating estrogen in the presence of high serum PRL was detrimental and resulted in accelerated albuminuria and premature anti-DNA (75% positive at 16 weeks of age). In contrast, disease was retarded in females with high estrogen levels who received bromocriptine. These high-estrogen, low-PRL females had delayed albuminuria and delayed anti-DNA (10% positive at 16 weeks of age).

E. Hyperprolactinemia and Immunologic Abnormalities in Humans

Hyperprolactinemic humans have immunologic abnormalities. Healthy women, made temporarily hyperprolactinemic by treatment with domperidone, had transient responses in which theophylline-sensitive T cells were increased, CD4+ lymphocytes were decreased, and mitogenic responses to concanavalin A were stimulated [39]. Chronic elevation of serum PRL did not, however, have consistent effects on the immune system. Cytokine levels were normal in patients with hyperprolactinemia [40]. Lymphocyte subsets were either normal (41) or were characterized by increased numbers of CD4+ cells [42]. Natural killer (NK) cell activity was either decreased [43] or normal [44]. Bromocriptine treatment to lower serum prolactin resulted in normalization of increased numbers of CD4+ TQ1+ cells [42] and increased efficiency and recycling capacity of NK cells [43].

F. Stimulation of Autoantibodies

Hyperprolactinemia stimulates autoantibodies in individuals who do not have clinically apparent autoimmune diseases. Pontiroli et al [45] studied 71 women with hyperprolactinemia, of whom 30 had evidence of prolactinomas by tomography. Three had antibodies directed against the pituitary, two had antithyroid antibodies, and three had antibodies to gastric parietal cells. In another series [46], women with prolactinomas had antimicrosomal antibodies and antithyroglobulin, each occurring in 21% of subjects. The autoantibodies were found in 8% and 5% of normal women, respectively. The occurrence of antithyroglobulin antibodies was 19% in men with hyperprolactinemia, compared with 2% in normal men. Reactivity against a number of autoantigens was found in a survey of 33 women with hyperprolactinemia; 82% had imaging studies showing pituitary adenomas. Of the women, 76% had at least one autoantibody, and eight had seven or more different autoantibodies. The most common antibody specificities were directed against single-stranded DNA, ds DNA, Sm, pyruvate dehydrogenase, and SSA/Ro. The subjects did not have clinical evidence of autoimmune disease [47]. Another survey found anticardiolipin antibodies in 5 of 23 (22%) women and men with serum prolactin concentrations above the norm [48].

Sera from patients who were hyperprolactinemic, but had no diagnosis of rheumatic disease, had multiple autoantibodies. Eight of 24 (33%) sera from women with hyperprolactinemia (serum PRL 26–253 ng/ml, normal 0–20 ng/ml) produced positive fluorescent antinuclear antibody (FANA) tests, and three of these sera contained either anti-Scl70, anti-SSB/La, or the Sm determinants B/B' and C. Sera from 8 of 15 men with hyperprolactinemia, including eight with prolactinomas, produced positive FANA tests. In comparison, FANA tests were positive in three of 15 age-matched men with normal prolactin concentrations ($p < 0.01$) [10].

G. Hyperprolactinemia Preceding the Onset of Autoimmune Diseases

In seven cases, serum PRL above the norm was documented before the onset of autoimmune disease. Elevated serum PRL was found in one patient 5 years before the appearance of Graves' disease. In a second patient, idiopathic hyperprolactinemia was present 2 years before dermatomyositis was diagnosed [49]. Two patients were hyperprolactinemic 12 years before the diagnosis of primary Sjögren's syndrome [50]. High serum PRL was present in three women at intervals of 3 months, 16 months, and 10 years before SLE was diagnosed. Lupus was expressed in these patients by prominent photosensitivity, malar rash, and antinuclear antibodies without involvement of the kidneys or central nervous system [51].

H. Hyperprolactinemia in Autoimmune Diseases

Elevated serum PRL concentrations are found commonly in autoimmune illness. One third of patients with multiple sclerosis had PRL elevations, and PRL was increased in the early stages of a multiple sclerosis flare [52]. Series containing small numbers of subjects verified the association between multiple sclerosis and hyperprolactinemia [53,54], and hyperprolactinemia was reported in the optic neuromyelitis variant of multiple sclerosis [55]. In contrast, a recent survey of 132 patients with multiple sclerosis found no difference in mean serum PRL concentrations and no difference in response to metoclopramide stimulation between the affected individuals and controls. There was no significant correlation between PRL levels and disease activity or classification [56]. PRL secretion, however, was increased in response to injection of thyroid-releasing hormone [57].

Four patients with autoimmune Addison's disease were hyperprolactinemic, and it was thought that deficient corticosteroids had caused PRL to rise above the norm [58]. Hashimoto's thyroiditis with autoimmune features (antinuclear antibodies, antibodies to smooth muscle, and antibodies to parietal cells) was associated with elevated PRL [59]. In a series of 92 women with hyperprolactinemia, 33 had evidence of a primary thyroid disorder. Antibodies to thyroglobulin were found in 26%, hyperplasia in 14%, and thyroid nodules in 3% [60].

PRL may be produced locally in the inflamed eye. Mean PRL concentration in the aqueous humor of 14 patients with previously documented anterior uveitis was 1.9 ng/ml ± 1 standard deviation (SD), a value that significantly exceeded the control value of 0.5 ± 0.5 ($p < 0.001$). Serum PRL levels did not, however, differ between the two groups [61] and patients with uveitis or severe iridocyclitis did not have elevated PRL concentrations in serum [62,63].

I. Prolactin in Rheumatic Diseases

Table 104-1 describes groups of patients with rheumatologic diseases who had significant serum PRL elevations in comparison with a normal control population. Hyperprolactinemia was found in 36% of patients with reactive arthritis [64] and in 34.8% and 59% of patients with scleroderma [65,66]. Identification of PRL-like proteins in cytoplasmic acinar epithelial cells of patients with Sjögren's syndrome raised the possibility that local production of PRL contributed to local inflammation [67], and hyperprolactinemia was reported in 46% of individuals with primary Sjögren's syndrome [68]. In a second survey, 55 patients with primary Sjögren's syndrome had higher mean serum PRL concentrations compared with 110 normal controls. PRL levels were highest in those diagnosed before the age of 45 years. Two patients developed primary Sjögren's syndrome 12 years after hyperprolactinemia was first detected. Both had unusually aggressive disease with systemic features [50].

The risk of rheumatoid arthritis (RA) is increased in women who breast-feed after the first pregnancy, and it was suggested that the propensity to develop RA was related to immune-stimulating PRL surges that accompany suckling [69]. PRL secretion was reported as either attenuated [70], normal [71], or upregulated in RA [72]. The proinflammatory cytokine, macrophage inflammatory protein-1 alpha, is produced by cells involved in the inflammatory rheumatoid process and may stimulate pituitary production of PRL [73]. Furthermore, the PRL gene is close to the human leukocyte antigen (HLA) region on the short arm of chromosome 6 and an interaction may exist between the HLA DR4 gene, which predisposes to RA and PRL [69].

These circumstances suggest that PRL has a role in initiating or sustaining inflammation in RA. Although the pathogenic stimulation may result from pituitary PRL, PRL of lymphocyte origin has the capacity to stimulate inflammation in affected rheumatoid joints [2]. PRL has been identified in tissue extracts from ankle joints of rats with acute adjuvant arthritis [74]. PRL is produced in the rheumatoid joint by fibroblast-like synovial cells and by lymphocytes that infiltrate the synovium, where it appears to stimulate collagenase activity and act as a growth factor for lymphocytes. It is believed that bromocriptine likely suppresses only pituitary PRL. In this instance, however, *in vitro*

Table 104-1
Hyperprolactinemia in Rheumatic Diseases

Diagnosis	Sex	N (% HPRL)	PRL, Rheumatic Disease*	PRL, Controls*	p**	Reference
Reactive arthritis	F,M	25 (36)	16.4±14.1†	8.7±4.5	<0.05	[64]
Scleroderma	F	24 (34.8)	16.75±9.06†	11.6±4.5	<0.001	[65]
	F	17 (59)	19.2±2.1‡	8.1±±1.1	<0.01	[66]
Sjögren's syndrome	F,M	11 (46)	25.2±20†	10.4±7.2	<0.04	[68]
	F,M	55 (4)	271.5±209.2†	205.9±ND	<0.02	[50]
Rheumatoid arthritis	M	29 (7)	13.14±1.62‡	7.48±0.51	<0.001	[76]
	M,F	22(22)	34.6	ND	0.001	[77]
	M	91 (40)	249±16†	189±85	0.0015	[78]
Prepubertal ANA-Positive Chronic Juvenile Arthritis	F	8 (38)	10.9±1.9§	5.8±1.3	0.048	[89]
Early Onset ANA-Positive Pauciarticular Chronic Juvenile Arthritis	F	11 (0)	8.9±4.0†	4.6±1.7	0.006	[90]
Late-Onset ANA-Negative Pauciarticular Chronic Juvenile Arthritis	F	8 (0)	7.8±2.4†	4.6±1.7	0.006	[90]

PRL, prolactin; N, number studied; HPRL, hyperprolactinemic; ANA, antinuclear antibodies; ND, no data.

*Normal values for serum PRL concentrations were <20 ng/ml [64,68], 2.6–20.6 ng/ml based on mean PRL concentration in controls ± standard deviation [65], 1.4–14.6 µg/L [66], <500 mIU/l [50], 5–20 ng/ml [76], upper limit of normal 20 ng/ml [77], 109–224 mU/l [78], 3–12 µg /L [89]. Normal values were not given for PRL concentrations in reference 90.

**p for mean PRL concentration in rheumatic disease vs mean PRL in controls.

†Mean ± standard deviation.

‡Mean ± standard error of the mean.

§This number was not defined as representing either standard deviation or standard error of the mean.

(Adapted with permission from Walker SE, Jacobson JD. [2000]. Roles of prolactin and gonadotropin-releasing hormone in rheumatic diseases. *Rheum Dis Clin North Am.* 26:713–736.)

application of bromocriptine to RA synovial cells and infiltrating lymphocytes suppressed the expression of mRNA for PRL and for tumor necrosis factor-alpha [75].

It would be anticipated that circulating levels of PRL are high in RA, but this is not always true. A study of 29 men with RA revealed that PRL was elevated compared to normal controls [76] (see Table 104-1), and 22% of 22 women and men with RA had modest hyperprolactinemia [77] (see Table 104-1). Mateo *et al* [78] did find that 40% of men with RA had serum PRL that exceeded the population norm, and the subjects' serum PRL concentrations had positive correlations with duration and functional stage of disease. In other studies, however, RA patients had PRL levels that were within normal limits and comparable to normal controls [79,80]. In a study of PRL bioactivity in RA, serum PRL concentrations were normal but the serum had impaired PRL activity on PRL-sensitive Nb2 cells [81]. In two series, serum PRL was significantly *lower* in both men and women with RA compared to controls [81,82].

Hyperprolactinemia has not been identified in surveys of patients with ankylosing spondylitis, fibromyalgia, or Behçet's syndrome. Serum PRL was said to be normal in 17 women [83] and 55 men with ankylosing spondylitis [84,85], but the PRL values were not given. Twenty-one women with hyperprolactinemia were tested for tender points, and 15 (71%) met American College of Rheumatology criteria for the classification of fibromyalgia [86]. Nevertheless, detailed studies of hormonal status in 12 premenopausal women who were selected because they had the primary diagnosis of fibromyalgia showed that both serum PRL and PRL responses to hypoglycemia were similar to healthy premenopausal controls [87]. PRL levels were normal in surveys of patients with Behçet's syndrome [88,89].

J. Hyperprolactinemia in Chronic Juvenile Arthritis

Table 104-1 shows that serum PRL concentrations were relatively high in a group of prepubertal girls (mean age 8.2 years) who had juvenile chronic arthritis and positive antinuclear antibody tests. PRL values in these girls were elevated significantly, compared with seronegative girls with juvenile chronic arthritis and age-matched controls [90]. In another survey, younger girls (mean age 4.5 years) with antinuclear antibody-positive pauciarticular juvenile chronic arthritis had increased serum PRL levels compared to controls (see Table 104-1). Serum IL-6 was increased significantly in the children with juvenile chronic arthritis and spondyloarthropathy, and there was positive correlation between levels of PRL and IL-6 [91].

K. Hyperprolactinemia in Systemic Lupus Erythematosus

There is currently great interest in the possibility that PRL influences SLE, and surveys have shown that the occurrence of hyperprolactinemia is increased in patients with SLE. Of serum samples submitted to an antinuclear antibody reference laboratory, 12% had abnormal elevations of PRL. The expected

Table 104-2

Hyperprolactinemia in Systemic Lupus Erythematosus

Sex	N (% HPRL)	PRL in SLE*	PRL in Controls*	p**	Reference
F, M	46 (22)	17.2 (3.6–188)†	8.4 (2.0–17.5)	ND	[95]
F, M	82 (19.5)	ND (5–58)†	ND	ND	[96]
F	29 (30)	19.4±15.6‡	9.5±6.8	<0.05	[97]
F, M	83 (15.9)	ND (5–57)†	ND	ND	[98]
F, M	30 (40)	19.4±11.3‡	12.0±7.5	<0.01	[99]
F, M	34 (31)	20±2§	ND	ND	[100]
F	36 (28)	17.1±12.9‡	9.9±3.5	<0.01	[101]
F, M	78 (26.9)	15.2±19.1‡	8.9±3.2	ND	[102]
F, M	60 (28.3)	17.4±15.1‡	6.3±3.2	<0.0001	[103]

PRL, prolactin; SLE, systemic lupus erythematosus; N, number of subjects with SLE studied; HPRL, hyperprolactinemic; ND, no data.

*Normal values for serum PRL concentrations were 2–20 ng/ml [95,102], 5–20 ng/ml [96,101], <25 ng/ml [97], <20 ng/ml [98–100], <20 ng/ml for females, and <15 ng/ml for males [103].

**p for mean PRL concentration in SLE vs mean PRL in controls.

†Parentheses enclose range.

‡Mean ± standard deviation.

§Mean ± standard error.

(Adapted with permission from Walker SE, Jacobson JD. [2000]. Roles of prolactin and gonadotropin-releasing hormone in rheumatic diseases. *Rheum Dis Clin North Am.* 26:713–736.)

occurrence of hyperprolactinemia was 1.3%. Hyperprolactinemia clustered in two groups: (1) sera from women 50 years of age and younger who were anti-ds DNA positive (20% hyperprolactinemic) and were thought to have SLE, and (2) sera from women older than 50 years who had antibodies to both Ro and La [92].

Eight men with SLE had serum PRL above the mean [93], and five pregnant patients with lupus had PRL greater than the expected values for gestation [94]. In additional groups, 16–40% of SLE subjects had serum PRL concentrations above the norm [95–103] (Table 104-2). In other surveys, PRL was not elevated in SLE. Ostendorf *et al* [104] found that only four women (2%) in a cohort of 182 patients with SLE had elevated PRL, and Munoz *et al* [105] reported decreases in serum PRL in 14 women with SLE during the luteal phase.

Some investigators found no relationship between PRL levels and disease activity in SLE [96,98–101], but current evidence supports the contention that elevated PRL levels correlate with clinical and/or serologic evidence of active disease [94,95,97, 100,102,103,106,107]. A study of 78 unselected patients with SLE found active lupus in 29 of the patients. PRL concentrations (measured by immunoradiometric assay and biologic assay) in the active patients were significantly greater compared with the patients with inactive disease, and the Toronto SLE Disease Activity Index (SLEDAI) scores had positive correlation with PRL levels. Increased prevalence of malar rash and central nervous system manifestations were significantly more common in patients with hyperprolactinemia compared to those with normal levels of circulating PRL [102]. A second survey compared 60 patients with SLE with 47 normal healthy subjects. Anti-ds DNA antibody levels correlated in a positive manner with serum PRL concentrations, and hyperprolactinemia was associated with fatigue, fever, anemia, elevated erythrocyte sedimentation

rate, decreased C3, and renal manifestations of SLE [103]. Miranda *et al* [108] classified 26 patients with SLE as having mild, moderate, or severely active lupus glomerulonephritis. The individuals with severe renal activity had mean serum PRL concentration of 24.7 ng/ml; this value was significantly greater than serum PRL in the patients with mild renal activity (18.6 ng/ml; $p < 0.05$). Those with severe renal activity also had elevated levels of urine PRL.

In juvenile SLE, one study found no relationship between serum PRL and disease. PRL did not differ between 37 children with SLE and 51 healthy children [109]. Another survey of 33 prepubertal children revealed hyperprolactinemia in three (9%). All three of the children with hyperprolactinemia had central nervous system complications of SLE (one with psychosis, two with cognitive dysfunction). In contrast, only 10% of patients with normal PRL had central nervous system involvement [110].

L. Causes of Hyperprolactinemia in Systemic Lupus Erythematosus

It is not known if the pituitary or activated lymphocytes [111] are the source of excessive circulating PRL in SLE. Certainly, the anterior pituitary contributes much of the circulating hormone. Some individuals with hyperprolactinemia and SLE have prolactinomas [51,112], and others have hyperprolactinemia secondary to recognized causes such as drugs, hypothyroidism, or renal insufficiency [10,92]. It has been suggested that low levels of homovanillic acid in SLE reflect impaired dopamine turnover and altered dopaminergic tone, which can affect pituitary PRL secretion [113]. Circulating cytokines that pass through SLE-damaged cerebral vessels and cross the blood–brain barrier in SLE may also stimulate the anterior pituitary to release excessive PRL [10].

Circulating antibodies to PRL contribute to hyperprolactinemia in SLE. These antibodies were identified in 5% of 259 consecutive SLE patients [107]. Of patients with hyperprolactinemia and SLE, 41% had macroprolactinemia consisting of circulating IgG PRL complexes, thought to represent PRL–anti-PRL [114]. The presence of anti-PRL antibodies has not been found to correlate with increased disease activity in SLE. Rather, antibody-positive individuals had low indices of active lupus [107,114]. The attenuation of disease could have resulted from anti-PRL antibodies interfering with PRL binding to receptors on lymphocytes, leading to functional inactivation of PRL. Anti-PRL antibody-positive individuals with SLE did, however, have significantly higher serum PRL (mean, 33.2 ng/ml) compared to patients with SLE without anti-PRL (mean, 11.6 ng/ml; $p = 0.0001$) [107]. Hyperprolactinemia in these cases could have resulted from anti-PRL interference with feedback mechanisms involved in regulation of pituitary secretion of PRL. PRL bound to anti-PRL has the potential to present a falsely low concentration of circulating PRL to the hypothalamus and anterior pituitary, resulting in compensatory oversecretion of the hormone.

High–molecular-weight immunoglobulin-PRL complexes may be retained within the vascular system, so that the PRL has limited access to targets in the central nervous system and the immune system. A longitudinal study of a pregnant woman with SLE showed that bioactive 150-kDa PRL (big big PRL) was the predominant circulating form of PRL. In contrast, healthy pregnant women had circulating monomeric PRL. When the patient's serum was injected into rats, the IgG-PRL complex was cleared more slowly than serum that contained predominantly monomeric PRL [115].

M. Prolactin-Lowering Therapy for Autoimmune Diseases

Some autoimmune diseases respond favorably to treatment with bromocriptine, an ergot derivative with potent dopamine receptor agonist activity that selectively inhibits secretion of PRL from the anterior pituitary. These responses support the contention that PRL can stimulate autoimmune responses. Bromocriptine therapy causes a prompt and marked decrease in serum PRL and is used to treat microprolactinoma, acromegaly, symptomatic hyperprolactinemia, and parkinsonism. Undesirable side effects include nausea, orthostatic hypotension, headache, fatigue, abdominal cramps, nasal congestion, and constipation. Serious adverse events have been almost completely limited to those instances in which bromocriptine was either used to suppress postpartum lactation or given in high doses to treat Parkinson's disease [116–119].

II. Immunosuppressive Effects of Bromocriptine

It has been proposed that bromocriptine suppresses immunity through decreased pituitary secretion of PRL [120,121]. Macrophages from bromocriptine-treated mice had deficient production of IFN-gamma that was reversed by treating the animals with ovine PRL [122]. However, bromocriptine can suppress cells of the immune system directly. Bromocriptine inhibited proliferation and immunoglobulin production in mitogen-stimulated cultures of human tonsil B cells and inhibited T-cell activation in a system in which the inhibition was independent of the extracellular PRL concentration [123,124].

Neidhart [125] provided convincing evidence that the immunosuppressive effects of bromocriptine were directly related to its ability to suppress pituitary secretion of PRL in an animal model of autoimmune disease. Bromocriptine did suppress proliferation of mitogen-stimulated mouse splenocytes. The lowest suppressive bromocriptine concentration, however, was 200 ng/ml. In contrast, the circulating level of bromocriptine in autoimmune F_1 hybrid NZB/NZW mice was 2–6 ng/ml. In the presence of this low level of bromocriptine, the mice had amelioration of autoimmune disease with reduced severity of renal disease. Because the bromocriptine concentration that suppressed in vitro immune responsiveness was 33–100 times greater than the serum bromocriptine concentration in treated mice, it was concluded that suppression of autoimmune disease was achieved by decreasing pituitary PRL secretion, not by directly suppressing lymphocyte proliferation.

A. Prevention of Autoimmune Disease in Animal Models

Prophylactic treatment with bromocriptine decreased the incidence of experimental autoimmune uveitis in female Lewis rats [126] and inhibited experimental allergic encephalomyelitis (EAE) and adjuvant arthritis (AA) [127–130]. Early treatment with bromocriptine ameliorated the severity of spontaneous SLE in female NZB/NZW mice. McMurray et al [34] used a bromocriptine dose that had been shown to suppress serum PRL to 8 ng/ml in swim-stressed NZB/NZW females, compared with 76 ng/ml in stressed female controls. Treatment began before the appearance of overt autoimmune disease and continued throughout the lifespans of the mice. At the age of 24 weeks, anti-ds DNA antibodies were decreased in treated mice compared to controls, and survival was prolonged significantly in the bromocriptine-treated mice. The protective effects of bromocriptine were confirmed by Elbourne et al [38]. Oophorectomized NZB/NZW mice that received bromocriptine from the age of 6 weeks developed autoimmune disease of intermediate severity. Concurrent treatment with high-dose estrogen did not accelerate disease in the bromocriptine-treated mice, a result implying that PRL was a more important determinant of disease severity than estrogen in NZB/NZW mice.

B. Treatment of Established Autoimmune Disease in Animal Models

In some experimental models, bromocriptine treatment was effective after clinical signs of disease appeared. EAE was suppressed in Lewis rats that received bromocriptine either 1 week after immunization or after clinical signs were noted [131,132]. The spontaneously diabetic BB rat had decreased severity of disease following treatment with both bromocriptine and cyclosporine [130,133]. Nonobese diabetic (NOD) mice had varying responses to bromocriptine therapy. Early treatment with bromocriptine, 200 µg injected daily from the age of 21 days, reduced the incidence of diabetes [134]. In contrast, long-term treatment with a higher dose (300 µg, 5 days a week) accelerated the onset of diabetes and increased islet inflammation in NOD mice [135].

Bromocriptine suppressed the severity of spontaneous peri-arteritis in aged Sprague-Dawley rats [130] and effectively treated animal models of SLE after signs of autoimmunity were present. BALB/c mice with two separate induced autoimmune states—either SLE induced by injected human anti-ds DNA monoclonal antibody or antiphospholipid syndrome induced by injected monoclonal mouse anti-cardiolipin antibody—responded to bromocriptine. The SLE mice had decreased glomerular deposition of immunoglobulin, and mice with antiphospholipid syndrome had decreased activated partial thromboplastin time and fewer resorbed fetuses [136]. Neidhart [125] reported that a PRL-suppressing dose of bromocriptine was beneficial in mature NZB/NZW females. Treatment was started at 36 weeks of age when the mice were expected to have clinical SLE and proteinuria and histologic evidence of glomerulonephritis were suppressed.

III. Bromocriptine Treatment of Autoimmune Diseases in Humans

Bromocriptine has been effective in treating autoimmune illnesses in humans. Hedner and Bynke [137] were the first to report success with bromocriptine in four individuals with iridocyclitis and ankylosing spondylitis, iritis with reactive arthritis, and iridocyclitis. In another series 14 individuals with sight-threatening, corticosteroid-resistant uveitis received bromocriptine combined with cyclosporine. Serum prolactin levels were suppressed below 2 ng/ml, and visual acuity improved markedly in eight patients [138]. In a double-blind study of 15 patients with recurrent anterior uveitis, seven subjects were randomized to receive bromocriptine, 5 mg/day, and eight subjects received placebo for 48 weeks. Two bromocriptine-treated patients and five controls had recurrences [139].

Four men with severe reactive arthritis responded dramatically to bromocriptine treatment [140]. In contrast, PRL-lowering therapy did not consistently benefit patients with RA. Only four of nine women treated with bromocriptine had improved RA according to American College of Rheumatology criteria [141]. A dopamine agonist, quinagolide, was given to nine subjects for 24 weeks, and serum PRL concentrations were suppressed to levels below detection within 4 weeks of starting treatment. Two patients met European League Against Rheumatism criteria for moderate response, but there was no improvement in the erythrocyte sedimentation rate or C-reactive protein [142]. The failure of RA to respond to dopamine agonists may indicate that PRL is not associated with disease activity. It is also possible that lymphocyte PRL, which has the potential to promote intraarticular inflammation [74,75], is not suppressed by bromocriptine.

Results from one older study suggested that hyperprolactinemia might benefit patients with RA. Thirteen patients with rheumatic disease (thought to be RA) received intramuscular ovine PRL in an uncontrolled study. Seven improved rapidly, three had moderate improvement, and three did not improve [143].

Although bromocriptine was effective in treating EAE [131,132] and diabetes mellitus [133–135] in experimental animals, it was not effective in humans with multiple sclerosis or diabetes mellitus. An open-label study of bromocriptine treatment in multiple sclerosis gave disappointing results. Patients with either the relapsing-remitting or chronic-progressive form of multiple sclerosis received 5 mg/day. Clinical relapses, new lesions on magnetic resonance imaging (MRI) of the brain and brainstem, and increased visual or auditory evoked responses showed progression in 14 of the 15 subjects who completed 1 year of treatment [144]. Bromocriptine was given to 15 diabetic subjects in a 16-week double-blind study, and seven subjects received placebo. Treatment was associated with small but significant decreases of hemoglobin A1c and fasting plasma glucose. There were, however, no changes in body composition, body fat distribution, oral glucose tolerance, insulin-mediated glucose disposal, or endogenous glucose production [145]. Atkison [146] found no advantage in combining bromocriptine with cyclosporine treatment of insulin-dependent diabetes.

IV. Bromocriptine Treatment of Human Systemic Lupus Erythematosus

Several case reports have described the successful use of bromocriptine to treat active SLE. A patient with SLE who was not reported to be hyperprolactinemic had central nervous system lupus and was resistant to conventional therapy. She improved after treatment with bromocriptine and intravenous IgG. In two instances, the disease flared after bromocriptine was discontinued [147, L. Schanberg, personal communication]. Four women with symptomatic hyperprolactinemia had mild SLE characterized by photosensitivity, malar rash, arthralgias, and positive FANA tests with titers ranging from 1:320 to 1:640. Two had antibodies to ds-DNA. None had renal involvement. Three of these patients had pituitary microadenomas, all had normal serum concentrations of 17-beta estradiol, and two had suppressed serum testosterone. In two cases, SLE flared after bromocriptine was stopped [51].

Funauchi et al [148] reported concordance between serum PRL concentrations and SLE disease activity in a 31-year-old woman with SLE who had a prolactinoma. Her disease manifestations included polyarthralgia, facial erythema, low-grade fever, thrombocytopenia, and antinuclear antibodies. She became amenorrheic 12 years after the onset of signs and symptoms of SLE. The plasma PRL was 39 ng/ml (normal concentration 2.9–30.5), and MRI of the brain showed a hyperintense lesion in the pituitary gland. The patient was treated with bromocriptine 2.5 followed by 5 mg/day. Once, bromocriptine was discontinued and circulating PRL increased and the patient experienced a lupus flare. Over a period of 6 years, 29 serial measurements of PRL had positive correlation with levels of anti-DNA antibodies.

A. Bromocriptine Trials in Systemic Lupus Erythematosus

McMurray et al [149] treated seven patients with SLE with mild to moderately active disease with bromocriptine in an open-label study. At entry, six patients had normal serum PRL and one had a microprolactinoma and borderline hyperprolactinemia (20.6 ng/ml; normal 2 to 18.5). Each patient received a dose of bromocriptine (3.75–7.5 mg/day) that was adjusted to keep serum PRL below 3 ng/ml. Treatment continued for 6–9 months, and results of the first 6 months of treatment were analyzed. The SLE Activity Measure (SLAM) and the SLEDAI were suppressed significantly, and constitutional symptoms, skin involvement, Raynaud's phenomenon, arthralgias, and arthritis improved. Three of four patients who took prednisone at entry were able to reduce the dose during treatment. After bromocriptine was stopped, five patients became hyperprolactinemic and all subjects had increased lupus activity. In six individuals, changes in medication were required to control lupus activity during the follow-up period.

The patients with SLE treated with bromocriptine experienced improvement in mood states, as measured by the Symptom Questionnaire survey. Total distress scores improved, and this improvement correlated positively with improvement in both the SLAM and the SLEDAI. The anger-hostility measure decreased during bromocriptine treatment. Improvement in this measure did not correlate with improved disease activity, and this observation raised the question that bromocriptine may have exerted favorable psychotropic effects [150].

In a double-blind study, Alvarez-Nemeguei et al [151] showed that treatment with a fixed low dose of bromocriptine (2.5 mg/day) reduced lupus flares. Thirty-six of 66 consecutive patients with SLE were randomized to receive a daily low dose of bromocriptine, 2.5 mg, and 30 controls received placebo. Patients entered the study without regard to disease activity, although those with organ failure were excluded. Modest hyperprolactinemia was found at entry in 51% of subjects in the bromocriptine treatment group and 40% of the controls. Subjects were followed prospectively for 2–17 months (mean 12.5 months). Serum PRL was reduced significantly in the bromocriptine treatment group, and there was evidence of clinical improvement after 5 months of treatment. The mean number of flares/patient/month in bromocriptine-treated patients was reduced to 0.08±0.1 vs 0.18±0.2 in controls ($p = 0.03$).

In a separate double-blind study, bromocriptine was compared to hydroxychloroquine in treatment of active but not life-threatening SLE. Patients were randomized to receive either bromocriptine, in a dose designed to suppress serum prolactin to a level less than 1 ng/ml, or hydroxychloroquine, 6 mg/kg for 1 year. Bromocriptine treatment was associated with significantly reduced serum PRL concentrations, and disease activity was decreased significantly compared to entry after 1 year of treatment. Similar improvement occurred in the patients with SLE who were randomized to receive hydroxychloroquine [152].

V. Suggestions for Further Investigations

- How does PRL exert its immunostimulatory effects in inflammatory disease—by distribution of pituitary PRL through the circulatory system or via local overproduction by stimulated lymphocytes?
- Why are some individuals with autoimmune disease hyperprolactinemic?
- Does bromocriptine exert its immunosuppressive effects solely through suppression of pituitary secretion of PRL?

Acknowledgement

This work was supported by the Office of Research and Development, Medical Research Service, Department of Veterans Affairs and grants from the Lupus Foundation of America; The Kansas City, Kansas Chapter of the Lupus Foundation of America; and the American Autoimmune Related Diseases Association, Inc.

References

1. Neill JD, Nagy GM. (1994). Prolactin and its secretion. In: Knobil E, Neill JD, eds. *The physiology of reproduction*. New York: Raven Press. 1833–2860.
2. Montgomery DW. (2001). Prolactin production by immune cells. *Lupus*. 10:665–675.
3. Weigent DA. (1996). Immunoregulatory properties of growth hormone and prolactin. *Pharmacol Ther*. 69:237–257.
4. Yu-Lee LY. (2002). Prolactin modulation of immune and inflammatory responses. *Recent Prog Horm Res*. 57:35–55.
5. Dogusan Z, Hooghe R, Verdood P, et al. (2001). Cytokine-like effects of prolactin in human mononuclear and polymorphonuclear leukocytes. *J Neuroimmunol*. 120:58–66.
6. Matera L, Mori M, Galetto A. (2001). Effect of prolactin on the antigen presenting function of monocyte-derived dendritic cells. *Lupus*. 10:728–734.
7. Walker SE, Jara L, eds. (1998). Special Issue. Prolactin in SLE. *Lupus*. 7:371–420.
8. Walker SE, Yu-Lee LY, eds. (2001). Special Issue. Prolactin and systemic lupus erythematosus: Mechanisms and clinical studies. *Lupus*. 10:659–762.
9. Matera L, Rapaport R, eds. (2002). *Neuroimmune Biology. Vol. 2: Growth and Lactogenic Hormones*. Amsterdam: Elsevier.
10. Walker SE, McMurray RW, Houri JM, et al. (1998). Effects of prolactin in stimulating disease activity in systemic lupus erythematosus. *Proc N Y Acad Sci*. 840:762–772.
11. Walker SE, Jacobson JD. (2000). Roles of prolactin and gonadotropin-releasing hormone in rheumatic diseases. *Rheum Dis Clin North Am*. 26:713–736.
12. Thoreau E, Petridou B, Kelly PA, et al. (1991). Structural symmetry of the extracellular domain of the cytokine/growth hormone/prolactin receptor family and interferon receptors revealed by hydrophobic cluster analysis. *FEBS Lett*. 282:26–31.
13. Dardenne M, Savino W, Gagnerault MC, et al. (1989). Neuroendocrine control of thymic hormonal production. I. Prolactin stimulates *in vivo* and *in vitro* the production of thymulin by human and murine thymic epithelial cells. *Endocrinology*. 125:3–12.
14. De Mello-Cuelho V, Villa-Verde DMS, Dardenne M, et al. (1997). Pituitary hormones modulate cell–cell interactions between thymocytes and thymic epithelial cells. *J Neuroimmunol*. 76:39–49.
15. Mukherjee P, Mastro AM, Hymer WC. (1990) Prolactin induction of interleukin-2 on rat splenic lymphocytes. *Endocrinology*. 126:88–94.
16. Montgomery DW, Shen GK, Ulrich ED, et al. (1992). Human thymocytes express a prolactin-like messenger ribonucleic acid and synthesize bioactive prolactin-like proteins. *Endocrinology*. 131:3019–3026.
17. DiMattia GE, Gellersen B, Bohnet HG, et al. (1988). A human B-lymphoblastoid cell line produces prolactin. *Endocrinology*. 122:2508–2517.
18. Gado K, Rimanoczi E, Hasitz A, et al. (2001). Elevated levels of serum prolactin in patients with advanced multiple myeloma. *Neuroimmunomodulation*. 9:231–236.
19. Hatfill SJ, Kirby R, Hanley M, et al. (1990). Hyperprolactinemia in acute myeloid leukemia and indication of ectopic expression of human prolactin in blast cells of a patient of subtype M4. *Leuk Res*. 14:57–62.
20. Nagy E, Berczi I. (1978). Immunodeficiency in hypophysectomized rats. *Acta Endocrinol*. 89:530–537.
21. Berczi I, Nagy E, Kovacs K, et al. (1981). Regulation of humoral immunity in rats by pituitary hormones. *Acta Endocrinol*. 98:506–513.
22. Berczi I, Nagy E, de Toledo SM, et al. (1990). Pituitary hormones regulate c-myc and DNA synthesis in lymphoid tissue. *J Immunol*. 146:2201–2206.
23. Cross RJ, Campbell JL, Roszman TL. (1989). Potentiation of antibody responsiveness after the transplantation of a syngeneic pituitary gland. *J Neuroimmunol*. 25:29–35.
24. Bryant HU, Holaday JW, Bernton EW. (1989). Cysteamine produces dose-related bidirectional immunomodulatory effects in mice. *J Pharm Exp Ther*. 249:424–429.
25. Grimaldi CM, Michael DJ, Diamond B. (2001). Cutting Edge: Expansion and activation of a population of autoreactive marginal zone B cells in a model of estrogen-induced lupus. *J Immunol*. 167:1886–1890.
26. Peeva E, Grimaldi C, Spatz L, et al. (2000). Bromocriptine restores tolerance in estrogen-treated mice. *J Clin Invest*. 106:1373–1379.

27. Peeva E, Michael D, Cleary J, *et al.* (2003). Prolactin modulates the naïve B cell repertoire. *J Clin Invest.* 111:275–283.

28. Hahn BH. (2002). Animal models of systemic lupus erythematosus. In: Wallace DJ, Hahn BH, eds. *Dubois' Lupus Erythematosus*, Sixth edition. Baltimore: Williams & Wilkins. 339–388.

29. Theofilopoulos AN, Koundouris S, Kono DH, *et al.* (2001). The role of IFN-gamma in systemic lupus erythematosus: a challenge to the Th1/Th2 paradigm in autoimmunity. *Arthritis Res.* 3:136–141.

30. Matera L, Mori M, Geuna M, *et al.* (2000). Prolactin in autoimmunity and antitumor defence. *J Neuroimmunol.* 109:47–55.

31. Tada Y, Ho A, Matsuyama T, *et al.* (1997). Reduced incidence and severity of antigen-induced autoimmune diseases in mice lacking interferon regulatory factor-1. *J Exp Med.* 185:231–238.

32. Walker SE, McMurray RW, Besch-Williford CL, *et al.* (1992). Premature death with bladder outlet obstruction and hyperprolactinemia in New Zealand Black X New Zealand White mice treated with ethinyl estradiol and 17 beta-estradiol. *Arthritis Rheum.* 35:1387–1392.

33. Roubinian JR, Talal N, Greenspan JS, *et al.* (1978). Effect of castration and sex hormone treatment on survival, anti-nucleic acid antibodies and glomerulonephritis in NZB/NZW F1 mice. *J Exp Med.* 147:1568–1583.

34. McMurray R, Keisler D, Kanuckel K, *et al.* (1991). Prolactin influences autoimmune disease activity in the female B/W mouse. *J Immunol.* 147:3780–3787.

35. Walker SE, Allen SH, McMurray RW. (1993). Prolactin and autoimmune disease. *Trends Endocrinol Metabol.* 4:47–151.

36. McMurray RW, Keisler D, Izui S, *et al.* (1994). Hyperprolactinemia in male NZB/NZW (B/W) F1 mice: Accelerated autoimmune disease with normal circulating testosterone. *Clin Immunol Immunopathol.* 71:338–343.

37. McMurray RW, Keisler D, Izui S, *et al.* (1993). Effects of parturition, suckling, and pseudopregnancy on variables of disease activity in the B/W mouse model of systemic lupus erythematosus. *J Rheum.* 20:1143–1151.

38. Elbourne KB, Keisler D, McMurray RW. (1998). Differential effects of estrogen and prolactin on autoimmune disease in the NZB/NZW F1 mouse model of systemic lupus erythematosus. *Lupus.* 7:420–427.

39. Rovensky J, Buc M, Jojda Z, *et al.* (1995). Effect of domperidone-induced hyperprolactinemia on selected immune parameters in healthy women. *Arch Immunol Ther Exp.* (Warsz) 43:221–227.

40. Clodi M, Svoboda T, Kotzmann H, *et al.* (1992). Effect of elevated serum prolactin concentrations on cytokine production and natural killer cell activity. *Neuroendocrinology.* 56:775–779.

41. Koller M, Kotzmann H, Clodi M, *et al.* (1997). Effect of elevated serum prolactin concentrations on the immunophenotype of human lymphocytes, mitogen-induced proliferation and phagocytic activity of polymorphonuclear cells. *Eur J Clin Invest.* 27:662–666.

42. Gerli R, Riccardi C, Nicoletti I, *et al.* (1987). Phenotypic and functional abnormalities of T lymphocytes in pathological hyperprolactinemia. *J Clin Immunol.* 7:463–470.

43. Vidaller A, Guadarrama F, Llorente L, *et al.* (1992). Hyperprolactinemia inhibits natural killer (NK) cell function *in vivo* and its bromocriptine treatment not only corrects it but makes it more efficient. *J Clin Immunol.* 12:210–215.

44. Matera L, Ciccarelli E, Cesano A, *et al.* (1989). Natural killer activity in hyperprolactinemic patients. *Immunopharmacology.* 18:143–146.

45. Pontiroli AE, Falsetti L, Bottazzo G. (1987). Clinical, endocrine, roentgenographic, and immune characterization of hyperprolactinemic women. *Int J Fertil.* 32:81–85.

46. Ishibashi M, Kuzuya N, Sawada S, *et al.* (1991). Anti-thyroid antibodies in patients with hyperprolactinemia. *Endocrinol Jpn.* 38:517–522.

47. Buskila D, Berezin M, Gur H, *et al.* (1995). Autoantibody profile in the sera of women with hyperprolactinemia. *J Autoimmun.* 8:415–424.

48. Toubi E, Gabriel D, Golan TD. (1997). High association between hyperprolactinemia and anticardiolipin antibodies. *J Rheumatol.* 24:1451 (letter).

49. Kawai T, Katoh K, Tani K. (1996). Hyperprolactinemia preceding development of autoimmune disease. *J Rheumatol.* 23:1483–1484.

50. Haga HJ, Rygh T. (1999). The prevalence of hyperprolactinemia in patients with primary Sjögren's syndrome. *J Rheumatol.* 26:1291–1295.

51. McMurray RW, Allen SH, Braun AL, *et al.* (1994). Longstanding hyperprolactinemia associated with systemic lupus erythematosus: Possible hormonal stimulation of an autoimmune disease. *J Rheumatol.* 21:843–850.

52. Draca S, Levic Z. (1996). The possible role of prolactin in the immunopathogenesis of multiple sclerosis. *Med Hypotheses.* 47:89–92.

53. Grinsted L, Heltberg A, Hagen C, *et al.* (1989). Serum sex hormone and gonadotropin concentrations in premenopausal women with multiple sclerosis. *J Intern Med.* 226:241–244.

54. Yamasaki K, Horiuchi I, Minohara M, *et al.* (2000). Hyperprolactinemia in multiple sclerosis. *Intern Med.* 39:296–299.

55. Vernant JC, Cabre P, Smadja D, *et al.* (1997). Recurrent optic neuromyelitis with endocrinopathies: A new syndrome. *Neurology.* 48:58–64.

56. Heesen C, Gold SM, Bruhn M, *et al.* (2002). Prolactin stimulation in multiple sclerosis—an indicator of disease subtypes and activity? *Endocr Res.* 28:9–18.

57. Azar ST, Yamout B. (1999). Prolactin secretion is increased in patients with multiple sclerosis. *Endocr Res.* 25:207–214.

58. Lever EG, McKerron CG. (1984). Auto-immune Addison's disease associated with hyperprolactinaemia. *Clin Endocrinol.* (Oxford) 21:451–457.

59. Legakis I, Petroyianni V, Saramantis A, *et al.* (2001). Elevated prolactin to cortisol ratio and polyclonal autoimmune activation in Hashimoto's thyroiditis. *Horm Metab Res.* 33:585–589.

60. Ferrari C, Boghen M, Paracchi A, *et al.* (1983). Thyroid autoimmunity in hyperprolactinemic disorders. *Acta Endocrinol.* 104:35–41.

61. Pleyer U, Gupta D, Weidle EG, *et al.* (1991). Elevated prolactin levels in human aqueous humor of patients with anterior uveitis. *Graefes Arch Clin Exp Ophthalmol.* 229:447–451.

62. Hedner LP, Bynke G. (1985). Endogenous iridocyclitis relieved during treatment with bromocriptine. *Am J Ophthalmol.* 100:618–619.

63. Palestine AG, Nussenblatt RB, Gelato M. (1988). Therapy for human autoimmune uveitis with low-dose cyclosporine plus bromocriptine. *Transpl Proc Suppl.* 20:131–135.

64. Jara LJ, Silveira LH, Cuellar ML, *et al.* (1994). Hyperprolactinemia in Reiter's syndrome. *J Rheumatol.* 21:1292–1297.

65. Shahin AA, Abdoh S, Abdelrazik M. (2002). Prolactin and thyroid hormones in patients with systemic sclerosis: correlations with disease manifestations and activity. *Z Rheumatol.* 61:703–709.

66. Kucharz EJ, Jarczyk R, Jonderko G, *et al.* (1996). High serum level of prolactin in patients with systemic sclerosis. *Clin Rheumatol.* 15:314.

67. Steinfeld S, Rommes S, Francois C, *et al.* (2000). Big prolactin 60 kDa is overexpressed in salivary glandular epithelial cells from patients with Sjögren's syndrome. *Lab Invest.* 80:239–247.

68. Gutierrez MA, Anaya JM, Scopelitis E, *et al.* (1994). Hyperprolactinaemia in primary Sjögren's syndrome. *Ann Rheum Dis.* 53:425–428.

69. Brennan P, Ollier B, Worthington J, *et al.* (1996). Are both genetic and reproductive associations with rheumatoid arthritis linked to prolactin? *Lancet.* 348:106–109.

70. Rovensky J, Bakosova J, Koska J, *et al.* (2002). Somatotropic, lactotropic and adrenocortical responses to insulin-induced hypoglycemia in patients with rheumatoid arthritis. *Ann N Y Acad Sci.* 966:263–270.

71. Eijsbouts A, van den Hoogen F, Laan R, *et al.* (1998). Similar response of adrenocorticotrophic hormone, cortisol and prolactin to surgery in rheumatoid arthritis and osteoarthritis. *Br J Rheumatol.* 37:1138–1139.

72. Zoli A, Ferlisi EM, Lizzio M, *et al.* (2002). Prolactin/cortisol ratio in rheumatoid arthritis. *Ann N Y Acad Sci.* 966:508–512.

73. Kullich WC, Klein G. (1998). High levels of macrophage inflammatory protein-1alpha correlate with prolactin in female patients with acute rheumatoid arthritis. *Clin Rheumatol.* 17:263–264.

74. Elhassan AM, Adem A, Suliman IA, *et al.* (1999). Prolactin, growth hormone, and IGF-1 in ankles and plasma of adjuvant arthritic rats. *Scand J Rheumatol.* 28:368–373.

75. Nagafuchi H, Suzuki N, Kaneko A, *et al.* (1999). Prolactin locally produced by synovium infiltrating T lymphocytes induces excessive synovial cell functions in patients with rheumatoid arthritis. *J Rheumatol.* 26:1890–1900.

76. Seriolo B, Ferretti V, Sulli A, *et al.* (2002). Serum prolactin concentrations in male patients with rheumatoid arthritis. *Ann N Y Acad Sci.* 966:258–262.

77. Lieberman S, Gurfinkiel M, Damilano S, *et al.* (2002). Prolactin and IgG-prolactin complex levels in patients with rheumatic arthritis. *Ann N Y Acad Sci.* 966:252–257.

78. Mateo L, Nolla JM, Bonnin MR, *et al.* (1998). High serum prolactin levels in men with rheumatoid arthritis. *J Rheumatol.* 25:2077–2082.

79. Templ E, Koeller M, Riedl M, *et al.* (1996). Anterior pituitary function in patients with newly diagnosed rheumatoid arthritis. *Br J Rheumatol.* 35: 350–356.

80. Gutierrez MA, Garcia ME, Rodriguez JA, *et al.* (1999). Hypothalamic–pituitary–adrenal axis function in patients with active rheumatoid arthritis: A controlled study using insulin hypoglycemia stress test and prolactin stimulation. *J Rheumatol.* 26:277–281.

81. Nagy E, Chalmers IM, Barager FD, *et al.* (1991). Prolactin deficiency in rheumatoid arthritis. *J Rheumatol.* 18:1662–1668.

82. Cutolo M, Balleari E, Giusti M, et al. (1986). Sex hormone status in women suffering from rheumatoid arthritis. J Rheumatol. 13:1019–1023.

83. Jiminez-Balderas FJ, Tapia-Serrano R, Madero-Cervera JI, et al. (1990). Ovarian function studies in active ankylosing spondylitis in women. Clinical response to estrogen therapy. J Rheumatol. 17:497–502.

84. Gordon D, Beastall GH, Thomson JA, et al. (1986). Androgenic status and sexual function in males with rheumatoid arthritis and ankylosing spondylitis. Quart J Med. 60:671–679.

85. Tapia-Serrano R, Jimenez-Balderas FJ, Murrieta S, et al. (1991). Testicular function in active ankylosing spondylitis. Therapeutic response to human chorionic gonadotrophin. J Rheumatol. 18:841–848.

86. Buskila D, Fefer P, Harman-Boehm I, et al. (1993). Assessment of non-articular tenderness and prevalence of fibromyalgia in hyperprolactinemic women. J Rheumatol. 20:2112–2115.

87. Adler GK, Kinsley BT, Hurwitz S, et al. (1999). Reduced hypothalamic–pituitary and sympathoadrenal responses to hypoglycemia in women with fibromyalgia syndrome. Am J Med. 106:534–543.

88. Keser G, Oksel F, Ozgen G, et al. (1999). Serum prolactin levels in Behçet's syndrome. Clin Rheumatol. 18:351–352.

89. Apaydin KC, Duranoglu Y, Ozgurel Y, et al. Serum prolactin levels in Behçet's disease. (2000). Jpn J Ophthalmol. 44:442–445.

90. McMurray RW, Allen SH, Pepmueller PH, et al. (1995). Elevated serum prolactin levels in children with juvenile rheumatoid arthritis and antinuclear antibody seropositivity. J Rheumatol. 22:1577–1580.

91. Picco P, Gattorno M, Buoncompagni A, et al. (1998). Prolactin and interleukin 6 in prepubertal girls with juvenile chronic arthritis. J Rheumatol. 25:347–351.

92. Allen SH, Sharp GC, Wang G, et al. (1996). Prolactin levels and antinuclear antibody profiles in women tested for connective tissue disease. Lupus. 5:30–37.

93. Lavalle C, Loto E, Paniagua R, et al. (1987). Correlation study between prolactin and androgens in male patients with systemic lupus erythematosus. J Rheumatol. 14:268–272.

94. Jara-Quezada L, Graef A, Lavalle C. (1991). Prolactin and gonadal hormones during pregnancy in systemic lupus erythematosus. J Rheumatol. 18:349–353.

95. Jara LJ, Gomez-Sanchez C, Silveira LH, et al. (1992). Hyperprolactinemia in systemic lupus erythematosus: Association with disease activity. Am J Med Sci. 303:222–226.

96. Pauzner R, Urowitz MB, Gladman DD, et al. (1994). Prolactin in systemic lupus erythematosus. J Rheumatol. 21:2064–2067.

97. Neidhart M. (1996). Elevated serum prolactin or elevated prolactin/cortisol ratio are associated with autoimmune processes in systemic lupus erythematosus and other connective tissue diseases. J Rheumatol. 23:476–481.

98. Buskila D, Lorber M, Neumann L, et al. (1996). No correlation between prolactin levels and clinical activity in patients with systemic lupus erythematosus. J Rheumatol. 23:629–632.

99. Huang CM, Chou CT. (1997). Hyperprolactinemia in systemic lupus erythematosus. Zhonghua Yi Xue Za Zhi (Taipei). 59:37–41.

100. Rovensky J, Jurankova E, Rauova L, et al. (1997). Relationship between endocrine, immune, and clinical variables in patients with systemic lupus erythematosus. J Rheumatol. 24:2330–2334.

101. Jimena P, Aguirre MA, Lopez-Curbelo A, et al. (1998). Prolactin levels in patients with systemic lupus erythematosus: a case controlled study. Lupus. 7:383–386.

102. Pacilio M, Migliaresi S, Meli R, et al. (2001). Elevated bioactive prolactin levels in systemic lupus erythematosus—Association with disease activity. J Rheumatol. 28:2216–2221.

103. Jacobi AM, Rohde W, Ventz M, et al. (2001). Enhanced serum prolactin (PRL) in patients with systemic lupus erythematosus: PRL levels are related to the disease activity. Lupus. 10:554–561.

104. Ostendorf B, Fischer R, Santen R, et al. (1996). Hyperprolactinemia in systemic lupus erythematosus. Scand J Rheumatol. 25:97–102.

105. Munoz JA, Gil A, Lopez-Dupla JM, et al. (1994). Sex hormones in chronic systemic lupus erythematosus. Correlation with clinical and biological parameters. Ann Med Interne (Paris). 145:459–463.

106. Zoli A, Ferlisi EM, Pompa A, et al. (1999). Basal and after-stimuli test for prolactinemia in systemic lupus erythematosus. Ann N Y Acad Sci. 876:155–158.

107. Leanos-Miranda A, Pascor-Lira D, Chavez-Rueda KA, et al. (2001). Antiprolactin autoantibodies in systemic lupus erythematosus: frequency and correlation with prolactinemia and disease activity. J Rheumatol. 28:1546–1553.

108. Miranda JM, Prieto RE, Paniagua R, et al. (1998). Clinical significance of serum and urine prolactin levels in lupus glomerulonephritis. Lupus. 7:387–391.

109. Athreya BH, Rafferty JH, Sehgal GS, et al. (1993). Adenohypophyseal and sex hormones in pediatric rheumatic diseases. J Rheumatol. 20:725–730.

110. El-Garf A, Salah S, Shaarawy M, et al. (1996). Prolactin hormone in juvenile systemic lupus erythematosus: A possible relationship to disease activity and CNS manifestations. J Rheumatol. 23:374–377.

111. Gutierrez MA, Molina JF, Jara LJ, et al. (1995). Prolactin and systemic lupus erythematosus: Prolactin secretion by SLE lymphocytes and proliferative (autocrine) activity. Lupus. 4:348–352.

112. Jara LJ, Alcala M, Vera-Lastra O, et al. (2003). Hyperprolactinemia secondary to microadenoma and systemic lupus erythematosus: An analysis of 36 cases. Accepted for presentation, 2003 Scientific Session, American College of Rheumatology.

113. Ferreira C, Paes M, Gouveia A, et al. (1998). Plasma homovanillic acid and prolactin in systemic lupus erythematosus. Lupus. 7:392–397.

114. Leanos A, Pascoe D, Fraga A, et al. (1998). Anti-prolactin autoantibodies in systemic lupus erythematosus patients with associated hyperprolactinemia. Lupus. 7:398–403.

115. Leanos-Miranda A, Pascoe-Lira D, Chavez-Rueda, KA, et al. (2001). Persistence of macroprolactinemia due to antiprolactin autoantibody before, during, and after pregnancy in a woman with systemic lupus erythematosus. Clin Endocrinol Metab. 86:2619–2624.

116. Parkes D. (1979). Bromocriptine. N Engl J Med. 301:873–878.

117. Vance ML, Evans WS, Thorner MO. (1984). Bromocriptine. Diagnosis and treatment. Drugs five years later. Ann Intern Med. 100:78–91.

118. McMurray RW. (2001). Bromocriptine in rheumatic and autoimmune diseases. Semin. Arthritis Rheum. 31:21–32.

119. Walker SE. (2002). Effectiveness of bromocriptine in the treatment of autoimmune diseases. In: Matera L, Rapaport R, eds. Neuroimmune Biology. Vol. 2: Growth and Lactogenic Hormones. Amsterdam: Elsevier. 287–296.

120. Hiestand PC, Mekler P, Nordmann R, et al. (1986). Prolactin as a modulator of lymphocyte responsiveness provides a possible mechanism of action for cyclosporine. Proc Natl Acad Sci U S A. 83:2599–2603.

121. Nagy E, Berczi I, Wren GE, et al. (1983). Immunomodulation by bromocriptine. Immunopharmacology. 6:231–243.

122. Bernton EW, Meltzer MS, Holaday JW. (1988). Suppression of macrophage activation and T-lymphocyte function in hypoprolactinemic mice. Science. 239:401–404.

123. Morikawa K, Oseko F, Morikawa S. (1993). Immunosuppressive property of bromocriptine on human B lymphocyte function in vitro. Clin Exp Immunol. 93:200–205.

124. Morikawa K, Oseko F, Morikawa S. (1994). Immunosuppressive activity of bromocriptine on human T lymphocyte function in vitro. Clin Exp Immunol. 95:514–518.

125. Neidhart M. (1997). Bromocriptine has little direct effect on murine lymphocytes, the immunomodulatory effect being mediated by the suppression of prolactin secretion. Biomed Pharmacother. 51:118–125.

126. Palestine AG, Muellenberg-Coulombre CG, Kim MK, et al. (1987). Bromocriptine and low dose cyclosporine in the treatment of experimental autoimmune uveitis in the rat. J Clin Invest. 79:1078–1081.

127. Neidhart M. (1996). Synergism between long-acting bromocryptine microcapsules and cyclosporine A in the prevention of various autoimmune diseases in rats. Experientia. 52:892–899.

128. Riskind PN, Massacesi L, Doolittle TH, et al. (1991). The role of prolactin in autoimmune demyelination: Suppression of experimental allergic encephalomyelitis by bromocriptine. Ann Neurol. 29:542–547.

129. Berczi B, Nagy E, Asa SL, et al. (1984). The influence of pituitary hormones on adjuvant arthritis. Arthritis Rheum. 27:682–688.

130. Neidhart M. (1989). Bromocriptine microcapsules inhibit ornithine decarboxylase activity induced by Freund's complete adjuvant in lymphoid tissues of male rats. Endocrinology. 125:2846–2852.

131. Dijkstra CD, Rouppe van der Voort E, De Groot CJA, et al. (1992). The therapeutic effect of bromocriptine on acute and chronic experimental allergic encephalomyelitis. Ann Neurol. 31:450–451.

132. Dijkstra CD, Rouppe van der Voort E, De Groot CJA, et al. (1994). Therapeutic effect of the D2-dopamine agonist bromocriptine on acute and relapsing experimental allergic encephalomyelitis. Psychoneuroendocrinology. 19:135–142.

133. Mahon JL, Gunn HC, Stobie K, et al. (1998). The effect of bromocriptine and cyclosporine on spontaneous diabetes in BB rats. Transplant Proc. 20(Suppl):197–200.

134. Hawkins TA, Gala RR, Dunbar JC. (1994). Prolactin modulates the incidence of diabetes in male and female NOD mice. Autoimmunity. 18:155–162.

135. Durant S, Alves V, Coulaud J, *et al*. (1995). Attempts to pharmacologically modulate prolactin levels and type 1 autoimmune diabetes in the non-obese diabetic (NOD) mouse. *J Autoimmun*. 8:875–885.

136. Blank M, Krause I, Busila D, *et al*. (1995). Bromocriptine immunomodulation of experimental SLE and primary anti-phospholipid syndrome via induction of nonspecific T suppressor cells. *Cell Immunol*. 162:114–122.

137. Hedner LP, Bynke G. (1985). Endogenous iridocyclitis relieved during treatment with bromocriptine. *Am J Ophthalmol*. 100:618–619.

138. Palestine AG, Nussenblatt RB, Gelato M. (1988). Therapy for human autoimmune uveitis with low-dose cyclosporine plus bromocriptine. *Transpl Proc*. 20:131–135.

139. Schaaf L, Zierhut M, Baur EM, *et al*. (1991). Bromocriptine in patients with chronic autoimmune-associated disorders. *Klin Wochenschr*. 69:943.

140. Bravo G, Zazueta B, Lavalle C. (1992). An acute remission of Reiter's syndrome in male patients treated with bromocriptine. *J Rheumatol*. 19:747–750.

141. Figueroa FE, Carrion F, Martinez ME, *et al*. (1997). Bromocriptine induces immunological changes related to disease parameters in rheumatoid arthritis. *Br J Rheumatol*. 36:1022–1023.

142. Eijsbouts A, van den Hoogen F, Laan R, *et al*. (1999). Treatment of rheumatoid arthritis with the dopamine agonist quinagolide. *J Rheumatol*. 26:2284–2285.

143. Ingvarsson CG. (1969). Prolactin in rheumatoid arthritis (A therapeutic test). *Acta Rheum Scand*. 15:4–17.

144. Bissay V, De Klippel N, Herroelen L, *et al*. (1994). Bromocriptine therapy in multiple sclerosis: an open label pilot study. *Clin Neuropharmacol*. 17:473–476.

145. Wasada T, Kawahara R, Iwamoto Y. (2000). Lack of evidence for bromocriptine effect on glucose tolerance, insulin resistance, and body fat stores in obese type 2 diabetic patients. *Diabetes Care*. 23:1040.

146. Atkison PR, Mahon JL, Dupre J, *et al*. (1990). Interaction of bromocriptine and cyclosporine in insulin dependent diabetes mellitus: results from the Canadian open study. *J Autoimmun*. 3:793–797.

147. Rabiniovich CE, Schanberg LE, Kredich DW. (1990). Intravenous immunoglobulin and bromocriptine in the treatment of refractory neuropsychiatric systemic lupus erythematosus. *Arthritis Rheum*. 33 (Suppl.), R22 (Abstract).

148. Funauchi M, Ikoma S, Enomoto H, *et al*. (1998). Prolactin modulates the disease activity of systemic lupus erythematosus accompanied by prolactinoma. *Clin Exp Rheumatol*. 16:479–482.

149. McMurray RW, Weidensaul D, Allen SH, *et al*. (1995). Efficacy of bromocriptine in an open label therapeutic trial for systemic lupus erythematosus. *J Rheumatol*. 22:2084–2091.

150. Walker SE, Smarr KL, Parker JC, *et al*. (2000). Mood states and disease activity in patients with systemic lupus erythematosus treated with bromocriptine. *Lupus*. 9:527–533.

151. Alvarez-Nemeguei J, Cobarrubias-Cobbs A, Escalante-Triay F, *et al*. (1998). Bromocriptine in systemic lupus erythematosus: A double-blind, randomized, placebo-controlled study. *Lupus*. 7:414–419.

152. Walker SE, Reddy GH, Miller D, *et al*. (1999). Treatment of active systemic lupus erythematosus (SLE) with the prolactin (PRL) lowering drug, bromocriptine (BC): Comparison with hydroxychloroquine (HC) in a randomized, blinded one-year study. *Arthritis Rheum*. 42, S282 (abstract).

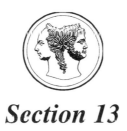

Section 13

AGING

Kevin C. Fleming, MD

Consultant, Division of General Internal Medicine, Mayo Clinic; Assistant Professor of Medicine,
CAQ and Fellowship, Geriatrics, Mayo Medical School, Rochester, MN

In the first decades of the new century, much of the developed world has already begun to experience a dramatically changed distribution by age. In America, the baby boomers have long dominated the population and its culture, and this cohort is now entering old age. Within 20 years, America will join nations such as Italy and Japan wherein the elderly comprise fully a fifth or more of its people. The "demographic imperative," the aging of first world societies, is predicted to have a profound impact on families, politics, and economics.

The graying of America will similarly alter health care for its aging citizens (if not for all of us). Interest in the medical aspects of old age has waxed and waned in the last 150 years, with the most recent renaissance spanning some 20 years. *Elderly* has been traditionally defined by the government, researchers, and employers as people older than the age of 65. However, in geriatric medicine, age alone often provides little useful information. There is considerable variation in the rate of aging in the human species, resulting in great differences among individuals. Nevertheless, disease accumulation, disability, and frailty increasingly characterize this cohort after age 75 or so.

Illness in old age differs from that in younger patients in many respects by reduced physiologic reserve, the atypical (or bland) presentation of disease, and multiple co-morbidities. It is well recognized that the medications used to address these illnesses can themselves result in further impairments. This is more likely in older patients who are taking numerous drugs for their many disorders and symptoms. In contrast to the rapid rebound seen among pediatric patients, delayed and incomplete recoveries among the elderly are often the rule. As a result, specialists in geriatrics have historically adopted the restoration and optimization of function as the primary goals of good care for older persons.

For the elderly of the modern era, it may be the best of times and the worst of times. Public health measures, medical treatments, and technologic advances have permitted great longevity for larger numbers of people than ever before, and often these years are spent in quite good health and physical function. For a significant proportion, however, these years can be spent in a lengthy decline marked by combined losses in social, economic, and health spheres. In contrast to a century ago, it is increasing wealth, rather than poverty, that now defines older Americans. However, for many baby boomers, personal savings and the safety net of social insurance may prove to be insufficient to fund old age.

Somewhat surprisingly, the role of gender in aging has not been long explored. This is surprising in that gender differences have been discussed and debated for decades in nearly all disciplines and in every possible sphere (e.g., economic, social, political, and health care). That old age would have thus far been less studied from the aspect of gender is not surprising because it is only within the latter half of the 20th century that significantly large numbers of people began to reach old age. As what was once rare becomes common, it is likely that interest in the various aspects of aging will further expand, including that of gender. Much as the effects of race and gender on medicine and medical care have been increasingly studied, the similarities and differences between male and female older adults will no doubt intensify.

In the following chapters, various aspects of the interplay between aging and gender are explored. It is notable that much of the current scientific literature has largely been focused on aging per se. Therefore, the knowledge about differences in aging between men and women is of a more limited nature than that known for younger cohorts (a condition unlikely to persist for long, no doubt). Regardless, there are already many useful distinctions to explore in the physiology, diseases, and socioeconomics of aging in the chapters to follow. It is this foundation on which the possible future of elder medicine will be built.

105

A History of Old Age in America

KEVIN C. FLEMING, MD

Consultant, Division of General Internal Medicine, Mayo Clinic; Assistant Professor of Medicine, CAQ and Fellowship,
Geriatrics, Mayo Medical School, Rochester, MN

I. Introduction

The looming increase in the population of older adults has been described as "the demographic imperative" or "the graying of America." These simply underscore the fact that a huge post World War II baby boom population is expected to survive well into their eighties and nineties. Whereas life expectancy at birth in 1900 was 49 years, in just a century this has reached 75 years. By the year 2020, one in five Americans will be older than 65. The last epoch in western history to experience a large percentage of elderly was during the Black Death in the Middle Ages, when 15% of the population was older than 60, because older adults were spared infection from bubonic plague [1].

To say "There will be many old people" is interesting, but what does it mean to individuals, families, and society? The lives of today's elderly have deep historical precedents by which one can better understand current social policies, health care, and retirement. In the following pages, I analyze America's past for its traditions and approaches to aging. The history of the elderly poor, long-term care, health care financing, and the regulatory environment have great relevance to current old age concerns and can inform discussions on aging's future.

II. Growing Old in Early America

A. A Small Minority

From 1650 to 1850, the elderly in America were few in number, comprising less than 2% of the population. In those times of high fertility and high mortality, old age was commonly defined as life after age 60. Many children did not survive the dangers of infancy and young adulthood. In some regions, 40% of all deaths were among children younger than 2 [2]. As late as 1870, only 3% of the U.S. population were 65 or older and just 0.37% were older than 80. The corresponding figures for England were 4.7% and 0.65% (in 1851), reflecting the large number of young immigrants in America [3].

In part because survival to old age was rare, older citizens were imbued with the mystique of wisdom. Most elderly in early America lived in nuclear households or with an unmarried child. The aged were generally treated with deference and respect, according to cultural norms and religious tradition. However, control of valuable farmland by elder patriarchs also contributed to economic, familial, and political authority through the potential for inheritance. However, there were few aged poor, because longevity was only possible among the privileged classes. Seen as a burden on the local taxes, the destitute elderly were not venerated but often despised and treated as outcasts [4–6].

1. The Status of Women

The Puritan patriarchy held and enforced traditional ideals that often regarded women as "one step above the beasts in the field" [7]. According to cultural norms, men were relied on to rule, protect, and provide for their wives, who were expected to remain subordinate. Ignorance of gynecology (e.g., associating evil with menstruation and childbirth) and fear of female sexuality were amplified by anxieties over novel inheritance patterns in the New World that permitted women a degree of independence not previously possible. Such concerns, for example, often lay at the heart of witchcraft accusations, the majority of which fell on middle-aged and elderly women on the periphery of society, including beggars, slaves, and unmarried women [8]. The independence of a wealthy widow, and the deference generally paid to the upper classes, contrasted markedly with the lives of most widows, who were usually quite poor. Impoverished older women were feared not only for their economic dependence but also for their physical appearance. The "twisted and gnarled" bodies and loss of youthful beauty were associated with satanic forces [9]. Notably, this view of the witch as an ugly old woman persists today.

Nevertheless, women in the colonial period from 1650 to 1740 experienced a stable and expanding economy and little crime. To augment family income, and consistent with the Protestant ethic of hard work and thrift, more women sought paid employment. They began moving into occupations previously dominated by men, such as teaching, weaving, and tailoring. In addition, widows and retirees were able to retain their independence (and continue to live in their own homes) through mortgages, bonds, and interest-bearing notes, securing a degree of financial freedom that had eluded many in Europe [10].

B. The Status of Elders

During the 17th and 18th centuries, most families and communities were dominated by religious and social principles endorsing male hierarchy, with economic dependence and reciprocal obligation between the generations. Frailty and decline in old age were considered to be natural and inevitable, part of man's punishment for original sin. However, this belief was coupled with the hope for redemption and a blessed afterlife. Survival into old age, infrequent as it was, signified a "distinguishing favor" from God. Aging was felt to be an integral component of life's journey, its final stage. Among Puritans, the male pilgrim faced the evils of the spiritual road quite alone, and the physical decay of aging was feared. For Puritan women, however, the traditional medieval pattern persisted. The ideal woman, a pilgrim on life's spiritual journey, accepted physical decline with grace and equanimity, using life experiences and nurturing relationships for spiritual progress. Thus, these "natural stages of life" provided religious meaning and social standing for aging men and women [11].

About the time of the American Revolution, a similar revolution in age relations occurred. Old age began to decline in status, and a new youth culture arose. From 1770 to 1820, the cultural shift away from an esteemed old age was reflected in language, dress, customs, and art. In meeting halls, front row seats were no longer reserved for the elderly. Fashion came to favor a more youthful look; white wigs were dropped in favor of toupees, and clothing ceased to flatter the older frame. Although people had once commonly pretended to be older than they actually were, claimed ages in the census drifted downward from this time on. Children were less frequently named after grandparents, and contempt for the old began to be expressed in terms like "old fogey," "codger," and "geezer." Around 1790, for the first time, retirement from public office at 60 or 70 became mandatory in many states. The ideal of age equality overthrew the "tyranny of age," and the exaltation of the old began to be replaced by the cult of youth [5].

Analysis of early American family structure reveals power relations between fathers and sons and the limits of the sons' autonomy determined by marriage, landholding, and inheritance. By the end of the 18th century however, patriarchal control was weakened in part by a land shortage, which led to the dispersal of sons and outmigration [12]. By common law, widows inherited one third of household goods and controlled one third of the real estate, usually generating sufficient maintenance income. Until the 20th century, property laws held greater protection for women's property obtained through parental inheritance or by gift. Authority vested in husbands and fathers thus left a woman with lesser control over property she had helped build in the course of a marriage. For additional security then, women exerted their collective moral and social authority within family and kin networks, developing places to turn for alternative support.

> "A woman who faced early death from childbirth counted on her sisters to protect her children from mistreatment . . . [and] elderly widows counted on their daughters and daughters-in-law to nurse them in reciprocity for prior care" [13].

Elderly women after the American Revolution sought to remain pious and to be useful by serving as models of moral integrity for the new nation. The female virtues accorded aged women of the day emphasized piety, submissiveness, domesticity, and service to others. Aged matriarchs were valued primarily in having set good examples for younger women by living the virtuous Christian life. Because motherhood was felt to be the most important female occupation among younger women, older women were thus revered for having been good mothers [14]. Elderly women were further esteemed for Christ-like submission, bearing the pain and suffering of old age with quiet and patient resignation. Physical decline as one grew old was considered part of one's spiritual atonement at the end of life. "Emphasizing sickness and dependency highlighted the elderly's proximity to death and was meant to spur efforts to prepare for future judgment" [15]. In addition, older women

were able to maintain continuity and connection among family and friends in their declining years. The lives of aging men, however, were more narrowly defined. A fall from power and loss of public status were often the primary markers of this stage in the life course of older men. Elderly men were thus seen as weaker, without authority, and more feminine. Although little documented, it is likely that most men never achieved significant public status in their lifetimes. Given the male yardstick of power and social achievement, their gendered experience in old age perhaps suffers in comparison to that of elderly women [16]. This issue is poignantly revisited in the 20th century in Arthur Miller's *Death of a Salesman:*

> "Willy Loman never made a lot of money. His name was never in the paper. . . . He's not to be allowed to fall into his grave like an old dog. Attention, attention must be finally paid to such a person" [17].

The Victorian era of the 19th century promoted the virtues of independence, success, and healthy living. The ideal self-made man practiced a strict regimen of self-denial and industriousness. The ideal Victorian woman followed a regimen of domestic and spiritual activities, relegated to the "woman's sphere." Longevity was no longer viewed as a gift from God but was rather felt to be a reward for proper behavior, hygiene, and self-discipline. Indeed a rising belief in human perfectibility led to popular health reform and a public movement that assumed all people were naturally healthy and that disease was caused by violation of fixed scientific laws [11]. However, around 1850, average life expectancy was a mere 39.5 years, and infant mortality claimed 22% of live births. Nearly half of all deaths occurred before age 15; less than 15% occurred after age 60 [18]. Pursuit of perfect health and longevity promised that good habits would lead to an old age characterized by good health and self-reliance. However, these beliefs had a darker implication. Physical decline and dependency in an elder meant a lack of discipline and implied that one's life had been immoral. Pain and suffering in old age now invoked feelings of shame and a sense of failure [11].

C. Age Stratification

In many ways, social customs and cultural expressions of early America often tended to ignore age distinctions. Although antebellum America recognized four loose stages of life (infancy, youth, maturity, and senescence), adults in preindustrial society were generally not segregated by age from farm work, social affairs, or community activities. Contemporary novels, diaries, autobiographies, and books on etiquette attest to the absence of age-based norms, often only recognizing childhood as a separate class, with manhood occurring as early as age 10. For example, birthdays were accorded no special observance until the latter half of the 19th century [2]. U.S. Census data confirm the lack of older age distinctions until 1830. At that time, older adults were blurred among those 45 years and over. Before 1850, blacks had even fewer age classifications than did whites (Table 105-1) [19].

By the end of the 19th century, however, stratification by age became institutionalized in American life. Cultural transitions

Table 105-1
Change in Categories in U.S. Census Over Time

U.S. Census	Age-Based Categories
1790	White males older than age 16
1800	Free whites ages younger than 10, 10–15, 16–25, 26–44, 45 yr and older
1820	Free whites ages younger than 10, 10–15, 16–25, 26–44, 45 yr and older
	Free colored and slaves ages younger than 14, 14–25, 26–44, 45 yr and older
1830	Free whites: younger than 5, 5–9, 10–14, 15–19, 20–29, 30–39, . . . , 90–99, 100+
	Free colored and slaves: younger than 10, 10–23, 24–35, 36–54, 55–99, 100+
1850	Free whites, free colored, and slaves: 1–4, 5–9, 10–14, 15–19, 20–29, . . . , 90–99, 100+
1880	Males and females 5–17, males 18–44; males 21 yr and older

such as school attendance, marriage, and retirement began to be based on age. This arose in part due to the needs of a modern industrial society for a different kind of economic order and social control. The relative timelessness of early America no longer served the new era, now based on science, time clocks, and calendars. Age categories would thus come to serve as an organizing principle for education, work, welfare, leisure, and retirement [2].

D. Old Age Devalued

By 1900, the failure of the Victorian vision of natural health to produce a good old age free of decay and dependence led to a backlash against the elderly. The universal optimism that strict adherence to natural health laws ensured a long and healthy life gave way to increasing pessimism about the prospect of aging. The rise of the industrial state compounded this rejection, reducing the value of the elderly (if not all individuals) to their mere capacity for production. In short order, the prevailing corporate view of "man as machine" found the elderly (primarily men at this time) to be burdensome, irrelevant, full of disease, and economically worthless [11]. Indeed, studies at the time suggested that intellectual and economic prowess peaked at age 40, declining quickly thereafter. This prompted physician William Osler's farewell comments at the 1905 Johns Hopkins University School of Medicine commencement on the absolute "uselessness of men above sixty years of age." He concluded that such men should be retired, and further mentioned (jokingly) a suggestion, attributed to Anthony Trollope's novel *The Fixed Period*, that men older than that age be chloroformed [20]. (These comments would be echoed 80 years later when Governor Richard Lamm of Colorado infamously stated that very ill elderly people "have a duty to die and get out of the way" [21].)

With the dawn of the 20th century, the status of seniors had reached a nadir. Reductions in mortality contributed to the presence of increasing numbers of older adults. The continued entry into the United States of young nonindustrial peoples

with distinctive cultures helped create the perception of an immigrant American working class comprised of "the depraved, the cesspool of Europe" [22]. However, despite the class and ethnic bias these prejudices generated, the massive influx of youthful laborers created enormous pressures on older workers in a highly competitive market. At the same time, advances in medicine, science, and big business led to a devaluation of the elderly, whose remaining years were now felt to be bounded by dependency, decay, and dementia. Old age itself was felt to be a disease. Not surprisingly, equating old age with obsolescence resulted in cultural ramifications such as job loss, early retirement, and segregation into rest homes [6,23].

The modern scientific and industrial era thus deemed old age "a problem to be solved," and elder obsolescence legitimated age discrimination and mandatory retirement. These concepts soon became embedded in government and workplace settings and created a life course sequence for men (i.e., education, then labor, then retirement) that persists to this day [24]. The principles of industrial scientific management were felt to be the modern solution to the old age problem. The elderly were felt to need management, by segregation out of the workplace and into retirement or a rest home. Old age also became increasingly medicalized, and the aging body was viewed as abnormal, a pathology of the natural state. The Victorian goal of perfect health and longevity was thus revived, and maximal physical functioning became the ideal of normal aging. The social sciences further stereotyped the elderly as sick, poor, and vulnerable and thus argued for their protection and management. Institutional approaches were increasingly favored, such as Social Security, home health assistance, and nursing home placement, much of which served to further segregate the elderly from a meaningful sociocultural presence.

By the 1970s, the legacy of Victorian optimism in boundless health and a now-dominant youth culture expanded the historic denial of death [25] to include a denial of aging. This process fostered the seemingly pro-elderly view that "old people are (or should be) healthy, sexually active, engaged, productive and self-reliant" [11]. This view persists today; however, the burgeoning elderly population and the vast dependency among those failing self-reliance have become cause for alarm as the welfare state approach to funding senescence (Social Security, Medicare, Medicaid) is increasingly threatened [26].

E. Elders Today

The historical forces of the fight for civil rights, the women's movement, and gay and disability rights, have marked the current cohort of elders but will likely modify the aging experiences of the baby boomers to a far greater degree. For example, the rapid rise of female employment in the 20th century, coupled with the shift toward a service economy and knowledge work, has transformed education and employment for both women and men. As a result, their gendered life courses are becoming increasingly similar. The woman's sphere of domestic labor has become by degrees less prominent, replaced in part by the previously male-dominated industrial-corporate structure. Thus, the pattern of education-then-labor-then-retirement is an experience increasingly shared between women and men [27].

Some differences remain, however. Older women today display greater social integration than do men, maintaining larger and more satisfying social networks of family, friends, and neighbors. Although men have more frequently sought paid employment after retirement, women have tended to perform more volunteer community service. However, this may be related to the fact that men have long derived their principal source of identity from the workplace, and retirement often begins a period of decline for many [28]. Notably, men older than 75 years have the highest rate of suicide in the U.S. population. Social isolation and depression are felt to be factors, an impaired resilience related in part to the loss of male cultural identifiers at retirement [29].

Women's lives have been thought to be more defined by relationships (e.g., wife, mother, sister, daughter, and friend), despite a lifetime of paid employment [30]. For example, the role of grandmother has served multiple roles in American culture. In the 19th century, the grandmother was a repository of traditional wisdom, but she also acted as a mediator in child-parent relations [31]. The modern family, however, has less experience with this facet of family life. When present, such grandparenting is more often custodial in nature, a form of surrogate parenting designed to accommodate working parents [32]. Indeed, elderly women (far more than older men) at present remain involved as caregivers for spouses, siblings, children, and grandchildren. Older employed daughters and daughters-in-law are often sought to provide needed care, whereas male family members prefer to managed finances or perform chores and repairs over more intimate activities such as bathing and toileting [33].

F. Summary

In early America, few survived to old age, but age was not the defining factor for work or social life in early America. The American Revolution and subsequent rise of industry was accompanied by a cultural shift favoring the young, and age divisions grew in importance. Notably, the elderly lost value as their numbers increased. The next section is devoted to the problem of poverty in late life and financing old age.

III. From Paupers to Pensioners: The Elderly Poor

Old age has long been a serious problem for all but the wealthy. In America's first 150 years, the prospect of old age frequently evoked fears of financial ruin, the poorhouse, and dependency. Until the latter half of the 19th century, most individuals were able to save little in a lifetime of work. In early American life, wages and income for most people were merely sufficient to meet daily expenses for food and shelter. Consequently, most elderly could not afford to retire and either moved in with children or worked until they could no longer (or were fired) [5].

A. Economic Stability and Decline

Following 60 years of war and rebellions that buffeted Europe, the period from 1650 to 1740 was marked by peace and economic stability. Wages rose, rents fell, and prices for food staples remained steady or declined. During this interval,

there was a modest improvement in the life expectancy for women and infants. As the economy improved, women began to marry at earlier ages and have more children. But after 1740, Europe and the colonies entered a long period of increasing prices that lasted 100 years and sparked numerous conflicts in the Western world, including the American Revolution. The poor were most severely affected, because the largest price increases occurred in staple commodities such as grain and beans and energy sources such as coal and firewood. Real wages began to fall behind the price of food. However, unlike similar periods in the 14th and 17th centuries, widespread famine did not occur. Although there was much suffering among the poor, increases in per capita income meant that fewer people were living near the edge. In addition, the growth of community welfare and increased charity from religious organizations contributed to the prevention of starvation [10]. In response to the plight of impoverished older citizens, Thomas Paine printed his 1795 pamphlet, *Agrarian Justice*, in which he advocated for national pensions "to live without wretchedness in Old Age, and go decently out of the World" [34]. But unlike his influential *Common Sense*, fellow citizens largely ignored these concerns.

By the mid-1800s, approximately $230 was needed to finance the expenditures for an older adult for 1 year. At this time, 70% of men older than 65 had less than $800 in assets; 30% had less than $100 to their names. In all, less than 20% of older men could finance 10 years of retirement without additional income. Poverty was even greater in the South, especially among widows and blacks [5,6]. Widows frequently inherited little or nothing. Without savings, pension, or family to care for them, old people continued to labor or found themselves destitute [35]. Even aging Presidents faced indigence, including Thomas Jefferson, James Monroe, and Ulysses S. Grant [36,37].

B. Aging for Minorities

Immigrants and African Americans had the fewest resources for old age. By 1850, 3.8% of blacks were older than 60, and 1.4% were older than 70 (Table 105-2). Most were slaves, unable to hold property or generate savings [19]. The "peculiar institution" of slavery further burdened aging blacks with the sudden and often unpredictable threat of sale and separation from family and community caregivers [38]. Elderly slaves were sometimes "freed" before becoming a burden to the plantation. Denied food and shelter, they were left to starve, their own children forbidden from providing assistance. Recalled one former slave

Table 105-2
Black Population in the United States in 1800 and 1850

U.S. Census	1800	1850
Slaves	887,612	3,200,600
"Free colored"	107,410	424,183
"Free colored" or slave older than 60 yr	NA	138,176
Total U.S. population	5,084,912	23,054,152

NA, not available.

"When my mother became old, she was sent to live in a little lonely log-hut in the woods. Aged and worn out slaves, whether men or women, are commonly so treated. No care is taken of them, except, perhaps, that a little ground is cleared about the hut, on which the old slave, if able, may raise a little corn. As far as the owner is concerned, they live or die as it happens; it is just the same thing as turning out an old horse. . . . . She was not treated worse than others: it is the general practice" [39].

Although abandonment was discouraged in some regions, senescence did not reduce the owner's demand for labor, and few were allowed to retire. Although some were given menial tasks, others were sold. Auction and plantation records document that elderly slaves were sold as mere fractions of a "full hand" [6].

C. The Poor Laws

There were no national or state programs for the poor in early America. In the tradition of English poor laws of the 1600s, townships assisted the poor elderly as their local duty, either in almshouses or with direct subsidies for food and housing. Local control of social welfare under these poor laws also meant local financing, with designated "overseers of the poor" given broad authority to levy taxes on town residents. Overseers provided relief for "the lame, impotent, old, blind, and such other among them, being poor and not able to work." Puritan beliefs became the foundation for early America's social welfare, emphasizing an ordered, hierarchical universe. The presence of a permanent underclass fit into this world view. Believing in predestination, Puritans could look at poverty as revealing a flaw in the poor person's character or a sign that one had sinned [35].

Tradition and legal prescription demanded kin responsibility. Thus relief was denied to elders who had family that could care for them, even when this introduced economic hardship. Communities placed elderly without kin among neighbors or in boarding houses [6]. In response to rising relief taxes, a number of towns rid themselves of the elderly poor by auctioning them off to farms for labor [40]. The low bidder would be paid to care for an indigent person in her home, with little financial incentive to provide quality care nor was any oversight required. This practice continued up to the 1820s, frequently accompanied by neglect, cruelty, and even torture. Some communities denied refuge to nonresidents, forcing the old and sick to wander from town to town in search of assistance, even in the middle of winter [35,41].

D. The Poorhouse

Almshouses, poorhouses and rural poorfarms had existed since colonial times as both a refuge for the helpless and a deterrent to the able-bodied. Assistance to the poor was based on the assumption that the recipient must be truly incapacitated for work. It was commonly held that the poor were poor because of immorality, laziness, or alcohol abuse. Thus, the able-bodied nonworking poor were deemed unworthy of assistance and needed to be disciplined and forced back into the labor market. The "worthy poor," however, were unable to support themselves because of sickness, disability, or old age (i.e., through no fault of their own). However, some felt that those who had not accumulated sufficient savings for their own later years were also unworthy [37].

This decentralized system of attending to the poor was called "outdoor" relief because funding was provided in the home, outside an institution. Although at times abused by its overseers, outdoor relief was also criticized for delivering service in homes, instead of motivating the needy to get out and help themselves. Early welfare reformers advocated governmental intervention for the social ills that were felt to be responsible for poverty, including laziness and alcoholism. As a result, many states created institutions for the impoverished, termed "indoor" relief, and the era of the poorhouse began.

Designed in part to dissuade the "undeserving poor" from seeking relief, poorhouses provided a meager existence. Residents were known as inmates, and labor was expected of all but the most frail. Fear of the poorhouse was felt key to maintaining the work ethic among laborers and the poor. Although few questioned that elderly paupers deserved public assistance, shame and fear stigmatized all those on relief, worthy or not. "Dread of life in an institution seems to be almost universal, although the most dreaded is, of course, the poorhouse" [42]. More than any other factor, the lack of family willing or able to care for an elder resulted in a move to the poorhouse [35].

Although there was a great deal of variability among poorhouses, public demands to keep expenses down frequently resulted in "wretched quarters" and "meager provisions." Respectable widows and unmarried mothers shared filthy poorhouse rooms with criminals, drunks, prostitutes, and the mentally infirm. Dreary, vermin-infested, and laden with human waste, poorhouses were dreaded as a last resort for the elderly poor; "one of humanity's great degradations." Residents suffered physical abuse and severe social stigma [43–45]. An 1897 investigation found just 12 cents per day expended toward each pauper, which was but a small fraction of the sum required for mere subsistence (typical estimates approached $1 a day) [46]. However, despite their alleged frugality—their principal selling point in Britain and America—it invariably cost more to keep paupers in poorhouses than to support them in their homes by direct income assistance [35]. Nevertheless, government and charitable organizations had improved welfare for the poor such that, combined with an increasingly global marketplace, the impoverished no longer starved during periods of scarcity such as with financial panics, repeated crop failures, and severe weather (e.g., 1816: "the year without a summer").

E. Economic Stability 1815 to 1896

In the decades following 1815, and until the election of President William Jennings Bryan in 1896, the cost of living in the United States remained remarkably steady. Despite the Civil War and brief financial panics, there were some 80 years of relative economic stability. This meant improved conditions for the elderly and poor, because food commodities, rents and energy costs were flat or even declined while wages increased [10].

F. The Rise of Pensions

In 1861, shortly after the start of the Civil War, Congress passed a military pension system. These pensions were intended as compensation for combat injuries, to recruit soldiers, and to bolster nationalist pride. The impact of the Civil War on manufactured goods, food availability, and labor costs resulted in a burst of inflation in the northern states and a period of hyperinflation in the South [10]. Five hundred thousand men were killed in the conflict or died from disease. Many of these were heads of households or adult children whose parents relied on them for financial support. Without pensions, the parents, widows, and children of these soldiers were frequently left without means and faced destitution [47].

Initially limited to the widows of Northern soldiers, Civil War pensions began to be approved for an expanding class of needy older claimants. In the decades following the end of the war, the military pension was thus transformed into a rudimentary old-age social insurance system for the respectable working class. In 1904, President Theodore Roosevelt expanded eligibility beyond war-related wounds by establishing old age itself as a disability [48].

By 1910, 93% of Northern white veterans, their widows or older parents received pensions, representing 25% of the elderly U.S. population. At this point, military pensions consumed 43% of all federal expenditures. In today's dollars, the stipend would be comparable to the average Social Security retirement benefit. However, this program did not lead to a national old age pension because of corruption, high costs, the financial panic of 1907, and a lack of political organization among the elderly. Although this first national experiment in disability and pension assistance died with the last Union veterans and their families, it marked a shift away from local relief for the elderly, and made acceptable a federal approach to welfare. In addition, the elderly receiving pensions did not experience the stigma associated with charity [49,50].

G. Sharecroppers

After Emancipation, elderly blacks who remained in the South continued to work as sharecroppers or became dependents of extended households. Economically and socially, the term *sharecropper* signified one of the lowest rungs on the Southern agricultural ladder. Lacking education and property rights, and rarely showing a profit from cotton, black, white, and Hispanic tenant farmers (males and females alike) labored well into old age. However, the advent of the mechanical cotton picker and the exclusion of blacks from loan programs eventually pushed sharecroppers off the land. As a result, older African Americans migrated to cities for employment. For those who remained, there were few government services and persistent poverty [6,51,52].

H. Preindustrial Families

Throughout the 19th century and the early part of the 20th, households were larger because they included more children boarders, servants, apprentices, and other unrelated individuals. They also contained different age configurations because of later marriage, later child bearing, higher fertility, and lower life expectancy. Indeed, approximately one half to one third of all households had boarders and lodgers at some point. These arrangements frequently provided young people in the transitional period between leaving home to getting married with surrogate family and the older couples who took them in with supplemental income and sociability. Strategies involving the care of relatives during critical life situations, including illness and infirmity in old age, were primarily in the domain of women. As a result of these cultural norms, the nurturing responsibilities of women permitted them to maintain ties with kin over the life course and geographic distance [53].

I. Expanding Rights and Women's Sphere

Although Revolution-era rights talk addressed the oppressive behavior that harmed all citizens (if not all persons) equally, the 19th and 20th century social movements expanded these rights to groups discriminated against on the basis of equally important differences. Nineteenth century America saw a marked broadening in rights for slaves, women, and children through the piecemeal growth of protections at common law and by statute, state or private regulation, and constitutional amendment [54].

Post-Civil War industrialization and immigration spurred enormous growth in American cities, largely in the north. Poorly skilled (and poorly paid) immigrants and southern blacks were often crowded into cramped and filthy tenements. In response to these woeful conditions, the middle-class women's culture of the 19th century began to further advance social change through the development of institutions defined and controlled by "the public female sphere." The women's suffrage movement, women's colleges, women's clubs, and women's trade unions created a gendered network separate from the male-dominated sphere. Similarly, the women's settlement house movement arose in the spirit of reform, establishing housing and mentoring especially for women and children. The settlement house movement sought to relieve the pressures of urban immigrant life by providing community social services in an informal, neighborly setting. The most notable example was Chicago's Hull House, founded by social reformer Jane Addams. Although concerned with providing moral improvement, Hull House also offered practical services to its community, like the first child care and kindergarten in Chicago [13]. These attempts at social progress and institutional reform would later characterize the approach to rights expansion for the elderly in the 20th century.

J. Status of the Elderly

According to some authors, urbanization, immigration, and the Industrial Revolution left many elders alone, without income and bereft of social status [5,23]. However, recent research suggests that, compared with spartan farm life, industrialization and more global markets improved the fortunes for most elderly. For poorer families, factory wages and living spaces were shared in households spanning three generations. However, a growing number of middle-class elderly could afford separate housing, avoiding the disharmony common to crowded city life [6]. The Industrial Age had raised per capita incomes for young and old alike. Poverty began to diminish for many elderly, although primarily among white males and their spouses. Single women, widows, minorities, and immigrants remained economically vulnerable with senescence. For these groups, continued labor and severe poverty marked old age. However, increasingly, many seniors were able to fulfill the growing desire to maintain independent households in their later years. This preference for independent living remains today.

K. Obsolete

With the 1920s, Americans increasingly viewed the elderly (primarily male laborers) as obsolete. Industry and scientific management theory regarded older workers as less productive, lacking the stamina, speed, and dexterity needed for factory work. In addition, they were more likely to be injured on the job, increasing a firm's liability. At the same time, organized labor wanted superannuated employees to make room for younger laborers. Increasing numbers of firms began to introduce mandatory retirement ages, and pensions were few. As a result, opportunities for employment after age 45 became limited. Without work, health benefits, or unemployment insurance, many people reached old age without sufficient savings [5,20,55].

L. The Safety Net

After World War I, efforts by welfare authorities and reformers to address the indignities of the almshouse gave rise to various programs to assist needy elderly. Charity and fraternal organizations, meager union pensions, and state and local government programs served in a piecemeal and incomplete fashion [23]. However, inflation and stock market losses in the 1920s and the Great Depression of the 1930s threatened this fragile safety net. Traditional estimates had suggested that around 1910, nearly one fourth of older Americans were in dependent poverty. By 1930, before the Depression began, fully 30% of elderly were thought to be in poverty. Estimates at the time claimed this proportion rose to 50% in 1935 and reached two thirds by 1940 [5,6]. The economic collapse of the Great Depression resulted in mass unemployment and social dislocation. Charitable donations dwindled and few families felt they could support their aging kin. The increasing numbers of poor throughout the country were viewed with alarm, raising fears that elder dependency would overwhelm state and county resources. Of the few states that could afford old age assistance, most offered paltry sums to live on. There was increasing concern that the middle-class elderly would soon face the poorhouse and "the stark terror of penniless, helpless old age" [56].

More recent data paint a somewhat different picture, however. From 1890 through 1950, real wages of older workers actually rose sharply. Combined with family economic strategies, a greater proportion of elderly began to experience economic security. In these decades, earnings increased as one grew older, permitting a gradual reduction in the common reliance on income transfers from work performed by adult and minor children. Furthermore, in contrast to claims that the elderly had been relegated to "the industrial scrap heap," older men and women had not reduced their workforce participation in the transition from agricultural to industrial labor. Instead, steep declines in elder employment did not occur until Social Security began public transfers to the elderly. Data obtained during the Great Depression demonstrated that economic status rose with age, peaking for those aged 60 to 64. According to internal Social Security Board data, at least 55% of the elderly were financially independent by 1941. Just 23% received Old Age Assistance (which did not require proof of need), a figure far below the two thirds poverty rate for the aged claimed by reformers. Instead, it was young children that were far more severely affected by the Great Depression [57].

As in prior eras, those elderly who were without family or had remained poor throughout life were most likely to become destitute with age. However, unlike the 15th and 16th centuries, poverty and bad times no longer meant mass starvation. Indeed, with each decade came gradual improvement in life at the margins, and with it grew expectations for quality of life in senescence. The overwhelming support for old age pensions in the form of Social Security was in part because of exaggerated claims of poverty among the elderly. However, it also arose from the desire among both young and old to avoid the acrimony created by multigenerational households and demands for direct monetary transfers from adult children to provide for their elderly parents. In addition, this fit with a trend toward increasing government provision of and control over welfare, as demonstrated in concurrent labor legislation limiting working hours for women and federal social policy providing grants to states promoting child and maternal health services [49].

M. Social Security

Widespread poverty and the resulting social unrest fostered increasing interest in the principles of socialist thought across the Western world. In the same vein, the Great Depression revived the old-age pension movement, a populist response that first arose as Civil War pensions began to disappear. Demands for a national pension became a decisive election-year issue in 1934 [50]. "For Roosevelt what mattered most was . . . trends that made the aged poor a running concern *now*, not earlier, [and] future years would determine whether or not the concern persisted" [58]. The basic theme of reformers became a widely held belief. For the majority, financial security in old age was not possible without governmental assistance, because destitution of the elderly was felt to be an inevitable outgrowth of an industrial economy. This mirrored a sentiment popular among scholars, reformers, and labor of the time that wages for all workers (young and old) were insufficient to meet basic needs, much less prepare for the future, such as saving for retirement. In reality, most elderly enjoyed relatively high standards of economic well being. A minority were impoverished, many of these were women without families to help care for them [50,57]. When President Franklin D. Roosevelt signed the Social Security Act of 1935, he said,

> "We can never insure one-hundred percent of the population against one-hundred percent of the hazards and vicissitudes of life. But we have tried to frame a law which will give some measure of protection to the average citizen and to his family against the loss of a job and against poverty-ridden old age." [59]

Amendments to include health care benefits with Social Security were first proposed in 1934. However, strong opposition from insurers, businessmen, and the American Medical Association defeated these measures. Unable to afford rising medical costs on Social Security incomes, a growing number of elderly relied on state assistance for payment of their medical bills, or on free care from hospitals and physicians. The high cost of medical care became the greatest single cause of economic dependency in old age, because only one in four elderly had adequate insurance. Hospitals increasingly bore the brunt of unpaid health expenses for older people, which came to be viewed as a threat to their very existence. By 1960, a bill for health insurance limited to social security obtained a floor vote in the U.S. Senate for the first time in its half century as a national issue, losing by a small margin [60].

N. Medicare

Pressure for relief persisted, and Senator John F. Kennedy made the newly termed "Medicare" a major issue in his run for president. With increasing numbers and entitlement financing, the elderly were fast becoming a significant political force. As a result, Congress was finally persuaded that older Americans needed help defraying medical costs [23,50]. As part of his vision of the Great Society, President Johnson signed Medicare and Medicaid into law in 1965. With these programs, the government had stepped in to fill an apparent void left by the marketplace, the uninsured (if not uninsurable) elderly.

O. Old Age, Retirement, and Poverty

The combination of income assistance in the form of Social Security and health insurance through Medicare made retirement increasingly attractive and, for the first time, financially feasible for a majority of elders. According to the impoverishment theory of industrialization and old age, few older men had the means to retire, and most left work only because of poor health or inability to find work, becoming dependent on their children or charity. However, large numbers of older men in the decades before the Great Depression did not work, for reasons unrelated to health or unemployment. This arose from the accumulation of sufficient family wealth across the lifespan to permit a formal retirement [58]. At the beginning of the 20th century, 21.5% of employed males age 55 or older were able to retire, despite the general absence of Social Security, employer pensions, and mandatory retirement. Contrary to previous views, the accumulation of significant life cycle savings was not infrequent, and occurred most often among self-employed males such as farmers, independent merchants, manufacturers, and professional service providers (e.g., lawyers). From 1900 to 1940, men increasingly sought industrial employment and retirement shifted from individual business wealth accumulation to work-related pensions, wage savings, and, eventually, social "insurance" [61].

Labor force participation fell more rapidly in the decades following passage of the Old Age Assistance and Social Security, and by 1950 just under half of older men were still working. Today, less than one fifth of men older than 65 work full or part time. Among men ages 55 to 64, labor force participation has also declined, from a peak of 95% in 1880 to 67% in 1990. In agriculture and early factory work, laborers reached peak earnings in their thirties. In contrast, contemporary birth cohorts have experienced steady gains in earnings until retirement. The trend toward retirement has resulted from relatively high levels of wealth and affordable leisure activities such as tourism [6,50].

P. Summary

Over its first 200 years, America has experienced the decline of elder pauperism, the demise of the poorhouse, and the rise of pensions and retirement. Surprisingly, many of these changes occurred during the 20th century, which was affected by progressively increasing prices throughout the world, engendering economic upheavals, political disorder, and social disruption and eventually leading to World Wars and horrific crimes against humanity. However, simultaneously, conditions for elderly Americans have slowly but consistently improved over time. Increases in quality of life became more widely prevalent, and expectations rose. Despite severe setbacks in the Great Depression and the World Wars, the expanding affordability of food, clothing, energy, and shelter for a greater and greater proportion of elderly is remarkable. Wider availability of modern health care and technology exists for all (or nearly all) elderly, where few if any such services were present for older adults before 1950.

In the next section, I deal with the sad history of nursing homes, through scandals, financing, and regulation.

IV. From Poorhouse to Nursing Home

A. Old Age Homes

By 1900, the county-run poorhouse was increasingly used as an old age home. The proportion of residents who were elderly grew from 33% in 1880, to 37% in 1900, and reached 66% by 1920 [62]. At the time, counties and local governments remained responsible for their own impoverished citizens. Thus, to transfer rising costs out of local treasuries, many senile elderly were moved from county-run almshouses to state-funded mental hospitals, eventually housing 70,000 elderly inmates [63]. Charitable "Homes for the Aged" also arose, frequently funded by churches, fraternal orders, benevolent societies, and ethnic organizations. These nonprofit facilities provided room and board primarily for the elderly poor without families, because kin responsibility remained a cultural assumption, although not a legal requirement. Proprietary nursing facilities also developed in the early 1900s, primarily serving the chronically ill or disabled. State licensure programs began in the 1920s, but standards and oversight were minimal, primarily focused on building and safety codes.

B. The Demise of the Poorfarm

Overall, county poorfarms accounted for the bulk of assistance provided to the elderly poor. Poorfarms were frequently selected on the basis of least cost to the county, a practice decried as "farming out the poor to the lowest bidder" (similar to the auctioning of the poor present in the 19th century). However, increasingly large numbers of disabled and chronically ill elderly were being admitted. Reports of abuse and inhumane conditions in poorhouses were common. The long-standing cultural stigmatization of poverty and fears of institutionalization in the poorhouse resulted in a provision of the Social Security Act (SSA) that was designed to deny funding to poorhouse residents. Despite their anecdotal reputation, many poorhouses provided a family atmosphere and supervision for elderly men and women who were often quite alone in the world. Without such funding, not surprisingly, these facilities soon died out. It was initially expected that Social Security income would promote independent living and significantly reduce the need for these aged citizens to live in congregational settings. However, this view betrayed an ignorance of the debilitating conditions common to the geriatric population, including dementia, functional impairments, and frailty. By the 1940s then, most poor-farm residents had relocated to private "rest homes," which were permitted to receive Social Security funds. In addition, numerous small private nursing homes also opened. Frequently, these were converted farmhouses, mansions, or motels with poor safety, fire, and access features, and the quality of care varied widely. Many were not equipped to care for frail or ill elderly, providing only a room and meals. During the Depression, unemployed nurses often ran these facilities, but most care remained custodial in nature. There are few data to show these facilities were demonstrably better than the poorfarms they had replaced, but by asserting entitlement over charity for these services, the stigma of poverty was no longer a factor for their residents or the public [5,64,65].

C. The Rise of the Nursing Home Industry

An unintended consequence of legislation directed against publicly funded poorhouses was the nurturing of an emerging for-profit nursing home industry. Social Security cash in citizen's hands helped transform long-term care into a largely proprietary endeavor. Subsequent legislation, taxes, and building codes continued to favor corporate dominance [65]. Charity, religious, and philanthropic organizations continued to operate facilities that cared for the elderly, but they frequently found themselves at a disadvantage compared with for-profit facilities. Organizational efficiencies, economies of scale, and access to superior management methods permitted greater success to the for-profits in a market that was becoming both increasingly regulated and more marginally profitable.

In the 1950s, states began to receive federal matching funds for direct payments to nursing home vendors providing resident care. This marked a shift toward a federal relationship with providers rather than with the elderly residents. (Notably, this method repeated the previous financial relationships with poorhouses, almshouses, and "overseers of the poor.") Nursing home construction followed closely on the heels of the boom in hospital construction. Indeed, nursing homes increasingly became viewed as alternatives to lengthy hospital stays, which could last weeks or months for many frail elderly, especially those without families able to provide care. Thus, federal loan guarantees served as an incentive to build more modern nursing homes, permitting earlier discharges and reducing costs. Government-backed construction loans coupled with the regularized income of vendor payments seemed to guarantee a secure return on investment. This attracted developers and real estate speculators, some of whose names would soon become synonymous with nursing home scandals. However, despite a 180% increase in spending on nursing home care, there was still a perceived shortage of a half million beds by the early 1960s [65].

Passage of Medicare and Medicaid resulted in the further development of commercial nursing homes and accelerated the trend away from nonprofit and government facilities. Congress had intended the limited Medicare nursing home benefit primarily as a mechanism to shorten hospital stays, thereby hoping to reduce Medicare costs. These programs provided considerable funds to the states, which agreed to minimum federal standards where none had previously existed. However, these regulations were rather lenient. At the time, providing a written plan of correction satisfied most violations, and penalties were few [66].

Providers were reimbursed for mortgage interest, depreciation, self-reported costs of care, and an added profit margin. Combined with apparently generous Medicaid and Medicare payments for care, much of the risk in this real estate venture appeared to be eliminated. The need for capital was enormous, however, because many new nursing homes were needed to meet existing shortages and replace obsolete facilities. Consequently, in the late 1960s Wall Street developed "a kind of frenzy" over corporate investment in nursing homes. Firms with backgrounds in construction, real estate, and the motel industry dominated this speculative market. As a result, bed supply increased from 460,000 to 1.1 million in less than a decade [65].

D. Nursing Home Scandals

However, complaints previously raised against almshouses and poorfarms were soon directed at nursing homes, forever altering their status in the public mind and memory. Recurrent scandals of theft, maltreatment, food poisonings, and deadly fires prompted hearings in the Senate Aging and Finance Committees. In 1971, President Nixon made speeches deploring nursing home conditions and presented a plan for tougher regulations [66]. Once the hottest stocks in the market, by 1972 nursing home stocks went bust. Corporate financial fraud, securities violations, and reports of inferior care and patient abuse fueled investor concerns. Far worse for stockholders, nursing home owners had badly misjudged Medicare funding. These seemingly generous posthospital payments actually covered less than 2% of expenses, and Medicaid accounted for nearly half of long-term care reimbursement and was far less lucrative. At times, conditions worsened as some homes cut back on food or staff to maintain profitability [64].

The expense of complying with new stricter building and safety standards forced many smaller "mom and pop" homes out of business. State restrictions on new bed construction encouraged corporate acquisition of existing facilities. Medicaid reimbursement of the costs of care further favored larger chains. Corporations were able to profit by selling goods and services to their own subsidiaries, such as food, laundry, management, and housekeeping services. In this manner, large nursing home chains came to control an increasing number of beds. Of the 16,700 nursing homes in the United States today, two thirds are for-profit, one fourth are nonprofit, and 8% are government owned. More than half belong to management or ownership chains [67].

V. Persistent Quality Concerns in Long-Term Care

A. Reform Through Regulation

In 1982, the Reagan Administration proposed deregulation of nursing homes in response to industry complaints. However, these plans were withdrawn under heavy public criticism [68]. Instead, the Institute of Medicine (IOM) was commissioned to study long-term care policies, and issued the 1986 report "Improving Quality of Care in Nursing Homes." It charged that many substandard nursing homes were allowed to operate and that residents frequently received inadequate, sometimes "shockingly deficient" care. Although abuse and neglect had declined in nursing homes, poor quality of life and inadequate medical care were "far too common" [66].

Rather than relaxing regulations, the IOM recommended far more stringent ones. These changes were enacted in the Nursing Home Reform Act of the Omnibus Budget Reconciliation Act of 1987, with far-reaching revisions to standards, inspection, and enforcement [68]. This legislation mandated more nurse's aide training and a broader array of care, including the provision of rehabilitative, physician, and social services. A uniform resident assessment instrument was implemented to ensure comprehensive evaluation, and states were now required to provide ombudsmen as resident advocates. Polypharmacy, restraint use, and resident rights issues were addressed. There is good evidence these regulations have improved the quality of care and created standards where few existed before. However, the expanded services (and paperwork) exacerbated budgetary pressures, conflicting with simultaneous cost-containment efforts [69,70].

B. The Medicaid Burden

In 1997, under pressure from states to reduce Medicaid spending, the federal government repealed the 1980 Boren amendment, which had required that Medicaid nursing home rates be "reasonable and adequate." The nursing home industry warned that Medicaid reimbursement levels were already too low and that further reductions would adversely affect quality of care [71,72]. These changing financial incentives soon led to the development of lower cost alternatives to the nursing home.

C. More Scandals

In 1997, scandal again erupted when a *Time* magazine article charged that California nursing home residents were being denied food and water and suffering from untreated infections. Blaming "greedy owners and slipshod facilities," the report claimed thousands of frail elderly were dying from neglect [73]. In response, the General Accounting Office later identified glaring quality of care deficiencies in fully one third of California nursing homes [74]. In 1999, the U.S. Senate Committee on Aging held critical hearings on nursing homes and their regulators, and President Clinton unveiled tougher enforcement standards [75–77]. The resulting surprise inspections and higher fines were decried by the industry as excessive and counterproductive, contributing to a financial crisis that had led to numerous nursing home bankruptcies.

In 2001, the IOM updated their seminal report, now entitled "Improving Quality of Care in Long Term Care" to encompass alternative services and settings. Quality of care in nursing homes overall was felt to have improved, primarily as a result of increased regulatory requirements and government scrutiny. Nevertheless, the report found that quality issues such as pressure sores, malnutrition, and pain continued to pose serious quality concerns. The report again called for more data, more penalties, and greater enforcement of standards. Of no small concern, low Medicaid reimbursement was also recognized as a potential source of quality problems [78].

VI. Summary

The history of America's elderly is more complex and varied than has been previously understood. The Revolutionary War not only brought forth a new nation but also heralded an overthrow of the cultural hierarchy where privilege was based on age, gender, race, and class. Subsequent changes have been slow and sorely incomplete but continue unrelentingly. Two hundred years of declining fertility and mortality has caused even extreme old age to become somewhat commonplace. Although no longer the rare and precious stones of history, today's aged are more robust and productive and promise to define their worth in ways beyond mere scarcity or wealth.

At a minimum, it is difficult to do justice to a gendered history of aging in the United States. It remains unclear whether or not one can reliably separate historical patterns that pertain solely to older women *qua* older women, or elderly men *qua* elderly men. Numerous historical tracts explain in far greater detail than possible herein the female experience in the American landscape. To no small degree, the effects of gender, race, class, religion, disability, ethnicity, and sexual orientation can further differentiate and inform the history of the elderly at each turn. However, it may not be necessary (or even desirable) to devise progressively finer distinctions among elders to draw some useful conclusions on gender and aging in America.

Among elderly Puritan women, piety, submissiveness, and domesticity were emphasized. A reputation as a good mother and for serving as an exemplary model of the Christian life was highly valued. In one's final days, the acceptance of suffering without becoming a bother was a component of this stage of life. Older men's lives appear to have been more circumscribed by their previous roles in the seeking of power and status. In old age, this power was maintained only as long as control over money and land persisted. Although this initially served to sustain a white male patriarchy, America's revolution against an unelected authority was soon echoed in a similar revolt against the family patriarch. Elderly men began to face the absence of a visible societal role and became viewed as weak and without authority (economic, moral, or otherwise). The dominant concerns of the Victorian era over success and self-control revealed in part the desires of a youth-oriented culture to avoid the travails of aging. Although the women's movement took the first of many steps toward equality, old age already appeared to have become increasingly defined less by gender than by physical function. Indeed, writings of the time focused more on women as women, whereas the prior gendered duties of older women and men began to disappear. Instead, the pursuit of health, longevity, and independence became the ultimate role for both older men and women, an optimistic view that persists today. However, this view neglects the experience of physical decline and dependency with aging and tends to negate a useful societal role for men and women in their final years of life, beyond the mere accumulation of health and wealth. In addition, as women and men increasingly share biographies marked by education, labor, and institutional care at the extremes of life, there may be more of a convergence of experience in old age, rather than a diverging, strictly gendered pattern.

Before the 19th century, early Americans accepted the infirmities and suffering of old age as an inevitable stage of life, to be borne with stoicism and a quiet grace. Religious faith, reciprocal family relations, and a social hierarchy supported the elderly, fellow pilgrims reaching the end of a spiritual journey. The dualism of inevitable loss and hope for redemption framed this final stage of life, and these few elderly were thus to be venerated. From the Victorian era to the present day, aging shifted from an existential concern to a medical and administrative problem, one that denied the inevitability of disease, decay, and dependency. However, a preoccupation with optimal health and normal functioning contributed to the devaluation of elders who did not achieve successful aging. These unsuccessful elderly, failing to control their bodies, are increasingly viewed as clients or patients, economically worthless, and requiring professional management [79].

The history of old age in the United States has also been marked by the search for economic security and the desire to live independently. In the agricultural economy of pre-industrial America, the standard of living was low for young and old alike. However, the commonly held beliefs that the elderly have always lived in poverty until the advent of social insurance and that the modern economy relegated the older worker to the industrial scrap heap appear to be incorrect. A surprising number of individuals were able to save sufficient resources for a period of retirement. But for a minority, the price of labor closely mirrored the cost of living, and these elderly either continued to work or lived in dependent poverty. More than any other factor, the lack of family willing or able to provide for an elder resulted in a move to the dreaded poorhouse. However, welfare and charity to the old were frequently condemned much as the poor in general were condemned, representing immoral, lazy, and spendthrift behaviors that should not be rewarded but corrected with training, reprimand, and shame.

The U.S. Civil War represented at least in part a conflict between state and federal power. One consequence, although perhaps unintended, was a change in the federal government's role in social welfare, particularly in public health. It made acceptable a federal approach to welfare for the elderly as a separate class and initiated the idea of entitlement to publicly funded pensions. The Industrial Era expanded the opportunity for economic and social independence among older Americans. The desire to live independently as long as possible has gained increasing importance since the 18th century. Indeed, the gradual decline of the extended-family dwelling was welcomed across the generations and the rise of the middle class made retirement a reality for more and more elderly. However, the progress toward independent living in old age may itself have contributed to a weakening of family bonds and kin responsibility as

living arrangements became increasingly separated by time and distance.

Although the Great Depression wiped out many economic gains among the poor and middle class (but far less so among the elderly), the cultural demands for a more secure and independent old age grew stronger. A larger national role evolved with the perceived failure of personal, family, state, and charitable resources. The era of governmental assurance of security in old age began with outdoor relief (Social Security), and later included health care (Medicare) and institutional long-term care (via Medicaid). This restated the social contract, such that each generation would support the elderly in return for similar support from subsequent generations. However, the merits of the economic argument for adopting social insurance (i.e., "the impoverished elderly") now appears less defensible. In addition, separation of kin from direct responsibility for their aging family members has helped foster the growth of institutional approaches to aging.

It is important to recognize that modern concerns about long-term care can be traced to its roots in the moral implications of poverty and welfare. The unresolved conflict over individual and societal responsibilities has shaped policies regarding retirement and old age dependency. In addition, discerning worthy from unworthy has been and remains problematic. However, precisely because the almshouse and poorfarm carried the stigma of unworthy dependency, underfunding and appalling care of the elderly were common. Nursing homes arose from their ashes by redefining dependent old age as medical and social work problems and asserting funds as entitlements rather than charity. Certainly, the stigma of shame attached to receiving charity and living at the poorfarm played some role in their demise. Unlike the poorfarm, rest homes, nursing homes, and group homes managed to remain free of the taint of poverty, because Social Security was an entitlement free of means testing, an important distinction that remains to this day. Indeed, a key concept to maintaining popular support for entitlement programs for the elderly has been avoiding associations with welfare and charity. Therefore, recipients prefer entitlement based on age and vigorously resist means testing or other methods of determining worthiness.

For nursing homes, the medical model and federal oversight were increasingly used to help solve the problem of aging. A hospital-like atmosphere supplanted the traditional board and care approach, creating an institutional quality of life. Regulations imposed architectural standards, care directives, and extensive documentation of nearly every activity, which increased the costs of care, all in the name of limiting error, neglect, and the risk of sanctions. Despite this, nursing home history is replete with the same scandals of abuse and neglect that made the poorhouse so fearsome, becoming a place where few care to go. Not surprisingly then, institutional elder care has long been marked by a core of mistrust, fostering the current regulatory approach. Thus, to ensure competent care, paid caregivers are required to adhere to numerous regulations and copiously document their activities. However, the institutional and management approach to eldercare frequently results in apathy and an impersonal bureaucracy but not often a home. This is precisely because the keys to high quality of life in long-term care, such as the nature of staff and resident interactions, cannot be achieved through regulation [80,81]. Seniors and their advocates demand expert health care services and a low risk environment but at the same time expect individual freedom, a residential atmosphere, and limited expense. These desires may be mutually exclusive, perhaps even unattainable, but a balance of goals may be achievable.

VII. Suggestions for Further Investigations

These quandaries remain because the central questions remain not only unanswered but as yet undiscussed.

- What kind of old age do we want for our parents and ourselves?
- What risks will we allow for the sake of individual autonomy?
- Given finite resources, what limits will we accept? What are we willing to pay for? Who should pay?
- To what degree must we prepare for our own futures?
- What level of financial burden can we demand of later generations?

As we approach a burgeoning elderly population, the long-delayed deliberations regarding the rights and responsibilities in funding retirement and health care are beginning to occur. That these issues, present to only a small degree in early America, have become increasingly important is evidence of our nation's expanding wealth, gains in health and longevity, and rising expectations for quality of life. However, they also expose concerns regarding family fragmentation, personal responsibility for old age planning, and the expansion of governmental influence in the lives of the elderly.

In addition, these questions represent unresolved tensions between generations and among economic classes. Conflicting values regarding autonomy, personal responsibility and the proper role of government contribute to the lack of consensus as well. Given these competing interests, it is not surprising that there has never been a national aging or long-term care policy in America. The present system seems to have arisen primarily while attempting to reduce expenses; "an afterthought, a side effect of decisions directed at other problems" [33]. Unless the debate expands beyond budgetary concerns, the historical pattern of scandal-reform-scandal in long-term care will likely continue to recur.

Knowledge of the history of aging in America can provide a useful touchstone, because awareness of what has gone before can expose what might arrive again, identify what is worthwhile to preserve from the past, and help to avoid relearning painful lessons [82]. It would be a mistake, however, to presume that this history merely repeats itself. The chronology of eldercare is indeed often bleak and sad, but the kind of care received today, although far from ideal, is a vast improvement over previous decades. An understanding of the issues in eldercare as they occurred *over time* can suggest limitations on future possibilities, identifying objectives that may be difficult to attain and at what cost. However, equally important, one must discern how the present diverges from the past, where making analogies with prior issues may be unwarranted or misleading. A more thorough analysis of the history of the elderly in the United States, along with revisiting our presumptions and common wisdom regarding

aging, gender, and long-term care, can permit a more prudent view of the future, perhaps one more feasible than fanciful.

References

1. Minois G. (1989). *History of Old Age: From Antiquity to the Renaissance*, pp. 210–217. Chicago: University of Chicago Press.
2. Chudacoff HP. (1989). *How Old Are You: Age Consciousness in American Culture*, p. 13. Princeton, NJ: Princeton University Press.
3. Posner RA. (1997). *Aging and Old Age*, pp. 32–33. Chicago: University of Chicago Press.
4. de Beauvoir S. (1972). *The Coming of Age*, pp. 134, 272. New York: Warner Books.
5. Fischer DH. (1978). *Growing Old in America*, pp. 64, 77–102, 174, 208, 228. New York: Oxford University Press.
6. Haber C, Gratton B. (1994). *Old Age and the Search for Security: An American Social History*, pp. 21–47, 69–79, 91–95, 110–114, 122–123, 174–179. Bloomington, IN: Indiana University Press.
7. Lindholdt P. (1988). Crimes of gender in Puritan America. *Am Q.* 40:563–568.
8. Main G, Main J. (1999, Jan). The red queen in New England? *William Mary Q.* pp. 121–150.
9. Fraser A. (1984). *The Weaker Vessel*, pp. 101–103. New York: Vintage Books.
10. Fischer DH. (1996). *The Great Wave: Price Revolutions and the Rhythm of History*, p. 117. Oxford, UK: Oxford University Press.
11. Cole TR. (1992). *The Journey of Life: A Cultural History of Aging in America*, pp. 87–240. Cambridge, UK: Cambridge University Press.
12. Hareven TK. (1991, Feb). The history of the family and the complexity of social change. *Am Hist Rev.* 96(1)95–124.
13. Kerber L. (1988, June). Separate spheres, female worlds, woman's place: The rhetoric of women's history. *J Am Hist.* pp. 9–39.
14. Welter B. (1966, Summer). The cult of true womanhood: 1820–1860. *Am Q.* 18:151–74.
15. Scott P. (1997). *Growing Old in the Early Republic: Spiritual, Social and Economic Issues, 1790–1830*, pp. 22–30. New York: Garland Publishing.
16. Premo T. (1990). *Winter Friends: Women Growing Old in the New Republic, 1785–1835*, p. 10. Urbana: University of Illinois Press.
17. Miller A. (1998). *Death of a Salesman: Certain Private Conversations in Two Acts and a Requiem*, Act 1, Part 8, p. 40. New York: Penguin Books, originally published in 1949.
18. U.S. Bureau of the Census. (1975). *Historical Statistics of the United States*. Washington DC: GPO, and U.S. Bureau of the Census. (1992). *Statistical Abstract of the United States*. Washington DC: GPO.
19. Inter-University Consortium for Political and Social Research. Study 00003: Historical Demographic, Economic, and Social Data: U.S., 1790–1970. Ann Arbor, MI: ICPSR. Available at http://fisher.lib.virginia.edu/census/ (accessed 1/2/03).
20. Hirshbein LD. (2001). William Osler and *The Fixed Period*: Conflicting medical and popular ideas about old age. *Arch Intern Med.* 161:2074–2078.
21. Life & Career, Richard Douglas Lamm, Mar. 29, 1984; available at http://www.cnn.com/ALLPOLITICS/1996/conventions/long.beach/lamm/life.career.shtml(accessed 1/12/03).
22. Gutman HG. (1973). Work, culture, and society in industrializing America, 1815–1919. *Am Hist Rev.* 78:531–588.
23. Achenbum WA. (1978). *Old Age in the New Land: The American Experience Since 1790*, pp. 29, 46–48, 60, 91, 113–125, 146. Baltimore, MD: Johns Hopkins University Press.
24. Moen P. (2001). The Gendered Life Course. In *Handbook of Aging and Social Sciences*, 5th Edition (Binstock R, George L, eds.), p. 189. San Diego, CA: Academic Press.
25. Becker E. (1997). *The Denial of Death*. New York: Touchstone Books, originally published in 1974.
26. Binstock RH. (1999). Older Persons and Health Care Costs. In *Life in Older America* (Butler RN, Grossman LK, Oberlink MR, eds.), p. 78. New York: Century Foundation Press.
27. Han SK, Moen P. (1999). Work and family over time: A life course approach. *Ann Am Acad Polit Soc Sci.* 562:98–110.
28. Hearn J. (1995). Imaging the Aging of Men. In *Images of Aging: Cultural Representations of Later Life* (Featherstone M, Wernick A, eds.), pp. 97–115. London: Routledge.
29. Pearson JL. (2002). Recent research on suicide in the elderly. *Curr Psychiatry Rep.* 4(1):59–63.

30. Moen P. (2001). The Gendered Life Course. In *Handbook of Aging and Social Sciences*, 5th Edition (Binstock R, George L, eds.), p. 181–182. San Diego, CA: Academic Press.

31. Smith P. (1970). *Daughters of the Promised Land: Women in American History*, pp. 314–315. Boston: Little, Brown and Company.

32. Ferraro K. (2001). Aging and Role Transitions. In *Handbook of Aging and Social Sciences*, 5th Edition (Binstock R, George L, eds.), pp. 318–319. San Diego, CA: Academic Press.

33. Carstensen LL. (2002). Aging in the 21st Century; Difficult Dialogues Program, Consensus Report, p. 12. Stanford, CA: Institute for Research on Women and Gender, Stanford University.

34. Paine T. (1797). *Agrarian Justice*. Philadelphia: R. Folwell. Available at http://www.ssa.gov/history/tpaine3.html (accessed.)

35. Katz MB. (1996). *In the Shadow of the Poorhouse*, pp. 9–209. New York: Basic Books, originally published in 1986.

36. Saltow L. (1975). *Men and Wealth in the United States, 1850–1870*, pp. 72–73. New Haven, CT: Yale University Press.

37. Katz MB. (2001). *The Price of Citizenship*, pp. 232–233. New York: Metropolitan Books.

38. Wyatt-Brown B. (1988). The mask of obedience: Male slave psychology in the Old South. *Am Hist Rev.* 3(5):1228–1252.

39. Grandy M. (1996). *Narrative of the Life of Moses Grandy; Late a Slave in the United States of America* (originally published in 1843). Electronic Edition. Academic Affairs Library, UNC-CH. University of North Carolina at Chapel Hill, pp. 51–52. Available at http://docsouth.unc.edu/grandy/grandy.html (accessed February 24, 2004).

40. Gans HJ. (1995). *The War Against the Poor: The Underclass and Antipoverty Policy*. Cambridge, MA: Perseus Books.

41. Newton J. (1975). *History of the Pan-Handle; Being Historical Collections of the Counties of Ohio, Brooke, Marshall and Hancock, West Virginia*. (Originally published by Wheeling, WV: JA Caldwell, 1879). Evansville, IN: Unigraphic Inc. p. 382. Available at http://www.rootsweb.com/~wvmarsha/poorhouse.htm (accessed February 24, 2004).

42. Solenberger A. (1911). *One Thousand Homeless Men: A Study of Original Records*, p. 314. New York: Russell Sage.

43. Brammer R. (1994). *A Home for the Homeless: Remembering the Pleasants County Poor Farm*. Goldenseal. Fall, 1994. Available at http://www.rootsweb.com/~wvpleasa/poor.htm (accessed February 24, 2004).

44. Evans HC. (1926). *The American Poorfarm and Its Inmates*, p. 5. Mooseheart, IL: Fraternal Congress and Loyal Order of the Moose.

45. The Almshouse: Testimony of Last Night's Meeting of the Investigating Committee. *Philadelphia North American and United States Gazette*. Jan 11, 1882. Available at http://poorhousestory.com/PA_PHIL_Scandal.htm (accessed February 24, 2004).

46. A disgrace to humanity: Shocking condition of affairs that exists at the Sheldon Poor House. *St Albans Weekly Messenger (Vermont)*. 4 Feb, 1897. Available at http://poorhousestory.com/VT_st_albans_weekly_messenger_1897.htm (accessed February 24, 2004).

47. McClintock MJ. (1996, Sept). Civil War pensions and the reconstruction of Union families. *J Am Hist.* 83(2):456–480.

48. Blanck P. (2001). Civil War pensions and disability. *Ohio State Law J.* 62:109–238. Available at http://moritzlaw.osu.edu/lawjournal/621.htm (accessed February 25, 2004).

49. Sapiro V. (1986). The gender basis of American social policy. *Polit Sci Q.* 101(2):221–238.

50. Costa DL. (1998). *The Evolution of Retirement: An American Economic History 1880–1990*, pp. 1–8, 162–169, 176–177, 195–196. Chicago: University of Chicago Press.

51. Grim V, Effland A. (1997). Sustaining a rural Black farming community in the South. *Rural Develop Perspect.* 12(3):45–52.

52. Kester H, Lichtenstein A. (1997). *Revolt Among the Sharecroppers*. Knoxville, TN: University of Tennessee Press.

53. Hareven TK. (1991). The history of the family and the complexity of social change. *Am Hist Rev.* 96(1):95–124.

54. Clark EB. (1995). The sacred rights of the weak: Pain, sympathy, and the culture of individual rights in antebellum America. *J Am Hist.* 82:463–493.

55. McClure E. (1968). *MORE THAN A ROOF. The Development of Minnesota Poor Farms and Homes for the Aged*, pp. 102, 128–129. St. Paul, MN: Minnesota Historical Society.

56. Eliot TH. The legal background of the Social Security Act: from a speech at Social Security Administration 1961. Available at http://www.ssa.gov/history/eliot2.html (accessed February 27, 2004).

57. Gratton B. (1996, Mar). The poverty of impoverishment theory: The economic well-being of the elderly, 1890–1950. *J Econ Hist.* 56:39–61.

58. Neustadt R, May E. (1982). *Thinking in Time: The Uses of History for Decision Makers*, p. 102. New York: Free Press.

59. Social Security Administration. (2000). *A Brief History of Social Security*. Social Security Administration Publication No. 21–059. Washington, DC: U.S. Government Printing Office.

60. Corning PA. (1969). *The History of Medicare*. Available at http://www.ssa.gov/history/corning.html (accessed 9/29/01).

61. Carter SB, Sutch R. (1996). Myth of the industrial scrap heap: A revisionist view of turn-of-the-century American retirement. *J Econ Hist.* 56:5–38.

62. Gratton B. (1986). *Urban Elders: Family, Work, and Welfare Among Boston's Aged, 1890–1950*, pp. 39–61. Philadelphia: Temple University Press.

63. Vogel RJ, Palmer HC. (1985). *Long-Term Care: Perspectives from Research and Demonstrations*. Rockville, MD: Aspen Systems Corp.

64. Gray BH, ed. (1986). *For-Profit Enterprise in Health Care*, p. 494. Washington DC: National Academy Press.

65. Vladeck BV. (1980). *Unloving Care*, pp. 115–121. New York: Basic Books.

66. Institute of Medicine, Committee on Nursing Home Regulation. (1986). *Improving the Quality of Care in Nursing Homes*, Appendix A pp. 1–44, 241–243. Washington DC: National Academy Press.

67. Giacalone JA. (2001). *The U.S. Nursing Home Industry*, pp. 80–81, 121–130. Armonk, NY: ME Sharpe.

68. Hawes C. (1997–1998). Regulation and the politics of long term care. *Generations.* 21(4):5–14.

69. Giacalone JA. (2001). *The U.S. Nursing Home Industry*, pp. 130–132. Armonk, NY: ME Sharpe.

70. Institute of Medicine, Committee on Nursing Home Regulation. (1986). *Improving the Quality of Care in Nursing Homes*, pp. 1–44. Washington DC: National Academy Press.

71. Wiener JM, Stevenson DG. (1998). *Repeal of the "Boren Amendment": Implications for Quality of Care in Nursing Homes*, number A-30 in series, *New Federalism: Issues and Options for States*. The Urban Institute. Available at http://newfederalism.urban.org/html/anf30.html (accessed March 1, 2004).

72. Clark, LW. (1998). The Demise of the Boren Amendment: What Comes Next in the Struggle Over Hospital Payment Standards Under the Medicaid Act? *Health Law Digest*. January 01, 1998. Available at http://www.duanemorris.com/publications/pub14.html (accessed February 12, 2004).

73. Thompson M. (1997). FATAL NEGLECT: In possibly thousands of cases, nursing-home residents are dying from a lack of food and water and the most basic level of hygiene. *TIME Magazine* October, 27, 1997. Available at http://www.time.com/time/archive/preview/0,10987,1101971027-136745,00.html (accessed March 1, 2004).

74. U.S. General Accounting Office. (1998). California Nursing Homes: Care Problems Persist Despite Federal and State Oversight. Washington, DC: GAO/HEHS-98-202.

75. Hearing before the United States Senate Special Committee on Aging. (1998). Betrayal: The Quality of Care in California Nursing Homes; Senator Charles E. Grassley, Chairman, July 28, 1998. Available at http://aging.senate.gov/events/hr23.htm (accessed March 1, 2004).

76. Hearing before the United States Senate Special Committee on Aging. (1999). Residents at Risk? Weaknesses Persist in Nursing Home Complaint Investigation and Enforcement; Senator Chuck Grassley, Chairman, March 22, 1999. Available at http://aging.senate.gov/events/hr28.htm (accessed March 1, 2004).

77. Hearing before the United States Senate Special Committee on Aging. (1999). The Nursing Home Initiative: Results at Year One; Senator Charles E. Grassley, Chairman, June 30, 1999. Available at http://aging.senate.gov/events/hr35.htm (accessed March 1, 2004).

78. Wunderlich GS, Kohler PO, eds. (2001). Institute of Medicine. *Improving the Quality of Care in Long Term Care*, pp. 1–20. Washington DC: Institute of Medicine; National Academy Press.

79. Cole TR. (1992). *The Journey of Life: A Cultural History of Aging in America*, pp. 227–238. Cambridge, UK: Cambridge University Press.

80. Howard PK. (2001). *The Lost Art of Drawing the Line: How Fairness Went Too Far*, pp. 78–171. New York: Random House.

106

Breast Diseases in Older Women and Men

SANDHYA PRUTHI, MD* AND SHILPA H. AMIN, MD**

*Consultant, Division of General Internal Medicine, Mayo Clinic; Assistant Professor of Medicine,
Mayo Medical School, Rochester, MN
**Women's Health Fellow in Endocrinology, Diabetes, Metabolism, Nutrition, and Internal Medicine,
Mayo Clinic, Rochester, MN

Abstract

Breast disease and breast cancer in older women and men is an area of great interest and potential for future research, especially because of the dramatic growth in the elderly population. This chapter provides a concise review of methods to detect, evaluate, and treat both benign and malignant diseases of the breast. The relationship of key lifestyle risk factors to the development of breast cancer are reviewed. The role of screening with use of breast self-examination (BSE), clinical breast examination, and mammography to prevent and detect breast cancer are discussed. The final section provides new understanding about the future of genomics research, breast cancer risk, and detection and prevention of breast cancer in the elderly.

I. Occurrence of Benign Breast Conditions in Older Women

A. Detection and Evaluation of a Breast Lump

Breast tissue is naturally nodular, and irregularity to palpation is not necessarily abnormal. This is the case for most premenopausal women because of hormonal fluctuations in women's menstrual cycle and the effect of these fluctuations on breast tissue. Perimenopausal and postmenopausal women have a predominance of fatty tissue with a decrease in the glandular nodularity of breast tissue. This decrease in nodularity is attributable to less estrogenic stimulation of breast tissue with increasing age.

A palpable mass is defined as a dominant mass distinct from surrounding tissue and asymmetrical relative to the other breast. A smooth, well-defined mass is more likely to be associated with a benign lesion. Worrisome for malignancy is a firm lesion with irregular margins and associated skin changes such as dimpling and retraction of the nipple or areolar region. The presence or absence of pain should not influence the need for further evaluation of a palpable mass.

In older women, the presence of a mass requires further evaluation to exclude malignancy.

The workup of a palpable mass begins with diagnostic mammography and ultrasonography. Figure 106-1 presents an algorithm to evaluate a palpable breast mass [1]. Normal mammographic findings do not preclude the need for further evaluation of a palpable breast mass.

B. Incidence and Management

1. Mastalgia

Mastalgia or breast pain is encountered more commonly in premenopausal women than in postmenopausal women. Less than 10% of female breast cancer patients present with mastalgia as their primary symptom. Whether these patients have mastalgia that leads to further evaluation and detection of an asymptomatic cancer or whether the mastalgia was caused by their breast cancer is not clear [2]. The cause of mastalgia in most patients is unknown. It may be related hormonally to fluctuations in estrogens, progesterone, and prolactin levels, and these hormonal fluctuations may even cause premenstrual water retention in breasts. Fibrocystic disease has been observed in women with mastalgia, although no evidence supports a direct relationship between them [3].

Mastalgia is often grouped into two categories: cyclic mastalgia in premenopausal women occurs in relation to the menstrual cycle, and noncyclic mastalgia is seen more commonly in postmenopausal women.

Cyclic mastalgia is usually bilateral and not well localized. In younger women, the pain is described as a soreness that extends into the axillary areas and arms. It may last for several days before onset of menses and is relieved usually after menses begins or is completed. Menstrual irregularity, emotional stress, and change in medications and physiology can trigger mastalgia [4].

Noncyclic mastalgia occurs most often in women during their perimenopausal or menopausal years. It is usually unilateral and associated with a sharp, burning, localized pain. The most common causes include chest wall disorders involving the bone, muscles, or costochondral joints; pleural disease; and cardiac disease. Uncommonly, a breast malignancy may present with symptoms of pain. History taking should include specific questions regarding palpable breast changes, menstrual irregularity, emotional stress, and medication changes. Determining the frequency, nature of the pain, and severity by using a pain scale is important to assess the degree of symptoms. A complete physical examination should include a detailed breast examination to note changes in the breast and new mass lesions. Diagnostic mammography, target ultrasonography, or both are recommended for those with high risk of breast disease, age older than 35 years, or both [5]. Most women have no findings of breast disease after a complete evaluation and can be reassured that there is no cause for serious concern. Breast pain in most women has a spontaneous remission rate of 22% in women with cyclical mastalgia,

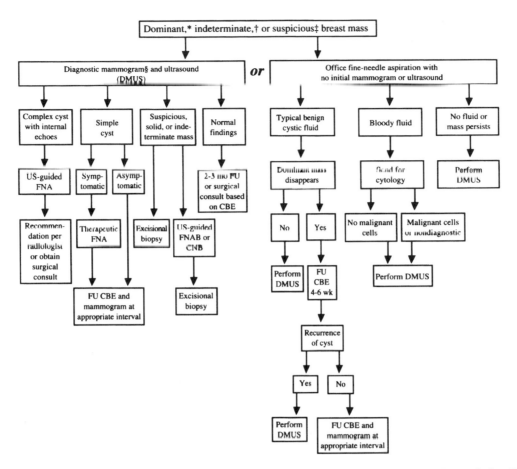

Fig. 106-1 Algorithm to evaluate a palpable mass. CBE, clinical breast examination; CNB, core needle biopsy; consult, consultation; FNA, fine needle aspiration; FNAB, FNA biopsy; FU, follow-up; US, ultrasonography. *Three-dimensional mass that is distinct from surrounding tissue. †Vague nodularity or thickening that differs from surrounding tissue. ‡Mass that is firm, irregular, immobile, and fixed to surrounding tissue or with associated skin changes such as dimpling. §Perform diagnostic mammography if not done in the past 6 months. For women younger than 40 years with a dominant mass, ultrasonography is initially performed, and obtaining a diagnostic mammogram is the radiologist's decision. (From Pruthi S. [2001]. Detection and evaluation of a palpable breast mass. *Mayo Clin Proc.* 76:641–648, with permission.)

and approximately 42% experience resolution at or around menopause [6].

Treatment should be focused on counseling the older woman regarding the normal physiology of her breasts as she ages and the importance of performing routine BSE as a way to monitor symptoms and note any observable changes over time. Nearly 10% of women with mastalgia require more intervention because of persistent pain. These women should be counseled on treatment options available [7].

Nonpharmacologic treatment options, including heating pads, gentle massage, and soft-cup bra support, may alleviate intermittent symptoms. Caffeine avoidance has shown minimal benefit in patients with mastalgia but no documented therapeutic improvement in randomized clinical trials [8].

Pharmacologic treatment options include vitamin E supplementation, which has shown limited benefit in some patients [9]. Two double-blind, placebo-controlled randomized trials have demonstrated no clear benefit of vitamin E, however [10,11]. Orally administered evening primrose oil (gamma-linolenic acid) has shown benefit to mastalgia patients in randomized

controlled trials [12,13] and has improved mastalgia in 40 to 60% of patients with less than 5% experiencing adverse effects [14]. Danazol is an antigonadotropin and the only prescription-required drug approved by the U.S. Food and Drug Administration for treatment of severe activity-limiting mastalgia. Patients with cyclical mastalgia report that symptoms improved by 50 to 75% at a dose of 100 to 400 mg per day [15,16]. In women with noncyclic mastalgia, symptoms improve by 75%. Adverse effects occur 20% of the time and include menstrual irregularity, acne, weight gain, and hirsutism [3,4,7].

2. Atypical Ductal and Lobular Hyperplasia

Atypical hyperplasias are proliferative lesions that are considered markers for increased risk of developing breast cancer. The combined relative risk of breast cancer resulting from atypical hyperplasias has ranged from 3.4 to 5.3 (average 6.8) in case-control trials [2,4]. Mammographic screening identifies microcalcifications in asymptomatic women without a palpable lesion. Subsequent biopsy detects atypical hyperplasia in 12 to 17% [2,3].

Atypical hyperplasia is either ductal or lobular. Atypical ductal hyperplasia refers to pathologic changes in the breast ducts of uniform epithelial cells and monomorphic, hyperchromatic round nuclei. Changes are uniform with smooth spaces or micropapillae with a narrow base as the proliferating cells maintain their orientation to one another within the duct. The relative risk of breast cancer associated with ductal hyperplasia is 2.4 to 4.7 [2,4]. Atypical lobular hyperplasia involves the lobular acini of the breast tissue and may involve the ducts. It is characterized by polygonal or cuboidal cells that are monotonous and hyperchromatic and form a noncohesive pattern of cells throughout the tissues. The relative risk of breast cancer associated with lobular hyperplasia is 5.3 to 5.8 [2,4].

The risk of breast cancer in patients with atypical hyperplasia is modified according to family history, time since biopsy, and menopausal status. A family history of breast cancer is associated with a 2- to 5-fold increased risk of disease in patients with atypical hyperplasia. The risk of breast cancer among women with atypical hyperplasia is greatest in the first 10 years after benign biopsy result reaching nearly 10-fold in some studies and decreases to that of women without a history of atypical hyperplasia after 10 years [2,3]. The Nurses' Health Study showed that the relative risk of breast cancer in patients with benign atypical hyperplasia is lower in postmenopausal women (3.7) than in premenopausal women (5.3), and the use of hormone replacement therapy (HRT) does not increase this risk [2,3].

In summary, the increased risk of breast cancer associated with benign atypical hyperplasia diagnosed by biopsy reinforces the need to continue close follow-up and annual screening of these patients. Because this condition is a marker for increased risk for breast cancer, these women should be counseled about risk reduction options.

Lobular carcinoma in situ (LCIS) is another lesion that is found incidentally during evaluation of microcalcifications seen on mammography or when breast tissue is removed for another indication. No specific clinical or mammographic findings are associated with LCIS. As a marker for increased risk for breast cancer, LCIS suggests a relative risk of 5.7 and in women with a family history, the relative risk increases to 8.5 [17]. Treatment options include observation (clinical breast examination every 6 to 12 months with annual mammography), chemoprevention with tamoxifen, participation in prevention trials, or bilateral prophylactic mastectomy.

3. Fibrocystic Breast Changes

Fibrocystic changes refer to an overall condition in which palpable thickening and tender lumpiness are symmetrical and bilateral. These changes are usually associated with cyclic pain and tenderness. Thus, in elderly women this condition is uncommon. The peak age incidence is during the mid thirties to forties. The pain associated with fibrocystic breast disease may worsen over time until the woman reaches menopause. In summary, the term *fibrocystic breast changes* is more descriptive than diagnostic. Preventive measures, as outlined previously, are recommended as routine monitoring of these changes for the development of breast cancer [3].

4. Intraductal Papilloma

This broad category includes lesions that have a papillary configuration on gross or microscopic evaluation. Lesions can be solitary intraductal papillomas or multiple papillomas. This discussion focuses on solitary intraductal papillomas, lesions of the subareolar lactiferous ducts that primarily occur in women in their thirties to fifties but can occur in elderly women too. The patient may complain of unilateral serosanguineous or frank bloody nipple discharge from one duct, and the secretion is always from the same point on the nipple. Papillary hyperplasia is another lesion in the duct lobular units and can cause similar bloody discharge and should be differentiated from a papilloma.

On physical examination, a mass may be palpable in 33% of women, and sometimes the papilloma may be seen at the orifice of the duct in the nipple. The papillary-appearing friable fibrovascular tumor of central myoepithelial cells has a cuboidal lining located within a duct and may have a stalklike or even sessile base in its attachment to the duct wall [2,3,5]. This tumor measures less than 1 cm in diameter. The increased risk of breast cancer associated with intraductal papillomas is slight (less than the risk associated with the finding of atypical hyperplasias). The main concern is to rule out the possibility of a breast cancer that can also present with bloody nipple discharge. If mammography shows a mass lesion or possible malignancy, a core biopsy and surgical excision are recommended [3]. Duct exploration and incision is the treatment of choice in patients older than 45 years with these new findings and persistent discharge more than a few times per week. The surgical procedure includes excision of the lesion and duct system. In women older than 50 years, careful investigation with duct excision is necessary because of the increased risk of breast cancer.

II. Risk Factors for Breast Cancer in Older Women

A. Age

Breast cancer is one of the most common cancers occurring in elderly women. The incidence of breast cancer increases with age, with about 50% of breast cancer cases occurring in women aged 65 years or older and more than 30% occurring in those older than 70 years [18]. The breast cancer incidence and mortality in the United States has begun to decrease in recent years [19]. This has been the result of the early detection from increased use of mammographic screening and successful adjuvant treatment of breast cancer. Increasing age appears to be a major risk factor for the development of breast cancer. One in eight women develops breast cancer by the age of 80 years, at which time the incidence appears to plateau [20]. If the current incidence rates remain constant, projections estimate a 72% increase in the number of elderly women in the United States diagnosed with breast cancer by 2025 [21]. Breast cancer mortality is second to lung cancer mortality. Increasing incidence and mortality from breast cancer in elderly women have profound economic implications for cancer care in the United States. As age increases, so do the number of co-morbid conditions. Innovative measures to provide access to care, detection of breast cancer at an early stage, and effective treatment options will have a substantial positive effect on the health care system.

B. Hormonal Risk Factors

A woman's endocrine history is associated with a number of risk factors for the development of breast cancer. The role of estrogen use, both exogenous and endogenous, in the pathogenesis of breast cancer is widely accepted. Risk factors associated with an increased risk of developing breast cancer include age at menarche, age at menopause, late age of first completed pregnancy, and HRT use.

1. Age at Menarche and Menopause

Early onset of menarche and late age at menopause result in greater lifetime exposure to estrogen because of longer duration of ovarian activity. Thus, they are associated with increased risk of breast cancer. Studies have shown a decrease in breast cancer risk after a bilateral oophorectomy by about 50% compared with natural menopause [22].

2. Pregnancy

Late age of first pregnancy, especially after age 30 years, also increases the risk for breast cancer [23]. It is theorized that the early age at first birth results in less cell turnover, therefore making the tissue less susceptible to DNA damage [24]. The data regarding the effects of spontaneous or induced abortion are equivocal [24].

3. Hormone Replacement Therapy

The Women's Health Initiative study is the largest and best prospective, randomized, placebo-controlled trial published on combination HRT [25]. The findings from this study revealed that HRT use resulted in an increased risk of coronary heart disease, thromboembolism, stroke, and invasive breast cancer. The study enrolled 16,608 healthy, postmenopausal women who were randomly assigned to receive HRT or placebo. The study was halted after 5.2 years by the trial's data and safety monitoring board because of small increases in the risk of invasive breast cancer. It was concluded that overall health risks exceeded benefits from use of combined estrogen plus progestin, although the all-cause mortality was not increased.

The U.S. Preventive Services Task Force (USPSTF) also reviewed the evidence of the effects of HRT in November 2002 and recommended against routine use of estrogen and progestin for the prevention of chronic conditions in postmenopausal women [26]. The known benefits of taking estrogen replacement therapy or combination HRT include relief of hot flashes, sleep disturbance, and vaginal dryness. Estrogen does have a favorable effect on restoring and preserving bone health. Other possible benefits include decrease in the risk of colorectal cancer and protection against macular degeneration. Results of clinical trials [27] have not been consistent with regard to use of HRT to slow progression of Alzheimer's disease, and studies are ongoing to evaluate the effect of HRT and other selective estrogen receptor modulators on memory loss and cognition.

Overall, there appears to be a small increase in breast cancer risk from HRT, primarily attributable to long-term use. Conversely, short-term use for the management of vasomotor symptoms is most likely safe. The decision to use HRT must be individualized. The balance of benefits and risks for an elderly woman need to focus on her personal preferences, risks for specific chronic health conditions, and severity of vasomotor symptoms.

III. Prevention of Breast Cancer in Older Women

A. Lifestyle Factors

1. Diet and Nutrition and Physical Exercise

Encouraging elderly women to pursue a healthy lifestyle plays a central role in their overall sense of well-being. Obesity is common in elderly women, and effective counseling on healthy approaches to diet and exercise is important. Evidence from case-control and cohort studies [28] reveals that postmenopausal obesity is associated with an increased risk of breast cancer. The conversion of adipose tissue to estrogen results in an increase in circulating levels of estrogen [28]. Dietary fat is believed to accelerate mammary tumorigenesis [29]. However, different types of fat seem to have different effects. Mediterranean diets including olive oil seem to be associated with lower risk of breast cancer [10]. Diets high in fat or animal products are associated with a greater risk of breast cancer [30]. Conversely, fruits and vegetables seem to have a protective effect, possibly because of the increase in bioactive compounds such as isoflavones and lignans [30].

The Iowa Women's Health Study of postmenopausal breast cancer interestingly showed no benefit of diet and exercise among active women in reducing the risk of breast cancer [28]. More importantly, regular physical exercise has benefits for elderly women by increasing bone density, controlling weight, and limiting the risk of heart disease [31].

2. Smoking

Studies of the association of active and passive smoking on breast cancer risk have yielded conflicting results [32,33]. Smoking is a well-known risk factor for the development of lung cancer. The effect of tobacco constituents in breast carcinogenesis and possible mutagenic activity is unknown. However, other hypotheses that have been entertained are the antiestrogen effect of smoking and lower risk of breast cancer [32].

3. Alcohol Consumption

Alcohol intake has been associated specifically with an increased risk of breast cancer and with other forms of cancer as well [34]. The mechanism by which alcohol exerts its effect on the breast is unclear. Proposed mechanisms [35] include cytotoxic effect, interference with DNA repair, and alteration in circulating steroid hormone levels. A study in 44,187 postmenopausal women reported that both alcohol consumption and postmenopausal HRT increased breast cancer risk [36]. Alcohol consumption is a modifiable risk factor, and women need to be informed about limiting their intake to no more than one alcoholic drink per day [36]. It would be advisable to ensure an adequate daily intake of folate and folate-containing foods in women who use alcohol.

B. Breast Self-examination

New doubts have arisen about the benefits of teaching women to perform BSE. A large study in Shanghai, China, compared the benefit of teaching women to do BSE to reduce mortality from breast cancer with no screening at all [37]. Participants were not screened with mammography or clinical breast examination. The study reported that intensive instruction in BSE did not reduce mortality from breast cancer. It was concluded that women who choose to practice BSE should be made aware that the efficacy of BSE is unproven, and use of BSE may lead to an increased number of biopsies. Because mammography is the standard of care for breast cancer screening, the results of this study are not generalizable to women in North America.

The American Cancer Society recommends annual use of the triad of screening mammography, clinical breast examination, and monthly BSE for early detection of breast cancer. Breast self-examination alone cannot reduce breast cancer mortality, but it can alert women if changes occur in their breasts. Women should be made aware that the technique can help detect a change that must be evaluated further to exclude the possibility of breast cancer. Finding a lump or the occurrence of a suspicious change provokes anxiety for most women. Women should be encouraged to feel comfortable notifying their health care provider promptly about any breast changes that occur. Further evaluation may include a clinical breast examination, directed ultrasonography of the area of concern, and diagnostic mammography. The imaging findings should be correlated with the clinical examination findings, and further workup with image-directed biopsies, surgical consultation, or both may be necessary to exclude malignancy.

C. Screening Mammography in Older Women

Breast cancer occurrence and mortality increase with age. Annual mammography is recommended as a tool to screen for breast cancer and in turn to reduce breast cancer–related deaths in women older than 50 years. The decision to pursue screening mammography is most often at the recommendation of a health care professional. However, use of screening mammography has declined in older women. Factors that have been described [38] to explain this are the limited number of studies that have evaluated the effectiveness of screening mammography among women aged 75 years or older, age-associated declines in health status, lack of interest about breast cancer control practices, poor health status, and competing health care needs and priorities. However, it is well known that anticipated life expectancy for the average 75-year-old woman is approximately 12 years. Thus, for a healthy 75-year-old woman, age alone should not be the deciding factor to forgo screening mammography.

A study by Burack et al [38] assessed the extent to which an age-associated reduction in mammography use could be explained by declining or poor health status. They concluded that an observed decline in recent mammography use with advancing age was not explained by variation in health status or poor health. Even for those reporting good or better health, the odds of recent mammography were 40% lower among women aged 75 years or older compared with those aged 50 to 64 years.

Another segment of the population in which screening mammography use has decreased is women who are considered frail and have multiple chronic illnesses requiring some assistance with activities of daily living. A study by Walter et al [39] studied the outcomes of screening mammography in a population of community-living women who wished to stay at home rather than enter nursing homes. The mean age of the 216 women was 81 years. Screening mammography identified four cases of breast cancer (one ductal carcinoma in situ [DCIS], three local breast cancers); in two cases the disease was clinically insignificant and would not have caused symptoms in the women's lifetime. These women died of unrelated causes within 2 years of diagnosis. A large proportion (42%) reported pain or psychologic distress as a result of screening. Walter et al concluded that screening mammography in frail older women resulted in workups that were not beneficial and that screening in this group should be individualized. In general, 5 years is the approximate span of time required before screened people have a lower disease-specific mortality rate than unscreened people [40].

The USPSTF in 2002 published the recommendations and rationale for screening for breast cancer [41]. The evidence of benefits for reducing mortality from breast cancer is strongest for women aged 50 to 69 years to continue screening every 12 to 33 months. The USPSTF further concluded that, for women aged 70 years or older whose life expectancy is not compromised by comorbid disease, the evidence of benefit is generalizable. As women age, the balance of benefits and potential risks is more favorable because of the higher absolute risk of breast cancer.

With regard to screening differences between older black and older white women, a 1998 study [42] demonstrated older black women are less likely to undergo mammography and more often receive a late-stage diagnosis of breast cancer than older white women. This study demonstrates the importance of encouraging regular mammography use for all older women because it provides the same benefit irrespective of race.

D. Chemoprevention

Chemoprevention has evolved considerably in the past several years as a promising way to prevent breast cancer. Selective estrogen receptor modulators such as tamoxifen and raloxifene can block the binding of estrogen at the breast, reduce estrogenic stimulation, and thus decrease the risk of developing breast cancer [43].

Four large randomized clinical trials that have examined the benefits of chemoprevention of breast cancer included women with no history of breast cancer. The studies of tamoxifen are Royal Marsden Hospital (United Kingdom [UK]) Tamoxifen Chemoprevention Trial [44]; the Italian Tamoxifen Prevention Study [45]; the National Surgical Adjuvant Breast and Bowel Project P-1 Study, known as the Breast Cancer Prevention Trial (BCPT) [46]; and the International Breast Study (IBIS) [47]. The largest study, BCPT, found that the incidence of invasive breast cancer decreased by 50% during a median follow-up of 54.6 months. The relative risk reduction was similar for all age groups (35 to 49 years, 50 to 59 years, and ≥60 years) and all risk levels. Risks included endometrial cancer, which was significant for women aged 50 years or older (relative risk, 4.01; 95% confidence interval, 1.70 to 10.90), pulmonary embolism, stroke, and deep venous thrombosis.

The UK study and the Italian study, in contrast to the BCPT, failed to demonstrate a significantly reduced breast cancer risk. It has been suggested that tamoxifen's ineffectiveness in these trials may be attributable to differences in the study population, trial design, and conduct. The main differences in the three randomized trials were size (BCPT, $n = 13,388$; UK, $n = 471$; Italian, $n = 5,408$); breast cancer events (BCPT, $n = 368$; UK, $n = 70$; Italian, $n = 41$), and HRT use (UK study). Furthermore, the study populations had different risk inclusion criteria (BCPT, >1.66% Gail model; UK, increased risk based on family history; Italian, no increased risk) [48].

The Multiple Outcomes of Raloxifene trial [49] studied raloxifene use among postmenopausal women with a history of osteoporosis. Although assessing the osteoporosis fracture risk was the primary aim, breast cancer incidence was also assessed. Raloxifene reduced the incidence of estrogen receptor–positive breast cancer by 90% (relative risk, 0.10; 95% confidence interval, 0.17 to 0.46).

Ongoing is the Study of Tamoxifen and Raloxifene, the second largest chemoprevention trial in North America, for the prevention of invasive breast cancer [43]. The study opened in July 1999 and will continue to accrue women at high risk for breast cancer through 2004 with a goal of enrolling 19,000 postmenopausal women.

The USPSTF reviewed the evidence with regard to chemoprevention and recommended that clinicians discuss chemoprevention with women at high risk for breast cancer [50]. The most commonly used tool to assess risk is the Gail model [51]. Use of this tool is becoming a routine part of general health care, and women who are identified as being at high risk are reviewing the risks and benefits of tamoxifen with their primary care providers. In BCPT, all women older than 60 years were eligible for tamoxifen treatment on the basis of the Gail model calculated risk of 1.66% or higher as the 5-year risk of developing invasive breast cancer. In older women, understanding the risks and benefits of tamoxifen requires appropriate time spent counseling on this topic.

IV. Malignant Diseases of the Breast and Treatment Options in Older Women

A. Phyllodes Tumor

Phyllodes tumor is a rapidly growing lesion that appears similar to a fibroadenoma because there is proliferation of stromal and glandular elements. It is the most common stromal tumor of the breast (rare stromal tumors include angiosarcoma, leiomyosarcoma, and malignant fibrous histiocytoma). This tumor usually occurs in women in the fifth decade of life and has been diagnosed in women as old as 70 years. It often presents as a rather large lesion that requires removal if detected; otherwise recurrence is likely. A simple mastectomy in older women may be recommended because of the large size of the phyllodes tumor [5,52] and to exclude the possibility of a malignant phyllodes tumor. Malignant phyllodes tumors can metastasize hematogenously and are locally invasive.

B. Ductal Carcinoma in Situ

This noninvasive lesion presents typically as a unilateral breast cancer located within the ducts. Ductal carcinoma in situ accounts for nearly 20% of all new breast cancers. Carcinomas in situ are lobular (15%) or ductal (85%). Nearly 50% of women diagnosed with DCIS by biopsy develop invasive cancer if they receive no follow-up treatment. The risk of local recurrences is higher with larger sized tumors (≥2.5 cm).

Ductal carcinoma in situ can be treated with wide local excision (lumpectomy) followed by radiation therapy or with simple mastectomy. In patients who choose breast-conserving surgery, multiple randomized clinical trials have shown conclusively that breast irradiation markedly reduces risk for local recurrence [53]. For older women, breast irradiation optimizes local control unless disabling comorbid conditions preclude an expected survival of reasonable length. The benefits of irradiation need to be balanced against its morbidity and cost. If breast irradiation is administered properly, then morbidity is low. Common short-term toxic effects include fatigue and skin irritation during radiation treatments. Long-term toxic effects include radiation pneumonitis, rib fracture, and cardiac injury (<1%). The breast carcinoma is in situ, and, therefore, lymph node dissection is not required.

Tamoxifen can be considered for some women as prevention of invasive breast cancer in patients with DCIS, but this discussion must weigh the risks and benefits of this drug for the individual patient [52,54,55].

C. Invasive Ductal Carcinoma

Between 80% and 90% of breast cancers are infiltrating ductal carcinomas (IDCs) [2,4,7]. Most arise in the intermediate duct systems and have varied histologic configurations of medullary, colloid (mucinous), tubular, or papillary patterns of growth. Bilateral breast cancers occur in less than 1% of cases with nearly 8% recurrence rate in the contralateral breast, an incidence rate of 1% per year after the initial breast cancer. The presenting symptoms usually are a palpable mass or mammographic abnormality. Histologic examination reveals a heterogeneous growth pattern of tumor cells arranged in nests, trabeculae, sheets, or cords. Pathologic appearance of IDC ranges from normal-appearing epithelial cells to marked cellular pleomorphism and nuclear atypia [2,5,52]. The cancers receive a histologic grade according to nuclear appearance, tubular formation, and mitotic activity. The sum of these three factors can determine a grade of well, moderately, or poorly differentiated IDC. Biologic markers such as estrogen, progesterone, growth factors, and oncogene and tumor-suppression gene products are helpful in differentiating appropriate treatment for the patient [3]. The conventional options of lumpectomy with radiation and simple mastectomy are effective for IDC [56]. For older patients, sentinel lymph node staging has been a step forward because it is less morbid and can provide important information about prognosis.

Tamoxifen has been shown to be of benefit as adjuvant therapy for elderly women who are node positive, and it is the systemic therapy of choice [2,4,7,18]. This is substantiated by the fact that 80% of cancers occurring in women aged 70 years or older are hormone receptor positive. The National Surgical Adjuvant

Breast and Bowel B-24 study evaluated the combination of tamoxifen and radiotherapy and found that it was superior to either treatment modality used alone to prevent recurrence [57]. For women whose tumors are estrogen receptor negative or do not respond to tamoxifen, chemotherapy is another treatment option. The optimal duration of adjuvant therapy with tamoxifen is 5 years.

In women with a history of thromboembolic disease, which is a contraindication for the use of tamoxifen, treatment with an aromatase inhibitor is another option [2,18].

D. Invasive Lobular Carcinoma

Between 5% and 10% of breast cancers are invasive lobular carcinomas (ILCs) [2,7]. This histologic type of cancer is more likely to present unilaterally as a multifocal cancer. Lobular carcinoma in situ coexists in breasts with ILC 70 to 80% of the time. Clinical presentation may be a palpable mass or mammographic abnormality. There may be a diffuse area of thickening or induration of the breast tissue on examination with poorly defined areas of asymmetrical densities seen on mammography [52,58]. Findings on histologic examination of ILC are consistent with several types: linear strands of tumor cells infiltrating the stroma; sheets of uniform cells without stroma; cells in aggregations of 20 or more enclosed in a fibrovascular stroma; or a mixture of tubular and sheetlike tumor cells, pleomorphic in appearance. Biologic markers in ILC typically express estrogen and progesterone receptors and are negative to the HER-2/neu gene. Conservative surgery and radiation therapy or simple mastectomy are mainstays of treatment of ILC [2]. Sentinel node biopsy is less morbid than axillary node dissection and provides prognostic information.

V. Breast Conditions in Older Men

A. Benign Conditions

Gynecomastia is a glandular enlargement of the male breast. It is unilateral and may present as a tender sensation of the breast with diffuse enlargement of the breast tissue. It is particularly common in elderly men in physiologic aging or may be associated with weight gain, obesity, specific drugs (i.e., H_2 blockers, alcohol, tricyclic antidepressants, hormonal agents, narcotics, benzodiazepines, alkylating agents, diuretics, antiarrhythmics) or systemic conditions, such as chronic liver or renal diseases and secondary hypogonadism. It is important to discern gynecomastia from the fatty enlargement of the breasts seen with obesity or that of an underlying carcinoma of the breasts. Physical examination and clinical screening are important in the evaluation of gynecomastia [2,3,7]. Chest radiography can evaluate for underlying lung cancer or metastatic disease. Hyperprolactinemia and β-human chorionic gonadotropin (β-hCG) levels suggest the presence of a testicular tumor or other malignancy (lung or liver). Low levels (<5 mU/ml) of β-hCG and testosterone with a high luteinizing hormone level may be noted in men with primary hypogonadism. An elevated serum estradiol value also may indicate adrenal or testicular tumors. Biopsy specimens from areas of concern in the breast tissue may be taken for further clarification of the diagnosis. Treatment is targeted at the underlying cause. Tamoxifen may be prescribed at 10 mg twice a day to alleviate the tenderness associated with gynecomastia.

A reduction in breast size may occur in 50% of older men. Surgical evaluation should be considered in cases of symptomatic gynecomastia, and most often surgical treatment is a simple mastectomy [4].

B. Malignant Conditions

Breast cancer in men occurs at only about 1% [2,55] of the current incidence of women and occurs at an average age of 60 years. The prognosis for breast cancer in men is worse than that in women. Metastases are often present at the time of the initial presentation of the disease even though clinical presentation of metastatic breast cancer may be latent for years. Hormonal and environmental influences may contribute to the development of breast cancer in men. Clinical presentation consists of a painless hard lump beneath the areola with or without associated nipple discharge, retraction, erosion, or ulceration. A clinical history of gynecomastia before development of breast cancer has been described [3,7]. Biopsy confirms the diagnosis, and breast cancer staging and grade are similar to those of women. Treatment options include modified radical mastectomy and axillary node dissection, and radiotherapy reduces the risk for local recurrence [2,4,55]. Hormone receptor status is important to determine appropriate response to endocrine ablation with tamoxifen, 20 mg daily, or castration for palliative treatment. Castration is effective in reducing tumor growth in 60 to 70% [2,55] of men and may relieve bone pain in men with metastatic disease. Aminoglutethimide, an aromatase inhibitor (250 mg 4 times daily), is also used in the treatment as well as estrogen therapy (diethylstilbestrol, 5 mg 3 times a day). Chemotherapy is indicated similarly as for women. The 5- and 10-year prognosis for all stages of breast cancer in men are 36 and 17%, respectively [2]. Aggressive palliative treatment must be given for metastatic disease in these patients [2,3].

VI. Breast Cancer Treatment Options

In general, more older women have estrogen receptor–positive tumors that are more well differentiated and have lower proliferative rates and an overall beneficial histologic profile than younger women [52,55]. Grading and staging of the disease are as important in older women as they are in younger women. The evaluation should include a detailed assessment of the location and extent of the primary tumor, the presence of positive axillary nodes by radiolabeled isotope examination, and metastatic disease by liver function tests and chest radiography. Therapies for older women are similar to regimens given to younger women with breast cancer [58,59].

Clinicians designing treatment regimens for older patients should consider several factors that influence treatment. These include chronologic and physiologic differences, comorbid medical illness and functional status, social supports, accessibility of medical treatment, potential toxic effects related to pharmacologic treatment, and the patient's own feelings about what the diagnosis of breast cancer means [52,60,61].

Advanced age is not a contraindication to treatment of older women with breast cancer. Surgical options include simple mastectomy or lumpectomy and radiotherapy [5,52]. Localized excision, axillary node sampling, and external-beam radiotherapy have survival rates comparable to those of radical mastectomy in older women. Adjuvant radiotherapy, hormonal therapy, and chemotherapy reduce the rate of local recurrence and increase survival at rates similar to those in younger women [5,18,21]. Tamoxifen has been shown [5,18] to reduce the rate of recurrence of estrogen receptor–positive breast cancers in older women by 50%.

Adjuvant hormonal therapies, including estrogen antagonists (tamoxifen), progestins, and aromatase inhibitors, effectively reduce the recurrence of breast cancer in older women and help control the spread of metastatic disease [2,5,54]. Adjuvant chemotherapy is used for more advanced disease refractory to hormonal treatments at the risk of increased toxicity to patients aged 70 years or older. Corticosteroids ameliorate the symptomatic effects of central nervous system metastases, upper extremity lymphedema, lymphocytic proliferation, and peritumor edema in these patients.

In summary, as more older patients are diagnosed as having breast cancers, they should be treated in a manner similar to their younger counterparts without limiting management and treatment options solely on the basis of age. Studies have shown benefits in survival with adequate intervention in these patients [52,55].

VII. Genomics and Breast Cancer

About half of all breast cancers occur primarily in women aged 65 years or older. Cancer incidence may be higher in the older population because cancers are thought to develop over a long period of time, DNA repair mechanisms decline with aging, and immunity lessens with age [52,55,62]. Key questions surrounding the population aged 65 years or older with cancer have been various: Why are tumors more common in the elderly? What are the differences in tumor aggressiveness? How should treatment be structured for this population?

Older patients with breast cancer are more likely to have a more favorable histologic type, higher levels of estrogen and progesterone receptor expression, lower growth fractions, and fewer occurrences of metastases. Older patients appear to have a longer survival than younger patients with breast cancer. In turn, this raises the question of treatment choices in this age group [7,58]. Surveys have shown that older women tend to choose more life-extending treatments even when the risk of toxicity is higher. Controversial breast cancer treatments for older women include irradiation after lumpectomy, adjuvant hormonal treatment, and the management of metastatic breast disease [2,5,52]. Furthermore, the age at which screening mammography should stop has not been established. This ranges from 74 to 85 years, depending on the consensus statement of the specific organization (e.g., American Geriatrics Society [58], USPSTF [41,59,60], American Cancer Society [7,41,52,55,58–60], American College of Radiology [7,41,52,55,58–60], American Academy of Family Physicians) [7,41,52,55,58–60,63]. The area of geriatric oncology is becoming increasingly important in terms of addressing these areas of screening, diagnosis and histologic type, pattern of disease, and mortality and treatment.

Genetic marker therapy with DNA chip technology allows parallel expression to profile thousands of genes. Cellular transcriptional activities in normal physiology and disease are characterized. DNA microarrays are used to identify gene expression patterns, particularly in cancer tissues. This has been shown to be useful in classifying tumors on the basis of shared expression patterns [64]. Several studies have examined the gene expression patterns of breast cancers and their subtypes, including examining lesions that predict higher risk of recurrence. Of note, however, few studies show a direct correlation between clinical variables and activity of these gene expression patterns and necessary follow-up to determine the course of breast cancers in relation to these patterns. This may be attributable to interference with protein synthesis, posttranslational modification, or both. Proteomics profiling, a corollary to genomic microarrays, involves the systemic separation, identification, and characterization of proteins present in biologic specimens [64]. Normal and abnormal tissue samples can be compared to discern a difference in protein expression with use of automated techniques. Proteomic analysis of both tissue and bodily fluids (serum, urine, cerebrospinal fluid, and synovial fluid) is meaningful to identify disease processes, including risks of disease and responses to potential treatments.

In summary, the implications of genomics research and breast cancer risk and detection for prevention and treatment are promising.

VIII. Suggestions for Further Investigations

- Understanding gene expression patterns in cancer and response to treatment
- Combined screening modalities in reducing breast cancer mortality in the elderly
- Lifestyle modification and its role in prevention of disease in the elderly

References

1. Pruthi S. (2001). Detection and evaluation of a palpable breast mass. *Mayo Clin Proc.* 76:641–648.
2. Harris JR, Lippman ME, Morrow M, Osborne CK. (2000). *Diseases of the Breast*, 2nd Edition. Philadelphia: Lippincott Williams & Wilkins.
3. Marchant DJ. (2002). Benign breast disease. *Obstet Gynecol Clin North Am.* 29:1–20.
4. Morrow M. (2000). The evaluation of common breast problems. *Am Fam Physician.* 61:2371–2378, 2385.
5. Morrow M. (1994). Breast disease in elderly women. *Surg Clin North Am.* 74:145–161.
6. Davies EL, Gateley CA, Miers M, Mansel RE. (1998). The long-term course of mastalgia. *J R Soc Med.* 91:462–464.
7. Osuch JR. (1998). Breast Health and Disorders Over the Life Phases. In *Textbook of Women's Health* (Wallis LA, Kasper AS, Reader GG et al., eds.), pp. 295–313. Philadelphia: Lippincott-Raven.
8. Levinson W, Dunn PM. (1986). Nonassociation of caffeine and fibrocystic breast disease. *Arch Intern Med.* 146:1773–1775.
9. Abrams AA. (1965). Use of vitamin E in chronic cystic mastitis (letter). *N Engl J Med.* 272:1080–1081.
10. Ernster VL, Goodson WH III, Hunt TK et al. (1985). Vitamin E and benign breast "disease": A double-blind, randomized clinical trial. *Surgery.* 97:490–494.
11. London RS, Sundaram GS, Murphy L et al. (1985). The effect of vitamin E on mammary dysplasia: A double-blind study. *Obstet Gynecol.* 65:104–106.
12. Pashby NL, Mansel RE, Hughes LE et al. (1981). A clinical trial of evening primrose oil in mastalgia (abstract). *Br J Surg.* 68:801.
13. Preece PE, Mansel RE, Bolton PM et al. (1976). Clinical syndromes of mastalgia. 2:670–673.
14. Pye JK, Mansel RE, Hughes LE. (1985). Clinical experience of drug treatments for mastalgia. *Lancet.* 2:373–377.

15. Baker HW, Snedecor PA. (1979). Clinical trial of danazol for benign breast disease. *Am Surg.* 45:727–729.

16. Greenblatt B, Ben-Nun I. (1980). Danazol in the treatment of mammary dysplasia. *Drugs.* 19:349–355.

17. Haagensen CD, Bodian C, Haagensen DE Jr. (1981). *Breast Carcinoma: Risk and Detection.* Philadelphia: WB Saunders.

18. Balducci L, Extermann M, Carreca I. (2001). Management of breast cancer in the older woman. *Cancer Control.* 8:431–441.

19. American Cancer Society. Breast Cancer Facts & Figures 2001–2002. American Cancer Society, Inc., Atlanta. Available at http://www.cancer.org/downloads/STT/BrCaFF2001.pdf (accessed March 18, 2003).

20. Vogel VG. (2001). *Management of Patients at High Risk for Breast Cancer.* Malden, MA: Blackwell Science.

21. Alberg AJ, Singh S. (2001). Epidemiology of breast cancer in older women: Implications for future healthcare. *Drugs Aging.* 18:761–772.

22. Ragaz J. (2002). Hormone replacement therapy in patients with a prior breast cancer history: A critical review. In *Manual of Breast Diseases* (Jatoi I, ed.), pp. 389–415. Philadelphia: Lippincott Williams & Wilkins.

23. Kelsey JL, Gammon MD, John EM. (1993). Reproductive factors and breast cancer. *Epidemiol Rev.* 15:36–47.

24. Martin AM, Weber BL. (2000). Genetic and hormonal risk factors in breast cancer. *J Natl Cancer Inst.* 92:1126–1135.

25. Rossouw JE, Anderson GL, Prentice RL *et al.* (2002). Risks and benefits of estrogen plus progestin in healthy postmenopausal women: Principal results from the Women's Health Initiative randomized controlled trial. *JAMA.* 288:321–333.

26. U.S. Preventive Services Task Force (2002). Postmenopausal hormone replacement therapy for primary prevention of chronic conditions: Recommendations and rationale. *Ann Intern Med.* 137:834–839.

27. Ganz PA, Castellon SA, Silverman DH. (2002). Estrogen, tamoxifen, and the brain. *J Natl Cancer Inst.* 94:547–549.

28. Moore DB, Folsom AR, Mink PJ *et al.* (2000). Physical activity and incidence of postmenopausal breast cancer. *Epidemiology.* 11:292–296.

29. Freedman LS, Clifford C, Messina M. (1990). Analysis of dietary fat, calories, body weight, and the development of mammary tumors in rats and mice: A review. *Cancer Res.* 50:5710–5719.

30. Hunter DJ, Spiegelman D, Adami HO *et al.* (1996). Cohort studies of fat intake and the risk of breast cancer—A pooled analysis. *N Engl J Med.* 334:356–361.

31. Sellars TA, Grabrick DM. (2002). The Epidemiology of Breast Cancer. In *Manual of Breast Diseases* (Jatoi I, ed.), pp. 149–175. Philadelphia: Lippincott Williams & Wilkins.

32. Kropp S, Chang-Claude J. (2002). Active and passive smoking and risk of breast cancer by age 50 years among German women. *Am J Epidemiol.* 156:616–626.

33. Calle EE, Miracle-McMahill HL, Thun MJ, Heath CW Jr. (1994). Cigarette smoking and risk of fatal breast cancer. *Am J Epidemiol.* 139:1001–1007.

34. Longnecker MP. (1994). Alcoholic beverage consumption in relation to risk of breast cancer: meta-analysis and review. *Cancer Causes Control.* 5:73–82.

35. Reichman ME, Judd JT, Longcope C *et al.* (1993). Effects of alcohol consumption on plasma and urinary hormone concentrations in premenopausal women. *J Natl Cancer Inst.* 85:722–727.

36. Chen WY, Colditz GA, Rosner B *et al.* (2002). Use of postmenopausal hormones, alcohol, and risk for invasive breast cancer. *Ann Intern Med.* 137:798–804.

37. Thomas DB, Gao DL, Ray RM *et al.* (2002). Randomized trial of breast self-examination in Shanghai: Final results. *J Natl Cancer Inst.* 94:1445–1457.

38. Burack RC, Gurney JG, McDaniel AM. (1998). Health status and mammography use among older women. *J Gen Intern Med.* 13:366–372.

39. Walter LC, Eng C, Covinsky KE. (2001). Screening mammography for frail older women: What are the burdens? *J Gen Intern Med.* 16:779–784.

40. Welch HG, Albertsen PC, Nease RF *et al.* (1996). Estimating treatment benefits for the elderly: The effect of competing risks. *Ann Intern Med.* 124:577–584.

41. U.S. Preventive Services Task Force (2002). Screening for breast cancer: Recommendations and rationale. *Am Fam Physician.* 65:2537–2544.

42. McCarthy EP, Burns RB, Coughlin SS *et al.* (1998). Mammography use helps to explain differences in breast cancer stage at diagnosis between older black and white women. *Ann Intern Med.* 128:729–736.

43. Wickerham DL, Tan-Chiu E. (2001). Breast cancer chemoprevention: Current status and future directions. *Semin Oncol.* 28:253–259.

44. Powles T, Eeles R, Ashley S *et al.* (1998). Interim analysis of the incidence of breast cancer in the Royal Marsden Hospital tamoxifen randomised chemoprevention trial. *Lancet.* 352:98–101.

45. Veronesi U, Maisonneuve P, Costa A *et al.* (1998). Prevention of breast cancer with tamoxifen: preliminary findings from the Italian randomised trial among hysterectomised women. Italian Tamoxifen Prevention Study. *Lancet.* 352:93–97.

46. Fisher B, Costantino JP, Wickerham DL *et al.* (1998). Tamoxifen for prevention of breast cancer: report of the National Surgical Adjuvant Breast and Bowel Project P-1 Study. *J Natl Cancer Inst.* 90:1371–1388.

47. IBIS Investigators. (2002). First results from the International Breast Cancer Intervention Study (IBIS-I): A randomised prevention trial. *Lancet.* 360:817–824.

48. Chlebowski RT, Col N, Winer EP *et al.* for the American Society of Clinical Oncology Breast Cancer Technology Assessment Working Group (2002). American Society of Clinical Oncology technology assessment of pharmacologic interventions for breast cancer risk reduction including tamoxifen, raloxifene, and aromatase inhibition. *J Clin Oncol.* 20:3328–3343.

49. Cummings SR, Eckert S, Krueger KA *et al.* (1999). The effect of raloxifene on risk of breast cancer in postmenopausal women. Results from the MORE randomized trial. Multiple Outcomes of Raloxifene Evaluation. *JAMA.* 281:2189–2197.

50. U.S. Preventive Services Task Force (2002). Chemoprevention of breast cancer: Recommendations and rationale. *Ann Intern Med.* 137:56–58.

51. Gail MH, Costantino JP, Bryant J *et al.* (1999). Weighing the risks and benefits of tamoxifen treatment for preventing breast cancer. *J Natl Cancer Inst.* 91:1829–1846.

52. Balducci L, Phillips DM. (1998). Breast cancer in older women. *Am Fam Physician.* 58:1163–1172.

53. Marks LB, Prosnitz LR. (1997). Lumpectomy with and without radiation for early-stage breast cancer and DCIS. *Oncology (Huntingt).* 11:1361–1371.

54. Grube BJ, Hansen NM, Ye W *et al.* (2001). Surgical management of breast cancer in the elderly patient. *Am J Surg.* 182:359–364.

55. Apantaku LM. (2000). Breast cancer diagnosis and screening. *Am Fam Physician.* 62:596–602.

56. Fisher B, Anderson S, Bryant J *et al.* (2002). Twenty-year follow-up of a randomized trial comparing total mastectomy, lumpectomy, and lumpectomy plus irradiation for the treatment of invasive breast cancer. *N Engl J Med.* 347:1233–1241.

57. Fisher B, Dignam J, Wolmark N *et al.* (1999). Tamoxifen in treatment of intraductal breast cancer: National Surgical Adjuvant Breast and Bowel Project B-24 randomised controlled trial. *Lancet.* 353:1993–2000.

58. American Geriatrics Society Clinical Practice Committee (2000). Breast cancer screening in older women. *J Am Geriatr Soc.* 48:842–844.

59. U.S. Preventive Services Task Force (1996). *Guide to Clinical Preventive Services: Report of the U.S. Preventive Services Task Force,* 2nd Edition. Baltimore: Williams & Wilkins.

60. Humphrey LL, Helfand M, Chan BK, Woolf SH. (2002). Breast cancer screening: A summary of the evidence for the U.S. Preventive Services Task Force. *Ann Intern Med.* 137:347–360.

61. McCarthy EP, Burns RB, Freund KM *et al.* (2000). Mammography use, breast cancer stage at diagnosis, and survival among older women. *J Am Geriatr Soc.* 48:1226–1233.

62. Vanderford V. (1999). Older women and mammography: Factors influencing their attitudes. *Geriatr Nurs.* 20:257–259.

63. Miller AB, To T, Baines CJ, Wall C. (2002). The Canadian National Breast Screening Study-1: Breast cancer mortality after 11 to 16 years of follow-up: A randomized screening trial of mammography in women age 40 to 49 years. *Ann Intern Med.* 137:305–312.

64. Kennedy S. (2001). Proteomic profiling from human samples: The body fluid alternative. *Toxicol Lett (Amst).* 120:379–384.

107

Care of the Older Women: Practical Issues

CAROL L. KUHLE, DO

Mayo/Mercy Family Practice Residency; Instructor, Mayo Clinic Graduate School of Medical Education,
Des Moines, IA

I. Introduction

Physicians will be faced with a dramatic increase in the elderly population over the next 30 years. Individuals older than the age of 65 are estimated to represent 17 to 22% of the U.S. population by 2030. Seventy-two percent of individuals older than the age of 65 will be women [1–3]. The number of women older than 85 is expected to double between 2030 and 2050 [4].

Prevention of disability and promotion of wellness in elderly women has far reaching public health implications. Women older than 65 years are reported to see their physician less for routine screening and health maintenance compared with younger women [5]. Significant barriers to appropriate screening of elderly women involve issues with both the patient and the provider. Physician recommendation is the major predictor of compliance with preventative screening. Every office visit by an elderly women should become an opportunity to discuss routine health maintenance issues [6].

This chapter explores the core health screening issues that impact elderly women, reviews related risk factors, and develops a practical approach to preventative health maintenance in the older women based on available scientific evidence. Medicare reimbursement criteria for health maintenance screening are also examined (Table 107-1).

II. Clinical Decision Making in the Geriatric Patient

Clinical trials on preventative health screening in the elderly, both men and women, have been limited leaving clinicians without clear evidence to guide decisions. Along with the increase incidence of cancer in the elderly, there is an increase in the positive predictive value of the screening tests [7–9]. Important considerations that influence screening decisions are (Table 107-2) [10]:

- The life expectancy of the patient
- The condition being screened and the associated morbidity and mortality
- Effects of previous screening that may have eliminated the majority potential of the disease
- The effects of prevention on the general health and quality of life of the individual
- The desire of the individual to be screened

These questions are especially important in individuals older than 70 years because the prevalence of age-related changes increases dramatically between age 70 and 75 [10]. Frailty becomes a distinction in deciding that an individual is appropriate for screening, and influences decisions about whether treatment or palliative therapy is appropriate when there is a significant finding. Frailty denotes a reduction in functional reserve making

Table 107-1
Medicare Reimbursement for Screening Examinations

Test	MC Code	Frequency	Diagnosis	Comments	Waivers
Bone density ultrasound	76977	Every 24 months	256.3—Most commonly: postmenopausal/estrogen deficiency		Yes, if does not meet the local medical review policy
Breast/pelvic examination	G0101	Every 2 years screening	V76.2—Screening V76.49—No uterus/cervix screening	7 of 12 elements must be documented	Yes for frequency
		Every year for high-risk patients	V15.89—High risk		GA modifier
Pap smear	Q0091	Every 2 years screening	V76.2—Screening	Do not use with E/M with genitourinary DX	Yes—Pap waiver for frequency
		Every year for high-risk patients	V15.89—High risk		GA modifier
Mammography	N/A clinics	>39 and >11 months since last screening	V76.12—Screening V76.11—High risk		Yes for frequency GA modifier

DX, diagnosis; E/M, evaluation/management; GA, waiver of liability statement on file; N/A, not applicable.

Table 107-2

Consideration for Screening Individuals Older than Age 65 Years

Life expectancy of the patient

The condition being screened and associated morbidity and mortality

Effects of previous screening that eliminates potential of disease

Effects of prevention on the general health and quality of life

Effects of clinical status on potential treatment decisions

Desire of the individual to be screened

(From Balducci L, Extermann M. [2001]. A practical approach to the older patient with cancer. *Curr Prob Cancer*. Jan/Feb:7–76, with permission.)

Table 107-3

Elements of Frailty

Dependence in one or more ADLs

Presence of one or more geriatric syndrome

Presence of three or more moderately severe comorbid conditions or of a serious, life-threatening co-morbid condition

ADLs, activities of daily living.
(From Balducci L, Begne C. [2002]. Management of cancer in the older person. *Clin Geriatr*. 10:54–59, with permission.)

the person less able to withstand the stress of aggressive therapy. Frailty can be defined by the presence of at least one of the following (Table 107-3) [11]:

- Dependence in one or more activities of daily living (ADLs)
- Presence of one or more geriatric syndromes
- Presence of three or more moderately severe co-morbid conditions or of a serious, life-threatening co-morbid condition

The primary care physician must consider recent advances in treatment of cancer when making a decision about which individuals will benefit from screening and potential treatment. Development of safer approaches to anesthesia and reduction in the extent of many procedures have made surgery more tolerable in older patients. Standard external beam radiation therapy has proven to be well tolerated by individuals older than the age of 80 [12]. New hormonal therapies are reasonably safe even in the oldest patient, and recent advances in use of chemotherapy drugs may ameliorate complications that were once devastating to older individuals [10].

III. Gynecologic Cancers

The incidence of gynecologic tumors increases in elderly women. After age 65, the risk of developing uterine cancer is 2-fold and ovarian cancer is 3-fold. Cervical cancer risk increases by 10% compared with women aged 40 to 65 years old. Gynecologic cancers tend to be diagnosed at more advanced stages [13,14]. The epidemiology, assessment of risk factors, and screening recommendations for gynecologic cancers are reviewed in this section.

A. Ovarian Cancer

1. Epidemiology

Ovarian cancer is the fifth most common malignancy in U.S. women and accounts for about 4 to 6% of all cancer cases in women in developed countries [15,16]. Epithelial ovarian cancer peaks in the seventh and eight decade of life with greater than 50% of ovarian cancers in women older than 65 years [17]. The mortality rate from ovarian cancer is greater than all gynecologic malignancies combined [15].

The stage of disease at presentation is more advanced in the elderly. Data from the Surveillance, Epidemiology, and End Results (SEER) reported presentation with stage I disease in 50% of patients younger than age 45, whereas 74% of patients age 74 or older presented with stage III or IV disease [18]. This is consistent with data analyzed by the International Federation of Gynecologic and Obstetrics (FIGO) Staging System [14]. Survival rates in the elderly are consistent with advanced disease at presentation. Five-year survival rate in stage I disease exceeds 80% compared with a 10% 5-year survival rate for stage IV disease [19].

2. Assessing Risk

The mechanisms of carcinogenesis in ovarian cancer are thought to be related to factors that affect the lifetime number of ovulations. Early menarche, late menopause, nulliparity, and low parity have been consistently related to an increase in ovarian cancer risk in both the young and the old [16]. The protection afforded by oral contraception does not apply to our present generation of elderly but will have an impact on the baby boomer generation as they age. Hormone replacement, particularly for greater than 10 years, has been related to an increased risk for ovarian cancer in some studies [16,20].

3. Screening

Early diagnosis of ovarian cancer is difficult because of the nonspecific symptoms of bloating, abdominal pain, indigestion, and fatigue in the months preceding diagnosis [5]. Pelvic examination detection rate is low for adnexal masses, and present screening methods lack evidence of mortality reduction [21].

a. CA-125. Levels of Ca-125 remain within normal limits for many women with early disease. Although an elevated Ca-125 is found in 50% of stage I and 90% of stage II, III, and IV disease, it has low specificity with many other causes for elevation. Ca-125 is felt to be an inadequate screen for ovarian cancer and is best used in following established disease [5,15,22].

b. TRANSVAGINAL ULTRASOUND (TVU). Transvaginal ultrasound has a low yield for detecting ovarian cancer in asymptomatic women. In studies of asymptomatic women at low risk and with a family history of ovarian cancer, only a few cases of ovarian cancer were detected at a high cost [23,24]. Although morphologic scoring and color flow Doppler have increased the specificity in clinically suspected disease to 90%, TVU is not recommended for routine screening in the general population at any age [22].

Women with families carrying the BRCA1 and/or BRCA2 gene, are of Ashkenazi descent, or are from families with two first-degree relatives with ovarian cancer are more likely to develop ovarian cancer [15,16,19,25]. Some literature recommends that screening be started by age 25 to 35 years old in this high-risk population, but benefit for this approach has not been proven [22]. (Medicare does not reimburse for screening Ca-125 or TVU in the general population.)

B. Endometrial Cancer

1. Epidemiology

Endometrial cancer is the most commonly diagnosed cancer of the female genital tract in developed countries [26]. Although overall mortality is low, elderly women present at a more advanced stage with less well differentiated and more invasive endometrial tumors [27,28]. Five-year survival rates of 76% for stage I disease are markedly decreased to 10.3% for stage IV disease [21].

2. Assessing Risk

Unopposed estrogen has been hypothesized to increase the risk of endometrial cancer. Factors that contribute to increased concentrations of circulating estrogens include obesity, chronic anovulation, late menopause, nulliparity, and exogenous estrogen unopposed by progesterone [29]. Other factors that increase risk are diabetes, hypertension, and pelvic irradiation [30].

3. Screening

Ninety percent of women with endometrial cancer present with abnormal vaginal bleeding. The amount of bleeding does not always correlate with the severity of the disease. Two to 5% of asymptomatic women with endometrial cancer are diagnosed after finding endometrial cells on their Pap smear [30]. Fifty percent of women with endometrial cancer have suspicious cervical cytology when initially diagnosed [31–34]. Women with endometrial cancer and positive cervical cytology were found to be older and had a higher FIGO stage [33–35]. Although annual screening with endometrial biopsy and TVU have not been shown to be cost-effective, even in high risk women, an endometrial biopsy is indicated in women with endometrial cells on their Pap smear [30].

Women on tamoxifen (Nolvadex) are a special concern as they are at risk for developing endometrial cancer. The National Surgical Adjuvant Breast and Bowel Project B-14 Trial found that these cancers are usually diagnosed at an early stage with good survival and screening endometrial biopsy for women on tamoxifen is not indicated. These findings have been confirmed in several other trials [22,36,37]. (Medicare does not reimburse for screening TVU or endometrial biopsy for endometrial cancer screening.)

C. Cervical Cancer

1. Epidemiology

Although cervical cancer is the sixth most common cancer in women in developed countries, the incidence is low after the age of 65. Older women, however, are less likely to have been screened and present with more advanced disease compared with younger women [14,28,38]. Fifteen percent of women aged 65 to 74 and 38% older than age 75 have never had a Pap smear, and more than 75% older than age 65 have never had regular screening [39].

2. Assessing Risk

Assessing sexual history in older women may be difficult to obtain but is important. History of multiple sexual partners, intercourse at a young age, venereal warts, and smoking increase the risk of cervical cancer [40,41]. The highest percentage of late-stage cervical cancer is found in women older than 65 years regardless of race or ethnic background [42,43].

Human papillomavirus (HPV) is found in 93% of all cervical cancers [44]. It is thought that an exposure to an oncogenic strain of HPV 16, 18, 31, or 33 during the second or third decade of life will gradually progress to invasive disease over 10 to 15 years. Human papillomavirus causing cervical cancer in older women is similar to those found in younger women. The question is whether there is a longer latency for oncogenic HPV in the elderly or if it is a result of new exposure to sexually transmitted diseases into the seventh decade of life [45]. DNA testing for high-risk types of HPV should be considered in older women with abnormal Pap smears in accordance with the 2001 consensus guidelines for management of women with abnormal cervical cytology [46].

Evaluating Pap smears in the elderly can be challenging. Specimen adequacy is noted based on the presence/absence of endocervical/transformation zone component [46]. Older women may have stenotic atrophic cervices making identification of the squamous columnar junction difficult. In elderly patients with an abnormal Pap smear, cone biopsy or loop electrosurgical excision procedure (LEEP) is often necessary to make the diagnosis. Visible lesions should be biopsied regardless of the Pap smear results [23].

3. Screening

Triennial screening in the elderly can reduce cervical cancer mortality by 74% [39,47,48]. There is no consensus about cervical screening among professional organizations. Cervical screening is recommended throughout a women's life by the National Cancer Institute, the American College of Obstetrics and Gynecology, and the American Cancer Society. The United States Preventative Task Force (USPTF), the American Geriatrics Society, and Mayo Clinic recommend Pap smears every 1 to 3 years until age 65. With the lack of clear evidence to support continuing cervical screening beyond age 65, this seems a reasonable approach. Pap smears can then be discontinued if several have been normal. In women who have not been screened adequately, Pap smears should be done annually until there are three negative examinations. Pap smears can then be discontinued after age 65 to 69. Risk factors should be taken into consideration when making a decision to decrease or discontinue Pap smears [28,49–51].

Older women with Pap smears reporting atypical glandular cells of undetermined significance (AGUS) require special consideration. It is recommended that women older than age 45 with AGUS have colposcopy, endocervical curettage with appropriate cervical biopsies, and endometrial biopsy because there is a one in three chance that a significant abnormality will be found. Extrauterine cancers should also be considered. In one series, 6 out of 281 women studied had cancer involving the bladder, colon, breast, vagina, and ovary [52]. (Medicare covers cervical screening every 2 years.)

D. Vulvar Cancer

1. Epidemiology

Vulvar cancer accounts for 3 to 5% of female genital tract malignancies [53]. Recent evidence suggests that vulvar cancer affecting older women in the sixth or seventh decade of life is distinct from vulvar cancer in younger women. Vulvar cancer related to HPV is more prevalent in women younger than 50 years, whereas vulvar non-neoplastic epithelial disorders (VNED) lead to cellular atypia and cancer in advanced age as a result of chronic inflammation. The rate of vulvar cancer increases with age reaching a peak of 20 per 100,000 women by 75 years of age [54].

2. Assessing Risk

As compared with younger women, older women with vulvar cancer are more likely to have a history of pre-existing vulvar inflammation, lichen sclerosis, or squamous cell hyperplasia. There is a low association with cervical cancer and history of smoking, a rare association with sexually transmitted disease, and a more well-differentiated histology compared with women with vulvar cancer related to pre-existing vulvar intraepithelial neoplasia (VIN) from HPV. Other potential causes for vulvar cancer include melanoma, adenocarcinoma, verrucous carcinoma, Paget's disease, and sarcoma [55].

3. Screening

Long-standing pruritus of the vulva is a characteristic presentation of vulvar cancer. Vaginal bleeding, discharge, dysuria, and pain may also be present. Despite lack of supporting evidence, expert opinion recommends annual visual inspection of the vulva even if the patient is no longer receiving annual Pap smears [56].

Differentiating normal from abnormal findings of the vulva can be challenging. Any vulvar lesion that is not responding to therapy, is suspicious for neoplasia, or cannot be reliably diagnosed by visual inspection should be biopsied [57]. Multiple punch biopsies through the dermis should be taken to detect possible invasion. Colposcopic examination may aid in defining a vulvar lesion, but any acetowhite lesion is nonspecific and suspicious [58]. (Medicare does not reimburse for screening examinations.)

III. Breast Cancer

A. Epidemiology

Breast cancer is the most common female malignancy and the leading cause of cancer death among women in the United States [59–61]. Fifty percent of newly diagnosed breast cancers are in women older than age 65, accounting for an approximate 10-fold increase in incidence compared to women younger than 65 [59]. For unclear reasons, older black women experience higher rates of breast cancer mortality [62].

All women are at risk, with an estimated 60 to 70% of all breast cancer patients without any obvious risk factors [63]. Lifetime risk for breast cancer differs with age. The common projection of a 1 in 8 cumulative lifetime risk for breast cancer does not account for the risk at varying ages. Women aged 50 to 59 years have a 1 in 36 lifetime risk, whereas women aged 70 to 79 have a 1 in 24 lifetime risk of having breast cancer [64].

B. Assessing Risk

Modifiable and nonmodifiable risk factors should be taken into consideration when assessing risk for breast cancer mortality in older women. Evidence about potential modifiable risk factors has been mostly epidemiologic and conflicting. Some recent studies have attempted to clarify risk and their impact on the incidence of breast cancer.

Women who carry BRCA1 and BRCA2 mutations have a high risk for developing both breast and ovarian cancers. By age 70 years, breast cancer survivors with a documented BRCA1 mutation have a 64% chance and BRCA2 have a 50% chance of developing a second primary breast cancer [65]. A family history of breast cancer, with or without a mutation, should be considered in the decision to screen older women for breast cancer.

The question of whether hormone replacement therapy (HRT) causes breast cancer remains unclear. The recent findings in the Women's Health Initiative (WHI) demonstrated a statistically significant increase in rates of invasive breast cancer compared with placebo in the estrogen plus progesterone group after 4 years of treatment [66]. A recent multicenter, case-controlled study also examined the breast cancer risk with different hormone therapy regimens. Issues raised by the WHI study were again strengthened as current users of continuous combined estrogen-progesterone for at least 5 years were found to have a significantly greater risk for breast cancer (odds ratio 1.54) [67]. The Breast Cancer Detection Demonstration Project with 46,000 women followed for 15 years also demonstrated that combination therapy with estrogen and progestin increased breast cancer risk when compared with estrogen alone in lean women (body mass index [BMI] <23) or on cyclic therapy [68,69]. In contrast, a review of epidemiologic evidence between 1975 to 2000 did not support the hypotheses that HRT with estrogen alone or in combination with progesterone significantly increased the risk of breast cancer [70]. Certainly use of HRT and the duration of use should be taken into consideration when assessing risk of invasive breast cancer.

Some lifestyle modifications may reduce the incidence of breast cancer. In a prospective cohort study of 44,186 registered nurses followed 16 years (Nurse's Health Study), consumption of 10 to 19.9 g (1 drink) or >20 g (>2 drinks) daily were associated with increased risk for breast cancer compared with no alcohol use (relative risk [RR] 1.2 vs. 1.3) The breast cancer risk increased in women who were on HRT and consumed alcohol compared with nonusers who did not drink (5 to 9.9 g or 10 to 19 g of alcohol daily, >5 years of HRT: RR 1.6 and 1.9, respectively) [71]. Cigarette smoking data has been conflicting; however, a recent study of 544 families at highest genetic risk for breast cancer (each containing five breast and/or ovarian cancers) demonstrated a 5.8-fold greater risk among daughters and sisters in ever-smokers compared with nonsmokers [72]. One study on screening mammography in women aged 70 to 79 years found a small gain in life expectancy and moderate costs savings in screening women with high bone mineral densities (BMD) compared with women with low BMDs [73]. These risk factors along with family history and use of HRT should be taken into consideration when deciding on which women older than age 70 to continue screening for breast cancer.

C. Screening

Screening for breast cancer in women older than 65 years has been controversial. Organizations that make screening recommendations in elderly women are conflicting and based on trials that include too few women aged 70 or older to provide meaningful results. The methodology of older studies that provided scientific basis for screening recommendations has been challenged by Cochrane reviewers [74–77]. The United States Preventative Services Task Force (USPSTF) identified similar design flaws but felt there was fair methodologic quality in the studies reviewed with consistent evidence that screening with mammography reduces breast cancer mortality among women aged 40 to 74 years of age [78].

A recent retrospective study was published reviewing information obtained from the SEER program and Medicare claims databases looking at 12,038 women diagnosed with a diagnosis of breast cancer after age 65. Older women with breast cancer were less likely to have undergone screening mammograms within 2 years before their diagnoses compared with younger women (59% vs 67%). Women older than the age of 75 were more likely to be diagnosed with stage IIA or worse compared with younger women (44% vs 36%). Despite this information, the question whether the risks of mammography outweigh the benefits in elderly remains unanswered [79].

Recommendations for screening mammography vary among organizations. The American Cancer Society (ACS) recommends yearly mammograms and clinical breast examinations (CBEs) with no upper age limit. Recommendations for mammograms and CBE every other year are made up to age 85 by the American Geriatrics Society (AGS) [80]. The USPTF felt upper age limits for mammography were uncertain because of lack of scientific evidence after age 74 [78].

Women older than age 70 are a heterogeneous group. Benefit for screening mammography has been found when there is a high risk of death from breast cancer, when there is a low risk of death from other causes, when women perceive themselves to be in good health or attach a high value to avoiding death from breast cancer, and when they are not bothered by the prospect of false-positive screening tests result or of being diagnosed and treated for breast cancer [81]. Whether to continue screening mammograms for women older than the age of 70 requires a decision based on the benefit gained for the individual patient. Consideration for concluding screening should be when a women's life expectancy is less than 6 years resulting from non-breast cancer causes [51]. (Medicare reimburses for annual mammograms.)

IV. Osteoporosis

A. Epidemiology

A recent United States National Institutes of Health consensus conference redefined osteoporosis as " a skeletal disorder characterized by compromised bone strength predisposing a person to an increased risk of fracture." Osteoporosis is characterized by a compromise in both the density and quality of the bone [82]. Twenty-nine percent of U.S. women older than age 65 have osteoporosis by BMD determination, and 20 to 30% already have at least one osteoporosis related vertebral fracture [83–85]. Vertebral fractures causing severe pain have led to 150,000 hospital admissions and 161,000 physician office visits annually [86].

Osteoporosis, a largely preventable disease, causes significant morbidity and mortality. In the 6 months following a hip fracture, 12 to 20% will die. Fifty percent of survivors will require an assistance device for ambulation, and 25% will require either nursing home care or assisted living [87].

Vertebral fractures also cause significant morbidity and mortality. Vertebral fracture are reported to increase the risk of a second vertebral fracture 4-fold [88,89]. The combination of a vertebral fracture and low bone density is associated with a doubling of the 3-year risk of hip fracture in women older than age 70 [90].

Despite well-recognized advances in diagnosis and treatment, low rates of screening and treatment of women with osteoporosis is reported. The National Health and Nutrition Examination Survey III found that only 5% of women with osteoporosis on BMD were told by the physician that they had osteoporosis [91,92]. Understanding risk factors and recommended screening will reduce both the cost and related morbidity and mortality from osteoporosis.

B. Assessing Risk

Several excellent reviews have been done in assessing risk factors for osteoporosis. Age alone is considered a major risk factor. Kanis *et al* reported that the 10-year probability for a fracture of the forearm, humerus, spine, or hip increases 8-fold between the ages of 45 and 80 for women and 5-fold for men [88,89]. The data from the USPTF and the National Institutes of Health in their updated consensus reports agree with this assessment [82,93].

The 2002 clinical practice guidelines for the diagnosis and management of osteoporosis in Canada categorize risk factors as major and minor (Table 107-4) [94].

The USPSTF recommendations for screening women 60 to 64 was also on the basis of risk factor assessment. The exact risk factors were difficult to specify based on evidence, but low body weight (<70 kg) was felt to be the single best predictor of low bone density. Other risk factors such as smoking, family history alcohol, caffeine use, or low calcium or vitamin D intake had less evidence to support their use in assessing screening women younger than age 65 [95].

Race influences risk for osteoporosis. African-American women have higher BMD and half the fracture rates compared with white women. Asian women have lower BMD but 40 to 50% lower fracture risk compared with white women making

Table 107-4
Factors that Identify People Who Should Be Assessed for Osteoporosis

Major Risk Factors	Minor Risk Factors
Age >65 years	Rheumatoid arthritis
Vertebral compression fracture	Past history of clinical hyperthyroidism
Fragility fracture after age 40	Chronic anticonvulsant therapy
Family history of osteoporotic fracture(especially maternal hipfracture)	Low dietary calcium intake (see nutrition section)
Systemic glucocorticoid therapy of >3 months' duration	Smoker
Malabsorption syndrome	Excessive alcohol intake
Primary hyperparathyroidism	Excessive caffeine intake (see nutrition section)
Propensity to fall	Weight <57 kg
Osteopenia apparent on x-ray film	Weight loss >10% of weight at age 25
Hypogonadism	Chronic heparin therapy
Early menopause (before age 45)	

(From Brown JP, Josse RG. [2002]. 2002 clinical guidelines for the diagnosis and management of osteoporosis in Canada. *CMAJ.* 167[10 Suppl]:1–34, with permission.)

dual-energy x-ray absorptiometry (DXA) an inaccurate measure in Asian women [96].

C. Screening

Measurement of the central skeleton using DXA is the gold standard and the preferred method in diagnosing osteoporosis and monitoring response to therapy [94,97]. Quantitative ultrasound (QUS) of the calcaneus in the absence of availability of DXA appears effective in estimating risk of fracture in women older than 65 years. Quantitative ultrasound is not useful in monitoring response to treatment because of insufficient ability to demonstrate changes in mineral density over 1- to 3-year intervals [98,99].

The World Health Organization (WHO) defines osteoporosis as a bone density of 2.5 standard deviations (SDs) below the mean for young adult women (T-score at or below −2.5). Osteopenia or low bone mass is defined as BMD between 1 and 2.5 SD below the mean for young adult women (T-score between −1 and −2.5) [100]. Z-scores represent the standard deviation below the bone density of the average women, at the same age as the subject, with the same physique [96]. Although there is no standard, secondary causes for osteoporosis should be considered when a patient's Z-score is >1.5 SD below the mean [101]. The WHO study group identified "severe osteoporosis" in patients with a T-score below −2.5 and a history of a fragility fracture. Fragility fractures are defined as a fracture that occurs with minimal trauma such as from a standing height or less or with no trauma [102].

The National Osteoporosis Foundation (NOF), the USPSTF, the Canadian consensus group on osteoporosis, and WHO all recommend that all women older than the age of 65 be screened with a BMD test [82,93,94,100,102]. Women younger than 65 years should be considered for screening if they have one major or two minor risk factors [94]. Although women older than 70 with multiple risk factors are at enough risk to start therapy without BMD, a baseline screen helps guide therapy. Serial BMD should be done every 2 years for continued screening and evaluation of response to treatment. More frequent monitoring should be considered in the patient on glucocorticoid treatment [96]. (Medicare reimburses for screening BMD at age 65 and serial BMD every 23 months.)

V. Conclusion

Women make up a large proportion of our geriatric population. They are a heterogeneous group with varying levels of wellness. Women at age 65 years have a life expectancy of approximately 20 years compared with 15 years for men [103]. Preventative health maintenance becomes a complex issue with many factors to consider (Table 107-5). Anticipated life expectancy and level of frailty guide the physician in making decisions about which individuals older than 65 years to screen. With recent advancements in surgery, radiation, and chemotherapy, screening and treatment decisions should not be made on the basis of age alone.

Table 107-5
Screening Recommendations for Women Older than Age 65

	Population	Recommendations
Ovarian cancer	General population	No screening
	High risk	May be screened at young age
Endometrial cancer	General population	No screening even if starting HRT
	Tamoxifen use	No screening
Cervical cancer	Previously screened	Pap smears every 1–3 years until age 65 (assess RF prior to stopping)
	Unscreened or inadequately screened	Annual Pap smears until 3 negative examinations, then consider stopping at age 65
Vulvar cancer	General population	Annual genital examination
Breast cancer	General population	Annual mammography until age 75, thereafter based on an anticipated life expectancy greater than 6 years
	High risk	Annual mammograms
Osteoporosis	General population	Baseline screen at age 65, then every 2 years

HRT, hormone replacement therapy; RF, risk factors.

VI. Suggestions for Further Investigations

- Could the sensitivity of breast cancer screening be improved with the use of ultrasound or thermal detection monitors?
- Will the Prostate, Lung, Colorectal, and Ovarian Cancer (PLCO) Trial provide clearer insight into effectiveness of screening for these cancers?
- As the population of women older than the age of 65 dramatically increases over the next 10 to 20 years, how will we deal with primary and secondary prevention of cardiovascular disease in women?
- How will we help the aging population of women deal with quality of life issues such as female sexuality?

References

1. La Croix AZ, Newton KM, Levelille SG, Wallace J. (1997). Healthy aging: A women's issue. *J Med*. 167:220–232.
2. Reuben DB, Yoshikawa TT, Besdine RW. (1991–1992). General Principles of Aging. Geriatric Review Syllabus, pp. 1–29. Dubuque, IA: Kendall/Hunt Publishing Company.
3. Goldberg TH, Chavin SI. (1997). Preventative medicine and screening in older adults. *J Am Beriatr Soc*. 45:344–354.
4. US Bureau of the Census. (1998). Statistical Abstracts of the United States:1998, 118th Edition. Washington DC: New York Plenum Press.
5. Mirhashemi R, Nieves-Neura W, Averretee HE. (2000). Gynecologic malignancies in older women. *Oncology*. 15:580–597.
6. Mandelblatt JS, Yabroff KR. (2000). Breast and cervical cancer screening for older women: Recommendations and challenges for the 21st century. *J Am Med Womens Assoc*. 55:201–215.
7. Yancik R, Ries LAG. (2000). Aging and cancer in America: Demographic and epidemiologic perspectives. *Hematol Oncol Clin North Am*. 14:17–24.
8. Yancik RM, Ries L. (1994). Cancer and older persons: Magnitude of the problem. *Cancer*. 74:1995–2003.
9. Robinson B, Beghe C. (1997). Cancer screening in the older patient. *Clin Geriatr Med*. 13:97–118.
10. Balducci L, Beghe C. (2002). Management of cancer in the older person. *Clin Geriatr*. 10:54–60.
11. Balducci L, Stanta G. (2000). Cancer in the frail patient; a coming epidemic. *Hematol Oncol Clin North Am*. 14:235–250.
12. Zachariah B, Balducci L. (2002). Radiation therapy of the older patient. *Hematol Oncol Clin North Am*. 14:131–167.
13. Celentano DD, Sharpiro S, Weisman CS. (1982). Cancer preventative screening behavior among elderly women. *Prev Med*. 11:545–563.
14. Grover SA, Cook EF, Adam J *et al.* (1989). Delayed diagnosis of gynecologic tumors in elderly women: Relation to national medical practice patterns. *Am J Med*. 86:151.
15. Markman M. (2000). The genetics, screening and treatment epithelial ovarian cancer: An update. *Cleve Clin J Med*. 67:294–298.
16. La Vecchia C. (2001). Epidemiology of ovarian cancer: A summary review. *Eur J Cancer Prev*. 10:125–129.
17. Averette HE, Hoskins W, Nguyen HN *et al.* (1993). National survey of ovarian carcinoma: A patient care evaluation of the American College of Surgeons. *Cancer*. 71:1629s–1638s.
18. Yancik R, Ries LG, Yates JW. (1986). Ovarian cancer in the elderly: An analysis of surveillance, epidemiology, and end results program data. *Am J Geriatr Soc*. 154:639–647.
19. Runowicz CD, Fields AL. (1999). Screening for gynecologic malignancies: A continuing responsibility. *Surg Oncol Clin North Am*. 8:703–723.
20. Lacey JV Jr., Mink PJ, Lubin JH *et al.* (2002). Menopausal hormonal replacement therapy and risk of ovarian cancer. *JAMA*. 288:334–341.
21. Temrungruanglert W, Kudelka AP, Edwards CL *et al.* (1997). Gynecologic cancer in the elderly. *Clin Geriatr Med*. 13:363–379.
22. Daly MB, Markman M, Rubin SC. (2001). Ovarian cancer screening: An ongoing challenge. *Patient Care*. July 30, 2001:14–20.
23. De Priest PD, Van Bagell JR, Gallion HH *et al.* (1993). Ovarian cancer screening in asymptomatic postmenopausal women. *Gynecol Oncol*. 51:205–209.
24. Kennedy AW, Flaggs JS, Webster KD. (1989). Gynecologic cancer in the very elderly. *Gynecol Oncol*. 32:49–52.
25. Holschneider CH, Bered JS. (2000). Ovarian cancer: Epidemiology, biology, and prognostic factors. *Semin Surg Oncol*. 19:3–10.
26. Parker SL, Tong T, Boldern S, Wingo PA. (1997). Cancer statistics. *CA Cancer J Clin*. 47:5–27.
27. Hoffman K, Nekhlyudov L, Deligdisch L. (1995). Endometrial carcinoma in elderly women. *Gynecol Oncol*. 58:198–201.
28. Noe CA, Barry PP. (1996). Healthy aging: Guidelines for screening and immunizations. *Geriatrics*. 57:198–201.
29. Akhmedkhanov A, Zeleniuch-Jacquotte A, Toniolo P. (2001). Role of exogenous and endogenous hormones in endometrial cancer: Review of the evidence and research perspectives. *Ann N Y Acad Sci*. 943:296–315.
30. Murphy GP, Lawrence W Jr, Lenhard RE Jr. *American Cancer Society Textbook of Clinical Oncology*, 2nd Edition, Murphy GP, Lawrence W, Jr, Lehand, RE, Jr, eds. 556–560. Atlanta, GA: American Cancer Society, Inc.
31. Fukuda K, Mori M, Uchiyama M *et al.* (1999). Preoperative cervical cytology in endometrial carcinoma and its clinicopathologic relevance. *Gynecol Oncol*. 72:273–277.
32. Cherkis RC, Patten SF, Dickinson JC, Dekanich AS. (1987). Significance of atypical endometrial cells detected by cervical cytology. *Obstet Gynecol*. 69:786–789.
33. DuBeshter, Warshal DP, Angel C *et al.* (1997). Endometrial carcinoma: the relevance of cervical biology. *Obstet Gynecol*. 77:458–462.
34. Larson DM, Johnson KK, Peyes CN Jr, Broste SK. (1994). Prognostic significance of malignant cervical cytology in patients with endometrial cancer. *Obstet Gynecol*. 84:399–403.
35. Schneider MLl, Wortmann M, Weigle A. (1986). Influence of histologic and cytologic grade and the clinical and post surgical state of the rate of endometrial adenocarcinoma. *Acta Cytol*. 30:623–627.
36. Gerber B, Krause A, Muller H *et al.* (2000). Effect of adjuvant tamoxifen on the endometrium postmenopausal women with breast cancer: A prospective long-term study using transvaginal ultrasound. *J Clin Oncol*. 18:3464–3470.
37. Fischer B, Constantino JP, Redmond CK *et al.* (1994). Endometrial cancer in tamoxifen treated breast cancer patients: Findings from the National Surgical Adjuvant Breast and Bowel Project (NSABP) B-14. *J Natl Cancer Inst*. 86:527–537.
38. Costout BS, Persing DH, Apple RJ *et al.* (1995). Molecular analysis of cervical carcinoma in elderly women. *Proc Soc Gynecol Oncol*. 36:108A.
39. Mandelblatt JS, Phillips RN. (1996). Cervical cancer: How often and why to screen older women. *Geriatrics*. 51:445–448.
40. Averette HE, Nguyen H. Gynecologic Cancer. In *American Cancer Society Textbook of Clinical Oncology*, 2nd Edition, Murphy GP, Lawrence W, Jr, Lehand, RE, Jr, eds. 33:552–579. Atlanta, GA: American Cancer Society, Inc.
41. Morrow CP, Townsend DE. (1987). Tumors of the Cervix. In *Synopsis of Gynecologic Oncology*, 3rd Edition, pp. 107–125. New York: Wiley.
42. Chen F, Trapido EJ, Davis K. (1994). Differences in stage at presentation of breast and gynecologic cancers among white, blacks, and Hispanics. *Cancer*. 73:2838–2842.
43. Ferrante JM, Gonzalez EC, Roetzheim RG *et al.* (2000). Clinical and demographic predictors of late-stage cervical cancer. *Arch Fam Med*. 9:439–445.
44. Mandelblatt JS, Richart R, Thomas L *et al.* (1992). Is HPV associated with cervical neoplasia in the elderly? *Gynecol Oncol*. 46:6–12.
45. Gostout BS, Podratz KC, McGovern RM, Persing DH. (1998). Cervical cancer in older women: Molecular analysis of human papillomavirus types, HLA types and p53 mutations. *Am J Obstet Gynecol*. 179:56–61.
46. Wright TC, Cox JT, Massad LS *et al.* (2002). 2001 Consensus guidelines for the management of women with cervical cytological abnormalities. *JAMA*. 287:2120–2129.
47. Parazzini F, Negri E, La Vecchia C *et al.* (1990). Screening practices and invasive cervical cancer risk in different age strata. *Gynecol Oncol*. 38:46.
48. Walsh JM. (1992). Cancer screening in older adults. *West J Med*. 156:495–500.
49. Oddone EZ, Feussner JR, Cohen JH. (1992). Can screening older patients for cancer save lives? *Clin Geriatr Med*. 8:51–67.
50. Homesley HD, Bundy BN, Sedis A *et al.* (1991). Assessment of current International Federation of Gynecology and Obstetrics staging of vulvar carcinoma relative to prognostic factors for survival. *Am J Obstet Gynecol*. 164:997–1004.
51. Scheitel SM, Fleming KC, Chutka DS, Evans JM. (1996). Geriatric health maintenance. *Mayo Clin Proc*. 71:289–302.

52. Koonings PP, Price JH. (2001). Evaluation of atypical glandular cells of undetermined significance: Is age important? *Gynecol Oncol*. 184(7):1457–1461.

53. Joura EA, Losch A, Haider-Angeler MG *et al*. (2000). Trends in vulvar neoplasia: Increasing incidence of vulvar intraepithelial neoplasia and squamous cell carcinoma of the vulva in young women. *J Reprod Med*. 45:613–615.

54. Crum CP. (1992). Carcinoma of the vulva: Epidemiology and pathogenesis. *Obstet Gynecol*. 79:448–454.

55. Wilkinson E. (1995). Premalignant and Malignant Tumors of the Vulva. In *Blaustein's Pathology of the Female Genital Tract* (Kurman R, ed.), pp. 17–xx. New York: Springer-Verlag.

56. Canavan TP, Cohen D. (2002). Vulvar cancer. *Am Fam Physician*. 66:1269–1274.

57. Apgar BS, Cox JT. (1996). Differentiating normal from abnormal findings of the vulva. *Am Fam Physician*. 53:1171–1180.

58. Powell LC Jr, Dinh TV, Rajaraman S *et al*. (1986). Carcinoma in situ of the vulva: A clinicopathologic study of 50 cases. *J Reprod Med*. 31:808–814.

59. Muss HB. (1996). Breast cancer in older women. *Semin Oncol*. 23:82–88.

60. Parkin DM, Piasani P, Ferlay J. (1999). Estimates of the worldwide incidence of 25 major cancers in 1990. *Int J Cancer*. 8:827–841.

61. Landis SH, Murray T, Bolden S, Wingo PA. (1999). Cancer statistics. *CA Cancer J Clin*. 49:8–31.

62. Flaws JA, Newschaffer CJ, Bush TL. (1996). Breast cancer mortality in black and in white women: A historical perspective by menopause status. *J Womens Health*. 7:1007–1015.

63. Madigan MP, Ziefler RG, Benichour J *et al*. (1995). Protection of breast cancer cases in the United States explained by well-established risk factors. *J Natl Cancer Inst*. 87:1681.

64. National Cancer Institute. (2001). *Lifetime Probability of Breast Cancer in American Women*. Bethesda, MD: National Cancer Institute.

65. The Breast Cancer Linkage Consortium. (1999). Cancer risks in BRCA2 mutation carriers. *J Natl Cancer Inst*. 15:1310–1316. (page 20)

66. Writing Group for the Women's Health Initiative Investigators. (2002). Risks and benefits of estrogen plus progestin in healthy postmenopausal women: Principal results from the women's health initiative randomized controlled trial. *JAMA*. 288:321–333.

67. Weiss LK, Burkman RT, Cushing-Haugen KL *et al*. (2002). Hormone replacement therapy regimens and breast cancer risk. *Obstet Gynecol*. 100:1148–1158.

68. Smith RZ, Mettlin CJ, Davis KJ *et al*. (2000). American Cancer Society guidelines for the early detection of cancer. *Cancer J Clin*. 20:34–49.

69. Schairer C, Lubin J, Trisi R *et al*. (2000). Menopausal estrogen and estrogen-progestin replacement therapy and breast cancer risk. *JAMA*. 383:485–489.

70. Bush TL, Whiteman M, Flaws JA. (2001). Hormone replacement therapy and breast cancer: A qualitative review. *Am Coll Obstet Gynecol*. 98:498–508.

71. Chen WY, Colditz GA, Rosner B *et al*. (2002). Use of postmenopausal hormones, alcohol, and risk for invasive breast cancer. *Ann Intern Med*. 137:798–804.

72. Couch FJ, Cerhan JR, Vierkant RZ *et al*. (2001). Cigarette smoking increases risk for breast cancer in high-risk breast cancer families. *Ca Epidem Bio Prev*. 10:327–332.

73. Kerlikowske D, Salzmann P, Phillips KA *et al*. (1999). Continuing screening mammography in women aged 70–79 years: Impact of life expectancy and cost effectiveness. *JAMA*. 282:2156–2163.

74. Gotzsche PC, Olsen O. (2000). Is screening for breast cancer with mammography justifiable? *Lancet*. 355:129–134.

75. Lennarth N, Ingvar A, Nils B *et al*. (2002). Long-term effects of mammography screening: Updated overview of the Swedish randomised trials. *Lancet*. 359:909–919.

76. Olsen O, Gotsche PC. (2001). Cochrane review on screening for breast cancer with mammography. *Lancet*. 358:1340–1342.

77. Horton R. (2001). Screening mammography: An overview revisited. *Lancet*. 358:1284–1285.

78. Humphrey LL, Helfand M, Chan BKS, Woolf S. (2002). Breast cancer screening: A summary of the evidence of the U.S. Preventative Services Task Force. *Ann Intern Med*. 137:347–360.

79. Randolph WM, Goodwin JS, Mahnken JD, Freeman JL. (2002). Regular mammography use is associated with elimination of age-related disparities in size and stage of breast cancer at diagnosis. *Ann Intern Med*. 137:783–790.

80. Bush TL, Noftolin F, Sataloff DM. (2001). New issues in breast cancer. *Patient Care*. May:40–59.

81. Barratt A, Irwig L, Glasziou P *et al*. (2001). Benefits, harms, and costs of screening mammography in women 70 years and over: A systematic review. *Med J Aust*. 176:266–271.

82. NIH consensus statement. (2000). Osteoporosis, prevention, diagnosis and therapy. *American Family Physician* 17(1):1–45.

83. Melton IJ III, Lane AW, Cooper C *et al*. (1993). Prevalence and incidence of vertebral deformities. *Osteoporos Int*. 3:113–119.

84. Davies KM, Stegman MR, Heaney RP, Recker RR. (1996). Prevalence and severity of vertebral fracture: The Saunders Bone Quality Study. *Osteoporos Int*. 6:160–165.

85. Kado DM, Browner WS, Palerno I *et al*. (1999). Vertebral fractures and mortality in older women: Study of Osteoporotic Fracture Research Group. *Arch Intern Med*. 159:1215–1220.

86. Melton LJ 3rd. (1997). Epidemiology of spinal osteoporosis. *Spine*. 22:2S–11S (PMID:9431638).

87. Riggs BL, Melton LJ. (1995). The worldwide problem of osteoporosis: Insights afforded by epidemiology. *Bone*. 17(5 Suppl):505–511S.

88. Ettinger B, Black DM, Midak BH *et al*. (1999). Reduction of vertebral fractures in postmenopausal women with osteoporosis treated with raloxifene: Results from a 3-year randomized clinical trial. *JAMA*. 282:637–645.

89. Diack DM, Aarden MK, Polarmo J, Cummings SR. (1999). Prevalent vertebral deformities predict hip fracture and new vertebral deformities but no wrist fractures. *J Bone Miner Res*. 14:821–828.

90. Lindsay R, Silverman SL, Cooper C *et al*. (2001). Risk of new vertebral fracture in the year following a fracture. *JAMA*. 285:370–373.

91. Gehlbach SH, Fournier M, Bigelow C. (2002). Recognition of osteoporosis by primary care physicians. *Am J Public Health*. 92:271–273.

92. Centers for Disease Control and Prevention. (1998). Osteoporosis among estrogen-deficient women-United States, 1988–1994. *MMWR Morb Mortal Wkly Rep*. 47:969–973.

93. Nelson HD, Helfand M, Woolf SH, Allan JD. (2002). Screening for postmenopausal osteoporosis: A review of the evidence for the U.S. Preventive Services Task Force. *Ann Intern Med*. 137:529–541.

94. Brown JP, Josse RG, for the Scientific Advisory Council of the Osteoporosis Society of Canada. (2002). 2002 Clinical practice guidelines for the diagnosis and management of osteoporosis in Canada. *J Can Med Assoc*. 167(10):1–34.

95. U.S. Preventive Services Task Force (USPSTF). (2003). Screening for osteoporosis in postmenopausal women: Recommendations and rationale. *Am J Nurs*. 103:73–80.

96. Messinger-Rapport BJ, Thacker HL. (2002). Prevention for the older women: A practical guide to prevention and treatment of osteoporosis. *Geriatrics*. 57(4):16–27.

97. Torgeson DJ, Campbell MK, Thomas RE, Reid DM. (1996). Prediction of perimenopausal fractures by bone mineral density and other risk factors. *J Bone Miner Res*. 11:193–197.

98. Njeh CF, Hans D, Li J *et al*. (2000). Comparison of six calcaneal quantitative ultrasound devices: Precision and hip fractures. *Osteoporos Int*. 11:1051–1062.

99. Rosenthall L, Caminis J, Tenehouse A. (1996). Calcaneal ultrasonometry response to treatment in comparison with dual x-ray absorptiometry measurements of the lumbar spine and femur. *Calif Tissue Int*. 64:200–204.

100. World Health Organization. (1998). *Guidelines for Pre-clinical Evaluation and Clinical Trials in Osteoporosis*, pp. 59–126. Geneva: World Health Organization.

101. Nelson HD, Morris CD, Kraemer DF. (2001). Osteoporosis in postmenopausal women: Diagnosis and monitoring, summary, evidence report/technical assessment, number 28. AHRQ publication no. 01-E031. Rocky Mountain Agency for Healthcare Research Quality.

102. National Osteoporosis Foundation. (1998). Osteoporosis: Review of the evidence for prevention, diagnosis, and treatment and cost-effectiveness analysis. *Osteoporos Int*. 8:57–80.

103. Wei JY, Sheehan MN. (1987). Approach to the Older Patient. In *Geriatric Medicine: A Case Based Manual*, Sheehan NM, Wei JY, eds. pp. 1–12.

108

Cancer Management in Older Women

STACY D. JACOBSON, MD* AND LYNN C. HARTMANN, MD**

*University of California, Davis, CA
**Mayo Clinic, Rochester, MN

I. Epidemiology of Cancer

By 2030, one in five Americans will be older than age 65 [1]. Currently, 60% of all malignancies and 69% of all cancer deaths are in patients ≥65 years old [2]. Tables 108-1 and 108-2 show the most common cancers and the leading causes of cancer deaths [3]. In terms of gynecologic cancers, the most common malignancy is uterine cancer, followed by ovarian cancer and cervical cancer [3]. Age is a significant risk factor for the development of these gynecologic tumors, and age portends a worse prognosis. As the population ages, oncologists will be faced with increasing numbers of older patients with complex past medical histories, comorbidities, and limited functional abilities. Comorbidity generally increases with age, with the average geriatric patient suffering from three different diseases [4]. Yancik et al [5] have confirmed a high prevalence of comorbid conditions in elderly patients with a wide variety of tumor types using SEER data. In cancer patients, the percentage of patients with comorbid conditions increases with age, as shown in Table 108-3 [6]. The most common comorbid conditions in cancer patients include cardiovascular disease, hypertension, chronic obstructive pulmonary disease (COPD), arthritis, diabetes, dementia, other cancers, and gastrointestinal (GI) and renal disease [7–9]. In many cases, older patients with cancer will die because of these competing comorbid conditions. The most common causes of death by age group are listed in Table 108-4 [10].

Despite increasing comorbidity, most people older than 75 years are independent, and life expectancy for a patient this age without cancer is about 10 to 12 years. Fifty-five percent of patients older than 85 are also independent, and life expectancy for this group is about 5 to 6 years [11,12]. Older patients have been excluded from or under-represented in clinical trials, and the tolerability and benefits of treatment in this population are largely unknown [13,14]. There is even less known about the average older patient, who is generally treated in the community with either standard-of-care or no treatment. Population-based studies have shown that older patients with breast, colon, and ovarian cancer receive less chemotherapy or radiation compared with younger patients [15–19]. For example, in one study, multivariate analysis showed that age ≥75, along with Hispanic race, and the presence of two or more comorbid conditions was associated with less use of chemotherapy in patients with advanced ovarian cancer [19]. The geriatric patient population, however, is heterogeneous. Age alone should not preclude consideration by the physician(s), patient, and family members of standard therapy or investigational cancer treatment in most cases.

Table 108-1
Most Common Cancers in Women and Men, 2002

Men	Women
1. Prostate (30%)	1. Breast (31%)
2. Lung (14%)	2. Lung (12%)
3. Colorectal (11%)	3. Colorectal (12%)
4. Bladder (7%)	4. Uterus (6%)
5. Melanoma (5%)	5. Non-Hodgkin's lymphoma (NHL) (4%)

(From Jemal A, Thomas A, Murray T, Thun M. [2002]. Cancer statistics, 2002. *CA Cancer J Clin.* 52:23–47, with permission.)

Table 108-2
Leading Causes of Cancer Deaths for Men and Women, 2002

Estimated Deaths, 2002: Men	Estimated Deaths 2002: Women	Deaths in Women Ages 60–79, 1999	Deaths in Women ≥80, 1999
1. Lung	1. Lung	1. Lung	1. Lung
2. Prostate	2. Breast	2. Breast	2. Colorectal
3. Colorectal	3. Colorectal	3. Colorectal	3. Breast
4. Pancreas	4. Pancreas	4. Pancreas	4. Pancreas
5. NHL	5. Ovary	5. Ovary	5. NHL

NHL, non-Hodgkin's lymphoma.
(From Jemal A, Thomas A, Murray T, Thun M. [2002]. Cancer statistics, 2002. *CA Cancer J Clin.* 52:23–47, with permission.)

Table 108-3

Percentage of Cancer Patients with Comorbid Conditions by Age,
Eindhoven Cancer Registry, 1993–1996

	<45 Years	45–59 Years	60–74 Years	>75 Years
Percentage of patients with comorbid diseases	12%	28%	53%	63%

(From Coebergh JW, Janssen-Heijnen ML, Post PN, Razenberg PP. [1999]. Serious co-morbidity among unselected cancer patients newly diagnosed in the southeastern part of the Netherlands in 1993–1996. *J Clin Epidemiol*. 52:1131–1136, with permission.)

Table 108-4

Leading Causes of Death for Those 60–79
and for Those 80+ (1998)

Age 60–79	Age 60–79	Age 80+
Men	Women	All
Heart disease	Cancer	Heart disease
Cancer	Heart disease	Cancer
COPD	COPD	Cerebrovascular disease
CVD	CVD	Pneumonia
Diabetes	Diabetes	COPD
Pneumonia/flu	Pneumonia/flu	Diabetes

COPD, chronic obstructive pulmonary disease; CVD, cardiovascular disease.
(From Greenlee RT, Hill-Harmon MB, Murray T, Thun M. [2001]. Cancer Statistics, 2001. *CA Cancer J Clin*. 51:15–36, with permission.)

Table 108-5

Screening Tests for Older Patients

Problem	Test
Mental status	Folstein mini-mental state examination (MMSE) [31]
Functional status	Activities of daily living (ADL); Instrumental activities of daily living (IADL) [29,30]
Depression	Geriatric depression scale (GDS) [32]
Nutrition	Dietary history, amount of weight loss, albumin [33]
Other	Visual/hearing loss, incontinence, social support, transportation issues [20]

II. Geriatric Assessment and Syndromes

Older patients are at risk for common geriatric syndromes, which may affect their ability to tolerate treatment for cancer. These are problems such as mental status changes and dementia; incontinence; malnutrition; and functional impairment including gait difficulties/falls, vision, and hearing loss [20]. Frailty is generally defined as patients who are ≥85, are dependent in one or more activity of daily living, have three or more comorbid conditions, or have the presence of any geriatric syndrome. These patients have very limited functional and physiologic reserves and generally are treated with symptom palliation alone [20–22]. There are also logistical issues to consider when treating older cancer patients such as limited social support and access to transportation. Older women are often the primary caregivers of their elderly husbands or other family members, and this also may affect the patient's ability to receive treatment. Some authors have recommended a comprehensive geriatric assessment to determine if any of these geriatric syndromes are present and to treat them accordingly (Table 108-5) [23,24]. Functional status is very important in determining whether or not patients may tolerate or benefit from chemotherapy. Multiple studies have shown that patients with impaired performance status (PS) have increased toxicity with chemotherapy and may not benefit from treatment. Commonly used scales in the assessment of functional status in oncology include the Eastern Oncology Cooperative Group (ECOG) performance status or the Karnofsky Index [25,26]. Other functional assessment

scales have been predictive of prognosis in non-cancer patients and are widely used in geriatrics [22,27,28]. These include the activities of daily living (ADL) scale and the instrumental activities of daily living (IADL) scale, which assess basic functions [29,30]. Overall, these screening tests can generally be performed with limited effort and may point out problems that otherwise may be unrecognized. The presence of an underlying geriatric syndrome may complicate or affect the patient's ability to tolerate and/or benefit from chemotherapy. However, if assessment is performed and problems are recognized early, patients may benefit from treatment of underlying conditions or social support as needed so that they may receive the recommended treatment for their cancer.

III. Comorbidity

The effect of comorbid diseases on cancer treatment tolerance and benefit has not been well studied. As described previously, PS is routinely measured in practice and clinical trials. However, PS does not correlate with comorbid burden of disease [34]. Assessment of comorbid diseases and their effect on life expectancy is important when deciding treatment recommendations for older patients [35]. Current tools available for assessing comorbidity are not easily applied in routine practice, and more research is needed in this area to develop assessment tools and to integrate these assessments into oncologic practice and clinical trials. A few studies described here highlight the importance of comorbidity on treatment benefits and outcomes.

Satariano *et al* [36] studied the effect of comorbidity on 3-year survival in women with breast cancer. The frequency and severity of comorbid conditions increased with age. Adjusting for stage, age, and type of treatment, the number of comorbid conditions was strongly associated with an increased rate of death. Of the women who died, younger women (40 to 54) were almost six times more likely to die of breast cancer than older women.

Yancik et al [37] performed a retrospective review of colorectal cancer patients using the SEER database to describe comorbid burden and its effects in this population. Three age groups were identified: 55 to 64, 65 to 74, and >75. The most common comorbid conditions were hypertension, heart disease, GI problems, arthritis, and COPD. Overall, 40% of patients (both genders) had five or more comorbid conditions. The number of comorbid conditions increased with age. More than 50% of patients who died had stage IV disease; however, the cause of death was colon cancer in 73%, heart disease in 9%, and other cancers in 4%. Using regression analysis, taking into account age, sex, and stage of disease, the total number of comorbid conditions and certain types of severe chronic illness contributed to early mortality. The authors concluded that comorbidity increases the complexity of managing patients with colorectal cancer and affects survival.

Sabin et al [38] studied the records of 152 patients with laryngeal cancer to determine the effect of comorbidity on survival. Two groups of patients were identified: those with "high" burden of comorbid disease versus "low" comorbid disease. Median survival was 41 months in the low comorbidity group compared with 8 months in the high comorbidity group. When adjusting for comorbidity, age was not associated with survival. The authors suggest that comorbidity is an independent predictor of tumor-specific survival and consideration should be given to including comorbidity into the staging system to improve prognostic ability.

IV. Screening and Diagnosis

A. General Issues

The goals of screening for cancer are to detect cancer in an early stage, when treatment is more effective. Screening and detecting cancer in asymptomatic patients should ideally convey a survival advantage, and screening tests should have good sensitivity and specificity to reduce the number of false-negative and false-positive results. Despite the fact that older patients have the highest incidence of cancer, they are less likely to be screened than younger people. This may be due to age and gender biases (i.e., physicians may offer screening tests less often to patients resulting from age/gender), less patient knowledge about cancer risk factors, less knowledge about screening tests and recommendations, and more fatalism if cancer is detected [39–43]. There are factors in older patients that need to be taken into account before pursuing screening. These include patient life expectancy, presence of multiple or severe comorbidities that may prevent treatment, patient preferences, and patient quality of life (QOL). The decision to screen the oldest old patients (≥80) must be made on an individual basis. Many of the published guidelines for cancer screening do not specify an upper age at which time to stop screening. These are listed in Table 108-6, highlighting the few recommendations that do suggest age limits [44–46].

B. Specific Cancers

1. Breast Cancer

Approximately 40% of all newly diagnosed breast cancers in the United States occur in women older than the age of 65 [47]. The randomized trials that showed benefit with screening mammography did not include a sufficient number of elderly women to study the benefit in this population specifically. The University of Massachusetts Medical School sponsored the forum on "Breast Cancer Screening in Older Women" in 1990 with support from The National Cancer Institute and National Institute on Aging. For women aged 65 and older they recommended annual clinical breast examination and mammography every 2 years, along with monthly breast self-examination, for women aged 65 and older [48]. The optimal interval for screening in this age group remains a subject of debate (12 vs 24 months), as does the age at which mammography ceases to offer benefit. In the Netherlands, mammographic screening is continued at least up to age 75 and often to age 85 in otherwise healthy women [49].

Retrospective data support the efficacy of mammography in older women. Faulk et al [47] examined 10,914 women aged 65 years and older and 21,226 women aged 50 to 64 years. The cancer detection rate was substantially higher in the older group. The median size of cancers in the –older than 65 group was 11 mm versus 12 mm in the younger group, and nodal status was more commonly negative in the elderly versus the younger group. Thus, these authors concluded that screening was at least as effective in detecting favorable-prognosis cancers in women older than age 65 as in the group aged 50 to 64 years.

2. Gynecologic Cancer

In the United States, the prevalence of screening for cervical cancer is quite high. For women ages 18 to 44, 89% had a Pap test done within a 3-year period, whereas 83.9% of women older than age 45 had a test performed [50]. Screening may be done at less frequent intervals once there have been normal Pap smears as described in Table 108-6 [46]. However, older women are less likely to be screened on a regular basis, and a Pap smear could be considered if none has been performed within the past 10 years [51]. Perhaps in the future, testing for human papillomavirus (high-risk subsets) may identify women who are at higher risk for developing cervical cancer and thus may benefit from continued screening [52].

There are currently no recommendations for screening standard risk asymptomatic women for endometrial or ovarian cancer. Women with genetic syndromes at high risk for the development of uterine cancer (hereditary nonpolyposis colon cancer [HNPCC]) or ovarian cancer (BRCA 1/2) may benefit from more intensive screening programs [46,53,54].

3. Colorectal Cancer

Colon cancer screening is recommended for men and women older than age 50 or younger for special populations at higher risk [46]. Annual fecal occult blood testing along with flexible sigmoidoscopy every 5 years is the preferred method, but other methods are also available including double-contrast barium

Table 108-6
Recommended Screening Tests for Women

	ACS	Other
Breast cancer	Mammogram and CBE annually for women older than 40; clinical breast examination every 3 years in women aged 20–39; monthly BSE for all women aged 20 and older	U.S. Preventive Task Force: mammogram every 1–2 years with or without CBE for women aged 50–69
Cervical cancer	Pap test and pelvic examination annually for all women who are sexually active or have been or who have reached age 18. After three consecutive normal smears, may have Pap test less often at the discretion of the physician	U.S. Preventive Task Force: No upper age limit is defined, but discontinuing screening at age 65 can be defended in women with a history of normal/regular Pap tests
Colorectal cancer	For average-risk patients, one of the following for men and women age 50 and older: fecal occult blood test (FOBT) yearly and sigmoidoscopy every 5 years (preferred), OR flexible sigmoidoscopy every 5 years, OR FOBT annually, OR colonoscopy every 10 years; OR double-contrast barium enema every 5 years (DRE at the time of screening except for FOBT)	PDQ: FOBT annually or biennially in people ages 50–80 decreases mortality from colorectal cancer. Regular screening by sigmoidoscopy in people older than age 50 may decrease mortality from colorectal cancer
Cancer-related check-up	Examinations every 3 years from ages 20–39 and annually after age 40. The cancer-related check-up should include examination for cancers of the thyroid, testicles, ovaries, lymph nodes, oral cavity, and skin and health counseling about tobacco, sun exposure, diet and nutrition, risk factors, sexual practices, and environmental and occupational exposures	

ACS, American Cancer Society; BSE, breast self-examination; CBE, clinical breast examination; DRE, digital rectal examination; PDQ, physician data query.
(From Kramer BS. [1995]. The Screening Editorial Board of the Physician Data Query: NCI State of the Art Statement on Cancer Screening. Bethesda, MD: National Cancer Institute; US Preventive Task Force. [1996]. Guide to Clinical Preventive Services. Alexandria, VA: International Medical Publishing; and Smith RA, Cokkinides V, vonEschenbach AC *et al.* [2002]. American Cancer Society guidelines for the early detection of cancer. *CA Cancer J Clin.* 52:8–22, with permission.)

enema every 5 years, colonoscopy every 10 years, flexible sigmoidoscopy alone, or fecal occult blood testing alone. Because overall screening rates are very low, most guidelines do not specify the preferred method of screening but allow for flexibility in the choices of tests to increase compliance with screening. The prevalence of U.S. adults older than age 50 that have had a flexible sigmoidoscopy or colonoscopy is only 34.2% of men and 30.3% of women over a 5-year period. Women were slightly more likely to have had a fecal occult test done over this 5-year period (21.3%) than men (17.1%). Women are much less compliant with colon cancer screening than for other commonly employed tests, such as Pap smear and mammograms [55,56].

There have been a number of studies that do show an increase in the incidence of proximal (right-sided) colon cancer in older patients, especially in women [57–63]. These right-sided tumors may have a higher frequency of microsatellite instability but how this ultimately affects treatment decisions must be investigated further [64]. Specific screening recommendations for women have not been proposed; however, it may be reasonable to offer older women a full colonoscopy as an option, because flexible sigmoidoscopy alone would not detect proximal cancers.

V. Prognostic Differences

The behavior of some cancers appears to be age- and gender-related. It is well established that older patients with acute myelocytic leukemia (AML), lymphoma, and ovarian and brain cancer have a worse prognosis compared with younger patients [65–76]. On the other hand, women with lung cancer and melanoma have a better prognosis compared with men [77–80].

A. Breast Cancer

There are conflicting data regarding the effect of age on breast cancer prognosis, with some studies showing shorter survival for younger patients and others showing worse prognosis with increasing age [81]. U.S. statistics show an increasing mortality rate with increasing age [82]. In a careful study from Finland, Holli and Isola [81] looked at the effect of age on survival in all breast cancer patients diagnosed in Finland from 1977 to 1986. This included 17,856 female breast cancer patients, and results were controlled for disease stage. The best survival rates were seen in women aged 46 to 50 years. In node-positive disease, the poorest 10-year relative survival rates were in the oldest age group (>75 years) and the youngest group (<35 years). Also, the highest proportion of women presenting with metastatic disease was seen in those older than age 75 (10.3%). A population-based study in southeastern Netherlands showed a worse survival for women older than 74 years than for younger patients, and in multivariate analysis this appeared to be related to their having a less favorable stage distribution at diagnosis [83]. As expected, the presence of significant comorbidities significantly increases mortality in breast cancer patients, independent of tumor stage [36].

When looking at prognostic factors in the cancers of older women, one sees an increased proportion of estrogen receptor (ER)-positive tumors and a decreased likelihood of poor prognosis, c-erb- B2 overexpressing breast cancers [81,84]. Also, the indolent breast cancers with unique histologies such as papillary and mucinous cancers are more frequent in older women [85].

B. Leukemia and Lymphoma

Older patients with leukemia have a poor prognosis; they often have poor risk cytogenetics, which is a powerful predictor of outcome [65,66]. Older patients are also more likely to have leukemia arising out of an abnormal marrow (myelodysplasia), and cells are more likely to express the MDR-1 multidrug resistance phenotype leading to drug resistance. Older patients also do not tolerate intensive chemotherapy regimens as well as their younger counterparts and are not candidates for allogeneic bone marrow transplantation (BMT) [86].

A large population of cases of diffuse B-cell large lymphoma occur in those patients older than 60 years. Non-Hodgkin's lymphoma (NHL) is a less treatable and less curable malignancy in older patients [87]. Older patients with NHL may present with more extranodal disease, which is a poor prognostic factor [68,69]. One of the reasons that elderly patients may have a poor prognosis is that they do not tolerate chemotherapy as well as younger patients.

C. Ovarian Cancer

Older women with ovarian cancer generally have a worse prognosis compared with younger patients. Older patients may present with more advanced disease, have less aggressive surgery, and may not be offered or treated with appropriate chemotherapy [70–72,88,90]. However, age may be an independent prognostic factor, and older women have a worse prognosis stage for stage. For example, Kosary et al [88] showed that women with advanced ovarian cancer who are older than the age of 70 years old had 5-year survival much lower than that of women younger than 40 years. Older patients are most likely to have advanced stage disease and are less likely to be treated in an aggressive fashion with surgery and/or chemotherapy. In a study by Alberts et al [89] factors that were associated with a poor outcome included age, stage of disease, PS, and African-American race. Poor outcomes are observed even in patients that are treated aggressively. In one study, older patients who had optimal debulking surgery followed by platinum-based chemotherapy were compared with younger patients; older

Table 108-7
Different Types of Endometrial Cancer

Type I Endometrial Cancer	Type II Endometrial Cancer
Estrogen induced/ associated with hyperplasia	Unrelated to estrogen
Low grade	High grade
Endometrioid histology	Clear cell/serous cell (high-risk histology)

patients had significantly shorter survival than did younger patients (22 months vs 37 months) [90].

D. Endometrial Cancer

Older women with endometrial cancer generally have a worse prognosis compared with younger patients, stage for stage. This may be due to difference in the biology of cancers in older patients, who tend to have cancers that are higher grade and more aggressive (Table 108-7) [91]. The molecular biology of cancers occurring in older women may thus be different and may include more abnormal p53 mutations and more loss of another tumor suppressor gene called PTEN [92–94]. Older women may also do worse because of less aggressive treatment or competing comorbidities [95].

VI. General Treatment Issues

A. Clinical Trials in Cancer

Most of the treatment recommendations that oncologists make are based on the results from decades of clinical trials testing various treatments. Despite the fact that upper age limit for clinical trials are not set, there appears to be serious under-representation of patients 65 years of age or older in these cancer treatment trials. Hutchins et al [14] looked at the experience from SWOG trials from 1993 through 1996 in which 16,396 patients were enrolled. The overall enrollment rate for women was similar to the proportion of woman in the United States with cancer (41% enrolled on SWOG trials vs 43% overall). Trials for which women were slightly under-represented included those for colorectal cancer and for lymphoma. In terms of the age of patients, the authors found a significant under-representation of older patients. Overall, patients older than the age of 65 only accounted for 25% of patients enrolled in SWOG trials as compared with 63% of the population of the United States that has cancer. This is true for all types of cancer with the exception of lymphoma. This study did not attempt to answer why older patients are not put on clinical trials. The authors suggest that perhaps logistical problems such as transportation, financial barriers, or a low rate of referral to older patients to cancer centers may contribute to underenrollment of older patients. Given the aging of the United States population, more studies must be done to understand the under enrollment of elderly patients and to improve enrollment so that treatment recommendations can be appropriately made.

B. Chemotherapy in Older Patients

Chemotherapy for the treatment of cancer is given for a variety of goals. In a few situations, chemotherapy alone can be curative (germ cell, lymphoma, leukemia). It is often given after surgery (adjuvant) to eradicate micrometastases and decrease the risk of recurrence. This is commonly done in early stage breast cancer and stage III colon cancer. Sometimes chemotherapy is given in combination with radiation, for primary curative treatment or in the adjuvant setting. Most chemotherapy, however, is used to treat advanced or metastatic cancer in an attempt to prolong survival and palliate symptoms. There have been a number of studies over the years suggesting that older patients tolerate chemotherapy as well as younger patients [96,97]. However, many of these studies involved patients treated on clinical trials, which represent a very select population. Patients on clinical trials usually must have good performance status (PS) and limited comorbidity to be eligible for the treatments and, therefore, may not represent the status of most older patients in the community. Our knowledge about the tolerance and benefits of chemotherapy in this population is limited, and results from clinical trials need to be interpreted with caution. This is especially true for the frail elderly, those patients who are dependent in activities of daily living, and in those with geriatric syndromes.

Certainly some elderly patients are too frail to treat aggressively. The definition of frailty generally includes age ≥85, presence of multiple comorbidities, dependence in one or more ADLs, and presence of one or more geriatric syndromes (dementia, falls, incontinence, osteoporotic fractures, failure to thrive). The life expectancy of such a frail person still can exceed 2 years, however [21]. Thus, some form of treatment for cancer may be indicated as some may still derive some benefit from treatment of cancer. For example, hormonal therapy for breast cancer is generally very well tolerated and effective. Newer single agent chemotherapeutics such as taxanes, gemcitabine, and navelbine are also generally well tolerated, especially when given weekly lower doses. The patient's life expectancy and degree of symptoms should be taken into account before proceeding with chemotherapy, as certainly some older patients will die with their cancer, not from cancer. Symptomatic and supportive care, including aggressive treatment of pain should be given to all patients regardless of gender or age.

It is known that there are age-related changes that predispose older patients to excess drug toxicity. Glomerular filtration rate (GFR) declines with age, and many chemotherapeutic agents are metabolized by the kidneys [98]. Drugs that have potential for toxicity in the setting of renal dysfunction are listed in Table 108-8. Older patients may also have altered drug absorption, distribution, metabolism, and elimination [99]. There may also be drug-drug interactions that can be a major problem in older patients, because older patients are more likely to be taking multiple medications. Patients may have multiple physician prescribers, multiple old medications or duplicate medications, and limited knowledge about their medications. Patients may also be taking multiple over-the-counter medications and alternative/complementary medications [100]. There are many common drugs that are metabolized by the P450 enzyme system, including antidepressants, anticonvulsants, cardiac/antihypertensive, pain medications, and warfarin that may

Table 108-8
Renal Metabolized/Excreted Chemotherapy and Common Uses

Renal Metabolized Chemotherapy	Common Uses
Cisplatin	Ovarian, lung, bladder, cervical, head and neck, esophageal, and gynecologic cancers
Carboplatin	Ovarian and lung cancers
Methotrexate	Hematologic, bladder, cervical, and head and neck cancer
Capecitabine	Breast, colon
Fludarabine	Hematologic cancer
Topotecan	Ovarian cancer

interact with chemotherapy [99]. Important examples include chemotherapy drugs that are metabolized by the liver and may alter warfarin, digoxin, and phenytoin metabolism, resulting in subtherapeutic or supratherapeutic levels. For example, capecitabine can cause prolongation of the international normalized ration (INR) in those taking warfarin and lead to bleeding. Adriamycin may accelerate the metabolism of digoxin, leading to lowered digoxin levels [101].

In general, older patients may experience more myelotoxicity, mucositis/diarrhea, cardiac toxicity, and neurologic toxicity than younger patients [102,103]. Careful baseline assessments for pre-existing neurologic conditions such as neuropathy and cardiac dysfunction are essential because pre-existing conditions predispose to toxicity from many commonly used drugs. Anthracyclines are a common class of drugs that cause cardiac dysfunction, especially with advancing age or a history of cardiac conditions. Diabetes, or pre-existing neuropathy may place patients at risk for severe neurotoxicity from drugs such as cisplatin, paclitaxel, and vincristine.

For most drugs, there are no dose modifications based on age or sex alone. Reducing the dose of chemotherapy below standard dosing for any given regimen is not routinely recommended and may have suboptimal results. This has been shown in breast cancer and lymphoma [104–107]. Attenuated regimens used for elderly patients with AML have had inferior outcomes [65,108]. Dose modifications should be made based on patients renal function, liver function, with consideration given to PS and pre-existing medical problems. Doses are also modified based on the toxicities encountered with prior cycles.

C. Radiation in Older Patients

Radiation therapy is an important part of treatment for many cancers. It can be used as primary treatment for curative intent, with or without chemotherapy. Women are most commonly given radiation in the adjuvant setting for breast cancer after mastectomy and pelvic radiation or brachytherapy for endometrial cancer. Locally advanced gynecologic cancers are also often treated with radiation in combination with chemotherapy with curative intent. Radiation can be also useful in the palliative setting, to treat painful bony metastasis, spinal cord compression, brain metastasis, and obstructive GI lesions. Despite the benefits of radiotherapy, older patients are less likely to receive these treatments than younger patients, possibly because of fear of excess toxicity and lack of benefit [17,109]. Withholding treatment from patients on the basis of age alone is not supported by the literature, because data obtained from examining the experience of older patients on clinical trials suggest that, overall, radiation therapy is well tolerated in this population [110]. Radiation can be safely and effectively given to older patients with head and neck cancer, lung cancer, esophageal cancer, cervical cancer, and Hodgkin's disease [111–116].

Multiple retrospective series have shown that even the oldest old (i.e., ≥80) tolerate radiation for a variety of cancers as well as their younger counterparts [112,117]. Zachariah *et al* performed a retrospective review of 203 patients aged 80 to 94, in which patients received radiation for head and neck cancer, and lung, pelvic, and breast cancer, both in the curative and palliative setting. This study showed that older patients had side effects and benefits comparable to younger patients. Treatment interruptions because of diarrhea, dehydration, and weight loss were more frequent in patients with pelvic cancer. In another retrospective review of older patients, a full course of radiation was given to 80% of patients older than age 80. Major side effects included weight loss, skin changes, and mucositis. Many of these older patients had treatment breaks because of fatigue and transportation issues [118]. However, with supportive care, many older patients will complete their intended treatment.

D. Surgery for Older Cancer Patients

Surgery can be curative for many cancers if found at early stages. Significant palliation can also be achieved for patients with advanced disease, such as for obstructing GI cancers. Older patients should not be excluded from the potential benefits of surgery on the basis of age alone. Life expectancy, comorbid conditions, cognitive status, social support, and overall functional status need to be taken into account when deciding on surgical options for the treatment of cancer. Surgery is generally well tolerated by older people, and appropriate cancer surgery should be offered to all older patients who are medically fit [119–124]. However, older patients that have multiple comorbid conditions or have limited functional capacity may have increased morbidity and mortality from surgery [125–127]. In one study, for patients older than age 80 undergoing surgery for colorectal cancer the in-hospital mortality for sedentary patients was 38% compared with 8% in active patients [125]. Emergency surgery, as may be required for obstructing colon tumors, is also not as well tolerated in older patients [119,121,128]. In general, all older patients need careful preoperative evaluation with special attention to underlying diseases and unrecognized cardiac or pulmonary conditions because these contribute to the majority of postoperative problems. Older patients with cancer undergoing surgery are at high risk for thrombotic complications and should receive aggressive deep venous thrombosis (DVT) prophylaxis [120,128].

VII. Management of Specific Cancers

A. Breast Cancer Treatment

1. Primary Therapy

Numerous studies have shown that older women tend to be treated with less extensive surgeries and are less likely to receive adjuvant radiation [83,129,130]. This pattern is notable because several studies have shown that elderly women in good health tolerate operative procedures well [85]. It is generally agreed that comorbidities and disease stage, rather than age alone, should determine which patients are candidates for a potentially curative surgery for cancer [85]. For older women who have breast-conserving therapy, the use of radiation therapy declines markedly with increasing age, regardless of comorbidity status and disease stage. Ballard-Barbash *et al* [129] used SEER data for a cohort of 18,704 women aged 65 years and older diagnosed with breast cancer in the late 1980s. Comparing the age groups 65 to 69 years and 80 and older, radiation therapy declined from 77% in the younger group to 25% in the older group among women with no comorbid conditions. In a Canadian study of women 50 and over with newly diagnosed node-negative breast cancer, investigators found that those 70 and older were much less likely to receive definitive locoregional treatment [130]. They were less likely to undergo breast-conserving surgery, radiation therapy, axillary dissection, or chemotherapy; however, they were as likely to receive tamoxifen as the younger women in the cohort. These less aggressive patterns of care in the more elderly women occurred independent of comorbidities. A recent U.S. study showed that radiation therapy was more likely to be omitted after breast conservation in the oldest women (age 80 and older) and that these women were considerably less likely to receive chemotherapy after controlling for baseline health and functional status [131].

There has been some interest in the use of tamoxifen alone in the elderly. A prospective randomized trial tested the use of tamoxifen versus surgery (either wide local excision or mastectomy) as the preferred primary treatment in unselected patients older than age 70 with nonmetastatic disease [132]. More patients in the tamoxifen-only group developed local progression or relapse than in the surgical group. With a mean follow-up of 6 years, surgery alone was determined to be more effective than tamoxifen because of improved local control, although overall survival rates were similar. However, for the infirm patient who cannot tolerate surgery, tamoxifen alone or an aromatase inhibitor is justifiable. In patients with receptor-positive disease, approximately 60% of elderly women can be expected to have some degree of tumor regression [133]. It should be noted that the median time to response is on the order of 2 to 3 months. The use of tamoxifen alone following lumpectomy, without radiation, is under examination in a Cancer and Leukemia Group B prospective randomized trial for women ≥70. All are treated with lumpectomy and tamoxifen; half receive breast radiation and half do not. The use of a sentinel node biopsy should be used in older women, as it is in younger women. If positive nodes are found at the sentinel procedure, it remains standard care to proceed with a full axillary dissection, if it would change the treatment strategy. If a patient is not considered a candidate for chemotherapy and an adjuvant hormonal therapy will be used regardless of nodal status, then there is no absolute need to proceed with a sentinel node study or axillary dissection.

2. Adjuvant Therapy

In postmenopausal women with node-positive disease, the International Breast Cancer Study Group compared tamoxifen alone for 5 years (306 patients) with tamoxifen plus three cycles of cyclophosphamide, methotrexate, and 5-fluorouracil (CMF) every 28 days (302 patients) [134]. Of note, women receiving chemotherapy who were ≥65 had significantly more toxicity compared with those younger than age 65. In the 65 and older group, the 5-year disease-free survival rates were 63% for CMF plus tamoxifen and 61% for tamoxifen alone (p=0.99). For the younger postmenopausal patients, the corresponding 5-year disease-free survival rates were 61% and 53% (p=0.008). At present, given the limited numbers of elderly women who have been randomized in clinical trials, it remains unclear how much chemotherapy adds to tamoxifen for the adjuvant therapy of node-positive elderly women. Available data thus far demonstrate only minimal impact of chemotherapy in this group of women. Of note, in the Oxford meta-analysis of adjuvant chemotherapy in breast cancer, last updated in 1998, only about 600 women included in the trials (3% of the total) were 70 years or older [135]. The role of adjuvant chemotherapy in postmenopausal patients with node-negative disease was studied by the International Breast Cancer Study Group Trial IX. Patients were stratified by ER status and randomly assigned to three cycles of adjuvant CMF followed by tamoxifen or tamoxifen alone [136]. For those women with ER-positive disease, the addition of CMF provided no benefit in terms of disease-free or overall survival. In women whose cancer was ER-negative, their 5-year disease-free survival was 69% with tamoxifen alone versus 84% with CMF (→) tamoxifen (p=0.003).

Regardless of patient age, adjuvant tamoxifen demonstrates an absolute improvement in 10-year survival of 10.9% for node-positive breast cancer (61.4% vs 50.5%) and 5.6% for node-negative disease (78.9% vs 73.3%) [137]. The aromatase inhibitors, which block estrogen synthesis, are an alternative to tamoxifen for hormonal therapy and, unlike tamoxifen, are not associated with an increased risk of thromboembolic complications or endometrial cancer. However, in postmenopausal women, aromatase inhibitors elevate the rate of bone turnover [138] and increase fracture risk [139]. At present, a 5-year course of adjuvant tamoxifen remains the preferred standard for females with ER-positive disease [140].

3. Advanced Disease

Treatment for metastatic breast cancer is palliative, not curative, and thus one must balance improving symptoms from disease and maintaining optimal QOL. Hormonal agents generally represent the primary means for treating metastatic breast cancer in older women with ER-positive disease. In postmenopausal women with advanced ER breast cancer, tamoxifen and aromatase inhibitors have similar antitumor efficacy [141–143]. Chemotherapy is an option for ER-negative disease, rapidly progressive and life-threatening disease, or disease that is no longer responsive to hormonal management. In general, the likelihood of response and toxicity profiles for the standard chemotherapy

regimens for advanced disease are similar in younger and older women, assuming no excess of comorbidities [144].

Anthracyclines and taxanes are dependent on the liver for handling and caution should be exercised in patients with significant liver dysfunction before using these drugs at standard doses. Methotrexate excretion is dependent on renal function.

B. Colon Cancer

Colon cancer is the third most common cancer in women and ranks third in cancer deaths [3]. In women ≥80 years old, colorectal cancer is the second leading cause of death, surpassing even breast cancer [3]. The treatment for colon cancer is surgical resection of the tumor and surrounding lymph nodes, and, for stage III cancers, adjuvant chemotherapy is recommended [145]. The 5-year survival for resected stage III (node-positive) patients ranges from 26 to 66%, depending on the number of nodes involved [146]. Adjuvant chemotherapy provides a 40% relative reduction in the risk of recurrence and a 33% relative reduction in the risk of death [147]. The current standard adjuvant regimen is 5-FU based, generally given as weekly or monthly along with leukopenia. A recent study did show that women experience more toxicity with 5-FU based chemotherapy for colorectal cancer [148]. A pooled analysis of 2448 patients receiving 5-FU-based bolus chemotherapy in 12 different treatment arms of clinical trials run through a cooperative group showed that women experienced more toxicity than men consistently across all cycles of treatment and for all toxicity types. Specifically, women had more stomatitis, leukopenia, nausea/vomiting, and diarrhea compared with men. Older (≥60) patients more often experienced severe stomatitis. The mechanism for this increased toxicity with 5-FU-based regimens is unknown. Ongoing pharmacogenomic studies may help to shed some light on differences in drug metabolism. At this point, there are no upfront dose reductions recommended for women, but physicians should be aware of the increased risk of toxicity, especially in older women.

In a separately reported pooled analysis, older patients in general did not suffer excess toxicity from adjuvant 5FU-based therapy for colon cancer, and had the same benefits as younger patients [149]. Older patients with metastatic disease treated with 5-FU-based regimens did experience slightly increased rates of diarrhea and stomatitis but had similar response rates and overall survival compared with younger patients [150]. Performance status was an important predictor of toxicity and response in this study.

C. Ovarian Cancer

Ovarian cancer is the seventh most common cancer in women, but it is the number one cause of death from gynecologic cancer [3]. The median age for ovarian cancer is about 63 years and the incidence does increase with age, peaking in the age group 70 to 74 years old [151]. Unfortunately, most women present with late-stage ovarian cancer. Most of the symptoms are very nonspecific and there has been no effective screening method to detect disease at an early stage. The staging of ovarian cancer is based on findings at surgery. The goals of surgery are to accurately stage the patient and also to debulk tumor. Surgery includes hysterectomy, bilateral salpingo-oophorectomy (BSO), lymph node dissection, peritoneal washing, inspection of the abdomen, and tumor debulking [152].

Most patients with ovarian cancer do require further treatment after adequate surgery and debulking. Patients who have well-differentiated very early stage cancers may not need chemotherapy because their general survival is very good. However, all other patients do benefit from cisplatin-based chemotherapy [153,154]. Patients are generally treated with paclitaxel and carboplatin chemotherapy for six cycles after they have recovered from their surgery. In general, this regimen is fairly well tolerated, with myelosuppression, alopecia, myalgias, and mild nausea and vomiting being common side effects. Cisplatin has also been used but may not be first choice in the elderly patient given the potential side effects. A recent study has shown that carboplatin used as a single agent is equivalent in terms of overall survival compared with the combination of paclitaxel/carboplatin and is less toxic. Single-agent carboplatin could be considered for some older patients with impaired functional status or pre-existing neuropathy [155].

D. Endometrial Cancer

Endometrial cancer is the most common gynecologic cancer in women and is primarily a disease of postmenopausal women [3]. Risk factors include obesity, hypertension, diabetes, excess estrogen (nulliparity, unopposed estrogens, anovulation), tamoxifen use, genetic syndromes (HNPCC), and a history of atypical hyperplasia on biopsy [156–159]. Most women present with abnormal bleeding and are fortunately diagnosed at an early stage and have a good prognosis. The treatment for early stage uterine cancer is surgery, which includes hysterectomy, BSO, node dissection, pelvic fluid cytology, and exploration [160]. The staging is based on surgical findings. Radiation therapy is often used in the adjuvant setting to decrease the chance of local recurrence [161,162]. This may be offered to women with deep myometrial invasion, cervical/adnexal spread, nodal disease, serous/clear cell histology/high grade, and positive peritoneal washings [163,164]. Radiation therapy can be used as the primary treatment for women who cannot tolerate surgery [165,166].

The role of chemotherapy in patients with high-risk features is not defined. Chemotherapy or hormonal therapy can be used in patients with metastatic disease but outcomes remain poor, with median survival less than 17 months. Hormonal therapy with progestational agents or tamoxifen may be useful in women with ER-positive low-grade tumors [167]. Commonly used chemotherapeutic agents include adriamycin, cisplatin, and carboplatin [168]. Newer combination regimens using paclitaxel may provide higher response rates, but improvement in overall survival has not yet been proven [169–171].

E. Lung Cancer

1. Epidemiology and Risk Factors

Lung cancer is now the leading cause of cancer deaths in both men and women [3]. More than half of patients diagnosed with lung cancer and more than two thirds of lung cancer deaths occur in people older than the age of 65 [172a,172b].

The major risk factor for the development of lung cancer is cigarette smoking. The increased incidence of lung cancer in women is thought to be due to increased numbers of women smokers. Women have a 1.5-fold greater risk of developing lung cancer from smoking compared with men [173]. There are more than 200 million women smokers, and this number is expected to rise, because tobacco companies continue to direct marketing efforts toward women [174]. Men and women may smoke for different reasons. Women may smoke more for the sedating effects (anxiety reducing), which may relate to the menstrual cycle and hormonal changes [175]. There may also be physiologic, biologic, and social factors that are gender specific and affect the ability of women to quit smoking [176,177]. Women may be more susceptible to the effects of smoking-induced carcinogens than men, and this may be related to gender differences in the P450 system, nicotine metabolism, and hormonal effects. A recent study suggested that a specific difference in expression of the gastrin-releasing peptide gene is expressed more frequently in women than in men and is activated earlier in women because of smoking, which may increase susceptibility to the development of lung cancer [178].

Lung cancer is usually divided into two types: non-small cell lung cancer (NSCLC), and small cell carcinoma (SCLC). These types of tumors are biologically different and are treated differently. Women are more likely to get SCLC, and female gender is associated with a better prognosis [80,181]. Within the NSCLC group, there is an increasing incidence of adenocarcinomas, and women are more likely to have adenocarcinoma than men [79]. Squamous cell carcinoma is the most common subtype of cancer in older patients, and older patients may present with earlier stage disease [182,183].

2. Treatment

The treatment for lung cancer is dependent on the stage at diagnosis. For early stage tumors (I,II) that primarily involve the lung and regional lymph nodes, surgery alone is standard treatment, with survival rates 62 to 80% for stage I disease, and 38 to 48% for stage II disease [179,180]. In general, age alone should not affect the decision to pursue surgery. Many studies have shown that surgery can be performed safely in older patients, provided careful preoperative assessment is performed [183]. Guidelines exist to determine resectability [184]. For those patients that are not surgical candidates, primary radiation can be used and may provide cure for some patients [185].

Locally advanced cancers (stage III) include larger tumors and those that involve the mediastinal lymph nodes. Although sometimes these tumors are resectable, the outcome is poor. Combined therapy with chemotherapy, radiation, and surgery can be offered to some fit patients; however, older patients may not tolerate an aggressive combined modality approach [186,187]. Several trials have explored the use of combined chemotherapy and radiation for the treatment of unresectable lung cancer, but these have substantial toxicities and treatment for elderly patients must be individualized [188,189]. More trials designed for older, frailer patients with advanced lung cancer are needed.

Chemotherapy is the standard treatment for advanced stage or metastatic lung cancer. Patients do have a small survival benefit and improvement in QOL when treated with chemotherapy compared with best-supportive care [190]. The benefit from chemotherapy does not appear age-related. However, many of the common chemotherapy regimens use cisplatin as a component, which may be toxic for older patients with impaired renal function, pre-existing neuropathy, or hearing loss. Substitution with carboplatin may also have more hematologic toxicity in older patients [191]. Older patients with multiple medical problems may also not tolerate chemotherapy well.

There have been a number of trials designed for older patients with lung cancer. Gridelli [192] reported a trial of single agent vinorelbine versus best supportive care for patients 70 or older. Less than 15% of these patients were women. Older patients tolerated the chemotherapy very well, and the overall response rate was 20%. These treated patients had longer survival times and improved QOL scores overall. However, there were more problems with nausea, hair loss, neuropathy, and constipation in treated patients. Other single agents have been studies in older patients, such as gemcitabine, paclitaxel, and taxotere. These single-agent regimens are generally well tolerated and have response rates of 15 to 30%, with median survival times of 21 to 40 weeks [193–196].

F. Lymphoma

Although NHL is a relatively uncommon cancer, the incidence increases with age. In men aged 60 to 70 and women ≥80, NHL is the fifth leading cause of death. [3]. Non-Hodgkin's lymphoma is a less treatable and less curable malignancy in older patients. Standard chemotherapy without growth factor support is associated with increased toxic death rates [197]. One of the reasons for increased toxicity is that older patients experience more severe hematologic side effects. Attempts have been made to modify chemotherapy in older patients using less intensive regimens; however, this has been associated with lower response rates and survival [198,199]. With the use of growth factors, more patients are able to tolerate full doses of chemotherapy and complete their therapy. and many authors have recommended the upfront use of growth factors in patients receiving standard chemotherapy for lymphoma [200,201]. A landmark trial has been completed through a French group in which patients older than 60 years were randomized to receive either Cytoxan, doxorubicin, vincristine, prednisone (CHOP) chemotherapy or Rituximab-CHOP (R-CHOP) [202]. The median age of patients on the trial was 69 years and 60% of patients had poor prognostic features. The response rate and overall survival were superior in the group receiving R-CHOP. A subset analysis revealed that the older patients (age 70 to 80 years) had similar benefit from R-CHOP as did the younger patients. The incidence of grade III and IV toxicities were generally low. This trial has been the first trial in many years to show an improvement in survival by adding another agent to standard chemotherapy for lymphoma.

VIII. Quality of Life/Pain Control

Women who reach 65 years can expect to live another 18.8 years [203]. These remaining years for many women, however,

may be spent as caretakers for family members, widowed, or alone [204]. Women also age differently than men. Although older women do have cardiac conditions, women suffer more from osteoporosis, peripheral vascular disease, and arthritis, which may limit their ability to function [205]. Pain is a very common problem in cancer patients. Patients may present with pain, develop pain during the course of their treatments, or develop pain as cancer progresses or metastasizes. Moderate to severe pain may occur in 70% or more of patients with metastatic cancer and may be often inadequately treated [206,207]. Pain can be due to a variety of causes, including tumor invading or compressing on soft tissue, bone, nerves, or organs. Inadequate pain control impairs patients' ability to function and negatively affects QOL [208]. Cleeland et al [209] showed that women and people older than 70 were among those with inadequate pain control as measured by a pain-management index score. One of the predictors of this score was the discrepancy between the doctor's and patient's estimate of the severity of pain, and the authors speculated that accurate assessment of pain may be difficult when the patient is not of the same sex, age, or racial background as the physician. Other barriers to adequate pain control include concerns about potential addiction, limited expectations about pain control, difficulty in communicating discomfort, lack of knowledge about the use of narcotics, and inadequate assessment of the cause of pain [206,210].

Pain control can be achieved in almost all patients using published guidelines [211–214]. Determining pain intensity using validated scales, looking for underlying causes of pain, and performing frequent assessment is imperative. Adequate use of narcotics for moderate to severe pain is important. Other medications such as anti-inflammatory drugs, antidepressants, and gabapentin can be very useful. Radiation therapy is also frequently used to palliate bony metastasis and is quite effective. Nerve blocks, regional anesthetics (i.e., epidural catheters), or neurosurgical interventions can be used in refractory cases.

A. Quality of Life Issues

Quality of life is increasingly being studied in cancer patients, and, in some cases, measurement of QOL parameters is incorporated into clinical trials. Quality of life encompasses many areas, including physical, social, spiritual, and emotional aspects of a person's life. There are many tools used to assess these various domains [215–217]. Quality of life can be affected by the various treatments for cancer. For example, patients may experience physical symptoms such as nausea and vomiting from chemotherapy that may negatively affect QOL. However, pain or other symptoms may be alleviated by effectively treating the cancer, and overall QOL may improve. The measurement of QOL as an endpoint in clinical trials is very important, especially when treatment is palliative in nature. Quality of life assessment is especially important in older patients, who may have limited life expectancy.

There have been many studies performed evaluating the QOL of older women with gynecologic cancers. Women do experience significant negative changes in their QOL, often because of the extensive treatments required to treat their cancers (i.e., surgery, radiation and/or chemotherapy). Women frequently report significant anxiety, depression, and altered sexual and social functioning [218–225]. Pain and diminished level of functioning because of treatments are the major factors that contribute to these negative effects on QOL [226]. Some studies have suggested that older patients suffer less psychologic stress than younger patients [227,228].

IX. Suggestions for Further Investigations

As our population ages, we will be faced with increasing numbers of older cancer patients. This chapter highlights major issues facing the older woman with cancer. Age and gender do have prognostic implications. Overall, the literature supports treating fit older women in a similar manner to younger women, with surgery, radiation, chemotherapy, or a combination of these modalities to cure or palliate symptoms. Performance status, functional status, comorbid diseases/geriatric syndromes, and nutritional and social issues must be assessed, because some patients who are debilitated or frail will not tolerate or benefit from therapy. More research is needed in many areas to further define how best to treat the growing elderly population and to explore the biologic differences that appear to exist between older and younger patients and between women and men.

Areas that need further study include the following:

- How can we increase accrual of elderly patients to clinical trials?
- What are the biologic differences in cancer between older and younger patients and between men and women? How do tumor-host interactions change with age?
- Can we further define which older patients will suffer toxicity from treatment and which patients will most likely benefit from treatment?
- How can we improve the QOL in older patients, pain control, and palliative care?
- Who will be the caretakers when the caretakers are ill? Special studies are needed that focus on the needs of older women including social, transportation, and economic issues.

References

1. Campbell PR. (1996). Population Projections for States by Age, Sex, Race, and Hispanic Origin: 1995–2025. Washington, DC: US Bureau of the Census, Population Division, PPL-47, 86.
2. Ries LAG, Eisner MP, Kosary CL et al. (eds). (2001). SEER Cancer Statistics Review, 1973–1998. Bethesda, MD: National Cancer Institute.
3. Jemal A, Thomas A, Murray T, Thun M. (2002). Cancer statistics, 2002. CA Cancer J Clin. 52:23–47.
4. Fried LP, Bandeen-Roche K, Kasper JD, Guralnik JM. (1999). Association of comorbidity with disability in older women: The Women's Health and Aging Study. J Clin Epidemiol. 52:27–37.
5. Yancik R, Havlik RJ, Wesley MN et al. (1996). Cancer and comorbidity in older patients: A descriptive profile. Ann Epidemiol. 6:399–412.
6. Coebergh JW, Janssen-Heijnen ML, Post PN, Razenberg PP. (1999). Serious co-morbidity among unselected cancer patients newly diagnosed in the southeastern part of the Netherlands in 1993–1996. J Clin Epidemiol. 52:1131–1136.
7. Satariano WA. (1992). Comorbidity and functional status in older women with breast cancer: Implications for screening, treatment and prognosis. J Gerontol. 47:24–31.
8. Repetto L, Venturino A, Vercelli M et al. (1998). Performance status and comorbidity in elderly cancer patients compared with young patients with neoplasia and elderly patients without neoplastic conditions. Cancer. 82:760–765.
9. Bergman L, Kluck HM, van Leeuwen FE et al. (1992). The influence of age on treatment choice and survival of elderly breast cancer patients in south-eastern Netherlands: A population based study. Eur J Cancer. 28A:1475–1480.
10. Greenlee RT, Hill-Harmon MB, Murray T, Thun M. (2001). Cancer Statistics, 2001. CA Cancer J Clin. 51:15–36.
11. Kane RL, Ouslander JG, Abrass IB. (1999). The Elderly Patient: Demography and Epidemiology. In Essentials of Clinical Geriatrics, 4th Edition, Kane RL, Ouslander JG, Abrass IB, eds. pp. 19–42. New York: McGraw-Hill.
12. Furner SE, Brody JA, Jankowski LM. (1997). Epidemiology and Aging. In Geriatric Medicine, 3rd Edition, Cassel CK, ed. pp. 37–43. New York: Springer.
13. Trimble EL, Carter CL, Cain D et al. (1994). Representation of older patients in cancer treatment trials. Cancer. 74(7 Suppl):2208–2214.
14. Hutchins LF, Unger JM, Crowley JJ et al. (1999). Underrepresentation of patients 65 years of age or older in cancer-treatment trials. N Engl J Med. 341:2061–2067.
15. Shcrag D, Cramer LD, Bach PB, Begg CB. (2001). Age and adjuvant chemotherapy use after surgery for stage III colon cancer. J Natl Cancer Inst. 93:850–857.
16. Greenfield S, Blanco DM, Elashoff RM, Ganz PA. (1987). Patterns of care related to age of breast cancer patients. JAMA. 257:2766–2770.
17. Mor V, Masterson-Allen S, Goldberg RJ et al. (1985). Relationship between age at diagnosis and treatments received by cancer patients. J Am Geriatr Soc. 33:585–589.
18. Sundararajan V, Grann VR, Jacobson JS et al. (2001). Variations in the use of adjuvant chemotherapy for node-positive colon cancer in the elderly: A population-based study. Cancer J. 7:213–218.
19. Sundararajan V, Hershman D, Grann VR et al. (2002). Variations in the use of chemotherapy for elderly patients with advanced ovarian cancer: A population-based study. J Clin Oncol. 20:173–178.
20. Naeim A, Reuben D. (2001). Geriatric syndromes and assessment in older cancer patients. Oncology (Huntingt). 15:1567–1577.
21. Balducci L, Extermann M. (2000). Management of the frail person with advanced cancer. Crit Rev Oncol Hematol. 33:143–148.
22. Balducci L, Beghe C. (2001). Cancer and age in the USA. Crit Rev Oncol Hematol. 37:137–145.
23. Overcash J. (1998). The Case for a Geriatric Oncology Program in a Cancer Center. In Comprehensive Geriatric Oncology (Balducci L, Liman GH, Ershler WB, eds), pp. 813–824. Amsterdam: Harwood Academic Publishers.
24. Monfardini S, Balducci L. (1999). A comprehensive geriatric assessment (CGA) is necessary for the study and the management of cancer in the elderly. Eur J Cancer. 35:1771–1772.
25. Karnofsky DA. (1968). Determining the extent of the cancer in clinical planning for cure. Cancer. 22:730–734.
26. Oken MM, Creech RH, Tormey DC et al. (1982). Toxicity and response criteria of the Eastern Cooperative Oncology Group. Am J Clin Oncol. 5:649–655.
27. Siu AL, Moshita L, Blaustein J. (1994). Comprehensive geriatric assessment in day hospital. J Am Geriatr Soc. 42:1094–1099.
28. Applegate WB, Blass JP, Williams TF. (1990). Instruments for the functional assessment of older patients. N Engl J Med. 322:1207–1214.
29. Katz S, Ford AB, Moskowitz RW et al. (1963). Studies of illness in the aged. JAMA. 185:914–919.
30. Lawton MP, Brody EM. (1969). Assessment of older people: Self-maintaining and instrumental activities of daily living. Gerontologist. 9:179–186.
31. Folstein MF, Flostein SE, McHugh PR. (1975). "Mini-mental state". A practical method for grading the cognitive state of patients for the clinician. J Psychiatr Res. 12(3):189–198.
32. Yesavage JA. (1991). Geriatric depression scale: Consistency of depressive symptoms over time. Percept Motor Skills. 73(3 Pt 1):1032.
33. Tchekmedyian NS, Heber D. (1998). Nutritional Therapy. In Comprehensive Geriatric Oncology (Balducci L, Liman GH, Ershler WB, eds.), pp. 161–168. Amsterdam: Harwood Academic Publishers.
34. Extermann M, Overcash J, Lyman GH et al. (1998). Comorbidity and functional status are independent in older cancer patients. J Clin Oncol. 16:1582–1587.
35. Extermann M. (2000). Measurement and impact of comorbidity in older cancer patients. Crit Rev Oncol Hematol. 35:181–200.
36. Satariano WA, Ragland DR. (1994). The effect of comorbidity on 3-year survival of women with primary breast cancer. Ann Intern Med. 120:104–110.
37. Yancik R, Wesley MN, Ries LA et al. (1998). Comorbidity and age as predictors of risk for early mortality of male and female colon carcinoma patients: A population-based study. Cancer. 82:2123–2134.

38. Sabin SL, Rosenfeld RM, Sundaram K et al. (1999). The impact of comorbidity and age on survival with laryngeal cancer. Ear Nose Throat J. 78:578, 581–584.

39. Mamon JA, Shediac MC, Crosby CB et al. (1990). Inner-city women at risk for cervical cancer: Behavioral and utilization factors related to inadequate screening. Prev Med. 19:363–376.

40. Levy S, Dowling P, Boult L et al. (1992). The effect of physician and patient gender on preventive medicine practices in patients older than fifty. Fam Med. 24:58–61.

41. Fox SA, Roetzheim RG, Kington RS. (1997). Barriers to cancer prevention in the older person. Clin Geriatr Med. 13:79–95.

42. Sutton S, Eisner E, Burklow J. (1994). Health communications to older Americans as a special population. The National Cancer Institute's consumer based approach. Cancer. 74(7 Suppl):2194–2199.

43. Taplin SH, Montano DE. (1993). Attitudes, age, and participation in mammographic screening. A prospective analysis. J Am Board Fam Pract. 6:13–23.

44. Kramer BS. (1995). The Screening Editorial Board of the Physician Data Query: NCI State of the Art Statement on Cancer Screening. Bethesda, MD: National Cancer Institute.

45. US Preventive Task Force. (1996). Guide to Clinical Preventive Services. Alexandria, VA: International Medical Publishing.

46. Smith RA, Cokkinides V, vonEschenbach AC et al. (2002). American Cancer Society guidelines for the early detection of cancer. CA Cancer J Clin. 52:8–22.

47. Faulk RM, Sickles EA, Sollitto RA et al. (1995). Clinical efficacy of mammographic screening in the elderly. Radiology. 194:193–197.

48. Costanza ME. (1992). Breast cancer screening in older women: Overview. J Gerontol. 47(Spec No):1–3.

49. van Dijck JA, Broeders MJ, Verbeek AL. (1997). Mammographic screening in older women. Is it worthwhile? Drugs Aging. 10(2):69–79.

50. Holtzman D, Powell-Griner E, Bolen J, Rhodes L. (2000). State- and sex-specific prevalence of selected characteristics—Behavioral Risk Factor Surveillance System, 1996 and 1997. MMWR CDC Surveill Summ. 49(6):1–39.

51. Robinson B, Beghe C. (1997). Cancer screening in the older patient. Clin Geriatr Med. 13:97–118.

52. Mandelblatt J, Richart R, Thomas L et al. (1992). Is human papillomavirus associated with cervical neoplasia in the elderly? Gynecol Oncol. 46:6–12.

53. Scheuer L, Kauff N, Robson M et al. (2002). Outcome of preventive surgery and screening for breast and ovarian cancer in BRCA mutation carriers. J Clin Oncol. 20:1260–1268.

54. Laframboise S, Nedelcu R, Murphy J et al. (2002). Use of CA-125 and ultrasound in high-risk women. Int J Gynecol Cancer. 12:86–91.

55. Donovan JM, Syngal SS. (1998). Colorectal cancer in women: An under-appreciated but preventable risk. J Womens Health. 7:45–48.

56. Anderson LM, May DS. (1995). Has the use of cervical, breast, and colorectal cancer screening increased in the United States? Am J Public Health. 85:840–842.

57. Okamoto M, Shiratori Y, Yamaji Y et al. (2002). Relationship between age and site of colorectal cancer based on colonoscopy findings. Gastrointest Endosc. 55:548–551.

58. Jensen OM. (1984). Different age and sex relationship for cancer of subsites of the large bowel. Br J Cancer. 50:825–829.

59. Butcher D, Hassanein K, Dudgeon M et al. (1985). Female gender is a major determinate of changing subsite distribution of colorectal cancer with age. Cancer. 56:714–716.

60. Fleshner P, Slater G, Aufses AH Jr. (1989). Age and sex distribution of patients with colorectal cancer. Dis Colon Rectum. 32(2):107–111.

61. Dubrow R, Bernstein J, Holford TR. (1993). Age-period-cohort modelling of large-bowel-cancer incidence by anatomic sub-site and sex in Connecticut. Int J Cancer. 53:907–913.

62. Ikeda Y, Koyanagi N, Mori M. (1996). Increased incidence of proximal colon cancer in the elderly. J Clin Gastroenterol. 23(2):105–108.

63. Tomoda H, Taketomi A, Baba H et al. (1998). The clinicopathological characteristics and outcome of patients with right colon cancer. Oncol Rep. 5:481–483.

64. Elsaleh H, Joseph D, Grieu F et al. (2000). Association of tumor site and sex with survival benefit from adjuvant chemotherapy in colorectal cancer. Lancet. 355:1745–1750.

65. Hamblin TJ. (1995). Disappointments in treating acute leukemia in the elderly. N Engl J Med. 332:1712–1713.

66. Pinto A, Zagonel V, Ferrara F. (2001). Acute myeloid leukemia in the elderly: Biology and therapeutic strategies. Crit Rev Oncol Hematol. 39:275–287.

67. Author Unknown. (1997). Effect of age on the characteristics and clinical behavior of non-Hodgkin's lymphoma patients. The non-Hodgkin's Lymphoma Classification Project. Ann Oncol. 8:973–978.

68. Carbone A, Tirelli U, Volpe R et al. (1986). Non-Hodgkin's lymphoma in the elderly. A retrospective clinicopathologic study of 50 patients. Cancer. 57:2185–2189.

69. Carbone A, Volpe R, Gloghini A et al. (1990). Non-Hodgkin's lymphoma in the elderly. I. Pathologic features at presentation. Cancer. 66:1991–1994.

70. Yancik R, Ries LG, Yates JW. (1986). Ovarian cancer in the elderly: An analysis of Surveillance, Epidemiology, and End Results Program data. Am J Obstet Gynecol. 154:639–647.

71. Hightower RD, Nguyen HN, Averette HE et al. (1994). National survey of ovarian carcinoma. IV: Patterns of care and related survival for older patients. Cancer. 73:377–383.

72. Thigpen T, Brady MF, Omura GA et al. (1993). Age as a prognostic factor in ovarian carcinoma. Cancer. 71(2 Suppl):606–614.

73. Chang CH, Horton J, Schoenfeld D et al. (1983). Comparison of postoperative radiotherapy and combined postoperative radiotherapy and chemotherapy in the multidisciplinary management of malignant gliomas. A joint Radiation Therapy Oncology Group and Eastern Cooperative Oncology Group study. Cancer. 52:997–1007.

74. Fernandez PM, Brem S. (1997). Malignant brain tumors in the elderly. Clin Geriatr Med. 13:327–338.

75. Grant R, Liang BC, Page MA. (1995). Age influences chemotherapy response in astrocytomas. Neurology. 45:929–933.

76. Sneed PK, Prados MD, McDermott MW et al. (1995). Large effect of age on the survival of patients with glioblastoma treated with radiotherapy and brachytherapy boost. Neurosurgery. 36:898–903.

77. Miller JG, Mac Neil S. (1997). Gender and cutaneous melanoma. Br J Dermatol. 136:657–665.

78. Sridhar KS, Raub W, Duncan RC et al. (1991). Lung carcinoma in 1,336 patients. Am J Clin Oncol. 14:496–508.

79. Ferguson MK, Skosey C, Hoffman PC, Golomb HM. (1990). Sex-associated differences in presentation and survival in patients with lung cancer. J Clin Oncol. 8:4102–4107.

80. Johnson BE, Steinberg SM, Phelps R et al. (1988). Female patients with small cell lung cancer live longer than male patients. Am J Med. 85:194–196.

81. Holli K, Isola J. (1997). Effect of age on the survival of breast cancer patients. Eur J Cancer. 33:425–428.

82. Department of Health and Human Services, Centers for Disease Control and Prevention, National Center for Health Statistics (1997). Health United States 1996–1997 and Injury Chartbook. Hyattsville, MD: DHHS.

83. Bergman L, Kluck HM, van Leeuwen FE et al. (1992). The influence of age on treatment choice and survival of elderly breast cancer patients in southeastern Netherlands: A population-based study. Eur J Cancer. 28A:1475-1480.

84. Diab SG, Elledge RM, Clark GM. (2000). Tumor characteristics and clinical outcome of elderly women with breast cancer. J Natl Cancer Inst. 92:550–556.

85. Yancik R, Ries LG, Yates JW. (1989). Breast cancer in aging women. A population-based study of contrasts in stage, surgery, and survival. Cancer. 63:976–981.

86. Pinto A, Zagonel V, Ferrara F. (2001). Acute myeloid leukemia in the elderly: Biology and therapeutic strategies. Crit Rev Oncol Hematol. 39:275–287.

87. Bertini M, Boccomini C, Calvi R. (2001). The Influence of advanced age on the treatment and prognosis of diffuse large-cell lymphoma (DLCL). Clin Lymphoma. 1:278–284.

88. Kosary CL. (1994). FIGO stage, histology, histologic grade, age, and race as prognostic factors in determining survival for cancers of the female gynecological system: An analysis of 1973–1987 SEER cases of cancers of the endometrium, cervix, ovary, vulva, and vagina. Semin Surg Oncol. 10:31–46.

89. Alberts DS, Dahlberg S, Green SJ et al. (1993). Analysis of patient age as an independent prognostic factor for survival in phase III study of cisplatin-cyclophosphamide versus carboplatin-cyclophosphamide in stages III (suboptimal) and IV ovarian cancer. A Southwest Oncology Group study. Cancer. 71(2 Suppl):618–627.

90. Marchetti DL, Lele SB, Priore RL et al. (1993). Treatment of advanced ovarian cancer in the elderly. Gynecol Oncol. 49:86–91.

91. Bokhman JV. (1983). Two pathogenetic types of endometrial carcinoma. Gynecol Oncol. 15:10–17.

92. Sherman ME. (2000). Theories of endometrial carcinogenesis: A multi-disciplinary approach. *Mod Pathol.* 13:295–308.

93. Mutter GL, Lin MC, Fitzgerald JT *et al.* (2000). Altered PTEN expression as a diagnostic marker for the earliest endometrial precancers. *J Natl Cancer Inst.* 92:924–930.

94. Mutter GL, Ince TA, Baak JP *et al.* (2001). Molecular identification of latent precancers in histologically normal endometrium. *Cancer Res.* 61:4311–4314.

95. Chao CK, Grigsby PW, Perez CA *et al.* (1996). Medically inoperable stage I endometrial carcinoma: A few dilemmas in radiotherapeutic management. *Int J Radiat Oncol Biol Phys.* 34:27–31.

96. Begg CB, Cohen JL, Ellerton J. (1980). Are the elderly predisposed to toxicity from cancer chemotherapy? An investigation using data from the Eastern Cooperative Oncology Group. *Cancer Clin Trial.* 3:369–374.

97. Giovanazzi-Bannon S, Rademaker A, Lai G, Benson AB 3rd. (1994). Treatment tolerance of elderly cancer patients entered onto phase II clinical trials: An Illinois Cancer Center study. *J Clin Oncol.* 12:2447–2452.

98. Bennett WM. (1990). Geriatric pharmacokinetics and the kidney. *Am J Kidney Dis.* 16:283–288.

99. Catterson ML, Preskorn SH, Martin RL. (1997). Pharmacodynamic and pharmacokinetic considerations in geriatric psychopharmacology. *Psychiatr Clin North Am.* 20:205–218.

100. Corcoran ME. (1997). Polypharmacy in the older patient with cancer. *Cancer Control.* 4:419–428.

101. Perry MC, Anderson CM, Dorr VJ, Wilkes JD. (1999). *Companion Handbook to the Chemotherapy Sourcebook.* Baltimore: Williams & Wilkins.

102. Cova D, Beretta G, Balducci L. (1998). Cancer Chemotherapy in the Older Patient: Magnitude of the Problem. In *Comprehensive Geriatric Oncology* (Balducci L, Liman GH, Ershler WB, eds.), pp. 429–442. Amsterdam: Harwood Academic Publishers.

103. Balducci L, Mowry K. (1992). Pharmacology and organ toxicity of chemotherapy in older patients. *Oncology (Huntingt).* 6(Suppl 2):62–68.

104. Bonadonna G, Valagussa P. (1981). Dose-response effect of adjuvant chemotherapy in breast cancer. *N Engl J Med.* 304:10–15.

105. Frei E 3rd, Canellos GP. (1980). Dose: A critical factor in cancer chemotherapy. *Am J Med.* 69:585–594.

106. Kwak LW, Halpern J, Olshen RA, Horning SJ. (1990). Prognostic significance of actual dose intensity in diffuse large-cell lymphoma: Results of a tree-structured survival analysis. *J Clin Oncol.* 8:963–977.

107. Monfardini S, Carbone C. (1998). Non-Hodgkin's Lymphomas. In *Comprehensive Geriatric Oncology* (Balducci L, Liman GH, Ershler WB, eds.), pp. 577–594. Amsterdam: Harwood Academic Publishers.

108. Extermann M. (1997). Acute leukemia in the older patient. *Clin Geriatr Med.* 13:227–244.

109. Goodwin JS, Samet JM, Key CR *et al.* (1986). Stage at diagnosis of cancer varies with the age of the patient. *J Am Geriatr Soc.* 34:20–26.

110. Olmi P, Cefaro GA, Balzi M *et al.* (1997). Radiotherapy in the aged. *Clin Geriatr Med.* 13:143–168.

111. Chin R, Fisher RJ, Smee RI, Barton MB. (1995). Oropharyngeal cancer in the elderly. *Int J Radiat Oncol Biol Phys.* 32:1007–1016.

112. Hishikawa Y, Kurisu K, Taniguchi M *et al.* (1991). Radiotherapy for carcinoma of the esophagus in patients aged eighty or older. *Int J Radiat Oncol Biol Phys.* 20:685–688.

113. Pignon T, Horiot JC, Van den Bogaert W *et al.* (1996). No age limit for radical radiotherapy in head and neck tumors. *Eur J Cancer.* 32A:2075–2081.

114. Hayakawa K. (2001). High-dose radiation therapy for elderly patients with inoperable or unresectable non-small cell lung cancer. *Lung Cancer.* 32:81–88.

115. Zachariah B, Balducci L. (2000). Radiation therapy in the older patient. *Hematol Oncol Clin North Am.* 14:131–167.

116. Scalliet P, Pignon T. (1998). Radiotherapy in the Elderly. In *Comprehensive Geriatric Oncology* (Balducci L, Liman GH, Ershler WB, eds.), pp. 421–427. Amsterdam: Harwood Academic Publishers.

117. Zachariah B, Balducci L, Venkattaramanabalaji GV *et al.* (1997). Radiotherapy for cancer patients aged 80 and older: A study of effectiveness and side effects. *Int J Radiat Oncol Biol Phys.* 39:1125–1129.

118. Wasil T, Lichtman SM, Gupta V, Rush S. (2000). Radiation therapy in cancer patients 80 years of age and older. *Am J Clin Oncol.* 23:526–530.

119. Berger DH, Roslyn JJ. (1997). Cancer surgery in the elderly. *Clin Geriatr Med.* 13:119–141.

120. Fabri PJ. (1998). Surgical Approaches to the Older Person with Cancer. In *Comprehensive Geriatric Oncology* (Balducci L, Liman GH, Ershler WB, eds.), pp. 369–375. Amsterdam: Harwood Academic Publishers.

121. Kemeny MM, Busch-Devereaux E, Merriam LT, O'Hea BJ. (2000). Cancer surgery in the elderly. *Hematol Oncol Clin North Am.* 14:169–192.

122. Smith JJ, Lee J, Burke C *et al.* (2002). Major colorectal cancer resection should not be denied to the elderly. *Eur J Surg Oncol.* 28:661–666.

123. Wobbes T. (1985). Carcinoma of the colon and rectum in geriatric patients. *Age Ageing.* 14:321–326.

124. Bader TF. (1986). Colorectal cancer in patients older than 75 years of age. *Dis Colon Rectum.* 29:728–732.

125. Sunouchi K, Namiki K, Mori M *et al.* (2000). How should patients 80 years of age or older with colorectal carcinoma be treated? Long-term and short-term outcome and postoperative cytokine levels. *Dis Colon Rectum.* 43:233–241.

126. Kingston RD, Jeacock J, Walsh S, Keeling F. (1995). The outcome of surgery for colorectal cancer in the elderly: A 12-year review from the Trafford Database. *Eur J Surg Oncol.* 21:514–516.

127. Greenburg AG, Saik RP, Pridham D. (1985). Influence of age on mortality of colon surgery. *Am J Surg.* 150:65–70.

128. Irvin TT. (1988). Prognosis of colorectal cancer in the elderly. *Br J Surg.* 5:419–421.

129. Ballard-Barbash R, Potosky AL, Harlan LC *et al.* (1996). Factors associated with surgical and radiation therapy for early stage breast cancer in older women. *J Natl Cancer Inst.* 88:716–726.

130. Hebert-Croteau N, Brisson J, Latreille J *et al.* (1999). Compliance with consensus recommendations for the treatment of early stage breast carcinoma in elderly women. *Cancer.* 85:1104–1113.

131. Mandelblatt JS, Hadley J, Kerner JF *et al.* (2000). Patterns of breast carcinoma treatment in older women: Patient preference and clinical and physical influences. *Cancer.* 89:561–573.

132. Gazet JC, Ford HT, Coombes RC *et al.* (1994). Prospective randomized trial of tamoxifen vs surgery in elderly patients with breast cancer. *Eur J Surg Oncol.* 20:207–214.

133. Margolese RG, Foster RS Jr. (1989). Tamoxifen as an alternative to surgical resection for selected geriatric patients with primary breast cancer. *Arch Surg.* 124:548–550, discussion 550–551.

134. Crivellari D, Bonetti M, Castiglione-Gertsch M *et al.* (2000). Burdens and benefits of adjuvant cyclophosphamide, methotrexate, and fluorouracil and tamoxifen for elderly patients with breast cancer: The International Breast Cancer Study Group Trial VII. *J Clin Oncol.* 18:1412–1422.

135. Author Unknown. (1998). Tamoxifen for early breast cancer: An overview of the randomised trials. Early Breast Cancer Trialists' Collaborative Group. *Lancet.* 351:1451–1467.

136. Author Unknown. (2002). Endocrine responsiveness and tailoring adjuvant therapy for postmenopausal lymph node-negative breast cancer: A randomized trial. *J Natl Cancer Inst.* 94:1054–1065.

137. Author Unknown. (1998). Polychemotherapy for early breast cancer: An overview of the randomized trails. Early Breast Cancer Trialists' Collaborative Group. *Lancet.* 352:930–942.

138. Heshmati HM, Khosla S, Robins SP *et al.* (2002). Role of low levels of endogenous estrogen in regulation of bone resorption in late postmenopausal women. *J Bone Miner Res.* 17:172–178.

139. Author Unknown. (2002). Anastrozole alone or in combination with tamoxifen versus tamoxifen alone for adjuvant treatment of postmenopausal women with early breast cancer: First results of the ATAC randomised trial. *Lancet.* 359:2131–2139.

140. Winer EP, Hudis C, Burstein HJ *et al.* (2002). American Society of Clinical Oncology technology assessment on the use of aromatase inhibitors as adjuvant therapy for women with hormone receptor-positive breast cancer: Status report 2002. *J Clin Oncol.* 20:3317–3327.

141. Bonneterre J, Thurlimann B, Robertson JF *et al.* (2000). Anastrozole versus tamoxifen as first-line therapy for advanced breast cancer in 668 postmenopausal women: Results of the Tamoxifen or Arimidex Randomized Group Efficacy and Tolerability study. *J Clin Oncol.* 18:3748–3757.

142. Nabholtz JM, Buzdar A, Pollak M *et al.* (2000). Anastrozole is superior to tamoxifen as first-line therapy for advanced breast cancer in postmenopausal women: Results of a North American multicenter randomized trial. Arimidex Study Group. *J Clin Oncol.* 18:3758–3767.

143. Goss PE, Strasser K. (2001). Aromatase inhibitors in the treatment and prevention of breast cancer. *J Clin Oncol.* 19:881–894.

144. Christman K, Muss HB, Case LD, Stanley V. (1992). Chemotherapy of metastatic breast cancer in the elderly. The Piedmont Oncology Association experience. *JAMA.* 268:57–62.

145. Moore HC, Haller DG. (1999). Adjuvant therapy of colon cancer. *Semin Oncol.* 26:545–555.

146. Cohen AM, Tremiterra S, Candela F et al. (1991). Prognosis of node-positive colon cancer. *Cancer.* 67:1859–1861.

147. Moertel CG, Fleming TR, Macdonald JS et al. (1995). Fluorouracil plus levamisole as effective adjuvant therapy after resection of stage III colon carcinoma: A final report. *Ann Intern Med.* 122:321–326.

148. Sloan JA, Goldberg RM, Sargent DJ et al. (2002). Women experience greater toxicity with fluorouracil-based chemotherapy for colorectal cancer. *J Clin Oncol.* 20:1491–1498.

149. Sargent DJ, Goldberg RM, Jacobson SD et al. (2001). A pooled analysis of adjuvant chemotherapy for resected colon cancer in elderly patients. *N Engl J Med.* 345:1091–1097.

150. Jacobson SD, Cha S, Sargent DJ et al. (2001). Tolerability, Dose Intensity, and Benefit of 5FU-Based Chemotherapy for advanced colorectal cancer in the elderly. A North Central Cooperative Group Study. *Proc Am Soc Clin Oncol.* 20(1):384a (Abstract #1534).

151. Yancik R, Ries LG, Yates JW. (1986). Ovarian cancer in the elderly: An analysis of Surveillance, Epidemiology, and End Results Program data. *Am J Obstet Gynecol.* 154:639–647.

152. Moore DH. (1993). Primary Surgical Management of Early Epithelial Ovarian Cancer. In *Ovarian Cancer* (Rubin SC, Sutton GP, eds.), pp. 219–239. New York: McGraw Hill.

153. Young RC, Walton LA, Ellenberg SS et al. (1990). Adjuvant therapy in stage I and stage II epithelial ovarian cancer. Results of two prospective randomized trials. *N Engl J Med.* 322:1021–1027.

154. McGuire WP, Hoskins WJ, Brady MF et al. (1996). Cyclophosphamide and cisplatin compared with paclitaxel and cisplatin in patients with stage III and stage IV ovarian cancer (from the Gynecologic Oncology Group). *N Engl J Med.* 334:1–6.

155. Unknown Author. (2002). Paclitaxel plus carboplatin versus standard chemotherapy with either single-agent carboplatin or cyclophosphamide, doxorubicin, and cisplatin in women with ovarian cancer: The ICON3 randomised trial. *Lancet.* 360:505–515.

156. Fisher B, Costantino JP, Wickerham DL et al. (1998). Tamoxifen for prevention of breast cancer: Report of the National Surgical Adjuvant Breast and Bowel Project P-1 Study. *J Natl Cancer Inst.* 90:1371–1388.

157. Soler M, Chatenoud L, Negri E et al. (1999). Hypertension and hormone-related neoplasms in women. *Hypertension.* 34:320–325.

158. Aarnio M, Mecklin JP, Aaltonen LA et al. (1995). Life-time risk of different cancers in hereditary non-polyposis colorectal cancer (HNPCC) syndrome. *Int J Cancer.* 64:430–433.

159. Wharton JT, Mikuta JJ, Mettlin C et al. (1986). Risk factors and current management in carcinoma of the endometrium. *Surg Gynecol Obstet.* 162:515–520.

160. Huh WK, Straughn JM Jr, Kelly FJ, Kilgore LC. (2001). Endometrial carcinoma. *Curr Treat Options Oncol.* 2:129–135.

161. Anderson JM, Stea B, Hallum AV et al. (2000). High-dose-rate postoperative vaginal cuff irradiation alone for stage IB and IC endometrial cancer. *Int J Radiat Oncol Biol Phys.* 46:417–425.

162. Aalders J, Abeler V, Kolstad P, Onsrud M. (1980). Postoperative external irradiation and prognostic parameters in stage I endometrial carcinoma: Clinical and histopathologic study of 540 patients. *Obstet Gynecol.* 56:419–427.

163. Naumann RW. (2002). The role of radiation therapy in early endometrial cancer. *Curr Opin Obstet Gynecol.* 14:75–79.

164. Grigsby PW. (2002). Update on radiation therapy for endometrial cancer. *Oncology (Huntingt).* 16:777–786, 790, discussion 791, 794–795.

165. Rose PG, Baker S, Kern M et al. (1993). Primary radiation therapy for endometrial carcinoma: A case controlled study. *Int J Radiat Oncol Biol Phys.* 27:585–590.

166. Kupelian PA, Eifel PJ, Tornos C et al. (1993). Treatment of endometrial carcinoma with radiation therapy alone. *Int J Radiat Oncol Biol Phys.* 27:817–824.

167. Barakat RR, Park RC, Grigsby PW et al. (1997). Corpus: Epithelial Tumors. In *Principles and Practice of Gynecologic Oncology*, 2nd Edition (Hoskins WH, Perez CA, Young RC, eds.), p. 859. Philadelphia: Lippincott-Raven.

168. Deppe G, Malviya VK, Malone JM et al. (1994). Treatment of recurrent and metastatic endometrial carcinoma with cisplatin and doxorubicin. *Eur J Gynaecol Oncol.* 15:263–266.

169. Lissoni A, Zanetta G, Losa G et al. (1996). Phase II study of paclitaxel as salvage treatment in advanced endometrial cancer. *Ann Oncol.* 7:861–863.

170. Ball HG, Blessing JA, Lentz SS, Mutch DG. (1996). A phase II trial of paclitaxel in patients with advanced or recurrent adenocarcinoma of the endometrium: A Gynecologic Oncology Group study. *Gynecol Oncol.* 62:278–281.

171. Hoskins PJ, Swenerton KD, Pike JA et al. (2001). Paclitaxel and carboplatin, alone or with irradiation, in advanced or recurrent endometrial cancer: A phase II study. *J Clin Oncol.* 19:4048–4053.

172a. Gridelli C, Perrone F, Monfardini S. (1997). Lung cancer in the elderly. *Eur J Cancer.* 33:2313–2314.

172b. Havlik RJ, Yancik R, Long S et al. (1994). The National Cancer Institute on Aging and the National Cancer Institute SEER Collaborative Study on comorbidity and early diagnosis of cancer in the elderly. *Cancer.* 74(7 Suppl):2101–2106.

173. Zang EA, Wynder EL. (1996). Differences in lung cancer risk between men and women: Examination of the evidence. *J Natl Cancer Inst.* 88:183–192.

174. Ernster V, Kaufman N, Nichter M et al. (2000). Women and tobacco: Moving from policy to action. *Bull World Health Organ.* 78:891–901.

175. Craig D, Parrott A, Coomber JA. (1992). Smoking cessation in women: Effects of the menstrual cycle. *Int J Addict.* 27:697–706.

176. Gritz ER, Nielsen IR, Brooks LA. (1996). Smoking cessation and gender: The influence of physiological, psychological, and behavioral factors. *J Am Med Womens Assoc.* 51(1–2):35–42.

177. Hanson MJ. (1994). Sociocultural and physiological correlates of cigarette smoking in women. *Health Care Women Int.* 15:549–562.

178. Shriver SP, Bourdeau HA, Gubish CT et al. (2000). Sex-specific expression of gastrin-releasing peptide receptor: Relationship to smoking history and risk of lung cancer. *J Natl Cancer Inst.* 92:24–33.

179. Williams DE, Pairolero PC, Davis CS et al. (1981). Survival of patients surgically treated for stage I lung cancer. *J Thorac Cardiovasc Surg.* 82:70–76.

180. Martini N, Burt ME, Bains MS et al. (1992). Survival after resection of stage II non-small cell lung cancer. *Ann Thorac Surg.* 54:460–465, discussion 466.

181. Langer CJ. (2001). Staging and prognosis in lung cancer. *Cancer Treat Res.* 105:53–94.

182. Lee-Chiong TL Jr, Matthay RA. (1993). Lung cancer in elderly patient. *Clin Chest Med.* 14:453–478.

183. Antonia SJ, Robinson LA, Ruckdeschel JC, Wagner H. (1998). Lung Cancer. In *Comprehensive Geriatric Oncology* (Balducci L, Liman GH, Ershler WB, eds.), pp. 611–628. Amsterdam: Harwood Academic Publishers.

184. Author Unknown. (1997). Pretreatment evaluation of non-small cell lung cancer. The American Thoracic Society and The European Respiratory Society. *Am J Respir Crit Care Med.* 156:320–332.

185. Rosenthal SA, Curran WJ Jr, Herbert SH et al. (1992). Clinical stage II non-small cell lung cancer treated with radiation therapy alone. The significance of clinically staged ipsilateral hilar adenopathy (N1 disease). *Cancer.* 70:2410–417.

186. Roth JA, Fossella S, Komaki R et al. (1994). A randomized trial comparing perioperative chemotherapy and surgery with surgery alone in resectable stage IIIA non-small cell lung cancer. *J Natl Cancer Inst.* 86:673–680.

187. Rosell R, Gomez-Codina J, Camps C et al. (1994). A randomized trial comparing preoperative chemotherapy plus surgery with surgery alone in patients with non-small-cell lung cancer. *N Engl J Med.* 330:153–158.

188. Sause W, Kolesar P, Taylor S et al. (2000). Final results of phase III trial in regionally advanced unresectable non-small cell lung cancer: Radiation Therapy Oncology Group, and Eastern Cooperative Oncology Group, and Southwest Oncology Group. *Chest.* 117:358–364.

189. Dillman RO, Herndon J, Seagren SL et al. (1996). Improved survival in stage III non-small cell lung cancer: Seven-year follow-up of cancer and leukemia group B (CALGB) 8433 trial. *J Natl Cancer Inst.* 88:1210–1215.

190. Author Unknown. (1995). Chemotherapy in non-small cell lung cancer: A meta-analysis using updated data on individual patients from 52 randomised clinical trials. Non-small Cell Lung Cancer Collaborative Group. *BMJ.* 311:899–909.

191. Gridelli C, Rossi A, Scognamiglio F et al. (1997). Carboplatin plus oral etoposide in elderly patients with advanced non small cell lung cancer. A phase II study. *Anticancer Res.* 17(16D):4755–4758.

192. Gridelli C. (2001). The ELVIS trial: A phase III study of single agent vinorelbine as first-line treatment in elderly patients with advanced non-small cell lung cancer. *Oncologist.* 6(Suppl 1):4–7.

193. Nakamura Y, Sekine I, Furuse K, Saijo N. (2000). Retrospective comparison of toxicity and efficacy in phase II trials of 3-h infusions of paclitaxel for patients 70 years of age or older and patient under 70 years of age. *Cancer Chemother Pharmacol.* 46(2):114–118.

194. Hainsworth JD, Burris HA 3rd, Litchy S et al. (2000). Weekly docetaxel in the treatment of elderly patients with advanced nonsmall cell lung carcinoma. A Minnie Pearl Cancer Research Network Phase II Trial. *Cancer.* 89:328–333.

195. Ricci S, Antonuzzo A, Galli L et al. (2000). Gemcitabine monotherapy in elderly patients with advanced non small cell lung cancer: A multicenter phase II study. Lung Cancer. 27(2):75–80.

196. Shepherd FA, Abratt RP, Anderson H et al. (1997). Gemcitabine in the treatment of elderly patients with advanced non-small cell lung cancer. Semin Oncol. 24(Suppl 7):S7-50–S7-55.

197. Tirelli U, Zagonel V, Errante D et al. (1998). Treatment of non-Hodgkin's lymphoma in the elderly: An update. Hematol Oncol. 16:1–13.

198. Monfardini S, Carbone A. (1998). Non-Hodgkin's Lymphoma. In Comprehensive Geriatric Oncology (Balducci L, Liman GH, Ershler WB, eds.), pp. 577–594. Amsterdam: Harwood Academic Publishers.

199. Zagonel V, Monfardini S, Tirelli U et al. (2001). Management of hematologic malignancies in the elderly: 13-year experience at the Aviana Cancer Center, Italy. Crit Rev Oncol Hematol. 39:289–305.

200. Zagonel V, Babare R, Merola MC et al. (1994). Cost-benefit of granulocyte colony-simulating factor administration in older patients with non-Hodgkin's lymphoma treated with combination chemotherapy. Ann Oncol. 5(Suppl 2):127–132.

201. Coiffier B, Lepage E, Briere J et al. (2002). CHOP chemotherapy plus rituximab compared with CHOP alone in elderly patients with diffuse large-B-cell lymphoma. N Engl J Med. 346:235–242.

202. Taueber CM. (1993). Sixty-five Plus in America. Current Population Reports, Special Studies, pp. 23–178. Pittsburgh, PA: US Government Printing Office.

203. Ahronheim JC. (1997). End-of life issues for very elderly women. J Am Med Womens Assoc. 52:147–151.

204. Ettinger WH Jr, Fried LP, Harris T et al. (1994). Self-reported causes of physical disability in older people: The Cardiovascular Health Study. CHS Collaborative Research Group. J Am Geriatr Soc. 42:1035–1044.

205. Cleary JF, Carbone PP. (1997). Palliative medicine in the elderly. Cancer. 80:1335–1347.

206. Grossman SA, Sheidler VR. (2000). Cancer Pain. In Abeloff: Clinical Oncology, 2nd Edition, pp. 539–553. New York: Churchill Livingstone.

207. Cleeland CS. (1984). The impact of pain on patients with cancer. Cancer. 54(11 Suppl):2635–2641.

208. Ferrell BR, Rhiner M, Ferrell BA. (1993). Development and implementation of a pain education program. Cancer. 72:3426–3432.

209. Cleeland CS, Gonin R, Hatfield AK et al. (1994). Pain and its treatment in outpatients with metastatic cancer. N Engl J Med. 330:592–596.

210. Joranson DE. (1993). Availability of opioids for cancer pain: Recent trends, assessment of system barriers, New World Health Organization guidelines, and the risk of diversion. J Pain Symptom Manage. 8:353–360.

211. Author Unknown. (1995). Quality improvement guidelines for the treatment of acute pain and cancer pain. American Pain Society Quality of Care Committee. JAMA. 274:1874–1880.

212. Author Unknown. (1992). Cancer pain assessment and treatment curriculum guidelines. The Ad Hoc Committee on Cancer Pain. J Clin Oncol. 10:1976–1982.

213. Benedetti C, Brock C, Cleeland C et al. (2000). NCCN Practice Guidelines for Cancer Pain. Oncology (Huntingt). 14(11A):135–150.

214. Aaronson NK. (1988). Quality of life: What is it? How should it be measured? Oncology (Huntingt). 2(5):64, 69–76.

215. Kornblith AB, Holland JC. (1994). Handbook of Measures for Psychological, Social, and Physical Function in Cancer. Volume 1: Quality of Life. New York: Memorial Sloan-Kettering Cancer Center.

216. Sloan JA, Cella D, Frost M et al. (2002). Assessing clinical significance in measuring oncology patient quality of life. Introduction to the symposium, content overview, and definition of terms. Mayo Clin Proc. 77:367–370.

217. Anderson B, Lutgendorf S. (1997). Quality of life in gynecologic cancer survivors. CA Cancer Jo Clin. 47:218–225.

218. Pignata S, Ballatori E, Favalli G, Scambia G. (2001). Quality of life: Gynecologic cancers. Ann Oncol. 12(Suppl 3):337–42.

219. Guidozzi F. (1993). Living with ovarian cancer. Gynecol Oncol. 50:202–207.

220. Kornblith AB, Thaler HT, Wong G et al. (1995). Quality of life of women with ovarian cancer. Gynecol Oncol. 59:231–242.

221. Portenoy RK, Thaler HT. (1994). Symptom prevalence, characteristics, and distress in a cancer population. Qual Life Res. 3(3):183–189.

222. Lutgendorf SK, Anderson B, Rothrock N et al. (2000). Quality of life and mood in women receiving extensive chemotherapy for gynecologic cancer. Cancer. 89:1402–1411.

223. Anderson B. (1994). Quality of life in progressive ovarian cancer. Gynecol Oncol. 55(3 Pt 2):S151–155.

224. Cain EN, Kohorn EI, Quinlan DM et al. (1983). Psychosocial reactions to the diagnosis of gynecologic cancer. Obstet Gynecol. 62:635–641.

225. Rummans TA, Frost M, Suman VJ et al. (1998). Quality of life and pain in patients with recurrent breast and gynecologic cancer. Psychosomatics. 39:437–445.

226. Payne SA. (1992). A study of the quality of life in cancer patients receiving palliative chemotherapy. Soc Sci Med. 35:1505–1509.

227. Ganz PA, Schag CC, Heinrich RL. (1985). The psychosocial impact of cancer on the elderly: A comparison with younger patients. J Am Geriatr Soc. 33:429–435.

228. Sammarco A. (2001). Psychological stages and quality of life of women with breast cancer. Cancer Nurs. 24:272–277.

109

The Evaluation and Treatment of Urinary Incontinence

DARRYL S. CHUTKA, MD

Associate Professor of Medicine, Mayo Medical School, Rochester, MN

Urinary incontinence is a common condition. Although it occurs in men, it is much more common in women. It can have a significant effect on the quality of life and has medical and economic complications. Urinary incontinence is not a single entity; several types exist. Stress urinary incontinence is the most common form of incontinence in women. It is especially common in younger women, younger than the age of 60. In patients older than 60, urinary stress incontinence, urgency incontinence, and mixed incontinence are equally prevalent. Urge incontinence is the most common form of incontinence in men and is found primarily in older men. Stress urinary incontinence is uncommon in men unless there has been some damage to the internal urinary sphincter. The evaluation of the patient with incontinence can usually be accomplished in the office setting. The patient's history is the most important component of the evaluation. The physical examination and laboratory tests confirm the findings obtained from the history. Both simple office urodynamic studies and formal urodynamic testing are available but usually unnecessary. Treatment depends on the type of incontinence present; behavioral, pharmacologic, and surgical options are available. It is estimated that up to 70% of patients with urinary incontinence can be improved or cured with appropriate treatment.

I. Introduction

Urinary incontinence is a very common problem, especially in the geriatric population. It is more common in females at all ages except during early childhood. Before the age of 65, it is a condition seen almost exclusively in women. After age 65, the prevalence in men rises dramatically, and in those over the age of 85, the prevalence in men nearly equals that of women. Urinary incontinence can lead to multiple complications of a social, psychologic, economic and medical nature. The social impact can be significant for both the patient and the patient's family. It frequently changes the lifestyle of individuals, commonly resulting in an alteration of physical activity and social isolation. Many with incontinence stop going out in public and many give up physical activities that can result in urine loss. In the elderly, urinary incontinence is a common reason for nursing home placement. Other social complications include loss of self-esteem and limitation of sexual activities. The medical complications of incontinence can include urinary tract infections and increased risk of skin breakdown. More than $16 billion is spent each year on care related to urinary incontinence. It is estimated that more than $11 billion is spent on those living in the community, whereas more than $5 billion is spent on those in nursing homes [1]. Because additional nursing time is required for nursing home residents with incontinence, the cost

of care for an incontinent resident is significantly higher than for one who is continent. In addition to medications used for incontinence, these costs also include frequent linen and clothing changes and devices such as pads and diapers frequently used by those with incontinence [2,3]. A variety of treatments are available for those with urinary incontinence. Although behavioral and pharmacologic treatments are most commonly used, more than 400,000 surgical procedures are performed for urinary incontinence annually [2].

Urinary incontinence is defined by the International Continence Society as the involuntary loss of urine that is severe enough to be a social or hygienic problem and that is objectively demonstrable. The reported prevalence of incontinence has significant variability resulting from inconsistent definitions used by various authors. It is estimated that 10 to 25% of older men and between 20 to 40% of older women living independently in the community experience some degree of urinary incontinence [4]. The British literature reports a prevalence of 1.6 to 26% for those living in the community [5]. The prevalence of incontinence is higher in those with increased frailty and is 40 to 60% for those residing in nursing homes. An estimated 25 to 30% of elderly discharged from the hospital for acute medical problems have urinary incontinence [6]. Overall, urinary incontinence is thought to be twice as common in women than in men [7,8].

Urinary incontinence is not commonly identified by physicians as a medical problem. Patients are rarely asked about the presence of incontinence, and few patients with incontinence report the problem to their physicians. In older patients, many assume incontinence to be a normal change related to aging [9]. Therefore, if incontinence is to be recognized as a problem, physicians need to ask patients about its presence. The volume of urine lost is not always related to its perceived severity by the patient. Even occasional, small volumes of urine lost can result in clinically significant incontinence depending on the circumstances. Unfortunately, many primary care providers underestimate the significance of urinary incontinence and there are a substantial number who are not comfortable performing an incontinence evaluation.

Advanced age is a risk factor for urinary incontinence for both men and women. Additional risk factors for females include postmenopausal state, previous pelvic or genitourinary surgery, various medications, diabetes, and conditions resulting in increased intra-abdominal pressure such as obesity [10]. The development of incontinence in women is associated with conditions that result in an alteration of the normal pelvic anatomy, impaired innervation, or a diminished vascular supply. Childbirth, specifically vaginal deliveries, is one of the most important risk factors for urinary incontinence in women. This can result in damage to the pelvic floor during childbirth, especially with the use of vaginal forceps, with longer labors, and with larger babies [11]. In addition to age, incontinence in men is associated with damage to the internal urinary sphincter resulting from prostate surgery or radiation. It can also occur in those with prostatic enlargement and marked urinary outflow obstruction.

II. Anatomy

Maintaining continence requires a complex interaction between the bladder, pelvic muscles, connective tissue, and nerves. This is especially important in females. The urinary bladder is composed of three layers of muscle; each layer arranged perpendicular to one another. This allows the bladder to expand in all directions as urine fills the hollow organ, maintaining a low pressure within the bladder. Although the dome of the bladder is relatively thin-walled and quite compliant, the base of the bladder has a thick muscular wall. As a result, this portion of the bladder is less distensible. The bladder contains abundant parasympathetic innervation and significant amounts of acetylcholinesterase. The dome of the bladder also receives beta-adrenergic innervation. Urine fills the bladder through the ureters, which empty into the bladder at the superior corners of the urinary trigone. The trigone is unique from the remainder of the bladder and is composed of two layers of smooth muscle. The deeper layer is thick and indistinguishable from the detrusor, whereas the superficial layer is thin. The detrusor neck or outlet contains no significant cholinergic innervation and, therefore, no acetylcholinesterase. This portion of the bladder is innervated by the sympathetic nervous system via alpha-adrenergic nerves. Alpha-adrenergic receptors have been identified in the bladder neck and internal urinary sphincter. This area of the bladder plays a major role in promoting urine storage and inhibiting urine flow.

The pelvic anatomy plays an especially important role in maintaining continence in females. The female urethra is approximately 3 to 4 cm in length and 5 to 6 mm in diameter. As the urethra exits the bladder neck, it inclines (with the patient in a standing position) as it passes through the pelvic floor muscles to the perineum. The wall of the urethra contains both smooth and striated muscle. The inner lining is continuous with the bladder mucosa. The proximal urethra is lined by transitional epithelium, whereas the distal urethra is lined by stratified squamous epithelium. The urethral mucosa is sensitive to stimulation by estrogen and undergoes similar changes as the vaginal mucosa with estrogen deprivation. Urethral closure depends on the combined effects of smooth muscle, striated muscle, connective tissue, and urethral mucosa. The proximal urethra contains the internal urinary sphincter, composed of two layers of smooth muscle arranged longitudinally. These muscles are innervated by alpha-adrenergic sympathetic nerve fibers and are under involuntary control. Surrounding the internal sphincter and slightly distal to this lies an additional layer of striated muscles arranged in a circular manner around the urethra. These muscles are part of the pelvic floor and form the external urinary sphincter.

The external urinary sphincter is innervated by the pudendal nerve and under voluntary control. The muscles of the external sphincter are not able to sustain a long-standing contraction and rapidly fatigue when contracted. The urethra contains a prominent vascular supply that also assists in urethral closure.

The pelvic floor consists of three layers: the endopelvic fascia, the levator ani, and the perineal membrane or external anal sphincter. It forms a structure similar to a hammock for the bladder and abdominal and pelvic organs. The endopelvic fascia attaches several pelvic organs to the walls of the pelvis and is very closely associated with the levator ani muscle. The levator ani and pubococcygeus muscles within the pelvic floor play an important role in maintaining continence. They help occlude the urethra during times of increased intra-abdominal pressure such as coughing, sneezing, running, and so forth. The levator ani stretches across the pelvis forming a sheet of supportive tissue. One portion of this muscle attaches to the bony pelvis anteriorly, ischial spines laterally, and the sacrum and coccyx posteriorly. In the female, the levator ani also attaches to the lateral vaginal walls. When the levator ani is contracted, the urethra, vagina, and rectum are lifted anteriorly, effectively compressing the lumen of the urethra.

An understanding of the neurophysiology of the urinary bladder results in a better appreciation of the mechanisms and treatment of urinary incontinence. Information regarding the degree of bladder fullness originates in stretch receptors located within the wall of the bladder. This information is carried along sensory, proprioceptive fibers through the pelvic nerves to the sacral spinal cord. This information then ascends the spinal cord via the dorsal columns to the brainstem detrusor nucleus. Motor innervation of the urinary system involves the central nervous system (CNS), spinal cord, and peripheral nerves (both somatic and autonomic). The sympathetic system promotes bladder filling by relaxing the detrusor and contracting the internal urinary sphincter. The parasympathetic system promotes bladder emptying by producing detrusor contraction and relaxation of the internal urinary sphincter. The somatic system via the pudendal nerve innervates the external urethral sphincter, which voluntarily contracts during times of transient increases in intra-abdominal pressure. A detrusor nucleus is located in the brain stem between the pons and midbrain. It receives inhibitory input from the frontal lobe and thalamus. Information from the brainstem detrusor nucleus descends within the spinal cord to the detrusor motor nucleus.

The parasympathetic nerves from the second through the fourth sacral nerve roots of the spinal cord traverse through the pelvic plexus. Axons synapse in the pelvic ganglia, eventually reaching the detrusor muscle. These nerves innervate the bladder muscle with cholinergic nerves using acetylcholine as their neurotransmitter. When bladder filling is desired, inhibitory stimuli travel down the spinal cord, resulting in parasympathetic inhibition and detrusor relaxation. When bladder emptying is desired, parasympathetic stimulation produces detrusor contraction.

The sympathetic nerves exit the spinal cord from T10 to L2. They travel via the hypogastric nerve to the superior hypogastric plexus and the pelvic plexus. They innervate the bladder neck and internal sphincter located in the proximal urethra. This portion of the bladder contains alpha-adrenergic nerves. The sympathetic nerves are stimulated during bladder filling, resulting in contraction of the internal urinary sphincter. This results in increased resistance and obstruction to urinary outflow. The remainder of the detrusor has beta-adrenergic receptors. With sympathetic stimulation, beta-receptors assist in detrusor relaxation, allowing bladder filling.

The external urethra consists of striated muscle and is under voluntary control. It is innervated by the pudendal nerve that originates in somatic nerves arising from S2 to S4. The primary role of the external sphincter is to provide closure of the urethral lumen during transient, sudden increases in intra-abdominal pressure such as coughing, sneezing, running, and so forth. This supplements the resting urethral closure pressure. The rise in intravesical pressure would otherwise overwhelm the ability of the internal sphincter to provide closure of the urethra.

Normally, pressure within the urethra in women ranges from 40 to 80 cm H_2O. Baseline intra-abdominal pressure is usually around 5 to 10 cm H_2O. Activities that increase intra-abdominal pressure such as coughing, sneezing, running, or jumping can raise this pressure to as high as 100 cm H_2O. These pressures are transmitted to the bladder. Despite this tremendous increase in intra-abdominal and bladder pressures, urethral closure and continence is normally maintained. Under normal circumstances, the urethra in most women lies within the abdominal cavity, and this increased intra-abdominal pressure is transmitted to the urethra and the bladder. This results in a further increase in the intra-urethral resistance, maintaining urethral closure. In addition, the pelvic floor muscles contract as a reflex resulting in a further increase in urethral resistance.

III. Physiology of Micturition

Urine typically enters the bladder at a rate of 0.5 to 5 ml/minute. As the bladder fills with urine, there is initially very little increase in pressure within the bladder because of its significant elastic properties and ability to expand. As the bladder fills, the pressure within the bladder generally remains <15 cm H_2O. As urine continues to enter the bladder, the pressure within the bladder eventually rises very slowly. Stretch receptors are stimulated and send afferent impulses through the pelvic nerves to the sacral dorsal roots in the second through fourth sacral spinal cord segments. The afferent impulses ascend the spinal cord in the lateral spinothalamic tracts to the cerebral cortex as the brain receives information regarding bladder fullness. Normally the first sensation of bladder fullness occurs when the urine volume in the bladder approaches 150 to 200 cc. During this time, inhibitory signals from the brainstem detrusor nucleus travel down the spinal cord resulting in sympathetic nerve stimulation and parasympathetic inhibition. As a result, the detrusor is relaxed and the internal urinary sphincter is contracted, promoting bladder filling. If the bladder continues to fill and micturition is not desired, cortical impulses continue to suppress detrusor contraction. Once the bladder reaches a critical volume, the cortical suppression is supplemented by voluntary pelvic floor and external urinary sphincter contraction to help keep the urethra closed and prevent urinary loss.

As the urine volume in the bladder continues to increase and micturition is eventually desired, the sympathetic nerves are inhibited as the parasympathetic nerves are stimulated. This results in parasympathetic efferent impulses producing a detrusor contraction. The inhibition of the sympathetic stimulation produces internal urinary sphincter relaxation. In response, the urethra shortens because of contraction of longitudinal smooth muscle within the urethral wall. Pelvic floor muscles relax allowing the bladder and urethra to descend and decrease the intra-urethral resistance. This results in a funneling of the bladder neck. The lumen of the urethra opens, and once the pressure within the bladder exceeds the resistance within the urethra urine flows out of the bladder. Patients can voluntarily stop their urine flow in midstream by contracting the urethral striated muscle of the external urinary sphincter compressing the urethra. Once the bladder is empty, smooth muscle of the internal sphincter that encircles the urethra contracts and once again, closes the urethral lumen.

IV. Mechanisms of Incontinence

Changes in the urinary system typically occur with aging. Changes that occur in both men and women include a smaller bladder capacity, decreased ability to postpone urination, and a reduced urethral closing pressure. The bladder residual urine volume tends to increase and premature detrusor contractions commonly occur. In women, loss of estrogen results in a thinning of the urethral mucosa. In men, enlargement of the prostate commonly occurs producing some partial urinary outflow obstruction. Despite these changes, urinary incontinence should not be considered a normal consequence of aging. However, these changes do make incontinence more likely if an additional problem is inflicted on the urinary system. A common misconception is that urinary incontinence is a single entity. There are several types of incontinence, each with a different physiologic mechanism and treatment. Incorrect treatment can result in worsening of the incontinence. Therefore, it becomes important to evaluate each patient and establish an accurate diagnosis before initiating treatment.

V. Stress Urinary Incontinence

Stress urinary incontinence represents the most common form of urinary incontinence in women overall [12]. It is very uncommon in men unless there has been some damage to the internal and/or external sphincter, usually from a prostatectomy or following radiation therapy for the treatment of prostate cancer. Stress incontinence in women occurs because of one of two problems: (1) urethral hypermobility, inadequate urethral support with downward displacement of the urethra from the abdomen into the pelvis or (2) intrinsic sphincter deficiency, incomplete or inadequate closure of the internal urinary sphincter. It is not unusual for females with stress urinary incontinence to have a combination of urethral hypermobility and intrinsic sphincter deficiency.

A patient with pure urinary stress incontinence usually gives a very straightforward history. They describe loss of urine that occurs with transient, abrupt increases in intra-abdominal pressure. These activities may include coughing, sneezing, laughing, running, and so forth. When severe, some may lose urine just assuming a standing position. Typically patients lose small amounts of urine with each episode of incontinence. Patients do not typically have incontinence during the night. It is important to ask patients about the severity of symptoms and the effect on their lifestyle because this can vary from patient to patient.

Continence requires the resistance within the urethra to exceed the pressure within the bladder, both when the person is at rest and under stressed conditions. Adequate support of the urethra and a functional internal and external sphincter is necessary.

Relaxation of the pelvic floor muscles results in descent of the bladder neck and loss of the normal 90° to 100° posterior urethrovesical angle. As the bladder neck descends from the abdomen into the pelvis, it pulls away from the pubic bones. The pubovesical ligaments pull on the anterior bladder neck, opening the urethral sphincter. This descent into the pelvis also results in an inequality of pressure applied to the bladder with increased intra-abdominal pressure. Normally, the urethrovesical junction lies within the abdomen, above the muscular/fascial diaphragm. In this location, increased intra-abdominal pressure is transmitted to both the bladder and urethra resulting in a rise in resistance within the urethra equal to the pressure generated within the bladder, maintaining closure of the urethral lumen. In women who have hypermobility of the urethra and bladder neck, these structures descend into the pelvis allowing the intra-abdominal pressure to be transmitted disproportionately to the bladder base instead of the bladder neck. This results in an intravesical pressure that exceeds intra-urethra pressure, resulting in urine leakage.

Disorders of the urinary sphincters can also result in stress urinary incontinence. Age-related changes in the internal sphincter include a reduction in striated muscle content and an increase in connective tissue. These changes reduce the function of the internal sphincter, especially in women. The amount of smooth muscle does not tend to change with age [13,14]. The urethra must be compressible by an external force to promote urinary continence. A rigid urethra resulting from atrophy of the urethral mucosa or from prior surgery may result in inadequate urethral closure. In women, tissue vascularity tends to decrease with age because of a diminished amount of hormonal stimulation. This results in a decreased submucosal engorgement with blood, resulting in thinning of the urethral mucosa that can contribute to an increased urethral lumen diameter. Although estrogen receptors have been identified within the urethral mucosa, treatment with estrogen has not demonstrated significant increases in urethral resistance [15,16].

Factors that predispose women to stress urinary incontinence include pregnancy, vaginal deliveries, and obesity [17,18]. Risk is increased by a factor of 2.5 in women who have had one vaginal delivery compared with nulliparous women [19,20]. The severity of incontinence is also associated with the number of vaginal deliveries [21]. Traction injuries to the pudendal nerve can occur with vaginal deliveries, especially with prolonged deliveries and with larger babies [11]. Pelvic nerve damage can also occur when vaginal forceps are used. This may be due to the prolonged labor, which usually precedes the use of forceps or nerve damage caused by the forceps themselves. As a result, the tone of the external sphincter can be decreased. Previous pelvic surgery is also a risk factor [22]. Disorders of the lumbosacral spine can result in weakness of the internal sphincter. Stress urinary incontinence in men generally requires damage to the internal urinary sphincter.

VI. Urge Incontinence

This is a very common form of urinary incontinence in both men and women and becomes more common with advancing age. It is by far, the most common form of incontinence in men.

This type of incontinence has been called detrusor instability, unstable bladder, overactive bladder, uninhibited bladder, spastic bladder, and urge incontinence. It is due to early, forceful bladder contractions, occurring well before the bladder has filled. Patients with urge incontinence describe loss of urine associated with a sensation of a strong urge to void. Typically these patients lose moderate amounts of urine with each episode of incontinence, although the volume of urine lost can be quite variable. Some have symptoms only during the daytime, whereas many also have nocturia. No specific physical examination findings are characteristic of this type of incontinence, although on occasion there may be findings of CNS disease or conditions associated with bladder irritation.

There are several reasons detrusor overactivity may occur. Increased urinary urgency from premature detrusor contractions occurs commonly with normal aging in both men and women. This does not appear to be secondary to any specific neurologic condition. Early detrusor contractions can be associated with bladder outlet obstruction, such as benign prostatic hypertrophy (BPH) or may be due to impaired inhibitory signals from the brain. This can occur with disorders of the frontal lobe. It is felt that portions of the brain, specifically the medial portion of the frontal lobes and basal ganglia play a role in suppressing the micturition reflex originating from the pons. Diseases or damage to these portions of the brain (i.e., mass lesions such as tumors or aneurysms, stroke, previous trauma, multiple sclerosis, normal pressure hydrocephalus, Parkinson's disease, or Alzheimer's disease) can result in a loss of inhibition from the pontine micturition center [23]. Increased afferent stimulation can result from bladder irritation such as cystitis, atrophic or bacterial urethritis, fecal impaction, BPH, bladder cancer, pelvic tumors, or uterine prolapse. Detrusor overactivity can also occur in individuals with a spinal cord transection above T7.

Female patients often describe symptoms consistent with both stress incontinence and detrusor overactivity (urge incontinence). This is known as mixed incontinence. Urge and mixed incontinence increase in frequency with age. In women older than 60, urge, stress and mixed incontinence have an equal prevalence. Often the loss of a small volume of urine from stress incontinence precedes a strong detrusor contraction, producing greater urine loss. A patient who is a good historian may be able to separate each component, although it can often be difficult for the physician to make a diagnosis of mixed incontinence based purely on the patient's history.

VII. Overflow Incontinence

This is a very uncommon form of urinary incontinence, although it is very important to identify, because it can be associated with serious urologic complications including hydronephrosis and renal insufficiency. There are two basic mechanisms that can result in overflow incontinence: chronic, high-grade bladder outflow obstruction or inadequate detrusor contractions (hypotonic/atonic bladder). Obstruction is much more common in men and is usually due to prostatic enlargement from BPH or occasionally prostate cancer. Although outflow obstruction is uncommon in women, it can occasionally be seen in those with pelvic masses. Another cause of obstruction includes a urethral stricture. An uncommon cause of overflow incontinence resulting from obstruction is detrusor-sphincter dyssynergia. This represents simultaneous contraction of the bladder and the external urinary sphincter, producing a functional obstruction. This is most commonly seen in those with spinal cord disease. Overflow incontinence is associated with very large bladder volumes, often in excess of 900 cc. As urine continues to enter the bladder, the pressure within the bladder eventually exceeds the resistance within the urethra and urine leakage occurs. Clinically, patients with overflow incontinence have frequent urinary dribbling throughout the day and night with very low urinary flow rates. Patients often describe urinary stream hesitancy and the need to strain to urinate.

Impaired detrusor contraction can occur in either men or women with an autonomic peripheral neuropathy, as seen in diabetes mellitus or chronic alcoholism. Spinal cord disease, including cord tumors below T12 or lumbar disc lesions can also produce impaired detrusor contractions. Various medications can impair detrusor contractions including those with anticholinergic activity such as tricyclic antidepressants, antipsychotic medications, and antispasmodics. Other offending drugs include calcium channel antagonists and muscle relaxants. A hypotonic/atonic bladder can also be seen in elderly patients following various surgical procedures. The bladder tone eventually returns in most patients after several days. Physical examination findings in those with overflow incontinence include a distended, palpable bladder. A large bladder residual volume is characteristic; however, patients are often unaware of the degree of bladder fullness present.

VIII. Functional/Iatrogenic Incontinence

Functional incontinence occurs in both men and women with a normally functioning urinary system who have one or more limitations in mobility that impairs their ability to reach a toilet in time to void. A patient with urinary urgency resulting from detrusor overactivity may develop urge incontinence if they have significant impairments such as advanced arthritis, stroke, or muscle weakness that limit their ability to ambulate. It may also be caused by the use of physical restraints. As the name implies, iatrogenic urinary incontinence occurs secondary to some action directed toward the patient. Placing a patient with cognitive impairment in an unfamiliar environment or the use of various medications can produce iatrogenic incontinence (Table 109-1). These medications may include potent diuretics such as furosemide that may overwhelm a patient with rapid bladder filling. Many psychoactive medications such as sedative/hypnotics, especially when used in those with some degree of cognitive impairment, can impair the awareness of bladder filling. Medications with alpha-adrenergic agonist activity, such as pseudoephedrine, can result in urinary retention by increasing the tone of the internal urinary sphincter. This is most common in men with an enlarged prostate. Medications with alpha-adrenergic antagonist activity such as terazosin or doxazosin can decrease the tone of the internal urinary sphincter. Although this may be a desired effect in men with urinary outflow obstruction resulting from BPH, it can worsen stress urinary incontinence in women. Muscle relaxants, narcotics, and calcium channel antagonists can result in ineffective detrusor contractions. This is also true of medications with anticholinergic effects. Ethanol can produce a diuresis and also impair the recognition of bladder filling. Caffeine ingestion can produce early detrusor

Table 109-1
Medications and Urinary Function

Potent diuretics	Overwhelm patient with bladder filling, promotes urinary frequency
Muscle relaxants	Inadequate detrusor contractions, promotes urinary retention
Anticholinergics	Inadequate detrusor contractions, promotes urinary retention
Narcotics	Inadequate detrusor contractions, promotes urinary retention, can produce delirium with impaired recognition of bladder filling
Calcium channel antagonists	Inadequate detrusor contractions, promotes urinary retention
Alpha-adrenergic agonists	Increases internal sphincter tone, promotes urinary retention
Alpha-adrenergic antagonists	Decreases internal sphincter tone, promotes urinary stress incontinence
Alcohol	Can produce premature detrusor contractions, promotes urinary frequency and urgency
Angiotensin-converting enzyme inhibitors	Can produce a cough, promotes urinary stress incontinence
Caffeine	Promotes premature detrusor contractions, promotes urinary frequency and urgency
Sedative/hypnotics	Inadequate detrusor contractions, promotes urinary retention, delirium, impaired recognition of bladder filling. Can impair detrusor contraction, promotes urinary retention

contractions leading to symptoms of urinary frequency and urgency. Many individuals may not realize the variety of products that contain substantial amounts of caffeine, and care providers often may not appreciate the large caffeine intake of many individuals. Therefore it is important to evaluate and estimate the patient's quantity of caffeine use and assess its relationship to the incontinence.

IX. Evaluation

The evaluation of those with urinary incontinence begins with a thorough history, focusing on urologic, neurologic, and, in women, gynecologic problems. Other important components of the history include medication use, presence of current and past medical problems, previous surgical procedures (especially prostate surgery in men and pelvic surgery in women), and past obstetrical history. Self-administered patient questionnaires can be used to help evaluate a patient's urinary symptoms. A urinary voiding diary kept for 24 to 48 hours can also provide valuable information regarding the incontinence and should be given to every patient undergoing an incontinence evaluation. Measurements should include the number of voidings, volumes voided, severity of urinary leakage, and timing and number of incontinent episodes per day. Its also important to know the patient's activity at the time of urine loss and if there was a sensation of urge associated with the voiding. The type and amount of fluid ingested is also desired information. Although voiding diaries can be very useful, they need to be interpreted carefully. The frequency of voidings must be assessed in context of the volume of urine voided. Frequent voidings may be normal with larger output volumes. Patients with large urinary outputs may be taking diuretics or have a polyuric state resulting from hyperglycemia or hypercalcemia. Low-volume voidings indicate a low fluid intake, commonly seen in individuals with detrusor overactivity who intentionally minimize their fluid intake to reduce the volume of urine produced and subsequently their urinary frequency. This practice of low-volume voiding actually tends to worsen detrusor overactivity.

The patient's detailed description of the incontinence symptoms is a very important component of the history including factors that precipitate urine loss; volume of urine lost; duration of symptoms; and any obstructive symptoms, such as difficulty initiating voiding, weak urinary stream, stream hesitancy, urinary frequency, sensation of incomplete bladder emptying, or nocturia. Questions regarding fecal incontinence, hematuria, and irritative symptoms such as dysuria and urinary urgency are also important. If not apparent, the patient's ambulatory status should be assessed. Because urinary incontinence may result from other medical conditions, a thorough history of past and current medical problems should be obtained. In women, a gynecologic history is a very important component of the incontinence evaluation. Information should be sought regarding pelvic prolapse, vaginal dryness/pruritus, dyspareunia, dysmenorrhea, previous pelvic surgery, history of endometriosis, and number of pregnancies and vaginal deliveries. The date of menopause (either natural or surgical) and previous and current use of hormonal therapy is also important. A neurologic history should inquire about any CNS disorders including Parkinson's disease, stroke, brain trauma, or surgery. Other areas of importance include a history of spinal cord disease or trauma, peripheral neuropathy, or multiple sclerosis. The patient's cognitive status should also be assessed. A complete medication history is especially important in a patient with incontinence (see Table 109-1). It is also important to ask patients about a chronic cough. Chronic pulmonary diseases and the use of angiotensin-converting enzyme inhibitors are associated with a chronic cough and may contribute to symptomatic stress urinary incontinence. Rather than attempting to treat the incontinence, treatment of the cough may result in resolution of the incontinence. A change in bowel function may signal fecal impaction, which can predispose a patient to urinary incontinence. A history of fecal incontinence is also associated with urinary incontinence.

It is thought that up to one third of all incontinence is transient [11]. Those with recent onset of urinary incontinence have a much higher likelihood of cure than those with incontinence of long-standing duration. The mnemonic DIAPPERS lists those conditions commonly associated with recent onset of urinary incontinence:

D: delirium (or any other state of cognitive impairment)
I: infection of the lower urinary tract
A: atrophic urethritis/vaginitis
P: pharmaceuticals (medications taken by the patient)
P: psychologic (delirium, depression)
E: endocrine disorders (hypercalcemia, hyperglycemia, hypothyroidism)

Table 109-2
Voiding Diary

Time	Fluid Intake	Type of Fluid	Time Urinated in Toilet	Amount Urinated in Toilet	Time of Accidental Urine Loss	Severity of Urine Loss (1–3)	Urge Present (Y/N)
	oz			oz			
	oz			oz			
	oz			oz			
	oz			oz			
	oz			oz			
	oz			oz			
	oz			oz			
	oz			oz			
	oz			oz			
	oz			oz			
	oz			oz			
	oz			oz			
	oz			oz			
	oz			oz			
	oz			oz			
	oz			oz			
	oz			oz			
	oz			oz			
Total daily intake	oz		Total daily output	oz			

R: restricted mobility (use of restraints, history of advanced arthritis, previous stroke, or any condition that impairs one's ability to reach the bathroom)

S: stool (fecal) impaction

If any of these conditions are found in association with the recent onset of urinary incontinence, correction of the problem often results in resolution of the urinary symptoms [24].

Because the history is the most important component of the evaluation for urinary incontinence, care providers are at a major disadvantage when the patient is unable to give an adequate history. This is often the case when the patient is demented, hospitalized, or in a nursing home. Frequent checks of the patient by caregivers are necessary to determine the timing of the incontinent episodes. An assessment of amount of urine loss can also be determined by measuring the degree of wetness of pads or diapers.

A physical examination should focus on the urologic and neurologic systems. A pelvic examination should be performed in women to check for gynecologic abnormalities. Female patients should be assessed for evidence of pelvic relaxation and muscular support of the pelvic organs. Signs of estrogen deficiency such as atrophic vaginitis should also be noted. The urethra should be palpated for evidence of tenderness, pus, or the presence of a diverticulum. It is important to examine the patient not only in the dorsal lithotomy position but also while standing to assess the effect of gravity on the pelvic organs. The presence of pelvic relaxation, cystocele, or rectocele may be more apparent by having the patient perform a Valsalva maneuver. The patient's ability to contract and relax the pelvic floor muscles should be tested. The examiner should also check for funneling of the bladder and urethra by placing the index and second finger on each side of the urethra. The patient is then asked to cough or perform a Valsalva maneuver as the examiner assesses the degree of bladder and urethra descent. Excessive descent of the proximal urethra is associated with bladder funneling and stress urinary incontinence in women. Urethral mobility can also be tested in females using the "Q-tip test." With the patient in the dorsal lithotomy position, a lubricated Q-tip is placed within the urethra and the angle of the Q-tip is measured from the horizontal plane. The patient is then asked to perform a Valsalva maneuver and the change in the urethral angle is assessed. Upward movement of the Q-tip is expected. Movement greater than 30° indicates hypermobility of the urethra. Lack of urethral mobility with this test in a patient with stress urinary incontinence should raise the question of intrinsic sphincter deficiency. Rectal examination should also be performed to test the patient's anal sphincter tone. Pubococcygeus and levator ani muscle tone should also be tested.

A neurologic examination concentrates on the cranial nerves, lower extremities, gait, balance, and neurologic function in the perineal area. Strength and sensation of the lower extremities should be tested as well as deep tendon reflexes. The sensation of the perineum and the presence of an anal wink should be checked to assess the innervation of the sacral nerve roots.

Laboratory studies usually provide only limited information in the investigation of a patient with urinary incontinence. Studies that are commonly obtained include a urinalysis, assessment for a urinary infection with a urine culture or urine Gram stain. These are useful in checking for evidence of urinary infection or bladder/urethra inflammation. Serum electrolytes, calcium, and blood glucose can be obtained to check for evidence of polyuric states.

Simple office urinary cystometry can be performed without elaborate equipment and can usually be completed within 20 minutes. The test can document premature detrusor contractions and can be used to assess bladder compliance and capacity. It may also be useful in determining if the patient would benefit from formal urodynamic studies. Office cystometry may be the only option available to study patients for a nursing home resident. The patient should be instructed to empty her bladder and assume the dorsal lithotomy position. The patient is asked to void and the residual urinary volume is then measured by inserting a urinary catheter. A volume of less than 50 cc is considered normal. Higher volumes imply inadequate bladder emptying either because of impaired detrusor contraction or bladder outlet obstruction.

The distal end of the catheter is then connected to the barrel of a 60 to 100 cc catheter-tip syringe with the plunger removed. The bladder is then slowly filled with sterile water or saline as 50 ml increments are added to the syringe. The patient is asked to identify the volume resulting in the first sensation of bladder filling. Normally this occurs at approximately 150 cc. The patient then identifies the sensation of a full bladder, normally approximately 350 cc. Finally, maximum bladder capacity is measured, normally approximately 500 cc. If there is a contraction of the detrusor, the meniscus of the syringe will rise and the bladder volume is noted when this occurs. If this occurs at volumes less than 250 ml, it is consistent with an overactive bladder. Once the bladder is filled with saline, the urinary catheter is removed and the patient is asked to perform various stress maneuvers such as a cough or a Valsalva maneuver, watching for the presence of urinary leakage. This test should be performed with the patient in both the seated and standing position. A positive urinary stress test results in loss of urine simultaneous with the cough. If urine loss occurs after a brief delay, the cough may have triggered a bladder contraction. This is consistent with detrusor overactivity. The patient is then asked to void, and the force of the urinary stream and voided urinary volume is assessed.

Formal urodynamic tests can be helpful in documenting the objective function of the lower urinary tract and determining the underlying pathophysiology of the incontinence, although they are not required in most patients evaluated for urinary incontinence. These tests typically include a cystometrogram (CMG), measurement of urinary flow (both peak and mean), and urethral pressure profile. Bladder leak point pressure can be assessed and electromyography (EMG) can be performed to assess the innervation of the pelvic floor and urinary sphincter. Radiologic studies that are occasionally useful include an assessment of bladder filling and emptying.

Filling cystometry measures intravesical pressure and volume. Saline is infused into the bladder via a catheter. As the volume of saline is measured, the pressure within the bladder is recorded. Normally, a gradual increase in intravesical pressure occurs as infused saline fills the bladder. A measurement of the first sensation to void is noted, as is the initial sensation of bladder fullness. Patients with detrusor overactivity demonstrate a rise in bladder pressure from early detrusor contractions.

These occur at relatively low bladder volumes and cannot be inhibited by the patient. Many patients with detrusor overactivity typically have a smaller than average bladder capacity. Patients with overflow incontinence resulting from an atonic bladder show a very gradual rise in intravesical pressure without detrusor contractions, with very large volumes of saline infused into the bladder. Voiding cystometry combines the measurement of urinary flow and voiding detrusor pressure. This pressure/flow study can be useful in those with urinary outflow obstruction and for those with inadequate bladder contractions. Peak flow is useful, with values less than 15 ml/second indicating ineffective detrusor contraction or significant bladder outlet obstruction. Normally the peak flow should be greater than 25 ml/second with the average flow approximately one half of the peak flow. The urethral pressure profile assesses intraluminal pressure within the urethra. Leak point pressure gives a measure of competence of the urinary sphincter. The patient is asked to cough with increasing force until urine loss takes place, quantifying the pressure at which incontinence occurs. This test can give an assessment of the sphincter's ability to prevent urinary leakage due to either increased bladder pressure as seen in detrusor overactivity or stress urinary incontinence. When patients have some suggestion of neurologic dysfunction based on history or examination, a pelvic floor and urinary sphincter EMG may be useful. It can be used to assess patients with detrusor/sphincter dyssynergia or in those with a nonfunctioning external sphincter.

The information obtained from urodynamic testing may be useful in selected patients with confusing histories or when patients are describing a mixed incontinence. Occasionally urodynamic testing can give confusing information and some patients may have results that may not fit their clinical symptoms. This may be due to the uncomfortable recording devices and atypical voiding positions the patients must assume.

X. Treatment of Urinary Incontinence

The effective management of those with urinary incontinence depends on an accurate diagnosis. Although not all patients will be cured of their incontinence, with appropriate treatment the majority will experience significant improvement in their symptoms. Treatment with urinary catheterization or diapers should only be considered when all other treatment options have failed. For the majority with urinary incontinence, nonpharmacologic treatment should be attempted initially.

A. Detrusor Instability

The goal of treatment for those with detrusor instability is a reduction in the frequency or severity of the premature detrusor contractions and the subsequent loss of urine. A list of potential bladder irritants should be reviewed with the patient (Table 109-3) Common irritants include caffeine, sucralfate, alcohol, and citrus juices. The patient should sequentially eliminate one potential bladder irritant at a time from their diet for several days to determine if it may be triggering premature detrusor contractions. Often, patients with detrusor overactivity reduce their fluid intake, thinking that this will decrease their incontinence symptoms. Low bladder volume voiding and a concentrated urine actually promotes frequent detrusor contractions. Patients

should be instructed to maintain a generous fluid intake to keep their urine from becoming excessively concentrated.

After review of the patient's voiding diary, an attempt at timed voiding may be useful. Once the normal frequency of voidings is determined, the patient is instructed to void at intervals slightly below this frequency, (usually between 60 to 90 minutes) even if they have no sensation to empty their bladder. The patient then gradually increases the time between voidings, usually in 30-minute increments. Many remain continent up to 3 to 4 hours. Improvement or cure from timed voidings has been reported to be from 50 to 70% [13]. In nursing home residents with cognitive impairment, timed voiding can be very effective in reducing the incontinent episodes. Prompted voiding is another option for this population. The patient is asked about their need to urinate at fixed time intervals. If they respond positively, they are then toileted and given feedback and positive social reinforcement for voiding and maintaining their continence. Urge suppression techniques can also be taught to patients with overactive bladder. When the patient has a strong urge to void, they are instructed to stop their activity and tightly contract their pelvic floor muscles and external urinary sphincter. In most, the urge gradually resolves after several seconds.

If behavioral treatment is ineffective, pharmacologic therapy should then be considered. Urinary tract infections should be treated although an association between asymptomatic bacteriuria and urinary incontinence has not been demonstrated. Several medications are often effective in those with detrusor instability. Parasympathetic nerve fibers innervate the detrusor and produce bladder contractions via cholinergic receptors. Inhibiting early detrusor contractions is often accomplished with medications having anticholinergic properties. Anticholinergic treatment reduces both the urinary frequency and urgency. Anticholinergic therapy must be used with some caution in men, because they may have some degree of urinary outflow obstruction from BPH associated with detrusor overactivity. Anticholinergic medications can promote urinary retention in these individuals. The two most commonly used anticholinergic medications are oxybutynin and tolterodine. In addition to their effect on the bladder, both of these medications have the potential to produce peripheral anticholinergic effects including dry mouth, constipation, and blurred vision. They also have the potential to cause confusion, especially in the elderly with some degree of pre-existing cognitive impairment. Both medications are now

Table 109-3
Potential Bladder Irritants

Caffeine
Aspartame
Citrus drinks and fruits
Coffee (even decaffeinated)
Tea
Alcohol
Milk and milk products
Tomatoes and tomato juice
Highly spiced foods
Honey
Chocolate

available in an extended-release form, and oxybutynin is available in a transdermal preparation. These formulations produce fewer peripheral anticholinergic symptoms, while maintaining the efficacy of the immediate-release forms. Tricyclic antidepressants such as imipramine and nortriptyline can also be effective in those with detrusor overactivity although they tend to produce more peripheral anticholinergic adverse effects. Occasionally patients may be willing to tolerate urinary frequency and urgency while they are at home but want a reduction in urinary symptoms when they go out in public. Although not as effective as when taken chronically, some patients do well with pharmacologic treatment taken intermittently, as needed.

B. Stress Urinary Incontinence

Pelvic floor muscle training can be very useful in the management of stress urinary incontinence and was initially described by Dr. Arnold Kegel in the 1940s [25]. It may also demonstrate improvement in those with urge incontinence. This technique more typically results in symptom improvement rather than complete cure. Exercises improve the strength of the pelvic floor muscles, although the precise mechanism of how this improves urethral closure is not fully understood. Some feel that pelvic floor exercises result in muscular hypertrophy with improved pelvic floor support. Improvement in stress urinary incontinence requires several months of pelvic muscle training. Brief instructions or written material alone is often ineffective in teaching pelvic floor exercises and patients then frequently perform these exercises incorrectly. Success requires the patient to be able to identify and contract the correct muscles of the pelvic floor. This is often enhanced with instruction and training by a professional. The pelvic floor muscles should be contracted for 10 seconds, 10 times per session. The exercise should be performed 10 times per day. Many patients have difficulty performing pelvic floor exercises, and biofeedback can help these patients identify the correct muscles to contract. Biofeedback is usually performed under the guidance of a qualified physical therapist. Benefits of pelvic floor exercises include a lack of adverse effects and low cost. The primary disadvantage of pelvic floor exercises is the relatively low patient compliance, primarily because of the long duration of time necessary to show benefit. Pelvic floor exercises are not appropriate in those who have significant pelvic or bladder prolapse, if there is evidence of pelvic muscle denervation, or if the patient has intrinsic sphincter deficiency [26]. It is also known that pelvic floor exercises are less effective in those with more severe symptoms, although this has not been a universal finding [27]. Although benefits from pelvic floor exercises will usually be seen by 3 months, older patients often require a longer duration of time to achieve benefit.

In women with more severe stress urinary incontinence or in those who have not had significant benefit from pelvic floor exercises, surgery may be an option. It may also be an option for those with mixed incontinence if stress urinary incontinence makes up a significant component of the symptoms. A decision to perform surgery for stress urinary incontinence depends on several factors, including the significance of the incontinence, degree of impaired quality of life, pathology present, and overall health of the patient. Nearly 200 surgical procedures have been proposed for the treatment of stress urinary incontinence. The fact that so many different procedures exist suggests that no one procedure is associated with a high likelihood of cure and low risks of adverse effects. Cure rates vary considerably and range from 20 to 90% [28]. Bladder suspension surgery is useful for the treatment of stress urinary incontinence resulting from urethral hypermobility. It raises and provides support to the bladder neck and proximal urethra. The Marshall-Marchetti-Krantz procedure was first described in 1949 and became the first accepted surgical treatment for stress urinary incontinence. It is a bladder neck suspension procedure and restores the retropubic position of the bladder neck. The bladder neck and superior wall of the vagina, just lateral to the urethra is attached to the symphysis pubis cartilage and periosteum. The Burch procedure is similar to the Marshall-Marchette-Krantz procedure, although the perivaginal fascia is attached to Cooper's ligament at the bladder neck. Cure rates of more than 80% have been reported. More recently, procedures are performed that suspend the bladder neck with sutures attached to the abdominal fascia, optimizing the function of the external urinary sphincter. They restore the bladder neck to its original position in the pelvis. Urethral sling procedures stabilize the proximal urethra and increase outflow resistance by creating increased intra-urethral resistance.

In those who have intrinsic sphincter deficiency, treatment involves increasing periurethral resistance. This is done by increasing urethral compression. Several compounds have been used in this treatment including Teflon, glutaraldehyde cross-linked collagen (Contagen), cross-linked polydimethylsiloxane elastomer (Macroplastique), and carbon-coated zirconium beads (Durasphere). Although injection of these compounds is much less invasive than pelvic surgery, the long-term efficacy has not yet been established. In short-term analysis, both agents perform similarly with 70 to 80% success rates after 1 year. Although collagen tends to lose its effectiveness with time because of its degradation, it is expected that Durasphere will provide a longer duration of benefit to patients. Although local injection of these agents is very safe and serious adverse effects are uncommon, potential complications include hematuria, urinary retention, and urinary tract infection [29].

Urethral plugs are available for women who have stress urinary incontinence associated with vigorous activities. These individuals may require treatment only at the time of these activities. The devices can be irritating and difficult for some to insert properly. Vaginal pessaries can also be used to increase the resistance of the proximal urethra although these also tend to produce vaginal irritation and are not widely accepted by the patient. Occasionally even the insertion of a tampon is effective in producing adequate external urethral compression and increased intra-urethral resistance.

At this time there is no approved or highly effective pharmacologic therapy available for stress urinary incontinence. Alpha-adrenergic agonist medications such as pseudoephedrine have been used to increase the tone of the internal sphincter, but the results are usually disappointing. When effective, they tend to produce only short-term benefit. Tricyclic antidepressants have also been used because of their norepinephrine reuptake inhibition and subsequent alpha-adrenergic agonist properties. Their use is limited because of their significant side effect profile.

In women with evidence of atrophic vaginitis or atrophic urethritis, a trial of topical estrogen may be of limited benefit. High success rates are not usually seen.

C. Overflow Incontinence

The treatment for overflow incontinence varies depending on the cause of inadequate bladder emptying. Overflow incontinence resulting from significant anatomic obstruction is very rare in women. In men, it is usually due to an enlarged prostate from BPH or occasionally prostate cancer. Other causes of obstruction include pelvic tumors and urethral strictures. Because these are all generally surgical problems, appropriate surgical intervention should be considered. Overflow incontinence can also occur in those with impaired contractility usually resulting from an autonomic peripheral neuropathy and ineffective bladder innervation. Although cholinergic agonists such as bethanechol can result in improved bladder contractions, the medication is not very effective for long-term use and not well tolerated in the doses necessary to produce improvement in bladder emptying. In most cases, bladder catheterization is necessary. Patients can often be safely taught to perform clean, intermittent self-catheterization. A catheterized volume of 350 to 500 cc is optimal. This usually requires catheterization three to four times a day. Larger volumes require more frequent catheterizations. Self-catheterization does require a fair degree of manual dexterity and adequate vision to perform this procedure safely or a caregiver who is capable of performing the catheterization. In some situations, an indwelling catheter is required. Elderly patients occasionally develop a hypotonic bladder following a surgical procedure. The goal of treatment for these patients includes keeping the bladder as empty as possible, initially with an indwelling urinary catheter and eventually replacing this with intermittent catheterizations. The frequency of catheterizations is based on the volume of urine voided by the patient and the volumes of postvoid residual urines obtained. The frequency of catheterizations is decreased as bladder contractility returns, as it does in most cases.

D. Functional/Iatrogenic Incontinence

Every attempt should be made to maximize a patient's mobility. Sometimes, very simple treatments can restore continence to a patient. Moving a patient in a nursing home to a bed closer to the bathroom or using a bedside commode often improves incontinence in many with mobility problems. The use of any restraints should be minimized and call lights for nursing home residents should be answered promptly. Clothing that allows easy removal, such as elastic or Velcro fasteners, should replace clothing with buttons or zippers. If a fecal impaction is found, it should be treated, and, very often, the incontinence will improve significantly. Medications should be reviewed carefully to determine if any may have an effect on continence.

XI. Summary

Urinary incontinence is common in both elderly men and women. Despite this, urinary incontinence should never be considered a normal result of aging. In elderly men, this is usually due to urge incontinence, whereas in women it is due to a combination of urge incontinence, stress urinary incontinence, and mixed incontinence. Although incontinence is not often brought to the attention of the care provider, it can result in significant emotional, medical, and economic complications. In addition to being under-reported, urinary incontinence is also undertreated. Many primary providers are not comfortable

Table 109-4
Summary of Treatment Options for Urinary Incontinence

Detrusor overactivity/urge incontinence
Behavioral
Identification of urinary urgency triggers
Urge suppression
Identification and avoidance of urinary irritants
Timed voiding
Prompted voiding
Pelvic floor exercises
Pharmacologic
Oxybutinin
Tolterodine
Tricyclic antidepressants (imipramine, nortriptyline)
Antispasmodics
Calcium channel antagonists
Topical estrogen
Stress urinary incontinence
Nonpharmacologic
Pelvic floor exercises
Urethral plug
Vaginal pessary/tampon
Pharmacologic
Pseudoephedrine
Topical estrogen
Surgical
Bladder suspension procedures
Urethral sling procedures
Urinary sphincter injections
Overflow incontinence
Obstruction to urinary outflow
Surgery to relieve obstruction (e.g., transurethral resection of prostate [TURP])
Intermittent bladder catheterization
Indwelling bladder catheterization
Inadequate bladder contractility
Bethanechol
Intermittent bladder catheterization
Indwelling bladder catheterization
Functional/iatrogenic incontinence
Improve mobility
Remove restraints
Shorten distance to toilet/use of bedside commode or bedpan
Review medications
Treat fecal impaction if present

performing an evaluation for incontinence. This is unfortunate because the evaluation of a patient with urinary incontinence is not difficult, and appropriate treatment can result in a significant improvement in the lifestyle of a patient. Although absorbent undergarments and chronic indwelling catheters can be useful in the treatment of incontinence, they tend to be overused, especially in nursing home residents. Although not always cured, an accurate evaluation and diagnosis followed by appropriate treatment results in significant improvement in most patients.

References

1. Keller SL. (1999). Urinary incontinence: Occurrence, knowledge, and attitudes among women aged 55 and older in a rural Midwestern setting. *J Wound Ostomy Continence Nurs.* 26:30–38.
2. Norton PA. (1993). Pelvic floor disorders: The role of fascia and ligaments. *Clin Obstet Gynecol.* 36:926–938.
3. Blaivas JG. (1987). A modest proposal for the diagnosis of urinary incontinence in women. (Editorial). *J Urol.* 138:597–598.
4. Yarnell JWG, St. Leger AS. (1979). The prevalence, severity and factors associated with urinary incontinence in a random sample of the elderly. *Age Ageing.* 8:81–85.
5. Feneley RCL, Shepherd AM, Powell PH, Blannin J. (1979). Urinary incontinence: Prevalence and needs. *Br J Urol.* 51:493–496.
6. Weiss BD. (1998). Diagnostic evaluation of urinary incontinence in geriatric patients. *Am Fam Physician.* 57:2675–2683.
7. Djokno AC, Brock B, Brown MB *et al.* (1986). Prevalence of urinary incontinence and other urological symptoms in the non-institutionalized elderly. *J Urol.* 136:1022.
8. Hording U, Pederwin K, Sidenius K *et al.* (1986). Urinary incontinence in 45-year-old women. *Scand J Urol Nephrol.* 20:1838.
9. Cohen SJ, Dugan E, Howard G *et al.* (1999). Communication between older adults and their physicians about urinary incontinence. *J Gerontol.* 54A:M34–37.
10. Brown JS, Seeley DG, Fong J *et al.* (1996). Urinary incontinence in older women: Who is at risk? Study of Osteoporosis Fractures Research Group. *Obstet Gynecol.* 87:715–721.
11. Allen RE, Hosher GL, Smith, AR *et al.* (1990). Pelvic floor damage and childbirth: A neurophysiological study. *Br J Obstet Gynaecol.* 97:770–779.
12. Skoner MM, Thompson WD, Caron VA. (1994). Factors associated with risk of stress urinary incontinence in women. *Nursing Res.* 43:5:301–306.
13. Carlile A, Davies I, Rigby A, Brocklehurst JC. (1988). Age changes in the human female urethra: A morphometric study. *J Urol.* 139:532–535.
14. Strohbehn K, DeLancey JOL. (1997). The anatomy of stress incontinence. *Op Tech Gynecol Surg.* 2:5–16.
15. Iosif CS, Batra S, Ek A *et al.* (1981). Estrogen receptors in the female lower urinary tract. *Am J Obstet Gynecol.* 141:817–823.
16. Jackson S, Shepherd A, Abrams P. (1996). The effect of oestradiol on objective urinary leakage in postmenopausal stress incontinence: A double blind placebo controlled trial. *Neurourol Urodyn.* 15:322–323.
17. MacArthur C, Lewis M, Bick D. (1993). Stress incontinence after childbirth. *Br J Midwifery.* 1(5):207–215.
18. Wells M. (1996). Continence following childbirth. *Br J Nurs.* 5:353–360.
19. Jolleys JV. (1988). Reported prevalence of urinary incontinence in women in a general practice. *BMJ.* 296:1300–1302.
20. Sommer P, Bauer T, Nielsen KK *et al.* (1990). Voiding patterns and prevalence of incontinence in women: A questionnaire survey. *Br J Urol.* 66:12–15.
21. Sampselle C, DeLancey JOL, Ashton-Miller J. (1996). Urinary incontinence in pregnancy and postpartum. *Neurourol Urodyn.* 15:329–330.
22. Dolman M. (1997). Mostly Female. In *Promoting Continence*: *A Clinical and Research Resource* (Getliffe K, Dolman M, eds.), pp. 68–106. London: Balliere Tindall.
23. DeGroat VC, Booth AM, Yoshimura N. (1993). Neurophysiology of micturition and its modification in animal models of human disease. In *The Autonomic Nervous System*: *Nervous Control of the Urogenital System*, vol. 3 (Maggi CA ed.), pp. 227–290. London: Harwood Academic Publishers.
24. Resnick NM. (1986). Urinary incontinence in the elderly. *Hosp Prac.* 11:21.
25. Frewen W. (1979). Role of bladder training in the treatment of the unstable bladder in the female. *Urol Clin North Am.* 6:273–277.
26. Jozwik M, Jozwik M. (1998). The physiological basis of pelvic floor exercises in the treatment of stress urinary incontinence. *Br J Obstet Gynecol.* 105:1046–1051.
27. Cammu H, Van Nylen M. (1997). Pelvic floor muscle exercises in genuine urinary stress incontinence. *Int Urogynecol J.* 8:297–300.
28. Schmidt RA, Dirk-Henrick, Z, Ragi D. (1999). Urinary incontinence update: Old traditions and new concepts. *Adv Intern Med.* 4:19–57.
29. Lightner D, Calvosa C, Anderson R *et al.* (2001). A new injectable bulking agent for treatment of stress urinary incontinence: Results of a multicenter, randomized, controlled double-blind study of Durasphere. *Urology.* 58:12–15.

110

Effects of Aging on Gonadotropin/Ovarian and Growth Hormone/Ovarian Relationships in Normal Women

WILLIAM S. EVANS, MD*, KIMBERLY T. BRILL, PhD**,
AND JOHANNES D. VELDHUIS, MD†

*Departments of Internal Medicine and Obstetrics and Gynecology, General Clinical Research Center, Center for Biomathematical Technology, and the Center for Research in Reproduction, University of Virginia Health System, Charlottesville, VA
**Department of Internal Medicine and General Clinical Research Center, University of Virginia Health System, Charlottesville, VA
†Department of Internal Medicine, Mayo Medical and Graduate Schools of Medicine, Rochester, MN

Abstract

Concurrent with a markedly improved life expectancy for women, attention has been increasingly focused on both age-associated reproductive and metabolic issues. With regard to the *reproductive axis* it is clear that the ability to achieve and maintain a successful pregnancy declines as a function of age. Although much of this decrease in reproductive potential may reflect changes in the quality of oocytes, it is also possible that age-associated alterations in the reproductive components of the neuroendocrine axis may contribute to this process. However, whether changes in the function of hypothalamic gonadotropin-releasing hormone (GnRH) pulse generator activity and/or in the secretion of luteinizing hormone (LH) and follicle stimulating hormone (FSH) by anterior pituitary gonadotropes are a direct consequence of the aging process, or simply reflect changes in gonadal feedback is unclear. An improved understanding of just how the process of aging adversely affects hypothalamic-pituitary-ovarian function may allow for significantly improved methods with which to enhance fertility in the aging female population.

With regard to the *somatotropic axis*, both hypothalamo-pituitary disease and aging are associated with variable degrees of hypo-somatotropism, the latter defined as depletion of growth hormone (GH) and insulin-like growth factor-1 (IGF-1). Both contexts are accompanied by evident dyslipidemia, increased cardiovascular mortality, greater visceral adiposity, reduced bone and muscle mass, impaired psychosocial well-being, and restricted physical aerobic performance. Postmenopausal women manifest combined reductions in systemic GH and estrogen availability. Hypo-estrogenemia is relevant to progressive GH deprivation, because repletion of estradiol drives GH secretion in the ovariprival subject. Aggregate clinical data establish this precept in relation to normal and precocious puberty in girls; GnRH agonist-induced downregulation of the gonadal axis in young women; ovariectomy in premenopausal individuals; controlled ovulation induction; short-term administration of antiestrogens; and replacement therapy with diverse estrogens delivered via any of oral, transdermal, intravenous, intranasal, intravaginal, and intramuscular routes. This overview highlights specific neuroendocrine mechanisms by which estradiol stimulates pulsatile GH secretion in the postmenopausal woman.

I. Introduction

That women are living longer than ever before is clear, with current estimates of life expectancy suggesting that the average woman will reach 80 years of age [1]. At the same time that life expectancy has shown dramatic improvement, changes in the social and political climate have influenced the attention that women now devote to their own health and the choices that they make regarding reproduction. With regard to overall health, many women are committed to maintaining a high level of function, regardless of age. In particular, women wish to avoid the adverse consequences of age-associated problems such as osteoporosis, obesity and associated metabolic issues, and cardiovascular disease. With regard to reproductive health, many women are opting to postpone childbearing into the fourth decade of life. For reasons that are yet to be fully elucidated, such reproductively "older" women have much more difficulty in conceiving and are at significantly greater risk of miscarriage [2] despite the extraordinary advances that have taken place within the context of assisted reproductive technologies.

To enhance the quality of care that we provide to women as they age, a much improved understanding of fundamental age-associated alterations in the reproductive and somatotropic axes is clearly needed. We now review some of the available information in both women and appropriate animal models with an emphasis on the neuroendocrine components of both the reproductive and somatotropic axes. In doing so, many more questions will arise than will be answered. We hope that substantial investigative attention will be focused in the decades to come on such questions, thus providing for improved diagnostic and therapeutic strategies that are so needed to address both the reproductive and overall health needs of aging women.

II. Effects of Aging on the Reproductive Axis

A. *Overview: The Hypothalamic-Pituitary-Ovarian Axis*

For many years it has been appreciated that normal reproductive function requires a highly coordinated and complex interplay of events among the components of the reproductive axis, including the hypothalamus, anterior pituitary gland, and gonad (Fig. 110-1). Central to the reproductive axis are the LH and FSH synthesizing and secreting cells known as gonadotropes, which reside in the anterior pituitary gland. It is known that the primary stimulatory signal impinging on the gonadotropes is GnRH, a decapeptide synthesized and secreted by specialized neurons within the hypothalamus (i.e., the so-called GnRH pulse generator). That GnRH is secreted into the hypothalamic-hypophyseal portal circulation in a pulsatile fashion was inferred by the now classic studies of Knobil and colleagues [3] and the recognition that a pulse of GnRH typically stimulates, in a one-to-one fashion, the secretion of a pulse of LH was confirmed directly in animal models 2 decades ago [4–6].

Since that time, much investigative attention has focused on developing techniques with which to identify and characterize secretory episodes of hormones such as LH with the thought being that the frequency of pulsatile LH release may reflect the frequency with which the hypothalamus is discharging GnRH (i.e., the so-called Window to the Brain premise).

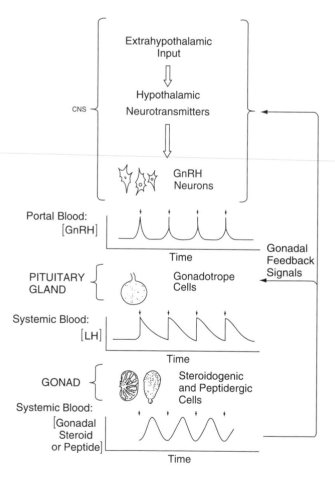

Fig. 110-1 Overall schema of the hypothalmic-pituitary-gonadal axis. Note that the secretion of the respective feedforward hormones is pulsatile in nature. Moreover, some components of the feedback signal may also be pulsatile (e.g., ovarian steroid and glycoprotein secretion). (Reproduced with permission from Evans WS, Sollenberger MJ, Booth RA, Jr. *et al.* [1992]. Contemporary aspects of discrete peak-detection algorithms:II. The paradigm of the luteinizing hormone pulse signal in women. *Endocrine Reviews.* 13:81–104.)

However, it must be recalled that other attributes of the LH secretory episode—such as mass of LH contained within each secretory event—may reflect not only the amount of GnRH impinging on the gonadotropes but also the response characteristics of the gonadotropes themselves. As discussed later, such response characteristics are modulated not only by the GnRH signal itself but by ambient concentrations of gonadal hormones bathing the gonadotropes at any given time. To add yet another layer of complexity, the activity of the GnRH pulse generator is influenced by both neurotransmitters of central nervous system (CNS) derivation and by feedback via gonadal products. Thus, any attempt to understand potential effects of aging on reproductive function requires that not only feedforward relationships be considered—for example, those of GnRH on gonadotropin secretion and of gonadotropins on ovarian function—but also that feedback relationships between gonadal products and hypothalamic-pituitary function be considered as well.

To appreciate the complexities of the potential effects of aging on the reproductive axis, a fundamental understanding of age-associated changes in ovarian function is needed. The number of oocytes declines significantly from a maximum of 6 to 7 million during fetal life to 1 to 2 million at birth, 300,000 to 600,000 at menarche, and a few hundred at the time of menopause [7–9] with atresia primarily accounting for this loss [8,10]. Moreover, oocytes obtained from older women engaging in assisted reproduction programs fertilize less well and exhibit more chromosomal abnormalities in comparison to those obtained from younger women [11]. Indeed, even fertilization of oocytes obtained from older women via intracytoplasmic sperm insertion often does not result in viable pregnancies [12]. It is therefore tempting to speculate that abnormalities intrinsic to the oocyte—with no associated hormonal abnormalities—may be responsible for the decrease in fertility rates, which fall progressively with aging. It would follow then that many if not all of the alterations in hypothalamic-pituitary function could well be secondary to age-related changes in ovarian function. For example, if it is the case that ovarian inhibin production falls early in the perimenopausal transition [13–16], then the well-recognized increase in the secretion of FSH may be an appropriate physiologic response to diminished negative feedback, with no primary age-related hypothalamic-pituitary alteration involved.

A significant body of evidence, however, obtained both in aging women and animal models has suggested that the reproductive components of the neuroendocrine axis may be affected not only indirectly by changes in ovarian function but also directly by the aging process. Thus, drawing on our knowledge of issues related to fertility in aging women, although chromosomal abnormalities and problems with fertilization and implantation tend to increase dramatically in the late thirties and early forties, overall fertility rates are already decreased significantly between the late twenties and early thirties [2]. Information obtained from donor egg programs suggests that embryos using eggs from younger women fail to implant in older women with the same efficiency as seen in the younger women [17]. Therefore, it would seem reasonable to hypothesize that age-related alterations in the CNS mechanisms that control hypothalamic function and/or in the hormonal milieu may adversely affect ovarian and/or uterine function.

B. Aging and the Reproductive Axis: Insights from the Rodent Model

That changes in the reproductive function may reflect direct effects of aging on the neuroendocrine axis has been strongly suggested by studies using animal models. More than 2 decades ago Peng et al [18] demonstrated that ovaries obtained from aging rats and subsequently transplanted into younger animals exhibit both follicular development and ovulation. The possibility that aging may directly compromise hypothalamic activity was evaluated early on by Huang et al [19] who reported that hypothalami obtained from fetal rats and transplanted into the third ventricles of older animals effect relatively normal ovarian activity. Subsequent studies focusing on hypothalamic-pituitary physiology in older versus younger rats have demonstrated both a decrease in episodic LH release in older animals [20] and attenuated LH surges prior to any apparent change in estrous cycle length [21]. More specifically, rats displaying attenuated LH surges lose regular cyclicity within 2 months, whereas those middle-aged rats with nonattenuated surges continue to cycle normally. Within this content, our laboratory has shown that the mass of LH secreted within individual LH bursts, which subserve the LH surge, is diminished in middle-aged rats with attenuated preovulatory LH surges [22]. Whether changes in LH release reflect alterations at the level of the hypothalamus and/or at the anterior pituitary remains unclear. Diminished pituitary responsivity to exogenously administered GnRH has been demonstrated in older rats under *in vivo* [20] and *in vitro* [23] conditions. Functional and irreversible defects have been documented in hypothalamic GnRH release mechanisms with demonstrable deficits in catecholamine turnover [24] and decreased GnRH neuronal c-fos expression [25]. A reduction or complete loss in ovarian steroid positive feedback also occurs in aging rats and mice [24]. Indeed, studies by Tsai et al [26] have revealed a progressive feedback loss to E_2 and P in aging rats. Although caution must be exercised in the interpretation of rodent data, the foregoing studies do suggest an effect of aging on the neuroendocrine components of the reproductive axis in these models.

C. Aging and the Reproductive Axis: Insights from the Human Model

1. Early Investigations of the Hypothalamic-Pituitary-Ovarian Axis

In contrast to the animal studies, considerably less detailed information is available with regard to the effects of aging on GnRH-gonadotropin-ovarian axis in women. Until recently much of our knowledge has been based on studies that have been primarily descriptive in nature and in many cases have yielded conflicting results. However, there is general agreement that serum concentrations of FSH increase in women as a function of age even when the menstrual cycle is ostensibly normal [27–30]. Whether there are concurrent changes in serum concentrations of LH is less clear with some authors reporting a simultaneous increase in serum LH together with FSH as a function of aging [27] and others documenting normal LH concentrations in the setting of regular menstrual cycles although serum FSH is increased [29,30]. Even more controversial are

reports concerning changes in serum estradiol concentrations in aging women. Whereas some investigators have found normal estradiol levels in perimenopausal women with raised gonadotropin levels [31,32] others have suggested that serum concentrations of this hormone may be increased [28,33,34] or decreased [29] in this group during certain phases of the menstrual cycle. Burger et al [15] have presented data from a large cross-sectional study of women in the perimenopausal age group who continue to have normal cycles, who had some menstrual irregularity, or who were becoming amenorrheic. Of particular interest, more than 40% of the women with normal cycles had serum FSH concentrations above the upper limit of the reference range. Moreover, between 20 to 25% of these women had serum estradiol concentrations below the lower limit of the normal range. The authors were careful to point out, however, that their study did not address potential mechanisms responsible for the observed alterations in gonadotropin, estradiol, and inhibin concentrations nor did the cross-sectional design allow for conclusions regarding the temporal nature of these changes. Similarly, serum concentrations of progesterone and/or its metabolites have been shown to be unchanged [29,31,34,35] or reduced [28,33] when measured during the midluteal phase of older versus younger women.

Based on these admittedly limited and somewhat inconsistent studies, many investigators have concluded that the hormone environment is in fact altered as a consequence of normal aging in healthy women and have begun to focus attention on the mechanisms that might subserve age-associated alterations in the reproductive hormone milieu. The fundamental question is whether the aging process is associated with (1) changes in the generation of the hypothalamic GnRH signal that prompts the secretion of LH and FSH by the pituitary, (2) changes in the pituitary response to GnRH, (3) changes in the ovarian response to the gonadotropin signal, and/or (4) changes in the inhibitory/facilitatory feedback effects of gonadal products on hypothalamic-pituitary function.

2. Potential Mechanisms Subserving Age-Associated Changes in Hypothalamic-Pituitary-Ovarian Function

a. EFFECTS OF AGING ON THE HYPOTHALAMIC GONADOTROPIN-RELEASING HORMONE PULSE GENERATOR. Several studies in the human have now suggested that the firing rate of the GnRH pulse generator is increased in the absence of the inhibitory effects of the gonadal hormones (i.e., after completion of the menopausal transition). Using the pulsatile secretion of LH [36,37], FSH [37], and alpha subunit [38] as markers of GnRH signaling, postmenopausal woman have been shown to exhibit increased frequencies in comparison to women in the early follicular and midluteal phases of the menstrual cycle but not above those seen in the late follicular phase of the cycle when the positive feedback effect of estradiol on gonadotropin secretion is maximal. Moreover, postmenopausal women demonstrate significantly reduced inter-LH pulse variability when compared with premenopausal women [39]. Taken as a group, it would seem as if there is an intrinsic GnRH secretory burst frequency, which can be maximal in the absence of gonadal hormones and in the setting of increased estrogen alone and suppressed by the combination of estrogen and progesterone (i.e., in the luteal phase).

Of particular interest are observations concerning GnRH pulse frequency in the pre-perimenopausal years and then during the years well after the menopausal transition. With regard to the former, there has been much interest in assessing reproductive function (i.e., potential for achieving pregnancy) in older but still ostensibly reproductively intact women. By the time that tests of ovarian reserve have become abnormal, reproductive potential is often already significantly decreased and attempts at pregnancy, even using aggressive assisted reproductive therapy techniques, are often unsuccessful. Assessment of older (42.6 years) women with normal menstrual function revealed a slowing of the GnRH pulse generator activity compared with their younger (mean age 27.7 years) colleagues [22]. Whether this slowing is consistent with a change in the CNS factors, which presumably set the intrinsic firing rate of the pulse generator as occurs in older rodents [20], or secondary to either enhanced estrogen production from the ovary [28,33,34] or enhanced sensitivity of the hypothalamus to estrogen remains unclear.

With regard the status of GnRH pulse frequency in younger versus older postmenopausal women an early study suggested that the frequency of LH pulses does not change in the years after the menopause [40]. However, more recent investigations using both LH [41] and alpha subunit [38] as surrogate markers of GnRH activity have revealed an effect of aging independent of gonadal hormone concentrations. Thus, in comparison to younger postmenopausal women, older postmenopausal women exhibit a slowing of the GnRH pulse generator in the setting of similar serum gonadal and adrenal hormone concentrations. The mechanisms subserving this apparent age-associated change in the GnRH neuronal firing rate are not understood.

As mentioned previously, in addition to the frequency of gonadotropin pulses, other attributes of such pulses can be assessed. Using robust biomathematical techniques such as deconvolution analysis with which to characterize gonadotropin secretory burst activity, the mass of hormone secreted within individual secretory bursts can be estimated. In comparison to premenopausal women in the early follicular phase of the menstrual cycle, secretory bursts of both LH and FSH identified in postmenopausal women have 3- to 4-fold more gonadotropin mass per burst, perhaps reflecting higher mean burst maximal secretory rates for both hormones. However, it is not possible to know whether higher gonadotropin burst mass reflects a greater amount of GnRH stimulating gonadotropes and/or enhanced responsivity of gonadotropes to the GnRH signal. Given that GnRH cannot be measured directly in the human, investigators have attempted to assess GnRH synthesis and secretion using other approaches. That GnRH content is diminished in hypothalami of postmenopausal versus premenopausal women has been recognized for some time [42]; however, whether this observation represents decreased synthesis or increased secretion of the decapeptide has been left unanswered. More recent studies have documented enhanced GnRH messenger RNA in hypothalami obtained from postmenopausal women [43]. These observations are consistent with increased GnRH synthesis in the setting of diminished inhibitory gonadal hormone feedback and would seem to support the premise that GnRH secretion is increased in postmenopausal women. To test the latter hypothesis, investigators have used a novel technique whereby the amount of GnRH secreted is estimated by the relationship between a

GnRH antagonist and degree of LH suppression (i.e., greater or lesser degrees of suppression should predict the strength of the GnRH signal) [44]. Such studies have suggested that GnRH secretion is almost certainly increased in postmenopausal women, a conclusion that is consistent with the notion that GnRH synthesis is also increased.

b. EFFECTS OF AGING ON LUTEINIZING HORMONE AND FOLLICLE STIMULATING HORMONE SECRETING GONADOTROPES WITHIN THE ANTERIOR PITUITARY GLAND. Given that changes in gonadotropin secretion with aging could reflect altered function at either the level of the hypothalamus or pituitary or both, studies have attempted to delineate whether the response characteristics of the gonadotropes change with aging. Primarily because of technical difficulties related to experimental design, this issue remains to be fully elucidated. Using the rodent as a model, both serum LH concentrations and LH beta mRNA levels within pituitary homogenates have been shown to be lower in older versus younger ovariectomized rats [45]. Gonadotropin-releasing hormone stimulated LH release appears decreased in older animals in vivo [24] and either unchanged [46] or decreased [23] using in vitro models. Relatively few studies have attempted to delineate the effect of aging on exogenously administered GnRH-stimulated gonadotropins in women. Indeed, whereas one study suggested that GnRH-stimulated LH release does not change as a function of aging in the postmenopausal years [40], another has suggested that older postmenopausal women respond to GnRH less well [41]. Again, it must be recalled that, even though the effects of gonadal hormone feedback at the level of the anterior pituitary have been minimized in postmenopausal women, the potential upregulating or downregulating effects of endogenously secreted GnRH are still present. Thus, any response to exogenously administered GnRH must be interpreted within this context.

The question as to whether there are age-associated alterations in the post-translational processing of the gonadotropins is of interest. We [37] and others [47] have shown that the half-life of LH is increased in postmenopausal women in comparison to that observed in premenopausal women during the early follicular, late follicular, and midluteal phases of the menstrual cycle (Fig. 110-2). The prolongation of gonadotropin half-life presumably reflects enhanced terminal sialic acid and sulfate residues, which correlate with relatively acidic (lower pI) isoforms as assessed by isoelectric and chromatofocusing [48,49]. However, it would appear that these alterations in post-translational processing may well relate to the effects of the gonadal hormone environment rather than the aging process (i.e., estrogen appears to inhibit the addition of sialic acid to the gonadotropin oligosaccharide chain, thus decreasing half-life but increasing in vitro biologic activity perhaps by stimulating glycosylation) [50]. Thus, although a primary effect of aging either on the synthesis, post-translational modification and/or secretion of the gonadotropins cannot be ruled out. Further studies are clearly needed to clarify which of these mechanisms, if any, are involved.

c. EFFECTS OF AGING ON GONADOTROPIN-STIMULATED OVARIAN FUNCTION. Whereas considerable work has focused on the putative effects of aging on the hypothalamic GnRH pulse

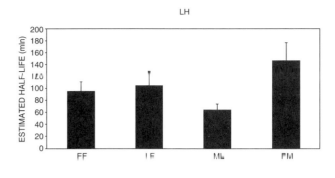

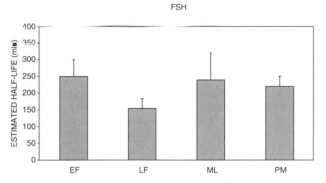

Fig. 110-2 Mean (±standard error of the mean [SEM]) endogenous gonadotropin half-lives estimated from deconvolution-resolved luteinizing hormone (LH) (upper panel) and follicle stimulating hormone (FSH) (lower panel) pulse profiles. Serum LH and FSH concentration-time scrics were obtained from premenopausal women during the early follicular, late follicular, and midluteal phases of the menstrual cycle and from postmenopausal women. For each experimental group, values identified with different superscripts differ significantly (p < 0.05). (From Booth RA Jr, Weltman JY, Yankov VI *et al.* [1996]. Mode of pulsatile follicle-stimulating hormone secretion in gonadal hormone-sufficient and -deficient women—a clinical research center study. *J Clin Endocrinol Metab.* 81:3208–3214, with permission.)

generator and on the hypothalamic-pituitary interactions, considerably fewer studies have examined the effects of aging on the feedforward effects of gonadotropins on ovarian function. In an earlier report, Jacobs *et al* [51] evaluated the effect of age on the ovarian response to human menopausal gonadotropin (hMG) in terms of follicular development and estrogen secretion. Overall, older women required relatively more hMG to effect the same degree of follicular development and estrogen secretion in older women compared with their younger peers. However, secondary analysis demonstrated that at the level of the individual follicle, estrogen secretion remained unaltered as a function of aging. Thus, the authors proposed that the age-associated decrease in hMG-stimulated estrogen secretion may reflect a decreased number of follicles available for recruitment rather than the response characteristics of individual follicles that have been successfully recruited. To evaluate in more detail such response characteristics of gonadotropin-stimulated ovarian hormone production, the ovary will need to be isolated from the confounding effects of endogenous gonadotropin secretion. The use of recently available GnRH antagonists should allow for

these sorts of studies to go forward. Indeed, it has recently been shown that the combination of ganirelix, a GnRH antagonist, together with the pulsatile administration of human recombinant LH, allows for the construction of LH/ovarian product dose-response relationships in normal women [52]. This approach should lend itself well to studies that will seek to determine whether there is a primary effect of aging on gonadotropin-stimulated ovarian hormone production.

d. EFFECTS OF AGING ON THE FEEDBACK OF OVARIAN PRODUCTS ON HYPOTHALAMIC-PITUITARY FUNCTION. As discussed previously, there is compelling evidence to suggest that alterations in the activity of the GnRH pulse generator could represent age-associated changes in feedback signaling by the ovary. It is entirely possible that the slowing of the GnRH pulse generator seen in preperimenopausal women is a consequence of altered gonadal hormone feedback rather than a reflection of changes in the CNS control of the system [22]. Whereas no good information is available related to the possibility that there is an age-associated change in the sensitivity of the hypothalamus to estrogen feedback in these women, it is certainly possible that increased secretion of estrogen may play a pivotal role. Conversely, the enhanced activity of the GnRH pulse generator with aging may primarily reflect diminished negative feedback by the gonadal hormones. However, whether estrogen sufficiency alone can slow the GnRH pulse generator-firing frequency and/ or suppress the amount of GnRH secreted per secretory episode remains somewhat unclear. In studies using a GnRH antagonist to estimate the amount of GnRH secreted in premenopausal versus postmenopausal women, the administration of estradiol was shown capable of diminishing the higher estimated GnRH secretion noted in postmenopausal women to the lower amounts observed in premenopausal women [44]. Whether estrogen alone can slow GnRH pulse frequency is less obvious, with some studies indicating that this does not occur [53] and others suggesting that estrogen can suppress GnRH pulse frequency but does so to a greater extent in younger versus older postmenopausal women [54]. The latter studies are consistent with the premise that the hypothalamic component of the reproductive axis may become less sensitive to gonadal hormone feedback with aging. Poorly understood, however, is how aging affects the ability of gonadal hormones to modulate LH and FSH secretion via direct effects on the pituitary. Although one study in rats has suggested that the facilitating effect of estrogen on the unstimulated secretion of LH by pituitary cells in culture obtained from young animals is not observed in cells obtained from older animals [46], studies addressing this issue in women will be exceedingly difficult to undertake because of the technical difficulties involved.

D. Summary

Given that the reproductive axis comprises a number of individual components that must function in a coordinated fashion with numerous feedforward and feedback relationships, any attempt to elucidate the effects of aging on this system is by definition challenging. Thus, whereas normal aging appears to associate with changes in hypothalamic GnRH pulse generator activity, it remains unclear as to whether such alterations reflect age-associated changes in CNS mechanisms, which control the pulse generator, and/or in the amount or response to age-associated changes in ovarian hormones. Although aging does appear to affect both basal and GnRH-stimulated pituitary function in animals, data concerning pituitary function in aging women are limited and inconsistent, leaving this issue unresolved and in need of further study. Similarly, although preliminary studies suggest that ovarian function at the level of the individual follicle may remain relatively unperturbed by the aging process, additional investigation using recently acquired pharmacologic tools is clearly necessary. Such studies will not only improve significantly our understanding of the physiologic effects of normal aging on the reproductive axis in women but will hopefully add to our diagnostic and therapeutic armamentarium related to the goal of achieving and maintaining successful pregnancies in older women.

III. Effects of Aging on the Somatotropic Axis

A. Overview: The Somatotropic Axis

Gonadal steroid hormones, age, body composition, aerobic fitness, and nutritional status modulate secretion of somatotropic hormones. Among diverse sex steroids, estradiol is a dominant positive regulator of GH secretion in the healthy human [55–71]. Indirect clinical studies suggest that estrogen may mediate a significant component of the gender contrast in GH secretion in young and older adults [55,56,58,66,72–82]. For example, premenopausal women exhibit a significantly (50%) lesser annual rate of age-related decline in daily GH production than men [68]. Combined GH and estradiol deficiency in postmenopausal individuals predicts unfavorable changes in body composition, lipid status, cardiovascular risk, cognitive function, muscle and bone mass, and perceived quality of life. Current concepts of the mechanistic basis for the foregoing associations embrace an ensemble of estrogen-dependent facets of neuroendocrine control of GH secretion (see later discussion).

B. Ensemble Notion of Somatotropic-Axis Control

The GH-IGF-1 axis operates via an array of specialized interactions (Fig. 110-3). Pivotal mechanisms include (1) pulsatile (feedforward) drive by hypothalamic growth hormone releasing hormone (GHRH), as established by *in vivo* GHRH immuno-neutralization and GHRH-receptor antagonist studies, analysis of GH secretion in the face of molecular mutations of the GHRH receptor, and/or direct sampling of GHRH release in hypothalamo-pituitary portal-venous blood; (2) reversible restraint of somatotrope-cell GH release, but not synthesis, by somatostatin (SS); (3) stimulation of GH secretion by the GHRP ghrelin; (4) negative feedback by the GH target-tissue product IGF-1; and (5) autoinhibition by GH itself via central-neural mechanisms [55,83–99]. A simplified network-like perspective of coordinate regulation of GH secretion provides a mechanistic platform that explicates the distinctive amplifying action of estrogen on GH pulse height or, more specifically, the mass of GH secreted per burst. Figure 110-4A gives the waveform to illustrate increased mass, and Figure 110-4B reports the numerical values of the increased burst mass.

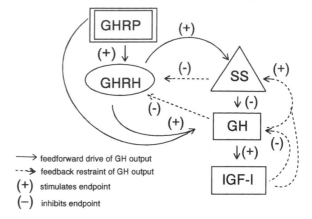

PRIMARY PEPTIDYL REGULATION OF GH-IGF-I AXIS

→ feedforward drive of GH output
---→ feedback restraint of GH output
(+) stimulates endpoint
(−) inhibits endpoint

Fig. 110-3 Concept of a network-like interaction (ensemble) among growth hormone releasing hormone (GHRH), growth hormone-releasing oligopeptide (GHRP)/ghrelin, and somatostatin under feedback modulation by (hypothalamo-pituitary-systemic) growth hormone (GH) and insulin-like growth factor-1 (IGF-1). (Unpublished schema.)

1. Growth Hormone-Releasing Oligopeptide

Modern knowledge of the novel class of peptides defined as GHRP began with *in vitro* analyses of synthetic pentapeptide (metenkephalin-derived) secretagogues more than 2 decades ago, several years before GHRH was isolated [100–102]. Known GHRP agonists include tripeptides, pentapeptides, hexapeptides, and heptapeptides, as well as nonpeptidyl mimetics of the GHRP-receptor signaling pathway [99,103–106].

The GHRP receptor is a G protein-coupled hepathelical transmembrane protein, which is expressed in the hypothalamus and pituitary gland (and nearly ubiquitously elsewhere) in the human, rat, rabbit, cow, pig, chicken, and puffer fish [99,107–110]. The GHRP receptor exhibits only modest (~30 to 33%) sequence identity with that of neurotensin and thyrotropin releasing hormone (TRH) and moderate (~50%) homology with that of motilin and galanin. Growth hormone-releasing oligopeptide activates G_{q11}-dependent release of inositol triphosphate, biphasic $[Ca^{2+}]_i$ elevations resulting from initial intracellular release and subsequent transmembrane uptake, and protein-kinase C-dependent signaling [111–113]. In contrast, SS opposes the actions of GHRP by inducing K^+ channel-driven membrane hyperpolarization, repressing $[Ca^{2+}]_i$ signal generation, and enforcing G_i-dependent inhibition of cAMP production. The unrelated GHRH receptor mediates stimulation of cAMP formation, GH gene transcription, *de novo* synthesis and rapid exocytotic release of GH [114].

Growth hormone-releasing oligopeptide (GHRP) acts by way of the CNS, the anterior pituitary gland, and diverse peripheral organs [115]. Cognate receptors are expressed by the majority of GHRH neurons in the arcuate nucleus and by approximately 50% of pituitary somatotropes in the adult rodent [99,107,116]. Central nervous system effects are diverse, and include *inter alia* enhancement of deep sleep, appetite, electrical firing of single GHRH neurons, c-fos gene activation in GHRH and NPY neurons, and the secretion of GHRH into cavernous-sinus blood [55,117–119]. At the pituitary level, GHRP drives *in vivo* GH

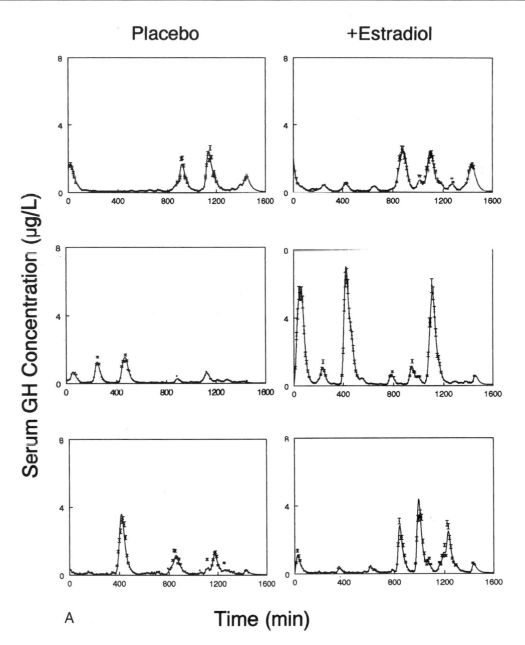

Fig. 110-4 Impact of oral estradiol versus placebo supplementation on growth hormone (GH) secretion in postmenopausal women. A, Responses of 10-min serum GH concentration profiles over 24 hours in three postmenopausal volunteers.

gene transcription in the infant rat, *in vivo* GH production at all ages, and *in vitro* GH secretion from neonatal and adult pituitary cells [102,103,106,109]. In the postmenopausal individual, GHRP-2 exerts marked agonistic effects on pulsatile GH release comparable to those of recombinant human (rh) GHRH (Fig. 110-5A).

2. Growth Hormone-Releasing Oligopeptide (GHRP) and Growth Hormone Releasing Hormone (GHRH)

Growth hormone-releasing oligopeptide achieves strong physiologic interactions with established effectors of the GH axis [55,83,120], including both SS (antagonistic) and GHRH (agonistic) [121–123]. A distinctive property of GHRP is synergy with GHRH [124]. The basis for synergy is multifactorial. For example, GHRP receptors are expressed on GHRH neurons [107], maximal GHRP stimulation requires functional (pituitary) GHRH receptors in the mouse (lit/lit mutation) and human (dwarfs of Sindh) [86,125], a high dose of a GHRH-receptor antagonist opposes acute GHRP drive in young adults [126], and GHRP will induce GHRH secretion from the hypothalamic tissue *in vitro* and into hypothalamo-pituitary portal blood *in vivo* [126,127]. The foregoing collection specialized interactions between GHRP and GHRH mediate supraadditive feedforward in the human, monkey, pig, sheep, and rodent [124,128,129].

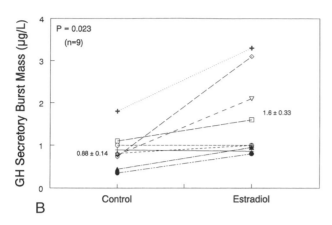

Fig. 110-4 B, Deconvolution estimates of the mass of GH secreted per burst in nine subjects studied as described in A. (Adapted from Shah N, Evans WS, Veldhuis JD. [1999]. Actions of estrogen on the pulsatile, nyctohemeral, and entropic modes of growth hormone secretion. *Am J Physiol.* 276:R1351–R1358, with permission.)

3. Growth Hormone-releasing Oligopeptide and Somatostatin

Growth hormone-releasing oligopeptide serves as a so-called functional SS antagonist. This term reflects the capability of GHRP to reduce SS's inhibition of GHRH stimulation by 2- to 3-fold *in vitro* and by 8- to 10-fold *in vivo* in the adult male rat [124]. The *in vitro* interaction reflects SSergic antagonism of $[Ca^{2+}]_i$ and K^+ signal generation via membrane receptor-coupled channels [99]. The *in vivo* interaction includes central-neural antagonism of hypothalamic gene activation [99,113,118]. Available experiments demonstrate that GHRPs do not directly inhibit SS binding or SS secretion into hypothalamo-pituitary portal blood [124,127].

4. Synergy Between Growth Hormone-Releasing Oligopeptide (GHRP) and Growth Hormone Releasing Hormone (GHRH) in the Human

Synergy between GHRP and GHRH requires a functionally connected hypothalamo-pituitary unit [55]. Indeed, supraadditive effects are not observed consistently *in vitro*. The magnitude of the *in vivo* synergy in postmenopausal women is marked (~100-fold) (Fig. 110-5B). Synergy is augmented in the rat and human by concomitant reduction in SSergic activity, which can be achieved by way of passive SS immunoneutralization or L-arginine infusion, respectively [55,99,122,130,131]. For example, in the adult male rat, concomitant infusion of GHRP-6, GHRH, and antiserum to SS elicits substantial GH release [124]. Likewise, in the human, simultaneous injection of hexarelin (a GHRP), GHRH and L-arginine evokes putatively maximal GH secretion, which appears to be independent of age [122,123,132]. In contrast, the individual efficacy of and joint synergy between GHRP and GHRH fall off markedly (by approximately 2-fold) in older individuals [55,122,124,132]. The precise basis for loss of responsivity to single or paired peptidyl secretagogue stimulation in aging is not established. However, the supra-addition effect of all three of SS withdrawal and GHRH and GHRP

stimulation in the hyposomatotropic aging individual illustrates the crucial tripeptidyl nature of the regulation of GH secretion [122,123,133].

An endogenous ligand for the GHRP-receptor effector system, ghrelin, was first cloned from the rat stomach and a human cDNA library in 1999 [84]. The naturally occurring agonist is a 28-residue 3-Ser-octanoylated peptide, which is expressed immunocytochemically in the hypothalamic arcuate nucleus and transcriptionally in the pituitary gland and gastrointestinal tract. *In vitro* potency is ~2.1 nM, which is comparable to that of GHRH, ~0.6 nM [134,135]. Circulating concentrations of ghrelin are in the potentially effectual range of 0.2 to 0.8 nM in the rodent and human. Native ghrelin mimics the majority of laboratory and clinical actions reported more extensively for synthetic GHRP-receptor agonists [136,137].

5. Autofeedback Control by Growth Hormone and Insulin-like Growth Factor-1

The foregoing trilogy of neuroregulatory peptides (GHRH, SS, and GHRP) mediates autonegative feedback of GH secretion in the experimental animal [83,87,138–140]. In particular, infusion or excessive production of GH or IGF-1 inhibits GHRH and GHRP-stimulated GH secretion by driving SS outflow and repressing GHRH and GHRP receptor and peptide expression acutely and chronically [138,141–145]. The rapid phase of reversible autoinhibition by GH unfolds over 1 to 2 hours and probably facilitates the suppression and then regeneration of recurrent GH pulses. Available data indicate that GH feedback-dependent pulse renewal may arise via reciprocal and time-delayed interactions between (at least) GHRH and SS [146–150]. Our concept of this dual-oscillator mechanism is illustrated schematically in Figure 110-6.

C. Specific Impact on Aging on Tripeptidyl Regulation of Growth Hormone Secretion

Clinical investigations based on intensive blood-sampling schedules and automated high-sensitivity immunoradiometric and chemiluminometric assays document 1.5- to 3-fold age-related damping of GH secretory-burst mass [64,65,67,151,152]. From a mechanistic vantage, attenuation of the mass of GH secreted per burst (and, thereby, GH pulse amplitude) would be a predicted outcome of excessive SSergic inhibition and/or diminished GHRP and GHRH stimulation [153]. In support of this thematic inference, first, peripheral infusion of SS or octreotide specifically reduces the calculated amount of GH released within individual bursts in young and older volunteers [89,154,155]. Second, the stimulatory effectiveness of single or multiple pulses of GHRH decreases asymptotically in aging men and women [65,83]. Third, the agonistic potency of GHRP declines in older humans [55,153,156]. However, more prolonged administration of GHRP-2 (by continuous subcutaneous infusion for 30 to 90 days) or of ipamorelin (an orally active nonpeptidyl secretagogue for 2 to 4 weeks) elevates 24-hour pulsatile GH secretion and the plasma IGF-1 concentration into the normal young-adult range in elderly men and women [157,158].

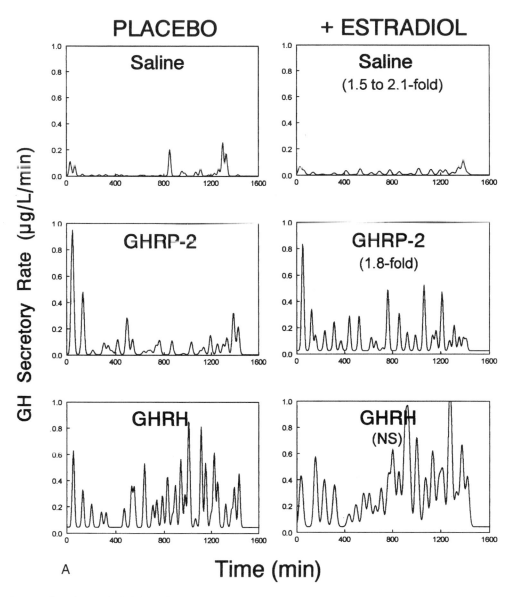

Fig. 110-5 A, Impact of continuous iv infusion of growth hormone-releasing oligopeptide-2 (GHRP-2) or growth hormone releasing hormone (GHRH) (1 μg/kg/hour) during oral placebo and estradiol replacement on growth hormone (GH) secretion rates in a healthy postmenopausal woman. The fold notation defines the ratio of the effect of estradiol to that of placebo.

D. Discrete Mechanisms of Estrogen Action in the Ovariprival Setting

1. Potentiation of Growth Hormone-Releasing Oligopeptide Stimulation

In cross-sectional studies, a (synthetic) GHRP evokes maximal secretagogue effects in mid-to-late puberty and more prominently in adolescent girls than boys [159–162]. The latter gender distinction is lost in early and middle adulthood [159], except in protracted critical illness [163]. Interventional studies in clinically prepubertal children indicate that administration of ethinyl estradiol orally for 3 days or single intramuscular injection of testosterone enanthate amplifies the GH secretory response

to hexarelin by approximately 2-fold [160]. Short-term supplementation of estradiol in postmenopausal women likewise doubles the stimulatory effect of GHRP-2 [164,165] (Fig. 110-7). Estrogen and/or gender impact ventromedial-nuclear GHRP receptor expression and feedforward efficacy of GHRP in the developing and adult animal [153,156,166]. From a molecular viewpoint, direct facilitative effects of estradiol on GHRP drive are putatively mediated via an estrogen-responsive *cis*-acting DNA regulatory element contained in the human GHRP-receptor gene promoter [166]. In addition, according to a tripeptidyl regulatory model, indirect estrogenic facilitation of GHRP feedforward drive *in vivo* could reflect nonexclusively: (1) reduction in SSergic activity and/or (2) amplification of endogenous GHRH outflow or (3) amplification of endogenous GHRH

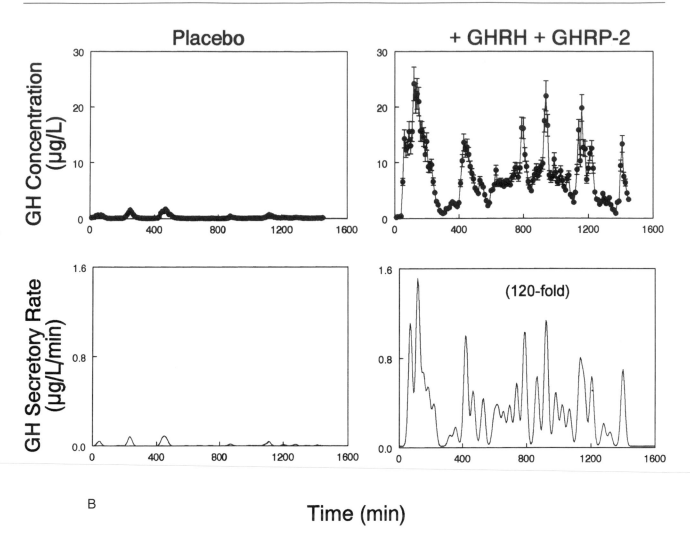

Fig. 110-5 B, One hundred and twenty-fold stimulatory effect of combined continuous intravenous infusion of GHRH and GHRP-2 (each 1 μg/kg/hour) over unstimulated daily GH secretion in a postmenopausal volunteer withdrawn from estrogen. Dual secretagogue drive maintains a normal frequency of GH pulses, thereby indicating that signals other than GHRH and GHRP (alone or combined) mediate the GH pulse-renewal process. (A, combined from Shah N, Evans WS, Bowers CY, Veldhuis JD. [2000]. Oral estradiol administration modulates continuous intravenous growth hormone [GH]-releasing peptide-2 driven GH secretion in postmenopausal women. *J Clin Endocrinol Metab*. 85:2649–2659 and Evans WS, Anderson SM, Hull LT *et al*. [2001]. Continuous 24-hour intravenous infusion of recombinant human growth hormone [GH]-releasing hormone-[1,44]-amide augments pulsatile, entropic, and daily rhythmic GH secretion in postmenopausal women equally in the estrogen-withdrawn and estrogen-supplemented states. *J Clin Endocrinol Metab*. 86:700–712; B, adapted from data in Veldhuis JD, Evans WS, Bowers CY. [2002]. Impact of estradiol supplementation on dual peptidyl drive of growth-hormone secretion in postmenopausal women. *J Clin Endocrinol Metab*. 87:859–866.)

action [153,156]. The first hypothesis is pertinent, because SS opposes the hypothalamic and pituitary actions of GHRP [118,122,124,130,131]. The second postulate is relevant, inasmuch as GHRP evokes hypothalamic GHRH secretion [127] and synergizes with exogenous GHRH (see previous discussion).

2. Attenuation the Suppressive Effects of Exogenous Somatostatin

Peripheral venous concentrations of SS do not reflect availability of this regulatory peptide into hypothalamo-pituitary portal blood. At central loci in the GH axis, SS is a pivotal inhibitor of the exocytotic release of GH and the hypothalamic secretion of GHRH [114,167–169]. In addition, albeit initially

viewed of paradoxical, short-term administration of a linear-hexapeptide antagonist of the SS receptor suppresses GH secretion and impairs linear growth in the juvenile rodent, thereby establishing a role for SS in maintaining pituitary responsiveness to repeated secretagogue stimulation *in vivo* [92,170,171]. Analogously, intermittent exposure of somatotropes to SS obviates agonist-induced phosphorylation-dependent downregulation of GHRH signaling *in vitro* [99,172]. Thus, SS has uniquely bipotential actions. In relation to this key effector peptide, a recent study indicates that estradiol repletion in postmenopausal women reduces the inhibitory potency of infused SS by 50% [154] (Fig. 110-8).

An unresolved mechanistic issue is whether estrogen restrains the hypothalamic secretion and/or CNS actions of SS. This

Double-Oscillator Model of GH Pulses

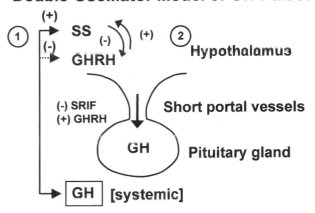

Fig. 110-6 Model of growth hormone (GH) pulse-renewal process in the human. One oscillator comprises systemic GH autofeedback via hypothalamic centers, thereby giving rise to volleys (clusters) of GH pulses. The other oscillator generates growth hormone releasing hormone (GHRH)-somatostatin (SS) cycles interneuronally, therein sustaining recurrent pulses within a volley. (Adapted from Farhy LM, Straume M, Johnson MJ *et al.* [2002]. Unequal autonegative feedback by growth hormone [GH] models the sexual dimorphism in GH secretory dynamics. *Am J Physiol.* 282:R753–R764, with permission.)

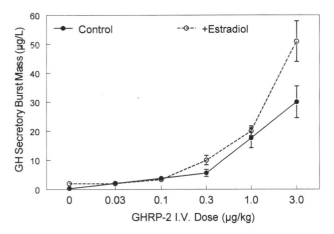

Fig. 110-7 Potentiating action of estradiol versus placebo administration on bolus intravenous growth hormone-releasing oligopeptide-2 (GHRP-2)-stimulated growth hormone (GH) secretory-burst mass in 11 healthy postmenopausal women. (From Anderson SM, Shah N, Patrie JT *et al.* [2000]. Short-term estradiol supplementation augments growth hormone [GH]-secretory responsiveness to dose-varying growth hormone-releasing peptide [GHRP-2] infusions in postmenopausal women. *J Clin Endocrinol Metab.* 86:551–560, with permission.)

consideration is particularly difficult to assess, given disparate inferences reported in the rodent and evident species differences in SS physiology [55,83]. For example, in the rat, testosterone and nonaromatizable androgens, but not estrogen, upregulate hypothalamic SS gene expression and stimulate GH secretion [173]. However, in the human, nonaromatizable androgens do not stimulate GH secretion [39,61,79,81,82]. Clinical studies become critical therefore to clarify how estrogen governs

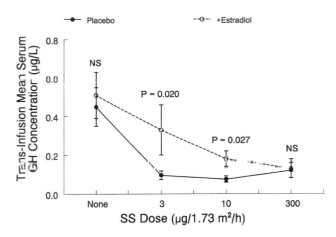

Fig. 110-8 Estrogen relieves submaximal inhibition of growth hormone (GH) release otherwise enforced by iv infusion of increasing doses of somatostatin (SS) in postmenopausal volunteers. p values denote within-subject statistical contrasts (p = NS defines p > 0.05). (Adapted from Bray MJ, Vick TM, Shah N *et al.* [2001]. Short-term estradiol replacement in postmenopausal women selectively mutes somatostatin's dose-dependent inhibition of fasting growth hormone secretion. *J Clin Endocrinol Metab.* 86:3143–3149, with permission.)

SS outflow, especially in aging individuals in whom SSergic inhibition may be accentuated [55,153,156,167].

Indirect clinical data are consistent with (but do not prove) the hypothesis that estradiol limits the suppressive effects of hypothalamic SS. First, in postmenopausal volunteers, estrogen replacement significantly augments daytime GH release, which is under greater inhibition by endogenous SS than nocturnal GH secretion [174,175]. Diurnal variation in SS outflow is inferred by continuing nycthemeral rhythmicity of GH output in the face of unvarying stimulation by GHRH, GHRP-2, or both agonists [65,128,164,165,176] (see Fig. 110-3A and 3B). Second, estrogen addback in leuprolide-suppressed young women reduces intermittent pituitary refractoriness to a pulse of GHRH, thus potentially signifying attenuation of SSergic activity [70]. Third, more irregular patterns of GH release in women than men are consistent with diminutive somatostatinergic restraint [59,61, 152,177,178].

3. Facilitation of Submaximal Stimulatory Effects of Growth Hormone Releasing Hormone (GHRH)

Diethylstilbestrol and estradiol administration in young men and postmenopausal women, respectively, and the estrogen-enriched preovulatory milieu in premenopausal women amplify the stimulatory effects of L-arginine, exercise, and insulin-induced hypoglycemia [56,57,66,71,130,131,179]. The foregoing secretagogues are notable, because each is believed to suppress hypothalamic SS release [55,83]. Accordingly, estrogenic stimulation of GH output under putatively SS-withdrawn conditions would signify that this sex steroid also exerts nonSSergic effects. Recent analyses of the dose-responsive actions of peptidyl secretagogues indicate that estradiol supplementation in postmenopausal women in fact enhances the stimulatory effect of (1) GHRP-2 (see previous discussion, Fig. 110-5) and (2) a submaximal dose of rh GHRH-1,44-amide [denoting increased GHRH potency] [180] (Fig. 110-9A). In contrast, estrogen does not alter the maximal effect of bolus or continuously infused GHRH, indicating unchanged efficacy [176,180] (Fig. 110-9B). The corollary consideration that estradiol may induce hypothalamic GHRH release or pituitary ghrelin expression in the human cannot be answered at present.

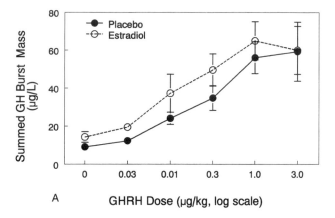

A

4. Muting of Growth Hormone-Dependent Autonegative Feedback

A single pulse of GH represses the subsequent response to GHRH and GHRP [141,144,145,167,181]. Autonegative feedback in the rodent is exerted via the CNS GH receptor, which drives hypothalamic SS synthesis and release [167,169,182,183]. Growth hormone concomitantly suppresses GHRH gene expression and GHRH outflow, in part by way of direct SSergic inhibitory synapses on arcuate-nucleus GHRH neurons [55,83,167,169, 181,182]. Thus, intracerebroventricular delivery of GH-receptor antisense oligonucleotides and systemic immunoneutralization of SS abrogate GH autofeedback [183,184]. Likewise, agents that putatively oppose SS release, such as L-arginine, relieve autoinhibition by GH [143]. Conversely, molecular defects in GH-receptor signaling and rare mutation of the IGF-1 peptide gene trigger marked GH hypersecretion [95,96].

A role for estrogen in muting GH autorestraint is plausible in the adult rat, inasmuch as the female animal is relatively resistant (but not insensitive) to GH feedback [185]. Analytically predicted consequences of feedback relief in the female include lesser episodicity of SS release, lower amplitude GH pulses, and greater disorderliness of the GH release process [146,147]. Experimental data corroborate these expectations [55,59,186].

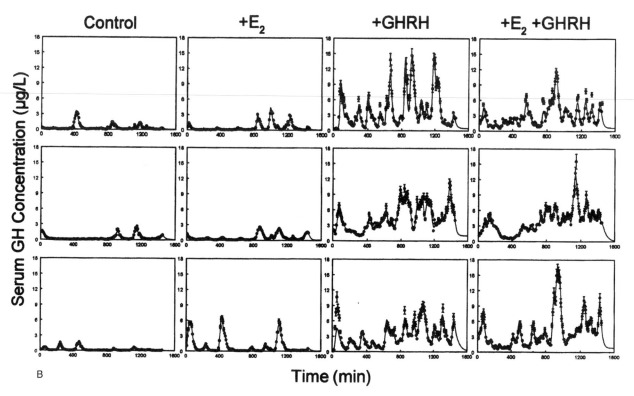

B

Fig. 110-9 A, Estradiol replacement augments dose-dependent drive of growth hormone (GH) secretion by randomly ordered, separate-day intravenous pulses of rh GHRH-1,44-amide in postmenopausal women. GH secretion is defined by the summed mass of GH released in pulses above basal secretion. Adapted from [180]. B, Impact of constant 24-hour intravenous infusion of saline or a near-maximally stimulatory dose (1 µg/kg/hour) of rh growth hormone releasing hormone (GHRH)-1,44-amide on pulsatile GH release monitored by sampling blood every 10 min after placebo versus estradiol replacement. (A, adapted from Evans WS, Bowers CY, Veldhuis JD. [2001]. Estradiol supplementation enhances pituitary sensitivity to recombinant human [RH] GHRH-1, 44-amide in somatostatin [SS]-withdrawn postmenopausal women. 83rd Annual Meeting of Endocrine Society, Abstract # P2-174; B, adapted from Evans WS, Anderson SM, Hull LT *et al.* [2001]. Continuous 24-hour intravenous infusion of recombinant human growth hormone [GH]-releasing hormone-[1,44]-amide augments pulsatile, entropic, and daily rhythmic GH secretion in postmenopausal women equally in the estrogen-withdrawn and estrogen-supplemented states. *J Clin Endocrinol Metab.* 86:700–712, with permission.)

For example, application of the approximate entropy statistic, which measures feedback-dependent regularity of secretory patterns, quantifies a less regular GH release process in the adult female than male rat and human [59,177,187,188]. In particular, approximate entropy analyses document more irregular GH secretory patterns in pubertal girls than boys, in women than men and after estrogen administration in postmenopausal individuals [59,61,152,175,177,178].

A recent clinical appraisal of GH autonegative feedback in the postmenopausal setting revealed that estradiol replacement selectively relieves autoinhibition of GHRP-2 (but not basal GHRH or exercise)-stimulated GH secretion [144] (Fig. 110-10). The complexity inherent in precisely dissecting the mechanistic basis of estrogenic regulation of GH autofeedback is made evident in complementary findings that (1) the number of hypothalamic (but not pituitary) binding sites for GHRP declines in the elderly human [110];

(2) the GHRP-receptor gene promoter is stimulated transcriptionally by estradiol *in vitro* [111]; (3) puberty, estrogen, and aromatizable androgens heighten GHRP effects and/or induce GHRP receptors in the rodent and/or human [160,161]; (4) brain GH-receptor density decreases in older men and women, thereby forecasting that GH autofeedback may wane in aging; (5) estrogen inhibits CNS GH-receptor expression in the rat [189]; and (6) the ovariprival state is associated with upregulation of hypothalamic estrogen-receptor gene expression [190].

5. Depletion of the Systemic Availability of Insulin-like Growth Factor-1

Earlier studies in the rat using partially purified somatomedin C suggested that IGF-1-like peptides suppress GH secretion via dual (hypothalamic and pituitary) sites of action [87]. In this regard, IGF-1 peptide and homonymous receptors are expressed in the hypothalamus and pituitary gland [191]. Recombinant IGF-1 directly inhibits pituitary GH gene expression and GH secretion *in vitro* [94], and, conversely, stimulates hypothalamic SS production *in vitro* and *in vivo* [139,168,192]. In the human, partial IGF-1 depletion resulting from fasting and profound IGF-1 deficiency resulting from rare partial truncation of the IGF-1 gene are accompanied by GH hypersecretion, which is suppressible by IGF-1 infusion [96,138,142,193]. In transgenic mice, postnatally inducible liver-specific disruption of the IGF-1

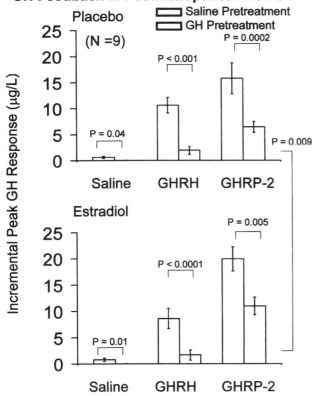

GH Feedback in Postmenopausal Women

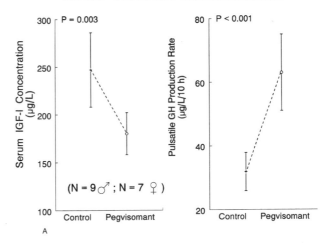

Reciprocal Effects of Pegvisomant on IGF-I and GH Concentrations

Fig. 110-10 Growth hormone (GH) concentration profiles depicting acute autofeedback by a single pulse of recombinant human growth hormone (rh GH) (10 µg/kg injected intervenous over 6 minutes) on each of basal (saline), GHRH (1 µg/kg), and growth hormone-releasing oligopeptide-2 (GHRP-2) (1 µg/kg)-stimulated GH release monitored 2 hours later in postmenopausal women (cohort mean ± standard error of the mean [SEM]) (top). Estradiol relieves autonegative feedback on GHRP-2 (but not basal or GHRH)-stimulated GH secretion in this setting (bottom). (From Anderson SM, Wideman L, Patrie JT *et al.* [2002]. Estradiol supplementation selectively relieves growth hormone [GH]'s autonegative feedback on GH-releasing peptide-2 [GHRP-2]-stimulated GH secretion. *J Clin Endocrinol Metab*. 86:5904–5911, with permission.)

Fig. 110-11 A, Pegvisomant-induced suppression of peripheral insulin-like growth factor-1 (IGF-1) concentrations and augmentation of overnight (10-hour mean) pulsatile growth hormone (GH) secretion. Data are individual values demarcated by gender in young men (*N* = 9) and women (*N* = 7). Pegvisomant is a recombinant (nine amino-acid mutated) GH molecule that selectively binds to and disables GH receptor-dependent cellular signaling. A single injection of drug (1 mg/kg subcutaneous) or placebo was given 72 hours earlier in a prospective, double-blind, within-subject crossover design. Growth hormone was assayed by double-monoclonal immunofluorometry, based on antigenic epitopes that do not cross-react with the modified GH protein, pegvisomant.

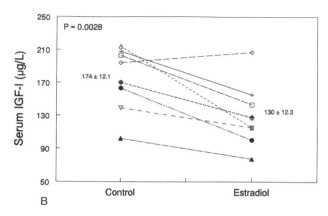

B

Fig. 110-11 B, Oral estradiol-induced decline in (fasting) serum total IGF-1 concentrations. (A, from Veldhuis JD, Bidlingmaier M, Anderson SM *et al.* [2001]. Lowering total plasma IGF-I concentrations by way of a novel, potent and selective GH-receptor antagonist, pegvisomant [B2036-PEG], augments the amplitude of GH secretory bursts and elevates basal/nonpulsatile GH release in healthy women and men. *J Clin Endocrinol Metab.* 86:3304–3310; B, adapted from Shah N, Evans WS, Veldhuis JD. [1999]. Actions of estrogen on the pulsatile, nyctohemeral, and entropic modes of growth hormone secretion. *Am J Physiol.* 276:R1351–R1358, with permission.)

gene lowers peripheral IGF-1 concentrations by 60 to 70% and stimulates GH secretion by 2- to 10-fold [194]. In a thematically analogous clinical context, a single subcutaneous dose of a selective and potent rh GH-receptor antagonist protein (pegvisomant, Trovert, B2036-PEG) reduces systemic IGF-1 concentrations by 30% and concomitantly doubles pulsatile and basal rates of GH secretion [195] (Fig. 110-11A). The degree of IGF-1 depletion induced by pegvisomant directly predicts the extent of rise in GH secretory-burst amplitude. The foregoing collective observations are important, because oral estrogen administration suppresses systemic IGF-1 concentrations by 25 to 35% putatively by repressing hepatic GH-receptor expression [175,196–198] (Fig. 110-11B). Therefore, a plausible but unproven mechanistic postulate is that estrogen replacement in postmenopausal women drives GH secretion in part by diminishing blood-borne IGF-1-dependent negative feedback.

E. Summary

Clinical studies almost 3 decades ago found that estrogen is a dominantly positive determinant of GH secretion and that age is a significantly negative determinant of GH secretion. Interim investigations have revealed important mechanisms of estradiol-dependent drive of GH secretion, as schematized in summary form in Figure 110-12. Continuing advances in the biology of SS, GHRH, and GHRP peptide action, expression, and regulation provide a broader investigative foundation to address this knowledge deficit in innovative and insightful ways. To this end, the this chapter highlights unique mechanisms by which estrogen directs the actions of and interactions among SS, GHRH, and GHRP in healthy postmenopausal women (Table 110-1).

Multifold Impact of Estradiol on Hypothalamo-Pituitary GH Axis

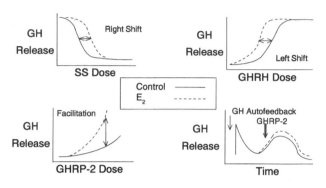

Fig. 110-12 Précis of estrogen-dependent mechanisms that amplify pulsatile growth hormone (GH) secretion in the gonadoprival woman exposed to a late follicular-phase concentration of estradiol-17 beta for 5 or more days. Line drawing. (Compiles concepts from references 144, 154, 165, 176, 180, and 199.)

Table 110-1

Précis of Significant Interactions between Estradiol and Somatostatin (SS), Growth Hormone Releasing Hormone (GHRH), and Growth Hormone-releasing Oligopeptide-2 (GHRP-2) in Postmenopausal Women

1. Estradiol enhances GHRH potency and somatotrope sensitivity to GHRH by 1.9- to 2.1-fold without altering peptide efficacy [176,180].
2. Estradiol potentiates the acute stimulatory effect of GHRP-2 by 1.8-fold [199].
3. Estradiol attenuates the inhibitory potency of infused SS by 50% [154].
4. Estradiol doubles the basal (interpulse) growth hormone (GH) secretory rate driven by continuous intravenous infusion of GHRP-2 but not by saline [164].
5. Estradiol amplifies the GHRP-2-stimulated amplitude of the 24-hpir rhythm in serum GH concentrations [164,165].
6. Estradiol normalizes the 24-hour variation in GHRP-2-damped GH interburst intervals [165].
7. Estradiol and GHRP-2 jointly increase the feedback-dependent irregularity (approximate entropy) of the GH secretory process [165].
8. GHRP-2 infusion overcomes oral estrogen's suppression of plasma insulin-like growth factor-1 (IGF-1) concentrations [165].
9. Estradiol relieves GH autonegative feedback on the GHRP-2 stimulus [144].

Acknowledgements

The authors thank Martha Burner and Jean Plote for excellent editorial support and David Boyd and Kandace Bradford for the graphics. This work was supported in part by the National Center for Research Resources via General Clinical Research Center grant RR-00847 (to the University of Virginia) and

RR-00585 (to the Mayo Clinic and Foundation) and NIH ROI AG 14799-05 and AG 19695-02.

References

1. Morley JE. (2002). Drugs, aging and the future. *J Gerontol.* 57:M2–M6.

2. Maroulis GB. (1995). Effect of aging on fertility and pregnancy. *Endocrinologist.* 5:364–370.

3. Nakai Y, Plant TM, Hess DL *et al.* (1978). On the sites of negative and positive feedback actions of estradiol in the control of gonadotropin secretion in the rhesus monkey (Macaca mulatto). *Endocrinology.* 102:1015–1018.

4. Levine JE, Ramirez VD. (1982). Luteinizing hormone-releasing hormone release during the rat estrous cycle and after ovariectomy, as estimated with push-pull cannulae. *Endocrinology.* 111:1439–1448.

5. Levine JE, Pau KY, Ramirez VD, Jackson GL. (1982). Simultaneous measurement of luteinizing hormone-releasing hormone and luteinizing hormone release in unanesthetized, ovariectomized sheep. *Endocrinology.* 111:1449–1455.

6. Clarke IJ, Cummins JT. (1982). The temporal relationship between gonadotropin releasing hormone (GnRH) and luteinizing hormone (LH) secretion in ovariectomized ewes. *Endocrinology.* 111:1737–1739.

7. Baker TG. (1963). A quantitative and cytological study of germ cells in human ovaries. *Proc R Soc Lond Series B Biol Sci.* 158:417–433.

8. Richardson SJ, Senikas V, Nelson JF. (1987). Follicular depletion during the menopausal transition: Evidence for accelerated loss and ultimate exhaustion. *J Clin Endocrinol Metab.* 65:1231–1237.

9. Block E. (1952). Quantitative morphological investigations of follicular system in women. *Acta Anat.* 14:108–123.

10. Gosden RG. (1987). Follicular status at the menopause. *Hum Reprod.* 2:617–621.

11. Plachot M, De Grouchy J, Junca AM *et al.* (1988). Chromosomal analysis of human oocytes and embryos in an *in vitro* fertilization program. *Ann N Y Acad Sci.* 541:384–397.

12. Silber SJ, Nagy Z, Liu J. (1995). The use of epididymal and testicular spermatozoa for intracytoplasmic sperm injection: The genetic implications for male infertility. *Hum Reprod.* 10:2031–2043.

13. Danforth DR, Arbogast LK, Mroueh J *et al.* (1998). Dimeric inhibin: A direct marker of ovarian aging. *Fertil Steril.* 70:119–123.

14. Seifer DB, Scott RT Jr, Bergh PA *et al.* (1999). Women with declining ovarian reserve may demonstrate a decrease in day 3 serum inhibin B before a rise in day 3 follicle-stimulating hormone. *Fertil Steril.* 72:63–65.

15. Burger HG, Dudley EC, Hopper JL *et al.* (1995). The endocrinology of the menopausal transition: A cross-sectional study of a population-based sample. *J Clin Endocrinol Metab.* 80:3537–3545.

16. Welt CK, McNicholl DJ, Taylor AE, Hall JE. (1999). Female reproductive aging is marked by decreased secretion of dimeric inhibin. *J Clin Endocrinol Metab.* 84:105–111.

17. Levran D, Ben Shlomo I, Dor J *et al.* (1991). Aging of endometrium and oocytes: Observations on conception and abortion rates in an egg donation model. *Fertil Steril.* 56:1091–1094.

18. Peng MT, Huang HH. (1972). Aging of hypothalamic-pituitary-ovarian function in the rat. *Fertil Steril.* 23:535–542.

19. Huang HH. (1988). Rejuvenation of the aging hypothalamic-pituitary axis with fetal hypothalamic graft. *Interdiscipl Top Gerontol.* 24:141–149.

20. Wise PM, Dueker E, Wuttke W. (1988). Age-related alterations in pulsatile luteinizing hormone release: Effects of long-term ovariectomy, repeated pregnancies and naloxone. *Biol Reprod.* 39:1060–1066.

21. Nass TE, LaPolt PS, Judd HL, Lu JK. (1984). Alterations in ovarian steroid and gonadotrophin secretion preceding the cessation of regular oestrous cycles in ageing female rats. *J Endocrinol.* 100:43–50.

22. Matt DW, Kauma SW, Pincus SM *et al.* (1998). Characteristics of luteinizing hormone secretion in younger versus older premenopausal women. *Am J Obstet Gynecol.* 178:504–510.

23. Brito AN, Sayles TE, Krieg RJ Jr, Matt DW. (1994). Relation of attenuated proestrous luteinizing hormone surges in middle-aged female rats to *in vitro* pituitary gonadotropin-releasing hormone responsiveness. *Eur J Endocrinol.* 130:540–544.

24. Wise PM. (1984). Estradiol-induced daily luteinizing hormone and prolactin surges in young and middle-aged rats: Correlations with age-related changes in pituitary responsiveness and catecholamine turnover rates in microdissected brain areas. *Endocrinology.* 115:801–809.

25. Lloyd JM, Hoffman GE, Wise PM. (1994). Decline in immediate early gene expression in gonadotropin-releasing hormone neurons during proestrus in regularly cycling, middle-aged rats. *Endocrinology.* 134:1800–1805.

26. Tsai HW, Hong LS, LaPolt PS, Lu JK. (1996). Gonadotropin surges elicited by progesterone after estradiol (E2)-priming, but not by E2 alone, in middle-aged, acyclic female rats exhibiting early persistence estrus. *Proc Tenth Annual Meeting of the Internat Cong Endocrinol.*

27. Metcalf MG, Livesey JH. (1985). Gonadotrophin excretion in fertile women: Effect of age and the onset of the menopausal transition. *J Endocrinol.* 105:357–362.

28. Reyes FI, Winter JS, Faiman C. (1977). Pituitary-ovarian relationships preceding the menopause. I. A cross-sectional study of serum follicle-stimulating hormone, luteinizing hormone, prolactin, estradiol, and progesterone levels. *Am J Obstet Gynecol.* 129:557–564.

29. Sherman BM, Korenman SG. (1975). Hormonal characteristics of the human menstrual cycle throughout reproductive life. *J Clin Invest.* 55:699–706.

30. Sherman BM, West JH, Korenman SG. (1976). The menopausal transition: Analysis of LH, FSH, estradiol, and progesterone concentrations during menstrual cycles of older women. *J Clin Endocrinol Metab.* 42:629–636.

31. Batista MC, Cartledge TP, Zellmer AW *et al.* (1995). Effects of aging on menstrual cycle hormones and endometrial maturation. *Fertil Steril.* 64:492–499.

32. Klein NA, Battaglia DE, Clifton DK *et al.* (1996). The gonadotropin secretion pattern in normal women of advanced reproductive age in relation to the monotropic FSH rise. *J Soc Gynecol Invest.* 3:27–32.

33. Santoro N, Brown JR, Adel T, Skurnick JH. (1996). Characterization of reproductive hormonal dynamics in the perimenopause. *J Clin Endocrinol Metab.* 81:1495–1501.

34. Reame NE, Kelche RP, Beitins IZ *et al.* (1996). Age effects of follicle-stimulating hormone and pulsatile luteinizing hormone secretion across the menstrual cycle of premenopausal women. *J Clin Endocrinol Metab.* 81:1512–1518.

35. Klein NA, Battaglia DE, Fujimoto VY *et al.* (1996). Reproductive aging: Accelerated ovarian follicular development associated with a monotropic follicle-stimulating hormone rise in normal older women. *J Clin Endocrinol Metab.* 81:1038–1045.

36. Rossmanith WG, Liu CH, Laughlin GA *et al.* (1990). Relative changes in LH pulsatility during the menstrual cycle; using data from hypogonadal women as a reference point. *Clin Endocrinol.* 32:647–660.

37. Booth RA Jr, Weltman JY, Yankov VI *et al.* (1996). Mode of pulsatile follicle-stimulating hormone secretion in gonadal hormone-sufficient and -deficient women—a clinical research center study. *J Clin Endocrinol Metab.* 81:3208–3214.

38. Hall JE, Lavoie HB, Marsh EE, Martin KA. (2000). Decrease in gonadotropin-releasing hormone (GnRH) pulse frequency with aging in postmenopausal women. *J Clin Endocrinol Metab.* 85:1794–1800.

39. Keenan BS, Richards GE, Ponder SW *et al.* (1993). Androgen-stimulated pubertal growth: The effects of testosterone and dihydrotestosterone on growth hormone and insulin-like growth factor-I in the treatment of short stature and delayed puberty. *J Clin Endocrinol Metab.* 76:996–1001.

40. Scaglia H, Medina M, Pinto-Ferreira AL *et al.* (1976). Pituitary LH and FSH secretion and responsiveness in women of old age. *Acta Endocrinol.* 81:673–679.

41. Rossmanith WG, Scherbaum WA, Lauritzen C. (1991). Gonadotropin secretion during aging in postmenopausal women. *Neuroendocrinology.* 54:211–218.

42. Rance NE, McMullen NT, Smialek JE *et al.* (1990). Postmenopausal hypertrophy of neurons expressing the estrogen receptor gene in the human hypothalamus. *J Clin Endocrinol Metab.* 71:79–85.

43. Rance NE, Uswandi SV. (1996). Gonadotropin-releasing hormone gene expression is increased in the medial basal hypothalamus of postmenopausal women. *J Clin Endocrinol Metab.* 81:3540–3546.

44. Gill S, Sharpless JL, Rado K, Hall JE. (2002). Evidence that GnRH decreases with gonadal steroid feedback but increases with age in postmenopausal women. *J Clin Endocrinol Metab.* 87:2290–2296.

45. Stewart DA, Blackman MR, Kowatch MA *et al.* (1990). Discordant effects of aging on prolactin and luteinizing hormone-beta messenger ribonucleic acid levels in the female rat. *Endocrinology.* 126:773–778.

46. Tang LK, Tang FY. (1981). LH responses to LHRH, DBcAMP, and 17 beta-estradiol in cultures derived from aged rats. *Am J Physiol.* 240:E510–E518.

47. Sharpless JL, Supko JG, Martin KA, Hall JE. (1999). Disappearance of endogenous luteinizing hormone is prolonged in postmenopausal women. *J Clin Endocrinol Metab.* 84:688–694.

48. Wide L. (1982). Male and female forms of human follicle-stimulating hormone in serum. *J Clin Endocrinol Metab.* 55:682–688.

49. Baenziger JU, Green ED. (1988). Pituitary glycoprotein hormone oligosaccharides: Structure, synthesis and function of the asparagine-linked oligosaccharides on lutropin, follitropin and thyrotropin. *Biochimica Biophysica Acta.* 947:287–306.

50. Liu TC, Jackson GL. (1977). Effect of *in vivo* treatment with estrogen on luteinizing hormone synthesis and release by rat pituitaries *in vitro. Endocrinology.* 100:1294–1302.

51. Jacobs SL, Metzger DA, Dodson WC, Haney AF. (1990). Effect of age on response to human menopausal gonadotropin stimulation. *J Clin Endocrinol Metab.* 71:1525–1530.

52. McCartney CR, Bellows AB, Hu Y *et al.* (2002). Heightened secretion of 17-hydroxyprogesterone in patients with polycystic ovary syndrome following sequential blockade of endogenous LH release and pulsatile IV infusions of exogenous. 84th Annual Meeting of the Endocrine Society, Abstract #P2–610.

53. Rossmanith WG, Handke-Vesely A, Wirth U, Scherbaum WA. (1994), Does the gonadotropin pulsatility of postmenopausal women represent the unrestrained hypothalamic-pituitary activity? *Eur J Endocrinol.* 130:485–493.

54. Santoro N, Banwell T, Tortoriello D *et al.* (1998). Effects of aging and gonadal failure on the hypothalamic-pituitary axis in women. *Am J Obstet Gynecol.* 178:732–741.

55. Giustina A, Veldhuis JD. (1998). Pathophysiology of the neuroregulation of GH secretion in experimental animals and the human. *Endocr Rev.* 19:717–797.

56. Frantz AG, Rabkin MT. (1965). Effects of estrogen and sex difference on secretion of human growth hormone. *J Clin Endocrinol Metab.* 25:1470–1480.

57. Merimee TJ, Fineberg SE. (1971). Studies of the sex-based variation of human growth hormone secretion. *J Clin Endocrinol Metab.* 33:896–902.

58. Mauras N, Rogol AD, Veldhuis JD. (1990). Increased hGH production rate after low-dose estrogen therapy in prepubertal girls with Turner's syndrome. *Pediatr Res.* 28:626–630.

59. Pincus SM, Gevers E, Robinson ICAF *et al.* (1996). Females secrete growth hormone with more process irregularity than males in both human and rat. *Am J Physiol.* 270:E107–E115.

60. van den Berg G, Veldhuis JD, Frolich M, Roelfsema F. (1996). An amplitude-specific divergence in the pulsatile mode of GH secretion underlies the gender difference in mean GH concentrations in men and premenopausal women. *J Clin Endocrinol Metab.* 81:2460–2466.

61. Veldhuis JD, Metzger DL, Martha PM Jr *et al.* (1997). Estrogen and testosterone, but not a non-aromatizable androgen, direct network integration of the hypothalamo-somatotrope (growth hormone)-insulin-like growth factor I axis in the human: Evidence from pubertal pathophysiology and sex-steroid hormone replacement. *J Clin Endocrinol Metab.* 82:3414–3420.

62. Wennink JMB, Delemarre-van de Waal HA, Schoemaker R *et al.* (1991). Growth hormone secretion patterns in relation to LH and estradiol secretion throughout normal female puberty. *Acta Endocrinol (Copenh).* 124:129–135.

63. Vahl N, Jorgensen JO, Skjaerback C *et al.* (1997). Abdominal adiposity rather than age and sex predicts the mass and patterned regularity of growth hormone secretion in mid-life healthy adults. *Am J Physiol.* 272: E1108–E1116.

64. Iranmanesh A, Grisso B, Veldhuis JD. (1994). Low basal and persistent pulsatile growth hormone secretion are revealed in normal and hyposomatotropic men studied with a new ultrasensitive chemiluminescence assay. *J Clin Endocrinol Metab.* 78:526–535.

65. Iranmanesh A, South S, Liem AY *et al.* (1998). Unequal impact of age, percentage body fat, and serum testosterone concentrations on the somatotropic, IGF-I, and IGF-binding protein responses to a three-day intravenous growth-hormone-releasing-hormone (GHRH) pulsatile infusion. *Eur J Endocrinol.* 139:59–71.

66. Veldhuis JD. (1998). Neuroendocrine control of pulsatile growth-hormone release in the human: Relationship with gender. *Growth Horm IGF Res.* 8:49–59.

67. Iranmanesh A, Lizarralde G, Veldhuis JD. (1991). Age and relative adiposity are specific negative determinants of the frequency and amplitude of growth hormone (GH) secretory bursts and the half-life of endogenous GH in healthy men. *J Clin Endocrinol Metab.* 73:1081–1088.

68. Weltman A, Weltman JY, Hartman ML *et al.* (1994). Relationship between age, percentage body fat, fitness and 24 hour growth hormone release in healthy young adults: Effects of gender. *J Clin Endocrinol Metab.* 78:543–548.

69. Veldhuis JD, Iranmanesh A, Weltman A. (1997). Elements in the pathophysiology of diminished growth hormone (GH) secretion in aging humans. *Endocrine.* 7:41–48.

70. Devesa J, Lois N, Arce V *et al.* (1991). The role of sexual steroids in the modulation of growth hormone (GH) secretion in humans. *J Ster Biochem Mol Biol.* 40:165–173.

71. Veldhuis JD. (1996). Gender differences in secretory activity of the human somatotropic (growth hormone) axis. *Eur J Endocrinol.* 134:287–295.

72. Bellantoni MF, Harman SM, Cho DE, Blackman MR. (1991). Effects of progestin-opposed transdermal estrogen administration on growth hormone and insulin-like growth factor-I in postmenopausal women of different ages. *J Clin Endocrinol Metab.* 72:172–178.

73. Mansfield MJ, Rudlin CR, Crigler JF Jr *et al.* (1988). Changes in growth and serum growth hormone and plasma somatomedin-C levels during suppression of gonadal sex steroid secretion in girls with central precocious puberty. *J Clin Endocrinol Metab.* 66:3–9.

74. Gourmelen M, Le Bouc Y, Girard F, Binoux M. (1984). Serum levels of insulin-like growth factor (IGF) and IGF binding protein in constitutionally tall children and adolescents. *J Clin Endocrinol Metab.* 59:1197–1203.

75. Friedman AJ, Rein MS, Pandian MR, Barbieri RL. (1990). Fasting serum growth hormone and insulin-like growth factor-I and -II concentrations in women with leiomyomata uteri treated with leuprolide acetate or placebo. *Fertil Steril.* 53:250–253.

76. De Leo V, Lanzetta D, D'Antona D, Danero S. (1993). Growth hormone secretion in premenopausal women before and after ovariectomy: Effect of hormone replacement therapy. *Fertil Steril.* 60:268–271.

77. van Kesteren P, Lips P, Deville W *et al.* (1996). The effect of one-year cross-sex hormonal treatment on bone metabolism and serum insulin-like growth factor-1 in transsexuals. *J Clin Endocrinol Metab.* 81:2227–2232.

78. Ho KKY, O'Sullivan AJ, Weissberger AJ, Kelly JJ. (1996). Sex steroid regulation of growth hormone secretion and action. *Horm Res.* 45:67–73.

79. Fryburg DA, Weltman A, Jahn LA *et al.* (1999). Androgenic Modulation of the Growth Hormone-IGF Axis and Its Impact on Metabolic Outcomes. In *Sex-Steroid Interaction with Growth Hormone* (Veldhuis JD, Giustina A, eds.), pp. 82–92. New York: Springer-Verlag.

80. Weissberger AJ, Ho KKY. (1993). Activation of the somatotropic axis by testosterone in adult males: Evidence for the role of aromatization. *J Clin Endocrinol Metab.* 1407:1412.

81. Metzger DL, Kerrigan JR. (1993). Androgen receptor blockade with flutamide enhances growth hormone secretion in late pubertal males: Evidence for independent actions of estrogen and androgen. *J Clin Endocrinol Metab.* 76:1147–1152.

82. Metzger DL, Kerrigan JR. (1994). Estrogen receptor blockade with tamoxifen diminishes growth hormone secretion in boys: Evidence for a stimulatory role of endogenous estrogens during male adolescence. *J Clin Endocrinol Metab.* 79:513–518.

83. Mueller EE, Locatelli V, Cocchi D. (1999). Neuroendocrine control of growth hormone secretion. *Physiol Rev.* 79:511–607.

84. Kojima M, Hosoda H, Date Y *et al.* (1999). Ghrelin is a growth-hormone-releasing acylated peptide from stomach. *Nature.* 402:656–660.

85. Jaffe CA, DeMott Friberg R, Barkan AL. (1993). Suppression of growth hormone (GH) secretion by a selective GH-releasing hormone (GHRH) antagonist. *J Clin Invest.* 92:695–701.

86. Baumann G, Maheshwari H. (1997). The dwarfs of Sindh: Severe growth hormone (GH) deficiency caused by a mutation in the GH-releasing hormone receptor gene. *Acta Pediatr Suppl.* 432:33–38.

87. Berelowitz M, Szabo M, Frohman LA *et al.* (1981). Somatomedin-C mediates growth hormone negative feedback by effects on both the hypothalamus and the pituitary. *Science.* 212:1279–1281.

88. Bowers CY. (1993). GH releasing peptides—structure and kinetics. *J Pediatr Endocrinol Metab.* 6:21–31.

89. Calabresi E, Ishikawa E, Bartolini L *et al.* (1996). Somatostatin infusion suppresses GH secretory burst number and mass in normal men: A dual mechanism of inhibition. *Am J Physiol.* 270:E975–E979.

90. Bertherat J, Bluet-Pajot MT, Epelbaum J. (1995). Neuroendocrine regulation of growth hormone. *Eur J Endocrinol.* 132:12–24.

91. Frohman LA, Jansson J-O. (1986). Growth hormone-releasing hormone. *Endocr Rev.* 7:223–253.

92. Baumbach WR, Carrick TA, Pausch MH *et al.* (1998). A linear hexapeptide somatostatin antagonist blocks somatostatin activity *in vitro* and influences growth hormone release in rats. *Mol Pharm.* 54:864–873.

93. Godfrey P, Rahal JO, Beamer WG et al. (1993). GHRH receptor of little mice contains a missense mutation in the extracellular domain that disrupts receptor function. Nat Genet. 4:227–232.

94. Yamashita S, Melmed S. (1986). Insulin-like growth factor I action on rat anterior pituitary cells: Suppression of growth hormone secretion and messenger ribonucleic acid levels. Endocrinology. 118:176–182.

95. Rosenbloom AL, Savage MO, Blum WF et al. (1992). Clinical and biochemical characteristics of growth hormone receptor deficiency (Laron syndrome). Acta Paediatr Scand. 81(Suppl 383):121–124.

96. Woods KA, Camacho-Hubner C, Savage MO, Clark AJ. (1996). Intrauterine growth retardation and postnatal growth failure associated with deletion of the insulin-like growth factor I gene. N Engl J Med. 335:1363–1367.

97. Bowers CY, Reynolds GA, Durham D et al. (1990). Growth hormone (GH)-releasing peptide stimulates GH release in normal men and acts synergistically with GH-releasing hormone. J Clin Endocrinol Metab. 70:975–982.

98. Argente J, Chowen JA, Zeitler P et al. (1991). Sexual dimorphism of growth hormone-releasing hormone and somatostatin gene expression in the hypothalamus of the rat during development. Endocrinology. 128:2369–2375.

99. Smith RG, van der Ploeg LH, Howard AD et al. (1997). Peptidomimetic regulation of growth hormone secretion. Endocr Rev. 18:621–645.

100. Bowers CY, Momany FA, Chang D et al. (1981). Structure-activity relationships of a synthetic pentapeptide that specifically releases GH in vitro. Endocrinology. 106:663–667.

101. Bowers CY, Chang J, Momany F, Folkers K. (1977). Effect of the enkephalins and enkephalin analogs on release of pituitary hormones in vitro. In Molecular Endocrinology (MacIntyre I, Szelke M, eds.), pp. 287–292. Amsterdam: Elsevier/North Holland.

102. Bowers CY, Momany FA, Reynolds A, Hong A. (1984). On the in vitro and in vivo activity of a new synthetic hexapeptide that acts on the pituitary to specifically release growth hormone. Endocrinology. 114:1537–1545.

103. Deghenghi R, Cananzi MM, Torsello A et al. (1994). GH-releasing activity of hexarelin, a new growth hormone releasing peptide, in infant and adult rats. Life Sci. 54:1321–1328.

104. Van den Berghe G, Veldhuis JD, de Zegher F et al. (1999). Growth hormone-releasing peptide-2 infusion synchronizes growth hormone, thyrotropin and prolactin release in prolonged critical illness. Eur J Endocrinol. 140:17–22.

105. Tiulpakov AN, Brook CG, Pringle PJ et al. (1995). GH responses to intravenous bolus infusions of GH releasing hormone and GH releasing peptide 2 separately and in combination in adult volunteers. Clin Endocrinol. 43:347–350.

106. Bowers CY, Sartor AO, Reynolds GA, Badger TM. (1991). On the actions of the growth hormone-releasing hexapeptide. Endocrinology. 128:2027–2035.

107. Tannenbaum GS, Lapointe M, Besudet A, Howard AD. (1998). Expression of growth hormone secretagogue-receptors by growth hormone-releasing hormone neurons in the mediobasal hypothalamus. Endocrinology. 139:4420–4423.

108. Guan XM, Yu H, Palyha OC et al. (1997). Distribution of mRNA encoding the growth hormone secretagogue receptor in brain and peripheral tissues. Brain Res. 48:23–29.

109. Locatelli V, Grilli R, Torsello A et al. (1994). Growth hormone-releasing hexapeptide is a potent stimulator of growth hormone gene expression and release in the growth hormone-releasing hormone-deprived infant rat. Pediatr Res. 36:169–174.

110. Muccioli G, Ghe C, Ghigo MC et al. (1998). Specific receptors for synthetic GH secretagogues in the human brain and pituitary gland. J Endocrinol. 157:99–106.

111. Korbonits M, Ciccarelli E, Ghigo E, Grossman AB. (1999). The growth hormone secretagogue receptor. Growth Horm IGF Res. 9(Suppl A):93–99.

112. Lei T, Buchfelder M, Fahlbusch R, Adams EF. (1995). Growth hormone releasing peptide (GHRP-6) stimulates phosphatidylinositol (PI) turnover in human pituitary somatotroph cells. J Mol Endocrinol. 14:135–138.

113. Herrington J, Hille B. (1994). Growth hormone-releasing hexapeptide elevates intracellular calcium in rat somatotropes by two mechanisms. Endocrinology. 1135:1100–1108.

114. Barinaga M, Bilezikjian LM, Vale WW et al. (1985). Independent effects of growth hormone releasing factor on growth hormone release and gene transcription. Nature. 314:279–281.

115. Tannenbaum GS, Epelbaum J, Bowers CY. (2003). Interrelationship between the novel peptide ghrelin, somatostatin and growth hormone-releasing hormone in regulation of pulsatile growth hormone secretion. Endocrinology. 144:967–974.

116. Kamegai J, Wakabayashi I, Miyamoto K et al. (1998). Growth hormone-dependent regulation of pituitary GH secretagogue receptor (GHS-R) mRNA levels in the spontaneous dwarf Rat. Neuroendocrinology. 68:312–318.

117. Dickson SM, Luckman SM. (1997). Induction of c-fos messenger ribonucleic acid in neuropeptide Y and growth hormone (GH)-releasing factor neurons in the rat arcuate nucleus following systemic injection of the GH secretagogue, GH-releasing peptide-6. Endocrinology. 138:771–777.

118. Fairhall KM, Mynett A, Robinson ICAF. (1995). Central effects of growth hormone-releasing hexapeptide (GHRP-6) on growth hormone release are inhibited by central somatostatin action. J Endocrinol. 144:555–560.

119. Locke W, Kirgis HD, Bowers CY, Abdoh AA. (1995). Intracerebroventricular growth-hormone-releasing peptide-6 stimulates eating without affecting plasma growth hormone responses in rats. Life Sci. 56:1347–1352.

120. Bennett PA, Thomas GB, Howard AD et al. (1997). Hypothalamic growth hormone secretagogue-receptor (GHS-R) expression is regulated by growth hormone in the rat. Endocrinology. 138:4552–4557.

121. Bowers CY, Granda-Ayala R. (1996). GHRP-2, GHRH and SRIF interrelationships during chronic administration of GHRP-2 to humans. J Pediatr Endocrinol Metab. 9:261–270.

122. Arvat E, Gianotti L, Grottoli S et al. (1994). Arginine and growth hormone-releasing hormone restore the blunted growth hormone-releasing activity of hexarelin in elderly subjects. J Clin Endocrinol Metab. 79:1440–1443.

123. Ghigo E, Arvat E, Gianotti L et al. (1998). Endocrine Response to Growth Hormone-Releasing Peptides Across Human Life Span. In Growth Hormone Secretagogues in Clinical Practice (Bercu BB, Walker RF, eds.), pp. 345–367. New York: Marcel Dekker.

124. Bowers CY. (1998). Synergistic Release of Growth Hormone by GHRP and GHRH: Scope and Implication. In Growth Hormone Secretagogues in Clinical Practice (Bercu BB, Walker RF, eds.), pp. 1–25. New York: Marcel Dekker.

125. Roelfsema F, Biermasz NR, Veldman RG et al. (2000). Growth hormone (GH) secretion in patients with an inactivating defect of the GH-releasing hormone (GHRH) receptor is pulsatile: Evidence for a role for non-GHRH inputs into the generation of GH pulses. J Clin Endocrinol Metab. 86:2459–2464.

126. Pandya N, DeMott-Friberg R, Bowers CY et al. (1998). Growth hormone (GH)-releasing peptide-6 requires endogenous hypothalamic GH-releasing hormone for maximal GH stimulation. J Clin Endocrinol Metab. 83:1186–1189.

127. Guillaume V, Magnan E, Cataldi M et al. (1994). Growth hormone (GH)-releasing hormone secretion is stimulated by a new GH-releasing hexapeptide in sheep. Endocrinology. 135:1073–1076.

128. Veldhuis JD, Evans WS, Bowers CY. (2002). Impact of estradiol supplementation on dual peptidyl drive of growth-hormone secretion in postmenopausal women. J Clin Endocrinol Metab. 87:859–866.

129. Pombo M, Barreiro J, Penalva A et al. (1995). Absence of growth hormone (GH) secretion after the administration of either GH-releasing hormone (GHRH), GH-releasing peptide (GHRP-6), or GHRH plus GHRP-6 in children with neonatal pituitary stalk transection. J Clin Endocrinol Metab. 80:3180–3184.

130. Wideman L, Weltman JY, Patrie JT et al. (2000). Synergy of L-arginine and growth hormone (GH)-releasing peptide-2 (GHRP-2) on GH release: Influence of gender. Am J Physiol. 279:R1455–R1466.

131. Wideman L, Weltman JY, Patrie JT et al. (2000). Synergy of L-arginine and GHRP-2 stimulation of growth hormone (GH) in men and women: Modulation by exercise. Am J Physiol. 279:R1467–R1477.

132. Micic D, Popovic V, Kendereski A et al. (1995). Growth hormone secretion after the administration of GHRP-6 or GHRH combined with GHRP-6 does not decline in late adulthood. Clin Endocrinol. 42:191–194.

133. Mueller EE, Cella SG, Parenti M et al. (1995). Somatotropic dysregulation in old mammals. Horm Res. 43:39–45.

134. Mayo KE, Godfrey PA, Suhr ST et al. (1995). Growth hormone-releasing hormone: Synthesis and signaling. Rec Prog Horm Res. 50:35–73.

135. Frohman LA. (1996). New insights into the regulation of somatotrope function using genetic and transgenic models. Metabolism. 45:1–3.

136. Bowers CY. (2001). Unnatural growth hormone-releasing peptide begets natural ghrelin. J Clin Endocrinol Metab. 86:1464–1469.

137. Muller AF, Lamberts SW, Janssen JA et al. (2002). Ghrelin drives GH secretion during fasting in man. Eur J Endocrinol. 146:203–207.

138. Berman M, Jaffe CA, Tsai W et al. (1994). Negative feedback regulation of pulsatile growth hormone secretion by insulin-like growth factor I: Involvement of hypothalamic somatostatin. J Clin Invest. 94:138–145.

139. Harel Z, Tannenbaum GS. (1992). Synergistic interaction between insulin-like growth factors-I and -II in central regulation of pulsatile growth hormone secretion. Endocrinology. 131:758–764.

140. Chomczynski P, Downs TR, Frohman LA. (1988). Feedback regulation of growth hormone releasing hormone gene expression by growth hormone in the rat hypothalamus. Mol Endocrinol. 2:236–241.

141. Massoud AF, Hindmarsh PC, Brook CG. (1995). Hexarelin induced growth hormone release is influenced by exogenous growth hormone. Clin Endocrinol. 43:617–621.

142. Chapman IM, Hartman ML, Pezzoli SS et al. (1997). Effect of aging on the sensitivity of growth hormone secretion to insulin-like growth factor-I negative feedback. J Clin Endocrinol Metab. 82:2996–3004.

143. Ghigo E, Arvat E, Valente F. (1991). Arginine reinstates the somatotrope responsiveness to intermittent growth hormone-releasing hormone administration in normal adults. Neuroendocrinology. 54:291–294.

144. Anderson SM, Wideman L, Patrie JT et al. (2002). Estradiol supplementation selectively relieves growth hormone (GH)'s autonegative feedback on GH-releasing peptide-2 (GHRP-2)-stimulated GH secretion. J Clin Endocrinol Metab. 86:5904–5911.

145. Richmond E, Rogol AD, Basdemir D et al. (2002). Accelerated escape from GH autonegative feedback in midpuberty in males: Evidence for time-delimited GH-induced somatostatinergic outflow in adolescent boys. J Clin Endocrinol Metab. 87:3837–3844.

146. Farhi LS, Straume M, Johnson ML et al. (2001). A construct of interactive feedback control of the GH axis in the male. Am J Physiol. 281: R38–R51.

147. Farhy LM, Straume M, Johnson MJ et al. (2002). Unequal autonegative feedback by growth hormone (GH) models the sexual dimorphism in GH secretory dynamics. Am J Physiol. 282:R753–R764.

148. Robinson ICAF. (1991). The growth hormone secretory pattern: A response to neuroendocrine signals. Acta Paediatr Scand (Suppl). 372:70–78.

149. Clark RG, Jansson JO, Isaksson OGP, Robinson ICAF. (1985). Intravenous growth hormone: Growth responses to patterned infusions in hypophysectomized rats. J Endocrinol. 104:53–61.

150. Zeitler P, Tannenbaum GS, Clifton DK, Steiner RA. (1991). Ultradian oscillations in somatostatin and growth hormone-releasing hormone mRNAs in the brains of adult male rats. Proc Natl Acad Sci U S A. 88:8920–8924.

151. Veldhuis JD, Liem AY, South S et al. (1995). Differential impact of age, sex-steroid hormones, and obesity on basal versus pulsatile growth hormone secretion in men as assessed in an ultrasensitive chemiluminescence assay. J Clin Endocrinol Metab. 80:3209–3222.

152. Hindmarsh PC, Dennison E, Pincus SM et al. (1999). A sexually dimorphic pattern of growth hormone secretion in the elderly. J Clin Endocrinol Metab. 84:2679–2685.

153. Veldhuis JD, Evans WS, Shah N et al. (1999). Proposed Mechanisms of Sex-steroid Hormone Neuromodulation of the Human GH-IGF-I Axis. In Sex-Steroid Interactions with Growth Hormone (Veldhuis JD, Giustina A, eds.), pp. 93–121. New York: Springer-Verlag.

154. Bray MJ, Vick TM, Shah N et al. (2001). Short-term estradiol replacement in postmenopausal women selectively mutes somatostatin's dose-dependent inhibition of fasting growth hormone secretion. J Clin Endocrinol Metab. 86:3143–3149.

155. Mulligan T, Jaen-Vinuales A, Godschalk M et al. (1999). Synthetic somatostatin analog (octreotide) suppresses daytime growth hormone secretion equivalently in young and older men: Preserved pituitary responsiveness to somatostatin's inhibition in aging. J Am Geri Soc. 47:1422–1424.

156. Veldhuis JD, Evans WS, Bowers CY, Anderson S. (2001). Interactive regulation of the postmenopausal growth hormone insulin-like growth factor axis by estrogen and growth hormone-releasing peptide-2. Endocrine. 14:45–62.

157. Granda-Ayala R, Bowers CY, Parulkar A et al. (2000). Continuous infusion of GHRP-2 for 30 days in elderly GH deficient subjects. Southern Society for Clinical Investigation, Abstract #84.

158. Chapman IM, Bach MA, Cauter EV et al. (1996). Stimulation of the growth hormone (GH)-insulin-like growth factor I axis by daily oral administration of a GH secretagogue (MK-0677) in healthy elderly subjects. J Clin Endocrinol Metab. 81:4249–4257.

159. Penalva A, Pombo M, Carballo A et al. (1993). Influence of sex, age, and adrenergic pathways on the growth hormone response to GHRP-6. Clin Endocrinol. 38:87–91.

160. Loche S, Colao A, Cappa M et al. (1997). The growth hormone response to hexarelin in children: Reproducibility and effect of sex steroids. J Clin Endocrinol Metab. 82:861–864.

161. Bellone J, Aimaretti G, Bartolotta E et al. (1995). Growth hormone-releasing activity of hexarelin, a new synthetic hexapeptide, before and during puberty. J Clin Endocrinol Metab. 80:1090–1094.

162. Arvat E, Ramunni J, Bellone J et al. (1997). The GH, prolactin, ACTH and cortisol responses to Hexarelin, a synthetic hexapeptide, undergo different age-related variations. Eur J Endocrinol. 1237:635–642.

163. Van den Berghe G, Baxter RC, Weekers F et al. (2000). A paradoxical gender dissociation within the growth hormone/insulin-like growth factor I axis during protracted critical illness. J Clin Endocrinol Metab. 85:183–192.

164. Shah N, Evans WS, Bowers CY, Veldhuis JD. (1999). Tripartite neuroendocrine activation of the human growth-hormone (GH) axis in women by continuous 24-hour GH-releasing peptide (GHRP-2) infusion: Pulsatile, entropic, and nyctohemeral mechanisms. J Clin Endocrinol Metab. 84:2140–2150.

165. Shah N, Evans WS, Bowers CY, Veldhuis JD. (2000). Oral estradiol administration modulates continuous intravenous growth hormone (GH)-releasing peptide-2 driven GH secretion in postmenopausal women. J Clin Endocrinol Metab. 85:2649–2659.

166. Kamegai J, Wakabayashi I, Kineman RD, Frohman LA. (1999). Growth hormone-releasing hormone receptor (GHRH-R) and growth hormone secretagogue receptor (GHS-R) mRNA levels during postnatal development in male and female rats. J Neuroendocrinol. 11:299–306.

167. Chihara K, Minamitani N, Kaji H et al. (1981). Intraventrically injected growth hormone stimulates somatostatin release into rat hypophyseal portal blood. Endocrinology. 109:2279–2281.

168. Aguila MC, Boggaram V, McCann SM. (1993). Insulin-like growth factor-I modulates hypothalamic somatostatin through a growth hormone releasing factor increased somatostatin release and messenger ribonucleic acid levels. Brain Res. 625:213–218.

169. Katakami H, Arimura A, Frohman LA. (1986). Growth hormone (GH)-releasing factor stimulates hypothalamic somatostatin release: An inhibitory feedback effect on GH secretion. Endocrinology. 118:1872–1877.

170. Stachura ME, Tyler JM, Farmer PK. (1988). Combined effects of human growth hormone (GH)-releasing factor-44 (GRF) and somatostatin (SRIF) on post-SRIF rebound release of GH and prolactin: A model for GRF-SRIF modulation of secretion. Endocrinology. 123:1476–1482.

171. Turner JP, Tannenbaum GS. (1995). In vivo evidence of a positive role for somatostatin to optimize pulsatile growth hormone secretion. Am J Physiol. 269:E683–E690.

172. Buscail L, Delesque N, Esteve JP et al. (1994). Stimulation of tyrosine phosphatase and inhibition of cell proliferation by somatostatin analogues: Mediation by human somatostatin receptor subtypes SSTR1 and SSTR2. Proc Natl Acad Sci U S A. 91:2315–2319.

173. Argente J, Chowen BJ, Steiner RA, Clifton DK. (1990). Somatostatin messenger RNA in hypothalamic neurons is increased by testosterone through activation of androgen receptors and not by aromatization to estradiol. Neuroendocrinology. 52:342–349.

174. Thorner MO, Vance ML, Hartman ML et al. (1990). Physiological role of somatostatin on growth hormone regulation in humans. Metabolism. 39: 40–42.

175. Shah N, Evans WS, Veldhuis JD. (1999). Actions of estrogen on the pulsatile, nyctohemeral, and entropic modes of growth hormone secretion. Am J Physiol. 276:R1351–R1358.

176. Evans WS, Anderson SM, Hull LT et al. (2001). Continuous 24-hour intravenous infusion of recombinant human growth hormone (GH)-releasing hormone-(1,44)-amide augments pulsatile, entropic, and daily rhythmic GH secretion in postmenopausal women equally in the estrogen-withdrawn and estrogen-supplemented states. J Clin Endocrinol Metab. 86:700–712.

177. Veldhuis JD, Straume M, Iranmanesh A et al. (2001). Secretory process regularity monitors neuroendocrine feedback and feedforward signaling strength in humans. Am J Physiol. 280:R721–R729.

178. Veldhuis JD, Roemmich JN, Rogol AD. (2000). Gender and sexual maturation-dependent contrasts in the neuroregulation of growth-hormone (GH) secretion in prepubertal and late adolescent males and females. J Clin Endocrinol Metab. 85:2385–2394.

179. Merimee TJ, Bergess JA, Rabinowitz D. (1966). Sex-determined variation in serum insulin and growth hormone response to amino acid stimulation. *J Clin Endocrinol Metab*. 26:791–793.

180. Evans WS, Bowers CY, Veldhuis JD. (2001). Estradiol supplementation enhances pituitary sensitivity to recombinant human (RH) GHRH-1, 44-amide in somatostatin (SS) withdrawn postmenopausal women. 83rd Annual Meeting of Endocrine Society, Abstract #P2–174.

181. Bertherat J, Timsit J, Bluet-Pajot M-T *et al*. (1993). Chronic growth hormone (GH) hypersecretion induces reciprocal and reversible changes in mRNA levels from hypothalamic GH-releasing hormone and somatostatin neurons in the rat. *J Clin Invest*. 91:1783–1791.

182. Tannenbaum GS. (1980). Evidence for autoregulation of growth hormone secretion via the central nervous system. *Endocrinology*. 107:2117–2120.

183. Patel Y. (1979). Growth hormone stimulates hypothalamic somatostatin. *Life Sci*. 24:1589–1594.

184. Pellegrini E, Bluet-Pajot MT, Mounier F *et al*. (1996). Central administration of a growth hormone (GH) receptor mRNA antisense increases GH pulsatility and decreases hypothalamic somatostatin expression in rats *J Neurosci*. 16:8140–8148.

185. Clark RG, Carlsson LMS, Robinson ICAF. (1987). Growth hormone secretory profiles in conscious female rats. *J Endocrinol*. 114:399–407.

186. Jansson J-O, Eden S, Isaksson OGP. (1985). Sexual dimorphism in the control of growth hormone secretion. *Endocr Rev*. 6:128–150.

187. Gevers E, Pincus SM, Robinson ICAF, Veldhuis JD. (1998). Differential orderliness of the GH release process in castrate male and female rats. *Am J Physiol*. 274:R437–R444.

188. Painson JC, Veldhuis JD, Tannenbaum GS. (2000). Single exposure to testosterone in adulthood rapidly induces regularity in the growth hormone release process. *Am J Physiol*. 278:E933–E940.

189. Gabrielsson BG, Carmignac DF, Flavell DM, Robinson ICAF. (1995). Steroid regulation of growth hormone (GH) receptor and GH-binding protein messenger ribonucleic acid in the rat. *Endocrinology*. 136:209–217.

190. Evans WS, Sollenberger MJ, Booth RA Jr *et al*. (1992). Contemporary aspects of discrete peak detection algorithms. II. The paradigm of the luteinizing hormone pulse signal in women. *Endocr Rev*. 13:81–104.

191. Goodyear CG, Stephano LD, Lai WH, Guyda HJ. (1984). Characterization of insulin like growth factor receptors in rat anterior pituitary hypothalamus and brain. *Endocrinology*. 114:1187–1195.

192. Korbonits M, Little JA, Camacho-Hubner C *et al*. (1996). Insulin-like growth factor-I and -II in combination inhibit the release of growth hormone releasing hormone from the rat hypothalamus *in vitro Growth Regul*. 6:110–120.

193. Hartman ML, Clayton PE, Johnson ML *et al*. (1993). A low dose euglycemic infusion of recombinant human insulin-like growth factor I rapidly suppresses fasting-enhanced pulsatile growth hormone secretion in humans. *J Clin Invest*. 91:2453–2462.

194. Sjogren K, Liu J-L, Blad K *et al*. (1999). Liver-derived insulin-like growth factor I (IGF-I) is the principal source of IGF-I in blood but is not required for postnatal body growth in mice. *Proc Natl Acad Sci U S A*. 96:7088–7092.

195. Veldhuis JD, Bidlingmaier M, Anderson SM *et al*. (2001). Lowering total plasma IGF-I concentrations by way of a novel, potent and selective GH-receptor antagonist, pegvisomant (B2036-PEG), augments the amplitude of GH secretory bursts and elevates basal/nonpulsatile GH release in healthy women and men. *J Clin Endocrinol Metab*. 86:3304–3310.

196. Domene HM, Marin G, Sztein J *et al*. (1994). Estradiol inhibits growth hormone receptor gene expression in rabbit liver. *Mol Cell Endocrinol*. 103:81–87.

197. Carmignac DF, Gabrielsson BG, Robinson ICAF. (1993). Growth hormone binding protein in the rat: Effects of gonadal steroids. *Endocrinology*. 133:2445–2452.

198. Friend KE, Hartman ML, Pezzoli SS *et al*. (1996). Both oral and transdermal estrogen increase growth hormone release in postmenopausal women—a Clinical Research Center study. *J Clin Endocrinol Metab*. 81:2250–2256.

199. Anderson SM, Shah N, Patric JT *et al*. (2000). Short term estradiol supplementation augments growth hormone (GH)-secretory responsiveness to dose-varying growth hormone-releasing peptide (GHRP-2) infusions in postmenopausal women. *J Clin Endocrinol Metab*. 86:551–560.

111
The Principle Syndromes of Dementia

DAVID KNOPMAN, MD

Professor of Neurology, Mayo Medical School, Consultant Mayo Clinic, Rochester, MN

Dementia is a common disorder in the elderly affecting both men and women with virtually no regard for the victim's gender. In the coming decades, dementia will continue to increase in prevalence as the numbers of elders increases. The diagnosis of dementia can be difficult as it emerges ordinary aging. Apart from other medical and neurologic conditions, however, the symptoms of dementia must be disentangled from the view held by lay people and physicians alike that growing old is synonymous with memory loss. Pervasive and worsening problems with cognition cannot be dismissed as simply representing aging. Thus, the great challenge in diagnosing dementia is recognizing the symptoms as distinct from the forgetting and mistakes that occur in everyday life.

I. The Definition of Dementia

Dementia is a syndrome defined by a subacute or insidious decline in cognition from a previously higher level [1]. The specificity of the diagnosis of dementia is enhanced by requiring that the patient's cognitive and behavioral deficits interfere "significantly" with daily function and independence.

Dementia, in contrast to disorders defined by deficits in only one cognitive or behavioral domain, is diagnosed when there are deficits in multiple domains. Some diagnostic criteria require three dysfunctional areas [2], whereas the *Diagnostic and Statistical Manual of Mental Disorders*, 4th Edition (DSM–IV) [1] and National Institute of Neurological, Communicative Disorders and Stroke—Alzheimer's Disease and Related Disorders Association (NINCDS-ADRDA) [3] criteria require only memory impairment plus one other cognitive or behavioral deficit to diagnose dementia. In addition to memory dysfunction, the other cognitive and behavioral manifestations of the dementia syndrome include abnormalities in speech/language, visuo-spatial function, abstract reasoning/executive function, and mood/personality.

Alzheimer's disease (AD) is the most common cause of dementia in the elderly. As a consequence, memory dysfunction in the form of frequent repeating of questions, forgetting of recent events and conversations, and misplacing of items are the most common symptoms of dementia that clinicians are likely to encounter.

The criteria for dementia resulting from AD from DSM-IV [1] and NINCDS-ADRDA [3] should not be considered as criteria for other forms of dementia. Disorders such as fronto-temporal dementia (FTD), primary progressive aphasia (PPA), or dementia with prominent visuo-spatial disorder have their own distinctive primary deficits and may not exhibit profound recent memory disturbances initially. Impaired judgment and dramatic changes in personality may be the initial manifestations of an FTD. Disturbances of language and speech are the initial manifestations of the progressive aphasias. In neither of these latter disorders will difficulties with learning new material be prominent.

Dementia is usually a disorder of the elderly but middle-aged and rarely younger adults may be affected. Cognitive aging and dementia are not synonymous nor does young age invalidate the use of the term dementia.

II. Alzheimer's Disease—The Prototypical Dementia with Prominent Anterograde Amnesia

A. Diagnostic Considerations

Alzheimer's disease is the most common of the dementias in the elderly in North America and Western Europe. Alzheimer's disease can be diagnosed clinically with confidence in a patient with the gradual and progressive impairment of recent memory and dysfunction in at least one other cognitive or behavioral domain [3].

Many clinical-pathologic studies have addressed the diagnostic accuracy of the clinical diagnosis of AD [4–14]. The mean sensitivity of the diagnosis of probable AD in these studies was 81% with a range of 49 to 100%. The mean specificity of the diagnosis of probable AD was 70% with a range of 47 to 100% [15].

In most instances in routine clinical practice, the diagnostic criteria of the NINCDS-ADRDA workgroup yield an accurate view of the diagnosis of AD [15]. When AD as a diagnosis is not correctly recognized (false negative), it is often because of atypical cognitive profiles or patterns of evolution. When AD is given as the clinical diagnosis erroneously (false positive), it is often because other pathologic entities in fact share considerable clinical similarity to AD.

1. Presentation of Alzheimer's Disease

Disturbances in recent memory function are the typical symptoms that lead to the suspicion and eventual diagnosis of AD. Patients repeat themselves in conversation, re-ask the same question, or forget recent conversations [16–19]. The symptoms may be so insidious in onset that they may be ignored or misinterpreted by family caregivers or physicians as insignificant, "normal aging," or depression. Patients with AD usually ignore their own shortcomings and deny or minimize their deficits [20–23]. Symptoms are typically present for 1 to 3 years before family members bring the patient to medical attention. Loss of the ability to carry out key daily tasks such as shopping, handling money, or doing chores around the house may be more powerful triggers than forgetfulness for seeking medical attention. Neuropsychiatric symptoms are more likely to prompt an evaluation than forgetfulness itself.

A deficit in memory is the hallmark of the cognitive disorder in AD. More precisely it is a deficit in new learning and encoding of information [18,24–27]. Although the ability to retrieve information from long-term memory is eventually impaired in AD, the important diagnostic feature is the deficit in new learning. It is sometimes referred to as short-term memory. Operationally, recall of information after a 5-minute delay is the measure of new learning in AD patients. In most patients with AD, memory complaints are the dominant set of symptoms. Memory complaints account for many of the symptoms that caregivers report [28].

Orientation is clearly impaired in patients with AD. Given the ubiquitous nature of impairment of orientation in dementia, as well as its ease of assessment, reference to orientation among the core deficits of dementia would seem warranted. To the extent that orientation is mediated by memory, attention, language, visuo-spatial function, and even executive functions, its impairment is a proxy for dysfunction in one or more of those domains.

Disturbances of language function, aphasia, are frequently seen in AD. Observational studies show that dementia patients exhibit deficits in naming [29,30] and word fluency at mild stages of disease [30,31].

Disturbances of visuo-spatial synthesis are well recognized symptoms in some AD patients [32–38].

Impairment of executive functions and attention may be demonstrable neuropsychologically in early AD [39–42], and the consequences of deficits in problem-solving, judgment, foresight and mental agility lead to loss of competence in daily living [43].

The spectrum of changes is protean, ranging from increased apathy and social withdrawal to disinhibition or irritability [44–50]. Recognition of the affective and behavioral symptoms of dementia should increase diagnostic sensitivity. So long as some other cognitive deficits are present, the inclusion of this domain should not reduce specificity of the diagnosis of dementia.

2. Age of Onset

There are some clinical features of the disease that co-vary with age. For example, the autosomal dominant form of AD occurs almost exclusively among those with very young age of onset. The effects of some susceptibility genes, such as APOE, have a strong age dependence. Clinically, several studies have shown that patients younger than age 65 to 70 years tend to have slightly different clinical presentations, either in terms of faster rates of progression or more language deficits at the time of diagnosis [51–55]. However, even if such differences are present in group analyses, age-related differences are hardly ever detectable on an individual basis [54].

3. Natural History

The natural history of AD is considerably variable from one individual to the next, but there are some approximate values that can be applied to the different phases of the illness. The average length of time from onset of symptoms until diagnosis is about 2 to 3 years [56–60]. The average duration of time from diagnosis to nursing home placement (a marker of severe dementia) is roughly 3 to 6 years [57,61–67]. Alzheimer's disease patients spend 3 years in nursing homes before death [68]. Thus, the total duration of AD is roughly 9 to 12 years.

A large number of studies have examined rate of progression of AD within the symptomatic phase using mental status examinations such as the mini-mental state examination (MMSE). Across patients whose initial MMSE scores ranged from 10 to 26, the average rate of change per year is about 3 points [69–75]. The variability is considerable as indicated by the standard deviation of ~4 of this value [70,76]. The rate of decline follows a curvilinear relationship to the initial cognitive test scores [77,78]. Faster rates of decline occur in the mid-portions of the scales, and slower rates occur among milder and more severe patients. Moreover, a decline over one 6-month or 1-year period does not predict the rate of decline over a subsequent time interval [75].

There are few predictors of rate of progression, but parkinsonian signs, hallucinations, and delusions have been shown to be associated with more rapid decline [79–81]. This set of observations are consistent with recent findings that patients with dementia with Lewy bodies have a faster rate of decline than comparably demented AD patients [82].

Another way of conceptualizing the progression of AD is to look at the time to reach key milestones of the disease such as deteriorating to a clinical dementia rating (CDR) of 3 or losing basic activities of daily living skills. In one large study of carefully diagnosed AD patients [83], these values can be used to discuss prognostic issues with families.

Mortality in AD averages less than 10% per year [56,57, 64,84–90]. Median survival for patients with AD is roughly 5 to 6 years [84,91–95]. Causes of death in AD include pneumonia, sepsis, and other common causes of mortality in the elderly such as cardiovascular disease and stroke [87,96]. Mortality in dementia is almost invariably worse for men than for women [84,93,97].

B. Stages of Alzheimer's Disease

1. Presymptomatic Phase

Currently, it is not possible to identify presymptomatic individuals who are at risk to develop AD except for those very rare individuals from families with known autosomal dominant AD. Several studies have shown that, in retrospect, individuals destined to develop AD are cognitively inferior, as a group, to those not destined to develop AD [98–104]. The group differences are not distinctive enough to be of use in prediction in individual instances, however.

2. Mild Cognitive Impairment

Between the state of normal cognitive and functional abilities and that of mild but definite dementia is a diagnostic grey zone that is now referred to as mild cognitive impairment (MCI) [100]. Others have referred to this state as possible dementia prodrome or very mild AD [16]. The term age-associated memory impairment appears to describe a similar group of patients, but the memory impairment is not age-associated but rather is disease-associated. Mild cognitive impairment is often a precursor of AD but not always [100,105]. Approximately 15% of MCI (or comparably defined) patients deteriorate and qualify for a diagnosis of AD per year [100,106–108]. Patients with MCI are sometimes identified because they are discovered coincidentally to have poor performance on mental status testing. Sometimes patients with MCI refer themselves to physicians because of concerns about their own memory. Mild cognitive impairment is an important condition to recognize not because it is itself a disease but rather because it is a risk-state for subsequently developing AD [109].

Diagnostic criteria [100] for MCI include a memory complaint, objective evidence of impaired recent memory, intact daily function, and intact nonmemory cognitive functions. The lack of significant impairment in functioning in daily affairs is perhaps the major distinction between early dementia and MCI. Individuals with MCI as defined previously show memory impairment comparable to AD patients but have scores on most nonmemory neuropsychologic tests that are comparable to normal elderly individuals [110].

As implied by the statistic of rate of conversion, not all MCI patients go on to develop AD. Thus, some individuals with the features of MCI have a static condition rather than a deteriorating one. Some of these individuals presumably have had impaired memory on a life-long basis. Others may have sustained brain injuries at an earlier age that have produced static dysfunction. Thus, the category of MCI, as currently conceptualized, is heterogeneous with respect to prognosis for future decline. Mild cognitive impairment is also heterogeneous with respect to the cognitive deficit that is most impaired. Some individuals may have predominantly language, visuo-spatial, or executive deficits, although memory deficits characterize most MCI individuals [111]. Attempts are ongoing to identify the subset of MCI patients who will invariably go on to AD. One predictor that has emerged is an increasing level of dysfunction in daily affairs as reported by an informant but not by the patient [112]. Hippocampal atrophy on magnetic resonance (MR) imaging together with neuropsychologic features hold considerable promise for identifying MCI patients who are at risk to progress to AD within a few years [113,114]. A study of patients with a syndrome nearly identically defined as MCI showed that positron emission tomography (PET) imaging abnormalities of the Alzheimer type (i.e., parietal hypometabolism) was usually seen in MCI patients who converted to AD during the follow-up period [115].

3. Mild Alzheimer's Disease

The syndrome of mild AD (which is CDR stage 1 [116] or GDS stages 3 or 4 [117]) is characterized by clear-cut deficits in recent memory, deficits in at least one of the other cognitive domains, and loss of functional independence. Functional loss might take the form of difficulties with financial affairs, difficulties with geographic orientation in their own homes and other familiar places [118], or an inability to do tasks such as those in one's job or around the home. Their ability to recall information from the past is often only minimally impaired at this stage of the illness. Changes in personality frequently are part of the presentation of mild AD. The spectrum of personality changes is protean, ranging from increased apathy and social withdrawal to disinhibition or irritability [44–50]. Depression also is common and can exacerbate cognitive deficits [119–121]. Paranoia and obsessions may become evident, although these are more likely to occur in later stages of the disease. Frank hallucinations and delusions occasionally occur in mild AD.

On mental status examination, patients with mild AD score between 20 and 26 on the MMSE. Memory performance may be the most abnormal portion of the cognitive examination. Patients recall nil after a short delay [18,24–26,122]. A mild AD patient may have largely intact conversational comprehension and spontaneous speech. However, mild patients and their families report word-finding difficulties that can be observed with naming tests that use less common objects [29,30]. Abstract reasoning deficits may be detectable with more difficult tasks that require mental agility to manipulate sequential mental tasks. However, prior intellectual and occupational achievement strongly affect how well a mild AD patient will do with naming or abstract reasoning. Most patients with mild AD have some constructional difficulties. On more detailed neuropsychologic testing, widespread deficits in visuo-spatial processing are often observed [32,123].

The motor neurologic examination is typically normal in patients with mild AD. Some subtle extrapyramidal signs may be seen [79,124,125].

4. Moderate Alzheimer's Disease

Patients with moderate AD (CDR stage 2) not only are dependent on others for higher level daily living activities such as finances, shopping, or transportation but may on occasion need to be reminded to bathe and to dress appropriately. Moderate AD patients may fail to recognize acquaintances that are not part of the patient's daily retinue. Patients at this stage of AD should no longer operate motor vehicles or devices such as lawn movers, power saws, or probably even stoves and ranges. Neuropsychiatric disturbances may become prominent. Delusions and hallucinations are common. Patients often begin to misrecognize their own homes as "home." Irritability and paranoia are common symptoms of moderate AD. Disrupted sleep may also occur.

On mental status examinations with the MMSE, moderately severe AD patients score between 10 and 19. Patients at this stage have word- and name-finding deficits that are obvious in conversation. Information or recent events are often almost instantly forgotten. Motor apraxia may be evident at this stage of AD [126].

If patients with moderate AD have reasonably competent spouse or child caregivers, they can often remain in the family residence. If not, moderate AD patients may need supervised living situations. Some assistance almost always becomes needed for solo caregivers in the later stages of moderate AD.

Even at this stage of the illness, the motor neurologic examination may be normal except for signs of mild rigidity or bradykinesia [79,124].

5. Severe Alzheimer's Disease

Patients with severe AD (CDR stage 3) need 24-hour supervision. They have negligible memory for events, conversations, and, unfortunately, even close family members. They have substantial word finding difficulties. Their spontaneous speech is impoverished. They may be virtually mute, or they may use jargon-filled speech that conveys no meaningful information

[127]. They need extensive assistance with bathing, dressing, eating, and toileting. They are more likely than milder patients to become aggressive when offered assistance with undressing or toileting, although some severe patients are very docile. Despite their fragmentary cognition, severely demented patients may experience depression, anxiousness, and fear. They typically score below 10 on the MMSE [127,128].

A minority of AD patients experience generalized seizures [129,130], often in the severe stage of the disease. Patients may also exhibit marked rigidity, bradykinesia, gait and balance difficulties, and masked facies [124,131].

C. The Lack of a Laboratory Marker to Confirm the Diagnosis

The diagnosis of AD cannot be verified with a laboratory test at present. A reliable noninvasive or minimally invasive marker of the brain neuropathology of AD is sorely needed. Criteria for evaluating future diagnostic markers have recently been formulated [132].

Structural neuroimaging with magnetic resonance imaging has the greatest potential for use in the diagnosis of AD [133–139]. Hippocampal atrophy [133,134] is increased substantially in AD, but there is overlap with nonimpaired elderly. Serial measurements of brain volume on neuroimaging may differentiate normal elderly from those with AD [135]. The high degree of technical precision needed to carry out such measurements may not be practical in the routine clinical diagnosis of AD. Magnetic resonance imaging can detect small infarctions that may have been clinically silent [140,141]. It is not clear whether identification of small infarctions has diagnostic value for estimating the burden of vascular pathology relevant to dementia.

Cerebrospinal fluid (CSF) markers lack diagnostic precision at present, but there may be instances in which abnormalities that appear specific for AD such as depressed levels of ABeta-42 and increased levels of tau or the AD7C protein will increase diagnostic certainty [142–146].

Genotyping for diagnostic purposes has been of intense interest since the discovery of the AD-APOE link [147,148]. APOE exhibits three allelic variations in humans. In AD patients, there is a disproportionate representation of the epsilon-4 (e4) allele compared with nondemented populations [147,148]. An early study claimed that, if a dementia patient possessed at least one APOE e4 allele, the probability that they had AD was extremely high [149,150]. This claim was subjected to a further test in 1170 patients with neuropathologically confirmed diagnoses [10]. Indeed the value of the presence of an APOE e4 allele was that 90% of those patients proved to have AD neuropathologically. On the other hand, among patients who were APOE e4 negative, 69% of those also had AD neuropathologically. Assuming that a competent clinical diagnostic assessment has already been completed, this study suggests that the addition of APOE testing increases diagnostic accuracy for a diagnosis of AD by about 4% if an APOE e4 allele is present (from 90 to 94%), and for a diagnosis of not-AD if an APOE e4 is absent by 8% (from 64 to 72%). The absence of APOE e4 allele increased specificity from 55 to 70.6% compared with the clinical diagnosis. For some patients, families, and physicians, this increase in diagnostic certainty may be desirable, whereas,

in most instances, it will be unnecessary. APOE testing also raises a number of other management issues such as genetic counseling that may complicate, rather than complement, the initial diagnostic approach [151–154].

D. Epidemiology of Dementia and Alzheimer's Disease

1. Prevalence

Prevalence refers to the number of cases in a population at any one time. The prevalence of dementia and AD increases with advancing age [155–165]. There is considerable consistency across recent prevalence surveys in North America and Europe, especially when case-finding methods for mild dementia is similar [166]. In 65 to 69 year olds the prevalence of dementia is approximately 1 per 100 individuals. With each subsequent 5-year increment, the prevalence of dementia and AD doubles [166]. Over age 85 years, estimates of the prevalence of dementia vary between 20% to nearly 50% [155–165]. Beyond age 85, it appears that dementia prevalence continues to rise. Some earlier studies found a decrease above this age, but most recent studies have confirmed that the proportion of individuals with dementia continues to rise over this age.

2. Incidence

The incidence of dementia, that is, the number of newly diagnosed cases in a certain time interval, also rises dramatically with advancing age [164,167–173]. The number of new cases of dementia, mainly AD, begins to exceed 1 per 100 individuals per year as early as the early seventies to the early eighties. It is not until the late seventies or mid-eighties that the rate of new cases reaches 2 per 100 individuals per year. The differences in definitions of dementia account for the variability in estimates of incidence rates between studies, with those studies using definitions that admit milder cases showing the higher incidence rates. Because patients with dementia tend to live for several years to as long as a decade or more, incidence rates are considerably lower than prevalence rates.

3. Gender

Most prevalence and incidence studies have shown a consistently higher rate of dementia in women over men [167]. This could represent a true biologic effect. Because of the excess premature mortality of males beginning at approximately age 45 years, the decreased survival of men could differentially influence the enumeration of men with dementia. In Rochester, Minnesota, perhaps because of the way that cases are ascertained, there was no increased risk for AD among women [174].

4. Conditions That Are Associated with Increase Risk for Alzheimer's Disease

Despite a large number of studies devoted to the detection of risk factors for dementia, only a few characteristics clearly increase an individual's risk for developing dementia. The two most prominent are advancing age and a family history of dementia. Genetic factors are covered in the next section. The remainder of this section is devoted to several characteristics that might potentially be risk factors.

Very low educational achievement (<eighth grade education) has been a consistently observed but modestly potent risk factor that increases a person's odds of developing AD by 2- to 3-fold [161,173,175–180]. There may be a threshold effect for education so that studies that do not include large numbers of subjects with less than an eighth-grade education may not detect the association [181]. Even when diagnostic methods are specifically modified to reduce educational or cultural biases, the education effect remains [177]. Snowdon and colleagues [182] have shown that cognitive performance at age 20 years was predictive of the subsequent development of dementia roughly 50 years later. Their hypothesis is that early life experiences contribute to the development of brain reserve. Increased numbers of neurons presumably acts as a buffer in ameliorating the deleterious effects of AD pathology. In general, enriched childhood environments will be associated with higher educational attainment, but in Snowdon's view it is the sum of all enriching experiences, not the least of which is good childhood nutrition, that protects from the subsequent development of dementia.

Cardiovascular disease confers a small to moderate increased risk for AD [159,183–187]. The cardiovascular risk factors associated with AD include atherosclerosis broadly defined, history of stroke, history of midlife hypertension, and carotid artery disease.

Several studies have shown that elevated homocysteine appears is associated with AD [188–191]. The most compelling study to date measured homocysteine levels in initially non-demented individuals [188]. Those individuals who subsequently became demented had higher levels of homocysteine at the baseline measurement.

The relationship between head injury and AD [192–195] has been the subject of serious concerns about recall bias among caregivers of diagnosed dementia patients. Because the putative head injury could have occurred 30 years before the development of dementia, prospective studies that allow minimization of recall bias have not yet been done. However, because of the link between boxing and AD [196,197], the importance of non-sport related head trauma to AD seems plausible. Mayeux *et al* [198] have proposed that the risk of head trauma for AD is mediated by APOE e4 genotype.

Occupational exposure to industrial solvents and agricultural chemicals have not shown consistent increases in risk for AD [199]. The evidence against aluminum [200–203] as a risk factor for AD outweighs suggestions [204,205] of a possible role for aluminum. Recent neuropathologic studies find no difference between AD and control brains in aluminum content, especially when exquisite attention is paid to analytic techniques [203,206]. In case control study comparing regions with high versus low aluminum levels in drinking water, the risk for AD in the high aluminum region was only trivially increased [202,207,208], except for one study [209].

5. Protective Factors

Interestingly, more success has been achieved in identifying factors that might protect against the subsequent development of AD. Several protective factors have been observed in incidence cohorts.

One is estrogen replacement therapy (ERT) [210–214]. The finding has been very consistent across studies and persisted even when socioeconomic status, education, and the presence of other health-promoting activities are factored in. However, doubt has been cast on the validity of the protective effects of estrogen with the publication of negative clinical trials of ERT in patients with AD [215,216].

The use of nonsteroidal anti-inflammatory agents (NSAIDs) [217–221] has also consistently been observed. In addition to simply showing an association with any use, a prospective, population-based epidemiologic study has shown that longer usage of NSAID use decreased risk for AD [222].

The use of statin-type cholesterol lowering drugs has been added to this list of agents that are associated with a lower risk of AD [223–225]. However, in a clinical trial of statins for secondary prevention of cardiovascular disease [226], statin therapy had no impact on cognition.

Cigarette smoking has appeared in most studies as a protective factor for AD [227–230], although in other studies it has been a risk factor [231–233]. Intuitively, it would appear more likely to be a risk factor because of its association with vascular disease. However, the putative mechanism by which smoking could be protective is via stimulation of nicotinic receptors in the brain. Nicotinic receptors on cholinergic neurons might mediate the production of trophic factors that promote survival of key neuronal populations in AD [234].

E. Genetics of Alzheimer's Disease

Family history of dementia is an important risk factor for the subsequent development of AD [235,236]. A large multicenter study that involved nearly 1700 patients found that the lifetime risk to first-degree relatives of clinically diagnosed AD patients was approximately 15% by age 80 years and 39% by age 96 years [235]. Women relatives were at greater risk for AD than men in this study. By age 93 years, women had a 13% higher risk than men. However, before age 70 the male to female difference was negligible. In another study [237], both African-American and white first-degree relative women had slightly greater risk for developing AD compared with men.

An additional genetic association of interest is between AD and Down syndrome. Bearing a child with Down syndrome is associated with an increased risk for AD in the mothers if they were younger than age 35 at the birth of the Down syndrome child [238].

There are two patterns of genetic risk for AD. One is through autosomal dominant transmission of mutations in one of three genes. The other pattern of genetic risk for AD is mediated by susceptibility genes, of which only one, the APOE gene, has been identified with certainty.

About 30 to 40% of early onset AD has been shown to be due to mutations in either the Alzheimer precursor protein (APP) located on chromosome 21, the presenilin 1 (PS1) gene located on chromosome 14, and its homolog presenilin 2 (PS2) located on chromosome 1 [239,240]. Approximately 150 families have been identified worldwide with mutations in one of these three genes.

The families with mutations in these genes have shown considerable consistency. The age of onset of affected individuals is in the 30- to 50-year range, with only some of the PS1 families showing a slightly later age of onset [241]. The clinical features of the dementia is generally indistinguishable from sporadic

AD [242,243]. Neuropathologically, the PS1, PS2, and APP genetic forms of AD appear similar by neuropathologic analysis except that the genetic forms of AD show greater severity [244]. All of the genetic forms of AD also result in overproduction of the amyloid beta (Abeta) peptide [245,246].

The families with APP mutations were the first to be identified [247]. Five mutations have been observed in APP [248]. The link between AD and Down syndrome anticipated the finding of the APP gene on chromosome 21. The extra dose of a chromosome 21 with the APP gene appears to accelerate the neuropathology of AD in Down syndrome patients, such that they demonstrate the pathology of AD roughly 30 years earlier than individuals with a normal number of chromosome 21 [249]. Mutations in this gene are quite rare [250].

The PS1 gene mutations causing autosomal dominant AD were the next to be linked to autosomal dominant AD [251]. A large number of mutations have been found [248,252]. PS1 is the most common gene involved in autosomal dominant AD.

PS2 mutations were first identified in one ethnic group, those of German descent who had emigrated to the western United States and Canada after residing in the Volga region of Russia in the 18th to 19th centuries [253]. The PS2 gene is approximately 70% homologous to the PS1 gene. PS2 mutations are much less common than ones in PS1.

Late-onset familial AD is mediated through susceptibility genes. APOE was the first of these genes to be identified. APOE is a lipid carrying protein present in serum and tissues [254]. In humans it is found in three allelic variations that differ from one another by two amino acid substitutions at positions 112 and 158. In Caucasian populations, the e3 allele is most common, whereas the other two variations e2 and e4 are less common [255]. In other ethnic groups, such as those of African descent, more individuals possess the e4 allele than in individuals of European descent [256]. Corder and colleagues [147] and Poirier and colleagues [148] independently showed that the e4 allele was substantially over-represented among AD patients. The observation has been replicated repeatedly. The homozygous state carries the most risk, mainly between the ages of 60 and 80 [256]. The heterozygous state is associated with a lower risk but between the same age range. Beyond these ages, the risk associated with APOE e4 declines. That the APOE e4 allele is a risk factor and not a typical autosomal dominant disease causing gene is illustrated by the roughly 50% cumulative incidence of AD in APOE e4 homozygotes in population studies [257–259]. Among individuals with the APOE genotype e3/e4, there was a slight increased risk for AD among women (odds ratio of 1.5). There were no other consistent interactions between gender and APOE genotypes.

Linkage to a gene or genes on chromosome 10 has been replicated in different datasets [260–262], making this gene the second susceptibility gene for AD. Prospects for the discovery of other susceptibility genes are good, although several candidate genes have not achieved replication to date.

III. Vascular Dementia: The Dementias Associated with Stroke

Cerebrovascular disease is very common in the elderly [263]. Dementia associated with stroke was previously referred to as multi-infarct dementia, but, more recently, the term vascular dementia (VaD) has been adopted. Hachinski [264] has suggested that even the name is misleading: he suggests "vascular cognitive impairment" as a more encompassing label than vascular dementia. The term *vascular dementia* is used here, acknowledging that *dementia* may be too restrictive a term for the range of cognitive dysfunction that occurs with stroke.

A. Diagnosis

Diagnostic criteria for VaD [1,265,266] first require that dementia be present as already defined. The key features that go into a clinical diagnosis of VaD are a strong temporal relationship between a stroke and dementia onset or worsening, neuroimaging evidence of bilateral or critical location infarctions, and focal neurologic signs on examination consistent with cerebrovascular disease lesions. There are several sets of consensus diagnostic criteria for VaD that embody these ideas. The NINDS-AIREN criteria [266] are the ones used in clinical trials. A more operational approach to the diagnosis of VaD can be found in the use of the Ischemic Scale [267]. The Hachinski Ischemic Scale has been validated neuropathologically [268,269]. A shortened form of it is widely used in clinical trials for its ability to exclude patients with vascular features. A serious deficiency in the Hachinski Ischemic scale is the lack of reference to imaging; silent cerebrovascular disease that may be etiologically important can often be documented only on imaging [141,270].

An important clue to the diagnosis of VaD is the temporal relationship between a documented stroke and the onset of cognitive impairment [271–274]. Abrupt onset of cognitive impairment is supportive of the diagnosis of VaD but by itself is not diagnostic [269]. The shorter the time difference between the two, the more likely it is that VaD is a serious diagnostic possibility. The more unlinked in time between the two, the less likely it is that the stroke was etiologically related to dementia.

The pleomorphic nature of VaD contributes to its definitional and diagnostic problems. Dementia resulting from a series of large cortical infarctions will have substantially different clinical manifestations than dementia resulting from arteriolar infarctions (lacunar infarctions) in the striatum and thalamus. The clinical deficits depend on location of the infarctions. Multiple lacunar infarctions may produce a pattern of cognitive impairment that is similar to FTD, because of the deafferentation and de-efferentation of the prefrontal regions by the subcortical infarctions [275]. Subcortical ischemic vascular disease, previously known as Binswanger's disease in its severest form, is due to both infarction of white matter plus arteriolar infarctions [276]. There is no unique cognitive profile of VaD [277]. Claims to the contrary lacked pathologic verification.

B. Neuroimaging in Vascular Dementia

The NINDS-AIREN criteria provide guidelines for what amount of infarct burden is sufficient for dementia [266]. These guidelines were generated by expert judgment rather than empiric studies, so there is some arbitrariness to them. Thus, it is a subjective judgment as to how much infarction—its volume, location, and degree of bilaterality—on neuroimaging is sufficient to make a diagnosis of VaD. The NINDS-AIREN criteria state that bilateral lesions of the cerebral cortex or deep grey matter structures of the cerebral hemispheres should be present for a diagnosis of VaD. Imaging changes in the white matter have also been difficult to link to clinical importance for VaD specifically as such lesions may also be seen in AD [278–282]. Features of white matter lesions on MR that are thought to be specific for VaD include confluent, "diffuse and extensive" hyperintensities on T2-weighted images and the presence of vascular-like lesions on T1-weighted images [266,280,283]. The VaD syndrome labeled as Binswanger's disease has extensive, confluent white matter lesions. White matter hyperintensities on MR images in nondemented individuals have been associated with cardiovascular risk factors, especially hypertension [284–287] and with lower scores on cognitive tests [285,288]. It is important to recall that not all cerebral infarctions are associated with clinical stroke events. Neuroimaging, especially with MR, plays an invaluable role in the diagnosis of VaD, because it detects infarcts that were clinically silent [141,270].

C. Epidemiology

Rates of VaD in clinical or epidemiologic contexts vary considerably. Studies in dementia clinics yield very low numbers of VaD patients [289]. Epidemiologic studies report proportions of VaD among prevalent dementia cases from a low of 5% [156] to as high as 40% [290]. Recent studies using consistent but defensible diagnostic criteria have found that VaD comprises 15 to 20% of prevalent dementias [155,156,158,163,165,291]. Proportions in incident cases is approximately the same [169,292–294]. In an autopsy study that drew from a population-based sample, the rate of pure VaD was 11% [4]. There are no gender-specific differences in the prevalence of VaD.

D. Treatment and Management

Clinical trials of anti-AD drugs in patients meeting NINDS-AIREN criteria for VaD (either probable VaD or AD with cerebrovascular disease) have shown that cholinesterase inhibitors (CEIs) were superior to placebo in cognitive assessments over 6 months [295].

Recognition of vascular disease in the setting of dementia has other therapeutic implications. Because individuals are occasionally found to have cerebral infarctions without antecedent clinical history [140,141], detection of "silent" infarctions in a dementia patient might prompt treatment with antiplatelet drugs. It might also induce a more careful look at other stroke risk factors such as hypertension, smoking, or possible embolic sources. Finally, the diagnosis of VaD might imply a lower genetic risk for dementia resulting from AD.

IV. The Dementias Associated with Extrapyramidal Features

Extrapyramidal signs are very common in the elderly [296]. Parkinson's disease itself is also common in the elderly. In roughly 30% of individuals with Parkinson's disease, dementia develops [297–299]. The proportion of patients with Parkinson's disease who are cognitively impaired is likely to be

under-recognized because of the overwhelming problems with the motor disturbances. Recognition of dementia in patients with extrapyramidal features is important because management and treatment issues are different from AD.

The most common disorder causing dementia associated with extrapyramidal features is one with a newly minted name, "dementia with Lewy bodies" (DLB) [300]. Other entities in the differential diagnosis of dementia with extrapyramidal features include progressive supranuclear palsy, corticobasal degeneration, striatonigral degeneration, Huntington's disease, and Wilson's disease.

A. Clinical Syndrome of Dementia with Lewy Bodies

The diagnostic criteria for DLB [300] include gait and balance disturbances, dementia, prominent visual hallucinations and delusions, fluctuations in cognitive status or arousal, sensitivity to dopaminergic blocking drugs such as first-generation antipsychotics, and other less consistently seen symptoms and signs.

The cognitive disorder differs in only subtle ways from that of AD [301,302]. Patients with DLB have slightly better recall [303,304] but somewhat worse executive functions than do AD patients. Patients with DLB have some of the cognitive deficits seen in FTDs, but they also have memory deficits and apathy. Both AD and DLB have impairment of visuo-spatial processing and constructions, but DLB patients may be slightly worse.

Fluctuations in levels of consciousness, alertness, and cognition also occur with DLB. Although AD patients are typically described as having good days and bad days, DLB patients seem to experience more dramatic variations in their status. An attractive hypothesis is that the fluctuations in DLB arise as a result of pathology in the arousal systems of the brain, that in turn give rise to disorders of night-time sleep (rapid eye movement [REM] sleep behavior disturbance) [305] and disorders of daytime arousal (fluctuations in mental focus or arousal) [306].

The visual hallucinations in DLB patients are dramatic, elaborate, and often quite outrageous. Delusional thinking often occurs. It is tempting to attribute the visual hallucinations to intrusion of REM sleep into wakefulness, as part of the pervasive disorder of arousal seen in DLB.

The diagnostic criteria proposed by the consensus conference on DLB [300] appear to imperfect sensitivity and specificity [4,307–312]. Among five non-population-based studies [308–312], the sensitivity of the clinical diagnostic criteria for DLB was low (58%, range 34 to 75%), although specificity was good (87%, range 71 to 94%). Recent clinical-pathologic studies have also failed to confirm a difference in pathology between patients with Parkinson's disease with dementia occurring greater than 1 year after the onset of the movement disorder versus patients meeting the DLB criteria in which the cognitive disorder occurred within 1 year of the onset of the parkinsonism [313].

B. Epidemiology

In the Framingham study [155], dementia with extrapyramidal features occurred in 7.7% of cases in an epidemiologic sample. We can infer that most of those patients may have had DLB. In autopsy series DLB (including both AD with Lewy bodies plus

Lewy body dementia lacking AD pathology) accounted for 25.5% of cases and ranked behind AD as the second most common dementing disorder [9]. The 3-fold discrepancy between epidemiologic and the neuropathologic estimates of DLB suggest that the spectrum of clinical manifestations of Lewy body pathology is too similar to AD to be distinguished. Alternatively, clinical assessments of patients with dementia fail to examine for subtle extrapyramidal findings or disturbances of arousal, both of which will lead to under-recognition of DLB. There are no gender-specific differences in the prevalence of DLB, although the problems with diagnosis make it possible that some true differences could be present but not detectable by current methods.

C. Treatment and Management

The diagnosis of dementia with extrapyramidal features has important management implications. First, antipsychotics such as haloperidol or thioridazine should be assiduously avoided in these individuals. Whether the disorder is due to DLB or progressive supranuclear palsy (PSP) predisposes the patient to dramatic worsening of the extrapyramidal signs and symptoms. Newer antipsychotics such as quetiapine and olanzapine that lack the dopaminergic blocking properties of traditional agents hold promise for treating the agitation that occurs in dementia with extrapyramidal features. Second, caregivers should be aware that hallucinations and delusions are quite common, but they can be successfully treated. Third, the impaired postural stability and tendency to fall should prompt extra supervision and aggressive use of L-dopa therapy in these patients. Finally, there appears to be a role for cholinomimetic agents in DLB [314].

V. The Fronto-temporal Dementias

The FTDs are much less common than either AD, VaD, or dementia associated with Parkinsonism. Fronto-temporal dementia is the preferred label for this clinical-pathologic entity because the FTDs encompass a broader neuropathologic spectrum than just Pick's disease. Fronto-temporal dementia is diagnosed on the basis of historical and mental status examination evidence of disproportionate impairment of reasoning and judgment relative to anterograde amnesia [315]. Primary progressive aphasia is a disorder with prominent expressive language disturbance relative to anterograde amnesia that shares the same neuropathologic differential diagnosis as FTD. Their clinical features are discussed separately, but the neuropathologic description of the two is combined.

A. Clinical Syndrome of Fronto-temporal Dementia

Patients with the behavioral-dysexecutive form of FTD have a disturbance of behavior, reasoning, and judgment. The term *dysexecutive syndrome* has been applied to the cognitive syndrome of patients with FTD who have grossly disturbed abstract reasoning, poor judgment, and reduced mental flexibility [315–318]. Behavioral disturbances are particularly prominent and may be erroneously attributed to primary psychiatric diseases. Patients may become very withdrawn and may be treated for depression to no avail. Alternatively, patients may become socially inappropriate, excessively ebullient, or inappropriately aggressive or may get themselves into trouble because of grossly impaired judgment. A misdiagnosis of the manic phase of bipolar disorder might be made in these instances.

Diagnostic criteria for FTD from a recent consensus conference [315] involve yet another attempt to standardize the diagnosis of FTD. The diagnostic criteria reflect the cognitive and behavioral characteristics of FTD observed in pathologically verified cases. The two dominant modes of presentation of FTD are that of a dramatic change in social comportment or that of a loss of intellectual ability. In the former case, patients with FTD show loss of empathy to the feelings of others, social withdrawal, and generally act out of prior character in interpersonal relationships. Cognitive testing in these individuals may reveal only subtle deficits. Other FTD patients present not so much with flamboyance or oddness but rather with histories of losing jobs because of cognitive difficulties. These cognitive difficulties take the form of impaired concentration, impaired organizational skills, failure to solve previously tractable problems, and an obvious loss of mental agility.

Psychometric testing plays an essential role in the diagnosis of FTD because the bedside mental status examination lacks sensitivity for early signs of executive dysfunction. Tests such as Trailmaking, the Wisconsin Card sorting task, digit symbol substitution, verbal fluency, and the Stroop task may all show impairment [319]. Neuroimaging may show evidence of frontal or anterior temporal atrophy, although not in all cases, especially early in the disease [320]. Functional imaging with single photon emission computed tomography (SPECT) or PET may be more sensitive for the early diagnosis of FTD [321–325], but there are still limited data on the actual clinical utility of functional imaging in the differential diagnosis of dementia and FTD.

Primary progressive aphasia is a disorder with similar pathology to FTD. The distinctive features of PPA, in contrast to AD, are the relative excess of dysfunction of language and the relative paucity of anterograde amnesia or other cognitive deficits [182,326–329]. The most common variant is a nonfluent type. In that disorder, conversational speech is nonfluent, hesitant, and filled with stammering and pauses for word finding. Comprehension is affected but sometimes only to a minor degree. Other cognitive functions may be difficult to test because of the speech disturbance, but, early in PPA, these other functions may be spared including affect and behavior. The mental status examination and the history of deficits are pivotal in the diagnosis of PPA. Patients with PPA are often misdiagnosed as having suffered a stroke, a diagnosis that becomes untenable as the patient continues to deteriorate. There is variability in the extent to which progressive aphasia progresses to global dementia. Progression to global dementia as an outcome of PPA is not a certainty, but it is likely.

A variant of progressive aphasia, often referred to as semantic dementia [330], is distinct in that speech is fluent, but their access to the meaning of words, objects, or faces is impaired. Whereas patients with the nonfluent PPA are often frustrated in their speaking, patients with semantic dementia are particularly unconcerned. Semantic dementia patients often have evidence of cognitive dysfunction in terms of judgment and reasoning abilities, and resemble FTD patients in these respects. Patients with semantic dementia often have deficits in visuo-spatial synthesis, emphasizing the overlapping nature of deficits that is possible.

As with FTDs, patients with PPA may show focal atrophy on structural imaging, especially of the dominant hemisphere's peri-Sylvian region. Similarly functional imaging may detect hypometabolism in that region. Neither feature is necessary for the diagnosis, however.

B. Epidemiology

There is limited data on the prevalence or incidence of FTD, because of its rarity and to concerns about accurate diagnosis. In autopsy series, the FTDs make up as few as 1% to as many as 10% of cases [9,320,331–334]. These disorders appear to be relatively more prevalent in younger dementia patients and less common in populations containing large numbers of individuals older than age 70 years. There are no gender-specific differences in the prevalence of FTD or PPA, although, once again, the rarity of disorders means that current information is incomplete.

C. Treatment and Management

Correct diagnosis of the FTDs spares the patient from futile attempts to treat depression or mania. If PPA patients are incorrectly diagnosed with stroke, they may be unnecessarily subjected to carotid angiography or surgery. Although a diagnosis of FTD carries the prognosis of inexorable decline, families of FTD patients appreciate the more accurate prognostication that comes with the proper diagnosis. When FTD patients are treated and labeled as AD, misdiagnosis becomes obvious to families who see how different their relative is from AD patients. The agitation that occurs in FTD patients may be treated in the same manner as AD patients. Nonpharmacologic behavior management is often sufficient to control the disruptive behaviors in FTD patients once the caregivers understand the nature of FTD.

Patients with PPA are managed quite differently from AD. Because their recent memory is not severely impaired, they may be given more independence than the typical AD patient.

VI. Creutzfeldt-Jakob Disease

Creutzfeldt-Jakob disease (CJD) is the prototypical neurologic disease that produces a rapidly progressive dementia. Most CJD patients are deceased in less than 1 year. The diagnosis of CJD is established based on the rapid onset of cognitive impairment. The dementia of CJD is pleomorphic. Anterograde amnesia, major affective disturbances, major behavioral disturbances, or progressive visual agnosia are common syndromes that may herald the onset of CJD. Global cognitive impairment rapidly ensues within months of onset. Creutzfeldt-Jakob disease is usually accompanied by motor deficits (cerebellar, pyramidal, or extrapyramidal) and eventually by seizures and electroencephalographic abnormalities [335]. The initial and subsequently appearing features of CJD include a dementia of variable nature and motor deficits of the cerebellar, extrapyramidal, or extraocular type. Diagnosis can be established with moderately high confidence on clinical grounds. However, autopsy confirmation is the gold standard. There should be no impediment to autopsy simply because of the suspicion of CJD.

Diagnostic aids include the electroencephalography (EEG), CSF examination, and MR scanning. The EEG is of limited value at the time of presentation. A CSF protein known as 14-3-3 has been found to have high predictive accuracy for CJD [336–338]. Its diagnostic failures (false positives) occurred in patients with acute strokes and viral encephalitis. Because these two disorders sometimes figure into the differential diagnosis of rapidly progressive dementia, the CSF immunoassay for the 14-3-3 protein might be most useful in subacute syndromes with very low stroke probability and no CSF pleocytosis. Some false-negative results also occurred, but the experience with the test is promising. Cerebrospinal fluid pleocytosis is very rare in CJD and should be considered as a strong indication that another process rather than CJD is present. Magnetic resonance abnormalities have been recognized in the past several years as valuable in diagnosis [339]. Magnetic resonance abnormalities on diffusion imaging that may also be seen with T2-weighted images include increased signal from subcortical grey matter and cortical ribbon structures. These findings are highly specific though somewhat insensitive, presumably earlier in the course of the disease [339]. Any other imaging abnormalities should suggest alternative diagnoses. At least 90% of patients have periodic electroencephalographic abnormalities eventually [340], but the detection level values are lower: 67% sensitivity at 86% specificity [341].

Creutzfeldt-Jakob disease generally behaves as a sporadic illness. The mechanism by which CJD develops in sporadic cases is unknown. The yearly incidence is about 1 case per million [335]. Cases of human to human transmission are well known to have occurred from dural transplants, a corneal transplant, and treatment with growth hormone extract [335]. New variant CJD has appeared in the United Kingdom in association with the bovine spongiform encephalopathy epidemic [342]. These patients are younger, have sensory complaints, and a have a somewhat more protracted course than the typical CJD patients. Whether the identification of these cases is the result of heightened interest in the disease or represents a truly new variant is unclear.

VII. Structural Brain Lesions and Dementia

Brain tumors, chronic subdural hematomas, and normal pressure hydrocephalus (NPH) make up this group of disorders. In general, brain tumors and chronic subdural hematomas are associated with relatively short courses before coming to medical attention. Furthermore, they are usually accompanied by other neurologic signs and symptoms—headaches, seizures, or motor disturbances—beyond dementia [343]. The justification for routine neuroimaging in newly diagnosed dementia patients is based on the empiric observations that tumors and subdural hematomas may rarely occur without other signs [344,345].

A. Normal Pressure Hydrocephalus

Normal pressure hydrocephalus is rare [343]. Most patients presenting with dementia and ventricular enlargement do not benefit from shunting. A population survey in the Netherlands estimated that 1 case in 2.2 million population per year respond successfully to shunt placement [346]. Despite these difficulties, diagnosis and treatment of an NPH patient can lead to gratifying results [347]. A recent study from a dementia clinic that served all of Denmark noted that most cases of dementias thought to be treatable represented NPH (15 or 18 potentially reversible dementias among 432 consecutive dementia cases) [348].

The clinical triad of NPH includes a gait disorder, dementia, and urinary incontinence. The gait disorder is one in which patients are unable to initiate gait, as if their feet are "glued to the floor." Patients with NPH also tend to have a wide base. In contrast, while sitting or laying, they are able to demonstrate the movements used in walking, for example, making a bicycling movement while laying on their backs. The terms "gait apraxia" or "magnetic gait" describe the locomotion problem in NPH. The gait disorder may be the symptom that is most predictive of a good response to shunting [349]. The dementia of NPH is nonspecific, but it is usually mild in patients who best respond to shunting. If there is any pattern to the dementia, it is characterized by apathy and a fronto-temporal pattern to the cognitive deficits. Urinary incontinence is probably the least reliable diagnostic feature of NPH. The incontinence occurs spontaneously, and patients may have no symptoms of urgency preceding the episodes of urination. Hydrocephalus on computed tomography (CT) or MR is necessary to consider the diagnosis. In addition to enlarged lateral and third ventricles, periventricular white matter hypointensity (on CT) or increased T2 signal (on MR) is usually seen. Short duration of dementia, less than 2 years, is also more likely to be associated with a beneficial response to shunting [349,350].

Normal pressure hydrocephalus is almost always idiopathic in origin, although hydrocephalic symptoms may occur following recovery from meningitis, subarachnoid hemorrhage, head injury, or some other process that leads to obstruction of CSF pathways. Patients with symptomatic hydrocephalus (i.e., after central nervous system [CNS] infections or subarachnoid hemorrhage) tend to respond more reliably than patients with no antecedent causal events.

The confirmation of the diagnosis of NPH by laboratory testing is inadequate, and clinical suspicion remains the strongest grounds for considering the diagnosis. Ventricular enlargement without cortical atrophy is suggestive of NPH but is highly nonspecific. Other tests have been proposed—measurement of CSF flow void in the aqueduct by MR, radioisotope cisternography, removal of more than 20 cc of CSF by lumbar puncture [351], resistance to CSF outflow [352], and various measurements of the third and lateral ventricles relative to the fourth ventricle—that all lack predictive power for identifying which patients will respond to shunting.

Treatment of NPH consists of the placement of a ventricular-peritoneal shunt neurosurgically. There are no pharmacologic therapies for NPH. In considering neurosurgical treatment of NPH, acute and chronic complications of shunting such as hemorrhage, infection, or shunt malfunction must be kept in mind.

VIII. Pharmacotherapy of Alzheimer's Disease

In the last few years, the number of potential therapeutic targets for AD has grown dramatically. The number of therapies for which there is actual clinical trial data has also been growing. The story is changing rapidly enough in this aspect of AD treatment that textbook treatments such as this one are likely to outdate within 6 to 12 months of their publication. Prevention, disease modification, or cure are future goals of anti-AD therapies. At the present, only palliative therapies exemplified by the CEIs are available.

A. Cholinesterase Inhibitors

The relevance of the cholinergic deficit in AD was reviewed in the section on pathogenesis of AD. Cholinesterase inhibitor drugs represent the only U.S. Food and Drug Administration (FDA)-approved primary treatment options for AD as of 2002. Based on theoretical and empiric grounds, CEI therapy is a reasonable, palliative approach to symptomatic AD [353].

Donepezil, rivastigmine, and galantamine are available by prescription in the United States. Tacrine [354] was the first of the CEIs to be marketed, but its short half-life and hepatotoxicity foiled its chances for success. Donepezil [355,356], rivastigmine [357,358], and galantamine [359,360] have been shown to have cognitive and clinical benefits in mild to moderate AD patients. The consistent efficacy shown with CEIs shows that the entire class of agents has similar effects on the symptoms of AD. In the clinical trials of the CEIs, the primary outcome measures have been the Alzheimer's Disease Assessment Scale-Cognitive section (ADAS-cog) [361] and some form of a Clinician's Global Rating scale [362,363]. Compared with the placebo groups, the ADAS-cog change over 24 to 30 weeks have ranged from slightly less than 3 points to about 5 points. For the global assessments [362,363], the 24- to 30-week ratings have yielded about 0.25 to 0.50 point improvement (where 3 points would be the maximal improvement) compared with the placebo groups. The MMSE change scores relative to placebo have ranged between 1 to 2 points.

In the clinical trials that were approximately 6 months in duration, the differences between the placebo treated patients and the CEI patients have fallen in a range of 2.5 to 5 points on the ADAS-cog [361]. The ADAS-cog is a widely used mental status assessment instrument that has been the standard in AD clinical trials over the years. From natural history studies and the clinical trials themselves, the drug-placebo differences correspond to about 6 to 9 months of delay of symptoms. Support for this general time frame as standing for the magnitude of the CEI effect size comes from open-label long-term extension studies with donepezil [364]. In these long-term extension studies, the group of patients treated with CEI had higher test scores on the ADAS-cog on follow-up compared with baseline until approximately 35 to 40 weeks of treatment. In contrast, the placebo groups in the earlier portions of the same studies declined below their baseline assessments of the ADAS-cog in about 6 weeks.

There are considerable differences in pharmacology between the various CEIs, but the differences in plasma half-life, mechanism of cholinesterase inhibition, mechanism of degradation, and so forth do not appear to distinguish the agents [357,365–368]. Gastrointestinal (GI) side effects such as nausea, diarrhea, and anorexia have been the most frequent type of adverse events that limit use of the CEIs. The GI side effects appear dose-dependent not pharmacology-dependent.

Although the cognitive effects in clinical trials correspond roughly in magnitude to the cognitive decline experienced by mildly to moderately demented AD patients over 6 to 9 months in natural history studies, extrapolation of these group effects on cognitive measures to improvements in the functioning of individual patients can be problematic. Indeed, substantial functional improvement is unusual with currently available CEIs. There also remains uncertainty about the duration of benefit of CEIs because these compounds have not been studied prospectively in controlled trials beyond about 6 months. Open-label studies of longer duration show about the same magnitude of effect as predicted by the 6-month studies [61].

B. Strategies Aimed at β-amyloid Processing

The production of the Abeta peptide is a key pathogenic event in AD. The Abeta peptide may be produced depending on the balance between three secretases that cleave the Alzheimer precursor protein into different fragments. Inhibition of either beta- or gamma-secretase is an obvious strategy aimed at reducing Abeta production. Initial human studies of beta- or gamma-secretase inhibitors are in phase I testing or on the verge of phase II investigations. Important questions about safety must of course first be answered. Concerns exist that the gamma secretase inhibitors may also affect notch signaling. Notch is a nuclear signaling receptor that could be involved in hematopoiesis [369]. Ultimately, if these agents prove to be safe, trials meant to prove efficacy will have to be designed and executed. Whether these will involve studies in symptomatic AD patients, those at risk for AD (MCI-type trials), or simply aged individuals (i.e., a prevention strategy) remains to be seen.

C. Antioxidants

The potential for antioxidant therapy in AD is another active area of investigation, based mainly on the neurochemical evidence of oxidative injury in the AD brain. Tocopherol is a fat-soluble substance that blocks lipid peroxidation and is the most widely used antioxidant. There is an extensive literature on α-tocopherol supporting its role as an antioxidant, with *in vitro* evidence of improved cell survival in the presence of toxins, including Abeta peptide [370]. On the other hand, there is no evidence of tocopherol deficiency in AD brain.

A clinical trial using the antioxidants selegiline (5 mg bid) and α-tocopherol (vitamin E) (1000 IU bid) was the first to report convincing benefits of this modality [371]. In this study, the median delay in appearance of the study endpoints of severe dementia was about 8 months, compared with the placebo group. There was no indication of superior improvement with the combination of tocopherol and selegiline. These preliminary findings, coupled with the very favorable safety and cost profile of α-tocopherol, suggest that it can be recommended to most patients with AD. The only safety concern with α-tocopherol is that it may exacerbate coagulopathies in some individuals. Although 1000 IU twice a day was well tolerated, it is not known whether lower doses are equally effective.

The modest success of α-tocopherol supports for the hypothesis that treatment with antioxidants represent a valid approach to the treatment of AD [353]. More potent antioxidants are needed. Furthermore, investigations of presymptomatic treatment with antioxidants are needed.

IX. Suggestions for Further Investigations

- Therapeutics: Since this chapter was written, memautine, a glutamate modulator, has been approved for the treatment of AD.
- Imaging: Refinement of quantitative MR imaging continues. Imaging of amyloid in the brains of AD patients is also coming closer to fruition.
- Genetics: Identification of genes that increase the risk for AD will continue to be a high priority.

Acknowledgement

This chapter is based on one entitled "Dementia" by D. Knopman that appears in *Baker's Clinical Neurology* (Joynt R, Griggs R eds.). Philadelphia: Lippincott, Williams & Wilkins, Philadelphia, 2002.

Dr. Knopman has served as a paid consultant to Pfizer Pharmaceuticals on one occasion and Bristol-Myers-Squibb on one occasion in the past 2 years. He participated in clinical trials sponsored by Lilly and Cortex.

References

1. American Psychiatric Association. (1994). *Diagnostic and Statistical Manual of Mental Disorders*, 4th Edition. Washington DC: American Psychiatric Association.
2. Cummings JL, Benson DF. (1992). *Dementia: A Clinical Approach*, 2nd Edition. Boston: Butterworths.
3. McKhann G, Drachman D, Folstein M *et al.* (1984). Clinical diagnosis of Alzheimer's disease: Report of the NINCDS-ADRDA Work Group under the auspices of Department of Health and Human Services Task Force on Alzheimer's Disease. *Neurology*. 34:939–944.
4. Holmes C, Cairns N, Lantos P, Mann A. (1999). Validity of current clinical criteria for Alzheimer's disease, vascular dementia and dementia with Lewy bodies. *Br J Psychiatry*. 174:45–50.
5. Jobst KA, Barnetson LP, Shepstone BJ. (1998). Accurate prediction of histologically confirmed Alzheimer's disease and the differential diagnosis of dementia: The use of NINCDS-ADRDA and DSM-III-R criteria, spect, X-ray CT, and apo E4 in medial temporal lobe dementias. Oxford Project to Investigate Memory and Aging. *Int Psychogeriatr*. 10:271–302.
6. Lim A, Tsuang D, Kukull W *et al.* (1999). Clinico-neuropathological correlation of Alzheimer's disease in a community-based case series. *J Am Geriatr Soc*. 47:564–569.
7. Wade JP, Mirsen TR, Hachinski VC *et al.* (1987). The clinical diagnosis of Alzheimer's disease. *Arch Neurol*. 44:24–29.
8. Victoroff J, Mack WJ, Lyness SA, Chui HC. (1995). Multicenter clinico-pathological correlation in dementia. *Am J Psychiatry*. 152:1476–1484.
9. Galasko D, Hansen LA, Katzman R *et al.* (1994). Clinical-neuropathological correlations in Alzheimer's disease and related dementias. *Arch Neurol*. 51:888–895.
10. Mayeux R, Saunders AM, Shea S *et al.* (1998). Utility of the apolipoprotein E genotype in the diagnosis of Alzheimer's disease. Alzheimer's Disease Centers Consortium on Apolipoprotein E and Alzheimer's Disease. *N Engl J Med*. 338:506–511.
11. Klatka LA, Schiffer RB, Powers JM, Kazee AM. (1997). Incorrect diagnosis of Alzheimer's disease. A clinicopathologic study. *Arch Neurol*. 53:35–42.
12. Blacker D, Albert MS, Bassett SS *et al.* (1994). Reliability and validity of NINCDS-ADRDA criteria for Alzheimer's disease. The National Institute of Mental Health Genetics Initiative. *Arch Neurol*. 51:1198–1204.
13. Gearing M, Mirra SS, Hedreen JC *et al.* (1995). The Consortium to Establish a Registry for Alzheimer's Disease (CERAD). Part X. Neuropathology confirmation of the clinical diagnosis of Alzheimer's disease. *Neurology*. 45:461–466.
14. Berg L, McKeel DW Jr, Miller JP *et al.* (1998). Clinicopathologic studies in cognitively healthy aging and Alzheimer's disease: Relation of histologic markers to dementia severity, age, sex, and apolipoprotein E genotype. *Arch Neurol*. 55:326–335.

15. Knopman DS, DeKosky ST, Cummings JL et al. (2001). Practice parameter: Diagnosis of dementia (an evidence-based review). Neurology. 56:1143–1153.

16. Rubin EH, Morris JC, Grant EA, Vendegna T. (1989). Very mild senile dementia of the Alzheimer type. I. Clinical assessment. Arch Neurol. 46:379–382.

17. Oppenheim G. (1994). The earliest signs of Alzheimer's disease. J Geriatr Psychiatry Neurol. 7:116–120.

18. Petersen RC, Smith GE, Ivnik RJ et al. (1994). Memory function in very early Alzheimer's disease. Neurology. 44:867–872.

19. Koss E, Patterson MB, Ownby R et al. (1993). Memory evaluation in Alzheimer's disease. Caregivers' appraisals and objective testing. Arch Neurol. 50:92–97.

20. Starkstein SE, Sabe L, Chemerinski E et al. (1996). Two domains of anosognosia in Alzheimer's disease. J Neurol Neurosurg Psychiatry. 61:485–490.

21. Lopez OL, Becker JT, Somsak D et al. (1994). Awareness of cognitive deficits and anosognosia in probable Alzheimer's disease. Eur Neurol. 34:277–282.

22. Seltzer B, Vasterling JJ, Yoder JA, Thompson KA. (1997). Awareness of deficit in Alzheimer's disease: Relation to caregiver burden. Gerontologist. 37:20–24.

23. Grut M, Jorm AF, Fratiglioni L et al. (1993). Memory complaints of elderly people in a population survey: Variation according to dementia stage and depression. J Am Geriatr Soc. 41:1295–1300.

24. Knopman DS, Ryberg S. (1989). A verbal memory test with high predictive accuracy for dementia of the Alzheimer type. Arch Neurol. 46:141–145.

25. Welsh K, Butters N, Hughes J et al. (1991). Detection of abnormal memory decline in mild cases of Alzheimer's disease using CERAD neuropsychological measures. Arch Neurol. 48:278–281.

26. Grober E, Kawas C. (1997). Learning and retention in preclinical and early Alzheimer's disease. Psychol Aging. 12:183–188.

27. Storandt M, Botwinick J, Danziger WL et al. (1984). Psychometric differentiation of mild senile dementia of the Alzheimer type. Arch Neurol. 41:497–499.

28. Vitaliano PP, Russo J, Breen AR et al. (1986). Functional decline in the early stages of Alzheimer's disease. Psychol Aging. 1:41–46.

29. Shuttleworth EC, Huber SJ. (1988). The naming disorder of dementia of Alzheimer type. Brain Lang. 34:222–234.

30. Faber-Langendoen K, Morris JC, Knesevich JW et al. (1988). Aphasia in senile dementia of the Alzheimer type. Ann Neurol. 23:365–370.

31. Green J, Morris JC, Sandson J et al. (1990). Progressive aphasia: A precursor of global dementia? Neurology. 40:423–429.

32. Mendez MF, Mendez MA, Martin R et al. (1990). Complex visual disturbances in Alzheimer's disease. Neurology. 40:439–443.

33. Graff-Radford NR, Bolling JP, Earnest FT et al. (1993). Simultanagnosia as the initial sign of degenerative dementia. Mayo Clin Proc. 68:955–964.

34. Levine DN, Lee JM, Fisher CM. (1993). The visual variant of Alzheimer's disease: A clinicopathologic case study. Neurology. 43:305–313.

35. Victoroff J, Ross GW, Benson DF et al. (1994). Posterior cortical atrophy. Neuropathologic correlations. Arch Neurol. 51:269–274.

36. Crystal HA, Horoupian DS, Katzman R, Jotkowitz S. (1982). Biopsy-proved Alzheimer disease presenting as a right parietal lobe syndrome. Ann Neurol. 12:186–188.

37. Hof PR, Bouras C, Constantinidis J, Morrison JH. (1990). Selective disconnection of specific visual association pathways in cases of Alzheimer's disease presenting with Balint's syndrome. J Neuropathol Exp Neurol. 49:168–184.

38. Giannakopoulos P, Gold G, Duc M et al. (1999). Neuroanatomic correlates of visual agnosia in Alzheimer's disease: A clinicopathologic study. Neurology. 52:71–77.

39. Kopelman MD. (1991). Frontal dysfunction and memory deficits in the alcoholic Korsakoff syndrome and Alzheimer-type dementia. Brain. 114:117–137.

40. Kanne SM, Balota DA, Storandt M et al. (1998). Relating anatomy to function in Alzheimer's disease: Neuropsychological profiles predict regional neuropathology 5 years later. Neurology. 50:979–985.

41. Lafleche G, Albert MS. (1995). Executive function deficits in mild Alzheimer's disease. Neuropsychology. 9:313–320.

42. Albert MS, Moss MB, Tanzi R, Jones K. (2001). Preclinical prediction of AD using neuropsychological tests. J Int Neuropsychol Soc. 7:631–639.

43. Marson DC, Cody HA, Ingram KK, Harrell LE. (1995). Neuropsychologic predictors of competency in Alzheimer's disease using a rational reasons legal standard. Arch Neurol. 52:955–959.

44. Mega MS, Cummings JL, Fiorello T, Gornbein J. (1996). The spectrum of behavioral changes in Alzheimer's disease. Neurology. 46:130–135.

45. Devanand DP, Jacobs DM, Tang MX et al. (1997). The course of psychopathologic features in mild to moderate Alzheimer disease. Arch Gen Psychiatry. 54:257–263.

46. Gilley DW, Wilson RS, Beckett LA, Evans DA. (1997). Psychotic symptoms and physically aggressive behavior in Alzheimer's disease. J Am Geriatr Soc. 45:1074–1079.

47. Patterson MB, Mack JL, Mackell JA et al. (1997). A longitudinal study of behavioral pathology across five levels of dementia severity in Alzheimer's disease: The CERAD Behavior Rating Scale for Dementia. The Alzheimer's Disease Cooperative Study. Alzheimer Dis Assoc Disord. 11(Suppl 2):S40–S44.

48. Reisberg B, Borenstein J, Salob SP et al. (1987). Behavioral symptoms in Alzheimer's disease: Phenomenology and treatment. J Clin Psychiatry. 48(Suppl):9–15.

49. Teri L, Larson EB, Reifler BV. (1988). Behavioral disturbance in dementia of the Alzheimer's type. J Am Geriatr Soc. 36:1–6.

50. Reichman WE, Coyne AC, Amirneni S et al. (1996). Negative symptoms in Alzheimer's disease. Am J Psychiatry. 153:424–426.

51. Raskind MA, Carta A, Bravi D. (1995). Is early-onset Alzheimer disease a distinct subgroup within the Alzheimer disease population? Alzheimer Dis Assoc Disord. 9(Suppl 1):S2–S6.

52. Becker JT, Huff FJ, Nebes RD et al. (1988). Neuropsychological function in Alzheimer's disease. Pattern of impairment and rates of progression. Arch Neurol. 45:263–268.

53. Heston LL, Mastri AR. (1982). Age at onset of Pick's and Alzheimer's dementia: Implications for diagnosis and research. J Gerontol. 37:422–424.

54. Huff FJ, Growdon JH, Corkin S, Rosen TJ. (1987). Age at onset and rate of progression of Alzheimer's disease. J Am Geriatr Soc. 35:27–30.

55. Lawlor BA, Ryan TM, Schmeidler J et al. (1994). Clinical symptoms associated with age at onset in Alzheimer's disease. Am J Psychiatry. 151:1646–1649.

56. Walsh JS, Welch HG, Larson EB. (1990). Survival of outpatients with Alzheimer-type dementia. Ann Intern Med. 113:429–434.

57. Knopman DS, Kitto J, Deinard S, Heiring J. (1988). Longitudinal study of death and institutionalization in patients with primary degenerative dementia. J Am Geriatr Soc. 36:108–112.

58. Thal LJ, Grundman M, Klauber MR. (1988). Dementia: Characteristics of a referral population and factors associated with progression. Neurology. 38:1083–1090.

59. Morris JC, Heyman A, Mohs RC et al. (1989). The Consortium to Establish a Registry for Alzheimer's Disease (CERAD). Part I. Clinical and neuropsychological assessment of Alzheimer's disease. Neurology. 39:1159–1165.

60. Galasko D, Klauber MR, Hofstetter CR et al. (1990). The Mini-Mental State Examination in the early diagnosis of Alzheimer's disease. Arch Neurol. 47:49–52.

61. Knopman D, Schneider L, Davis K et al. (1996). Long-term tacrine (Cognex) treatment: Effects on nursing home placement and mortality, Tacrine Study Group. Neurology. 47:166–177.

62. Stern Y, Tang MX, Albert MS et al. (1997). Predicting time to nursing home care and death in individuals with Alzheimer disease. JAMA. 277:806–812.

63. Colerick EJ, George LK. (1986). Predictors of institutionalization among caregivers of patients with Alzheimer's disease. J Am Geriatr Soc. 34:493–498.

64. Brodaty H, McGilchrist C, Harris L, Peters KE. (1993). Time until institutionalization and death in patients with dementia. Role of caregiver training and risk factors. Arch Neurol. 50:643–650.

65. Heyman A, Peterson B, Fillenbaum G, Pieper C. (1997). Predictors of time to institutionalization of patients with Alzheimer's disease: The CERAD experience, part XVII. Neurology. 48:1304–1309.

66. Scott WK, Edwards KB, Davis DR et al. (1997). Risk of institutionalization among community long-term care clients with dementia. Gerontologist. 37:46–51.

67. Severson MA, Smith GE, Tangalos EG et al. (1994). Patterns and predictors of institutionalization in community-based dementia patients. J Am Geriatr Soc. 42:181–185.

68. Welch HG, Walsh JS, Larson EB. (1992). The cost of institutional care in Alzheimer's disease: Nursing home and hospital use in a prospective cohort. J Am Geriatr Soc. 40:221–224.

69. Galasko D, Corey-Bloom J, Thal LJ. (1991). Monitoring progression in Alzheimer's disease. J Am Geriatr Soc. 39:932–941.

70. van Belle G, Uhlmann RF, Hughes JP, Larson EB. (1990). Reliability of estimates of changes in mental status test performance in senile dementia of the Alzheimer type. J Clin Epidemiol. 43:589–595.

71. Katzman R, Brown T, Thal LJ et al. (1988). Comparison of rate of annual change of mental status score in four independent studies of patients with Alzheimer's disease. Ann Neurol. 24:384–389.

72. Kraemer HC, Tinklenberg J, Yesavage JA. (1994). 'How far' vs 'how fast' in Alzheimer's disease. The question revisited. *Arch Neurol.* 51:275–279.

73. Ortof E, Crystal HA. (1989). Rate of progression of Alzheimer's disease. *J Am Geriatr Soc.* 37:511–514.

74. Schneider LS. (1992). Tracking dementia by the IMC and the MMSE. *J Am Geriatr Soc.* 40:537–538.

75. Salmon DP, Thal LJ, Butters N, Heindel WC. (1990). Longitudinal evaluation of dementia of the Alzheimer type: A comparison of 3 standardized mental status examinations. *Neurology.* 40:1225–1230.

76. Knopman D, Gracon S. (1994). Observations on the short-term 'natural history' of probable Alzheimer's disease in a controlled clinical trial. *Neurology.* 44:260–265.

77. Stern RG, Mohs RC, Davidson M *et al.* (1994). A longitudinal study of Alzheimer's disease: Measurement, rate, and predictors of cognitive deterioration. *Am J Psychiatry.* 151:390–396.

78. Morris JC, Edland S, Clark C *et al.* (1993). The consortium to establish a registry for Alzheimer's disease (CERAD). Part IV. Rates of cognitive change in the longitudinal assessment of probable Alzheimer's disease. *Neurology.* 43:2457–2465.

79. Stern Y, Albert M, Brandt J *et al.* (1994). Utility of extrapyramidal signs and psychosis as predictors of cognitive and functional decline, nursing home admission, and death in Alzheimer's disease: Prospective analyses from the Predictors Study. *Neurology.* 44:2300–2307.

80. Chui HC, Lyness SA, Sobel E, Schneider LS. (1994). Extrapyramidal signs and psychiatric symptoms predict faster cognitive decline in Alzheimer's disease. *Arch Neurol.* 51:676–681.

81. Lopez OL, Wisnieski SR, Becker JT *et al.* (1997). Extrapyramidal signs in patients with probable Alzheimer disease. *Arch Neurol.* 54:969–975.

82. Olichney JM, Galasko D, Salmon DP *et al.* (1998). Cognitive decline is faster in Lewy body variant than in Alzheimer's disease. *Neurology.* 51:351–357.

83. Galasko D, Edland SD, Morris JC *et al.* (1995). The Consortium to Establish a Registry for Alzheimer's Disease (CERAD). Part XI. Clinical milestones in patients with Alzheimer's disease followed over 3 years. *Neurology.* 45:1451–1455.

84. Heyman A, Peterson B, Fillenbaum G, Pieper C. (1996). The consortium to establish a registry for Alzheimer's disease (CERAD). Part XIV: Demographic and clinical predictors of survival in patients with Alzheimer's disease. *Neurology.* 46:656–660.

85. Martin DC, Miller JK, Kapoor W *et al.* (1987). A controlled study of survival with dementia. *Arch Neurol.* 44:1122–1126.

86. Katzman R, Hill LR, Yu ES *et al.* (1994). The malignancy of dementia. Predictors of mortality in clinically diagnosed dementia in a population survey of Shanghai, China. *Arch Neurol.* 51:1220–1225.

87. Kukull WA, Brenner DE, Speck CE *et al.* (1994). Causes of death associated with Alzheimer disease: Variation by level of cognitive impairment before death. *J Am Geriatr Soc.* 42:723–726.

88. Bowen JD, Malter AD, Sheppard L *et al.* (1996). Predictors of mortality in patients diagnosed with probable Alzheimer's disease. *Neurology.* 47:433–439.

89. Evans DA, Smith LA, Scherr PA *et al.* (1991). Risk of death from Alzheimer's disease in a community population of older persons. *Am J Epidemiol.* 134:403–412.

90. Barclay LL, Zemcov A, Blass JP, Sansone J. (1985). Survival in Alzheimer's disease and vascular dementias. *Neurology.* 35:834–840.

91. Molsa PK, Marttila RJ, Rinne UK. (1995). Long-term survival and predictors of mortality in Alzheimer's disease and multi-infarct dementia. *Acta Neurol Scand.* 91:159–164.

92. Aguero-Torres H, Fratiglioni L, Guo Z *et al.* (1999). Mortality from dementia in advanced age: A 5-year follow-up study of incident dementia cases. *J Clin Epidemiol.* 52:737–743.

93. Wolfson C, Wolfson DB, Asgharian M *et al.* (2001). A reevaluation of the duration of survival after the onset of dementia. *N Engl J Med.* 344:1111–1116.

94. Aevarsson O, Svanborg A, Skoog I. (1998). Seven-year survival rate after age 85 years: Relation to Alzheimer disease and vascular dementia. *Arch Neurol.* 55:1226–1232.

95. Helmer C, Joly P, Letenneur L *et al.* (2001). Mortality with dementia: Results from a french prospective community-based cohort. *Am J Epidemiol.* 154:642–648.

96. Beard CM, Kokmen E, Sigler C *et al.* (1996). Cause of death in Alzheimer's disease. *Ann Epidemiol.* 6:195–200.

97. Knopman D, Rocca WA, Cha RH *et al.* (2003). Survival study of vascular dementia in Rochester, Minnesota. *Arch Neurol.* 60:85–90.

98. Tierney MC, Szalai JP, Snow WG, Fisher RH. (1996). The prediction of Alzheimer disease. The role of patient and informant perceptions of cognitive deficits. *Arch Neurol.* 53:423–427.

99. Masur DM, Sliwinski M, Lipton RB *et al.* (1994). Neuropsychological prediction of dementia and the absence of dementia in healthy elderly persons. *Neurology.* 44:1427–1432.

100. Petersen RC, Smith GE, Ivnik RJ *et al.* (1995). Apolipoprotein E status as a predictor of the development of Alzheimer's disease in memory-impaired individuals. *JAMA.* 273:1274–1278.

101. Jacobs DM, Sano M, Dooneief G *et al.* (1995). Neuropsychological detection and characterization of preclinical Alzheimer's disease. *Neurology.* 45:957–962.

102. Katzman R, Aronson M, Fuld P *et al.* (1989). Development of dementing illnesses in an 80-year-old volunteer cohort. *Ann Neurol.* 25:317–324.

103. Howieson DB, Dame A, Camicioli R *et al.* (1997). Cognitive markers preceding Alzheimer's dementia in the healthy oldest old. *J Am Geriatr Soc.* 45:584–589.

104. Elias MF, Beiser A, Wolf PA *et al.* (2000). The preclinical phase of Alzheimer disease: A 22-year prospective study of the Framingham cohort. *Arch Neurol.* 57:808–813.

105. Hanninen T, Hallikainen M, Koivisto K *et al.* (1995). A follow-up study of age-associated memory impairment: Neuropsychological predictors of dementia. *J Am Geriatr Soc.* 43:1007–1015.

106. Tierney MC, Szalai JP, Snow WG *et al.* (1996). Prediction of probable Alzheimer's disease in memory-impaired patients: A prospective longitudinal study. *Neurology.* 46:661–665.

107. Devanand DP, Folz M, Gorlyn M *et al.* (1997). Questionable dementia: Clinical course and predictors of outcome. *J Am Geriatr Soc.* 45:321–328.

108. Daly E, Zaitchik D, Copeland M *et al.* (2000). Predicting conversion to Alzheimer disease using standardized clinical information. *Arch Neurol.* 57:675–680.

109. Petersen RC, Stevens JC, Ganguli M *et al.* (2001). Practice parameter: Early detection of dementia: Mild cognitive impairment (an evidence-based review): Report of the Quality Standards Subcommittee of the American Academy of Neurology. *Neurology.* 56:1133–1142.

110. Petersen RC, Smith GE, Waring SC *et al.* (1999). Mild cognitive impairment: Clinical characterization and outcome. *Arch Neurol.* 56:303–308.

111. Petersen RC, Doody R, Kurz A *et al.* (2001). Current concepts in mild cognitive impairment. *Arch Neurol.* 58:1985–1992.

112. Tabert MH, Albert SM, Borukhova-Milov L *et al.* (2002). Functional deficits in patients with mild cognitive impairment: Prediction of AD. *Neurology.* 58:758–764.

113. Jack CR, Petersen RC, Xu YC *et al.* (1999). Prediction of AD with MRI-based hippocampal volume in mild cognitive impairment. *Neurology.* 52:1397–1403.

114. Visser PJ, Verhey FR, Hofman PA *et al.* (2002). Medial temporal lobe atrophy predicts Alzheimer's disease in patients with minor cognitive impairment. *J Neurol Neurosurg Psychiatry.* 72:491–497.

115. Berent S, Giordani B, Foster N *et al.* (1999). Neuropsychological function and cerebral glucose utilization in isolated memory impairment and Alzheimer's disease. *J Psychiatr Res.* 33:7–16.

116. Hughes CP, Berg L, Danziger WL *et al.* (1982). A new clinical scale for the staging of dementia. *Br J Psychiatry.* 140:566–572.

117. Reisberg B, Ferris SH, de Leon MJ, Crook T. (1982). The Global Deterioration Scale for assessment of primary degenerative dementia. *Am J Psychiatry.* 139:1136–1139.

118. Henderson VW, Mack W, Williams BW. (1989). Spatial disorientation in Alzheimer's disease. *Arch Neurol.* 46:391–394.

119. Greenwald BS, Kramer-Ginsberg E, Marin DB *et al.* (1989). Dementia with coexistent major depression. *Am J Psychiatry.* 146:1472–1478.

120. Kramer SI, Reifler BV. (1992). Depression, dementia, and reversible dementia. *Clin Geriatr Med.* 8:289–297.

121. Levy ML, Cummings JL, Fairbanks LA *et al.* (1996). Longitudinal assessment of symptoms of depression, agitation, and psychosis in 181 patients with Alzheimer's disease. *Am J Psychiatry.* 153:1438–1443.

122. Buschke H, Sliwinski MJ, Kuslansky G, Lipton RB. (1997). Diagnosis of early dementia by the Double Memory Test: Encoding specificity improves diagnostic sensitivity and specificity. *Neurology.* 48:989–997.

123. Binetti G, Cappa SF, Magni E *et al.* (1998). Visual and spatial perception in the early phase of Alzheimer's disease. *Neuropsychology.* 12:29–33.

124. Galasko D, Kwo-on-Yuen PF, Klauber MR, Thal LJ. (1990). Neurological findings in Alzheimer's disease and normal aging. *Arch Neurol.* 47:625–627.

125. Funkenstein HH, Albert MS, Cook NR *et al.* (1993). Extrapyramidal signs and other neurologic findings in clinically diagnosed Alzheimer's disease. A community-based study. *Arch Neurol.* 50:51–56.

126. Rapcsak SZ, Croswell SC, Rubens AB. (1989). Apraxia in Alzheimer's disease. *Neurology.* 39:664–668.

127. Peavy GM, Salmon DP, Rice VA *et al.* (1996). Neuropsychological assessment of severely demented elderly: The severe cognitive impairment profile. *Arch Neurol.* 53:367–372.

128. Volicer L, Hurley AC, Lathi DC, Kowall NW. (1994). Measurement of severity in advanced Alzheimer's disease. *J Gerontol.* 49:M223–M226.

129. Romanelli MF, Morris JC, Ashkin K, Coben LA. (1990). Advanced Alzheimer's disease is a risk factor for late-onset seizures. *Arch Neurol.* 47:847–850.

130. Mendez MF, Catanzaro P, Doss RC *et al.* (1994). Seizures in Alzheimer's disease: Clinicopathologic study. *J Geriatr Psychiatry Neurol.* 7:230–233.

131. Clark CM, Ewbank D, Lerner A *et al.* (1997). The relationship between extrapyramidal signs and cognitive performance in patients with Alzheimer's disease enrolled in the CERAD Study Consortium to Establish a Registry for Alzheimer's Disease. *Neurology.* 49:70–75.

132. (1998). Consensus report of the Working Group on Molecular and Biochemical Markers of Alzheimer's Disease. The Ronald and Nancy Reagan Research Institute of the Alzheimer's Association and the National Institute on Aging Working Group. *Neurobiol Aging.* 19:109–116.

133. Jack CR Jr, Petersen RC, O'Brien PC, Tangalos EG. (1992). MR-based hippocampal volumetry in the diagnosis of Alzheimer's disease. *Neurology.* 42:183–188.

134. Fox NC, Warrington EK, Freeborough PA *et al.* (1996). Presymptomatic hippocampal atrophy in Alzheimer's disease. A longitudinal MRI study. *Brain.* 119:2001–2007.

135. Fox NC, Freeborough PA, Rossor MN. (1996). Visualisation and quantification of rates of atrophy in Alzheimer's disease. *Lancet.* 348:94–97.

136. Scheltens P, Launer LJ, Barkhof F *et al.* (1997). The diagnostic value of magnetic resonance imaging and technetium 99m-HMPAO single-photon-emission computed tomography for the diagnosis of Alzheimer disease in a community-dwelling elderly population. *Alzheimer Dis Assoc Disord.* 11:63–70.

137. Reiman EM, Uecker A, Caselli RJ *et al.* (1998). Hippocampal volumes in cognitively normal persons at genetic risk for Alzheimer's disease. *Ann Neurol.* 44:288–291.

138. Killiany RJ, Moss MB, Albert MS *et al.* (1993). Temporal lobe regions on magnetic resonance imaging identify patients with early Alzheimer's disease. *Arch Neurol.* 50:949–954.

139. Laakso MP, Soininen H, Partanen K *et al.* (1998). MRI of the hippocampus in Alzheimer's disease: Sensitivity, specificity, and analysis of the incorrectly classified subjects. *Neurobiol Aging.* 19:23–31.

140. Bryan RN, Wells SW, Miller TJ *et al.* (1997). Infarctlike lesions in the brain: Prevalence and anatomic characteristics at MR imaging of the elderly—data from the Cardiovascular Health Study. *Radiology.* 202:47–54.

141. Longstreth WT Jr, Bernick C, Manolio TA *et al.* (1998). Lacunar infarcts defined by magnetic resonance imaging of 3660 elderly people: The Cardiovascular Health Study. *Arch Neurol.* 55:1217–1225.

142. Galasko D, Clark C, Chang L *et al.* (1997). Assessment of CSF levels of tau protein in mildly demented patients with Alzheimer's disease. *Neurology.* 48:632–635.

143. Galasko D, Chang L, Motter R *et al.* (1998). High cerebrospinal fluid tau and low amyloid beta42 levels in the clinical diagnosis of Alzheimer disease and relation to apolipoprotein E genotype. *Arch Neurol.* 55:937–945.

144. de la Monte SM, Ghanbari K, Frey WH *et al.* (1997). Characterization of the AD7C-NTP cDNA expression in Alzheimer's disease and measurement of a 41-kD protein in cerebrospinal fluid. *J Clin Invest.* 100:3093–3104.

145. Kanai M, Matsubara E, Isoe K *et al.* (1998). Longitudinal study of cerebrospinal fluid levels of tau, A beta1-40, and A beta1-42(43) in Alzheimer's disease: A study in Japan. *Ann Neurol.* 44:17–26.

146. Andreasen N, Vanmechelen E, Van de Voorde A *et al.* (1998). Cerebrospinal fluid tau protein as a biochemical marker for Alzheimer's disease: A community based follow up study. *J Neurol Neurosurg Psychiatry.* 64:298–305.

147. Corder EH, Saunders AM, Strittmatter WJ *et al.* (1993). Gene dose of apolipoprotein E type 4 allele and the risk of Alzheimer's disease in late onset families. *Science.* 261:921–923.

148. Poirier J, Davignon J, Bouthillier D *et al.* (1993). Apolipoprotein E polymorphism and Alzheimer's disease. *Lancet.* 342:697–699.

149. Saunders AM, Hulette O, Welsh-Bohmer KA *et al.* (1996). Specificity, sensitivity, and predictive value of apolipoprotein-E genotyping for sporadic Alzheimer's disease. *Lancet.* 348:90–93.

150. Welsh-Bohmer KA, Gearing M, Saunders AM *et al.* (1997). Apolipoprotein E genotypes in a neuropathological series from the Consortium to Establish a Registry for Alzheimer's Disease. *Ann Neurol.* 42:319–325.

151. Post SG, Whitehouse PJ, Binstock RH *et al.* (1997). The clinical introduction of genetic testing for Alzheimer disease. An ethical perspective. *JAMA.* 277:832–836.

152. (1995). Statement on use of apolipoprotein E testing for Alzheimer disease. American College of Medical Genetics/American Society of Human Genetics Working Group on ApoE and Alzheimer disease. *JAMA.* 274:1627–1629.

153. (1996). Apolipoprotein E genotyping in Alzheimer's disease. National Institute on Aging/Alzheimer's Association Working Group. *Lancet.* 347:1091–1095.

154. McConnell LM, Koenig BA, Greely HT, Raffin TA. (1998). Genetic testing and Alzheimer disease: Has the time come? Alzheimer Disease Working Group of the Stanford Program in Genomics, Ethics & Society. *Nat Med.* 4:757–759.

155. Bachman DL, Wolf PA, Linn R *et al.* (1992). Prevalence of dementia and probable senile dementia of the Alzheimer type in the Framingham Study. *Neurology.* 42:115–119.

156. Evans DA, Funkenstein HH, Albert MS *et al.* (1989). Prevalence of Alzheimer's disease in a community population of older persons. Higher than previously reported. *JAMA.* 262:2551–2556.

157. Graves AB, Larson EB, Edland SD *et al.* (1996). Prevalence of dementia and its subtypes in the Japanese American population of King County, Washington state. The Kame Project. *Am J Epidemiol.* 144:760–771.

158. Hendrie HC, Osuntokun BO, Hall KS *et al.* (1995). Prevalence of Alzheimer's disease and dementia in two communities: Nigerian Africans and African Americans. *Am J Psychiatry.* 152:1485–1492.

159. Hofman A, Ott A, Breteler MM *et al.* (1997). Atherosclerosis, apolipoprotein E, and prevalence of dementia and Alzheimer's disease in the Rotterdam Study. *Lancet.* 349:151–154.

160. Kokmen E, Beard CM, Offord KP, Kurland LT. (1989). Prevalence of medically diagnosed dementia in a defined United States population: Rochester, Minnesota, January 1, 1975. *Neurology.* 39:773–776.

161. Ott A, Breteler MM, van Harskamp F *et al.* (1995). Prevalence of Alzheimer's disease and vascular dementia: Association with education. The Rotterdam study. *BMJ.* 310:970–973.

162. Pfeffer RI, Afifi AA, Chance JM. (1987). Prevalence of Alzheimer's disease in a retirement community. *Am J Epidemiol.* 125:420–436.

163. White L, Petrovitch H, Ross GW *et al.* (1996). Prevalence of dementia in older Japanese-American men in Hawaii: The Honolulu-Asia Aging Study. *JAMA.* 276:955–960.

164. Fillenbaum GG, Heyman A, Huber MS *et al.* (1998). The prevalence and 3-year incidence of dementia in older Black and White community residents. *J Clin Epidemiol.* 51:587–595.

165. (1994). Canadian study of health and aging: Study methods and prevalence of dementia. *CMAJ.* 150:899–913.

166. Hy LX, Keller DM. (2000). Prevalence of AD among whites: A summary by levels of severity. *Neurology.* 55:198–204.

167. Gao S, Hendrie HC, Hall KS, Hui S. (1998). The relationships between age, sex, and the incidence of dementia and Alzheimer disease: A meta-analysis. *Arch Gen Psychiatry.* 55:809–815.

168. Jorm AF, Jolley D. (1998). The incidence of dementia: A meta-analysis. *Neurology.* 51:728–733.

169. Bachman DL, Wolf PA, Linn RT *et al.* (1993). Incidence of dementia and probable Alzheimer's disease in a general population: The Framingham Study. *Neurology.* 43:515–519.

170. Hebert LE, Scherr PA, Beckett LA *et al.* (1995). Age-specific incidence of Alzheimer's disease in a community population. *JAMA.* 273:1354–1359.

171. Ott A, Breteler MM, van Harskamp F, Stijnen T, Hofman A. (1998). Incidence and risk of dementia. The Rotterdam Study. *Am J Epidemiol.* 147:574–580.

172. Rocca WA, Cha RH, Waring SC, Kokmen E. (1998). Incidence of dementia and Alzheimer's disease: A reanalysis of data from Rochester, Minnesota, 1975–1984. *Am J Epidemiol.* 148:51–62.

173. Stern Y, Gurland B, Tatemichi TK *et al.* (1994). Influence of education and occupation on the incidence of Alzheimer's disease. *JAMA.* 271:1004–1010.

174. Edland SD, Rocca WA, Petersen RC *et al.* (2002). The incidence of Alzheimer's disease does not vary by gender in Rochester, Minnesota. *Arch Neurol.* 59:1589–1593.

175. Callahan CM, Hall KS, Hui SL *et al.* (1996). Relationship of age, education, and occupation with dementia among a community-based sample of African Americans. *Arch Neurol.* 53:134–140.

176. Zhang MY, Katzman R, Salmon D *et al.* (1990). The prevalence of dementia and Alzheimer's disease in Shanghai, China: Impact of age, gender, and education. *Ann Neurol.* 27:428–437.

177. Stern Y, Tang MX, Denaro J, Mayeux R. (1995). Increased risk of mortality in Alzheimer's disease patients with more advanced educational and occupational attainment. *Ann Neurol.* 37:590–595.

178. Cobb JL, Wolf PA, Au R *et al.* (1995). The effect of education on the incidence of dementia and Alzheimer's disease in the Framingham Study. *Neurology.* 45:1707–1712.

179. Friedland RP. (1993). Epidemiology, education, and the ecology of Alzheimer's disease. *Neurology.* 43:246–249.

180. Katzman R. (1993). Education and the prevalence of dementia and Alzheimer's disease. *Neurology.* 43:13–20.

181. Beard CM, Kokmen E, Offord KP, Kurland LT. (1992). Lack of association between Alzheimer's disease and education, occupation, marital status, or living arrangement. *Neurology.* 42:2063–2068.

182. Snowdon DA, Kemper SJ, Mortimer JA *et al.* (1996). Linguistic ability in early life and cognitive function and Alzheimer's disease in late life. Findings from the Nun Study. *JAMA.* 275:528–532.

183. Carmelli D, Swan GE, Reed T *et al.* (1998). Midlife cardiovascular risk factors, ApoE, and cognitive decline in elderly male twins. *Neurology.* 50:1580–1585.

184. Kalmijn S, Feskens EJ, Launer LJ, Kromhout D. (1996). Cerebrovascular disease, the apolipoprotein e4 allele, and cognitive decline in a community-based study of elderly men. *Stroke.* 27:2230–2235.

185. Prince M, Cullen M, Mann A. (1994). Risk factors for Alzheimer's disease and dementia: A case-control study based on the MRC elderly hypertension trial. *Neurology.* 44:97–104.

186. Launer LJ, Masaki K, Petrovitch H *et al.* (1995). The association between midlife blood pressure levels and late-life cognitive function. The Honolulu-Asia Aging Study. *JAMA.* 274:1846–1851.

187. Elias MF, Wolf PA, D'Agostino RB *et al.* (1993). Untreated blood pressure level is inversely related to cognitive functioning: The Framingham Study. *Am J Epidemiol.* 138:353–364.

188. Seshadri S, Beiser A, Selhub J *et al.* (2002). Plasma homocysteine as a risk factor for dementia and Alzheimer's disease. *N Engl J Med.* 346:476–483.

189. Kalmijn S, Launer LJ, Lindemans J *et al.* (1999). Total homocysteine and cognitive decline in a community-based sample of elderly subjects: The Rotterdam Study. *Am J Epidemiol.* 150:283–289.

190. Clarke R, Smith AD, Jobst KA *et al.* (1998). Folate, vitamin B12, and serum total homocysteine levels in confirmed Alzheimer disease. *Arch Neurol.* 55:1449–1455.

191. McCaddon A, Davies G, Hudson P *et al.* (1998). Total serum homocysteine in senile dementia of Alzheimer type. *Int J Geriatr Psychiatry.* 13:235–239.

192. French LR, Schuman LM, Mortimer JA *et al.* (1985). A case-control study of dementia of the Alzheimer type. *Am J Epidemiol.* 121:414–421.

193. Graves AB, White E, Koepsell TD *et al.* (1990). The association between head trauma and Alzheimer's disease. *Am J Epidemiol.* 131:491–501.

194. Mortimer JA, van Duijn CM, Chandra V *et al.* (1991). Head trauma as a risk factor for Alzheimer's disease: A collaborative re-analysis of case-control studies. EURODEM Risk Factors Research Group. *Int J Epidemiol.* 20(Suppl 2):S28–S35.

195. Chandra V, Kokmen E, Schoenberg BS, Beard CM. (1989). Head trauma with loss of consciousness as a risk factor for Alzheimer's disease. *Neurology.* 39:1576–1578.

196. Jordan BD, Relkin NR, Ravdin LD *et al.* (1997). Apolipoprotein E epsilon4 associated with chronic traumatic brain injury in boxing. *JAMA.* 278:136–140.

197. Roberts GW, Allsop D, Bruton C. (1990). The occult aftermath of boxing. *J Neurol Neurosurg Psychiatry.* 53:373–378.

198. Mayeux R, Ottman R, Maestre G *et al.* (1995). Synergistic effects of traumatic head injury and apolipoprotein-epsilon 4 in patients with Alzheimer's disease. *Neurology.* 45:555–557.

199. Kukull WA, Larson EB, Bowen JD *et al.* (1995). Solvent exposure as a risk factor for Alzheimer's disease: A case-control study. *Am J Epidemiol.* 141:1059–1071.

200. Graves AB, White E, Koepsell TD *et al.* (1990). The association between aluminum-containing products and Alzheimer's disease. *J Clin Epidemiol.* 43:35–44.

201. Hachinski V. (1998). Aluminum exposure and risk of Alzheimer disease. *Arch Neurol.* 55:742.

202. Salib E, Hillier V. (1996). A case-control study of Alzheimer's disease and aluminium occupation. *Br J Psychiatry.* 168:244–249.

203. Bjertness E, Candy JM, Torvik A *et al.* (1996). Content of brain aluminum is not elevated in Alzheimer disease. *Alzheimer Dis Assoc Disord.* 10:171–174.

204. Crapper DR, Krishnan SS, De Boni U, Tomko GJ. (1975). Aluminum: A possible neurotoxic agent in Alzheimer's disease. *Trans Am Neurol Assoc.* 100:154–156.

205. Good PF, Perl DP, Bierer LM, Schmeidler J. (1992). Selective accumulation of aluminum and iron in the neurofibrillary tangles of Alzheimer's disease: A laser microprobe (LAMMA) study. *Ann Neurol.* 31:286–292.

206. Lovell MA, Ehmann WD, Markesbery WR. (1993). Laser microprobe analysis of brain aluminum in Alzheimer's disease. *Ann Neurol.* 33:36–42.

207. Forster DP, Newens AJ, Kay DW, Edwardson JA. (1995). Risk factors in clinically diagnosed presenile dementia of the Alzheimer type: A case-control study in northern England. *J Epidemiol Community Health.* 49:253–258.

208. Martyn CN, Barker DJ, Osmond C *et al.* (1989). Geographical relation between Alzheimer's disease and aluminum in drinking water. *Lancet.* 1:59–62.

209. McLachlan DR, Bergeron C, Smith JE *et al.* (1996). Risk for neuropathologically confirmed Alzheimer's disease and residual aluminum in municipal drinking water employing weighted residential histories. *Neurology.* 46:401–405.

210. Brenner DE, Kukull WA, Stergachis A *et al.* (1994). Postmenopausal estrogen replacement therapy and the risk of Alzheimer's disease: A population-based case-control study. *Am J Epidemiol.* 140:262–267.

211. Jacobs DM, Tang MX, Stern Y *et al.* (1998). Cognitive function in nondemented older women who took estrogen after menopause. *Neurology.* 50:368–373.

212. Kawas C, Resnick S, Morrison A *et al.* (1997). A prospective study of estrogen replacement therapy and the risk of developing Alzheimer's disease: The Baltimore Longitudinal Study of Aging. *Neurology.* 48:1517–1521.

213. Paganini-Hill A, Henderson VW. (1996). Estrogen replacement therapy and risk of Alzheimer disease. *Arch Intern Med.* 156:2213–2217.

214. Tang MX, Jacobs D, Stern Y *et al.* (1996). Effect of oestrogen during menopause on risk and age at onset of Alzheimer's disease. *Lancet.* 348:429–432.

215. Mulnard RA, Cotman CW, Kawas C *et al.* (2000). Estrogen replacement therapy for treatment of mild to moderate Alzheimer disease: A randomized controlled trial. Alzheimer's Disease Cooperative Study. *JAMA.* 283:1007–1015.

216. Henderson VW, Paganini-Hill A, Miller BL *et al.* (2000). Estrogen for Alzheimer's disease in women: Randomized, double-blind, placebo-controlled trial. *Neurology.* 54:295–301.

217. Andersen K, Launer LJ, Ott A *et al.* (1995). Do nonsteroidal anti-inflammatory drugs decrease the risk for Alzheimer's disease? The Rotterdam Study. *Neurology.* 45:1441–1445.

218. Breitner JC, Gau BA, Welsh KA *et al.* (1994). Inverse association of anti-inflammatory treatments and Alzheimer's disease: Initial results of a co-twin control study. *Neurology.* 44:227–232.

219. McGeer PL, Schulzer M, McGeer EG. (1996). Arthritis and anti-inflammatory agents as possible protective factors for Alzheimer's disease: A review of 17 epidemiologic studies. *Neurology.* 47:425–432.

220. Prince M, Rabe-Hesketh S, Brennan P. (1998). Do antiarthritic drugs decrease the risk for cognitive decline? An analysis based on data from the MRC treatment trial of hypertension in older adults. *Neurology.* 50:374–379.

221. Stewart WF, Kawas C, Corrada M, Metter EJ. (1997). Risk of Alzheimer's disease and duration of NSAID use. *Neurology.* 48:626–632.

222. In't Veld BA, Ruitenberg A, Hofman A *et al.* (2001). Nonsteroidal antiinflammatory drugs and the risk of Alzheimer's disease. *N Engl J Med.* 345:1515–1521.

223. Jick H, Zornberg GL, Jick SS *et al.* (2000). Statins and the risk of dementia. *Lancet.* 356:1627–1631.

224. Wolozin B, Kellman W, Ruosseau P *et al.* (2000). Decreased prevalence of Alzheimer disease associated with 3-hydroxy-3-methylglutaryl coenzyme A reductase inhibitors. *Arch Neurol.* 57:1439–1443.

225. Rockwood K, Kirkland S, Hogan DB *et al.* (2002). Use of lipid-lowering agents, indication bias, and the risk of dementia in community-dwelling elderly people. *Arch Neurol.* 59:223–227.

226. Heart Protection Study Collaborative Group. (2002). MRC/BHF Heart Protection Study of cholesterol lowering with simvastatin in 20,536 high-risk individuals: A randomised placebo-controlled trial. *Lancet.* 360:7–22.

227. Brenner DE, Kukull WA, van Belle G *et al.* (1993). Relationship between cigarette smoking and Alzheimer's disease in a population-based case-control study. *Neurology.* 43:293–300.

228. Ford AB, Mefrouche Z, Friedland RP, Debanne SM. (1996). Smoking and cognitive impairment: A population-based study. *J Am Geriatr Soc.* 44:905–909.

229. Graves AB, van Duijn CM, Chandra V *et al.* (1991). Alcohol and tobacco consumption as risk factors for Alzheimer's disease: A collaborative re-analysis of case-control studies. EURODEM Risk Factors Research Group. *Int J Epidemiol.* 20(Suppl 2):S48–S57.

230. Hebert LE, Scherr PA, Beckett LA *et al.* (1992). Relation of smoking and alcohol consumption to incident Alzheimer's disease. *Am J Epidemiol.* 135:347–355.

231. Ott A, Slooter AJ, Hofman A *et al.* (1998). Smoking and risk of dementia and Alzheimer's disease in a population-based cohort study: The Rotterdam Study. *Lancet.* 351:1840–1843.

232. Galanis DJ, Petrovitch H, Launer LJ *et al.* (1997). Smoking history in middle age and subsequent cognitive performance in elderly Japanese-American men. The Honolulu-Asia Aging Study. *Am J Epidemiol.* 145:507–515.

233. Prince M, Lewis G, Bird A *et al.* (1996). A longitudinal study of factors predicting change in cognitive test scores over time, in an older hypertensive population. *Psychol Med.* 26:555–568.

234. Whitehouse PJ, Kalaria RN. (1995). Nicotinic receptors and neurodegenerative dementing diseases: Basic research and clinical implications. *Alzheimer Dis Assoc Disord.* 9(Suppl 2):3–5.

235. Lautenschlager NT, Cupples LA, Rao VS *et al.* (1996). Risk of dementia among relatives of Alzheimer's disease patients in the MIRAGE study: What is in store for the oldest old? *Neurology.* 46:641–650.

236. Heston LL, Mastri AR, Anderson VE, White J. (1981). Dementia of the Alzheimer type. Clinical genetics, natural history, and associated conditions. *Arch Gen Psychiatry.* 38:1085–1090.

237. Green RC, Cupples LA, Go R *et al.* (2002). Risk of dementia among white and African American relatives of patients with Alzheimer disease. *JAMA.* 287:329–336.

238. Schupf N, Kapell D, Lee JH *et al.* (1994). Increased risk of Alzheimer's disease in mothers of adults with Down's syndrome. *Lancet.* 344:353–356.

239. Blacker D, Tanzi RE. (1998). The genetics of Alzheimer disease: Current status and future prospects. *Arch Neurol.* 55:294–296.

240. Tanzi RE, Bertram L. (2001). New frontiers in Alzheimer's disease genetics. *Neuron.* 32:181–184.

241. Bird TD, Levy-Lahad E, Poorkaj P *et al.* (1996). Wide range in age of onset for chromosome 1—related familial Alzheimer's disease. *Ann Neurol.* 40:932–936.

242. Lampe TH, Bird TD, Nochlin D *et al.* (1994). Phenotype of chromosome 14-linked familial Alzheimer's disease in a large kindred. *Ann Neurol.* 36:368–378.

243. Bird TD, Lampe TH, Nemens EJ *et al.* (1988). Familial Alzheimer's disease in American descendants of the Volga Germans: Probable genetic founder effect. *Ann Neurol.* 23:25–31.

244. Lippa CF, Saunders AM, Smith TW *et al.* (1996). Familial and sporadic Alzheimer's disease: Neuropathology cannot exclude a final common pathway. *Neurology.* 46:406–412.

245. Mann DM, Iwatsubo T, Nochlin D *et al.* (1997). Amyloid (Abeta) deposition in chromosome 1-linked Alzheimer's disease: The Volga German families. *Ann Neurol.* 41:52–57.

246. Mann DM, Iwatsubo T, Cairns NJ *et al.* (1996). Amyloid beta protein (Abeta) deposition in chromosome 14-linked Alzheimer's disease: Predominance of Abeta42(43). *Ann Neurol.* 40:149–156.

247. Goate A, Chartier-Harlin MC, Mullan M *et al.* (1991). Segregation of a missense mutation in the amyloid precursor protein gene with familial Alzheimer's disease. *Nature.* 349:704–706.

248. Hardy J. (1997). Amyloid, the presenilins and Alzheimer's disease. *Trends Neurosci.* 20:154–159.

249. Wisniewski KE, Wisniewski HM, Wen GY. (1985). Occurrence of neuropathological changes and dementia of Alzheimer's disease in Down's syndrome. *Ann Neurol.* 17:278–282.

250. Schellenberg GD, Anderson L, O'Dahl S *et al.* (1991). APP717, APP693, and PRIP gene mutations are rare in Alzheimer disease. *Am J Hum Genet.* 49:511–517.

251. Sherrington R, Rogaev EI, Liang Y *et al.* (1995). Cloning of a gene bearing missense mutations in early-onset familial Alzheimer's disease. *Nature.* 375:754–760.

252. Hutton M, Busfield F, Wragg M *et al.* (1996). Complete analysis of the presenilin 1 gene in early onset Alzheimer's disease. *Neuroreport.* 7:801–805.

253. Rogaev EI, Sherrington R, Rogaeva EA *et al.* (1995). Familial Alzheimer's disease in kindreds with missense mutations in a gene on chromosome 1 related to the Alzheimer's disease type 3 gene. *Nature.* 376: 775–778.

254. Boyles JK, Zoellner CD, Anderson LJ *et al.* (1989). A role for apolipoprotein E, apolipoprotein A-I, and low density lipoprotein receptors in cholesterol transport during regeneration and remyelination of the rat sciatic nerve. *J Clin Invest.* 83:1015–1031.

255. Hallman DM, Boerwinkle E, Saha N *et al.* (1991). The apolipoprotein E polymorphism: A comparison of allele frequencies and effects in nine populations. *Am J Hum Genet.* 49:338–349.

256. Farrer LA, Cupples LA, Haines JL *et al.* (1997). Effects of age, sex, and ethnicity on the association between apolipoprotein E genotype and Alzheimer disease. A meta-analysis. APOE and Alzheimer Disease Meta Analysis Consortium. *JAMA.* 278:1349–1356.

257. Hyman BT, Gomez-Isla T, Briggs M *et al.* (1996). Apolipoprotein E and cognitive change in an elderly population. *Ann Neurol.* 40:55–66.

258. Myers RH, Schaefer EJ, Wilson PW *et al.* (1996). Apolipoprotein E epsilon4 association with dementia in a population-based study: The Framingham study. *Neurology.* 46:673–677.

259. Henderson AS, Easteal S, Jorm AF *et al.* (1995). Apolipoprotein E allele epsilon 4, dementia, and cognitive decline in a population sample. *Lancet.* 346:1387–1390.

260. Bertram L, Blacker D, Mullin K *et al.* (2000). Evidence for genetic linkage of Alzheimer's disease to chromosome 10q. *Science.* 290:2302–2303.

261. Ertekin-Taner N, Graff-Radford N, Younkin LH *et al.* (2000). Linkage of plasma Abeta42 to a quantitative locus on chromosome 10 in late-onset Alzheimer's disease pedigrees. *Science.* 290:2303–2304.

262. Myers A, Holmans P, Marshall H *et al.* (2000). Susceptibility locus for Alzheimer's disease on chromosome 10. *Science.* 290:2304–2305.

263. Wolf PA, Cobb JL, D'Agostino RB. (1992). Epidemiology of Stroke. In *Stroke. Pathophysiology, Diagnosis and Management* (Barnett HJM, Mohr JP, Stein BM, Yatsu FM, eds.), pp. 3–27 New York: Churchill Livingstone.

264. Hachinski V. (1994). Vascular dementia: A radical redefinition. *Dementia.* 5:130–132.

265. Chui HC, Victoroff JI, Margolin D *et al.* (1992). Criteria for the diagnosis of ischemic vascular dementia proposed by the State of California Alzheimer's Disease Diagnostic and Treatment Centers. *Neurology.* 42:473–480.

266. Roman GC, Tatemichi TK, Erkinjuntti T *et al.* (1993). Vascular dementia: Diagnostic criteria for research studies. Report of the NINDS-AIREN International Workshop. *Neurology.* 43:250–260.

267. Hachinski VC, Lassen NA, Marshall J. (1974). Multi-infarct dementia. A cause of mental deterioration in the elderly. *Lancet.* 2:207–210.

268. Rosen WG, Terry RD, Fuld PA *et al.* (1980). Pathological verification of ischemic score in differentiation of dementias. *Ann Neurol.* 7:486–488.

269. Moroney JT, Bagiella E, Desmond DW *et al.* (1997). Meta-analysis of the Hachinski Ischemic Score in pathologically verified dementias. *Neurology.* 49:1096–1105.

270. Brott T, Tomsick T, Feinberg W *et al.* (1994). Baseline silent cerebral infarction in the Asymptomatic Carotid Atherosclerosis Study. *Stroke.* 25:1122–1129.

271. Kokmen E, Whisnant JP, O'Fallon WM *et al.* (1996). Dementia after ischemic stroke: A population-based study in Rochester, Minnesota (1960–1984). *Neurology.* 46:154–159.

272. Tatemichi TK, Desmond DW, Stern Y *et al.* (1994). Cognitive impairment after stroke: Frequency, patterns, and relationship to functional abilities. *J Neurol Neurosurg Psychiatry.* 57:202–207.

273. Pohjasvaara T, Mantyla R, Salonen O *et al.* (2000). MRI correlates of dementia after first clinical ischemic stroke. *J Neurol Sci.* 181:111–117.

274. Henon H, Durieu I, Guerouaou D *et al.* (2001). Poststroke dementia: Incidence and relationship to prestroke cognitive decline. *Neurology.* 57:1216–1222.

275. Wolfe N, Linn R, Babikian VL *et al.* (1990). Frontal systems impairment following multiple lacunar infarcts. *Arch Neurol.* 47:129–132.

276. Caplan LR. (1995). Binswanger's disease—revisited. *Neurology.* 45:626–633.

277. Looi JC, Sachdev PS. (1999). Differentiation of vascular dementia from AD on neuropsychological tests. *Neurology.* 53:670–678.

278. Mirsen TR, Lee DH, Wong CJ *et al.* (1991). Clinical correlates of white-matter changes on magnetic resonance imaging scans of the brain. *Arch Neurol.* 48:1015–1021.

279. Munoz DG, Hastak SM, Harper B *et al.* (1993). Pathologic correlates of increased signals of the centrum ovale on magnetic resonance imaging. *Arch Neurol.* 50:492–497.

280. Fazekas F, Kapeller P, Schmidt R *et al.* (1996). The relation of cerebral magnetic resonance signal hyperintensities to Alzheimer's disease. *J Neurol Sci.* 142:121–125.

281. Erkinjuntti T, Gao F, Lee DH *et al.* (1994). Lack of difference in brain hyperintensities between patients with early Alzheimer's disease and control subjects. *Arch Neurol.* 51:260–268.

282. Scheltens P, Barkhof F, Valk J *et al.* (1992). White matter lesions on magnetic resonance imaging in clinically diagnosed Alzheimer's disease. Evidence for heterogeneity. *Brain.* 115:735–748.

283. Liu CK, Miller BL, Cummings JL *et al.* (1992). A quantitative MRI study of vascular dementia. *Neurology.* 42:138–143.

284. Liao D, Cooper L, Cai J *et al.* (1997). The prevalence and severity of white matter lesions, their relationship with age, ethnicity, gender, and cardiovascular disease risk factors: The ARIC Study. *Neuroepidemiology.* 16:149–162.

285. Breteler MM, van Amerongen NM, van Swieten JC *et al.* (1994). Cognitive correlates of ventricular enlargement and cerebral white matter lesions on magnetic resonance imaging. The Rotterdam Study. *Stroke.* 25:1109–1115.

286. van Swieten JC, Geyskes GG, Derix MM *et al.* (1991). Hypertension in the elderly is associated with white matter lesions and cognitive decline. *Ann Neurol.* 30:825–830.

287. Longstreth WT, Jr., Manolio TA, Arnold A *et al.* (1996). Clinical correlates of white matter findings on cranial magnetic resonance imaging of 3301 elderly people. The Cardiovascular Health Study. *Stroke.* 27:1274–1282.

288. Kuller LH, Shemanski L, Manolio T *et al.* (1998). Relationship between ApoE, MRI findings, and cognitive function in the Cardiovascular Health Study. *Stroke.* 29:388–398.

289. Larson EB, Reifler BV, Sumi SM *et al.* (1985). Diagnostic evaluation of 200 elderly outpatients with suspected dementia. *J Gerontol.* 40:536–543.

290. Folstein MF, Bassett SS, Anthony JC *et al.* (1991). Dementia: Case ascertainment in a community survey. *J Gerontol.* 46:M132–138.

291. Lobo A, Launer LJ, Fratiglioni L *et al.* (2000). Prevalence of dementia and major subtypes in Europe: A collaborative study of population-based cohorts. Neurologic Diseases in the Elderly Research Group. *Neurology.* 54:S4–S9.

292. Fratiglioni L, Launer LJ, Andersen K *et al.* (2000). Incidence of dementia and major subtypes in Europe: A collaborative study of population-based cohorts. Neurologic Diseases in the Elderly Research Group. *Neurology.* 54:S10–S15.

293. Canadian Study of Health and Aging Working Group. (2000). The incidence of dementia in Canada. *Neurology.* 55:66–73.

294. Knopman D, Rocca WA, Cha RH *et al.* (2002). Incidence of vascular dementia in Rochester, Minnesota, 1985–1989. *Arch Neurol.* 59:1605–1610.

295. Erkinjuntti T, Kurz A, Gauthier S *et al.* (2002). Efficacy of galantamine in probable vascular dementia and Alzheimer's disease combined with cerebrovascular disease: A randomised trial. *Lancet.* 359:1283–1290.

296. Bennett DA, Beckett LA, Murray AM *et al.* (1996). Prevalence of parkinsonian signs and associated mortality in a community population of older people. *N Engl J Med.* 334:71–76.

297. Rajput AH, Offord KP, Beard CM, Kurland LT. (1987). A case-control study of smoking habits, dementia, and other illnesses in idiopathic Parkinson's disease. *Neurology.* 37:226–232.

298. Mayeux R, Denaro J, Hemenegildo N *et al.* (1992). A population-based investigation of Parkinson's disease with and without dementia. Relationship to age and gender. *Arch Neurol.* 49:492–497.

299. Aarsland D, Tandberg E, Larsen JP, Cummings JL. (1996). Frequency of dementia in Parkinson disease. *Arch Neurol.* 53:538–542.

300. McKeith IG, Galasko D, Kosaka K *et al.* (1996). Consensus guidelines for the clinical and pathologic diagnosis of dementia with Lewy bodies (DLB): Report of the consortium on DLB international workshop. *Neurology.* 47:1113–1124.

301. Hansen L, Salmon D, Galasko D *et al.* (1990). The Lewy body variant of Alzheimer's disease: A clinical and pathologic entity. *Neurology.* 40:1–8.

302. Salmon DP, Galasko D, Hansen LA *et al.* (1996). Neuropsychological deficits associated with diffuse Lewy body disease. *Brain Cogn.* 31:148–165.

303. Heyman A, Fillenbaum GG, Gearing M *et al.* (1999). Comparison of Lewy body variant of Alzheimer's disease with pure Alzheimer's disease: Consortium to Establish a Registry for Alzheimer's Disease, Part XIX. *Neurology.* 52:1839–1844.

304. Ferman TJ, Boeve BF, Smith GE *et al.* (1999). REM sleep behavior disorder and dementia: Cognitive differences when compared with AD. *Neurology.* 52:951–957.

305. Boeve BF, Silber MH, Ferman TJ *et al.* (1998). REM sleep behavior disorder and degenerative dementia: An association likely reflecting Lewy body disease. *Neurology.* 51:363–370.

306. Ballard C, O'Brien J, Gray A *et al.* (2001). Attention and fluctuating attention in patients with dementia with Lewy bodies and Alzheimer disease. *Arch Neurol.* 58:977–982.

307. Hohl U, Tiraboschi P, Hansen LA *et al.* (2000). Diagnostic accuracy of dementia with Lewy bodies. *Arch Neurol.* 57:347–351.

308. Luis CA, Barker WW, Gajaraj K *et al.* (1999). Sensitivity and specificity of three clinical criteria for dementia with Lewy bodies in an autopsy-verified sample. *Int J Geriatr Psychiatry.* 14:526–533.

309. Lopez OL, Litvan I, Catt KE *et al.* (1999). Accuracy of four clinical diagnostic criteria for the diagnosis of neurodegenerative dementias. *Neurology.* 53:1292–1299.

310. Mega MS, Masterman DL, Benson DF *et al.* (1996). Dementia with Lewy bodies: Reliability and validity of clinical and pathologic criteria. *Neurology.* 47:1403–1409.

311. Litvan I, MacIntyre A, Goetz CG *et al.* (1998). Accuracy of the clinical diagnoses of Lewy body disease, Parkinson disease, and dementia with Lewy bodies: A clinicopathologic study. *Arch Neurol.* 55:969–978.

312. Verghese J, Crystal HA, Dickson DW, Lipton RB. (1999). Validity of clinical criteria for the diagnosis of dementia with Lewy bodies. *Neurology.* 53:1974–1982.

313. Apaydin H, Ahlskog JE, Parisi JE *et al.* (2002). Parkinson disease neuropathology: Later-developing dementia and loss of the levodopa response. *Arch Neurol.* 59:102–112.

314. McKeith I, Del Ser T, Spano P *et al.* (2000). Efficacy of rivastigmine in dementia with Lewy bodies: A randomised, double-blind, placebo-controlled international study. *Lancet.* 356:2031–2036.

315. McKhann GM, Albert MS, Grossman M *et al.* (2001). Clinical and pathological diagnosis of frontotemporal dementia: Report of the Work Group on Frontotemporal Dementia and Pick's Disease. *Arch Neurol.* 58:1803–1809.

316. (1994). Clinical and neuropathological criteria for frontotemporal dementia. The Lund and Manchester Groups. *J Neurol Neurosurg Psychiatry.* 57:416–418.

317. Gustafson L. (1993). Clinical picture of frontal lobe degeneration of non-Alzheimer type. *Dementia.* 4:143–148.

318. Neary D, Snowden JS, Northen B, Goulding P. (1988). Dementia of frontal lobe type. *J Neurol Neurosurg Psychiatry.* 51:353–361.

319. Boone KB, Miller BL, Lee A *et al.* (1999). Neuropsychological patterns in right versus left frontotemporal dementia. *J Int Neuropsychol Soc.* 5:616–622.

320. Knopman DS, Mastri AR, Frey WH *et al.* (1990). Dementia lacking distinctive histologic features: A common non-Alzheimer degenerative dementia. *Neurology.* 40:251–256.

321. Read SL, Miller BL, Mena I *et al.* (1995). SPECT in dementia: Clinical and pathological correlation. *J Am Geriatr Soc.* 43:1243–1247.

322. Miller BL, Cummings JL, Villanueva-Meyer J *et al.* (1991). Frontal lobe degeneration: Clinical, neuropsychological, and SPECT characteristics. *Neurology.* 41:1374–1382.

323. Talbot PR, Lloyd JJ, Snowden JS *et al.* (1998). A clinical role for 99mTc-HMPAO SPECT in the investigation of dementia? *J Neurol Neurosurg Psychiatry.* 64:306–313.

324. Friedland RP, Koss E, Lerner A *et al.* (1993). Functional imaging, the frontal lobes, and dementia. *Dementia.* 4:192–203.

325. Kamo H, McGeer PL, Harrop R *et al.* (1987). Positron emission tomography and histopathology in Pick's disease. *Neurology.* 37:439–445.

326. Kertesz A, Hudson L, Mackenzie IR, Munoz DG. (1994). The pathology and nosology of primary progressive aphasia. *Neurology.* 44:2065–2072.

327. Snowden JS, Neary D. (1993). Progressive language dysfunction and lobar atrophy. *Dementia.* 4:226–231.

328. Kirshner HS, Tanridag O, Thurman L *et al.* (1987). Progressive aphasia without dementia: Two cases with focal spongiform degeneration. *Ann Neurol.* 22:527–532.

329. Mesulam MM. (2001). Primary progressive aphasia. *Ann Neurol.* 49:425–432.

330. Hodges JR, Patterson K, Oxbury S, Funnell E. (1992). Semantic dementia. Progressive fluent aphasia with temporal lobe atrophy. *Brain.* 115:1783–1806.

331. Risse SC, Raskind MA, Nochlin D *et al.* (1990). Neuropathological findings in patients with clinical diagnoses of probable Alzheimer's disease. *Am J Psychiatry.* 147:168–172.

332. Joachim CL, Morris JH, Selkoe DJ. (1988). Clinically diagnosed Alzheimer's disease: Autopsy results in 150 cases. *Ann Neurol*. 24:50–56.

333. Boller F, Lopez OL, Moossy J. (1989). Diagnosis of dementia: Clinico-pathologic correlations. *Neurology*. 39:76–79.

334. Brun A. (1993). Frontal lobe degeneration of non-Alzheimer type revisited. *Dementia*. 4:126–131.

335. Brown P. (1994). Infectious Cerebral Amyloidoses: Creutzfeldt-Jakob disease and the Gerstmann-Straussler-Scheinker Syndrome. In *Handbook of dementing illnesses* (Morris JC, ed.), pp. 353–377. New York: Marcel Dekker.

336. Hsich G, Kenney K, Gibbs CJ et al. (1996). The 14-3-3 brain protein in cerebrospinal fluid as a marker for transmissible spongiform encephalopathies. *N Engl J Med*. 335:924–930.

337. Zerr I, Bodemer M, Gefeller O et al. (1998). Detection of 14-3-3 protein in the cerebrospinal fluid supports the diagnosis of Creutzfeldt-Jakob disease. *Ann Neurol*. 43:32–40.

338. Aksamit AJ Jr, Preissner CM, Homburger HA. (2001). Quantitation of 14-3-3 and neuron-specific enolase proteins in CSF in Creutzfeldt-Jakob disease. *Neurology*. 57.728–730.

339. Schröter A, Zerr I, Henkel K et al. (2000). Magnetic resonance imaging in the clinical diagnosis of Creutzfeldt-Jakob disease. *Arch Neurol*. 57:1751–1757.

340. Chiofalo N, Fuentes A, Galvez S. (1980). Serial EEG findings in 27 cases of Creutzfeldt-Jakob disease. *Arch Neurol*. 37:143–145.

341. Steinhoff BJ, Racker S, Herrendorf G et al. (1996). Accuracy and reliability of periodic sharp wave complexes in Creutzfeldt-Jakob disease. *Arch Neurol*. 53:162–166.

342. Johnson RT, Gibbs CJJ Jr. (1998). Medical progress: Creutzfeldt-Jakob disease and related transmissible spongiform encephalopathies. *N Engl J Med*. 339:1994–2004.

343. Alexander EM, Wagner EH, Buchner DM et al. (1995). Do surgical brain lesions present as isolated dementia? A population- based study. *J Am Geriatr Soc*. 43:138–143.

344. Martin DC, Miller J, Kapoor W et al. (1987). Clinical prediction rules for computed tomographic scanning in senile dementia. *Arch Intern Med*. 147:77–80.

345. Freter S, Bergman H, Gold S et al. (1998). Prevalence of potentially reversible dementias and actual reversibility in a memory clinic cohort. *CMAJ*. 159:657–662.

346. Vanneste J, Augustijn P, Dirven C et al. (1992). Shunting normal-pressure hydrocephalus: Do the benefits outweigh the risks? A multicenter study and literature review. *Neurology*. 42:54–59.

347. Friedland RP. (1989). 'Normal'-pressure hydrocephalus and the saga of the treatable dementias. *JAMA*. 262:2577–2581.

348. Hejl A, Hogh P, Waldemar G. (2002). Potentially reversible conditions in 1000 consecutive memory clinic patients. *J Neurol Neurosurg Psychiatry*. 73:390–394.

349. Graff-Radford NR, Godersky JC. (1986). Normal-pressure hydrocephalus. Onset of gait abnormality before dementia predicts good surgical outcome. *Arch Neurol*. 43:940–942.

350. Graff-Radford NR, Godersky JC, Jones MP. (1989). Variables predicting surgical outcome in symptomatic hydrocephalus in the elderly. *Neurology*. 39:1601–1604.

351. Wikkelso C, Andersson H, Blomstrand C et al. (1986). Normal pressure hydrocephalus. Predictive value of the cerebrospinal fluid tap-test. *Acta Neurol Scand*. 73:566–573.

352. Boon AJ, Tans JT, Delwel EJ et al. (1997). Dutch normal-pressure hydro-cephalus study: Prediction of outcome after shunting by resistance to outflow of cerebrospinal fluid. *J Neurosurg*. 87:687–693.

353. Doody RS, Stevens JC, Beck C et al. (2001). Practice parameter: Management of dementia (an evidence-based review): Report of the Quality Standards Subcommittee of the American Academy of Neurology. *Neurology*. 56:1154–1166.

354. Knapp MJ, Knopman DS, Solomon PR et al. (1994). A 30-week randomized controlled trial of high dose tacrine in patients with Alzheimer's disease. The Tacrine Study Group. *JAMA*. 271:985–991.

355. Rogers SL, Farlow MR, Doody RS et al. (1998). A 24-week, double-blind, placebo-controlled trial of donepezil in patients with Alzheimer's disease. *Neurology*. 50:136–145.

356. Burns A, Rossor M, Hecker J et al. (1999). The effects of donepezil in Alzheimer's disease—Results from a Multinational Trial. *Dement Geriatr Cogn Disord*. 10.237–244.

357. Corey-Bloom J, Anand R, Veach J, for the ENA 713 B352 Study Group. (1998). A randomized trial evaluating the efficacy and safety of ENA 713 (rivastigmine tartrate), a new acetylcholinesterase inhibitor, in patients with mild to moderately severe Alzheimer's disease. *Int J Geriatric Psychophar-macol*. 1:55 65.

358. Rosler M, Anand R, Cicin-Sain A et al. (1999). Efficacy and safety of rivastigmine in patients with Alzheimer's disease: International randomised controlled trial. *BMJ*. 318:633–640.

359. Raskind MA, Peskind ER, Wessel T, Yuan W. (2000). Galantamine in AD: A 6-month randomized, placebo-controlled trial with a 6-month extension. *Neurology*. 54:2261–2268.

360. Tariot PN, Solomon PR, Morris JC et al. (2000). A 5-month, randomized, placebo-controlled trial of galantamine in AD. *Neurology*. 54:2269–2276.

361. Rosen WG, Mohs RC, Davis KL. (1984). A new rating scale for Alzheimer's disease. *Am J Psychiatry*. 141:1356–1364.

362. Knopman DS, Knapp MJ, Gracon SI, Davis CS. (1994). The Clinician Interview-Based Impression (CIBI): A clinician's global change rating scale in Alzheimer's disease. *Neurology*. 44:2315–2321.

363. Schneider LS, Olin JT, Doody RS et al. (1997). Validity and reliability of the Alzheimer's Disease Cooperative Study—Clinical Global Impression of Change. The Alzheimer's Disease Cooperative Study. *Alzheimer Dis Assoc Disord*. 11(Suppl 2):S22–S32.

364. Rogers SL, Friedhoff LT. (1998). Long-term efficacy and safety of donepezil in the treatment of Alzheimer's disease: An interim analysis of the results of a US multicentre open label extension study. *Eur Neuropsychopharmacol*. 8:67–75.

365. Davis KL, Powchik P. (1995). Tacrine. *Lancet*. 345:625–630.

366. Rogers SL, Doody RS, Mohs RC, Friedhoff LT. (1998). Donepezil improves cognition and global function in Alzheimer disease: A 15-week, double-blind, placebo-controlled study. Donepezil Study Group. *Arch Intern Med*. 158:1021–1031.

367. Morris JC, Cyrus PA, Orazem J et al. (1998). Metrifonate benefits cognitive, behavioral, and global function in patients with Alzheimer's disease. *Neurology*. 50:1222–1230.

368. Bryson HM, Benfield P. (1997). Donepezil. *Drugs Aging*. 10:234–239; discussion 240–241.

369. Selkoe DJ. (2001). Presenilin, Notch, and the genesis and treatment of Alzheimer's disease. *Proc Natl Acad Sci U S A*. 98:11039–11041.

370. Behl C, Davis J, Cole GM, Schubert D. (1992). Vitamin E protects nerve cells from amyloid beta protein toxicity. *Biochem Biophys Res Commun*. 186:944–950.

371. Sano M, Ernesto C, Thomas RG et al. (1997). A controlled trial of selegiline, alpha-tocopherol, or both as treatment for Alzheimer's disease. The Alzheimer's Disease Cooperative Study. *N Engl J Med*. 336:1216–1222.

112

Mechanisms Involved in Gender Differences in Alzheimer's Disease: The Role of Leuteinizing and Follicle Stimulating Hormones

RICHARD BOWEN, MD*, CRAIG S. ATWOOD, PhD**, GEORGE PERRY, PhD**,
AND MARK A. SMITH, PhD**

*Voyager Pharmaceutical Corporation, Raleigh, NC
**Institute of Pathology, Case Western Reserve University, Cleveland, OH

Abstract

Alzheimer's disease, the leading cause of senile dementia, is clinically characterized by progressive memory loss; impairments in behavior, language, and visual-spatial skills; and, ultimately, death. Unfortunately, at present, therapeutic management of the disease is primarily targeted toward palliative treatment of symptoms rather than forestalling the progression of the disease. As such, even with state of the art pharmaceutical intervention, continued and progressive cognitive decline in patients is inevitable. The major obstacle in managing the disease and designing rational therapeutic targets is our incomplete understanding of the pathogenesis of the disease. In fact to date, although we know that age, gender, genetics, and environment all play a role in the disease, there has been no single mechanistic hypothesis, aside from that discussed herein, that explains all of the known features and risk factors for the disease.

One of the most intriguing aspects concerning the epidemiology of Alzheimer's disease is that the prevalence rate in women is roughly twice that in men and this skewed sex ratio is specific for Alzheimer's disease but not other dementias. The goal of this review is to delve further into these gender differences and to examine potential mechanistic hypotheses that underlie such differences. Specifically, we focus on how hormones of the hypothalamic-pituitary-gonadal axis, in particular the gonadotropins, play a central and determining role in disease susceptibility and progression such that therapeutic interventions targeted at gonadotropins could both prevent disease in those patients currently asymptomatic or halt, and even reverse, disease in those currently afflicted.

I. Background and Epidemiology of Alzheimer's Disease

Alzheimer's disease is by far the most common cause of senile dementia such that, within the United States, 10% of the population older than 65 years and as many as 47% of those older than 85 years are afflicted. Following initial diagnosis, the course of the disease varies from a few years to more than 20 years, with an average of 4 to 8 years. In fact, death related to Alzheimer's disease is the fourth leading cause of death in the aged population of the United States and is responsible for more than half of the institutionalization of the aged. Given such statistics, it is not surprising that the annual social cost of Alzheimer's disease for the United States is more than $100 billion, and this figure is projected to increase with the greater longevity and increased average age of the population.

The disease is invariably associated with, and defined by, neuronal and synaptic loss and the presence of extracellular deposits of amyloid-ß senile plaques and the intracellular formation of tau as neurofibrillary tangles in the brain and cerebral blood vessels [1,2]. The etiologic events that lead to the generation of these pathologic hallmarks are not well understood. Nonetheless, a number of hypotheses have been touted as explaining Alzheimer's disease, with the amyloid hypothesis gaining most attention because of the findings that early onset Alzheimer's disease result from mutations in either the amyloid ß protein precursor or presenilin-1 and presenilin-2, proteins involved in the processing of amyloid-ß [1]. However, perturbation of these elements in cell or animal models does not result in the multitude of biochemical and cellular changes found in the disease. For example, there is little or no neuronal loss in transgenic rodent models that overexpress amyloid-ß protein precursor despite large depositions of amyloid-ß protein [3]. More importantly, however, there is now considerable evidence that amyloid-ß is a consequence rather than causative factor in disease pathogenesis [4–6]. This has led to a consideration of other theories to explain the mechanism of disease that include tau phosphorylation [7–9], oxidative stress [10], metal ion dysregulation [11], and inflammation [12]. However, although these aspects are all associated with Alzheimer's disease and almost certainly play a role in the disease process, not one of these theories is sufficient alone to explain the spectrum of abnormalities found in the disease.

II. Gender Differences and Sex Hormones

One of the most intriguing aspects concerning the epidemiology of Alzheimer's disease is a skewed predication based on gender. This aspect has led to a focus on the roles of estrogen and testosterone in disease pathogenesis, and there are a number of lines of evidence suggesting that estrogen deficiency, following menopause, may contribute to the cause of Alzheimer's disease in women. First, the prevalence rate of Alzheimer's disease in women is roughly twice that in men [e.g., 13,14], and this skewed sex ratio is specific for Alzheimer's disease but not other dementias. This is in line with the abrupt earlier loss of gonadal function in females compared with males. Second, positive correlation exists between Alzheimer's disease and decreased estrogen levels following menopause (levels below that of men) with postmenopausal women with higher endogenous estrogen levels having a decreased prevalence of Alzheimer's disease [15]. Third, there is a decreased incidence [16] and a delay in the onset [17] of Alzheimer's disease among women on hormone replacement therapy following menopause [18]. Interestingly, estrogen replacement in postmenopausal women is associated with improved cognitive function [19]. Fourth, one study has shown a higher incidence of amyloid-ß senile plaques in the brains of women [20]. Finally, estrogens have been shown to be potent neuroprotective agents in a variety of *in vivo* model systems including fimbria-fornix lesions and middle cerebral artery occlusion [21].

If, however, the decline in estrogen is responsible for Alzheimer's disease, then it might be expected that disease-like changes would be observed during the 12- to 14-year period before pubescence when circulating concentrations of sex steroids are low. Furthermore, a decline in estrogen or testosterone does not explain why males with Down syndrome are at significantly higher risk of developing Alzheimer's disease-type changes and at an earlier age than their female counterparts [22]. Indeed, the concentration of estrogen and testosterone in both sexes is similar in patients with Down syndrome to those in the general population. These points indicate major flaws in our current understanding of the role of estrogen and testosterone in Alzheimer's disease. Indeed, recent studies have cast doubt on estrogen-replacement therapy as being protective against Alzheimer's disease [23–27] with only prophylactic use of estrogen delaying the onset of Alzheimer's disease [e.g., 16–18].

III. The Hypothalamic-Pituitary-Gonadal Axis

As discussed previously, most research evaluating how differences in gender relate to disease is primarily focused on the sex steroids estrogen and testosterone. However, there are a number of other hormones involved in the hypothalamic-pituitary-gonadal axis that regulates reproductive function, and, importantly, receptors for these other hormones are expressed in many nonreproductive tissues including the brain. As discussed later, we suspect, and have supporting evidence, that other hormones of the hypothalamic-pituitary-gonadal axis may be playing a central role in the pathogenesis of Alzheimer's disease.

The hormones of the hypothalamic-pituitary-gonadal axis include gonadotropin-releasing hormone, luteinizing hormone, follicle stimulating hormone, estrogen, progesterone, testosterone, activin, inhibin, and follistatin. The level of each of these hormones is regulated by complex feedback loops with the loop being initiated in the hypothalamus, which secretes gonadotropin-releasing hormone [reviewed in 28]. This, in turn, stimulates the anterior pituitary to secrete the gonadotropins, luteinizing hormone, and follicle stimulating hormone, which then bind to receptors on the gonads and stimulate oogenesis/spermatogenesis and sex steroid production. The sex steroids

feedback to the hypothalamus and pituitary, resulting in a decrease in gonadotropin secretion.

Activin and inhibin, members of the TGFß family of proteins, also are involved in this axis [reviewed in 29]. Activin is produced by most tissues and binds to both pituitary and hypothalamic receptors stimulating the secretion of follicle stimulating hormone and, to a lesser extent, luteinizing hormone. Unlike activin, no inhibin receptors have been reported. However, inhibin, which is primarily produced in the gonads in association with oogenesis/spermatogenesis, is known to bind to and inactivate activin. Inhibin therefore indirectly controls gonadotropin synthesis. Follistatin is a monomeric protein unrelated to TGFß proteins and is expressed in many different tissues. It also irreversibly binds to and inactivates activin.

With menopause/andropause, there is an increase in the production of gonadotropins and the bioavailability of activin that results from the loss of negative feedback of the sex steroids on the hypothalamus/pituitary and a decrease in gonadal inhibin production. In women, the loss of this negative feedback by estrogen and inhibin [30] results in a 3- to 4-fold and a 4- to 18-fold increase in the concentrations of serum luteinizing hormone and follicle stimulating hormone, respectively [31]. Likewise, men also experience a greater than 2-fold, and 3-fold, increase in luteinizing hormone and follicle stimulating hormone, respectively, as their reproductive function deteriorates [32]. Surprisingly, the effects of increased circulating gonadotropins on the aging brain are largely unexplored.

Luteinizing hormone and follicle stimulating hormone are produced by the pituitary gland, whereas the luteinizing hormone homologue, human chorionic gonadotropin, originates from the placenta. These glycoprotein hormones (molecular mass 30 to 40 kDa) consist of a common α-subunit and a hormone-specific ß-subunit that are associated through noncovalent interactions. The α-subunit consists of 92 amino acid residues, containing 10 cysteines involved in intrasubunit disulfide linkages and two N-glycosylation sites, and is encoded by a single gene, comprising 4 exons, localized on chromosome 6q12.21. The ß-subunits confer functional specificity of the hormones even though they share considerable homology (e.g., 83% between luteinizing hormone and human chorionic gonadotropin). The human luteinizing hormone ß-subunit gene is located on chromosome 19q13.32 [33], and it is notable that polymorphisms on chromosome 19q13.2 are associated with increased penetrance in sporadic Alzheimer's disease cases [34,35].

Understanding the regional and temporal selectivity of neuronal death in Alzheimer's disease is of paramount importance to understanding disease pathogenesis and, in this regard, it is notable that the regional expression of luteinizing hormone receptor in brain corresponds to the regional vulnerability exhibited in Alzheimer's disease [36–38]. That such receptors have functional and mechanistic importance in Alzheimer's disease is highlighted by our recent finding of elevated luteinizing hormone in a regiospecific manner that is predictive of neuronal vulnerability [39]. There are more than 40 papers indicating that the neurons in the brain of a patient with Alzheimer's disease express many cell cycle related proteins [reviewed in 40,41]. Because the highest concentrations of human chorionic gonadotropin also correspond to the time of most rapid cell proliferation (i.e., the fetal period), we suspect that neuronal elevations in luteinizing hormone could play a major role in the mitogenic abnormalities that characterize the disease [39].

IV. Mitogenic Abnormalities in Alzheimer's Disease

Although not traditionally characterized as a disease of aberrant mitogenesis, the unscheduled initiation of a cell division cycle in a mature, normally postmitotic neuron has been postulated to lead to an abortive re-activation of a variety of cell cycle components and ultimately the demise of the cell [40,41]. Neuronal changes supporting the involvement of cell cycle related events in the cause of the disease include the ectopic expression of markers of the cell cycle [42], organellekinesis [43], and cytoskeletal alterations including tau phosphorylation [44]. However, perhaps most compelling is the reactivation of the mitotic signaling pathways ERK and MAPK [9,45,46], which are coincidentally also known to be upregulated by gonadotropins, including luteinizing hormone [47]. Importantly, such mitotic alterations not only are one of the earliest neuronal abnormalities in the disease [46,48] but also, from a mechanistic stance, could lead to all of the other pathologic changes reported in the disease [40]. This latter finding strongly suggests that therapeutic interventions targeted toward ameliorating mitotic changes could be predicted to have a profound and positive impact on disease progression. In this regard, we and others have made a concerted effort to elucidate the initiating factor that drives aberrant mitotic re-entry in Alzheimer's disease.

V. Alzheimer's Disease is Associated with Elevated Serum Gonadotropins

In earlier studies, we reported a 2-fold increase in circulating gonadotropins in individuals with Alzheimer's disease compared with age-matched control individuals [49,50]. Because, as discussed previously, the highest density of gonadotropin receptors in the brain are found within the hippocampus [36–38], a region devastated in Alzheimer's disease, and gonadotropins are known to cross the blood-brain-barrier [51], we speculated that elevated gonadotropins, particularly luteinizing hormone, may be a driving pathogenic force in Alzheimer's disease [39]. In support of such a notion, we found significant elevations of luteinizing hormone in vulnerable populations in individuals with Alzheimer's disease compared with aged control cases [39]. Notably, such increases in neuronal luteinizing hormone appear to be a very early change in disease history serving to predict neuronal populations at risk of degeneration and death. In fact, elevations in luteinizing hormone parallel the ectopic expression of cell cycle and oxidative markers that represent one of the initiating pathologic changes preceding neuronal degeneration by decades [52]. Because luteinizing hormone is likely a powerful mitogen [47], it is likely, given the temporal and spatial overlap with mitotic changes in Alzheimer's disease [39; unpublished observations], that elevations in luteinizing hormone are responsible for inappropriate cell cycle re-entry in neurons [39,40]. Obviously this does not preclude the involvement of the other hormones of the hypothalamic-pituitary-gonadal axis that also exhibit significant changes in serum concentrations later in life.

VI. Therapeutic Considerations: Gonadotropin-releasing Hormone Antagonists

The reason that estrogen replacement therapy has not been shown to be effective in the treatment of Alzheimer's disease [23,24] is likely because it does not restore the hypothalamic-pituitary-gonadal axis to its premenopausal state because the gonadotropin stimulating effect of activin is still increased due to the loss of inhibin after menopause. In addition, even the "normal" concentrations of luteinizing hormone exhibited earlier in life may be detrimental late in life. Therefore, leuprolide acetate, a gonadotropin-releasing hormone agonist that has been shown to suppress luteinizing hormone to undetectable levels by downregulating pituitary gonadotropin-releasing hormone receptors, might be an effective method of treatment for Alzheimer's disease. Although the use of leuprolide in premenopausal women has resulted in memory loss and depression [53], these adverse reactions were shown to be due to the secondary abrupt loss of estrogen production and memory and mood returned to normal after estrogen replacement [54]. Because women with Alzheimer's disease are postmenopausal and already have lost their ability to produce estrogen, leuprolide would be predicted to have no effect on their estrogen production.

Because gonadotropins are likely mitogenic and are implicated in cell cycle changes associated with Alzheimer's disease, we tested whether a gonadotropin-releasing hormone analogue (leuprolide) was able to downregulate gonadotropin releasing hormone receptors in neuroblastoma cells thereby inhibiting the mitogenicity of growth factors. Administration of leuprolide in humans has been shown to initially increase pituitary secretion of gonadotropins for 2 to 3 days, after which pituitary receptors are downregulated resulting in a significant decrease in luteinizing hormone secretion thereafter [54]. We found that leuprolide at concentrations equivalent to that present in the blood of individuals taking this drug for prostate cancer (~10 nM) dramatically decreased cell growth of neuroblastoma cells (unpublished observations). These results indicate that leuprolide is an effective gonadotropin-releasing hormone receptor antagonist in neurons and has great potential for use in diseases of aberrant cell cycle regulation such as Alzheimer's disease and neuroblastomas.

VII. Suggestions for Further Investigations

- What is the therapeutic efficacy of gonadotropin-lowering drugs (e.g., leuprolide) in patients with Alzheimer's disease?
- What role do other members of the hypothalamic-pituitary-gonadal axis play in Alzheimer's disease?
- What is the role of the hypothalamic-pituitary-gonadal axis in other neurodegenerative diseases and/or age-associated diseases?

References

1. Selkoe DJ. (1997). Alzheimer's disease: Genotypes, phenotypes and treatments. *Science.* 275:630–631.
2. Smith MA. (1998). Alzheimer disease. In *International Review of Neurobiology* (Bradley RJ, Harris RA, eds.), vol. 42, pp 1–54. San Diego, CA: Academic Press.
3. Irizarry MC, Soriano F, McNamara M *et al.* (1997). Aß deposition is associated with neuropil changes, but not with overt neuronal loss in the human

amyloid precursor protein V717F (PDAPP) transgenic mouse. *J Neurosci.* 17:7053–7059.

4. Perry G, Nunomura A, Raina AK, Smith MA. (2000). Amyloid-ß junkies. *Lancet.* 355:757.

5. Obrenovich ME, Joseph JA, Atwood CS *et al.* (2002). Amyloid-ß: A (life) preserver for the brain. *Neurobiol Aging.* 23.1097–1099.

6. Rottkamp CA, Atwood CS, Joseph JA *et al.* (2002). The state versus amyloid-ß: The trial of the most wanted criminal in Alzheimer disease. *Peptides.* 23:1333–1341.

7. Trojanowski JQ, Clark CM, Arai H, Lee VM. (1999). Elevated levels of tau in cerebrospinal fluid: Implications for the antemortem diagnosis of Alzheimer's disease elevated levels of tau in cerebrospinal fluid. *J Alzheimers Dis.* 1.297 305.

8. Avila J. (2000). Tau aggregation into fibrillar polymers: Taupathies. *FEBS Lett.* 476:89–92.

9. Zhu X, Perry G, Raina AK, Smith MA. (2002). The role of mitogen-activated protein kinase pathways in Alzheimer disease. *NeuroSignals.* 11:270–281.

10. Perry G, Castellani RJ, Hirai K, Smith MA. (1998). Reactive oxygen species mediate cellular damage in Alzheimer disease. *J Alzheimers Dis.* 1:45–55.

11. Perry G, Sayre LM, Atwood CS *et al.* (2002). The role of iron and copper in the aetiology of neurodegenerative disorders: Therapeutic implications. *CNS Drugs.* 16:339–352.

12. Atwood CS, Huang X, Moir RD *et al.* (2001). Neuroinflammatory responses in the Alzheimer's disease brain promote the oxidative post-translational modification of amyloid deposits. In *Alzheimer's Disease: Advances in Etiology, Pathogenesis and Therapeutics* (Iqbal K, Sisodia SS, Winblad B, eds.), pp. 341–361. Chichester, United Kingdom: John Wiley & Sons, Ltd.

13. Jorm AF, Korten AE, Henderson AS. (1987). The prevalence of dementia: A quantitative integration of the literature. *Acta Psychiatr Scand.* 76:465–479.

14. McGonigal G, Thomas B, McQuade C *et al.* (1993). Epidemiology of Alzheimer's presenile dementia in Scotland, 1974–88. *BMJ.* 306:680–683.

15. Manly JJ, Merchant CA, Jacobs DM *et al.* (2000). Endogenous estrogen levels and Alzheimer's disease among postmenopausal women. *Neurology.* 54:833–837.

16. Henderson VW, Paganini-Hill A, Emanuel CK *et al.* (1994). Estrogen replacement therapy in older women. Comparisons between Alzheimer's disease cases and nondemented control subjects. *Arch Neurol.* 51:896–900.

17. Tang MX, Jacobs D, Stern Y *et al.* (1996). Effect of oestrogen during menopause on risk and age at onset of Alzheimer's disease. *Lancet.* 348:429–432.

18. Kawas C, Resnick S, Morrison A *et al.* (1997). A prospective study of estrogen replacement therapy and the risk of developing Alzheimer's disease: The Baltimore Longitudinal Study of Aging. *Neurology.* 48:1517–1521.

19. Jacobs DR, Pereira MA Meyer KA, Kushi LH. (2000). Fiber from whole grains, but not refined grains, is inversely associated with all-cause mortality in older women: The Iowa women's health study. *J Am Coll Nutr.* 19:326S–330S.

20. Stam FC, Wigboldus JM, Smeulders AW. (1986). Age incidence of senile brain amyloidosis. *Pathol Res Pract.* 181:555–562.

21. Shi J, Zhang YQ, Simpkins JW. (1997). Effects of 17ß-estradiol on glucose transporter 1 expression and endothelial cell survival following focal ischemia in rat. *Exp Brain Res.* 117:200–206.

22. Schupf N, Kapell D, Nightingale B *et al.* (1998). Earlier onset of Alzheimer's disease in men with Down syndrome. *Neurology.* 50:991–995.

23. Mulnard RA. (2000). Estrogen as a treatment for Alzheimer disease. *JAMA.* 284:307–308.

24. Mulnard RA, Cotman CW, Kawas C *et al.* (2000). Estrogen replacement therapy for treatment of mild to moderate Alzheimer disease: A randomized controlled trial. Alzheimer's Disease Cooperative Study. *JAMA.* 283:1007–1015.

25. Wang PN, Liao SQ, Liu RS *et al.* (2000). Effects of estrogen on cognition, mood, and cerebral blood flow in AD: A controlled study. *Neurology.* 54:2061–2066.

26. Henderson VW, Paganini-Hill A, Miller BL *et al.* (2000). Estrogen for Alzheimer's disease in women: Randomized, double-blind, placebo-controlled trial. *Neurology.* 54:295–301.

27. Seshadri S, Zornberg GL, Derby LE *et al.* (2001). Postmenopausal estrogen replacement therapy and the risk of Alzheimer disease. *Arch Neurol.* 58:435–440.

28. Genazzani AR, Gastaldi M, Bidzinska B *et al.* (1992). The brain as a target organ of gonadal steroids. *Psychoneuroendocrinology.* 17:385–390.

29. Welt C, Sidis Y, Keutmann H, Schneyer A. (2002). Activins, inhibins, and follistatins: From endocrinology to signaling. A paradigm for the new millennium. *Exp Biol Med.* 227:724–752.

30. Couzinet B, Schaison G. (1993). The control of gonadotrophin secretion by ovarian steroids. *Hum Reprod Suppl.* 2:97–101

31. Chakravarti S, Collins WP, Forecast JD *et al.* (1976). Hormonal profiles after the menopause. *BMJ.* 2(6039):784–787.

32. Neaves WB, Johnson L, Porter JC *et al.* (1984). Leydig cell numbers, daily sperm production, and serum gonadotropin levels in aging men. *J Clin Endocrinol Metab.* 59:756–763.

33. Fiddes JC, Talmadge K. (1984). Structure, expression and evolution of the gene for the human glycoprotein hormones. *Recent Prog Horm Res.* 40:43–78.

34. Corder EH, Saunders AM, Strittmatter WJ *et al.* (1993). Gene dose of apolipoprotein E type 4 allele and the risk of Alzheimer's disease in late onset families. *Science.* 261:921–923.

35. Poirier J, Davignon J, Douthillier D *et al.* (1993). Apolipoprotein E polymorphism and Alzheimer's disease. *Lancet.* 342:697–699.

36. Lei ZM, Rao CV, Kornyei JL *et al.* (1993). Novel expression of human chorionic gonadotropin/luteinizing hormone receptor gene in brain. *Endocrinology.* 132:2262–2270.

37. Al Hader AA, Lei ZM, Rao CN. (1997). Novel expression of functional luteinizing hormone/chorionic gonadotropin receptors in cultured glial cells from neonatal rat brains. *Biol Reprod.* 56:501–507.

38. Al-Hader AA, Lei ZM, Rap CV. (1997). Neurons from fetal rat brains contain functional luteinizing hormone/chorionic gonadotropin receptors. *Biol Reprod.* 56:1071–1076.

39. Bowen RL, Smith MA, Harris PLR *et al.* (2002). Elevated luteinizing hormone expression colocalizes with neurons vulnerable to Alzheimer's disease pathology. *J Neurosci Res.* 70:514–518.

40. Raina AK, Zhu X, Rottkamp CA *et al.* (2000). Cyclin' toward dementia: Cell cycle abnormalities and abortive oncogenesis in Alzheimer disease. *J Neurosci Res.* 61:128–133.

41. Bowser R, Smith MA. (2002). Cell cycle proteins in Alzheimer's disease: Plenty of wheels but no cycle. *J Alzheimers Dis.* 4:249–254.

42. McShea A, Harris PLR, Webster KR *et al.* (1997). Abnormal expression of the cell cycle regulators p16 and CDK4 in Alzheimer's disease. *Am J Pathol.* 150:1933–1939.

43. Hirai K, Aliev G, Nunomura A *et al.* (2001). Mitochondrial abnormalities in Alzheimer's disease. *J Neurosci.* 21:3017–3023.

44. Zhu X, Rottkamp CA, Boux H *et al.* (2000). Activation of p38 kinase links tau phosphorylation, oxidative stress, and cell cycle-related events in Alzheimer disease. *J Neuropathol Exp Neurol.* 59:880–888.

45. Perry G, Roder H, Nunomura A *et al.* (1999). Activation of neuronal extracellular receptor kinase (ERK) in Alzheimer disease links oxidative stress to abnormal phosphorylation. *Neuroreport.* 10:2411–2415.

46. Zhu X, Castellani RJ, Takeda A *et al.* (2001). Differential activation of neuronal ERK, JNK/SAPK and p38 in Alzheimer disease: The "two hit" hypothesis. *Mech Ageing Dev.* 123:39–46.

47. Harris D, Bonfil D, Chuderland D *et al.* (2002). Activation of MAPK cascades by GnRH: ERK and Jun N-terminal kinase are involved in basal and GnRH-stimulated activity of the glycoprotein hormone LHß-subunit promoter. *Endocrinology.* 143:1018–1025.

48. Vincent I, Zheng JH, Dickson DW *et al.* (1998). Mitotic phosphoepitopes precede paired helical filaments in Alzheimer's disease. *Neurobiol Aging.* 19:287–296.

49. Bowen RL, Isley JP, Atkinson RL. (2000). An association of elevated serum gonadotropin concentrations and Alzheimer disease? *J Neuroendocrinol.* 12:351–354.

50. Short RA, Bowen RL, O'Brien PC, Graff-Radford NR. (2001). Elevated gonadotropin levels in patients with Alzheimer disease. *Mayo Clin Proc.* 76:906–909.

51. Lukacs H, Hiatt ES, Lei ZM, Rao CV. (1995). Peripheral and intracerebroventricular administration of human chorionic gonadotropin alters several hippocampus-associated behaviors in cycling female rats. *Horm Behav.* 29:42–58.

52. Nunomura A, Perry G, Aliev G *et al.* (2001). Oxidative damage is the earliest event in Alzheimer disease. *J Neuropathol Exp Neurol.* 60:759–767.

53. Varney NR, Syrop C, Kubu CS *et al.* (1993). Neuropsychologic dysfunction in women following leuprolide acetate induction of hypoestrogenism. *J Assist Reprod Genet.* 10:53–57.

54. Sherwin BB, Tulandi T. (1996). "Add-back" estrogen reverses cognitive deficits induced by a gonadotropin-releasing hormone agonist in women with leiomyomata uteri. *J Clin Endocrinol Metab.* 81:2545–2549.

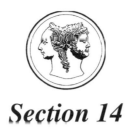

Section 14

FUTURE AREAS TO EXPAND

113

Gender Differences in Dermatology

MARY GAIL MERCURIO, MD

Associate Professor of Dermatology, University of Rochester School of Medicine, Rochester, NY

This chapter summarizes the current state of the literature regarding gender differences in dermatology. The skin is just one of the many tissues capable of metabolizing hormones, and many of the sexual dimorphisms can be attributed to the effects of distinctive hormonal milieus between the sexes. The abrupt and often dramatic evidence of structural and functional changes appearing at the time of menopause and the reversibility with replacement therapy give credence to the impact of estrogen on the skin. Sex steroids influence the development and function of cells of the immune system resulting in females having higher immunoglobulin levels and prevalence of autoimmune diseases including systemic lupus, which is discussed elsewhere in this text. In contrast, the gender discrepancy in melanoma survival is not clearly explicable at the present time on the basis of hormones. Although there is increasing research directed at women's health, conditions not unique to the female sex or reproduction need further exploration. The dearth of gender-specific research in dermatology has primarily arisen as an incidental finding in studies with an alternate focus. An increased emphasis on gender-specific basic science, clinical, and epidemiologic research highlighting dissimilarities should result in improvements in illness prevention and optimal health care delivery for both women and men.

I. Structure and Function of Skin

Human skin consists of three distinct layers: (1) the outer multilayered epidermis, which serves as a barrier to precisely control both ingress of noxious substances and egress of water; (2) the underlying dermis rich in connective tissue to maintain strength and structure; and (3) the innermost layer, the adipose tissue, which functions as a thermoregulator, energy source and insulator and provides a cushion or, as is often the case, too much of a cushion.

A. Epidermis

In its important barrier function, the skin limits inward migration of environmental substances and outward migration of water to maintain homeostasis. Measurements of the functional state of the barrier include transepidermal water loss (TEWL) and percutaneous absorption. Early dermatologic literature erroneously suggests that women react more intensely to irritants than men. Multiple studies have demonstrated no significant gender-related differences in barrier integrity or barrier recovery following perturbation in adult skin [1,2]. In addition, no difference in TEWL has been demonstrated between men and women, and both sexes demonstrate an increase in TEWL with age that correlates clinically with increased skin dryness [3]. These clinical characteristics are consistent with studies that have shown that the stratum corneum in adult males and females is of equivalent thickness and lipid composition, although in females the percentage composition of various sphingolipid species does change from childhood to adulthood and remains stable in males over this time period [4,5]. The perception that women have more sensitive skin than men probably relates to their increased use of cosmetics and skin care items rather than any physiologic gender difference [6].

Gender differences in the survival of premature infants have long been recognized, with males displaying increased morbidity and mortality. Sex differences in rates of the epidermal barrier development have been demonstrated, and delayed skin maturation in males is a possible contributor to this prognostic dissimilarity. Studies have shown that ontogeny of the epidermal permeability barrier and lung occur in parallel in the fetal rat, and sex differences in maturation have been demonstrated whereby testosterone inhibits and estrogen enhances barrier development [7,8]. These oppositional effects of testosterone and estrogen on help to explain the increased mortality in premature male versus female infants [9].

B. Dermis

The old adage that men are "thicker skinned" is structurally accurate. Total skin collagen content is less in females resulting in thinner skin compared with males [10,11]. With aging, the collagen content decreases in both sexes; the decline is more gradual in men occurring throughout adulthood, whereas in women there is a significant and sometimes dramatic thinning commencing at the time of menopause [12]. Nearly one third of skin collagen is lost in the first 5 years after menopause [13]. In adult skin, the features of aging, such as increased slackness and wrinkling, are closely linked to the total collagen content. Estrogen deficiency particularly affects the fibroblasts of the dermis decreasing collagen production. Similar to skin, type 1 collagen is abundant in bone and its correlative decrease in this tissue reduces bone mineral content with age culminating in osteoporosis [14].

Hormone replacement therapy (HRT) has been demonstrated in multiple studies to have beneficial effects on the various sequelae of menopause, including the skin. Estrogen supplementation preserves skin collagen content in postmenopausal women, thereby supporting the hypothesis that estrogen decline plays a causal role in critical cutaneous ageing phenomenon [15–17]. Aging related to the failure of estrogen production at the menopause accelerates intrinsic aging and, together with photoaging, may dramatically increase the apparent age of a woman; women with higher levels of estrogen subjectively appear younger than their chronologic age, whereas those with low levels of the hormone appear older [18]. In addition to increasing collagen and decreasing slackness and wrinkling of skin, other benefits of estrogen are substantial and include decreased dry skin and improved barrier function [19,20], increased wound healing [21], and decreased risk of venous ulcers [22]. Recent results from the Women's Health Initiative study highlighting the coronary disadvantages of HRT have already abruptly curtailed its use in postmenopausal women who will no longer be able to benefit from the cutaneous effects [23]. The combination of these new limitations on widely prescribing HRT along with the obvious cutaneous benefits will likely prompt further study to better define the applicability of topical estrogen for direct application to facial skin to harness the known advantages. Limited research has shown that topical estrogen acts like oral HRT in preserving skin thickness and increasing collagen and maintaining moisture content of the skin [24–26]. Because life expectancy is increasing and women are spending one half to one third of their lives after menopause, and the use of HRT is diminishing, and a greater awareness of the impact of menopause on the skin is imperative.

Cigarette smoking is the most preventable cause of significant morbidity and mortality in the United States. In addition to ultraviolet light exposure, smoking is an important exogenous contributor to premature skin aging. Cigarette smoking is an independent risk factor for the early onset of wrinkling resulting in the distinctive "smoker's face" with deep furrows radiating from the corner of the mouth. The mechanism is multifactorial but primarily related to elastic fiber damage [27]. A recent study suggests that women may be more susceptible to the wrinkling effects of smoking, demonstrating the relative risk of moderate-to-severe wrinkling for current smokers was 2.3 in men and 3.1 in women [28]. Given the overwhelming quest by both men and women to maintain a youthful appearance, knowledge of the association between cigarette smoking and skin aging may be an effective motivator for smoking cessation, and dermatologists have an ideal vantage point for delivery of this potentially life-saving message.

C. Adipose Tissue

The dermis is attached to the subcutaneous fat layer, which is involved in thermoregulation, energy provision, support, nutrition, and cosmetic appearance. The adipose tissue is composed of multiple layers of fat interspersed with connective tissue. The connective tissue compartmentalizes the fat cells into chambers. It has been demonstrated that the shape of the chambers differ in men and women such that protrusion of these chambers readily occurs in women causing the "mattress phenomenon" or cellulite, but in men the chambers more securely contain the fat preventing protrusion [29]. Men with androgen deficiency demonstrate these same findings as women suggesting that this sexual dimorphism in the structural characteristics of subdermal connective tissue may be due to the proliferative effect of androgens on the mesenchyme [30].

Profound gender differences in fat accumulation are obvious; women tend to have greater subcutaneous fat distribution involving the gluteal and femoral regions and men tend to accumulate a greater proportion of visceral adipose tissue in the abdominal region. These patterns of fat distribution result in the terms "pear" and "apple" body habitus used to describe women and men, respectively. These regionally differing fat depots also demonstrate different adipocyte metabolic behaviors including triglyceride deposition and lipoprotein lipase activity [31]. Women with hyperandrogenemia in the setting of polycystic ovary syndrome (PCOS) often have a distribution of fat resembling that of a man—which along with this male habitus also antagonizes their cardiac risk gender advantage. Independent of the general overweight level, the ratio of waist-to-hip circumferences (WHR) is associated with adverse levels of lipids, lipoproteins, and insulin and is predictive of heart disease [32].

II. Skin Cancer

Ultraviolet radiation from the sun is a major etiologic event in the development of skin cancer, and individuals with fairer skin complexion are at greatest risk. Dermatologists and others have long been striving through vigorous educational campaigns to raise public awareness of the detrimental impact of ultraviolet light exposure as a means of preventing skin cancer. Males have a higher incidence of all three major forms of skin cancer— basal cell carcinoma, squamous cell carcinoma, and melanoma. Sunlight exposure and genetic factors influence the risk for skin cancer. Sunscreens have been advocated as an important means of skin cancer prevention. A reduced incidence of precancerous skin lesions has been demonstrated with regular use of sunscreen [33]. Females use sunscreen more frequently than males and are more knowledgeable than men about the long-term effects of sun exposure [34,35]. A study identifying predictors of sunscreen use in males and females revealed that men are more likely to use sunscreen because they fear cancer, whereas women are primarily motivated by cosmetic concerns [36].

A. Melanoma

Melanoma is the most serious form of skin cancer accounting for the majority of skin cancer deaths. In the United States, the incidence of melanoma is rising more rapidly than any other cancer increasing 120% between 1973 and 1994 [37]. Lifetime risk for melanoma in the United States is about 1 in 70, with males developing melanoma at a higher rate than females. The distribution of melanoma incidence by age range and sex varies. Up until age 40, women are diagnosed with melanoma at a higher rate than men. After 40, however the rate increases with increasing age for both sexes but more dramatically in men. In contrast to men, women demonstrate a more gradual age-related increase in incidence with a plateau beginning at menopause [38].

The sites of predilection for the development of melanoma reflect gender differences in sun exposure patterns, namely clothing and hairstyles. Intermittent sun exposure, often recreational rather than occupational, is more closely linked to melanoma [39]. Multiple studies have shown that sites of predilection for melanoma differ between the sexes with men most likely to develop melanoma on the trunk and women on the lower extremities [37]. This correlates with the regional differences in sites with greatest tendency for melanocytic nevi, a risk factor for the development of melanoma [40,41]. The development of melanoma on parts of the body that are not exposed to the sun indicate that a direct effect of ultraviolet radiation is not the only causative factor in the development of this cancer.

Mortality rates from melanoma are increasing more gradually than incidence rates; this has been attributed to educational programs aimed at early detection resulting in an increased proportion of thinner melanomas at the time of diagnosis. It is well documented that females show a higher survival rate than males rendering gender an accepted prognostic parameter in melanoma assessment independent of any other risk factor [42,43]. The survival advantage is particularly apparent among patients with advanced stage disease suggesting that the putative factor is exerted at the level of metastasis inhibition [44]. Mechanisms by which gender might be accountable for prognostic differences are not entirely clear, but further insight is critical to better hone prevention and treatment strategies. Evidence linking female hormones to melanoma has been controversial; however, the battery of data suggest that sex steroids themselves are not the mediator of this survival advantage [45]. Estrogen receptors do exist on melanoma cells, although they are low affinity receptors differing from the type 1 estrogen receptors seen in breast and prostate tumors. In addition, antiestrogenic agents do not appear to have an antiproliferative effect on melanoma cell lines [45]. Neither exogenous nor endogenous hormones contribute significantly to an increased risk of melanoma [46,47]. The inferior prognosis previously linked with pregnancy likely stems from increased tumor thickness as a result of delayed diagnosis from attributing clinical atypia to physiologic changes of pregnancy [48]. Despite the popularity of the notion that moles change during pregnancy, the relation between changing melanocytic nevi and pregnancy had not been clearly studied until the recent demonstration that the size of nevi do not appear to change during this time and any change should, therefore, be highly suspect [49].

Lifestyle modification and early detection are the principal means of improving mortality from this disease. One of the most critical factors in melanoma prognosis is depth of the cancer so that early diagnosis is critical, and patients play a very important role in early detection. At diagnosis, males have more invasive and fatal melanomas than women. Screening and education are shown to be particularly useful in individuals with a high risk of melanoma [50], and those patients who were informed to be at risk of melanoma had thinner tumors at the time of diagnosis [51]. Professional screening and conscientious self-examination should decrease the melanoma incidence and mortality. Women have been shown to be better informed about melanoma than men, and women are more likely than men to examine their skin and identify melanoma in themselves [52,53].

B. Cutaneous Lymphomal

Primary cutaneous lymphomas are a heterogeneous group of disorders of T and B cell origins, the most prevalent of which is the T-cell lymphoma, mycosis fungoides. Male gender is an epidemiologic risk factor for developing cutaneous lymphoma, and further investigation is necessary to determine what role, if any, sex hormones are involved in the pathogenesis of lymphoproliferative disorders [53a].

III. Pilosebaceous Unit

The pilosebaceous unit, comprised of the hair follicle and sebaceous gland, is the most thoroughly elucidated androgen-sensitive skin component. Androgen receptors are found in the hair follicle and sebaceous glands. Androgen stimulation of the hair follicle can have one of two diametrically opposed effects: (1) miniaturization of the terminal hair as occurs in the setting of androgenetic alopecia (AGA) in men and women or (2) conversion of a vellus hair to a terminal hair as occurs in the setting of hirsutism, a condition afflicting women only. Androgen stimulation of the sebaceous gland causes secretion of sebum, a complex mixture of lipids that play an important role in the overall pathogenesis of the disease. Sebaceous gland secretion is higher in males than females at all ages, peaking at puberty in both sexes. In men, sebum levels remain essentially unchanged from young adulthood until the eighth decade; in contrast, women experience a sharp decline in sebum production in the sixth decade [54]. The explanation for the pattern of decreasing sebaceous gland secretion with age in both men and women is a concomitant decrease in the endogenous production of androgens, although the glands themselves actually enlarge.

A. Acne

Acne is one clinical condition arising from an aberration of this important endocrine target. The sebaceous glands are highly responsive to hormones, the most active of which is dihydrotestosterone (DHT), a potent androgen arising from conversion of serum testosterone by the enzyme 5α reductase. There are two distinct forms of 5α-reductase, type I and type II, which differ in their tissue distributions. Isoenzyme type I predominates in the sebaceous gland. Circulating testosterone is locally converted to DHT in the sebaceous gland, and DHT stimulates production of sebum. The activity of the type 1 isozyme is greater in skin from acne-prone regions such as the face compared with areas not prone to the development of acne [55]. Although DHT is essential for attainment of adult levels of sebum secretion, additional factors are operative; there is a wide degree of overlap between males and females in their sebum secretion rates despite significant differences in circulating androgen levels [56].

Although acne mainly affects adolescents, it also occurs in a significant portion of adults older than 25 years, the majority of whom are women [57]. In the adult women who develop this variant of acne, it may either be a continuum of teenage acne or arise de novo in those without a history of acne. The effect of androgens, more than other etiologic factors in the causation of acne, seems to be particularly important in adult females. In one study, serum levels were found to be significantly higher in women with acne than women without acne; serum androgens appear to be less important than nonhormonal factors in the pathogenesis of acne in men, and these authors speculate that this may be because sebaceous gland enzyme activity in men may already be maximally stimulated by their serum levels of androgens [58]. Clinically, the adult female variety of acne has a predilection for the jaw-line region and lesions tend to be inflammatory in nature; premenstrual exacerbations and mild coexistent facial hirsutism are common. Hormonal interventions for acne are particularly valuable in the adult female setting, including estrogen and antiandrogens, which have a net effect of reducing androgen expression and are for obvious reasons not a treatment option for males. There are no hormonal therapies presently available that specifically target androgen metabolizing enzymes within the sebaceous gland, namely 5α-reductase type I.

B. Androgenetic Alopecia

The pathogenesis of AGA, also known as pattern baldness, involves a genetic predisposition and adequate androgen levels. In both sexes, it is characterized both clinically and histologically by progressive, nonscarring miniaturization of the hair follicle. Dihydrotestosterone is the androgen primarily implicated in the development of AGA; testosterone is converted to DHT by the enzyme 5α-reductase type II residing in the inner root sheath of the hair follicle. Recognition of the important role of androgens on hair growth occurred decades ago when it was demonstrated that castrated males did not develop AGA, but those with a genetic predilection subsequently developed AGA if supplemented with testosterone [59]. The androgen hypothesis was honed further making DHT the putative androgen by the demonstration that individuals born with a genetic deficiency of 5a-reductase did not develop AGA [60].

In men with AGA, the hair loss generally involves bilateral recession at the temples and thinning at the vertex. In the most extensive cases, there is complete loss on the top of the head with a residual horse-shoe shaped fringe of hair along the occipital scalp from ear-to-ear. In contrast, most women with AGA, demonstrate a characteristic retention of the frontal hairline with thinning of the midscalp that is most accentuated frontally giving a central part the appearance of a Christmas tree [61]. Variations in distribution and density of 5α-reductase on the scalp reflect the differing presentations of AGA in men and women [62]. It is a very important distinction to note when bitemporal/vertex ("male pattern") hair loss is present in a woman because a systemic hyperandrogenic state should be sought. In this situation, there may be increased levels of testosterone arising from the adrenal glands or ovaries, and the hair loss may be the first clinical evidence of a tumor. Most women with AGA have normal levels of circulating androgens, and are therefore, by definition, not hyperandrogenic; in simpler terms, the hair follicles in most men and women with AGA have an increased sensitivity to normal levels of circulating androgens because of increased local 5α-reductase activity. A genetic relationship between PCOS and early male pattern baldness has been documented suggesting that these are female and male phenotypes, respectively, of the same gene abnormality [63].

The putative role of DHT in the pathogenesis of AGA provide a strong rationale for the use of the 5α-reductase type 2 inhibitor, finasteride, in the treatment. Finasteride is effective in the treatment of males with AGA [64]. A small study has shown it to be ineffective in postmenopausal females with AGA [65]. It may, however, be beneficial in the small subset of females with AGA who have elevated circulating androgens—a situation more closely resembling the male hormonal milieu

[66]. Clearly large-scale studies are needed to determine the efficacy of 5α-reductase inhibitors in women of all ages and particularly the majority of females with hair loss in the setting of normal circulating androgens. These data are slow to come by because of the reluctance to use finasteride in women of child-bearing age; DHT is necessary during embryogenesis, and there is potential for incomplete masculinization of the external genitalia of an unborn male fetus exposed to the drug through maternal intake. It has long been assumed by dermatologists that all female AGA is the same and that female and male AGA are the same entity with differing clinical presentations. These perceptions are only recently being challenged, in part, because of their divergent treatment responses to 5α-reductase inhibition [67–69].

IV. Conclusion

Sex steroids perform many functions apart from reproduction resulting in widespread impact on multiple systems and tissues including the skin. There are no doubt numerous additional structural, functional, and disease-specific cutaneous gender differences yet to be identified. As more gender-specific research is performed, the findings will translate into improved comprehension of the pathogenesis of cutaneous disorders to the benefit of all patients.

V. Suggestions for Further Investigations

More exacting research is necessary to further delineate gender differences in prevalence of cutaneous malignancies and disparate presentations of numerous dermatologic conditions.

References

1. Lammintausta K, Maibach H, Wilson D. (1987). Irritant reactivity in males and females. *Contact Dermatitis.* 17:275–280.
2. Reed JT, Ghadially R, Elias PM. (1995). Skin type, but neither race nor gender, influence epidermal permeability barrier function. *Arch Dermatol.* 131:1134–1138.
3. Cua AB, Wilhelm KP, Maibach HI. (1990). Frictional properties of human skin: Relation to age, sex, anatomic region, stratum corneum hydration and transepidermal water loss. *Br J Dermatol.* 123:473–479.
4. Denda M, Koyama J, Hori J et al. (1993). Age- and sex-dependent change in stratum corneum sphingolipids. *Arch Dermatol Res.* 285:415–417.
5. Lock-Andersen J, Therkildsen P, de Fine Olivarius F et al. (1997). Epidermal thickness, skin pigmentation and constitutive photosensitivity. *Photoderm Photoimmunol Photomed.* 13(4):153–158.
6. Draelos ZD. (1999). Variability in skin parameters and sensitive skin. *Cosmetic Dermatol.* Aug:11–14.
7. Hanley K, Rassner U, Jiang Y et al. (1996). Hormonal basis for the gender difference in epidermal barrier formation in the fetal rat. *J Clin Invest.* 97:2576–2584.
8. Kao JS, Garg A, Mao-Qiang Man et al. (2001). Testosterone perturbs epidermal permeability barrier homeostasis. *J Invest Dermatol.* 116:443–451.
9. LaPine TR, Jackson JC, Bennett FC. (1995). Outcome of infants weighing less than 800 grams at birth: 15 years' experience. *Pediatrics.* 96:479–483.
10. Seidenari S, Pagnoni A, Di Nardo A et al. (1994). Echographic evaluation with image analysis of normal skin: Variations according to age and sex. *Skin Pharmacol.* 7:201–209.
11. Escoffier C, de Rigal J, Rochefort A et al. (1989). Age-related mechanical properties of human skin: An *in vivo* study. *J Invest Dermatol.* 93: 353–357.
12. Pierard-Franchimont C, Dehavay CF, Delexhe-Mauhin R et al. (1999). Climacteric skin ageing of the face: A prospective longitudinal comparative trial on the effect of oral hormonal replacement therapy. *Maturitas.* 32:87–95.

13. Lobo RA. (2001). In *Medscape Clinical Update: Menopause Management for the Millennium*. Ftr5 *Medscape General Medicine* 2001. Available at www.medscape.com/viewarticle/413064.

14. Whitmore SE, Levine MA. (1998). Risk factors for reduced skin thickness and bone density: Possible clues regarding pathophysiology, prevention, and treatment. *J Am Acad Dermatol*. 38:215–255.

15. Brincat M, Moniz CF, Kabalan S *et al.* (1987). Decline in skin collagen content and metacarpal index after the menopause and its prevention with sex hormone replacement. *Br J Obstet Gynaecol*. 94:126–129.

16. Castel-Branco C, Duran M, Gonzalez-Merlo J. (1992). Skin collagen changes related to age and hormone replacement therapy. *Maturitas*. 15:113–119.

17. Maheux R, Naud F, Rioux M *et al.* (1994). A randomized double-blind, placebo controlled study on the effect of conjugated estrogens on skin thickness *Am J Obstet Gynecol*. 170:642–649.

18. Wildt L, Sir-Peterman T. (1999). Oestrogen and age estimations of perimenopausal women. *Lancet*. 354:224.

19. Dunn LB, Damesyn M, Moore A *et al.* (1997). Does estrogen prevent skin aging? *Arch Dermatol*. 133:339–342.

20. Pierard-Franchimont C, Letawe C, Goffin V *et al.* (1995). Skin water-holding capacity and transdermal estrogen therapy for menopause: A pilot study. *Maturitas*. 22:151–154.

21. Ashcroft GS, Dodsworth J, Van Boxtel E *et al.* (1997). Estrogen accelerates cutaneous wound healing associated with an increase in TGF-B1 levels. *Nat Med*. 3:1209–1215.

22. Margolis DJ, Knauss J, Bilker W. (2002). Hormone replacement therapy and prevention of pressure ulcers and venous leg ulcers. *Lancet*. 359:675–677.

23. Manson JE, Hsia J, Johnson KC *et al.* (2003). Estrogen plus progestin and the risk of coronary heart disease. *N Engl J Med*. 349:523–534.

24. Schmidt JG, Binder M, Demschik G *et al.* (1996). Treatment of skin aging with topical estrogens. *Int J Dermatol*. 35:669–674.

25. Creidi P, Faivre B, Agache P *et al.* (1994). Effect of a conjugated oestrogen cream on ageing facial skin. *Maturitas*. 19:211–223.

26. Varila E, Rantala I, Oikarinen A *et al.* (1995). The effect of topical oestradiol on skin collagen of postmenopausal women. *Br J Obstet Gynaecol*. 102:985–989.

27. Smith JR, Fenske NA. (1996). Cutaneous manifestations and consequences of smoking. *J Am Acad Dermatol*. 34:717–732.

28. Ernster VL, Grady D, Mike R *et al.* (1995). Facial wrinkling in men and women, by smoking status. *Am J Pub Health*. 85:78–82.

29. Rosenbaum M, Prieto V, Hellmer J *et al.* (1999). An exploratory investigation of the morphology and biochemistry of cellulite. *Plast Reconstr Surg*. 101:1934–1939.

30. Nurnberger F, Miller G. (1978). So-called cellulite: An invented disease. *J Dermatol Surg Oncol*. 4(3):221–229.

31. Pedersen SB, Morten J, Richelsen B. (1994). Characterization of regional and gender differences in glucocorticoid receptors and lipoprotein lipase activity in human adipose tissue. *J Clin Endocrinol Metab*. 78:1354–1359.

32. Freedman DS, Jacobsen SJ, Barboriak JJ *et al.* (1990). Body fat distribution and male/female differences in lipids and lipoproteins. *Circulation*. 81: 1498–1506.

33. Naylor MF, Boyd A, Smith DW *et al.* (1995). High sun protection factor sunscreens in the suppression of actini neoplasia. *Arch Dermatol*. 131: 170–175.

34. Reintgen D. (1998). A meeting of the minds: Highlights on the melanoma program of the seventh world congress on cancers of the skin. *Skin Cancer Foundation J*. 16:30–31.

35. McCarthy ED, Ethridge KP, Wagner RF. (1999). Beach holiday sunburn: The sunscreen paradox and gender differences. *Cutis*. 64:37–42.

36. Hourani LL, La Fleur B. (1995). Predictors of gender differences in sunscreen use and screening outcome among skin cancer screening participants. *J Behav Med*. 18:461–468.

37. Hall HI, Miller DR, Rogers JD *et al.* (1999). Update on the incidence and mortality from melanoma in the United States. *J Am Acad Dermatol*. 40:35–42.

38. Beddingfield F, Litwack S, Ziogas A *et al.* (2001). A population-based study of gender differences in melanoma epidemiology: 1988–1997 (abstract). *J Invest Dermatol*. 117:539.

39. Gilchrist BA, Eller MS, Geller AC, Yaar M. (1999). The pathogenesis of melanoma induced by ultraviolet radiation. *N Engl J Med*. 340:1341–1348.

40. Gallagher RP, Mclean DI, Yang CP *et al.* (1990). Anatomic distribution of acquired melanocytic nevi in white children. *Arch Dermatol*. 126:455–471.

41. MacLennan R, Kelly JW, Rivers JK *et al.* (2003). The Eastern Australian Childhood Nevus Study: Site differences in density and size of melanocytic nevi in relation to latitude and phenotype. *J Am Acad Dermatol*. 48:367–375.

42. Karkousis CP, Driscoll DL. (1995). Prognostic parameters in localized melanoma: Gender versus anatomical location. *Eur J Cancer*. 31A:320–324.

43. Streetly A, Markowe H. (1995). Changing trends in the epidemiology of malignant melanoma: Gender differences and their implications fro public health. *Int J Epidemiol*. 24:897–907.

44. Kememy MM, Busch, E Stewart A *et al.* (1998). Superior survival of young women with malignant melanoma. *Am J Surg*. 175:437–445.

45. Miller JG, MacNeil S. (1997). Gender and cutaneous melanoma. *Br J Dermatol*. 136:657–665.

46. Smith MA, Fine JA, Barnhill RL, Berwick M. (1998). Hormonal and reproductive influences and risk of melanoma in women. *Int J Epidemiol*. 27:751–757.

47. Grin CM, Drisoll MS, Grant-Kels JM. (1998). The relationship of pregnancy, hormones, and melanoma. *Semin Cut Med Surg*. 17:167–171.

48. Daryanani D, Plukker JT, De Hullu JA *et al.* (2003). Pregnancy and early-stage melanoma. *Cancer*. 97:2130–2133.

49. Pennoyer JW, Grin CM, Driscoll MS *et al.* (1997). Changes in size of melanocytic nevi during pregnancy. *J Am Acad Dermatol*. 36:378–382.

50. Masri GD, Clark WH, Guerry IV *et al.* (1990). Screening and surveillance of patient at high risk for malignant melanoma result in detection of earlier disease. *J Am Acad Dermatol*. 22:1042–1048.

51. Cassileth BR, Temoshok L, Frederick BE *et al.* (1988). Patient and physician delay in melanoma diagnosis. *J Am Acad Dermatol*. 18:591–598.

52. Richard MA, Grob JJ, Avril MF *et al.* (2000). Delays in diagnosis and melanoma prognosis: The role of patients. *Int J Cancer*. 89:272–279.

53. Schwartz JL, Wang TS, Hamilton TA *et al.* (2002). Thin primary cutaneous melanoma: Associated detection patterns, lesion characteristics, and patient characteristics. *Cancer*. 95:1562–1568.

53a Wohl Y, Golan H, Brenner S. (2003). Cutaneous lymphomas and association to sex hormones. *SKINmed*. 2(5):312–315.

54. Pochi PE, Strauss JS, Downing DT. (1979). Age-related changes in sebaceous gland activity. *J Invest Dermatol*. 73:108–111.

55. Thiboutot D, Harris G, Iles V *et al.* (1995). Activity of the type 1 5α-reductase exhibits regional differences in isolated sebaceous glands and whole skin. *J Invest Dermatol*. 105:209–214.

56. Downing DT, Stewart ME, Strauss JS. (1986). Changes in sebum secretion and the sebaceous gland. *Dermatol Clin*. 4:419–423.

57. Goulden V, Stables GI, Cunliffe WJ. (1999). Prevalence of facial acne in adults. *J Am Acad Dermatol*. 41:577–580.

58. Thiboutot D, Gilliland K, Light J *et al.* (1999). Androgen metabolism in sebaceous glands from subjects with and without acne. *Arch Dermatol*. 135:1041–1045.

59. Hamilton JB. (1960). Effect of castration in adolescent and young adult males upon further changes in the proportions of bare and hairy scalp. *J Clin Endocrinol*. 20:1309–1318.

60. Imperato-McGinley J. (1997). 5α-reductase-2 deficiency. *Curr Ther Endocrinol Metab*. 6:384–387.

61. Olsen EA. (2001). Female pattern hair loss. *J Am Acad Dermatol Suppl*. 45(3):S70–S80.

62. Sawaya ME, Price VH. (1997). Different levels of 5α-reductase type 1 and 2, aromatase, and androgen receptor in hair follicles of women and men with androgenetic alopecia. *J Invest Dermatol*. 109:296–300.

63. Govind A, Obhrai AM, Clayton RN. (1999). Polycystic ovaries are inherited as an autosomal dominant trait. *J Clin Endocrinol Metab*. 84:38–43.

64. Kaufman KD, Olsen EA, Whiting D *et al.* (1998). Finasteride in the treatment of men with androgenetic alopecia. *J Am Acad Dermatol*. 39:578–588.

65. Price VH, Roberts JL, Hordinsky M *et al.* (2000). Lack of efficacy of finasteride in postmenopausal women with androgenetic alopecia. *J Am Acad Dermatol*. 43:768–776.

66. Shum KW, Cullen DR, Messenger AG. (2002). Hair loss in women with hyperandrogenism: Four cases responding to finasteride. *J Am Acad Dermatol*. 47:733–739.

67. Orme S, Cullen DR, Messenger AG. (1999). Diffuse female hair loss: Are androgens necessary? *Brit J Dermatol*. 141:521–523.

68. Olsen EA, Hordinsky M, Roberts JL, Whiting DA. (2002). Female pattern hair loss. *J Am Acad Dermatol*. 47:795.

69. Norwood OT, Lehr B. (2000). Female androgenetic alopecia: A separate entity. *Dermatol Surg*. 26:679–682.

Index